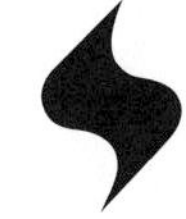

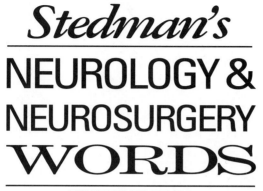

Stedman's NEUROLOGY & NEUROSURGERY WORDS

FOURTH EDITION

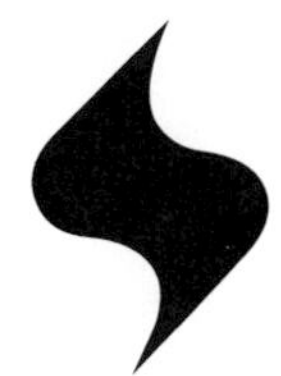

Stedman's NEUROLOGY & NEUROSURGERY WORDS

FOURTH EDITION

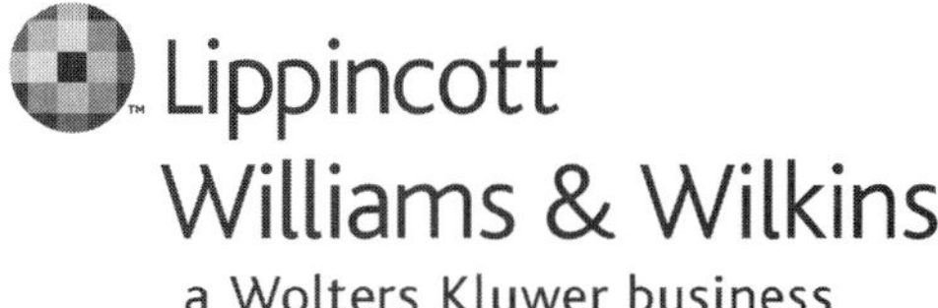

Lippincott Williams & Wilkins
a Wolters Kluwer business

Publisher: Julie K. Stegman
Senior Product Manager: Eric Branger
Managing Editor: Amy Millholen
Typesetter: Josephine Bergin
Printer & Binder: Malloy Litho, Inc.

351 West Camden Street
Baltimore, Maryland 21201-2436

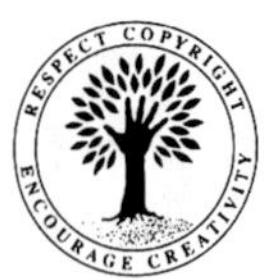

Printed in the United States of America

Fourth Edition, 2006

Library of Congress Cataloging-in-Publication Data
Stedman's neurology & neurosurgery words. — 4th ed.
p. ; cm. ^ (Stedman's word books)
Includes bibliographical references.
ISBN 978-0-7817-9642-2
ISBN 0-7817-9642-3 (alk. paper)
1. Neurology—Dictionaries. 2. Nervous system—Surgery—Dictionaries. I. Stedman, Thomas Lathrop, 1853-1938. II. Title: Stedman's neurology and neurosurgery words. III. Title: Neurology & neurosurgery words. IV. Series.
[DNLM: 1. Neurology—Terminology—English. 2. Neurosurgery —Terminology--English. WL 15 S8115 2007]
RC334.S74 2007
616.8'003--dc22

2005035949

07
2 3 4 5 6 7 8 9 10

Contents

Acknowledgments

An important part of our editorial process is the involvement of medical transcriptionists—as advisors, reviewers, and editors.

We extend special thanks to Kathy Hess, CMT, and Jeanne Bock, CSR, MT, for editing the manuscript and helping to resolve many difficult questions. Our appreciation also goes to Janet West for revising and developing the appendices. We are grateful to advisory board members Sue Bartolucci, L. Ann Hall, Angela Kelly, Andrea Linderman, Beth Pessetto, and Janet West, who were instrumental in the development of this edition. Special thanks to Nicola Ho for sharing her genetics expertise.

Our appreciation goes to Pat Forbis for helping to enhance the A-to-Z content for this edition. We also extend thanks to Jeanne Bock for her assistance with the Sample Reports appendix. Additional thanks to Helen Littrell for performing the final prepublication review.

Special thanks to Barb Ferretti, who played an integral role in the process by reviewing the content files for format and updating the database.

As with all our *Stedman's* word references, this resource incorporates the suggestions and expertise of our many contacts in the medical transcriptionist community. Thanks to all of our advisory board participants, reviewers, and editors; AAMT meeting attendees; and others who have written us with requests and comments—keep talking, and we'll keep listening.

Editors' Preface

As we find ourselves in yet another Olympic year, I (Kathy) am reminded of an editor's preface that I wrote for another Word Book published in a prior Olympic year in which MTs were compared to Olympic athletes. I think that analogy is as true today as it was when I wrote it. Just as the Olympic athletes dedicate their lives to training for their game, we as MTs must continually train, learn, and grow in order to remain successful and at the top of our "game." To that end, Lippincott Williams & Wilkins is dedicated to publishing only the finest Word Books to assist us in our training and in doing our jobs as accurately and efficiently as possible.

We believe you will find this newest edition of *Stedman's Neurology & Neurosurgery Words* to be a useful and complete compilation of the latest terms being used in these medical specialties. Also contained in this fourth edition is a vast collection of common anatomical terminology, radiologic terminology, and related nomenclature, as well an appendix section that includes anatomic illustrations, various tables, and sample reports that will be of great assistance to the user.

Although at first glance neurology and neurosurgery bring to mind "brain surgery" (no pun intended), the diseases related to these specialties can impact all parts of the human body—from the head (brain dysfunction) to the toes (gait impairment). Because of that, we have included a variety of terms in this book that relate to conditions caused or exacerbated by neurological disorders but not necessarily classic neurological terminology. For terms that are more specific to another specialty, please refer to the variety of Stedman's Word Books that cover the various specialties.

Over the years, we have had the pleasure of working with several managing editors at Stedman's. Thank you to Amy Millholen, the managing editor on this Word Book. Amy has been incredibly responsive to our needs throughout the process with this book, ensuring that our job of editing the publication went smoothly. We thank Barb Ferretti, the database editor for this book, for her attention to detail in fully incorporating our edits into this book's database. We also thank all the content cullers who reviewed medical journals, textbooks, and internet web sites to provide the most current and comprehensive terminology available. Finally, we thank you, the customer, for continuing to let us know about new terms, equipment, and ways in which we can improve our products for you.

Jeanne Bock, CSR, MT

Kathy Hess, CMT

Publisher's Preface

Stedman's Neurology & Neurosurgery Words, Fourth Edition, offers an authoritative assurance of quality and exactness to the wordsmiths of the healthcare professions—medical transcriptionists, medical editors and copyeditors, health information management personnel, court reporters, and the many other users and producers of medical documentation.

Stedman's Neurology & Neurosurgery Words, Fourth Edition, contains comprehensive neurology and neurosurgery terminology, including the areas of sleep medicine, Alzheimer disease, epilepsy, and other neurological disorders, as well as neurosurgical procedures and equipment. The updated and expanded appendix sections provide anatomical illustrations with useful captions and labels, all new sample reports and common terms by procedure, as well as a table of nerves, types of brain and spinal cord tumors, sleep medicine terminology, and drugs by indication. New for this edition are appendices on cranial nerve functions and tests, common neurologic disorders, and manual muscle testing.

This fourth edition, with the addition of more than 3,000 new terms, includes the Stedman's Word Book Series trademarks: cross-referencing by first and last word, A-Z format with main entries and subentries, and appendix material for additional comprehension and application of the terminology.

We at Lippincott Williams & Wilkins strive to provide you with the most up-to-date and accurate word references available. Your use of this Word Book will prompt new editions, which we will publish as often as updates and revisions justify. We welcome your suggestions for improvements, changes, corrections, and additions—whatever will make this *Stedman's* product more useful to you. Please complete the postage-paid card in this book with your comments, suggestions, and recommendations, or visit us online at www.stedmans.com.

Explanatory Notes

Medical transcription is an art as well as a science. Both approaches are needed to correctly interpret the dictation of a physician, whose language is a product of education, training, and experience. This variety in medical language means that there are several acceptable ways to express certain terms, including jargon. *Stedman's Neurology & Neurosurgery Words, Fourth Edition*, provides variant spellings and phrasings for many terms. These elements, in addition to complete cross-indexing, make *Stedman's Neurology & Neurosurgery Words, Fourth Edition*, a valuable resource for determining the validity of terms as they are encountered.

Alphabetical Organization

Alphabetization of main entries is letter by letter as spelled, ignoring punctuation, spaces, prefixed numbers, or other special characters. For example:

hydroxychloroquine
17-hydroxycorticosteroid
6-hydroxydopamine

Terms beginning or ending with Greek letters show the Greek letters spelled out and listed alphabetically. For example:

beta
  b. activity
  interleukin b.
  b. wave

In subentry alphabetization, the abbreviated singular form or the spelled-out plural form of the noun main entry word is ignored.

Format and Style

All main entries are in **boldface** to expedite locating a sought-after term, to enhance distinction between main entries and subentries, and to relieve the textual density of the pages.

Irregular plurals and variant spellings are shown on the same line as the singular or preferred form of the word. For example:

ala, pl. alae
akathisia, acathisia

Hyphenation

As a rule of style, multiple eponyms (e.g., Mears-Rubash approach) are hyphenated. Also, hyphens have been added between a manufacturer and one or more eponyms (e.g., Vital-Metzenbaum dissecting scissors). Please note that in many cases, hyphenation is a question of style, not of accuracy, and thus is a matter of choice.

Possessives

Possessive forms have been dropped in this reference for the sake of consistency and conformance with the guidelines of the American Association for Medical Transcription (AAMT) and other groups. Please note, however, that in many cases, retaining the possessive, like hyphenating, is a question of style, not of accuracy, and thus is a matter of choice. To form the possessive of a word, simply add the apostrophe or apostrophe "s" to the end of the word.

Cross-indexing

The word list is in an index-like main entry-subentry format that contains two combined alphabetical listings:

(1) A noun main entry-subentry organization, which is typical of the A-Z section of medical dictionaries like Stedman's:

abasia
 atactic a.
 ataxic a.
 choreic a.

efficacy
 clinical e.
 drug e.
 lack of e.

(2) An adjective main entry-subentry organization, which lists words and phrases as you hear them. The main entries are the adjectives or modifiers in a multiword term. The subentries are the nouns around which the terms are constructed and to which the adjectives or modifiers pertain:

epidemiological
e. research
e. study

ankle
a. clonus
a. jerk

This format provides the user with more than one way to locate and identify a multiword term. For example:

Fukuyama
F. congenital muscular dystrophy

dystrophy
Fukuyama congenital muscular d.

blank
b. gaze

gaze
blank g.

It also allows the user to see together all terms that contain a particular descriptor, as well as all types, kinds, or variations of a noun entity. For example:

lip
l. reflex
rhombic l.
l. smacking automatism

typhus
epidemic t.
t. fever
murine t.

Wherever possible, abbreviations are separately defined and cross-referenced. For example:

ANS
autonomic nervous system

autonomic
a. nervous system (ANS)

system
autonomic nervous s. (ANS)

Note on gene terms: Conventionally, all letters in human gene names are capitalized and the entire term is italicized *(TSC1, TSC2)*. It is also acceptable to write gene names as "TSC1 gene" or "TSC2 gene." Roman (non-italicized) text indicates a protein, but the addition of the word "gene" indicates that one is referring to the gene encoding that protein. So, it is appropriate to write "*TSC1*" or "TSC1 gene" but *not* "*TSC1* gene." In this Word Book, we have listed gene names without the italics and followed by the word "gene" so that these terms could be cross-referenced.

References

In addition to the lists of our MT Editorial Advisory Board members (from their daily transcription work), we used the following sources for new terms in *Stedman's Neurology & Neurosurgery Words, Fourth Edition.*

Books

The AAMT Book of Style, 2nd Edition. Modesto, CA: AAMT, 2002.

Agur AM, Lee MJ. Grant's Atlas of Anatomy, 10th Edition. Baltimore: Lippincott Williams & Wilkins, 1999.

Arnoff G. Evaluation and Treatment of Chronic Pain. Philadelphia: Lippincott Williams & Wilkins, 1998.

Bear M, Connors B, Paradiso M. Neuroscience: Exploring the Brain, 2nd Edition. Baltimore: Lippincott Williams & Wilkins, 2000.

Biller J. Practical Neurology, 2nd Edition. Philadelphia: Lippincott Williams & Wilkins, 2002.

Brazis PW, Masdeu JC, Biller J. Localization in Clinical Neurology, 4th Edition. Baltimore: Lippincott Williams & Wilkins, 2001.

Brillman J, Kahan S. In A Page Neurology. Malden, MA: Blackwell Publishing, 2005.

Browne TR, Holmes GL. Handbook of Epilepsy, 3rd Edition. Philadelphia: Lippincott Williams & Wilkins, 2004.

Campbell WW, Pridgeon RM. Practical Primer of Neurology. Philadelphia: Lippincott Williams & Wilkins, 2001.

Carney PR, Berry RB, Geyer JD. Clinical Sleep Disorders. Philadelphia: Lippincott Williams & Wilkins, 2005.

Dorland's Neurology Word Book for Medical Transcriptionists. Philadelphia: Saunders, 2001.

Drake E. Sloane's Medical Word Book, 4th Edition. Philadelphia: Saunders, 2001.

Fairbanks DNF, Mickelson SA, Woodson BT. Snoring and Obstructive Sleep Apnea. Philadelphia: Lippincott Williams & Wilkins, 2002.

Howard MA, III. Clinical Neurosurgery: A Publication of the Congress of Neurological Surgeons. Philadelphia: Lippincott Williams & Wilkins, 2001.

Lance LL. Quick Look Drug Book. Baltimore: Lippincott Williams & Wilkins, 2002.

Levy RH, Mattson RH, Meldrum BS, Perucca E. Antiepileptic Drugs, 5th Edition. Baltimore: Lippincott Williams & Wilkins, 2002.

Mazzoni P, Rowland LP. Merritt's Neurology Handbook. Philadelphia: Lippincott Williams & Wilkins, 2001.

Menkes JH, Sarnat HB, Maria BL. Child Neurology, 7th Edition. Philadelphia: Lippincott Williams & Wilkins, 2006.

Moore SP, Psarros TG. The Definitive Neurological Surgery Board Review. Malden, MA: Blackwell Publishing, 2005.

Orthopedic/Neurology Words and Phrases, 2nd Edition. Modesto, CA: Health Professions Institute, 2000.

Pillitteri A. Maternal and Child Health Nursing, 3rd Edition. Philadelphia: Lippincott Williams & Wilkins, 1998.

Rosdahl DB. Textbook of Basic Nursing, 7th Edition. Philadelphia: Lippincott Williams & Wilkins, 1999.

Samuels MA (ed.). Manual of Neurologic Therapeutics, 7th Edition. Philadelphia: Lippincott Williams & Wilkins, 2004.

Sirven JI, Malamut BL. Clinical Neurology of the Older Adult. Philadelphia: Lippincott Williams & Wilkins, 2002.

Stedman's Medical Dictionary, 27th Edition. Baltimore: Lippincott Williams & Wilkins, 2000.

Vera Pyle's Current Medical Terminology, 9th Edition. Modesto, CA: Health Professions Institute, 2003.

Weiner HL, Levitt LP, Rae-Grant A. Neurology, 7th ed. Philadelphia: Lippincott Williams & Wilkins, 2004.

Wyllie E. The Treatment of Epilepsy, 3rd Edition. Baltimore: Lippincott Williams & Wilkins, 2001.

Images

Agur, AMR, Lee, MJ. Grant's Atlas of Anatomy, 10th Edition. Baltimore: Lippincott Williams & Wilkins, 1999.

Anatomical Chart Company. All rights reserved.

LifeART Emergency Collection 2, CD-ROM. Baltimore: Lippincott Williams & Wilkins.

LifeART Nursing Collection 1, CD-ROM. Baltimore: Lippincott Williams & Wilkins.

LifeART Nursing Collection 2, CD-ROM. Baltimore: Lippincott Williams & Wilkins.

LifeART Super Anatomy Collection 3, CD-ROM. Baltimore: Lippincott Williams & Wilkins.

LifeART Super Anatomy Collection 7, CD-ROM. Baltimore: Lippincott Williams & Wilkins.

LifeART Super Anatomy Collection 7, CD-ROM. Baltimore: Lippincott Williams & Wilkins. Neil O. Hardy. Westport, CT. From Stedman's Medical Dictionary, 27th Edition. Baltimore: Lippincott Williams & Wilkins, 2000.

LifeART Super Anatomy Collection 8, CD-ROM. Baltimore: Lippincott Williams & Wilkins.

LifeART Super Anatomy Collection 9, CD-ROM. Baltimore: Lippincott Williams & Wilkins.

MediClip Human Anatomy 1-3, CD-ROM. Baltimore: Lippincott, Williams & Wilkins.

Michael Schenk, Jackson, MS. From Stedman's Medical Dictionary, 27th Edition. Baltimore: Lippincott Williams & Wilkins, 2000.

Mikki Senkarik, San Antonio, TX. From Pillitteri A. Maternal & Child Health Nursing: Care of the Childbearing & Childrearing Family, 3rd Edition. Philadelphia: Lippincott Williams & Wilkins, 1998.

Neil O. Hardy. Westport, CT. From Rosdahl DB. Textbook of Basic Nursing, 7th Edition. Philadelphia: Lippincott Williams & Wilkins, 1999.

Neil O. Hardy. Westport, CT. From Stedman's Medical Dictionary, 27th Edition. Baltimore: Lippincott Williams & Wilkins, 2000.

Smeltzer SC, Bare BG. Brunner & Suddarth's Textbook of Medical-Surgical Nursing, 9th Edition. Baltimore: Lippincott Williams & Wilkins, 2000.

Stedman's Medical Dictionary, 27th Edition. Baltimore: Lippincott Williams & Wilkins, 2000.

Stedman's Orthopaedic & Rehab Words, 4th Edition. Baltimore: Lippincott Williams & Wilkins, 2003.

Stedman's Psychiatry/Neurology/Neurosurgery Words, 2nd Edition. Baltimore: Lippincott Williams & Wilkins, 1999. Susan Caldwell. Pikesville, MD. From Stedman's Medical Dictionary, 27th Edition. Baltimore: Lippincott Williams & Wilkins, 2000.

Journals

Alzheimer Disease and Associated Disorders. Philadelphia: Lippincott Williams & Wilkins, 2004-2005.

Clinical Neuropharmacology. Philadelphia: Lippincott Williams & Wilkins, 2004-2005.

Cognitive and Behavioral Neurology. Philadelphia: Lippincott Williams & Wilkins, 2004-2005.

Current Opinion in Neurology. Baltimore: Lippincott Williams & Wilkins, 2002-2005.

Journal of Cerebral Blood Flow and Metabolism. Baltimore: Lippincott Williams & Wilkins, 2002.

Journal of Spinal Disorders & Techniques. Philadelphia: Lippincott Williams & Wilkins, 2004-2005.

Latest Word. Philadelphia: Saunders, 1999-2002.

The Neurologist. Baltimore: Lippincott Williams & Wilkins, 2002-2005.

Neurology. Baltimore: Lippincott Williams & Wilkins, 2004-2005.

NeuroReport. Baltimore: Lippincott Williams & Wilkins, 2001.

Neurosurgery. Baltimore: Lippincott Williams & Wilkins, 1999-2005.

Neurosurgery Quarterly. Baltimore: Lippincott Williams & Wilkins, 2002-2005.

Perspectives on the Medical Transcription Profession. Modesto, CA: Health Professions Institute, 2001.

Spine. Philadelphia: Lippincott Williams & Wilkins, 2004-2005.

Stroke. Baltimore: Lippincott Williams & Wilkins, 2002.

Websites

http://emedicine.com/neuro

http://neurosurgery.ucla.edu/Diagnoses/BrainTumor/BrainTumorDis_Intro.html

http://www.americanspine.com

http://www.biomedcentral.com

http://www.centerwatch.com/patient/drugs/druglist.html

http://www.childneurologysociety.org

http://www.foxhollowtech.com

http://www.medlink.com/medlinkcontent.asp

http://www.medtronicssofamordanek.com

http://www.mtdesk.com/lstpsych.shtml

http://www.mtdesk.com/psychdef.shtml

http://www.neurologychannel.com

http://www.neurology.org

http://www.neurosurgery.org/

http://www.promedproducts.com

http://www.thejns-net.org

http://www.thesaundersgroup.com

A
A band
A fiber
A wave
A1 adenosine receptor
A1, A2 segment of anterior cerebral artery
AA
amino acid
anterograde amnesia
AAAS
achalasia, adrenocortical insufficiency, alacrimia syndrome
triple A syndrome
AADC
aromatic amino acid decarboxylase
AAGP
American Association for Geriatric Psychiatry
AANS/CNS
American Association of Neurological Surgeons/Congress of Neurological Surgeons
AANS/CNS Joint Committee of Military Neurosurgeons
AANS/CNS Joint Section Lumbar Disc Herniation Study
AANS/CNS Outcomes Committee
AAO
alert and oriented
Aarskog-Scott syndrome (ASS)
AB
alertness behavior
abacavir
Abadie
A. sign
A. sign of tabes dorsalis
ABAER
automated brainstem auditory evoked response
abarognosis
abasement
abasia
atactic a.
ataxic a.
choreic a.
frontal a.
spastic a.
abasia-astasia
abasic, abatic
abatardissement
abaxial, abaxile
Abbokinase
Abbott fluorescence polarization immunoassay technique
abbreviated
A. Injury Score
A. Life Event Questionnaire
ABC
angry backfiring C
atomic, biologic, chemical
ABC anterior cervical plating system
ABC cervical plating system
ABC E-Plate
ABC syndrome
ABC warfare
abciximab
abdomen
anterior cutaneous nerves of a.
carinate a.
navicular a.
abdominal
a. aortic plexus
a. aura
a. brain
a. compartment syndrome
a. epilepsy
a. migraine
a. neuralgia
a. reflex
a. trauma
abdominalis
plexus aorticus a.
abdominocardiac reflex
abdominopelvic splanchnic nerve
abducens
a. eminence
a. nerve
a. nerve palsy
a. nerve paralysis
a. nerve paresis
nervus a. [CN VI]
a. nucleus
a. pathway
abducentis
eminentia a.
nucleus nervi a.
abducent nerve [CN VI]
abduction
a. nystagmus
a. weakness
abductor pollicis brevis (APB)
Abercrombie neuronal cell count formula
aberrant
a. artery
a. autocrine control
a. bundle
a. carotid

aberrant *(continued)*
a. gamma burst pattern
a. ganglion
a. laboratory parameter
a. motor behavior
a. neuron
a. regeneration
aberration
chromosomal a.
intersegmental a.
Abeta
beta-amyloid
A. fibril
A. molecule
A. peptide
A. protein
Abeta-centered neuritic plaque
abetalipoproteinemia
ABG
arterial blood gas
ABI
acquired brain injury
auditory brainstem implant
multichannel ABI
ability
abstracting a.
bathing and dressing a.
conceptual a.
construction a.
constructional a.
fluid a.
intellectual a.
nonverbal abstractive a.
nonverbal synthesizing a.
Porch Index of Communicative A.
positive a.
premorbid a.
a. test
verbal a.
visuoconstructional a.
walking a.
working a.
abirritation
ablation
choroid plexus a.
stereotactic surgical a.
thermal a.
total pituitary a.
ablative
a. central neurosurgical procedure
a. spinal cord procedure
abnegate
abneural
abnormal
a. epileptic neuron
a. fluency
a. illness behavior
A. Involuntary Movement Scale
A. Involuntary Movement Score
a. joint motion
a. metabolism
a. muscle response
a. nocturnal respiratory reflex
a. personality
a. reaction
a. respiratory drive
a. response to sensory stimulation
a. sleep-wake schedule disorder
a. sweating
a. tactile sensation
a. thinking
a. trait
a. trunk movement
a. ventilation
a. waveform
abnormality
active interictal a.
behavioral a.
bony a.
brain growth a.
brainstem a.
branchial cleft a.
bulbar a.
central nervous system a.
channel kinetic a.
C-nociceptor filter-evoked central a.
CNS a.
concordant interictal epileptiform a.
convergence a.
cranial nerve a.
CSF tau protein a.
cutaneous a.
cytoarchitectonic a.
cytoskeletal a.
endogenous a.
filter-evoked central a.
focal slow-wave a.
frontal plane growth a.
gain-of-function a.
gait a.
G-protein a.
hallucal a.
ictal epileptiform a.
immunologic a.
interictal epileptiform a.
mesocorticolimbic dopaminergic a.
metabolic a.
migration a.
morphometric a.
motor a.
motoric a.
neuritic cytoskeletal a.
neuroanatomic a.
neuronal migration a.
occult a.
ocular a.
oculomotor a.
personality a.

polysomnographic a.
pons a.
posture reflex a.
psychomotor a.
pupillary a.
radiologic a.
saccadic a.
segmental conduction a.
sex chromosome a.
sleep hygiene a.
slow-wave a.
soft tissue a.
spinal cord injury without radiographic a. (SCIWORA)
striatal dopaminergic a.
structural a.
subcortical/frontal lobe a.
subtle structural a.
torsional a.
trait-level region a.
transient signal a.
white matter signal a.
X-linked a.

abnormal-shaped cell
ABO antigen compatibility
abolic syndrome
abolition
concentration-dependent a.
aborted procedure
abortive
a. neurofibromatosis
a. poliomyelitis
a. therapy
abortus
Brucella a.
aboulia (*var. of* abulia)
ABPN
American Board of Psychiatry and Neurology
ABR
auditory brainstem response
abradant
Abrams heart reflex
Abramson catheter
abreact
abrogate
abrupt loss of vision
abscess
actinomycotic brain a.
arthrifluent a.
Aspergillus brain a.
Aspergillus cerebral a.
bacterial brain a.
brain a.
cerebellar a.
cerebral a.
cervical epidural a.
cranial epidural a.
daughter a.
encapsulated brain a.
epidural a.
extradural a.
a. formation
frontal lobe a.
intracranial epidural a.
intradural a.
nocardial brain a.
otic a.
parasitic brain a.
periapical a.
pituitary a.
Pott a.
psoas a.
pyogenic brain a.
retropharyngeal a.
spinal cord a.
spinal epidural a.
sterile a.
subdural a.
subgaleal a.
temporal lobe a.
thecal a.
tuberculous a.
absence
atonic a.
a. attack
atypical a.
automatic a.
complex a.
a. of emotional responsiveness
enuretic a.
epileptic a.
hypertonic a.
muscle a.
myoclonic a.
protein induced by vitamin K a. (PIVKA)
pure a.
retrocursive a.
a. seizure
simple a.
a. status epilepticus
sternutatory a.
subclinical a.

NOTES

absence *(continued)*
tussive a.
vasomotor a.
absent
a. ataxia
a. pupil
a. speech
a. spinous process
a. state
absentia
epileptica a.
absolute
a. agraphia
a. band amplitude
a. construction of phase
a. EP amplitude
a. flow
a. hemostasis
a. metabolic activity
a. neutrophil count (ANC)
a. refractory period
a. scale
a. terminal innervation ratio
a. threshold
absorbable
a. gelatin film
a. gelatin sponge
absorbefacient
absorptiometry
dual-energy x-ray a. (DEXA, DXA)
dual-photon a.
absorption
cerebrospinal fluid a.
erratic a.
intramuscular a.
a. velocity
abstemious
abstract
a. behavior
a. versus representational
a. versus representational dimension
abstracting
a. ability
a. disability
abstraction
level of a.
a. skill
abstruse
abterminal
abubble
abulia, aboulia
abulic mental change
abuse
a. field
a. potential
substance a.
abysm
AC
alternating current
ACA
acute cerebellar ataxia
acalculia
aphasic a.
visuospatial a.
acamprosate
acanthamebiasis
Acanthamoeba
A. infection
A. meningitis
acanthesthesia
acanthocytosis with chorea
acapnia
acarbose
ACAT
acylcholestrol acyl transferase
automated computerized axial tomography
acataphasia
acathectic
acathexia
acathisia (*var. of* akathisia)
acaudal
acaudate
accelerans
accelerated aging
accelerating center
acceleration
a. extension injury
rotatory a.
acceleration-deceleration forces in craniocerebral trauma
accelerator
Bevatron a.
a. fiber
isocentric linear a.
linear a. (LINAC)
a. nerve
Philips linear a.
Racetrack Microtron MM50 a.
stereotactic linear a.
accelerometry
ambulatory a.
Accell Total Bone Matrix
acceptance strategy
access
arterial a.
lexical a.
accession
accessorii
nervi phrenici a.
nuclei oculomotorii a.
nucleus spinalis nervi a.
pars spinalis nervi a.
pars vagalis nervi a.
radix cranialis nervi a.
radix spinalis nervi a.

rami musculares rami externi nervi a.
ramus externus nervi a.
ramus internus nervi a.
truncus nervi a.
accessorius
nervus obturatorius a.
nervus peroneus profundus a.
nucleus cuneatus a.
a. willisii
accessory
a. basal amygdaloid nucleus
a. conduction pathway (ACP)
a. cramp
a. cuneate nucleus
a. flocculus
Isola spinal implant system a.
a. middle cerebral artery
a. nerve [CN XI]
a. nerve lymph node
a. nerve paresis
a. nerve trunk
a. nucleus of optic tract
a. oculomotor nucleus
a. olivary nucleus
a. olive
a. phrenic nerve
a. portion of spinal cord
accident
a. behavior
cerebrovascular a. (CVA)
a. neurosis
vascular a.
accidental
a. image
a. injury
accident-prone
acclimation
cold a.
acclimatize
accommodation
a. curve
a. disorder
a. of nerve
accompaniment
late-life migraine a.
psychopathologic a.
accompanying vein of hypoglossal nerve
accoucheur's hand
accretion
Accu-Flo
A.-F. CSF reservoir
A.-F. dura film
A.-F. polyethylene bur hole cover
A.-F. silicone rubber bur hole cover
A.-F. ventricular catheter
Acculink stent
accumbens
nucleus a.
accumbentis
pars lateralis nuclei a.
pars medialis nuclei a.
accumulation
cholesterol a.
galactose-1-phosphate a.
galactosylsphingosine a.
glucosylsphingosine a.
ketoacid a.
psychosine a.
sulfatide a.
accuracy of memory
Accura shunt
Accurate Surgical and Scientific Instruments (ASSI)
Accuray
A. CyberKnife
A. Neurotron 1000 machine
Accusway balance measurement system
Ace
A. halo-cast assembly
A. halo pelvic girdle
A. Hershey halo jig
A. low-profile MR halo
A. Mark III halo
A. Trippi-Wells tong cervical traction
A. universal tong cervical traction
acebutolol
acedia
acellular human dermal graft
acenesthesia
acephalgic migraine
acephaly
acerbic, acerb
acerbophobia
aceruloplasminemia
acervuline
acervulus
acetaldehyde
acetate
butyl a.
cortisone a.
cortone a.

NOTES

acetate *(continued)*
desmopressin a.
desoxycorticosterone a.
ethylene-vinyl a. (EVAc)
glatiramer a.
Hydrocortone A.
leuprolide a.
medroxyprogesterone a.
methylprednisolone a.
potassium a.
sodium a.
zinc a.
acetazolamide
acetohexamide
acetonemia
acetonemic
acetonide
acetrizoate
acetrizoic acid
acetyl
a. cholinesterase inhibitor
a. coenzyme A
a. coenzyme A carboxylase
acetylase
***N*-acetylaspartate**
***N*-acetylaspartic acid**
acetylcholine (ACH, ACh)
a. esterase
a. receptor (AChR)
acetylcholine-binding protein
acetylcholinesterase (AChE, AChEIs)
a. collagen tail
***N*-acetylgalactosamine-4-sulfate sulfatase**
***N*-acetylglucosamine-6-sulfate sulfatase**
***N*-acetylglutamate synthetase deficiency**
***N*-acetylneuraminic acid**
acetylphosphate
acetylsalicylic
a. acid
a. acid patch
acetyltransferase
choline a.
dihydrolipoamide a.
ACF
asymmetrical crying facies
ACH, ACh
acetylcholine
ACH receptor
AChA
anterior choroidal artery
achaete-scute gene
achalasia
a., adrenocortical insufficiency, alacrimia syndrome (AAAS)
cricopharyngeal a.
esophageal a.
AChE
acetylcholinesterase
acheiria
AChEIs
acetylcholinesterase
AChEIs receptor antagonist
Achilles
A. reflex
A. tendon reflex time
achlorhydria
achondroplasia
AChR
acetylcholine receptor
achromasia
neuronal a.
achromatic response
achromatopsia
achromia
cortical a.
achromians
incontinentia pigmenti a.
acid
acetrizoic a.
N-acetylaspartic a.
N-acetylneuraminic a.
acetylsalicylic a.
adenosine monophosphate a. (AMPA)
alpha-amino-3-hydroxy-5-methylisoxazole-4-propionic a.
amidotrizoic a.
amino a. (AA)
aminocaproic a.
arachidonic a.
atractylic a.
benzoic a.
carbonic a.
cerebrospinal fluid lactic a.
chenodeoxycholic a.
cis-parinaric a.
cis-retinoic a. (CRA)
13-*cis*-retinoic a. (13-CRA)
clavulanic a.
complementary deoxyribonucleic a. (cDNA)
cyclic deoxyribonucleic a.
deoxyribonucleic a. (DNA)
diatrizoic a.
diethylenetriamine pentaacetic a. (DTPA)
differential display of messenger ribonucleic a.
dihomogammalinolenic a.
docosahexaenoic a. (DHA)
double-stranded deoxyribonucleic a. (dsDNA)
eicosapentaenoic a.
epsilon-aminocaproic a.
ethacrynic a.
ethyl-eicosapentaenoic a.
ethylenediaminetetraacetic a.
excitatory amino a.

folic a.
folinic a.
gadolinium diethylenetriamine pentaacetic a. (Gd-DTPA)
gamma-aminobutyric a. (GABA)
gamma-aminobutyric a. type A (GABA-A)
gamma-aminolevulinic a.
gamma-linolenic a.
ganglioside monosialic a.
glucuronic a.
glutaric a.
a. hematoxylin
hepatoiminodiacetic a. (HIDA)
heteronuclear ribonucleic a. (hnRNA)
highly unsaturated fatty a. (HUFA)
homocysteine a.
homovanillic a. (HVA)
hyaluronic a.
5-hydroxyindoleacetic a.
hypochlorous a. (HOCI)
inhibitory amino a.
iobenzamic a.
iobutoic a.
iocarmic a.
iodoalphionic a.
iodoxamic a.
ioglicic a.
ioglycamic a.
iopanoic a.
iophenoxic a.
iopronic a.
iosefamic a.
ioseric a.
iosumetic a.
ioteric a.
iothalamic a.
iotroxic a.
ioxaglic a.
ioxithalamic a.
ipodate a.
kainic a.
kynurenic a.
L-alanine a.
L-glutamic a.
a. lipase
a. lipase deficiency
L-lysine a.
long-chain fatty a.
L-tyrosine a.
a. maltase deficiency
mefenamic a.
messenger ribonucleic a.
metrizoic a.
mitochondrial deoxyribonucleic a. (mtDNA)
myristic a.
neuroactive amino a.
nitric a.
okadaic a.
Owsley a.
oxolinic a.
palmitic a.
paraisopropyliminodiacetic a. (PIPIDA)
plasma fatty a.
polyanhydroglucuronic a.
polylactic a.
potassium citrate and citric a.
quinolinic a.
quisqualic a.
retinoic a.
rho-aminosalicylic a.
ribonucleic a. (RNA)
serum folic a.
sialic a.
thiobarbituric a.
tolfenamic a.
tranexamic a.
tricarboxylic a. (TCA)
triiodobenzoic a.
tyropanoic a.
uric a.
valerianic a.
valproic a.

acid-base
a.-b. disturbance
a.-b. imbalance

acidemia
methylmalonic a.
organic a.
propionic a.

acid-fast
a.-f. bacilli smear
a.-f. stain

acidophil adenoma

acidophilic pituitary tumor

acidosis
brain tissue a.
extracellular a.
hypokalemic metabolic a.
lactic a.
metabolic a.

NOTES

acidosis *(continued)*
myoclonus epilepsy with ragged red fibers-lactic a. (MERRLA)
respiratory a.
acid-Schiff
periodic a.-S. (PAS)
aciduria
alpha-aminoadipic a.
alpha-ketoadipic a.
alpha-methylacetoacetic a.
argininosuccinic a.
ethylmalonic a.
glutaric a. type I-III
4-hydroxybutyric a.
2-hydroxyglutaric a.
3-hydroxyisobutyric a.
3-hydroxy-3-methylglutaric a.
isovaleric a.
3-methylglutaconic a.
methylmalonic a.
mevalonic a.
organic a.
propionic a.
pyroglutamic a.
Acinetobacter calcoaceticus
acinic cell carcinoma
Acland clip
ACM
acute cerebrospinal meningitis
acmesthesia
ACoA, AComA
anterior communicating artery
aconative
aconite
aconitine
acoria, akoria
acorn
a. bit
a. drill
acoustic
a. agraphia
a. ambiguity
a. aphasia
a. area
a. bone window
a. crest
a. evoked potential
a. lemniscus
a. nerve
a. nerve complex
a. nerve disorder
a. nerve sheath tumor
a. neurilemoma
a. neurinoma
a. neuroma
A. Neuroma Association
A. Neuroma Registry
a. neuroma surgery
a. noise
a. nucleus
a. papilla
a. radiation
a. reflex
a. schwannoma
a. signature event
a. spot
a. startle reflex
a. stria
a. tubercle
a. tuberculum
acoustical shadowing
acousticofacial
a. crest
a. ganglion
acousticopalpebral reflex (APR)
ACP
accessory conduction pathway
AC-PC
anterior commissure-posterior commissure
AC-PC line
acquired
a. antibody
a. brain injury (ABI)
a. cardiac disease
a. childhood aphasia
a. dementia
a. demyelinative neuropathy
a. drive
a. epileptic aphasia
a. epileptiform opercular syndrome
a. fluent aphasia
a. hepatocerebral degeneration
a. hepatocerebral syndrome
a. hydrocephalus
a. immunodeficiency syndrome (AIDS)
a. immunodeficiency syndrome dementia complex
a. myopathy
a. nystagmus
a. pandysautonomia
a. reflex
a. spinal stenosis
a. toxoplasmosis
a. vertical diplopia
acquisita
myotonia a.
acquisition
3-dimensional a.
target a.
a. time
Acra-Cut
A.-C. blade
A.-C. cranial perforator
A.-C. cranioblade
A.-C. wire pass drill
Acragun system

acral
acrid
acroagnosis
acroanesthesia
acroasphyxia
acroataxia
acrobrachycephaly
acrocallosal syndrome
acrocephalia (*var. of* acrocephaly)
acrocephalic
acrocephalosyndactyly
acrocephalous
acrocephaly, acrocephalia
acrocinesia, acrocinesis
acrodynia
acrodysesthesia
acroedema
acroesthesia
acrognosis
acrohypothermia
acrolect
acromegalia (*var. of* acromegaly)
acromegalic neuropathy
acromegaloid-hypertelorism-pectus carinatum syndrome
acromegaly, acromegalia
  hypothalamic a.
acromial
  a. dimple
  a. reflex
acromicria
acronarcotic
acroneurosis
acroparalysis
acroparesthesia syndrome
acropathy
  mutilating a.
acrophase
acrosclerosis
acrotrophodynia
acrotrophoneurosis
acrylaldehyde
acrylamide
  a. monomer
  a. peripheral neuropathy
acrylic
  a. cranioplasty
  a. glue
  a. prosthesis
act
  Individuals with Disabilities Education A. (IDEA)
  instrumental a.
actamathesia
ACTH
  adrenocorticotropic hormone
Acthar
ACTH-producing adenoma
ACTH-secreting pituitary tumor
ActiGraph
actigraphy
actin filament
Actinomadura madurae
actinomycetoma
actinomycosis lymphocytic meningitis
actinomycotic brain abscess
actinoneuritis
action
  drug a.
  dual mechanism of a.
  a. dystonia
  hypnotic a.
  local vasoconstrictive a.
  a. potential
  reflex a.
  A. Research Arm Test
  scotomata of a.
  a. tremor
  vasoconstrictive a.
  viscoelastic a.
Activa
  A. tremor control system
  A. tremor control system implant
  A. tremor control therapy
activated
  a. epilepsy
  a. estrogen receptor
  a. macrophage
activating condition
activation
  amygdala a.
  anterior hippocampal a.
  antigen-driven cell a.
  ascending reticular a.
  brain a.
  brainstem a.
  caspase-3 a.
  cerebellar a.
  complement a.
  a. defect
  EEG a.

NOTES

activation *(continued)*
electroencephalogram a.
emotion-related a.
enzyme a.
functional a.
GFAP gene a.
glial fibrillary acidic protein a.
hippocampal a.
ipsilateral cortical a.
latency of tibialis anterior a.
limbic a.
metabolic a.
neural a.
neuronal a.
nociceptor a.
parahippocampal a.
peripheral nociceptor a.
posterior hippocampal a.
prefrontal cortex a.
a. procedure
right ventricular a. (RVA)
activator
plasminogen a. (PA)
recombinant tissue plasminogen a. (RTPA)
a. table
tissue plasminogen a. (TPA, t-PA)
urokinase-type plasminogen a. (u-PA)
active
a. integral range of motion (AIROM)
a. interictal abnormality
a. metabolite
a. pathophysiologic process
a. sleep
a. sleep characteristic
a. state
a. surface electrode
a. technique
a. zone
active-phase
activities
activity
absolute metabolic a.
adrenal nerve a.
adrenomedullary a.
alpha frequency a.
antimuscarine cholinergic a.
anxiolytic a.
asymmetrical generalized epileptiform a.
background a.
barbiturate-induced spindle-like a.
beta a.
bilateral a.
bimanual neuronal a.
biochemical a.
blocking a.
burst of delta a.
calmodulin-independent neuronal nitric oxide synthase a.
cerebral antioxidant a.
C-fiber a.
cholinergic a.
cortical a.
daily living a.'s
a.'s of daily living (ADL)
decreased interest in a.
decremental a.
delta a.
desynchronization a.
diffuse distribution of a.
disruption of normal a.
dopaminergic a.
efferent sympathetic a.
electrical a.
electrocerebral a.
electrographic seizure a.
endplate a.
epileptiform a.
excessive diffuse low- and medium-wave beta a.
extracellular calcium a.
extracerebral a.
focal delta slow-wave a.
focal epileptiform a.
forebrain a.
frenzied psychomotor a.
frontal intermittent rhythmic delta a. (FIRDA)
gamma-aminolevulinic acid dehydratase a.
high-frequency a.
high-voltage slow and sharp a.
hypersynchronous a.
hypnotic a.
ictal epileptiform a.
insertional a.
intensive motor a.
interictal EEG a.
interictal epileptiform a.
intermittent rhythmic delta a. (IRDA)
lambdoid a.
language-specific brain a.
lateralized a.
level of a.
Lewis blood group a.
A. Loss Assessment
low-amplitude a.
low-frequency a.
low physical a.
low-voltage a.
lysosomal enzymatic a.
masticatory muscle a.
metabolic a.
MFD a.

monomorphic a.
monorhythmic frontal delta a.
monorhythmic sinusoidal delta a.
motor a.
muscle a.
myorelaxant a.
neuronal spike a.
noncerebral a.
nonepileptiform a.
occipital dominant intermittent rhythmic delta a.
occipital intermittent rhythmic delta a. (OIRDA)
orbitofrontal a.
oscillatory brain a.
paroxysmal alpha a.
pathologic spontaneous a.
peripheral cholinergic a.
peripheral electromyographic a.
photic-induced epileptiform a.
physical a.
polymorphic delta a. (PDA)
polyrhythmic a.
polyspike-and-wave a.
posterior dominant a.
postganglionic efferent a.
posttraumatic epileptiform a.
preganglionic efferent a.
primary headache associated with sexual a.
progestational a.
propagation of a.
reflex neurologic a.
rhythmic delta a.
rhythmic spindle-shaped a.
runs of a.
scalp-derived EEG a.
scattered dysrhythmic slow a.
sedative a.
seizure a.
seizurelike a.
semipurposeful a.
serotonergic a.
sigma a.
sleep a.
slow-wave a. (SWA)
social a.
spectral peak frequency of a.
spike-and-wave a.
spiking a.
spontaneous a.
synaptic a.
synchronous epileptiform a.
thermoeffector a.
theta a.
tonic-clonic a.
triphasic slow-wave a.
uncontrollable motor a.
unilateral epileptiform a.
unilateral focus of a.
whole-body a.
widespread beta a.
widespread distribution of a.

ACU-dyne antiseptic

acuity
central vision a.
temporal processing a. (TPA)
visual a.

acuology

acupoint

acupressure

acupuncture
a. analgesic
a. anesthesia
a. point
a. treatment

acustica
area a.
radiatio a.

acusticae
striae medullares a.
taeniae a.

acustici
trigonum nervi a.

acusticus
nervus a. [CN VIII]
nucleus a.
porus a.

acustimulation

acute
a. acquired hemiplegia
a. African sleeping sickness
a. alcohol poisoning
a. angular kyphosis
a. anoxia
a. anterior poliomyelitis
a. aphonia
a. ascending paralysis
a. atrophic paralysis
a. axonal motor neuropathy
a. brachial radiculitis
a. bulbar poliomyelitis
a. burst injury

NOTES

acute *(continued)*
a. central cervical spinal cord injury
a. cerebellar ataxia (ACA)
a. cerebellar hemispheric lesion
a. cerebral infarction
a. cerebrospinal meningitis (ACM)
a. change in mental status
a. chorea
a. confusional migraine
a. confusional state
a. decubitus ulcer
a. delirium
a. demyelinating encephalomyelitis
a. disconnection syndrome
a. disseminated encephalitis
a. disseminated encephalomyelitis (ADE)
a. disseminating encephalomyelitis
a. dystonic reaction (ADR)
a. epidemic leukoencephalitis
a. febrile polyneuritis
a. foot shock stress
a. fulminating meningococcemia
a. generalized headache
a. genomic response
a. hemorrhagic encephalitis
a. hydrocephalus
a. idiopathic demyelinating polyradiculoneuritis (AIDP)
a. idiopathic polyneuritis
a. inclusion body encephalitis
a. infective polyneuritis
a. inflammatory demyelinating polyneuropathy (AIDP)
a. inflammatory demyelinating polyradiculoneuropathy
a. inflammatory demyelinating polyradiculopathy
a. inflammatory polyneuropathy
a. intermittent porphyria
a. ischemic brachial neuropathy
a. lateral poliomyelitis
a. lateral sclerosis (ALS)
a. life-threatening event (ALTE)
a. localized headache
a. Marchiafava-Bignami disease
a. motor sensory axonal sensory neuropathy
a. mountain sickness (AMS)
a. necrotizing encephalitis
a. necrotizing hemorrhagic encephalomyelitis
a. necrotizing hemorrhagic leukoencephalitis
a. necrotizing myelitis
a. neuronal damage
a. neuronal toxicity
a. neuropsychologic disorder
a. nociceptive response
a. organic brain syndrome
a. organic reaction
a. pain disorder
a. painful polyneuropathy
a. pandysautonomia
a. paralytic poliomyelitis
a. partial myelopathy
a. perivascular myelinoclasis
a. physiologic assessment and chronic health evaluation (APACHE)
A. Physiology Score
a. posterior multifocal placoid pigment
a. postinfectious polyneuropathy
a. postinfective polyneuritis
a. posttraumatic neurosis
a. primary hemorrhagic meningoencephalitis
a. psychoorganic syndrome
a. purulent meningitis
a. purulent meningitis infection
a. recurrent headache
a. reflex bone atrophy
a. relapse
a. rheumatic fever
a. rheumatic fever vasculitis
a. sensory motor axonal neuropathy
a. severe hypotension
a. spinal cord compression
a. steroid quadriplegic myopathy
a. stroke
a. subdural hematoma
a. thrombosis
a. transverse myelitis
a. transverse myelopathy
a. trypanosomiasis
a. tubular necrosis
a. whiplash

acutely acquired hemiplegia
acute-onset paraparesis
acyclovir
acylcholestrol acyl transferase (ACAT)
acyl-CoA
acyl-CoA dehydrogenase deficiency
acyl-CoA oxidase deficiency

AD
Alzheimer disease
autonomic dysreflexia

AD7C cerebrospinal fluid test
Adamantiades-Behçet disease
adamantinoma
pituitary a.

adamantinomatous craniopharyngioma
Adamkiewicz artery
Adams-Stokes
A.-S. disease

A.-S. syncope
A.-S. syndrome
adaptation
a. dynamic
fascicular a.
adaptational approach
adapted reference clamp
adapter
Brown-Roberts-Wells ring a.
halo ring a.
sleeve a.
Telestill photo a.
adaptive
a. control of thought system
a. equipment
a. functioning
ADAS
Alzheimer Disease Assessment Scale
ADAS noncognitive subscale
ADAS-Cog
Alzheimer Disease Assessment Scale–Cognition
ADC
AIDS dementia complex
Alzheimer Disease Center
apparent diffusion coefficient
axiodistocervical
Adcon-L adhesion control
addiction
neonatal drug a.
Addison disease
addisonia
encephalopathia a.
additive neurotoxicity
add-on drug
adduction weakness
adductor
a. dysphonia
a. foot reflex
a. thigh reflex
ADE
acute disseminated encephalomyelitis
A-delta fiber
adendritic, adendric
adenine arabinoside
adenocarcinoma
mucin-secreting a.
adenohypophyseal (*var. of* adenohypophysial)
adenohypophysectomy
adenohypophyseos
intermedia a.
pars distalis a.
pars intermedia a.
adenohypophysial, adenohypophyseal
a. cell
a. compromise
a. neoplasia
adenohypophysis
agranular chromophobe cell in a.
intermediate part of a.
adenohypophysitis
allergic a.
lymphocytic a.
adenoid cystic carcinoma
adenoid-type adenoma
adenoma
acidophil a.
ACTH-producing a.
adenoid-type a.
basophil a.
basophilic a.
choroid plexus a.
chromophil a.
chromophobe a.
chromophobic a.
cutaneous a.
ectopic pituitary a. (EPA)
endocrine-inactive pituitary a.
eosinophil a.
fetal a.
follicle-stimulating/luteinizing hormone a.
giant pituitary a.
glycoprotein-secreting a.
gonadotropin-producing a.
growth hormone-producing a.
growth-hormone-secreting a.
hypersecretory a.
intraspinal a.
invasive pituitary a.
islet cell a.
mammosomatotroph cell a.
mixed growth hormone-prolactin cell a.
nonfunctioning a.
null cell a.
pituitary a.
pleomorphic a.
prolactin-producing a.
prolactin-secreting pituitary a.
sebaceous a.
a. sebaceum
suprasellar a.

NOTES

adenoma *(continued)*
thyrotropin-producing a.
undifferentiated cell a.
adenomatoid odontogenic tumor
adenomectomy
transsphenoidal selective a.
adenoneural
adenopathy
hilar a.
adenopituicyte
adenosine
a. 3′,5′-cyclic monophosphate (cAMP)
a. diphosphate (ADP)
endogenous a.
a. monophosphate acid (AMPA)
a. monophosphate deaminase deficiency
nucleoside a.
a. 5′-phosphosulfate (APS)
a. receptor
a. triphosphatase (ATPase)
a. triphosphate
a. 5′-triphosphate (ATP)
a. triphosphate-dependent potassium channel
a. triphosphate synthesis
adenosylcobalamin
***S*-adenosylmethionine (SAM, SAMe)**
***S*-adenosyl-*l*-methionine**
adenovirus
adenylate cyclase
adenyl cyclase
adenylosuccinate lyase deficiency
adenylyl cyclase
adequate stimulus
ADH
antidiuretic hormone
adherence
diet a.
exercise a.
adhesio, pl. **adhesiones**
a. interthalamica
a. interthalamica tumor
adhesion
arachnoid a.
interthalamic a.
matrix a.
a. molecule
motility a.
neuronal a.
adhesive arachnoiditis
adiabatic fast passage
adiadochokinesis, adiadochocinesia, adiadochocinesis
adiaphoria
Adie
A. tonic pupil
A. tonic pupil syndrome
Adie-Holmes pupil
adipocellular
adipogenic, adipogenous
adiposalgia
adipose
a. graft
a. tissue
adiposis cerebralis
adiposity
cerebral a.
pituitary a.
adiposogenital
a. degeneration
a. dystrophy
a. syndrome
adiposogenitalis
dystrophia a.
aditus
a. ad aqueductum cerebri
a. ad infundibulum
adjacent
a. instability
a. level disease
a. segment
adjunct
neuroleptic a.
adjunctive
a. amphetamine
a. medication
a. screw fixation
a. strategy
a. therapy
adjuration
adjustability
3D positional a.
adjustable pedicle connector
adjustment sleep disorder
adjuvanticity
adjuvant whole-brain radiation therapy
Adkins spinal fusion
ADL
activities of daily living
extended ADL
ADL index
instrumental ADL
ADL test
Adlone Injection
ADmark Assay
administration
chronic a.
compulsive drug a.
drug a.
intracisternal a.
intramuscular a.
leptomeningeal enhancement postcontrast a.
longstanding corticosteroid a.
methylphenidate a.
oral a.

standard dose a.
systematic drug a.
admonition
adneural
adolescence
myoclonic epilepsy of a.
adolescent narcolepsy
adolescent-onset epilepsy
ADP
adenosine diphosphate
ADPR
Alzheimer Disease Patient Registry
ADP-ribosylation
pertussis-toxin-catalyzed ADP-r.
ADR
acute dystonic reaction
ADRC
Alzheimer Disease Research Center
AD-related dementia
adrenal
a. androgen
a. androgen production
a. androstenedione
a. axis
a. body transplant
a. chromaffin cell
a. cortex
a. crisis
a. gland
a. insufficiency
a. leukodystrophy
a. medulla graft
a. medulla transplantation
a. nerve activity
a. segment
adrenaline-Mecholyl test
adrenergic
a. blockade
a. fiber
a. hyperstimulation
a. innervation
a. neuronal blocking agent
a. neurotransmission
a. neurotransmitter
a. receptor
a. system
2-adrenergic
alpha 2-a.
adrenoceptive
adrenoceptor
adrenochrome
adrenocortical
a. coma
a. hyperfunction
a. insufficiency
adrenocorticotropic
a. compromise
a. hormone (ACTH)
a. hormone-secreting pituitary tumor
adrenocorticotropin
adrenoleukodystrophy (ALD)
neonatal a.
X-linked a.
adrenoleukodystrophy/adrenomyeloneuropathy (ALD/AMN)
a.-a. complex
adrenoleukomyeloneuropathy
adrenolytic
adrenomedullary
a. activity
a. component
adrenomimetic
adrenomyelodystrophy (AMD)
adrenomyeloneuropathy
adrenoreceptor
ADRS
Alzheimer Disease Rating Scale
Adson
A. bipolar forceps
A. brain-exploring cannula
A. brain-extracting cannula
A. brain suction tip
A. brain suction tube
A. clip-introducing forceps
A. conductor
A. cranial rongeur
A. cup forceps
A. dissecting hook
A. dressing forceps
A. dural hook
A. dural knife
A. dural needle holder
A. dural protector
A. dural protector guide
A. elevator
A. enlarging bur
A. ganglion scissors
A. hemilaminectomy retractor
A. hemostatic forceps
A. hypophysial forceps
A. knot tier
A. laminectomy chisel
A. modified maneuver

NOTES

Adson *(continued)*
A. needle
A. nerve hook
A. perforating bur
A. right-angle knife
A. scalp clip
A. test
A. tissue forceps
A. wire saw
Adson-Anderson cerebellar retractor
Adson-Brown forceps
Adson-Mixter neurosurgical forceps
Adson-Rogers cranial bur
Ad-Tech
A.-T. electrode guide
A.-T. electrode strip
A.-T. Spencer platinum depth electrode
adterminal
adult
a. acid maltase deficiency
General Ability Measure for A.'s (GAMA)
a. granulosa cell tumor (AGCT)
hemispheric asymmetry reduction in older a.'s (HAROLD)
a. lipofuscinosis
a. neural stem cell
a. polyglucosan body disease
a. pseudohypertrophic muscular dystrophy
a. respiratory distress syndrome
a. Reye syndrome (ARS)
a. scoliosis
a. scoliosis patient
a. scoliosis surgery
subclinical rhythmic EEG discharge of a.'s (SREDA)
subclinical rhythmic epileptiform discharge of a.
a. Wada testing
adultomorphic
a. behavior
a. behavior role
a. stance
adult-onset
a.-o. combined methylmalonic aciduria and homocystinuria
a.-o. dystonia
a.-o. epilepsy
a.-o. movement disorder
a.-o. myasthenia gravis
a.-o. nemaline myopathy
a.-o. spinal muscular atrophy
advanced
a. cortical disease
a. design LINAC radiosurgery
a. glycation end-product (AGE)
a. imaging technique
a. sleep-phase syndrome (ASPS)
a. sleep staging rule
a. wakefulness theory
advance directive
advancement
bimaxillary a.
frontoorbital a.
genioglossus a.
hyoid a.
maxillomandibular a. (MMA)
monobloc a.
transcranial frontofacial a.
advantage
psychometric a.
right ear a.
therapeutic a.
adventitial neuritis
adverse
a. autonomic response
a. negative immunosuppressive effect
a. neurologic complication
a. side effect
adversity
early life a.
adynamia episodica hereditaria
Aeby plane
AED
antiepileptic drug
Aedes aegypti
AEEG
ambulatory electroencephalogram
ambulatory electroencephalography
aegypti
Aedes a.
aerobic exercise
aerocele
epidural a.
intracranial a.
aerodigestive tract
aerophilus
Haemophilus a.
aerosolized droplet nucleus
aeruginosa
Pseudomonas a.
Aesculap
A. bipolar cautery
A. skull perforator
Aesculap-Miethke valve
aesthetics
afebrile seizure
affability
surface a.
affect
cognitive generation of a.
a. elicitation
evoked a.
generation of a.
hyperactive a.

hypoactive a.
a. spasm
a. trauma model
affective
a. arousal theory
a. process
a. processing
a. prodrome of epilepsy
a. prodrome of migraine
a. property
a. reaction
a. schematic mental model
a. startle reflex
a. state
a. symptom
a. symptom of seizure
affectomotor
affect-related
a.-r. processing
a.-r. schematic mental model
affectualization
afferent
a. digital lesion
a. digital nerve
excitatory a.
general somatic a. (GSA)
general visceral a. (GVA)
a. input
a. limb
a. motor unit
a. nerve fiber
a. nerve lesion
a. neurofiber
a. neuron
a. pathway
a. pupillary defect
a. relation
special somatic a. (SSA)
a. thermosensory information
affiliation drive
affiliative drive
affinity
receptor a.
affixa
lamina a.
A-fiber evoked response
afibrinogenemia
AFP
alpha fetoprotein
A-frame electrode
African
A. sleeping sickness
A. trypanosomiasis
AFT
attractor field therapy
afterbrain
aftercontraction
aftercurrent
afterdischarge
amygdala-kindled a.
myotonic a.
photic a.
a. threshold
afterhyperpolarization
afterimage
afterimpression
afterloading catheter
aftermovement
afternystagmus
cycles of a.
optokinetic a. (OKAN)
afterperception
afterpotential
negative a.
positive a.
aftersensation
aftersound
aftertaste
aftertouch
aftervision
agalactiae
Streptococcus a.
aganglionic
aganglionosis
agapism
agarose
a. gel electrophoresis
low-melt temperature a.
agastroneuria
AGCT
adult granulosa cell tumor
AGE
advanced glycation end-product
arterial gas embolism
age
a. effect
a. of onset
A.'s and Stages Questionnaires
age-appropriate strategy
age-associated
a.-a. memory failure

NOTES

age-associated *(continued)*
a.-a. memory impairment
a.-a. sensitivity
age-dependent
a.-d. epilepsy
a.-d. epilepsy syndrome
a.-d. length
a.-d. slowing
Agee
3M A. carpal tunnel release system
A. technique
agenesia corticalis
agenesis
callosal a.
carotid artery a.
a. of corpus callosum
corpus callosum a.
nuclear a.
Pang-type a.
partial a.
sacral a.
sacrococcygeal a.
total a.
agent
adrenergic neuronal blocking a.
alerting a.
alkylating a.
alpha-adrenergic blocking a.
anticholinergic a.
antidipsotropic a.
antidyskinetic a.
antifibrinolytic a.
antimicrobial a.
antineoplastic a.
antiparkinsonism a.
antispastic a.
beta-adrenergic receptor blocking a.
bioterrorism a.
N-butyl 2-cyanoacrylate with lipiodol adhesive a.
calcium channel blocking a.
cerebral blood flow a.
cerebral vasodilating a.
chemosensitivity-enhancing a.
chimpanzee coryza a. (CCA)
conventional neuroleptic a.
cytotoxic a.
disease-modifying a. (DMA)
endogenous neuroprotective a.
fast-acting a.
fibrinolytic a.
FloSeal hemostatic a.
ganglionic blocking a.
5-HT releasing a.
hyperosmotic a.
hypnotic a.
immunotherapeutic a.
lipid-lowering a.
monoamine oxidase inhibitor-serotonergic a.
mood-stabilizing a.
natural chemotherapy a.
neuromuscular blocking a.
neuronal stabilizing a.
nonionic contrast a.
noxious a.
Onyx liquid embolic a.
oral antiviral a.
osmotic dehydrating a.
pharmacologic a.
pharmacological a.
phrenotropic a.
Proceed hemostatic a.
psychopharmacologic a.
psychotomimetic a.
psychotropic a.
reinforcing a.
second-line a.
serotonergic a.
short-acting hypnotic a.
susceptibility a.
sympathomimetic a.
tantalum powder contrast a.
therapeutic a.
traditional neuroleptic a.
tumor differentiating a.
in utero teratologic a.
age-related
a.-r. brain change
a.-r. comorbidity
a.-r. deterioration process
a.-r. developmental process
a.-r. epileptogenesis
a.-r. maturation
a.-r. memory impairment
a.-r. pharmacodynamic change
a.-r. pharmacokinetic change
a.-r. sleep physiology
age-specific
a.-s. cumulative incidence
a.-s. risk factor
ageusia, ageustia
ageusic aphasia
agger nasi cell
agglomerate
heterotopia a.
agglutination
latex a.
aggrandize
aggrecan proteoglycan
aggregate
epileptic neuronal a.
fibrillary a.
gaze-coordinating a.
neuronal a.
nuclear a.

aggregated
technetium-99m albumin a.
Aggrenox
aggression
pathological a.
aggressive papillary middle ear tumor
aging
accelerated a.
amyloidosis of a.
brain a.
Duke Twins Study of Memory in A.
neuroanatomy of a.
agitans
Hunt juvenile paralysis a.
paralysis a.
spasmus a.
agitated
a. delirium syndrome
a. depression
a. reaction
agitation
Caitlin a.
a. level
marked motor a.
motor a.
nocturnal a.
overlapping a.
overt a.
a. response
agitolalia
agitophasia
aglomerular
agnate
agnea
agnosia
apperceptive visual a.
associative visual a.
auditory a.
autotopagnosia a.
color a.
corporal a.
facial a.
finger a.
generalized auditory a.
gustatory a.
ideational a.
localization a.
object a.
optic a.
position a.
posture a.
selective auditory a.
somatagnosia a.
tactile a.
topographical a.
verbal auditory a.
visual a.
visuospatial a.
agonadism
agonist
alpha a.
alpha-2 a.
beta adrenergic a.
dopamine a.
D2-selective dopamine a.
ergot-derivative dopamine a.
GABA a.
gamma aminobutyric acid a.
high-dose dopaminergic a.
5-HT a.
low-dose dopaminergic a.
M1 a.
a. muscle
serotonin 5-HT receptor a.
vasopressin receptor a.
agrammatism agraphia
agrammatologia
agranular
a. chromophobe cell in adenohypophysis
a. cortex
agranulocytosis
agraphia
absolute a.
acoustic a.
agrammatism a.
a. alexia
alexia with a.
alexia without a.
amnemonic a.
aphasic a.
apraxic a.
atactic a.
atactica a.
cerebral a.
constructional a.
lexical a.
literal a.
mental a.
motor a.
musical a.
paretic a.
perseverative a.

NOTES

agraphia *(continued)*
phonological a.
pure a.
spatial a.
verbal a.
agraphic
agrypnodal coma
agyria
AH
autonomic hyperreflexia
AHA-SOC
American Heart Association Stroke Outcome Classification
AHI
apnea-hypopnea index
AHSCT
autologous hematopoietic stem cell transplantation
ahylognosia
ahypnia
AI
apnea index
AI adenosine receptor
AI, AII area
AICA
anterior inferior cerebellar artery
Aicardi-Goutières
A.-G. disease
A.-G. syndrome
Aicardi syndrome
aid
ergogenic a.
external memory a.
walking a.
AIDP
acute idiopathic demyelinating polyradiculoneuritis
acute inflammatory demyelinating polyneuropathy
autoimmune demyelinating polyneuropathy
AIDS
acquired immunodeficiency syndrome
AIDS dementia
AIDS dementia complex (ADC)
AIDS encephalopathy
AIDS neuropathy
AIDS-associated vacuolar myelopathy
AIDS-related
AIDS-r. myelopathy
AIDS-r. toxoplasmosis
AIF
apoptosis-inducing factor
ailment
neurologic a.
AION
anterior ischemic optic neuropathy
air
a. blade
a. blast
a. cell
a. conduction test
a. contrast study
a. drill
a. embolism
a. embolus
a. gun pellet
intracranial a.
a. plasma spray
a. plethysmography
a. tube
a. ventriculography
air-bone gap
airborne arthroconidia
air-brain interface
air-fluid level
AIROM
active integral range of motion
air-powered drill
air-stepping
airstream mechanism
airway
artificial a.
a. control
a. edema
esophageal a.
a. mucosal receptor
a. muscle tone
a. obstruction
pharyngeal a.
a. protection
Starling resistor model of upper a.
upper a.
akathisia, acathisia
focal a.
treatment-emergent a.
akinesia, akinesis
a. algera
a. amnestica
early morning a.
akinesthesia
akinetic, akinesic
a. apraxia
a. drop attack
a. drop spell
a. epilepsy
a. mutism
a. patient
akinetic-rigid
a.-r. Huntington disease
a.-r. syndrome
Akineton
akoria (*var. of* acoria)
Akros
A. extended-care mattress
A. pressure mattress
AK-Taine

Akureyri disease
ala, pl. **alae**
a. of central lobule
a. cerebelli
a. cinerea
alae lingulae cerebelli
a. lobuli centralis
a. lobulis centralis
Alagille syndrome
Alajouanine syndrome
alalia
alalic
alanine
a. transaminase
a. tRNA
alanyl
alanyl-tRNA synthetase
alar
a. lamina of neural tube
a. ligament
a. plate
a. screw
a. soft tissue collapse
alaris
lamina a.
alarm
a. clock headache
ventilator a.
alba
commissura ventralis a.
substantia a.
Albee
A. lumbar spinal fusion
A. olive-shaped bur
A. shelf procedure
albendazole therapy
Albert Grass Heritage PSG
albicans
Candida a.
Cryptococcus a.
albinism
oculocutaneous a.
albocinereous
Albright syndrome
albumin
low serum a.
a. metabolism
serum a.
technetium-99m macroaggregated a.
a. transfusion
albuminocytologic dissociation
albuterol
Alcadd Test, Revised Edition
alcaptonuria, alkaptonuria
alchemy
Alcock test
alcohol
allyl a.
a. dehydrogenase
intermediate brain syndrome due to a.
a. metabolism
a. neurolysis
a. persisting dementia
polyvinyl a.
saliva screen for a.
a. toxicity
a. withdrawal
a. withdrawal seizure
alcohol-dependent sleep disorder
alcoholic
a. amblyopia
a. amnesia
a. classification
a. coma
a. delirium tremens
a. encephalopathy
a. epilepsy
a. myopathy
a. peripheral neuropathy
a. poisoning
a. polyneuropathy
a. withdrawal tremor
alcoholica
amblyopia a.
alcohol-induced
a.-i. depression
a.-i. insomnia
a.-i. peripheral neuropathy
alcoholism
Collaborative Study on the Genetics of A. (COGA)
alcohol-precipitated epilepsy
alcohol-related
a.-r. ataxia
a.-r. phenotype
a.-r. seizure
ALD
adrenoleukodystrophy
ALD/AMN
adrenoleukodystrophy/adrenomyeloneuropathy
ALD/AMN complex
aldehyde dehydrogenase

NOTES

aldose reductase
aldosterone deficiency
Aldrich syndrome
alemmal
alemtuzumab humanized monoclonal antibody
alendronate
alert
oriented and a.
a. and oriented (AAO)
Alertec
alerting
a. agent
a. maneuver on electroencephalogram
a. stimulus on electroencephalogram
alertness
a. behavior (AB)
level of a.
mental a.
phasic a.
state of a.
Alexander disease
alexia
agraphia a.
a. allochiria
anterior a.
central a.
incomplete a.
motor a.
musical a.
optical a.
posterior a.
pure a.
sensory a.
tactile a.
visual a.
a. with agraphia
a. without agraphia
alexic
alexithymic
alfentanil hydrochloride
algera
akinesia a.
dyskinesia a.
algesia (*var. of* algesthesia)
algesic
algesichronometer
algesimeter (*var. of* algesiometer)
algesimetry
algesiogenic
algesiometer, algesimeter, algometer
Aly a.
Björnström a.
Boas a.
pressure a.
algesthesia, algesia, algesthesis
algetic
algica
synesthesia a.
algiomotor
algiomuscular
algodystrophy
algogenesis, algogenesia
algogenic
algologist
algology
algometer (*var. of* algesiometer)
algometry
algoneurodystrophy
algophobia
algorithm
bone a.
Fourier transform a.
hydrophobicity a.
interpolation a.
algospasm
ALI
argon laser iridotomy
aliasing on electroencephalogram
Alice in Wonderland syndrome
alien
a. hand sign
a. hand syndrome
a. limb phenomenon
a. limb sign
alienation
body a.
sense of a.
ALIF
anterior lumbar interbody fusion
alignment
ocular a.
sagittal anatomic a.
stable a.
alimentary
a. edema
a. seizure
alimentation
parenteral a.
alinjection
aliphatic
aliquot
alkaline phosphatase
alkaloid
a. neuropathy
vinca a.
alkalosis
metabolic a.
respiratory a.
tetany of a.
alkaptonuria (*var. of* alcaptonuria)
alkylamine
alkylating
a. agent
a. chemotherapy
allachesthesia (*var. of* allesthesia)

allantoic bladder
allantoidean
allantois
allele
ApoE e4 a.
Asp risk a.
e4 a.
fukutin a.
wild-type a.
allelic
a. heterogeneity
a. loss
allelism
allelomorph
Allen
A. and Ferguson classification system
A. maneuver
A. picture
A. rule
A. test
allergic
a. adenohypophysitis
a. angiitis
a. encephalomyelitis
a. reaction
allesthesia, allachesthesia, allochesthesia, alloesthesia
visual a.
Allevyn dressing
Allgrove syndrome
alliance
contractual a.
relational a.
Tuberous Sclerosis A.
allied reflex
alligator cup forceps
all-median nerve hand
allochesthesia (*var. of* allesthesia)
allochiria, allocheiria
alexia a.
allocortex
AlloDerm acellular dermal matrix
allodynia
brush-evoked a.
brush-induced a.
cold-induced a.
cutaneous a.
static a.
alloesthesia (*var. of* allesthesia)
allogenic transplant
allograft
a. bone grafting
fibular a.
a. iliac bone
Puros Accugraft a.
A. spacer
a. strut
Tutoplast processed a.
allokinesis
allokinetic
allolalia
Allomatrix bone substitute
allomeric function
allonomous
allopatric species
allophasis
allophone tabulation
alloplastic
a. cranioplasty
a. material
allosteric manner
allotriosmia
allotropic
all-ulnar nerve hand
allyl
a. alcohol
a. isothiocyanate
allylglycine
almond nucleus
almotriptan malate
Alnico
A. Magneprobe magnet
A. Magneprobe magnet alpha
alobar holoprosencephaly
alogia
alopecia
a. capitis totalis
a. disseminata
a. follicularis
Johnston a.
a. liminaris frontalis
lipedematous a.
moth-eaten a.
a. neurotica
patterned a.
a. prematura
a. triangularis congenitalis
alosetron
Alpers disease
alpha
a. 2-adrenergic
a. agonist

NOTES

alpha *(continued)*
Alnico Magneprobe magnet a.
a. antagonist
a., beta, gamma hypothesis
a. beta peptide
a. blocking
a. cell of anterior lobe of hypophysis
a. coefficient
Cronbach a.
a. ET
a. ethyltryptamine
a. fetoprotein (AFP)
a. fiber
a. frequency activity
a. frequency band
a. frequency coma
a. frequency range
a. galactoside A, B
a. glucosidase
a. index
a. interferon
a. latrotoxin
a. mannosidase
a. mannosidosis
a. motoneuron
a. motor neuron
obsessional compulsive inventory a.
occipital a.
a. pattern
a. response
a. rhythm
a. rhythm frequency
a. rhythm generator
a. secretase
a. spindle
a. state
a. test
a. tocopherol
a. transient
a. wave
a. wave strain
alpha-1 adrenergic antagonist
alpha-2
a.-2 adrenergic receptor
a.-2 agonist
a.-2 globulin
alpha-*N*-acetylgalactosaminidase
alpha-*N*-acetylglucosaminidase
alpha-adrenergic
a.-a. blocking agent
a.-a. receptor
alpha-adrenoceptor antagonist
alpha-amino-3-hydroxy-5-methylisoxazole-4-propionic acid
alpha-aminoadipic aciduria
alpha-arc
***dl*-alpha-difluoromethylornithine**
alpha-*L*-iduronidase
alpha-ketoadipic aciduria
alpha-ketoglutarate oxidation
alpha-methylacetoacetic aciduria
alphamimetic
alphaprodine hydrochloride
alpha-synuclein
a.-s. gene
a.-s. haplotype
a.-s. pathology
a.-s. protein
Alphavirus
Alport syndrome
alprazolam
ALS
acute lateral sclerosis
amyotrophic lateral sclerosis
Guamanian ALS
sporadic ALS
ALSA
Amyotrophic Lateral Sclerosis Association
ALS-like syndrome
ALS-PD
amyotrophic lateral sclerosis-Parkinson dementia
ALS-PD complex
Alstrom-Hallgren syndrome
ALTE
acute life-threatening event
alteplase
alteration
awareness a.
behavior a.
cyclic a.
genetic a.
genomic a.
language a.
a. of memory structure
metabolic a.
neurocognitive a.
selective speech perception a.
sleep and dream a.
speech processing a.
speech tracking a.
altered
a. axonal excitability
a. cognition
a. cognitive function
a. immune response
a. level of consciousness
a. mental status
a. sensation
a. sleep schedule
a. spatial perception
a. tau processing
a. time perception
alternans
hemiplegia a.

alternate
a. binaural loudness balance
a. binaural loudness balance test
a. hemianesthesia
a. motion rate (AMR)
alternating
a. current (AC)
a. hemiplegia of childhood
a. hypoglossal hemiplegia
a. mydriasis
a. nystagmus
a. skew deviation
a. tremor
alternation
genetic a.
alternative
graft material a.
a. occipital artery middle cerebral artery
a. therapy
a. tremor
althesin
altitude insomnia
altitudinal
a. hemianopia
a. visual field defect
altophobia
Altropane
altruism
aluminum
brain a.
a. contouring template set
a. cranioplasty
a. glycinate
a. hydroxide with magnesium hydroxide and simethicone
a. intoxication
a. master rod
a. toxic disorder
a. toxicity
alvear fasciculus
alvei (*pl. of* alveus)
alveolar
a. hypoventilation syndrome
a. nerve
alveolus, pl. **alveoli**
alveus, pl. **alvei**
a. of hippocampus
Aly algesiometer
Alzheimer
A. Association
A. atrophic dementia
A. basket
A. cell
A. disease (AD)
A. Disease Assessment Scale (ADAS)
A. Disease Assessment Scale–Cognition (ADAS-Cog)
A. Disease Assessment Scale-Cognition subscale
A. Disease Center (ADC)
A. disease neuropathology
A. disease noncognitive subscale
A. Disease Patient Registry (ADPR)
A. Disease Rating Scale (ADRS)
A. disease-related dementia
A. Disease and Related Disorders Association
A. Disease Research Center (ADRC)
A. neurofibrillary degeneration
A. precursor protein (APP)
A. sclerosis
A. senile dementia (ASD)
A. survivor
A. type I, II astrocyte
Alzheimer-like pathology
Alzheimer-type senile dementia
amacrine cell
amantadine hydrochloride
amaurosis
cat's-eye a.
central a.
a. centralis
cerebral a.
a. fugax
gaze-evoked a.
Leber congenital a.
uremic a.
amaurotic idiocy
ambageusia
ambenonium
ambidexterity, ambidextrism
ambidextrous
Ambien
ambiens
cisterna a.
ambient cistern
ambiguity
acoustic a.
diagnostic a.

NOTES

ambiguous
a. external stimulus
a. nucleus
ambiguus
nucleus a.
ambilevous
AmBisome
amblyaphia
amblygeustia
amblyogenic period
amblyope
amblyopia
alcoholic a.
a. alcoholica
a. ex anopsia
tobacco-alcohol a.
toxic a.
ambulation
brace-free a.
a. skill
violent a.
ambulatory
a. accelerometry
a. automatism
a. EEG recording
a. electroencephalogram (AEEG)
a. electroencephalography (AEEG)
AMD
adrenomyelodystrophy
amebiasis
cerebral a.
Entamoeba histolytica cerebral a.
Iodamoeba buetschlii cerebral a.
amebic
a. aneurysm
a. infection
a. meningoencephalitis
ameboid
a. astrocyte
a. cell
ameboidism
ameloblastoma
pituitary a.
ameloblastomatous craniopharyngioma
AME microcurrent TENS unit
amenorrhea
hypothalamic a.
primary a.
amentia
eclamptic a.
nevoid a.
America
Autism Society of A.
Huntington Disease Society of A. (HDSA)
American
A. Academy of Cerebral Palsy
A. Academy of Sleep Medicine
A. Association of Directors of Psychiatric Residency Training
A. Association for Geriatric Psychiatry (AAGP)
A. Association of Neurological Surgeons/Congress of Neurological Surgeons (AANS/CNS)
A. Association for the Psychophysiological Study of Sleep
A. Board of Psychiatry and Neurology (ABPN)
A. Brain Tumor Association
A. Council for Headache Education
A. Epilepsy Society
A. Heart Association Stroke Outcome Classification (AHA-SOC)
A. Musculoskeletal Tumor Society rating scale
A. Optical Hardy-Rand-Rittler color plate
A. Pain Society
A. Parkinson Disease Association
A. silk suture
A. Sleep Disorders Association
A. Spinal Cord Injury Association classification
A. Spinal Injury Association (ASIA)
A. Spinal Injury Association/International Medical Society of Paraplegia (ASIA/IMSOP)
A. Spinal Injury Association/International Medical Society of Paraplegia Impairment Scale
A. Sterilizer operating table
A. Stroke Association
The A. Society of Pediatric Neurosurgeons
A. Thoracic Society
A. trypanosomiasis
Ames demonstration
A-methaPred Injection
Amicar
amiculum, pl. **amicula**
a. of inferior olive
a. olivare
amidotrizoic acid
Amikin
amine
biogenic a.
a. precursor uptake decarboxylase (APUD)
amineptine
aminergic

amino
a. acid (AA)
a. acid metabolic disorder
a. acid neurotransmitter
a. acid transporter
aminoacidopathy
aminoaciduria
arginase deficiency a.
argininosuccinic a.
cystathioninuria a.
a. deficiency
dicarboxylic a.
histidinemia a.
hydroxyisovaleric a.
hyperlysinemia a.
hyperprolinemia a.
isovaleric acidemia a.
methylmalonic a.
neonatal tyrosinemia a.
primary a.
sulfite oxidase deficiency a.
tyrosinemia a.
aminobenzoate
butyl a.
sodium a.
aminocaproic acid
Aminoff
A. disability score
A. Scale
aminoglutethimide
aminoglycoside
intratympanic a.
aminopenicillin
4-aminopyridine
aminotransferase
aspartate a. (AST)
kynurenine a.
ornithine-ketoacid a.
Amipaque
Amitone
amitriptyline
a. hydrochloride
a. hydrochloride and chlordiazepoxide
Ammon
A. horn
A. horn sclerosis
ammonia
a. blood level
a. intoxication
ammonis
cornu a.
subiculum cornu a.
ammonium
a. chloride
a. chloride delirium
a. tetrathiomolybdate
ammonotelic
amnemonic
a. agraphia
a. aphasia
amnesia
alcoholic a.
amnesic a.
antegrade a.
anterograde a. (AA)
a. for attack
auditory a.
basal forebrain a.
Broca a.
circumscribed a.
concussion a.
confabulatory a.
continuous a.
dense a.
dissociative a.
emotional a.
episodic a.
executive deficit transient global a.
functional retrograde a.
generalized a.
global a.
hippocampal a.
hysterical a.
ictal a.
infantile a.
Korsakoff a.
korsakoffian a.
lacunar a.
localized a.
olfactory a.
organic a.
patchy retrograde a.
postconcussion a.
postconcussive a.
posthypnotic a.
posttraumatic a.
pretraumatic a.
psychogenic a.
retroactive a.
selective a.
shrinking retrograde a.

NOTES

amnesia *(continued)*
tactile a.
transient global a. (TGA)
a. for trauma
traumatic a.
verbal a.
visual a.
amnesic, amnestic
a. amnesia
a. aphasia
a. apraxia
a. disorder
a. disorder due to general medical condition
a. dysnomia
a. memoration
a. patient
a. state
a. syndrome
amnestica
akinesia a.
amniocentesis
amniote
amobarbital-induced hemiparesis
amobarbital test
amodiaquine
amoral personality
amorphagnosia
amorphosynthesis
amorphous fraction of adrenal cortex
Amostat
amotivation
amount
maximum tolerable a.
amoxapine
AMPA
adenosine monophosphate acid
AMPA receptor
AMPA receptor-mediated response
Ampalex
amperometric response
amphetamine
adjunctive a.
a. and dextroamphetamine
gamma hydroxybutyrate and a.
a. intoxication
a. sulfate
a. withdrawal
amphetamine/methamphetamine
analog of a./m.
phencyclidine and a./m.
amphicrania
amphicyte
amphiphysin autoantibody
amphotonia, amphotony
Amplatz exchange length wire
amplification
a. reaction
symptom a.
amplifier
Botox injection a.
compression a.
DAM-80 a.
gradient a.
NeuroProbe a.
power a.
Ampligen
amplitude
absolute band a.
absolute EP a.
asymmetry a.
CMAP a.
compound muscle action potential a.
high a.
local reduction in a.
peak-to-peak a.
percentage of error in a. (PEA)
reduction of a.
relative band a.
respiratory effort a.
saccade a.
sensory compound action potential a.
sensory nerve action potential a.
SNAP a.
very low a.
waveform a.
ampullaria
crura membranacea ampullaria ductuum a.
a. ductuum
ampullaris
crista a.
cupula cristae a.
neuroepithelium cristae a.
ampullar nerve
ampullary
a. crest
a. cupula
a. limb of semicircular duct
amputation neuroma
AMR
alternate motion rate
AMS
acute mountain sickness
Amsler grid testing
AMTR
anterior mesial temporal resection
amusia
instrumental a.
motor a.
sensory a.
vocal motor a.
amyelencephalia
amyelia
amyelic
amyelinated

amyelination
amyelinic
amyelous, amyeloic, amyelonic
amygdala, pl. **amygdalae**
a. activation
a. atrophy
a. cerebelli
a. damage
a. fear circuitry
a. kindling
nucleus amygdalae
a. nucleus group
a. response
a. seizure
a. subnucleus
a. volume
a. volumetric loss
amygdala-kindled afterdischarge
amygdala-prefrontal cortex-locus ceruleus interaction
amygdalar epilepsy
amygdaline
amygdaloclaustral area
amygdaloclaustralis
area a.
amygdalofugal
a. fiber
a. pathway
amygdalohippocampectomy
amygdaloid
a. body
a. complex
a. nucleus
a. tubercle
amygdaloidectomy
amygdaloidei
pars basolateralis corporis a.
pars corticomedialis corporis a.
pars olfactoria corporis a.
rami corporis a.
amygdaloideum
corpus a.
amygdalopiriformis
area transitionis a.
amygdalopiriform transition area
amygdalotomy
amyl
a. hydrate
a. nitrite
amylase plaque
amylene
a. chloral
a. hydrate
amyloid
a. angiopathy
a. beta peptide
a. beta protein
a. body
congophilic a.
a. deposition
a. neuropathy
a. plaque
a. plaque deposition
a. polyneuropathy
a. precursor protein (APP)
a. precursor protein gene
amyloidoma
amyloidosis
a. of aging
cerebrovascular a.
familial a.
hereditary neuropathic a.
heredofamilial a.
a. peripheral neuropathy
skeletal a.
transthyretin-associated neuropathic a.
amyloidosis-Dutch type
amyoesthesia, amyoesthesis
amyoplasia congenita
amyotonia congenita
amyotrophic
a. lateral sclerosis (ALS)
A. Lateral Sclerosis Association (ALSA)
a. lateral sclerosis-Parkinson dementia (ALS-PD)
a. lateral sclerosis-Parkinson dementia complex
a. type of spongiform encephalopathy
amyotrophy, amyotrophia
Aran-Duchenne a.
asthmatic a.
benign focal a.
brachial a.
diabetic a.
dystonic a.
hemiplegic a.
hereditary neuralgic a.
juvenile a.
monomelic a.

NOTES

amyotrophy *(continued)*
neuralgic a.
a. parkinsonism
primary progressive a.
progressive nuclear a.
progressive spinal a.
syphilitic a.
amytal
sodium a.
anacamptometer
anacatesthesia
anachronism
EEG a.
anacoluthon
anacusis
Anafranil
anaglyphoscope
anal
a. nerve
a. reflex
a. sphincter
a. verge
a. wink
analeptic
analgesia
a. dolorosa
interpleural a. (IPA)
intrathecal morphine a.
paretic a.
patient-controlled a. (PCA)
reverse a.
analgesic, analgetic
acupuncture a.
a. cuirass
migraine neuralgia a.
narcotic a.
a. rebound headache
analgesimeter
analgosedation
analog, analogue
a. of amphetamine/methamphetamine
a. domain
a. filter
I-labeled cocaine a.
meperidine a.
a. of phencyclidine thiophene
prion a.
analogous brain mechanism
analog-to-digital converter
analogue (*var. of* analog)
analysis, pl. **analyses**
autoregressive model for signal a.
behavior a.
best-fit a.
bioelectrical impedance a.
biomechanical a.
cephalometric a.
cluster a.
3-color FACScan a.
complex segregation a.
compressed spectral a.
computer-aided image a.
computer-assisted EEG signal a.
computerized EEG signal a.
conventional factor a.
Courtship A.
Cox regression a.
CSF a.
deformity a.
densitometric a.
digital signal a.
3-dimensional vector a.
DNA a.
3D relationship a.
electrooculographic a.
FACScan a.
finite element a.
Fourier a.
functional a.
gender-specific a.
genetic linkage a.
group a.
haplotype a.
high-resolution chromosome a.
a. of homonomy
immunocytochemical a.
imprinting center mutation a.
intent-to-treat a.
interaction process a.
Kaplan-Meier survival a.
linear least-square regression a.
linkage a.
logistic regression a.
microsatellite marker a.
mitochondrial deoxyribonucleic acid a.
morphometry a.
Northern blot a.
perception a.
post hoc a.
power spectral a.
preliminary a.
principal-components a.
a. procedure
quantitative EEG a.
quantitative motor unit potential a.
regression a.
Sassouni a.
shape a.
signal a.
sleeplessness a.
spatiotemporal source a.
SPECT a.
spectral a.
spinal fluid a.
state-of-the-art a.
total body neutron activation a.
a. variance

a. of variance (ANOVA)
volumetric a.
voxel-by-voxel a.
voxel-wise a.
Western blot a.
analytical therapy
analytic therapy
analyzer
Axon Sentinel-4 a.
Beckman Coulter CEQ8000 fluorescent DNA a.
fast Fourier transformation spectrum a.
immunoturbidimetry a.
Octopus visual field a.
wave a.
anamnestic
ananastasia
anapeiratic
anaphia, anhaphia
anaphylactic
a. shock
a. shock prophylaxis
anaphylactogenesis
anaphylactoid reaction
anaphylaxis
anaplasia
anaplastic
a. astrocytoma
a. ependymoma
a. focus
a. meningioma
a. mixed glioma
a. oligodendroglioma
a. zone
anaplerosis
pyruvate-mediated a.
Anaprox
anaptic
anaptyxis
anarithmia
anarthria
anastomosing fiber
anastomosis, pl. **anastomoses**
carotid-basilar a.
carotid-vertebral a.
cross-face a.
cross-facial nerve graft a.
end-to-end a.
excimer laser-assisted nonocclusive a. (ELANA)
extradural a.
Galen a.
grafting a.
hypoglossal-facial nerve a.
Hyrtl a.
intradural a.
intraterritorial a.
jump-graft hypoglossal-facial nerve a.
leptomeningeal a.
Martin-Gruber a.
microneurovascular a.
microvascular a.
persistent primitive carotid-basilar artery a.
persistent trigeminal artery a.
primary end-to-end a.
Riche-Cannieu a.
spinal accessory nerve-facial nerve a.
STA-MCA a.
superior temporal artery-middle cerebral artery a.
temporal-cerebral arterial a.
traumatic a.
anastomotic
a. fiber
a. leak
anatomic
a. fact
a. hook
a. localization
a. pathology
a. rule
anatomical
a. correlate
a. evidence
a. hemispherectomy
a. snuffbox
a. variant
anatomic-functional
anatomicoclinical syndrome
anatomy
cervicothoracic pedicle a.
MRI-based brain a.
pediatric spinal a.
pedicle a.
surgical a.
ANC
absolute neutrophil count
ANCA
antineuronal cytoplasmic autoantibody

NOTES

ANCA-positive granulomatous giant cell arteritis
anchor
Isola spinal implant system a.
traction a.
anchorage-dependent signal
anchoring point
ancillary test
ancyroid, ankyroid
Andermann syndrome
Andersch
A. ganglion
A. nerve
Andersen
A. disease
A. syndrome
Anderson-Adson scalp retractor
Andrade syndrome
André anatomical hook
Andrews frame
androgen
adrenal a.
circulating a.
a. receptor
a. secretion
androgenic property
androgenous
androgynous
androstenedione
adrenal a.
anecdotal
a. data
a. evidence
anechoic chamber
anelectrotonic state
anelectrotonus
Anel method
anemia
congenital aplastic a.
congenital hemolytic a.
Fanconi a.
myelophthisic a.
pernicious a.
sideroblastic a.
anemic
a. anoxia
a. hypoxia
a. polyneuritis
a. polyneuropathy
anemometer
warm-wire a.
anencephalic, anencephalous
anencephaly, anencephalia
a. dysraphism
a. screening
anergasia
anergastic
anergic
anergy
aneroid chest bellows
anesthekinesia, anesthecinesia
anesthesia
acupuncture a.
angiospastic a.
barbiturate burst-suppression a.
bulbar a.
compression a.
conduction a.
continuous intravenous regional a. (CIVRA)
contralateral a.
corneal a.
crash induction of a.
crossed a.
diagnostic a.
dissociated a.
dissociative a.
doll's head a.
a. dolorosa
facial a.
gauntlet a.
general endotracheal a.
general orotracheal a.
girdle a.
glove a.
gustatory a.
halothane a.
hysterical a.
intravenous regional a. (IVRA)
isoflurane a.
local a.
Mayo block a.
muscular a.
olfactory a.
painful a.
perineural a.
pharyngeal a.
pressure a.
ring block a.
SAB a.
saddle-shaped a.
segmental a.
sevoflurane a.
spinal a.
splanchnic a.
stocking a.
stocking-glove a.
tactile a.
thalamic hyperesthetic a.
thermal a.
thermic a.
unilateral a.
visceral a.
anesthesimeter
anesthetic
dissociative a.
eutectic mixture of local a.'s (EMLA)

a. leprosy
a. monitoring
short-acting local a.
volatile a.

anethopathy

aneuploidy

aneurogenic

aneurolemmic

aneurysm

amebic a.
anterior circulation intracranial a.
anterior communicating artery a.
arterial a.
arteriosclerotic intracranial a.
arteriovenous a.
aspergillotic a.
asymptomatic intracranial a.
atherosclerotic a.
bacterial a.
basilar apex a.
basilar artery trunk a.
basilar bifurcation a.
basilar tip a.
berry a.
bilobed a.
blisterlike a.
blood blister-like a.
brain a.
carotid artery a.
carotid cave a.
carotid-ophthalmic artery a.
cavernous carotid a.
cavernous sinus a.
cerebral arterial a.
cerebral artery a.
cerebrovascular a.
Charcot-Bouchard intracerebral a.
circle of Willis a.
cirsoid a.
classic dissecting a.
clinoidal a.
a. clip
a. clip applicator
clip ligation of a.
clipped a.
a. clipping
coating of a.
coexisting a.
congenital cerebral a.
cranial a.
de novo a.
dissecting a.
distal anterior cerebral artery a.
distal lenticulostriate artery a.
dolichoectatic a.
dome of a.
extracerebral a.
extracranial a.
familial intracranial a. (FIA)
feeding artery of a.
a. formation
fundus of a.
fusiform a.
a. of Galen vein
giant basilar a.
giant cervical carotid artery a.
giant intracranial a.
giant saccular a.
great cerebral vein of Galen a.
hunterian ligation of a.
Hunt-Kosnik classification of a.
hypophysial a.
a. incidence
incidental a.
infectious a.
infraclinoid a.
internal carotid artery a.
International Study of Unruptured Intracranial A.'s (ISUIA)
intracavernous carotid a.
intracerebral a.
intracranial a.
intradural a.
intranidal a.
a. location
lower basilar a.
luetic a.
miliary a.
M1 segment a.
multiple intracranial a.'s
mycotic intracranial a.
neck of a.
a. neck dissector
a. needle
neoplastic a.
nongiant a.
a. obliteration
a. occlusion
ophthalmic artery a.
ophthalmic segment a.
paraclinoid internal carotid artery a.
partially clipped a.
a. of persistent trigeminal artery
PICA a.

NOTES

aneurysm *(continued)*
posterior circulation a.
posterior communicating a.
posterior fossa a.
posterior inferior communicating artery a.
precursor sign to rupture of a.
prerupture of a.
rebleeding of a.
remaining a.
rerupture of a.
residual a.
ruptured saccular a.
a. sac
saccular a.
sellar a.
serpentine a.
a. size
spirochetal a.
supraclinoid a.
suprasellar a.
a. surgery
thrombosed giant a.
a. trapping
trapping of a.
traumatic intracranial a. (TICA)
unruptured intracranial a.
unspecified a.
vein of Galen a.
venous a.
vertebrobasilar a.
wide-necked a.
Willis circle a.
wrapping of a.
aneurysmal
a. bleeding
a. bone cyst
a. bruit
a. bulging
a. characteristic
a. clipping operation
a. coiling
a. dilation
a. dome
a. rebleed
a. rest
a. rupture
a. subarachnoid hemorrhage
aneurysm-associated disorder
aneurysmectomy
aneurysmoplasty
aneurysmorrhaphy
aneurysmotomy
aneusomy syndrome
Anexsia
Angeles
University of California Los A. (UCLA)
Angell James dissector
Angelman syndrome (AS)
Angelucci syndrome
anger
unprovoked a.
angiitis
allergic a.
granulomatous a.
isolated a.
necrotizing a.
primary a.
angina
nocturnal a.
angioblastic meningioma
angioblastoma
angiocentric immunoproliferative lesion
AngioConray contrast medium
angiodysgenetic myelomalacia
angioedema
angioendothelioma
malignant endovascular papillary a.
angioendotheliomatosis
neoplastic a.
angiofibroma
juvenile a.
nasopharyngeal a.
Vogt triad of seizures, mental retardation, and facial a.
angiogenesis
glioma a.
angiogenic
a. inducer
a. inhibitor
a. response
angioglioma
angiogliomatosis
angiogliosis
angioglomoid tumor
Angiografin
angiogram
blush of dye on a.
carotid a.
cerebral digital a.
digital subtraction a.
innominate a.
intercostal artery a.
internal carotid a.
intraarterial digital subtraction a.
magnetic resonance a.
MR a.
postembolization a.
postoperative a.
preoperative a.
Seldinger a.
small-angle double-incidence a.
vertebral a.
4-vessel cerebral a.
angiogram-negative SAH

angiographic
a. catheter
a. finding
a. recanalization
a. reference system
a. road-mapping technique
a. targeting
a. targetry
a. vasospasm
angiographically
a. confirmed
a. occult intracranial vascular malformation (AOIVM)
a. visualized vascular malformation (AVVM)
angiography
baseline a.
cerebral a.
cerebrovascular a.
closed a.
contrast echocardiography magnetic resonance a.
contrast-enhanced magnetic resonance a.
contrast-enhanced MR a.
cut-film a.
2DFT time-of-flight MR a.
digital intravenous a.
digital subtraction a. (DSA)
digital subtraction venous a.
3-dimensional computed tomographic a. (3D-CTA)
gadolinium-enhanced MR a. (Gd-MRA)
helical CT a.
intraarterial catheter a.
intraarterial catheterization a.
intraarterial digital subtraction a. (IADSA)
intracranial MR a.
intraoperative a.
magnetic resonance a. (MRA)
nuclear cerebral a. (NCA)
open a.
orthogonal a.
phase-contrast magnetic resonance a. (PCMRA)
postoperative a.
preoperative a.
spinal a.
stereomagnification a.
stereotactic a.
superselective a.
time-of-flight a.
transradial cerebral a.
vertebral a.
angioid streak
AngioJet rapid thrombectomy system
angiokeratoma corporis diffusum
angiokinetic
angiolipoma
epidural a.
infiltrating spinal a.
spinal epidural a.
angiolithic sarcoma
angioma, pl. **angiomata**
arteriovenous interhemispheric a.
capillary a.
cavernous a.
cerebral cavernous a.
cerebral vein a.
cerebrovascular a.
cutaneous a.
encephalic a.
extracerebral cavernous a.
intracranial cavernous a.
intradermal a.
leptomeningeal venous a.
pontine a.
retinal a.
spinal cord a.
supratentorial cavernous a.
venous a.
vertebral a.
angiomatosis
cephalotrigeminal a.
cerebral a.
cerebroretinal a.
congenital dysplastic a.
corticomeningeal a.
cutaneomeningospinal a.
Divry-van Bogaert familial corticomeningeal a.
encephalofacial a.
encephalotrigeminal a.
leptomeningeal capillary-venous a.
meningeal a.
mesencephalooculofacial a.
neurocutaneous a.
neuroretinal a.
oculoencephalic a.
Rendu-Osler a.
retinocerebral a.
telangiectatic a.

NOTES

angiomatous meningioma
angionecrosis
angioneurectomy
angioneuredema
angioneuropathic
angioneuropathy
angioneurosis
angioneurotic edema
angioneurotomy
angioparalysis
angioparalytic neurasthenia
angioparesis
angiopathic
a. neurasthenia
a. vertigo
angiopathy
amyloid a.
cerebral amyloid a. (CAA)
congenital dysplastic a.
congophilic amyloid a.
radiation a.
angiophacomatosis, angiophakomatosis
angioplastic meningioma
angioplasty
stent-assisted carotid a.
angioreticuloma
angiosarcoma
Angio-Seal closure device
angiospastic anesthesia
angiostatin
angiostrongyliasis
Angiostrongylus costaricensis
angiotomomyelography
angiotropic lymphoma
angle
cephalic a.
cephalomedullary a.
cephalometric a.
cerebellopontine a. (CPA)
cervicothoracic pedicle a.
Citelli a.
Cobb a.
craniofacial a.
flip a.
Gardner a.
a. measurement device
a. meningioma
pedicle axis a.
phase a.
pontine a.
a. position potentiometer
pulse flip a.
Rolando a.
sagittal flexion a.
sagittal pedicle a.
Schmidt-Fischer a.
sinodural a.
sylvian a.
Sylvius a.
tentorial a.
torso flexion a.
transverse pedicle a.
venous a.
angled
a. aneurysm clip
a. awl
a. needle
a. nerve root retractor
angled-lens endoscope
angled-shaft endoscope
angry
a. backfiring C (ABC)
a. backfiring C nociceptor
angular
a. bundle
a. convolution
a. frequency
a. gyrus
a. gyrus syndrome
a. knife
a. momentum
a. position
angularis
gyrus a.
angulation
radius of a.
screw a.
angulus pontocerebellaris
anhaphia (*var. of* anaphia)
anhidrosis
anhidrotic ectodermal dysplasia
anhydrase
carbonic a.
anhydration
anhydrous
anhypnia
ani (*pl. of* anus)
animal
A. Naming test
a. venom
anion
peroxynitrite a.
superoxide a.
aniracetam
aniridia
anisocoria
anisodont
anisomastia
anisonucleosis
anisotropic
a. band
a. 3DFT
a. diffusion
anisotropy
chemical shift a.
fractional a. (FA)
nonaxial a.
a. of white matter

ankle
a. clonus
a. jerk
a. reflex
a. reflex measurement
ankle-brachial index
ankyloglossia
ankylosing spondylitis
ankylosis
cricoarytenoid a.
ankyroid (*var. of* ancyroid)
annectent gyrus
Annett test
annular (*var. of* anular)
annulus (*var. of* anulus)
anochlesia
anococcygeal nerve
anococcygeus
nervus a.
anodal block
anodmia
anoesis
anoetic
anomalous
a. branching
a. cerebral artery
a. innervation
a. nonrecurrent right inferior laryngeal nerve
a. origin
a. parental vocal pattern
a. result
anomaly, pl. **anomalies**
Aristotle a.
autosomal chromosomal a.
chromosomal a.
coloboma, heart disease, atresia choanae, retarded growth, genital anomalies, ear anomalies (CHARGE)
congenital a.
cranial a.
duplication a.
facial nerve congenital a.
Klippel-Feil a.
megadolichobasilar a.
megadolichovertebrobasilar a.
multiple congenital anomalies
sellar a.
structural autosomal a.
subtelomeric a.
Willis circle developmental a.
anomia
color a.
finger a.
gustatory a.
tactile a.
word-selection a.
anomic aphasia
anophthalmia
X-linked a.
anopsia
amblyopia ex a.
anorectal function
anorexia nervosa
anorexigenic
anorthography
anosmia
essential a.
functional a.
a. gustatoria
hypogonadism with a.
ipsilateral a.
mechanical a.
preferential a.
reflex a.
respiratory a.
true a.
anosmic aphasia
anosodiaphoria
anosognosia
anosognosic
a. epilepsy
a. seizure
anospinal center
anosteoplasia
anostosis
ANOVA
analysis of variance
global ANOVA
anoxemia
anoxia
acute a.
anemic a.
birth a.
cerebral a.
corneal a.
perinatal a.
perioperative a.
terminal a.
anoxic
a. damage
a. hypoxia

NOTES

anoxic *(continued)*
a. injury
a. ischemia
anoxic-ischemic encephalopathy
ANP
atrial natriuretic peptide
ANS
autonomic nervous system
ansa, pl. **ansae**
a. cervicalis
Haller a.
a. hypoglossi
lenticular a.
a. lenticularis
ansae nervorum
ansae nervorum spinalium
peduncular a.
a. peduncularis
Reil a.
a. sacralis
a. subclavia
Vieussens a.
anserinus
pes a.
ansiform lobule
ansoparamedian fissure
ansotomy
Anspach
A. craniotome
A. 65K drill
A. 65K instrument system
A. 65K neuro system
Anstie test
antagonism
central dopaminergic a.
pharmacological a.
physiological a.
antagonist
AChEIs receptor a.
alpha a.
alpha-1 adrenergic a.
alpha-adrenoceptor a.
beta-adrenoreceptor a.
calcium channel a.
dopaminergic a.
a. drug
excitotoxic neurotransmitter a.
Glu-receptor a.
glutamate receptor a.
histamine a.
histamine-2 a.
5HT1A a.
N-methyl-D-aspartate receptor a.
a. muscle
NMDA receptor a.
serotonin a.
serotonin/dopamine a.
antagonistic
a. effect
a. reflex
a. thermoeffector
antalgic limp
antapoplectic
antebrachial cutaneous nerve
antebrachium
antegrade amnesia
antephialtic
anterior
a. abdominal cutaneous branch of intercostal nerve
a. acoustic stria
a. alexia
a. ampullary nerve
a. amygdaloid area
a. antebrachial nerve
a. aphasia
a. apraxia
area amygdaloidea a.
arteria cerebelli inferior a.
arteria cerebri a.
arteria choroidea a.
arteria spinalis a.
a. ascending ramus
a. auricular nerve
a. basal encephalocele
a. branch of axillary nerve
a. branch of thoracic nerve
a. bulb syndrome
a. callosotomy
a. canaliculus of chorda tympani
a. cavernous sinus space
a. C1-C2 screw approach
a. central convolution
a. central gyrus
a. cerebellar notch
a. cerebral artery
a. cerebral artery plexus
a. cerebral vein
a. cervical approach to cervicothoracic junction
a. cervical cord syndrome
a. cervical discectomy and fusion
a. cervical surgery vocal cord damage
a. cervicothoracic junction surgery
a. cheek electrode
a. choroidal artery (AChA)
a. cingulate cortex
a. cingulate flow
a. cingulate gyrus
a. cingulate gyrus tumor
a. cingulate prefrontal syndrome
a. circulation
a. circulation intracranial aneurysm
a. circulation stroke
a. clinoid
a. clinoid process
a. colliculus

columna a.
a. column disruption
a. column fracture
a. column of medulla oblongata
a. column osteosynthesis
a. column of spinal cord
commissura alba a.
commissura grisea a.
a. commissure-posterior commissure (AC-PC)
a. commissure-posterior commissure line
a. commissure-posterior commissure reference point
a. communicating artery (ACoA, AComA)
a. communicating artery aneurysm
a. communicating artery distribution infarction
a. construct
a. cord impingement
a. cornual syndrome
a. corpectomy
a. correction
a. cortex penetration
a. corticospinal tract
a. cranial base
a. cranial fossa
a. cranial fossa surgery
a. craniofacial resection
a. cutaneous branch of femoral nerve
a. cutaneous branch of iliohypogastric nerve
a. cutaneous branch of intercostal nerve
a. cutaneous nerves of abdomen
a. decompression
decussatio tegmentalis a.
a. discectomy
a. distraction
a. distraction instrumentation
ductus semicircularis a.
a. ethmoidal nerve
a. external arcuate fiber
a. extradural clinoidectomy
a. extremity of caudate nucleus
fasciculus corticospinalis a.
a. fasciculus proprius
fasciculus proprius a.
fasciculus pyramidalis a.
a. femoral cutaneous nerve
forceps a.
a. fovea
a. frontal
a. funiculus
a. gray column
a. gray commissure
a. ground bundle
gyrus paracentralis a.
gyrus temporalis transversus a.
a. head region
a. hippocampal activation
a. horizontal ramus
a. horn
a. horn cell
a. horn cell disease
a. horn cell isolation
a. horn cell motor impairment
a. horn index
a. hypothalamic area
a. hypothalamic nucleus
a. hypothalamic region
a. hypothalamus
incisura cerebelli a.
a. inferior cerebellar artery (AICA)
a. inferior cerebral artery
a. inferior communicating artery
a. insula region
a. intercavernous sinus
a. interhemispheric approach
a. intermediate groove
a. intermediate sulcus
a. internal fixation device
a. internal stabilization
a. interosseous nerve
a. interosseus syndrome
a. interpositus nucleus
a. ischemic optic neuropathy (AION)
a. jugular vein
a. Kostuik-Harrington distraction system
a. limbic association area
a. limb of internal capsule
a. lobe of hypophysis
a. longitudinal ligament
a. lower cervical spine surgery
a. lumbar interbody fusion (ALIF)
a. lumbar spine interbody fusion
a. lunate lobule
a. median fissure of medulla oblongata
a. median fissure of spinal cord

NOTES

anterior *(continued)*
a. medullary velum
a. meningeal artery
a. mesial temporal resection (AMTR)
a. metallic fixation
nervus ampullaris a.
nervus ethmoidalis a.
nervus interosseus antebrachii a.
a. neuropore
a. neutralization
a. notch of cerebellum
nucleus cochlearis a.
nucleus hypothalamicus a.
nucleus interpositus a.
nucleus olfactorius a.
a. nucleus of thalamus
a. nucleus of trapezoid body
nucleus ventralis a.
a. occipital artery-middle cerebral artery bypass
a. olfactory nucleus
a. paracentral gyrus
a. paracentral lobule
a. parietal lesion
a. parolfactory sulcus
pars a.
a. part of anterior commissure of brain
a. part of pons
a. pectoral cutaneous branch of intercostal nerve
a. peduncle of thalamus
a. perforated substance
a. periventricular nucleus
a. pillar of fornix
a. piriform gyrus
a. pituitary hormone
a. pituitary insufficiency
a. plate fixation
a. poliomyelitis
a. pontomesencephalic vein
a. primary division
a. pulmonary branch of vagus nerve
a. pyramid
a. pyramidal fasciculus
a. pyramidal tract
a. quadrigeminal body
radiatio thalami a.
a. radical surgery
radix a.
a. ramus of cervical nerve
a. ramus of lateral sulcus of cerebrum
a. ramus of lumbar nerve
a. ramus of sacral nerve
a. ramus of spinal nerve
a. ramus of thoracic nerve
a. raphespinal tract
a. recess
a. recess of interpeduncular fossa
recessus a.
regio hypothalamica a.
a. rhizotomy
a. root
a. root of spinal nerve
a. scalene muscle
a. screw fixation
a. serratus muscle
a. short-segment stabilization
sinus intercavernosus a.
a. skull base malignancy
spina bifida a.
a. spinal artery
a. spinal artery syndrome
a. spinal cord syndrome
a. spinal fixation
a. spinal plating
a. spinocerebellar tract
a. spinothalamic tract
a. stabilization procedure
stria cochlearis a.
a. subscapular approach
substantia perforata a.
sulcus intermedius a.
sulcus lateralis a.
sulcus parolfactorius a.
a. superior alveolar branch of infraorbital nerve
a. surgical exposure
a. tegmental decussation
a. temporal artery
a. temporal atrophy
a. temporal branch
a. temporal focal spike
a. temporal lobectomy
a. thalamic radiation
a. thalamic tubercle
a. thalamotomy
a. tibialis sign
tractus corticospinalis a.
tractus pyramidalis a.
tractus raphespinalis a.
tractus reticulospinalis a.
tractus spinocerebellaris a.
tractus spinothalamicus a.
tractus trigeminothalamicus a.
a. transverse temporal gyrus
a. triangle approach
a. trigeminothalamic tract
truncus vagalis a.
a. tubercle of thalamus
a. vagal trunk
a. vein of septum pellucidum
vena cerebri a.
vena pontomesencephalica a.
vena septi pellucidi a.

a. vermis
a. vermis syndrome
a. white commissure

anteriores
fibrae arcuatae externae a.
nervi auriculares a.
nervi labiales a.
nervi scrotales a.
nuclei tegmentales a.
rami temporales a.

anterioris
nuclei interstitiales hypothalami a.
pars anterior commissurae a.
pars anterior lobuli quadrangularis a.
pars dorsalis lobuli quadrangularis a.
pars posterior commissurae a.
pars posterior lobuli quadrangularis a.
pars precommunicalis arteriae cerebri a.
pars ventralis lobuli quadrangularis a.
rami gastrici anteriores trunci vagalis a.
rami hepatici trunci vagalis a.
rami nasales interni laterales nervi ethmoidalis a.
rami nasales interni mediales nervi ethmoidalis a.
rami nasales nervi ethmoidalis a.
ramus nasalis externus nervi ethmoidalis a.

anterior-posterior
a.-p. fusion with segmental spinal instrumentation
a.-p. fusion with SSI

anterius
cornu a.
corpus quadrigeminum a.
tuber a.

anterochiasmatic lesion

anterocollis dystonia

anterodorsal
a. nucleus of thalamus
a. thalamic nucleus

anterodorsalis
nucleus a.

anterograde
a. amnesia (AA)
a. axonal transport
a. fast component neuropathy
a. memory

anterolateral
a. central artery
a. column
a. column of spinal cord
a. cordotomy
a. groove
a. sulcus
a. system
a. tract
a. tractotomy

anterolaterales
arteriae thalamostriatae a.
tractus a.

anterolateralis
nucleus a.
sulcus a.

anterolisthesis
traumatic a.

anteromedial
a. central branch
a. nucleus of thalamus
a. retropharyngeal approach
a. temporal lobe resection
a. thalamic nucleus

anteromediales
arteriae thalamostriatae a.
rami centrales a.

anteromedialis
nucleus a.
ramus frontalis a.

anteromedian groove

anteromesial temporal lobectomy

anteroposterior (AP)
a. fracture
a. hypothalamic sleep
a. projection
a. talocalcaneal

anteroventralis
nucleus a.

anteroventral thalamic nucleus

anthelix (*var. of* antihelix)

anthophilous

anthrax
cerebral a.
concentrated a.
cutaneous a.
inhalation a.
meningeal a.
a. meningoencephalitis

anthropomorphic face

NOTES

anthroponomy
anthroposcopy
anthroposomatology
anthroposophy
anti-33-kDa antibody
antiabsence antiepileptic drug
antiacetylcholine receptor antibody
anti-AChE
antiactin antibody
antiadrenergic
antiadrenogenic
antialias filtering
antianalytic
antianaphylaxis
antiapoptotic protein
antiarrhythmic
antibasal ganglia antibody
antibiotic
intrathecal a.
a. neurotoxicity
ototoxic a.
a. penetration
a. powder
antibody
acquired a.
alemtuzumab humanized monoclonal a.
antiacetylcholine receptor a.
antiactin a.
antibasal ganglia a.
anti-GFP polyclonal a.
antigliadin a.
anti-GQ1b a.
anti-Hu a.
antihuman a.
anti-I-kBa a.
anti-33-kDa a.
anti-Ma2 a.
anti-MAG a.
antineuronal a.
antineutrophil cytoplasmic a.
antinuclear a.
antiphospholipid a.
anti-Ri a.
antiribosomal P a.
anti-Ro a.
anti-tau monoclonal a.
antitoxoplasmic a.
anti-Yo a.
autoreactive a.
disease-associated a.
Hu a.
human antimouse a. (HAMA)
influenza A a.
monoclonal a.
MuSK a.
OKT3 monoclonal a.
polyclonal a.
antibody-mediated disorder
anticardiolipin
anticatalyst
anticipatory a.
anticataplectic
anticephalalgic
anticholinergic
a. agent
a. for bruxism
a. dose
a. drug
a. effect
a. medication
a. for night terror
a. for sleepwalking
anticholinesterase
anticipatory
a. anticatalyst
a. saccade
a. vomiting (AV)
anticoagulant
lupus a.
anticoagulation therapy
anticonvulsant
a. effect
a. effect on sleep
a. intoxication
a. medication-induced postural tremor
a. prophylaxis
a. therapy
anticonvulsant-induced dyskinesia
anticonvulsive
anticus
locus perforatus a.
a. reflex
scalenus a.
a. sign
tetanus a.
antidipsotropic agent
antidiuretic hormone (ADH)
antidopaminergic
a. effect
a. potency
antidote drug
antidromic
a. conduction
a. response
a. stimulation
a. volley
antidyskinetic agent
antiepilepsirine
antiepileptic
a. drug (AED)
a. drug hypersensitivity syndrome
a. drug-induced bone disease
enzyme-inducing a.
antiepileptogenesis
antiferromagnetism

A

antifibrinolytic
a. agent
a. therapy
antiganglioside
antigen
bacterial a.
carcinoembryonic a. (CEA)
CD44 a.
cryptococcal a.
histocompatibility a.
Histoplasma polysaccharide a.
HLA-CW2 a.
HLA-DR2 a.
human lymphocyte a. (HLA)
33-kDa a.
prostate-specific a. (PSA)
tuberculous a.
varicella-zoster virus a.
antigen-antibody complex
antigen-driven cell activation
antigen-specific
a.-s. T-cell response
a.-s. T-suppressor cell
anti-GFP polyclonal antibody
antigliadin antibody
antiglial fibrillary acidic protein
anti-GM$_1$ antibody test
anti-GQ1b antibody
antigravity reflex
anti-GT1a IgA
antihelix, anthelix
double a.
antihemophilic factor A, C
antihistamine
a. neurotoxicity
sedative a.
antihistaminergic effect
anti-Hu antibody
antihuman
a. antibody
a. transferrin
anti-I-kBa antibody
antilethargic
anti-Lewisite
British a.-L.
anti-Ma2 antibody
anti-Ma2-associated encephalitis
anti-MAG antibody
antimetabolite
antimicrobial
a. agent
a. prophylaxis
a. susceptibility test
a. therapy
antimigraine therapy
antimongoloid slant
antimuscarine cholinergic activity
antimuscarinic
a. drug
a. effect
antimyasthenic
antineoplastic agent
antineuralgic
antineuritic
antineurofilament
antineuronal
a. antibody
a. cytoplasmic autoantibody (ANCA)
antineutrophil cytoplasmic antibody
antinociceptive effect
antinodal behavior
antinomian
antinomianism
antinuclear
a. antibody
a. antibody test
antioncogene
antioxidant
a. effect
endogenous a.
a. system
a. therapy
antiparasympathomimetic
antiparkinsonian response
antiparkinsonism agent
antiphospholipid
a. antibody
a. antibody in stroke study
a. syndrome
antiplatelet
a. drug
a. therapy
antipyrine
antireflux therapy
antiretroviral
a. medication
a. therapy
a. toxic neuropathy
anti-Ri antibody
antiribosomal P antibody
anti-Ro antibody
antisaccade task

NOTES

antiseizure
a. effect
a. medication
antisense
a. oligonucleotide
a. strategy
antiseptic
ACU-dyne a.
antiserum
nerve growth factor a.
antisiphon device
antispasmodic
antispastic agent
antisympathetic
anti-tau monoclonal antibody
antitetanic
antithrombin
a. III (AT III)
a. III deficiency
antitonic
antitoxin
botulinum a.
tetanus a.
antitoxoplasmic antibody
antitrismus
Antivert
antiviral
chemotherapy a.
a. medication
a. therapy
antivivisection
anti-Yo antibody
Antley-Bixler syndrome
Anton
A. symptom
A. syndrome
Anton-Babinski syndrome
Antoni
A. A, B cell
A. A, B tissue
A. A neurinoma classification
A. type A, B neurilemoma
A. type A, B pattern
Antopol disease
antra (*pl. of* antrum)
Antrizine
antrochoanal polyp
antrophose
antrostomy
antrum, pl. **antra**
mastoid a.
maxillary a.
Anturane
Antyllus method
anular, annular
a. plexus
a. protrusion
a. radial rupture
a. tear
anulospiral
a. ending
a. fiber
a. organ
anulus, annulus, pl. **anuli**
a. fibrosus fiber
a. fibrous disci intervertebralis
fissure of a.
a. thickness
a. of Vieussens
a. of Zinn
anus, pl. **ani**
Bartholin a.
a. cerebri
anxiety control training
anxiogenic stimulus
anxiolytic
a. activity
a. drug
a. property
a. stimulus
anxiolytic-induced
anxiolytic/sedative
anxious
a. delirium
a. somatic depression
AO
Arbeitsgemeinschaft für Osteosynthesefragen
AO dynamic compression plate
AO dynamic compression plate construct
AO fixateur interne
AO fixateur interne instrumentation
AO gouge
AO group
AO guide pin
AO internal fixator
AO notched instrumentation
AO reconstruction plate
AO Scale
AO stopped-drill guide
AO-ASIF
Arbeitsgemeinschaft für Osteosynthesefragen-Association for the Study of Internal Fixation
AO-ASIF fixateur interne
AOIVM
angiographically occult intracranial vascular malformation
aorta, pl. **aortae**
a. coarctation
pars thoracica aortae
thoracic part of a.
aortic
a. arch syndrome
a. body
a. body tumor

a. insufficiency
a. nerve
aorticorenal ganglion
aorticorenalia
ganglia a.
aorticum
corpus a.
glomus a.
aortobifemoral bypass graft
aortocranial disease
AP
anteroposterior
Apacet
APACHE
acute physiologic assessment and chronic health evaluation
APACHE II measure of disease severity
apallesthesia
apallic
a. state
a. syndrome
APAP
autoadjusting positive airway pressure
APAP Plus
aparalytic
apathetic
a. akinetic mutism
a. hyperthyroidism
a. mood
a. thyrotoxicosis
apathism
APB
abductor pollicis brevis
ape
a. fissure
a. hand
a. hand of syringomyelia
aperiodic
a. complex
a. wave
aperta
rhinolalia a.
spina bifida a.
Apert syndrome
apertura, pl. **aperturae**
a. aqueductus cerebri
a. aqueductus mesencephali
a. lateralis ventriculi quarti
a. mediana ventriculi quarti
aperture
lateral a.
median a.
apex, pl. **apices**
basilar a.
a. cornus dorsalis medullae spinalis
a. cornus posterioris
a. cornus posterioris medullae spinalis
a. of dorsal horn of spinal cord
petrous a.
a. of posterior horn
a. of posterior horn of spinal cord
Apfelbaum retractor
Apgar score
aphagia
aphagopraxia
aphanisis
aphasia
acoustic a.
acquired childhood a.
acquired epileptic a.
acquired fluent a.
ageusic a.
amnemonic a.
amnesic a.
anomic a.
anosmic a.
anterior a.
associative a.
ataxic a.
auditory a.
Benson-Geschwind classification of a.
Broca a.
cerebrovascular a.
combined a.
commissural a.
conduction a.
contiguity disorder a.
cortical a.
crossed a.
A. Diagnostic Profile
dynamic a.
expressive a.
expressive-receptive a.
fluent a.
frontocortical a.
frontolenticular a.
functional a.
gibberish a.
global a.

NOTES

aphasia *(continued)*
graphic a.
graphomotor a.
Grashey a.
hypophonic a.
impressive a.
induced a.
intellectual a.
jargon a.
Kussmaul a.
A. Language Performance Scale
lenticular a.
a. lethica
Lichtheim a.
major motor a.
mixed a.
motor a.
nominal a.
nonfluent a.
optic a.
partial nominal a.
pathematic a.
pictorial a.
posterior a.
primary progressive a. (PPA)
progressive nonfluent a.
psychosensory a.
pure a.
receptive a.
semantic a.
sensory a.
subcortical motor a.
subcortical sensory a.
syntactical a.
tactile a.
temporoparietal a.
thalamic a.
total a.
transcortical a.
true a.
visual a.
Wernicke a.
aphasiac, aphasic
aphasiologist
aphasiology
aphemesthesia
aphemia
aphonia
acute a.
functional a.
hysterical a.
nonorganic a.
a. paralytica
spastic a.
aphonic
aphonogelia
aphonous
aphorism
hippocratic a.
aphorize
aphrasia
apical
a. dendrite
a. distraction
a. ectodermal ridge
a. process
a. turn of cochlea
apices (*pl. of* apex)
apicoectomy
apiculate waveform
apiospermum
Scedosporium a.
apituitarism
aplasia
cerebellar a.
cerebral a.
cochlear a.
a. cutis congenita
labyrinthine a.
nuclear a.
vertebral a.
APLD
automated percutaneous lumbar discectomy
apnea
central sleep a. (CSA)
Cheyne-Stokes central a.
idiopathic central sleep a.
a. index (AI)
induced hypocapnic central a.
mixed a.
obstructive sleep a. (OSA)
positional obstructive sleep a.
sleep a.
sleep-induced a.
apnea-hypopnea
a.-h. index (AHI)
obstructive sleep a.-h. (OSAH)
apnea-like spell
apneic
a. pause
a. threshold
apneusis
apneustic
a. breathing
a. center
a. period
apocalyptic
apocrine
a. cystadenoma
a. gland
apodemialgia
APOe4
apolipoprotein epsilon 4
ApoE
apolipoprotein epsilon
ApoE e4 allele
ApoE genotype

apoenzyme
apoferritin
Apofix interlaminar clamp
apogeotropic nystagmus
apokemnophilia
Apokyn
apolar cell
apolegamic
apolipoprotein
  a. E genotype
  a. epsilon (ApoE)
  a. epsilon 4 (APOe4)
  a. gene cluster
apomorphine
aponeurectomy
aponeurorrhaphy
aponeurotica
  galea a.
aponeurotic reflex
apophysary point
apophysial, apophyseal
  a. joint
  a. point
  a. ring
apophysis cerebri
apoplectic
  a. coma
  a. cyst
  a. hemorrhage
  a. vertigo
apoplecticus
  habitus a.
apoplectiform
apoplectoid
apoplexy
  bulbar a.
  cerebellar a.
  cerebral a.
  chiasmal a.
  delayed a.
  embolic a.
  functional a.
  ingravescent a.
  labyrinthine a.
  neonatal a.
  pituitary a.
  pontine a.
  posttraumatic a.
  Raymond a.
  serous a.
  spasmodic a.
  spinal a.
  thrombotic a.
apoptosis
  neuronal cell a.
  a. suppression
  thymocyte a.
apoptosis-inducing factor (AIF)
apoptosome
apoptotic
  a. body
  a. cell death
  a. nigral neuron
  a. stage
aporioneurosis
apotentiality
  cerebral a.
apothanasia
APP
  Alzheimer precursor protein
  amyloid precursor protein
apparatus
  Brown-Roberts-Wells a.
  C-arm fluoroscopic a.
  halo a.
  heat-loss a.
  Horsley-Clarke stereotactic a.
  Kandel stereotactic a.
  Leksell a.
  Mayfield-Kees skull fixation a.
  mitotic spindle a.
  Perroncito a.
  Reichert-Mundinger a.
  Spiegel-Wycis human a.
  subneural a.
  sucker a.
  Todd-Wells a.
  vestibular a.
  Vienna reaction a.
  Wells stereotactic a.
apparent
  a. diffusion coefficient (ADC)
  a. origin
appearance
  axon torpedo a.
  beaten metal a.
  de novo a.
  histologic a.
  meningothelial a.
  pearl chain a.
  ping-pong a.
  posterior beaten copper a.

NOTES

appearance *(continued)*
thumbprinting a.
tuberous sclerosis railroad track a.
Appedrine
appendicular
apperceptive
a. disorder
a. visual agnosia
appetitive
a. disturbance
a. state
appliance
Herbst a.
Klearway oral a.
mandibular advancing oral a.
monobloc-type a.
oral a.
application
clip a.
force a.
halo a.
Harrington rod instrumentation force a.
Isola spinal implant system a.
paraspinal rod a.
transverse fixator a.
vertebral plate a.
applicator
aneurysm clip a.
NeuroAvitene a.
scalp clip a.
applied relaxation
applier
bayonet clip a.
clip a.
Crockard transoral clip a.
Ligaclip a.
Mayfield miniature clip a.
Mayfield temporary aneurysm clip a.
mini a.
Olivecrona clip a.
Raney scalp clip a.
Sano clip a.
Vari-Angle clip a.
apprehension
pain a.
approach
adaptational a.
anterior C1-C2 screw a.
anterior interhemispheric a.
anterior subscapular a.
anterior triangle a.
anteromedial retropharyngeal a.
Bailey-Badgley anterior cervical a.
basal interhemispheric a.
basal pterional a.
basal subfrontal a.
bilateral occipital transtentorial a.
bottom-up a.
buccopharyngeal a.
cerebellopontine angle a.
cholinergic a.
Cloward cervical disc a.
combined anterior and posterior a.
combined low cervical and transthoracic a.
combined presigmoid-transtransversarium intradural a.
combined supra/infratentorial-transsinus a.
combined transsylvian and middle fossa a.
computer-assisted volumetric stereotactic a.
condylar a.
continuous a.
contralateral transcallosal a.
costotransversectomy a.
empirical a.
endoscopic a.
extended subfrontal a.
extreme lateral inferior transcondylar a.
extreme lateral transcondylar a.
far lateral inferior suboccipital a.
foraminal a.
frontotemporal a.
functional a.
glabellar a.
Hardy a.
Harmon cervical a.
holistic a.
inferior extradural a.
inferior transvermian a.
inferolateral endonasal transsphenoidal a.
infratemporal a.
infratentorial lateral supracellular a.
integrative a.
interfascial a.
interforniceal a.
intradural a.
intraforaminal a.
intratentorial supracerebellar a.
ipsilateral a.
Kanavel a.
labioglossomandibular a.
labiomandibular a.
laparoscopic transperitoneal a.
lateral extracavitary a.
lateral intradural a.
low cervical a.
medial extradural a.
middle cranial fossa a.
middle fossa craniotomy a.
middle fossa transtentorial translabyrinthine a.

midline spinal a.
mini-open a.
molecular a.
multimodal therapeutic a.
multiple-tracer a.
multisystemic therapy a.
neuroimaging a.
oblique transcorporeal a.
occipital bitranstentorial/falcine a.
occipital interhemispheric a.
occipital transtentorial a.
orbital venous a.
orbitofrontal a.
orbitozygomatic temporopolar a.
partial labyrinthectomy petrous apicectomy a.
patient-centered a.
percutaneous a.
petrosal a.
pharmacological a.
posterior fossa a.
posterior occipitocervical a.
posterior subscapular a.
posterior transcallosal a.
posterolateral a.
presigmoid a.
primary pharmacological a.
psychotherapeutic a.
pterional a.
resection of pituitary tumor, transfacial a.
retrolabyrinthine-presigmoid a.
retrolabyrinthine-transsigmoid a.
retromastoid a.
retroperitoneal a.
retropharyngeal a.
retrosigmoid a.
rhinoseptal a.
sacral foraminal a.
screw plate a.
sensate focus a.
Smith-Robinson a.
stabilization a.
staged surgical a.
standard retroperitoneal flank a.
stereotactic microsurgical a.
sternum-splitting a.
subchoroidal a.
subfrontal transbasal a.
sublabial midline rhinoseptal a.
sublabial transseptal transsphenoidal a.
suboccipital posterior fossa a.
suboccipital transmeatal a.
subtemporal basal a.
subtemporal infratemporal a.
subtemporal keyhole a.
superior intradural a.
superior ophthalmic vein a.
suprabrow a.
supracerebellar a.
supraclavicular a.
supraorbital pterional a.
supratentorial a.
sylvian a.
targeted a.
therapeutic a.
thoracoabdominal a.
thoracolumbar retroperitoneal a.
transantral ethmoidal a.
transaxillary a.
transcallosal interforniceal-transforaminal microsurgical a.
transcallosal interhemispheric a.
transcallosal transforaminal a.
transcavernous transpetrous apex a.
transcerebellar hemispheric a.
transchoroidal a.
transcochlear a.
transcortical transventricular a.
transcranial frontotemporoorbital a.
transcubital a.
transfacial transclival a.
transfrontal a.
transfrontonasoorbital a.
translabyrinthine suboccipital a.
translabyrinthine transotic a.
transmandibular glossopharyngeal a.
transmaxillosphenoidal a.
transnasal a.
transnasoorbital a.
transoral a.
transpalatal a.
transpedicular a.
transperitoneal a.
transpetrosal a.
transsinus a.
transsphenoidal a.
transsylvian a.
transtemporal a.
transtentorial a.
transthoracic a.
transtorcular a.
transuncodiscal a.

NOTES

approach *(continued)*
transvenous a.
transventricular a.
transzygomatic a.
ultrasound-guided transfrontal transventricular a.
Wiltberger anterior cervical a.
Wiltse paraspinal a.
zygomatic resection a.
approbation
approximating closure
approximation
method of successive a.
vocal fold a.
approximator
Neuromeet nerve a.
APR
acousticopalpebral reflex
apractagnosia
apractic (*var. of* apraxic)
aprataxin gene mutation
apraxia
akinetic a.
amnesic a.
anterior a.
a. battery
Bruns gait a.
buccofacial a.
buccolingual a.
callosal a.
cerebral mapping of a.
classic a.
Cogan oculomotor a.
congenital ocular motor a.
construction a.
constructional a.
cortical a.
developmental articulatory a.
diagnostic a.
disconnection a.
dressing a.
a. of eyelid opening
facial a.
gait a.
ideational a.
ideatory a.
ideokinetic a.
ideomotor a.
innervation a.
innervatory a.
left-sided a.
Liepmann a.
limb-kinetic a.
magnetic a.
motor a.
oculomotor a.
oral a.
A. Profile: A Descriptive Assessment Tool for Children
pure limb a.
repellent a.
sensory a.
speech a.
transcortical a.
verbal a.
visuospatial constructional a.
apraxia-ataxia
truncal a.-a.
apraxic, apractic
a. agraphia
a. disorder
a. dysarthria
apraxic-ataxic
aprepitant
Apresazide
Apresoline
a priori criterion
aprobarbital
aproctia
aprophoria
aprosencephaly
aprosexia
aprosody, aprosodia
speech a.
a. of speech
aprotinin
APS
adenosine 5′-phosphosulfate
APS hydroxyapatite
aptiganel hydrochloride
APUD
amine precursor uptake decarboxylase
APUD cell
apurinic
apyknomorphous
apyretic tetanus
apyrimidinic
AquaMEPHYTON Injection
Aquaplast mask
Aquatensen
aquatic rehabilitation
aqueduct
cerebral a.
a. cerebrum
cochlear a.
Cotunnius a.
forking of sylvian a.
gliosis of a.
mesencephalon a.
a. of midbrain
Monro a.
opening of cerebral a.
sylvian a.
a. of Sylvius
a. veil
ventricular a.
vestibular a.

aqueductal
a. gliosis
a. gliosis with hydrocephaly
a. intubation
a. occlusion
a. stenosis
aqueductoplasty
aqueductus
a. cerebri
a. cochlea
a. cotunnii
a. mesencephali
a. sylvii
a. vestibuli
aqueous
a. humor deficiency
a. povidone-iodine
arabinoside
adenine a.
cytosine a. (ara-C)
ara-C
cytosine arabinoside
arachidonic
a. acid
a. acid cascade
a. acid metabolism
arachnitis
arachnodactyly
congenital a.
contracture a.
arachnoid
a. adhesion
a. of brain
a. canal
a. cell
a. cistern
cranial a.
a. cyst
a. fibrosis
a. foramen
a. granulation
a. granulation villus
a. knife
a. mater cranialis
a. mater encephali
a. membrane
a. nerve root sheath dilation
a. plane
a. sheath
a. sleeve
a. space
spinal a.
a. of spinal cord
a. trabecula
a. of uncus
arachnoidal
a. cyst
a. gliomatosis
a. granulation
a. hyperplasia
a. root sleeve
arachnoidea, arachnoides
a. mater cranialis
a. mater encephali
a. mater spinalis
arachnoiditis
adhesive a.
basilar a.
chiasmal a.
chronic adhesive a.
fibrosing a.
neoplastic a.
obliterative a.
a. of opticochiasmatic cistern
optochiasmic a.
ossifying a.
postoperative a.
spinal cord a.
arachnoid-shape Beaver blade
Aramine
Arana-Iniquez
A.-I. intracranial cyst removal
A.-I. intracranial cyst removal technique
Aran-Duchenne
A.-D. amyotrophy
A.-D. disease
A.-D. muscular atrophy
A.-D. muscular dystrophy
Arantius ventricle
araphia
ARAS
ascending reticular activating system
Arbeitsgemeinschaft
A. für Osteosynthesefragen (AO)
A. für Osteosynthesefragen-Association for the Study of Internal Fixation (AO-ASIF)
arbor, pl. **arbores**
dendritic a.
a. vitae
a. vitae cerebelli
arborea
Datura a.

NOTES

arborescent white substance of cerebellum
arborization
dendrite a.
arboviral encephalitis
arbovirus, arborvirus
a. meningoencephalitis
arc
dynamic reference a.
a. guidance system
Leksell a.
monosynaptic reflex a.
neural a.
a. radius system
reflex a.
Sceratti a.
spinal reflex a.
stereotactic a.
Y-shaped reference a.
arcade
a. of Frohse
trabecular a.
arc-centered guidance system
arch
lamina of vertebral a.
neural a.
archaeocerebellum (*var. of* archicerebellum)
archaeopsychic
archaism
archeokinetic
archicortex
Archimedes spiral
archipallium
archistriatalis
nucleus robustus a.
archistriatum
architectonics
architecture
focal cortical a.
nuclear a.
sleep a.
arciform wave
Arclite light source
arc-quadrant stereotactic system
arcuate
a. eminence
a. fasciculus
a. fiber
a. fiber of cerebrum
a. nucleus
a. nucleus of thalamus
a. visual field defect
arcuatus
nucleus a.
arcus parietooccipitalis
ardanesthesia
area, pl. **areae**
acoustic a.
a. acustica
AI, AII a.
amygdaloclaustral a.
a. amygdaloclaustralis
a. amygdaloidea anterior
amygdalopiriform transition a.
anterior amygdaloid a.
anterior hypothalamic a.
anterior limbic association a.
association a.
auditory association a.
auditory cortical a.
Betz cell a.
bilateral contralateral primary sensorimotor areas
bilateral secondary sensorimotor areas
brain a.
Broca motor speech a.
Broca parolfactory a.
Brodmann a. 6,7,9,24,32,34,41,43,44,46
Brodmann cortical a.
a. CA4-1
callosal a.
a. centralis
cingulate motor a. (CMA)
cortical a.
cross-sectional a. (CSA)
dermatomic a.
diencephalic transition a.
dominant hemisphere parietal a.
dominant hemisphere temporal a.
dorsal hypothalamic a.
dorsolateral prefrontal cortical a.
entorhinal a.
excitable a.
a. of facial nerve
first somatosensory a.
first visual a.
Flechsig a.
a. of Forel
frontocortical a.
frontoorbital a.
fusiform face a. (FFA)
gasserian ganglion a.
gray matter a.
gustatory receiving a.
head a.
high-density a.
hypothalamic a.
a. hypothalamica dorsalis
a. hypothalamica intermedia
a. hypothalamica lateralis
a. hypothalamica posterior
a. hypothalamica rostralis
inferior vestibular a.
insular a.
intermediate hypothalamic a.

language a.
lateral hypothalamic a.
lateral rostral supplementary motor a.
low-density a. (LDA)
medial preoptic a.
medial rostral supplementary motor a.
a. medullovasculosa
mesencephalic transition a.
mesial prefrontal cortical a.
motor speech a.
neocortical association a.
a. nervi facialis
neuropsychologic a.
noneloquent a.
nuclei areae H, H1, H2
nucleus arcuatus of intermediate hypothalamic a.
occipital association cortical a.
olfactory a.
orbitofrontal a.
paraolfactory cortical a.
parastriate a.
parietal neocortical association a.
parietotemporal a.
parolfactory a.
periamygdaloid a.
perifornical a.
peristriate a.
periventricular gray matter a.
piriform a.
postcentral a.
posterior hypothalamic a.
a. postrema
postrolandic a.
precentral a.
precommissural septal a.
prefrontal cortical a.
premotor a.
preoptic a.
a. preoptica
prestriate a.
pretectal a.
a. pretectalis
primary motor a.
primary receiving a.
primary receptive a.
primary somatomotor a.
primary somatosensory a.
primary visual a.
processing a.
projection a.
receptive a.
retrochiasmatic a.
a. retrochiasmatica
rolandic a.
Rolando a.
rostral supplementary motor a.
sclerotic a.
sclerotome a.
secondary somatosensory a.
secondary visual a.
second somatosensory a.
second visual a.
sensorial a.
sensorimotor a.
sensory association a.
sensory processing a.
septal a.
silent a.
somatesthetic a.
somatosensory a.
somesthetic a.
striate a.
stripe a.
a. subcallosa
subcallosal a.
subcortical gray matter a.
superior temporal auditory cortical a.
superior vestibular a.
supplementary motor a. (SMA)
suppressor a.
suprasellar a.
taste receiving a.
temporal neocortical association a.
temporolimbic a.
temporoparietal association a.
third visual a.
a. transitionis amygdalopiriformis
trigger a.
a. under curve
vagus a.
ventral regimental a.
ventral tegmental a. (VTA)
vestibular a.
a. vestibularis
a. vestibularis inferior
a. vestibularis superior
visual association a.
visual cortical a.
visual receiving a.
visuopsychic a.

NOTES

area *(continued)*
visuosensory a.
watershed a.
Wernicke second motor speech a.
areal stimulation
arecoline
areflexia
detrusor a.
upper limb a.
arenacea
corpora a.
arenavirus infection
Arenberg-Denver inner ear valve implant
areolar tissue
Argentinian hemorrhagic fever
arginase
a. deficiency
a. deficiency aminoaciduria
arginine
a. vasopressin
a. vasotocin
argininemia
arginine-vasopressin (AV, AVP)
argininosuccinic
a. acid synthase deficiency
a. aciduria
a. aminoaciduria
argininosuccinicaciduria
arginosuccinate lyase deficiency
argon
a. ion
a. laser
a. laser iridotomy (ALI)
Argyll
A. Robertson pupil
A. trocar catheter
argyrophil
a. organizer region protein
a. plaque
arhinencephaly (*var. of* arrhinencephaly)
Aricept
Ariel computerized exercise system
aripiprazole
Aristotle anomaly
arithmetica
epilepsia a.
ARJP
autosomal recessive juvenile parkinsonism
arm
a. dystonia
fixed dosing a.
phantom a.
a. phenomenon
a. weakness
Yasargil Leyla retractor a.
armamentarium
clinical a.
pharmacological a.
Armstrong disease
Army-Navy retractor
Arnold
A. bundle
A. canal
A. ganglion
A. nerve
A. nerve reflex cough syndrome
A. tract
Arnold-Chiari
A.-C. deformity
A.-C. malformation
A.-C. syndrome
aromatic
a. amino acid decarboxylase (AADC)
a. hydrocarbon
aromatization
peripheral a.
arousal
a. category
a. component of consciousness
confusional a.
cortical a.
a. defect
a. disorder
flow-limitation a.
a. mechanism
mental a.
physiological a.
psychological/physiological a.
a. reaction
respiratory effort-related a.
respiratory event a.
respiratory-related a.
sleeplessness associated with conditional a.
a. symptom
a. threshold
array
compressed spectral a.
density-modulated spectral a. (DSA)
percutaneous electrode a.
rostrocaudal contact a.
rostrocaudal epidural a.
star a.
subdural electrode a.
surface coil a.
a. of symptom
transverse tripolar epidural a.
arrest
deep hypothermic circulatory a.
sinus a.
speech a.
arrested hydrocephalus
arrhaphia

arrhigosis
arrhinencephaly, arhinencephaly, arrhinencephalia
arrhythmia
cardiac a.
fatal a.
obstructive a.
torsades de pointes a.
arrhythmogenic
arrhythmokinesis
ARS
adult Reye syndrome
arsenic
a. peripheral neuropathy
a. poisoning
a. polyneuropathy
a. toxic disorder
a. toxicity
arsenical
a. polyneuropathy
a. tremor
Arsobal
Artane
artefacta
self-induced dermatitis a.
arteria, pl. **arteriae**
a. basilaris
a. calcarina
a. cerebelli inferior anterior
a. cerebelli inferior posterior
a. cerebelli superior
a. cerebri anterior
a. cerebri media
a. cerebri posterior
a. choroidea
a. choroidea anterior
a. choroidea posterior
arteriae encephali
a. inferior anterior cerebelli
a. inferior posterior cerebelli
a. occipitalis
a. occipitalis lateralis
a. occipitalis medialis
a. orbitofrontalis lateralis
a. orbitofrontalis medialis
arteriae parietooccipitalis
a. precunealis
a. radicularis magna
a. recurrens
a. spinalis anterior
a. spinalis posterior
a. superior cerebelli
a. temporalis posterior
arteriae thalamostriatae anterolaterales
arteriae thalamostriatae anteromediales
arterial
a. access
a. aneurysm
a. biopsy
a. blood gas (ABG)
a. border zone
a. bruit
a. circle of cerebrum
a. circle of Willis
a. dissection
a. gas embolism (AGE)
a. groove
a. hemorrhage
a. inflammation
a. occlusive disease
a. occlusive retinopathy
a. oxygen
a. oxygen desaturation
a. oxygen saturation
a. photothrombosis
a. plasma input
a. thoracic outlet syndrome
a. thrombosis
a. vasospasm
arterialization
arterialized leptomeningeal vein
arteriograph bath
arteriography
carotid a.
cerebral a.
spinal a.
arteriolar infarction
arteriolopathy
retinocochleocerebral a.
arteriolosclerosis
arteriopathy
autosomal dominant a.
arteriosclerosis
cerebral a.
eccentric a.
hyaline a.
arteriosclerotic
a. brain disease
a. encephalopathy
a. intracranial aneurysm
paranoid-type a.
a. vertigo

NOTES

arteriosus
truncus a.
arteriovenous (AV)
a. aneurysm
a. crossing
a. fistula
a. interhemispheric angioma
a. malformation (AVM)
a. malformation nidus definition
a. malformation radiosurgery
a. nicking
arteritica
polymyalgia a.
arteritis, pl. **arteritides**
ANCA-positive granulomatous giant cell a.
Aspergillus a.
a. cardiovascular disease
cranial a.
extracranial a.
giant cell a. (GCA)
granulomatous a.
Heubner a.
Horton giant cell a.
intracranial granulomatous a.
necrotizing granulomatous systemic a.
neurocranial granulomatous a.
obliterative a.
pediatric stroke from Takayasu a.
rheumatoid a.
spinal cord a.
Takayasu a.
temporal a.
viral intracerebral a.
artery
A1, A2 segment of anterior cerebral a.
aberrant a.
accessory middle cerebral a.
Adamkiewicz a.
alternative occipital artery middle cerebral a.
aneurysm of persistent trigeminal a.
anomalous cerebral a.
anterior cerebral a.
anterior choroidal a. (AChA)
anterior communicating a. (ACoA, AComA)
anterior inferior cerebellar a. (AICA)
anterior inferior cerebral a.
anterior inferior communicating a.
anterior meningeal a.
anterior spinal a.
anterior temporal a.
anterolateral central a.
ascending cervical a.
ascending frontoparietal a.
auditory a.
axillary a.
basal cerebral a.
basilar a.
Bernasconi-Cassinari a.
bilateral segmental a.'s
a. of brain
calcarine a.
callosomarginal a.
caroticotympanic a.
carotid a.
a. of central sulcus
cerebellar a.
cerebral a.
a. of cerebral hemorrhage
Charcot a.
choroidal pericallosal a.
cingulothalamic a.
collicular a.
common carotid a. (CCA)
communicating branch of fibular a.
communicating branch of peroneal a.
contralateral temporary a.
costocervical a.
cranial a.
distal medial striate a.
dolichoectatic internal carotid a.
dynamic entrapment of vertebral a.
en passage feeder a.
external carotid a.
extracranial carotid a. (ECA)
extradural vertebral a.
facial a.
feeding a.
friable a.
frontal a.
frontopolar a. (FPA)
giant tortuous basilar a.
Global Utilization of Streptokinase and t-PA for Occluded Coronary A.'s (GUSTO-1)
great anterior medullary a.
a. of Heubner
inferior cerebellar a.
inferolateral pontine a.
innominate a.
intercostal a.
internal carotid a. (ICA)
intracranial a.
ipsilateral middle cerebral a.
lateral occipital a.
lateral posterior choroidal a.
left common carotid a.
lenticulostriate a. (LSA)
lumbar a.
maxillary a.
maxillomandibular a.
medial occipital a.

medial striate a.
medullary a.
meningeal a.
midbrain perforating a.
middle cerebral a. (MCA)
middle meningeal a. (MMA)
M2 segment of right middle cerebral a.
nodular induration of temporal a.
occipital a.
ophthalmic a.
paramedian thalamopeduncular a.
parent a.
periarterial plexus of choroid a.
pericallosal azygos a.
petrous carotid a.
pial a.
plexus of choroid a.
plexus of medial cerebral a.
polar a.
pontine a.
popliteal a.
a. of postcentral sulcus
posterior cerebellar a.
posterior cerebral a.
posterior choroidal a.
posterior communicating a. (PComA)
posterior inferior cerebellar a. (PICA)
posterior inferior communicating a. (PICA)
posterior spinal a.
posterolateral spinal a.
a. of precentral sulcus
primitive otic a.
primitive trigeminal a.
primordial inferior hypophysial a.
radial a.
radiculospinal a.
recurrent perforating a.
spinal cord a.
splenial a.
stapedial a.
subclavian a.
sulcocommissural a.
superficial temporal a. (STA)
superficial temporal artery-middle cerebral a. (STA-MCA)
superficial temporal artery-posterior cerebral a. (STA-PCA)
superficial temporal artery-superior cerebellar a. (STA-SCA)
superior cerebellar a.
superior hypophysial a.
superior laryngeal a.
superior thyroid a.
supraclinoid internal carotid a.
supreme intercostal a.
telencephalic ventriculofugal a.
temporal a.
temporopolar a. (TPA)
thalamocaudate a.
thalamogeniculate a.
thalamoperforating a.
thyrocervical trunk of subclavian a.
trifurcation of middle cerebral a.
trigeminocerebellar a.
ventriculofugal a.
vermian a.
vertebral a. (VA)
vertebrobasilar a.
vidian a.
zygomaticoorbital a.

artery-artery embolus
artery-to-artery embolism
artery-to-vein shunt
Artha-G
arthralgia
migratory a.
subtalar a.
temporomandibular joint a.
arthresthesia
arthrifluent abscess
arthritic general pseudoparalysis
arthritidis
Mycoplasma a.
arthritis, pl. **arthritides**
cervical spine a.
degenerative a.
enteropathic a.
gouty a.
hypertrophic a.
juvenile rheumatoid a.
neuropathic a.
psoriatic a.
rheumatoid a.
arthroconidia
airborne a.
arthrodesis
atlantoaxial a.
Brooks atlantoaxial a.
C1-C2 posterior a.

NOTES

arthrodesis *(continued)*
cervical a.
Cloward cervical a.
extension injury posterior atlantoaxial a.
flexion injury posterior atlantoaxial a.
lumbar interbody a.
occipitocervical a.
posterior atlantoaxial a.
surgical a.
arthrogryposis congenita multiplex
arthropathy
calcium pyrophosphate dihydrate a.
Charcot a.
diabetic a.
neurogenic a.
neuropathic a.
sensory neurogenic a.
tabetic a.
Arthus reaction
articular
a. branch of deep fibular nerve
a. corpuscle
a. cortex
a. leprosy
a. mass separation
a. mass separation fracture
a. sensibility
articulare
corpusculum a.
articularia
corpuscula a.
articularis
nervus a.
ramus a.
articulating disc prosthesis
articulation
atlantoaxial a.
a. disorder
disrupted occipitocervical a.
Vermont spinal fixator a.
artifact
asymmetric a.
ballistocardiographic a.
beam hardening a.
blink a.
cardiac pacemaker a.
cardioballistic a.
chemical shift a.
edge a.
electrode-pop a.
electrode-popping a.
electromyographic a.
eye blink a.
eye movement a.
ferromagnetic a.
fried egg a.
Gibbs a.
glossokinetic a.
imaging a.
impedance a.
lateralized a.
line a.
loose belt a.
machine a.
magnetic susceptibility a.
misplaced thermocouple a.
motion a.
movement a.
muscle a.
nonbiological a.
nonphysiologic a.
oculographic a.
a. on x-ray
paper stop a.
perspiration a.
physiological a.
pulsation a.
pulse wave a.
rectus spike a.
rhythmic a.
spikelike a.
statistical a.
stimulus a.
susceptibility a.
swallow a.
sweat a.
tissue magnetic susceptibility a.
truncation a.
vibration a.
artifactual clearing
artificial
a. airway
a. blood substrate
a. disc modeling
a. endplate
a. intervertebral disc
a. spinal disc
a. vertebral body
artiodactylous
aryepiglottic fold neurofibroma
arylsulfatase
a. A
a. A deficiency
AS
Angelman syndrome
asbestosis
ascending
a. cervical artery
a. current
a. degeneration
a. frontal convolution
a. frontal gyrus
a. frontoparietal (ASFP)
a. frontoparietal artery
a. myelitis
a. neuritis

a. neurotransmitter system
a. paralysis
a. paresis
a. parietal convolution
a. parietal gyrus
a. pharyngeal plexus
a. poliomyelitis
a. ramus of lateral sulcus of cerebrum
a. reticular activating system (ARAS)
a. reticular activation
a. reticular arousal system
a. tract

ascension phase

ascorbate
quinine a.
sodium a.

ASCVD
atherosclerotic cardiovascular disease

ASD
Alzheimer senile dementia

Asendin

asepsis

aseptic
a. meningeal reaction
a. meningoencephalitis
a. necrosis
a. uremic meningitis

ASFP
ascending frontoparietal

ashen
a. tubercle
a. wing

Asher physical build assessment technique

ashi point

ash-leaf
a.-l. spot
a.-l. spot in tuberous sclerosis

Ashworth
A. scale
A. score of muscle spasticity

ASIA
American Spinal Injury Association
ASIA grading system

ASIA/IMSOP
American Spinal Injury Association/International Medical Society of Paraplegia

Asian alcohol flush reaction

ASIF
Association for the Study of Internal Fixation
ASIF broad dynamic compression
ASIF broad dynamic compression bone plate
ASIF T plate

Aslan endoscopic scissors

asleep-awake-asleep surgical resection

asomatognosia

aspartate aminotransferase (AST)

aspartic proteinase

aspartoacylase deficiency

aspartylglycosaminidase

aspartylglycosaminuria

Asp/Asp genotype

aspect
associative a.
diagnostic a.
immunologic a.
laminar cortex posterior a.
molecular genetic a.
normative a.
perceptual a.

aspen
A. electrocautery
A. laparoscopy electrode
A. ultrasound system

Asperger
A. disorder
A. syndrome

aspergilloma

aspergillosis

aspergillotic aneurysm

Aspergillus
A. arteritis
A. brain abscess
A. cerebral abscess
A. fumigatus
A. glaucus
A. nidulans
A. niger
A. terreus
A. ustus

asphyxia
birth a.
intrapartum a.
lactic acid production in perinatal a.
Myers model of perinatal a.
neonatal a.

NOTES

asphyxia *(continued)*
neonate a.
perinatal a.
aspiny neuron
aspiration
bone plate a.
Integra Selector ultrasonic a.
needle a.
negative a.
stereotactic needle a.
ultrasonic a.
aspirator
Cavitron Ultrasonic Surgical A. (CUSA)
Selector ultrasonic a.
Sharplan Ultra ultrasonic a.
Sonocut ultrasonic a.
ultrasonic surgical a.
aspirin
Carotid Artery Stenosis with Asymptomatic Narrowing: Operation Versus A. (CASANOVA)
a. therapy
Asp risk allele
ASPS
advanced sleep-phase syndrome
ASS
Aarskog-Scott syndrome
assault
brain a.
assay
ADmark A.
autoantibody a.
a. buffer
CH50 a.
clonogenic cell a.
enzyme-linked immunosorbent a. (ELISA)
5-HT receptor a.
5-hydroxytryptamine receptor a.
immunocytochemical a.
immunofluorescence a.
limulus amebocyte lysate a.
MAO spectrophotometric a.
nephelometric a.
plaque reduction a.
radiobinding a.
serotonin receptor a.
spectrophotometric a.
TaqMan a.
tissue-based monoamine oxidase a.
assembly
Ace halo-cast a.
Brown-Roberts-Wells arc-ring a.
cryocooler a.
multiple-hook a.
tubulin a.
assessment
Activity Loss A.
A. of Aphasia and Related Disorders, Second Edition
Baycrest Neurocognitive A.
Behavioural Neurology A. (BNA)
closed-chain functional a.
cognitive function a.
competency a.
complement symptom-focused a.
comprehensive a.
concussion a.
cross-sectional a.
diagnostic a.
environmental a.
Fugl-Meyer a.
functional a.
injury severity a.
longitudinal a.
long-term disability a.
a. method
Moire topographic scoliosis a.
multidimensional a.
neuroimaging a.
neuropsychological a.
objective a.
outcome a.
Performance Oriented Balance and Mobility A.
A. for Persons Profoundly or Severely Impaired
presurgical a.
a. procedure
risk-benefit a.
Rivermead Motor A.
shunt a.
SQUID array for reproductive a. (SARA)
standardized a.
symptom a.
vision a.
in vivo stereological a.
ASSI
Accurate Surgical and Scientific Instruments
ASSI coagulator
assimilative factor
assisted ventilation
assistive technology device
associated movement
association
Acoustic Neuroma A.
Alzheimer A.
Alzheimer Disease and Related Disorders A.
American Brain Tumor A.
American Parkinson Disease A.
American Sleep Disorders A.
American Spinal Injury A. (ASIA)

American Stroke A.
Amyotrophic Lateral Sclerosis A. (ALSA)
a. area
Batten Disease Support and Research A. (BDSRA)
Children's Hemiplegia and Stroke a.'s (CHASA)
clang a.
conditioned fear a.
contextual a.
a. cortex
A. of Directors of Medical Student Education in Psychiatry
fear a.
a. fiber
haplotype a.
International Rett Syndrome A. (IRSA)
laws of a.
a. mechanism
multiple a.'s
National Aphasia A. (NAA)
National Mental Health A. (NMHA)
National Rehabilitation A.
National Stroke A.
National Tuberous Sclerosis A. (NTSA)
a. neurofiber
occipital a.
A. of Sleep Disorder Center
Stroke and the Alzheimer Disease and Related Disorders A.
A. for the Study of Internal Fixation (ASIF)
a. system
The Stroke Council of The American Heart A.
a. time
Tourette Syndrome A. (TSA)
a. tract

associationis
neurofibra a.

associative
a. aphasia
a. aspect
a. visual agnosia

associativity
criterion of a.

assumption
Hodgkin-Huxley a.
variance a.

AST
aspartate aminotransferase

astasia

astasia-abasia

astatic seizure

astereognosis

asterion

asterixis

asteroides
Nocardia a.

asthenia
myalgic a.
neurocirculatory a.
treatment-emergent a.

asthenic type

asthenopia
nervous a.

asthma
sleep-related a.
a. treatment

asthmatic amyotrophy

astigmatism

astragalectomy

astral body

astroblast

astroblastoma

astrocyte
Alzheimer type I, II a.
ameboid a.
fibrillary a.
fibrous a.
gemistocytic a.
peripapullar a.
protoplasmic a.
reactive a.
stellate a.
suspended embryonic a.
wedge-shaped a.

astrocytic
a. change
a. end foot
a. gliosis
a. reaction
a. signal
a. tumor

astrocytoma
anaplastic a.
brainstem a.
cerebellar a.

NOTES

astrocytoma *(continued)*
cerebral anaplastic a.
chiasmatic-hypothalamic pilocytic a.
cystic a.
desmoplastic cerebral a.
diencephalic a.
diffuse cellular a.
fibrillary a.
gemistocytic a.
giant cell a.
grade I–IV a.
hypothalamic a.
intracranial a.
juvenile cerebellar a.
juvenile pilocytic a. (JPA)
low-degree a.
low-grade diffuse a.
malignant a.
optic nerve a.
pilocytic juvenile a.
piloid a.
pilomyxoid a.
a. protoplasmaticum
protoplasmic a.
pseudopalisading a.
subcortical protoplasmic a.
subependymal giant cell a.
subependymal glomerate a.
supratentorial a.
thalamic a.
xanthomatous a.
astrocytosis cerebri
astroependymoma
astroglia cell
astrogliosis
astrotactin protein
asymbolia
pain a.
asymmetric
a. artifact
a. flaccid weakness
a. hyperreflexia
a. motor neuropathy
a. optokinetic nystagmus
a. tonic neck reflex
a. tonic seizure
a. visual distractor
asymmetrical
a. crying facies (ACF)
a. generalized epileptiform activity
a. palatal paresis
asymmetry
a. amplitude
cytoarchitectural a.
encephalic a.
facial a.
left/right a.
nasal-temporal a.
planum temporale a.
Wada memory a.
asymptomatic
a. carotid artery stenosis
a. carotid atherosclerosis study
a. carotid bruit
a. hydrocephalus
a. intracranial aneurysm
a. neck bruit
a. neurosyphilis
a. visual field defect
asynchronism
asynchronous blinking
asynchrony
impulse a.
asynergic
asynergy, asynergia
AT
ataxia-telangiectasia
AT III deficiency
AT III
antithrombin III
atactic
a. abasia
a. agraphia
a. ataxia
atactica agraphia
atactiform
atactilia
ataractic
Atarax
ataraxic
Atavi atraumatic spine fusion system
atavistic
ataxia, ataxy
absent a.
acute cerebellar a. (ACA)
alcohol-related a.
atactic a.
autosomal dominant cerebellar a.
Biemond a.
Briquet a.
Bruns frontal a.
buccolingual a.
cerebellar degeneration a.
cerebral a.
Charlevoix-Saguenay a.
chronic a.
crural a.
diabetes-related a.
early-onset a.
echovirus infection a.
episodic a. type 2 (EA-2)
equilibratory a.
familial episodic a.
familial paroxysmal kinesigenic a.
familial spastic a.
Ferguson-Critchley a.
Friedreich hereditary a.

frontal a.
gait a.
a. gene
gluten a.
Greenfield classification of spinocerebellar a.
hand a.
hereditary cerebellar a.
hereditary posterior column a.
hereditary spinal a.
hysterical a.
infantile-onset spinocerebellar a.
infantile X-linked a.
inherited a.
ipsilateral cerebellar a.
kinesigenic a.
kinetic a.
late-onset a.
Leyden a.
locomotor a.
Marie a.
Menzel a.
motor a.
multiple sclerosis a.
myxedema a.
neoplastic a.
oculomotor a.
olivopontocerebellar a.
optic a.
pancerebellar a.
periodic vestibular a. (PVA)
pes cavus in Friedreich a.
polyQ a.
progressive a.
respiratory a.
Sanger Brown a.
sensory a.
spastic a.
spinal a.
spinocerebellar a. (SCA)
spinocerebellar a. 1–7
spinocerebellar a. gene encoding types 1–7 (*SCA1–7*)
sporadic a.
static a.
truncal a.
trunk a.
vasomotor a.
vestibulocerebellar a.

ataxiadynamia

ataxiagram

ataxiagraph

ataxiameter

ataxiaphasia

ataxia-telangiectasia (AT)
a.-t. syndrome

ataxic
a. abasia
a. aphasia
a. breathing
a. cerebral palsy
a. dysarthria
a. gait
a. hemiparesis
a. lymphopathy
a. neuropathy
a. paramyotonia
a. paraplegia
a. respiration

ataxin-1 protein

ataxiophemia

ataxy (*var. of* ataxia)

Ateles
cerebral cortex of A.

atenolol

atheroembolism
diffuse disseminated a.

atheroma

atheromatosis

atheromatous disease

atherosclerosis
carotid a.
cerebral a.
coronary a.
vertebrobasilar a.

atherosclerotic
a. aneurysm
a. cardiovascular disease (ASCVD)
a. infarction
a. plaque

athetoid
a. cerebral palsy
a. dysarthria
a. spasm

athetosic, athetotic
a. dysarthria
a. dystonia
a. idiocy

athetosis
double-congenital a.
posthemiplegic a.

athymic

athyreosis

Ativan

NOTES

atlantal fracture
Atlantis anterior cervical plate system
atlantoaxial
a. arthrodesis
a. articulation
a. dislocation
a. fixation
a. fusion
a. instability
a. interval
a. joint
a. rotatory subluxation
a. separation
a. stabilization
atlantodental
atlantoepistrophic ligament
atlantomastoid
atlantooccipital
a. joint
a. separation
a. stabilization
atlas
a. burst fracture
A. of polysomnography
Schaltenbrand-Wahren stereotactic a.
stereotactic a.
a. of Talairach and Tournoux
atlas-axis combination fracture
atomic, biologic, chemical (ABC)
atonia
choreatic a.
muscle a.
atonic
a. absence
a. bladder
a. cerebral palsy
a. drop attack
a. epilepsy
a. seizure
atonic-astatic diplegia
atopognosia, atopognosis
atopy
atorvastatin
ATP
adenosine 5′-triphosphate
ATPase
adenosine triphosphatase
sodium-potassium ATPase
atractylic acid
atracurium besylate
atraumatic Sprotte needle
atresia
aural a.
choanal a.
laryngeal a.
oral a.
atrial
a. fibrillation
a. myxoma
a. natriuretic peptide (ANP)
a. ring
atrophedema
atrophia (*var. of* atrophy)
atrophic
a. lesion
a. neuroarthropathy
atrophica
myotonia a.
atrophicans
atrophoderma neuriticum
atrophy, atrophia
acute reflex bone a.
adult-onset spinal muscular a.
amygdala a.
anterior temporal a.
Aran-Duchenne muscular a.
basal forebrain a.
Behr complicated optic a.
brain a.
cerebellar vermian a.
cerebral peduncular a.
Charcot-Marie-Tooth a.
circumscribed cerebral a.
congenital cerebellar a.
cortical a.
corticospinal a.
Cruveilhier a.
Dejerine-Sottas a.
Dejerine-Thomas a.
denervated muscle a.
dentatorubral a.
dentatorubropallidoluysian a. (DRPLA)
diffuse brain a.
disuse a.
dorsum sellae a.
Duchenne-Aran spinal muscular a.
Eichhorst a.
entorhinal cortex a.
Erb a.
facial progressive a.
facioscapulohumeral a.
familial spinal muscular a.
Fazio-Londe a.
focal muscular a.
frontal temporal a.
gray matter a.
Gudden a.
gyral a.
hereditary cerebellar a.
hippocampal formation a.
Hoffmann muscular a.
Hunt a.
idiopathic muscular a.
infantile progressive spinal muscular a.
intermediate spinal muscular a.
intratentorial a.

ischemic muscular a.
juvenile spinal muscular a.
Kugelberg-Welander distal muscular a.
Kugelberg-Welander juvenile spinal muscle a.
Landouzy-Dejerine a.
Leber hereditary optic a.
lobar a.
Marie-Foix-Alajouanine cerebellar a.
Menzel olivopontocerebellar a.
monomelic muscular a.
multiple system a.
multisystem a. (MSA)
muscle a.
muscular fiber a.
myelopathic muscular a.
myopathic a.
neocortical a.
neuritic muscular a.
neurogenic a.
neuromuscular a.
neuropathic a.
neurotrophic a.
nutritional-type cerebellar a.
olivopontocerebellar a.
optic nerve a.
pallidal a.
parenchymatous a.
perifascicular a.
peroneal muscular a.
Pick a.
postneuritic a.
primary optic a.
progressive circumscribed cerebral a.
progressive facial a.
progressive infantile spinal muscular a.
progressive neuromuscular a.
progressive neuropathic muscle a.
progressive postpolio muscle a. (PPPMA)
pseudohypertrophic muscular a.
scapulohumeral a.
scapuloperoneal muscular a.
segmental sensory disassociation with brachial muscular a.
spinal muscular a. type 1–4 (SMA)
subcortical a.
Sudeck a.
sulcal a.
temporal horn a.
temporal lobe a.
testicular a.
tooth a.
transneuronal a.
trophoneurotic a.
urogenital a.
vermian a.
Vulpian a.
Vulpian-Bernhardt spinal muscular a.
Werdnig-Hoffmann spinal muscular a.
white a.
whole-brain a.
X-linked spinobulbar muscular a.
Zimmerlin a.

atropine

AT/RT

atypical teratoid/rhabdoid tumor

attached

a. cranial section
a. craniotomy

attachment

cerebellar a.
collodion a.
dural a.
a. dynamic
Hardy a.
Hudson cerebellar a.
Mayfield-Kees table a.
neuromuscular a.
a. relationship
side-to-end hypoglossal-facial nerve a.
University Plate spinal a.
a. versatility

attack

absence a.
akinetic drop a.
amnesia for a.
atonic drop a.
autoimmune a.
brain a.
cataleptic a.
cephalgic a.
a. characteristic
crescendo transient ischemic a.
cryptogenic drop a.
drop a.
epileptic drop a.

NOTES

attack *(continued)*
factitious a.
jackknife a.
kinesigenic a.
limited symptom a.
masticatory a.
motor jacksonian a.
oxygen radical a.
physical a.
position of a.
psychomotor a.
recurrent panic a.
salaam a.
sensory jacksonian a.
sleep a.
spontaneous panic a.
Stokes-Adams a.
tonic drop a.
transient hemisphere a.
transient ischemic a. (TIA)
uncinate a.
vagal a.
vasospastic a.
vasovagal a.
vertebrobasilar transient ischemic a.
vertigo a.
Attenade
attentional cueing
attenuation
a. of alpha rhythm on EEG
a. coefficient on MRI scan
intraaural a.
a. reflex
a. value on MRI scan
attitudinal
a. reflex
a. risk factor
attitudinize
attonita
cephalea a.
attractor
a. field therapy (AFT)
A. retrieval device
attritional stage
atypia
histologic a.
atypical
a. absence
a. absence seizure
a. antipsychotic drug
a. cleft
a. curve pattern
a. facial neuralgia
a. facial pain
a. gait disorder
a. giant cell tumor
a. idiopathic scoliosis
a. lymphocytosis
a. meningioma
a. parkinsonism
a. petit mal seizure
a. sleep pattern
a. somatoform disorder
a. stereotyped movement disorder
a. teratoid/rhabdoid tumor (AT/RT)
a. teratoma
a. tic disorder
a. trigeminal neuralgia
audiofrequency eddy current
audiogenic
a. epilepsy
a. seizure
audiogram
pure-tone a.
audiologic study
audiometric study
audiometry
average evoked response a.
brainstem electrical response a.
cortical a.
impedance a.
pure-tone a.
audiovestibular syndrome
audiovisual
a. electroencephalogram
a. stimulation
audiovisual-tactile stimulation
audition
chromatic a.
gustatory a.
auditivae
ostium tympanicum tubae a.
auditory
a. agnosia
a. amnesia
a. aphasia
a. arteriovenous malformation
a. artery
a. association area
a. association cortex
a. aura
a. brainstem evoked response
a. brainstem implant (ABI)
a. brainstem response (ABR)
a. canal
a. compound action potential
a. continuous performance task
a. cortical area
a. cue
a. evoked potential
a. evoked response
a. fatigability
a. ganglion
a. hair
a. hallucination
a. hyperalgesia
a. hyperesthesia
a. illusion

a. koniocortex
a. lemniscus
a. memory
a. nerve
a. neuropathy
a. nucleus
a. oculogyric reflex
a. organ
a. pathway
a. perception
a. perceptual disorder
a. prosthesis
a. radiation
a. receptor cell
a. region
a. responsive naming task
a. seizure
a. span
a. stimulus
a. stria
a. synesthesia
a. system
a. threshold
a. tract
a. transfer deficit
a. tubercle
a. visual-evoked response
a. vocabulary
a. word center
a. word/nonword discrimination task

auditus
organum a.

Auerbach
A. ganglion
A. plexus

augmentor
a. fiber
a. nerve

aura, pl. **aurae**
abdominal a.
auditory a.
complex intellectual a.
consistent a.
a. continua
defined a.
déjà vu a.
epigastric a.
epileptic a.
experiential a.
gustatory a.
intellectual a.
kinesthetic a.
migraine with a.
migraine without a. (MwoA)
migrainous a.
motor a.
olfactory a.
painless a.
a. procursiva
psychical a.
reminiscent a.
residual a.
sensory a.
shimmering light with a.
simple primitive a.
somatosensory a.
status a.
tingling with a.
uncinate a.
vertiginous a.
visceral a.
visually sparkling with a.
visual shimmering with a.
visual shining with a.
wavering light with a.

aural
a. atresia
a. fullness
a. vertigo

aureus
Staphylococcus a.

auricular
a. branch of vagus nerve
a. ganglion
a. lesion

auricularis
ramus anterior nervi a.

auriculopalpebral reflex

auriculotemporal
a. nerve
a. nerve syndrome

auriculotemporali
ramus communicans nervi glossopharyngei cum nervo a.

auriculotemporalis
nervus a.
rami parotidei nervi a.
rami temporales superficiales nervi a.
ramus membranae tympani nervi a.

aurique
grippe a.

auropalpebral reflex

NOTES

Australian
A. Council for Education Research
A. X disease
A. X encephalitis
autism
A. Diagnostic Interview
A. Diagnostic Observation Schedule
infantile a.
a. screening
A. Screening Questionnaire
A. Society of America
a. spectrum
a. tendency
a. with regression
autism-related symptom
autistic psychopathy
auto
REMstar A.
autoadjusting positive airway pressure (APAP)
autoantibody
amphiphysin a.
antineuronal cytoplasmic a. (ANCA)
a. assay
a. assay testing
brain-associated a.
striational a.
autocerebral cooling
autochthonous graft
autoecholalia
autofluorescence focal fluorescence
autogenous
a. bone graft
a. cable graft interposition VII-VII neuroanastomosis
a. iliac bone
autograft
a. bone
a. bone grafting
autoimmune
a. attack
a. chorea
a. demyelinating polyneuropathy (AIDP)
a. disease
a. illness
a. process
a. reaction
a. thyroiditis
autoimmunity
pituitary a.
autoinduction
enzyme a.
autokinesia, autokinesis
autokinetic
autologous
a. adrenal medullary tissue
a. blood transfusion
a. bone marrow rescue
a. fat graft
a. fibrin sealant glue
a. hematopoietic stem cell transplantation (AHSCT)
automated
a. brainstem auditory evoked response (ABAER)
a. computed axial tomography
a. computerized axial tomography (ACAT)
a. percutaneous lumbar discectomy (APLD)
a. test target calibration
automatic
a. absence
a. auditory brainstem response
a. chorea
a. decompensation EMG
a. epilepsy
a. positioning system
automatism
ambulatory a.
chewing a.
epileptic a.
facial expression a.
gestural a.
ictal a.
immediate posttraumatic a.
lip smacking a.
mumbling a.
oral alimentary a.
patting a.
scratching a.
spinal a.
swallowing a.
automotor seizure
autonomic
a. affective law
a. arousal disorder
a. change in sleep
a. column of spinal cord
a. denervation
a. disruption
a. division of nervous system
a. dysfunction
a. dysreflexia (AD)
a. epilepsy
a. failure
a. function
a. ganglion
a. hyperreflexia (AH)
a. hyperventilation
a. imbalance
a. impairment
a. instability
a. motor neuron
a. nerve
a. nerve fiber
a. nervous system (ANS)

a. neurofiber
a. neurogenic bladder
a. neuropathy
a. oculomotor nucleus
a. part
a. part of peripheral nervous system
a. plexus
a. seizure
a. varicosity
a. visceral motor nucleus

autonomica
pars abdominalis a.
pars pelvica a.
pars thoracica a.

autonomicae
neurofibrae a.

autonomici
nuclei oculomotorii a.
pars pelvica systematis a.
pars thoracica systematis a.
plexus a.

autonomicorum
ganglia plexuum a.

autonomicum
systema nervosum a.

autonomicus
nervus a.
plexus a.
ramus a.

autonomotropic

autonomous
a. function
a. functional component

autonomy
bodily a.
patient a.

auto-PAP

autophagy

autophony

autoplastic

autopsy-based neurochemical study

autopsychic

autopsy-confirmed diagnosis

autoradiographic
a. image
a. localization
a. study

autoradiography
DAT a.
dopamine transporter a.
quantitative receptor a.

autoreactive antibody

autoreceptor

autoregressive model for signal analysis

autoregulation
a. of cerebral blood flow
cerebral pressure a.
pressure a.

autoscope

autoscopy

autosomal
a. chromosomal anomaly
a. dominant
a. dominant arteriopathy
a. dominant cerebellar ataxia
a. dominant febrile convulsion
a. dominant genetic defect
a. dominant inheritance
a. dominant migraine
a. dominant movement disorder
a. dominant nocturnal frontal lobe epilepsy
a. dominant temporal lobe epilepsy
a. dominant transmission
a. recessive
a. recessive inheritance
a. recessive juvenile parkinsonism (ARJP)
a. recessive syndrome of encephalopathy

autosomatognosis

autosympathectomy secondary to neuropathy

autotitrating continuous positive airway pressure

autotopagnosia agnosia

auxiliary valve

AV
anticipatory vomiting
arginine-vasopressin
arteriovenous
AV shunt

avalanche
a. conduction
a. theory

Avanti sheath

avascular necrosis

Avellis
palatopharyngeal paralysis of A.
A. paralysis
A. syndrome

Aventyl

NOTES

average
a. evoked response
a. evoked response audiometry
pure-tone a.
a. velocity
avidin-biotin
a.-b. peroxidase complex
a.-b. stain technique
avidin-biotin-complex-peroxidase method
avis
calcar a.
nidus a.
unguis a.
avitaminosis B_{12} peripheral neuropathy
Avitene
A. microfibrillar collagen
A. microfibrillar collagen hemostat
A. packing
A. powder
AVM
arteriovenous malformation
AVM nidus definition
Avonex
AVP
arginine-vasopressin
avulsion
brachial plexus a.
bypass coaptation for cervical nerve root a.
cauda equina a.
conus medullaris root a.
a. injury
nerve root a.
peripheral a.
root a.
sacral plexus a.
third nerve a.
AVVM
angiographically visualized vascular malformation
awake
a., alert, and oriented
a. brain surgery
a. craniotomy
a. language paradigm
awakening
early final a.
nighttime a.
nocturnal a.
awareness alteration
awl
angled a.
hemostat a.
pedicle a.
pointed a.
reaming a.
rectangular a.
Swanson scaphoid a.
T-handle bone a.

axes (*pl. of* axis)
axial
a. burst fracture
a. compression
a. compression stability
a. gradiometer
a. gripping strength
a. load
a. loading
a. loading fracture
a. magnetic resonance image
a. manual traction test
a. musculature
a. myopia
a. neuritis
a. pattern scalp flap
a. plane angular deformity biomechanics
a. posturing
a. projection
a. rotation
a. section
a. spinal system
a. spin-echo image
a. stiffness
a. traction
axial-occipital ligament
axifugal
axile corpuscle
axilemma
axilla, pl. **axillae**
axillaris
nervus a.
axillary
a. artery
a. nerve
a. sheath
AxioCam camera
axiodistocervical (ADC)
axiom
axiomatic
axion
axioplasm
axipetal
axiramificate
axis, pl. **axes**
adrenal a.
basicranial a.
cerebrospinal a.
a. corpuscle
corticotrophic a.
a. cylinder
encephalomyelonic a.
endocrine a.
a. function
hip a.
horizontal a.
hypothalamic-hypophysial-gonadal a.
hypothalamic-pituitary a.

hypothalamic-pituitary-adrenal a.
longitudinal a.
neural a.
spinal a.
thyrotrophic a.
time a.
vertical a.
visual a.

axis-atlas combination fracture
3-axis gradient coil
axoaxonic synapse
Axocet
axodendritic synapse
axodendrosomatic synapse
axofugal
axogenesis
axoid
Axokine
axolemma
axolemmal ion channel
axolysis
axon

bifurcating a.
cervix of a.
corticospinal a.
a. degeneration
extending a.
a. flare
fusimotor a.
giant a.
granule cell a.
a. guidance
a. hillock
intracortical a.
lamprey spinal a.
a. loss polyneuropathy
motor unit a.
myelinated a.
myelination of a.
naked a.
a. reaction
a. reflex
a. reflex test
a. regeneration
a. regrowth
a. response
rostral spinal a.
Schaffer collateral a.
sensory a.
A. Sentinel-4 analyzer
swollen a.
a. terminal
thalamocortical a.
a. torpedo appearance
transected a.
unmyelinated a.
a. wave

axonal

a. conduction
a. cytoskeleton
a. damage
a. degeneration
a. diameter
a. distal neuropathy
a. growth
a. injury
a. lesion
a. loss
a. mechanism
a. plasticity
a. polyneuropathy
a. process
a. reaction
a. regeneration
a. shearing injury
a. spheroid
a. swelling
a. terminal bouton
a. transport
a. transport disruption

axonography
axonopathic neurogenic thoracic outlet syndrome
axonopathy

cerebral a.
distal a.
multifocal acquired motor a.
proximal a.

axonotmesis
axonotmetic injury
axopetal
axophage
axoplasm degeneration
axoplasmic

a. flow
a. flow and papilledema
a. transport

axosomatic synapse
Axostim nerve stimulator
axotomize
axotomy

delayed a.
instantaneous a.
peripheral nerve a.

NOTES

axotomy *(continued)*
- primary a.
- secondary a.

Axsain

Ayala
- A. disease
- A. index
- A. quotient

Ayers needle holder

Ayer test

Ayer-Tobey test

azacyclonol hydrochloride

azamethonium bromide

azaperone

azaspirodecanedione

azidothymidine

Azilect

aziridinylbenzoquinone

Azorean disease

Azorean-Joseph-Machado disease

aztreonam

azurophilic granule

azygos vein

B
B amyloid protein
B cell
B fiber
B vitamin deficiency neuropathy
B1
vitamin B1
B6
vitamin B6
B12
serum vitamin B12
vitamin B12
Babcock forceps
Babès
B. node
B. nodule
B. tubercle
Babinski
B. percussion hammer
B. phenomenon
B. reflex
B. response
B. sign
B. syndrome
B. test
Babinski-Nageotte syndrome
bacampicillin
bacillary layer
***Bacilles anthracis* meningitis**
bacilliformis
Bartonella b.
bacillus, pl. **bacilli**
gram-negative b.
tubercle b.
back
b. of foot reflex
b. pain
b. pain predictor
background
b. activity
b. alpha frequency
b. disorganization
b. factor
b. rhythm
Backhaus towel clip
Backlund
B. biopsy needle
B. stereotactic instrument
backout
screw b.
backpack
b. palsy
b. paralysis
backward
digit span b. (DSB)
b. progression
spatial span b. (SSB)
baclofen
Bacon cranial rongeur
bacterial
b. aneurysm
b. antigen
b. brain abscess
b. cell wall component
b. encephalitis
b. infection
b. meningitis
b. meningitis treatment
b. meningoencephalitis
b. peripheral neuropathy
b. toxin
b. wound contamination
bactericidal
bacteriostatic
Bacteroides
B. fragilis
B. non-fragilis
Bactiseal antimicrobial-impregnated catheter system
baculovirus infection
Baddeley model
Badgley
B. iliac wing resection
B. laminectomy retractor
BAEP
brainstem auditory evoked potential
BAER
brainstem auditory evoked response
bag
nuclear b.
Bailey
B. conductor
B. rib spreader
Bailey-Badgley
B.-B. anterior cervical approach
B.-B. cervical spine fusion
Baillarger
B. band
exterior band of B.
external band of B.
external line of B.
inner band of B.
inner line of B.
interior band of B.
internal band of B.
internal line of B.
B. line
outer band of B.
outer line of B.
B. sign

Bailliart ophthalmodynamometer
BAK cage
BAK/cervical interbody fusion system
BAK/C interbody fusion system
baked brain phenomenon
Baker point
balance
alternate binaural loudness b.
Clinical Test of Sensory Interaction and B. (CTSIB)
b. deficit
b. disorder
b. disturbance
dopaminergic-cholinergic b.
dynamic ambulatory b.
dynamic standing b.
B. Error Scoring System
fluid b.
genic b.
homeostatic b.
b. impairment
magnesium b.
B. Master-training and assessment system
measure of b.
poor b.
Secure B.
sitting b.
standing b.
static and dynamic sitting b.
static and dynamic standing b.
sudden loss of b.
balancer
MMS-900 microscope b.
balancing subdural hematoma
Balint syndrome
ball
Marchi b.
B. operation
tantalum b.
Ballantine hemilaminectomy retractor
Baller-Gerold syndrome
Ballet disease
8-ball hemorrhage
ball-in-cone valve
ballismus, ballism
ballistic material
ballistocardiographic artifact
balloon
b. catheter
b. cell
b. compression
detachable silicone b.
elastomeric b.
electrodetachable b.
Endeavor b.
extradural b.
b. kyphoplasty
latex b.
Magic B1 b.
metrizamide-filled b.
nondetachable endovascular b.
nondetachable occlusive b.
b. occlusion-aspiration embolus entrapment device
occlusion balloon catheter with silicone b.
b. occlusion test
silicone b.
Solstice b.
Spiegelberg epidural b.
Symmetry angioplasty b.
b. test occlusion
ballooned floor of ventricle
ballooning
b. of sella
b. of vertebral interspace
ball-tip nerve hook
ball-type disc prosthesis
Baló
B. concentric sclerosis
B. disease
Baltic
B. myoclonus
B. myoclonus disease
B. myoclonus epilepsy
B. syndrome
Baltimore Therapeutic Equipment (BTE)
Bamberger
B. disease
B. sign
Bamberger-Pins-Ewart sign
bamboo spine
Bancaud phenomenon on EEG
band
A b.
alpha frequency b.
anisotropic b.
Baillarger b.
Bechterew b.
b. of Broca
Broca diagonal b.
Büngner b.
dentate b.
diagonal b.
dysferlin b.
Essick cell b.
furrowed b.
Gennari b.
b. of Giacomini
b. heterotopia
I b.
isotropic b.
b. of Kaes-Bechterew
b. keratopathy
negative oligoclonal b.
normal-frequency b.
oligoclonal b.

Osborn b.
peritumoral b.
piezoelectric b.
reelin immunoreactive b.
Reil b.
transcallosal b. (TCB)
Vicq d'Azyr b.
bandage
Comperm tubular elastic b.
Dressinet netting b.
fibrin b.
hammock b.
bandaletta diagonalis
banding
Giemsa b.
quinacrine fluorescent b.
bandwagon effect
bandwidth
data acquisition b.
receiver b.
banging
head b.
bank
Traumatic Coma Data B.
Bankson Language Test 2
Bannayan syndrome
Bannister disease
Bannwarth syndrome
bar
distraction b.
Dynamic mesh pre-angled connecting b.
Greenberg-type b.
Leyla self-retaining tractor b.
longitudinal spinal b.
screw alignment b.
baragnosis, barognosis
Bárány
B. chair
B. maneuver
B. pointing test
positional vertigo of B.
barber chair syndrome
Barbita
barbiturate
b. burst-suppression anesthesia
b. peripheral neuropathy
b. poisoning
barbiturate-induced spindle-like activity
Barbour technique
Bardeen disc
Bardet-Biedl syndrome
baresthesia
baresthesiometer
barium
b. ferrite
b. sulfate
Barker point
Barkhof MRI criteria
Barkman reflex
Barlow syndrome
Barnes
B. dystrophy
B. global score
baroceptor
barognosis (*var. of* baragnosis)
baroreceptor nerve
baroreflex
barostat
barotrauma
Barouk microstaple
Barr body
barrel
b. bur
b. field
b. staved graft
Barré-Lieou syndrome
Barré pyramidal sign
barrier
blood-brain b. (BBB)
blood-brain tumor b. (BBTB)
blood-cerebral b.
blood-cerebrospinal fluid b.
blood-CSF b.
blood-thymus b.
hematoencephalic b.
intrablood-brain b. (IBBB)
Bartel criteria
Bartelmez
club ending of B.
Barthel
B. Activities of Daily Living Scale
B. Index
Bartholin
B. anus
B. gland
Barth syndrome
Bartonella
B. bacilliformis
B. henselae
bartonellosis
Bartter syndrome
basal
b. cell nevus syndrome

NOTES

basal *(continued)*
b. cerebral artery
b. cistern
b. cistern effacement
b. encephalocele
b. endothelium-derived relaxing factor
b. forebrain amnesia
b. forebrain atrophy
b. forebrain cholinergic pathway
b. forebrain region
b. ganglia calcification
b. ganglia classification
b. ganglia syndrome
b. ganglia-thalamocortical motor circuit
b. ganglion
b. ganglionic lesion
b. gland
b. interhemispheric approach
b. joint reflex
b. lamella
b. lamina
b. lamina of choroid
b. lamina of cochlear duct
b. lamina of neural tube
b. layer of choroid
b. line
b. meningoencephalocele
b. nucleus
b. nucleus of Ganser
b. nucleus of Meynert
b. plate
b. plate of neural tube
b. pterional approach
b. skull fracture
b. subfrontal approach
b. substantia
b. vein
b. vein of Rosenthal (BVR)

basales
nuclei b.

basalis
cisterna b.
lamina b.
substantia b.
vena b.

base
anterior cranial b.
b. of brain
data b.
b. of dorsal horn of spinal cord
lateral skull b.
phantom b.
b. of posterior horn of spinal cord
skull b.

Basedow pseudoparaplegia

baseline
b. angiography
b. cognitive functioning
b. EEG
b. measure
b. rating
Reid b.
b. scan
b. severity
b. study
b. test
b. visit

baseline-to-endpoint change

basement
b. laboratory
b. membrane
b. membrane protein

bases (*pl. of* basis)

basiarachnitis

basiarachnoiditis

basic
b. brain mechanism
b. brain pathway
b. fibroblast growth factor
b. impairment
B. Living Skills Scale
b. skill

basicranial
b. axis
b. flexure

basilar
b. apex
b. apex aneurysm
b. arachnoiditis
b. artery
b. artery migraine
b. artery migraine headache
b. artery thrombosis syndrome
b. artery trunk aneurysm
b. bifurcation
b. bifurcation aneurysm
b. crest of cochlear duct
b. ectasia
b. impression
b. invagination
b. lamina
b. leptomeningitis
b. membrane
b. membrane of cochlear duct
b. meningitis
b. meninx
b. part of pons
b. pontine sulcus
b. skull fracture
b. subdental synchondrosis
b. tip aneurysm

basilaris
arteria b.
glandula b.
membrana b.
sulcus b.

basilar-type migraine
basilar-vertebral artery disease
basiocciput tumor
basis, pl. **bases**
compassionate-use b.
b. cornus dorsalis medullae spinalis
b. cornus posterioris medullae spinalis
empirical b.
genetic b.
idiosyncratic b.
pathophysiological b.
b. pedunculi cerebri
b. pedunculus
b. pontis
presumptive b.
basket
Alzheimer b.
b. cell
fibrillar b.
Moss-Harms b.
basolateral amygdaloid nucleus
basomedial amygdaloid nucleus
basophil
b. adenoma
b. substance
basophilia
Cushing b.
pituitary b.
substantia b.
basophilic
b. adenoma
b. pituitary tumor
b. substance
basophilism
Cushing b.
Bassen-Kornzweig
B.-K. disease
B.-K. peripheral neuropathy
B.-K. syndrome
Basser syndrome
Bassett electrical stimulation device
Bastian-Bruns
B.-B. law
B.-B. sign
Bastian law
bath
arteriograph b.
bathing
b. and dressing ability
perilymph b.
bathmotropic
negatively b.
positively b.
bathmotropism
bathyanesthesia
bathyesthesia
bathyhyperesthesia
bathyhypesthesia
batimastat protease inhibitor
Batson plexus
Batten
B. disease
B. Disease Support and Research Association (BDSRA)
Batten-Mayou disease
battery
apraxia b.
brief cognitive test b.
cognitive test b.
Dementia Assessment B.
neuropsychological test b.
Rand Functional Limitations B.
Rand Physical Capacities B.
Rivermead Perceptual Assessment B.
Western Aphasia B.
battledore incision
Battle sign
BAVM
brain arteriovenous malformation
Baxter disease
Baycrest Neurocognitive Assessment
Bayesian technique
Bayle disease
bayonet
b. aneurysm clip
b. clip applier
b. forceps
b. handle
BBB
blood-brain barrier
BBBD
blood-brain barrier disruption
BBS
Berg Balance Scale
BBTB
blood-brain tumor barrier
bcl-2 gene
Bcl-xL gene
BCNU
1,3-bis(2-chlorethyl)-1-nitrosourea

NOTES

BCNU *(continued)*
bischloroethylnitrosourea
bischloronitrosourea
BCNU-impregnated polymer wafer
BD
brain damage
brain dead
brain death
BDI
Beck Depression Inventory
BDNF
brain-derived neurotrophic factor
BDSRA
Batten Disease Support and Research Association
beaked tectum
BEAM
brain electrical activity method
brain electrical activity monitoring
beam
b. hardening artifact
high-energy X-ray b.
laser b.
particle b.
proton b.
radiation b.
beaten
b. copper cranium
b. copper pattern
b. metal appearance
beating-heart brain-dead donor
beaver
B. discission blade
B. keratome blade
Bechterew
B. band
B. deep reflex
B. disease
B. layer
layer of B.
line of B.
B. nucleus
B. reaction
B. sign
B. test
B. tract
Bechterew-Mendel reflex
Beck Depression Inventory (BDI)
Becker
B. disease
B. myotonia
B. variant
B. variant of Duchenne dystrophy
Becker-Kiener dystrophy
Becker-type tardive muscular dystrophy
Beckman
B. Coulter CEQ8000 fluorescent DNA analyzer
B. Coulter QuickStart
B. retractor
Beckman-Adson laminectomy blade
Beckman-Eaton
B.-E. laminectomy
B.-E. laminectomy blade
B.-E. laminectomy retractor
Beckman-Weitlaner
B.-W. laminectomy
B.-W. laminectomy retractor
Beckwith-Wiedemann syndrome
bed
BioDyne b.
Burke Bariatric b.
Cardiopulmonary Paragon 8500 b.
CircOlectric b.
Clinitron air b.
dynamic b.
Flexicair b.
high air loss b.
high muscular resistance b.
Keane Mobility b.
KinAir b.
Lapidus b.
low air loss b.
Magnum 800 b.
Medicus b.
Mega-Air b.
Mega Tilt and Turn b.
b. nucleus of stria terminalis
Restcue b.
Skytron b.
Stryker b.
Thera Pulse b.
Tilt and Turn Paragon b.
tumor b.
bedbound
bedrest
bedridden
bedside
B. Evaluation Screening Test, Second Edition
b. multimodality monitoring
b. testing
Beery developmental test of visuomotor integration
Beevor sign
Begbie disease
BEHAB
brain-enriched hyaluronan binding
behavior
aberrant motor b.
abnormal illness b.
abstract b.
accident b.
adultomorphic b.
alertness b. (AB)
b. alteration
b. analysis

antinodal b.
catatonic motor b.
Center for Ecology, Evolution and B. (CEEB)
chain b.
chewing b.
chronic illness b.
b. deficit
b. disorder
drive b.
estrous b.
frontal lobe seizure with complex b.
hyperenergetic b.
interictal b.
b. mapping
b. modification therapy
molar b.
molecular b.
nonfunctional and repetitive motor b.
B. Pathology in Alzheimer Disease Rating Scale
pattern of repetitive b.
rapid eye movement-sleep b.
b. reflex
REM-sleep b.
seizure-related b.
semipurposeful b.
sensorimotor b.
Society for Quantitative Analyses of B.
sundowning b.
b. system
B. Therapy and Research Society
time-dependent b.
unusual sleep b.
violent b.
visuomotor b.

behavioral
b. abnormality
b. assessment measure
b. desensitization
b. difference
b. disorder
b. effect
b. function
b. improvement
b. inactivity
b. input
b. manifestation
b. neuroscience
b. perspective
b. symptom
b. trajectory

behavior-orientation

Behavioural Neurology Assessment (BNA)

Behçet
B. disease
B. syndrome

Behr
B. complicated optic atrophy
B. disease

Beimer-Clip aneurysm clip

Bell
B. law
B. nerve
B. Object Relations and Reality Testing Inventory
B. palsy
B. phenomenon
B. sign
B. spasm

Bellatal

Bell-Magendie law

bellows
aneroid chest b.

belly dancer dyskinesia

Belmont collar

benazepril and hydrochlorothiazide

Bence Jones protein

benchmark measure

bender
French rod b.
B. Gestalt Visual Motor test

bending
rod b.
b. strength

bendroflumethiazide

beneceptor

Benedek reflex

benediction hand

Benedikt
B. ipsilateral oculomotor paralysis
B. syndrome

Benemid

benign
b. adult familial myoclonic epilepsy
b. angiopathy of CNS vasculitis
b. capillary hemangioblastoma
b. childhood epilepsy with centrotemporal spike

NOTES

benign *(continued)*
b. childhood partial epilepsy
b. coital cephalalgia
b. congenital hypotonia
b. cranial nerve tumor
b. epilepsy with occipital focus
b. epileptiform transients of sleep (BETS)
b. epileptiform variant
b. exertional headache
b. familial chorea
b. familial essential tremor
b. familial infantile convulsion
b. familial neonatal convulsion
b. fasciculation with cramp
b. focal amyotrophy
b. focal epilepsy
b. functional vertigo
b. hereditary chorea
histologically b.
b. infantile familial convulsions plus paroxysmal choreoathetosis
b. infantile myoclonus
b. intracranial hypertension
b. lymphocytic choriomeningitis
b. lymphocytic meningitis
b. lymphoepithelial parotid tumor
b. maturation delay
b. meningioma
b. monoclonal gammopathy
b. myalgic encephalitis
b. myalgic encephalomyelitis
b. neonatal sleep myoclonus
b. occipital epilepsy
b. paroxysmal positional vertigo
b. paroxysmal torticollis
b. paroxysmal vertigo of childhood
b. partial epilepsy of childhood
b. partial epilepsy with centrotemporal spike (BPECTS)
b. positional paroxysmal vertigo
b. postural vertigo
b. rolandic epilepsy
b. senescent forgetfulness
b. stupor
b. tetanus
b. X-linked recessive muscular dystrophy

benserazide
benserazide-L-dopa
Benson-Geschwind classification of aphasia
Benton
B. Naming Test
B. Visual Form Discrimination Test
B. Visual Retention Test (BVRT)

Bentson exchange length wire
Bentyl
benzamide
substituted b.

benzedrine
benzenepropanamine
benzilate
quinuclidinyl b.

benznidazole
benzoate
rizatriptan b.

benzodiazepine
b. discontinuation syndrome
b. postsynaptic receptor
short-acting b.

benzoic acid
benzothiadiazide
benzothiazine
dibenzepin b.

benzoylecgonine
benztropine mesylate
Berardinelli syndrome
Berenstein guiding catheter
Berg Balance Scale (BBS)
Berger
B. paresthesia
B. rhythm
B. sign

Bergeron chorea
Bergmann
B. cord
B. fiber
B. glial cell

Bergman rule
Bergstrom cannula
beriberi, beri beri
cerebral b.
dry b.
infantile b.
wet b.

Berliner percussion hammer
Berlin Sleep Questionnaire
Bernard
B. puncture
B. syndrome

Bernard-Horner syndrome
Bernard-Soulier disease
Bernasconi-Cassinari artery
Bernhardt
B. disease
B. paresthesia

Bernhardt-Roth syndrome
Bernoulli law
Bero test
berry aneurysm
Bertillon cephalometer
Bessman-Baldwin syndrome
best-fit
b.-f. analysis
b.-f. curve

best registration error

besylate
atracurium b.
beta
b. activity
b. adrenergic agonist
b. adrenergic receptor blocker
b. amyloid protein
b. B-sheet conformation
b. fiber
b. galactosidase
b. glucuronidase
b. hemolytic streptococcus meningitis
b. histine
b. human chorionic gonadotropin
b. hydroxybutyrate
b. hydroxylase
interleukin b.
b. latrotoxin
b. mannosidase
b. mannosidosis
b. methylcrotonylglycinuria
b. motoneuron
b. myosin heavy chain
b. rhythm
b. secretase
b. subunit of human chorionic gonadotropin (beta HCG)
transforming growth factor b.
b. wave
beta-1a
interferon b.-1a
beta-adrenergic receptor blocking agent
beta-adrenoreceptor antagonist
beta-alpha-theta-delta discharges
beta-amyloid (Abeta)
b.-a. fibril
b.-a. oligomer
b.-a. pathology
b.-a. plaque
b.-a. processing
beta-amyloid-related epitope
beta-1b
interferon b.-1b
beta-blocker
beta-B-structure sheet
beta-B-TP
betaB-Trace protein
betaB-Trace protein (beta-B-TP)
beta-emitting radiation
Betaferon
beta HCG
beta subunit of human chorionic gonadotropin
beta-hexosaminidase A deficiency
beta-lactam antibiotic neurotoxicity
betamethasone
beta$_2$ microglobulin
beta-pleated sheet
Betaseron needle-free delivery system
bethanechol
BETS
benign epileptiform transients of sleep
between-brain
Betz
B. cell
B. cell area
Beuren syndrome
Bevan-Lewis cell
Bevatron accelerator
Beyer laminectomy rongeur
Bezold ganglion
Bezold-Jarisch reflex
BHI
brain-heart infusion
breath-holding index
bias
cytokine b.
spatial b.
bias-free evidence
bibrachial paresis
BICAP
Bipolar Circumactive Probe
BICAP cautery
BICAP unit
bicarbonate
potassium b.
serum b.
sodium b.
bicaudate ratio
biceps
b. femoris reflex
b. jerk
bicerebral infarction
Bichat
B. canal
B. fissure
B. foramen
bicisate
technetium-99m b.
Bickerstaff
B. migraine
B. migraine headache

NOTES

bicoronal scalp flap
Bidder organ
bidentate ligand
bidirectionally
Biedl-Moon-Laurence syndrome
Bielschowsky
B. disease
B. head tilt test
B. maneuver
Bielschowsky-Jansky disease
Biemond
B. ataxia
B. disease
B. syndrome
Bier
B. block
B. lumbar puncture needle
B. saw
Biernacki sign
bifid
b. cranium
b. hook
b. uvula
bifida
cranial b.
spina b.
bifidum
cranium b.
bifilar needle electrode
bifrontal
b. craniotomy
b. headache
b. incision
b. malignant meningioma
bifunctional
b. protein
b. protein deficiency
bifurcating axon
bifurcation
basilar b.
carotid b.
cervical carotid b.
b. cone
intracranial b.
Bigelow calvaria clamp
bigemina
corpora b.
bigeminal body
bigeminum
biglycan proteoglycan
bilateral
b. acoustic neuromas syndrome
b. activity
b. arachnoid cysts
b. centrocecal scotoma
b. choroid plexus cysts
b. contralateral primary sensorimotor areas
b. craniectomies
b. eyelid blinking
b. gaze palsy
b. hemisphere dysfunction
b. homonymous hemianopia
b. hydrocephalus
b. hyperreflexia
b. independent periodic lateralized epileptiform discharges (BIPLEDs)
b. ligamentectomies
b. medial orbital ecchymoses
b. mesial temporal lobe epilepsy
b. motor phenomena
b. occipital infarctions
b. occipital transtentorial approach
b. periventricular nodular heterotopia
b. pupil dilation
b. secondary sensorimotor areas
b. segmental arteries
b. spastic hemiplegia
b. synchrony
b. temporary tarsorrhaphies
b. temporoparietal emphasis
b. tonic stiffening
b. upper brainstem infarctions
b. vagotomies
b. variable screw placement system
b. ventral rhizotomies
bilaterally synchronous epileptic discharges
bilayer
lipid b.
lipid-protein b.
bilevel positive airway pressure (BiPAP)
bilharziasis
biliary dyskinesia
Biligrafin
Biligram
bilious headache
bilirachia
bilirubin
b. encephalopathy
b. serum level
Bilivistan
Billroth disease
biloba
gingko b.
bilobed aneurysm
Bilopaque
Biloptin
bimanual
b. coordination deficit
b. neuronal activity
bimastoid line
bimaxillary advancement
bimedial frontal leukotomy
bimodal distribution
binaural distorted speech test

binding
brain-enriched hyaluronan b. (BEHAB)
H-imipramine b.
protein b.
serum protein b.
b. site
in vivo benzodiazepine receptor b.
Bing-Horton syndrome
Bing-Neel syndrome
Bing reflex
binocular
b. acuity change
b. flash stimulus
b. loupe
Binswanger
B. dementia
B. disease
B. encephalopathy
B. type
bioamine
bioaminergic
bioavailability
neuroleptic b.
Biobond
biocalibration
bioccipital headache
bioceramic
calcium phosphate b.
biochemical
b. activity
b. change
b. genetics
b. information
b. oxygen demand (BOD)
b. pathway
b. phenotypic marker
b. study
b. tumor marker
BioCleanse tissue sterilization process
Biocoral graft material
biocycle
BioDyne bed
bioelectrical impedance analysis
bioelectricity
bioenergetic deficiency
bioethics bionics
biofeedback
EMG b.
b. therapy
Biogel Sensor surgical glove
biogenic amine
biohydraulic
Biojector 2000 needle-free injection management system
biolinguistic
biologic
b. correlate
b. determinant
b. dysregulation
b. evidence
b. intervention
b. marker
b. pathogenesis
b. perspective
b. reductionism
b. research
b. response modifier
b. risk factor
b. substrate
b. time
b. training
b. window on CNS function
biologically quiescent glioma
biological stressor
biomagnetometer
BTi b.
37-channel b.
biomechanical
b. analysis
b. factor
b. model
b. stability
b. testing
biomechanics
axial plane angular deformity b.
distraction instrumentation b.
Dwyer instrumentation b.
posterior fixation system b.
Roy-Camille posterior screw plate fixation b.
spine b.
biomedical model
biometric result
bionics
bioethics b.
bionomics
biopercular syndrome
biophysical study
biophysiology
bioplastic
biopsy
arterial b.
brain b.

NOTES

biopsy *(continued)*
contralateral b.
CT-guided b.
endoscopic sphenoidal b.
image-guided stereotactic brain b.
leptomeningeal/wedge cortical b.
lumbar spine b.
meningeal b.
muscle b.
nerve b.
PET-guided stereotactic b.
quadriceps muscle b.
stereotactic b.
sural nerve b.
targeted brain b.
temporal artery b.
thoracic spine b.
transnasal b.
Tru-Cut needle b.
vastus lateralis muscle b.
biopterin deficiency
biosynthesis
heme b.
Biot
B. breathing
B. breathing sign
B. respiration
bioterrorism agent
biothesiometer
biotin
b. holocarboxylase synthetase deficiency
b. metabolic disorder
biotinidase deficiency
BioTrainer exercise meter
bioweapon
BiPAP
bilevel positive airway pressure
BiPAP Pro II with heated humidification
biparietal
b. enlargement
b. hypoperfusion
b. lesion
bipedal walking
biperiden
biphasic
b. action potential
b. locomotor response
Biphetamine
biplane roentgenogram
BIPLEDs
bilateral independent periodic lateralized epileptiform discharges
bipolar
b. bayonet forceps
b. cautery
b. cautery probe
b. cautery scissors
B. Circumactive Probe (BICAP)
b. coagulating forceps
b. coagulator
b. diathermy forceps tip
b. diathesis
b. electrocautery
b. electrocautery forceps
4F b. electrode
b. gradient
b. I disorder
b. long-shaft forceps
b. montage
b. needle electrode
b. neuron
b. patient
b. polysomnographic finding
b. retinal cell
b. stimulating electrode
b. vertebral traction
biportal technique
Birbeck granule
birdcage resonator
bird-headed dwarf
birdlike facies
birefringence
crystalline b.
flow b.
form b.
intrinsic b.
b. in polarized light
strain b.
streaming b.
birefringent
birth
b. anoxia
b. asphyxia
b. injury
b. palsy
b. trauma
b. trauma theory
birth-related spinal cord injury
1,3-bis(2-chlorethyl)-1-nitrosourea (BCNU)
bischloroethylnitrosourea (BCNU)
bischloronitrosourea (BCNU)
Bischof myelotomy
bisection
vertical line b.
bis(guanylhydrazone)
methylglyoxal b.
Bishop putty
bispectral EEG monitor
bisphosphonate
bisulfate
clopidogrel b.
bit
acorn b.
cannulated drill b.
diamond b.
drill guide with drill b.

Howmedica microfixation system drill b.
Leibinger Micro Imlants drill b.
Luhr microfixation system drill b.
Storz Microsystems drill b.
Synthes Microsystem drill b.

bitartrate
metaraminol b.

bitemporal
b. headache
b. hemianopia
b. hypoperfusion

biundulant meningoencephalitis

bivalved speculum

biventer
b. lobule
lobulus b.

biventralis
lobulus b.

biventral lobule

bizarre
b. asynchronous movement
b. high-frequency discharge
b. high-frequency potential
b. posturing
b. repetitive discharges
b. symptom
b. variant

Björeson syndrome

Björnström algesiometer

black
b. box warning
b. eye
B. grading scale
b. hole
b. mass
B. Max high-speed drill
b. substance

bladder
allantoic b.
atonic b.
autonomic neurogenic b.
cord b.
b. disturbance
nervous b.
neurogenic b.
b. reflex
reflex neurogenic b.
stammering of b.
uninhibited neurogenic b.
b. urgency

blade
Acra-Cut b.
air b.
arachnoid-shape Beaver b.
Beaver discission b.
Beaver keratome b.
Beckman-Adson laminectomy b.
Beckman-Eaton laminectomy b.
double-vector b.
Komet K-2000 surgical saw b.
K-2000 surgical saw b.
Meyerding laminectomy b.
Meyerding-Scoville b.
Micro-Aire b.
retractor b.
ribbon b.
Scoville b.
tapered b.

Blair-Ivy loop

Blake pouch

Blandin ganglion

bland myopathy

blank
b. gaze
Strong Vocational Interest B. (SVIB)

blast
air b.
b. effect
stoma b.

blastocyte

blastoderm

Blastomyces dermatitidis

blastomycosis
nasopharyngeal b.
spinal b.

blastomycotic meningitis

bleed
ipsilateral b.

bleeding
aneurysmal b.
b. disorder
gastrointestinal b.
intraabdominal b.
intracranial b.
intrathoracic b.
b. rate
b. risk
short-term b.
b. time

blennorrhagic swelling

NOTES

blennorrhagicum
keratoderma b.
Blenoxane
bleomycin sulfate
blepharitis
blepharoconjunctivitis
blepharophimosis
blepharoplast
blepharoptosis
blepharospasm, blepharospasmus
essential b.
blepsopathia
Blessed Dementia Scale
Blessed-Roth Dementia Scale
Bleulerian schizophrenia
blind
b. headache
ipsilaterally b.
b. spot
b. test
blindness
cerebral b.
cortical b.
gaze-evoked b.
hysterical b.
ipsilateral monocular b.
letter b.
mind b.
monocular b.
object b.
psychic b.
sight b.
sign b.
smell b.
space-form b.
syllabic b.
taste b.
text b.
total monocular b.
transient monocular b. (TMB)
word b.
blindsight
blink
b. artifact
eye b.
b. reflex
b. reflex latency
b. response
blinking
asynchronous b.
bilateral eyelid b.
eye b.
rapid eye movement-onset b.
REM-onset b.
blisterlike aneurysm
bloater
blue b.
blob
b. cell
b. channel
bloc
en b.
Bloch equation
Bloch-Sulzberger syndrome
block
anodal b.
Bier b.
cervical steroid epidural nerve b.
clonic b.
conduction b.
depolarization b.
diagnostic b.
dynamic b.
epidural b.
exit b.
hydroxyapatite b.
intracellular calcium b.
local diagnostic b.
methylmethacrylate b.
monolithic adult b.
motor conduction b.
motor point b.
nerve root b.
neurolytic b.
paraspinal muscle b.
phenol motor point b.
sham b.
short-acting b.
somatic b.
spinal subarachnoid b.
stellate ganglion b.
subarachnoid b. (SAB)
sympathetic b.
tonic b.
trigger point muscle b.
ventricular b.
b. vertebra
voltage-sensitive b.
blockade
adrenergic b.
D2 b.
dopamine receptor b.
intravenous regional sympathetic b.
muscarinic cholinergic b.
neuromuscular b.
pharmacological b.
reuptake b.
sympathetic b.
blockage
shunt b.
blocker
beta adrenergic receptor b.
calcium channel b.
dopamine receptor b.
voltage-gated sodium channel b.

blocking
b. activity
alpha b.
EEG alpha b.
Blocq disease
blood
b. blister-like aneurysm
b. cell
b. culture
b. donor
b. feud
b. flow
b. flow change
b. flow measurement
b. flow velocity
b. flow volume
b. loss
b. oxygenation level dependent (BOLD)
b. oxygenation level-dependent contrast technique
b. oxygen level dependent (BOLD)
b. oxygen level-dependent functional magnetic resonance imaging
b. patch
b. pool (BP)
b. pool imaging
b. screening
b. thinning
b. and thunder retina
b. urea nitrogen (BUN)
b. velocity
b. vessel
b. viscosity
blood-brain
b.-b. barrier (BBB)
b.-b. barrier disruption (BBBD)
b.-b. barrier disruption chemotherapy
b.-b. transcytosis
b.-b. tumor barrier (BBTB)
blood-cerebral barrier
blood-cerebrospinal fluid barrier
blood-CSF barrier
blood-gas exchange
blood/injection phobia
bloodless decerebration
blood-nerve barrier breakdown
blood-thymus barrier
blood-tissue exchange
bloody tap
Bloom
B. disease
B. syndrome
Bloomer Learning test
blot
Southern b.
Blount laminar spreader
blown pupil
blow-out fracture
blue
b. bloater
b. diaper syndrome
b. edema
Histoacryl b.
methylene b.
blue-stained
toluidine b.-s.
Blumenau nucleus
Blumenbach clivus
blunt
b. K-wire
b. nerve hook
b. obturator
b. spike-and-wave complex on EEG
b. suction tube
blunt-ring curette
blurred vision
blurring
visual b.
blush
choroidal b.
b. of dye on angiogram
BMI
body mass index
B-mode
B-m. image
B-m. ultrasonography
BMP
bone morphogenetic protein
bone morphogenic protein
BNA
Behavioural Neurology Assessment
BNCT
boron neutron capture therapy
BNP
brain natriuretic peptide
Boas algesiometer
Bobath response
bobbing
head b.
inverse ocular b.

NOTES

bobbing *(continued)*
ocular b.
reverse ocular b.
bobble-head doll syndrome
Bobechko
B. sliding barrel hook
B. spreader
Bochdalek
flower basket of B.
B. ganglion
B. pseudoganglion
Bock
B. ganglion
B. nerve
BOD
biochemical oxygen demand
Bodian silver impregnation
bodily
b. autonomy
b. symptom
body
b. alienation
amygdaloid b.
amyloid b.
anterior nucleus of trapezoid b.
anterior quadrigeminal b.
aortic b.
apoptotic b.
artificial vertebral b.
astral b.
Barr b.
bigeminal b.
Bunina b.
carotid b.
b. of caudate nucleus
b. of cerebellum
b. coil
b. concept
b. of corpus callosum
cortical Lewy b.
Cowdry inclusion b. type A, B
Cowdry-type intranuclear inclusion b.
cytoid b.
dementia with Lewy b. (DLB)
dorsal nucleus of trapezoid b.
b. ego damage
foreign b.
b. of fornix
geniculate b.
glomus b.
Golgi b.
habenular b.
Harting b.
Herring b.
Hirano b.
b. image
b. image distortion
inclusion b.
infundibular b.
b. jerk
juxtarestiform b.
Kelvin b.
Lafora b.
lateral geniculate b.
lateral nucleus of mammillary b.
lateral nucleus of trapezoid b.
b. of lateral ventricle
b. lateropulsion
Lewy b.
Luys b.
b. of Luys syndrome
mamillary b.
mammary b.
b. mass index (BMI)
medial geniculate b.
medial nucleus of trapezoid b.
metallic foreign b.
b. modification
b. movement detector
myelin b.
Negri b.
nerve cell b.
neuronal ceroid lipofuscinosis curvilinear b.
newtonian b.
Nissl b.
nucleus of lateral geniculate b.
nucleus of mamillary b.
nucleus of medial geniculate b.
nucleus of trapezoid b.
olivary b.
pacchionian b.
paraphysial b.
paraterminal b.
parietal b.
parolivary b.
PAS-positive circular b.
peduncle of mamillary b.
pedunculus of pineal b.
Pick b.
pineal b.
pontobulbar b.
b. position
posterior quadrigeminal b.
psammoma b.
pseudopsammoma b.
quadrigeminal b.
Reilly b.
Renaut b.
restiform b.
rhinencephalic mamillary b.
b. righting reflex
Rohon-Beard cell b.
sand b.
b. schema
b. schema distortion
Schwann cell b.

b. sense
serotoninergic cell b.
b. spatial orientation
striate b.
b. sway
tigroid b.
Todd b.
trapezoid b.
Vater-Pacini b.
ventral nucleus of trapezoid b.
Verocay b.
Weibel-Palade b.
b. weight-supported treadmill training
Wolf-Orton b.
zebra b.

body-related obsessive-like symptom

Bogaert-Bertrand spongy dystrophy

Bohlman
B. anterior cervical vertebrectomy
B. cervical fusion technique

Bohr effect

Bohr-Haldane effect

BOLD
blood oxygenation level dependent
blood oxygen level dependent
BOLD f-MRI

Bolivian hemorrhagic fever

Bollinger
posttraumatic apoplexy of B.

bolt
Camino microventricular b.
Camino ventricular b.
ICP Camino b.
Philly b.
Richmond b.
subarachnoid b.

Boltzmann
B. distribution
B. distribution law

bolus dosing

bombesin

Bondek suture

bone
b. algorithm
allograft iliac b.
autogenous iliac b.
autograft b.
bone in b.
calvarial b.
cancellous b.
b. conduction
congenital defect of cranial b.
b. core
b. curette
b. cyst
b. density scan
b. density screening
b. dissection
b. flap
b. fragment
b. graft
b. graft collapse
b. graft decompression
b. graft extrusion
b. graft harvest site
b. grafting
b. graft placement
b. health
hyoid b.
increased Wormian b.
b. loss
magic b.
b. marrow
b. marrow rescue
b. marrow stem cell
b. marrow stromal cell
b. marrow suppression
b. marrow transplantation
b. marrow transplantation graft-versus-host disease
b. matrix formation
b. mineral content
b. mineral density
b. morphogenetic protein (BMP)
b. morphogenetic protein-2
b. morphogenic protein (BMP)
occipital b.
b. pain
petrous b.
b. plate
b. plate aspiration
b. plate selection
b. punch
b. reflex
b. remodeling
b. screw
b. sensibility
spongy b.
b. stock
temporal b.
trabecular b.
trigeminal impression of temporal b.

NOTES

bone *(continued)*
b. tumor
Tutoplast b.
b. wax
b. window CT scan
wormian b.
bone-biting rongeur
bone/ligament dissection
bone-screw interface strength
BoneSource hydroxyapatite cement
Bonferroni-Dunn procedure
Bonhoeffer
B. sign
B. symptom
B. syndrome
Bonnet-Dechaume-Blanc syndrome
Bonnet sign
Bonnevie-Ullrich syndrome
Bonnier syndrome
bony
b. abnormality
b. canal
b. dissection
b. dysplasia
b. element destruction
b. endplate
b. exposure
b. facet
b. landmark
b. overhang
b. purchase
b. spinal column
Bookwalter retractor
booster clip
boost irradiation technique
boot
thigh-high alternating compression air b.
Borchardt olive-shaped bur
border
b. cell
vermilion b.
borderline
b. pathology
b. patient
borderzone infarction
boric acid neurotoxicity
Börjeson-Forssman-Lehmann syndrome
Bornholm disease
boron neutron capture therapy (BNCT)
Borrelia
B. burgdorferi
B. hermsii
borreliosis
Lyme b.
Bosin disease
bossing
occipital b.
Boston
B. brace system
B. Classification System
B. Diagnostic Aphasia Exam-Cookie Theft Card
B. Diagnostic Aphasia Examination
B. LINAC
B. Naming Test
B. neurosurgical couch
Bosworth spinal fusion
Botox
B. injection amplifier
B. injection amplifier brace
Böttcher
B. cell
B. ganglion
bottom-up approach
botulinum
b. antitoxin
Clostridium b.
b. toxin
b. toxin injection
b. toxin type A, B
botulinus neurotoxin (BTX)
botulism
food-borne b.
human b.
infantile b.
b. peripheral neuropathy
b. toxin
b. with paralysis
bouche de tapir
Bouchet-Gsell sign
Bouin-Hollande fixative
boundary
diagnostic b.
B. Shift Integral (BSI)
B. Shift Integral calibration
B. Shift Integral method
whole-brain b.
Bourneville
B. disease
B. tuberous sclerosis
Bourneville-Pringle disease
bouton
axonal terminal b.
synaptic b.
terminal b.
bovine
b. chromaffin cell
b. pericardium for dural graft
b. spongiform encephalopathy
Bowditch law
bowel disturbance
Bower model of mood-congruent memory
bowing reflex
bow-tie nystagmus

box
B. and Block timed manipulation test
BTE bolt b.
cyclin b.
boxcar effect
boydii
Pseudallescheria b.
BP
blood pool
Imagent BP
BPECTS
benign partial epilepsy with centrotemporal spike
BPI
brain perfusion index
Braak
B. & Braak staging
B. neurofibrillary staging
B. stage
brace
Botox injection amplifier b.
halo b.
Hudson b.
kyphosis b.
Milwaukee b.
SOMI Jr. b.
System-Loc back b.
Yale b.
brace-free ambulation
bracelet
Nageotte b.
brachial
b. amyotrophy
b. birth palsy
b. cutaneous nerve
b. diplegia
b. locomotion
b. plexitis
b. plexopathy
b. plexus
b. plexus avulsion
b. plexus avulsion injury
b. plexus exploration
b. plexus lesion
b. plexus neuritis
b. plexus neuropathy
brachial-basilar insufficiency syndrome
brachialgia
b. and cord syndrome
b. statica paresthetica
brachialis
divisiones anteriores plexus b.
divisiones posteriores plexus b.
fasciculus lateralis plexus b.
pars infraclavicularis plexus b.
pars supraclavicularis plexus b.
plexus b.
radices plexus b.
trunci plexus b.
truncus inferior plexus b.
truncus medius plexus b.
truncus superior plexus b.
brachiocephalic vein
brachiocrural involvement
brachiofacial cortical hypesthesia
brachioradialis
b. reflex
b. transfer for wrist extension
brachioradial reflex
brachium
b. of caudal colliculus
b. colliculi caudalis
b. colliculi inferioris
b. colliculi rostralis
b. colliculi superioris
b. conjunctivum cerebelli
b. of inferior colliculus
inferior quadrigeminal b.
b. opticum
b. pontis
b. quadrigeminum inferius
b. quadrigeminum superius
b. of rostral colliculus
b. of superior colliculus
superior quadrigeminal b.
Brachmann-de Lange syndrome
brachybasia
brachycephalia (*var. of* brachycephaly)
brachycephalic, brachycephalous
brachycephalism
brachycephaly, brachycephalia
brachycranic
brachytherapy
high-energy b.
interstitial b.
remote afterloading b. (RAB)
b. seed implantation
stereotactic b.
volumetric interstitial b.
bracing
external b.
postoperative b.

NOTES

Bracken Basic Concept Scale, Revised
Brackmann suction irrigator
Bradbury-Eggleston syndrome
Braden flushing reservoir
bradyarthria
bradycardia
sinus b.
bradycinesia (*var. of* bradykinesia)
bradyesthesia
bradyglossia
bradykinesia, bradycinesia
end-of-dose b.
bradykinesia/akinesia
bradykinesis
bradykinetic
bradykinin
bradylalia
bradylexia
bradylogia
bradyphagia
bradyphasia
bradyphemia
bradyphrenia
bradypnea
bradypsychia
bradyteleokinesis, bradyteleocinesia
Bragard
B. sign
B. sign test
Bragg
B. ionization peak
B. peak proton beam therapy
B. peak radiation
B. peak radiosurgery
Brahmanism
braided
b. occlusion device
b. Spectra UHMWPE surgical cable
b. titanium cable
brain
abdominal b.
b. abscess
b. abscess with headache
b. abscess with hemiparesis
b. activation
b. aging
b. aluminum
b. aneurysm
anterior part of anterior commissure of b.
arachnoid of b.
b. area
b. areas generating sleep
b. arteriovenous malformation (BAVM)
artery of b.
b. assault
b. atrophy
b. attack
base of b.
b. biopsy
b. biopsy needle
b. blood flow
b. central pain
b. cicatrix
b. circuitry
b. clip forceps
b. compression
compression of b.
b. concussion
b. congestion
contrecoup injury of b.
b. contusion
b. cooling
b. cooling system
coup injury of b.
b. cryolesion
b. cyst
b. damage (BD)
b. dead (BD)
b. death (BD)
b. death protocol
b. development
b. differentiation
b. disease
b. disorder
b. dopamine
b. dopaminergic pathway
b. dopaminergic system
dura mater of b.
b. dysfunction
b. dysplasia
b. edema
b. electrical activity map
b. electrical activity mapping
b. electrical activity method (BEAM)
b. electrical activity monitoring (BEAM)
b. engorgement
enlarged b.
b. epitope
fetal b.
b. functional failure
b. function disruption
b. functioning
b. gene therapy
glucose metabolism in b.
b. glucose metabolism
b. growth abnormality
hemangioma of b.
hemosiderin-stained b.
b. herniation
hypoxic-ischemic b.
b. illness
b. imaging
b. imaging method

b. infarction
b. infusion
injured b.
b. injury
b. insult
b. involvement
b. ischemia
b. isoform
b. laceration
b. lactate
lateral fossa of b.
b. lesion
b. location
b. mantle
B. Matters Stroke Initiative Edinburgh Artery Study
medullary artery of b.
b. metabolic effect
b. metabolic mechanism
b. metabolic response
b. metastasis
b. morphometry
b. MRI
b. murmur
b. natriuretic peptide (BNP)
b. neurochemical system
b. nucleus
olfactory b.
b. overgrowth
b. oxygenation
b. oxygen consumption
b. parenchyma
b. perfusion index (BPI)
b. perfusion study
planar stereotaxic atlas of human b.
b. plasticity
b. potential
b. potential study
prefrontal cortex of b.
b. process
b. prolyl oligopeptidase
b. puncture
b. purpura
b. radiation necrosis
b. reflex
b. region for sleep
b. relaxation score
respirator b.
b. retention
b. retraction
b. retractor
b. revascularization
b. sand
b. shift
smell b.
softening of b.
b. space
b. spatula
b. spatula forceps
b. SPECT scan
split b.
b. spoon
b. stem
b. stimulation
b. structure
b. structure study
b. substrate
supratentorial b.
b. swelling
b. synaptic membrane
b. synaptosome
b. target
tight b.
b. tissue
b. tissue acidosis
b. tissue oxygen
b. transplantation
b. trocar
b. tumor
b. tumor forceps
B. Tumor Registry
B. Tumor Study Group (BTSG)
b. tumor with headache
ventricle of b.
ventromedial prefrontal cortex of b.
Virchow-Robin space of b.
visceral b.
b. volume
b. voyager 4.0
b. wart
b. wave
b. wave complex
b. wave cycle
wet b.

brain-age quotient

brain-associated autoantibody

brain-behavior relationship

brain-blood partition

braincase

brain-derived

b.-d. HVA concentration
b.-d. neurotrophic factor (BDNF)
b.-d. neurotropic factor

NOTES

brain-enriched
b.-e. hyaluronan binding (BEHAB)
b.-e. hyaluronan binding protein
brain-heart infusion (BHI)
BrainLAB VectorVision neuronavigational system
BrainMap
Couples B.
BrainSCAN
B. computer planning system
B. LINAC radiosurgery system
brainstem, brain stem
b. abnormality
b. activation
b. astrocytoma
b. auditory evoked potential (BAEP)
b. auditory evoked response (BAER)
b. cavernous malformation
b. compression
b. diencephalic mapping
b. edema
b. electrical response audiometry
b. encephalitis
b. evoked potential
b. evoked response
b. glioma
b. hemorrhage
b. infarction
b. injury (BSI)
b. ischemia
b. lesion
b. morphogenesis
b. neuron
b. reflex
b. reticular formation
reticular nucleus of b.
rostral b.
rudimentary b.
b. structure
b. syndrome
b. tumor
BrainVoyager software
branch
anterior temporal b.
anteromedial central b.
b. of auriculotemporal nerve to tympanic membrane
callosal marginal b.
carotid sinus b.
choroid b.
circumferential b.
communicating b.
b. to coracobrachialis
descending b.
facial nerve b.
frontal polar b.
b. of glossopharyngeal nerve to stylopharyngeus muscle
b. to internal capsule, genu
b. to internal capsule, posterior limb
b. to internal capsule, retrolentiform limb
b. of internal carotid artery to trigeminal ganglion
lingual b.
b. of lingual nerve to isthmus of fauces
M2 b.
meningohypophysial b.
b. of oculomotor nerve to ciliary ganglion
orthosympathetic b.
peripheral trigeminal nerve b.
b. to sternocleidomastoid
superior laryngeal nerve external b.
trigeminal b.
branched-chain ketoaciduria
brancher enzyme deficiency disease
branchial
b. cleft
b. cleft abnormality
b. efferent column
branching
anomalous b.
branchiomotor nucleus
Brasdor method
brasiliensis
Paracoccidioides b.
Brauch-Romberg
B.-R. symptom
B.-R. syndrome
Braun-Yasargil right-angle clip
Bravais-jacksonian epilepsy
Brawner decision
BrDu
bromodeoxyuridine
BrDu immunohistochemistry
BrDu immunolabeling cell
BrDu-positive cell
breach rhythm
break
major b.
b. shock
strand b.
breakage
pedicle screw b.
screw b.
breakdown
blood-nerve barrier b.
myelin b.
skin b.
breakpoint
sequencing deletion b.

breakthrough
depressive b.
normal perfusion pressure b. (NPPB)
b. phenomenon
breath
gasping for b.
breath-holding
b.-h. index (BHI)
b.-h. spell
breathing
apneustic b.
ataxic b.
Biot b.
Cheyne-Stokes b.
cluster b.
b. control
b. difficulty
b. pattern
periodic b.
b. retraining
sleep b.
sleep-disordered b.
underlying sleep-disordered b.
breathy dystonia
bregma
bregmocardiac reflex
Bremer
B. AirFlo halo vest
B. halo
B. halo crown
B. halo crown system
B. halo crown traction
B. halo crown traction set
B. torque-limiting cap
Breschet sinus
Brescia-Cimino fistula
breves
nervi ciliares b.
Brevibloc
brevican proteoglycan
breviradiate
brevis
abductor pollicis b. (APB)
fibrae associationes b.
wrist-to-abductor pollicis b.
Brevital
Bricklin Perceptual Scale
bridegroom's palsy
bridge
caudolenticular gray b.
b. region
transcapsular gray b.
bridging vein
brief
B. Cognitive Rating Scale
b. cognitive test battery
b. ischemic insult
B. Pain Inventory
B. Symptom Inventory
B. Test of Head Injury
bright
b. light exposure
b. light exposure for jet lag
b. light reexposure for shift work
b. light therapy
b. thalamus syndrome
Brill-Zinsser disease
brim sign
Briquet
B. ataxia
B. disease
B. syndrome
brisk jaw jerk
Brissaud
B. disease
B. reflex
B. syndrome
Brissaud-Marie syndrome
Brissaud-Sicard syndrome
Bristol
B. disc prosthesis
B. disc replacement
British
B. Ability Scale
B. anti-Lewisite
broad
b. AO dynamic compression plate
b. phonemic transcription
broad-based
b.-b. gait
b.-b. gait with swaying
Broadbent law
Broca
B. amnesia
B. aphasia
band of B.
B. center
B. convolution
B. diagonal band
B. dysphasia
B. field
B. fissure

NOTES

Broca *(continued)*
B. gyrus
B. motor speech area
B. parolfactory area
B. region
B. syndrome
Brodie disease
Brodmann
B. area 6,7,9,24,32,34,41,43,44,46
B. classification
B. cortical area
B. cytoarchitectonic field
broken existing implant
bromazepan
bromfenac sodium capsule
bromide
azamethonium b.
calcium b.
ethidium b. (EB)
b. intoxication
ipratropium b.
pancuronium b.
perfluorooctyl b.
potassium b.
pyridostigmine b.
serum b.
sodium b.
vecuronium b.
brominated oil
bromisoval
bromocriptine
b. mesylate
b. test
bromodeoxyuridine (BrDu)
Bronx Aging Study
brooding personality
Brooks
B. atlantoaxial arthrodesis
B. cervical fusion
B. technique
Brooks-Gallie cervical operation
Brooks-Jenkins
B.-J. atlantoaxial fusion
B.-J. cervical operation
brow-down position
Brown-Adson forceps
Brown-Goodwin scale
brownian motion
Browning vein
Brown-Roberts-Wells
B.-R.-W. apparatus
B.-R.-W. arc-ring assembly
B.-R.-W. arc system
B.-R.-W. base ring
B.-R.-W. computer
B.-R.-W. computerized tomography stereotactic guidance
B.-R.-W. floor stand
B.-R.-W. head frame
B.-R.-W. headrest
B.-R.-W. head ring halo
B.-R.-W. ring adapter
B.-R.-W. stereotactic system
B.-R.-W. technique
Brown-Séquard
B.-S. paralysis
B.-S. sign
B.-S. syndrome
Brown syndrome
Brown-Vialetto-van Laere syndrome
brow pang
brucei
Trypanosoma b.
Brucella
B. abortus
B. melitensis
B. meningitis
brucellosis
cerebral b.
b. peripheral neuropathy
Bruce tract
Bruch membrane discontinuity
Brudzinski
B. reflex
B. sign
Brueghel syndrome
Brugada syndrome
bruit
aneurysmal b.
arterial b.
asymptomatic carotid b.
asymptomatic neck b.
carotid b.
intracranial b.
Bruker
B. Biospec system
B. S 200 MR system
Brunner modified incision
Bruns
B. frontal ataxia
B. gait apraxia
B. nystagmus
B. sign
B. syndrome
brush
Cragg thrombolytic b.
brush-evoked allodynia
Brushfield spot
Brushfield-Wyatt
B.-W. disease
B.-W. syndrome
brush-induced allodynia
bruxism
anticholinergic for b.
secondary b.
sleep b.
SSRI-induced b.

Bryan
B. cervical disc prosthesis
B. cervical disc system
BSI
Boundary Shift Integral
brainstem injury
BTE
Baltimore Therapeutic Equipment
BTE bolt box
BTE work simulator
B_2-TFn
BTi biomagnetometer
B_2-transferrin
BTSG
Brain Tumor Study Group
BTX
botulinus neurotoxin
bubbly bone lesion
buccal
b. frenulum
b. nerve
buccalis
nervus b.
buccinator nerve
buccofacial apraxia
buccolingual
b. apraxia
b. ataxia
b. dyskinesia
buccopharyngeal approach
Buck
B. neurological hammer
B. percussion hammer
buckling sign
buckthorn
b. ingestion
b. polyneuropathy
bucrylate
Bucy
B. cordotomy knife
B. laminectomy rongeur
Bucy-Frazier
B.-F. coagulation cannula
B.-F. suction cannula
bud
gustatory b.
taste b.
Budde
B. halo retractor system
B. halo ring
B. halo ring retractor
B. surgical system
Budde-Greenberg-Sugita stereotactic head frame
Budge center
buffer
assay b.
phosphate b.
Buffex
buffy coat homogenate
bulb
b. dynamometer
end b.
glomerular layer of olfactory b.
Held end b.
jugular b. (JB)
Krause end b.
Krause terminal b.
molecular layer of olfactory b.
b. of occipital horn
b. of occipital horn of lateral ventricle
olfactory b.
b. of posterior horn of lateral ventricle
bulbar
b. abnormality
b. anesthesia
b. apoplexy
b. cephalic pain tractotomy
b. corticonuclear fiber
b. dysfunction
b. hereditary motor neuropathy
b. involvement
b. muscle weakness
b. musculature
b. myelitis
b. nucleus
b. palsy
b. paralysis
b. poliomyelitis
b. syndrome
b. tract
bulbi (*pl. of* bulbus)
bulbocavernosus
b. reflex
b. reflex evaluation
bulboid corpuscle
bulboidea
corpuscula b.
bulbomimic reflex
bulbonuclear
bulbopontine sulcus

NOTES

bulbopontis
sulcus b.
bulboreticulospinalis
tractus b.
bulboreticulospinal tract
bulborum
pars intermedia commissura b.
bulbosacral system
bulbospinal
bulbospongiosus reflex
bulbus, pl. **bulbi**
b. cornus occipitalis ventriculi lateralis
b. cornus posterioris
b. cornus posterioris ventriculi lateralis
b. encephali
fibrae corticonucleares b.
b. olfactorius
phthisis b.
pyramis b.
stratum pigmenti b.
bulging
aneurysmal b.
bulk
b. flow transcytosis
tumor b.
bulky leptomeningeal deposit
bulldog response
bullet
b. caliber
copper-jacketed b.
ferromagnetic b.
nickel-jacketed b.
steel-containing b.
b. trajectory
bull's-eye
b.-e. deformity
b.-e. rash
bullying
b. culture
b. target
Bumke pupil
BUN
blood urea nitrogen
bunamiodyl
bundle
aberrant b.
angular b.
anterior ground b.
Arnold b.
cingulum b.
comb b.
b. of fibrils
Flechsig ground b.
Gierke respiratory b.
Gowers b.
ground b.
Held b.
Helweg b.
Hoche b.
Krause respiratory b.
lateral ground b.
lateral proprius b.
Lissauer b.
Loewenthal b.
longitudinal medial b.
longitudinal pontine b.
maculoneural b.
medial forebrain b.
medial longitudinal b.
Meynert retroflex b.
Monakow b.
b. nailing method
olfactory b.
olivocochlear b.
b. of Oort
Pick b.
posterior longitudinal b.
precommissural b.
predorsal b.
Probst b.
b. of Rasmussen
Rasmussen olivocochlear b.
Schütz b.
solitary b.
thalamomamillary b.
tumor-nerve b.
Türck b.
Vicq d'Azyr b.
Büngner band
Bunina body
Bunnell
B. dissecting probe
B. forwarding probe
bunyavirus encephalitis
buphthalmia, buphthalmos, buphthalmus
bupivacaine
buprenorphine HCl
bupropion metabolite
bur, burr
Adson enlarging b.
Adson perforating b.
Adson-Rogers cranial b.
Albee olive-shaped b.
barrel b.
Borchardt olive-shaped b.
Cushing cranial b.
dermabrasion b.
D'Errico enlarging drill b.
D'Errico perforating drill b.
diamond b.
Doyen cylindrical b.
Doyen spherical b.
enlarging b.
finish b.
flame-tip b.
high-torque b.

b. hole
b. hole cover
b. hole drainage
b. hole neuroendoscopic fenestration
b. hole transducer
Hudson brace b.
Lindermann b.
McKenzie enlarging b.
pear b.
perforating b.
right-angle b.
Rosen b.
Rotablator rotating b.
round b.
Shannon b.
spherical b.
Stille b.

Burdach
B. column
B. cuneate fasciculus
B. fiber
B. fissure
B. nucleus
B. tract

burden
caregiver b.

Burdick Eclipse ECG machine
Burford-Finochietto rib spreader
Burford retractor
burgdorferi
Borrelia b.

Burke Bariatric bed
Burke-Fahn-Marsden Dystonia Rating Scale
burner
b. injury
b. syndrome

burning
b. feet syndrome
b. hands syndrome

Burn and Rand theory
Burns Brief Inventory of Communication and Cognition
burr (*var. of* bur)
burst
b. of delta activity
epileptiform b.
epileptogenic b.
b. fracture
b. injury
b. neuron
b. suppression
sympathetic nerve b.
b. temporal lobe

bursting
b. cell
epileptiform b.
paroxysmal b.

Burundanga intoxication
Buschke
B. disease
B. Free and Cued Selective Reminding Procedure
B. Free and Cued Selective Reminding Test

Buschke-Fuld Selective Memory test
Bush-Francis Catatonia Rating Scale
Busse-Buschke disease
butaclamol hydrochloride
Butalan
butalbital
butethal
Butisol
butorphanol
b. tartrate
b. tartrate nasal spray

butterfly
b. coil
b. distribution
b. needle
b. rash
b. vertebra

butterfly-shaped
b.-s. monobloc
b.-s. monobloc vertebral plate

butterfly-type glioma
button
rubber b.
subdural b.

buttress response
butyl
b. acetate
b. aminobenzoate
b. chloride
b. formate
b. hydride
b. nitrate

***N*-butyl**
N-b. cyanoacrylate
N-b. 2-cyanoacrylate with lipiodol adhesive agent

butylcholinesterase
butyrophenone
Buzzard maneuver

NOTES

buzz group
BVR
basal vein of Rosenthal
BVRT
Benton Visual Retention Test
bypass
anterior occipital artery-middle cerebral artery b.
b. coaptation for cervical nerve root avulsion
EC-IC arterial b.
extracranial-intracranial b.
Fukushima cavernous b.
b. graft
IC-IC b.
intracranial-intracranial b.
STA-MCA b.
STA-PCA b.
STA-SCA b.
superficial temporal artery to middle cerebral artery b.
superficial temporal artery to posterior cerebral artery b.
superficial temporal artery to superior cerebral artery b.
vertebral plate b.
bystander effect

C
angry backfiring C (ABC)
C fiber
C2
medial branch C2
C2 syndrome
C4
fourth cervical nerve
c
cytochrome *c*
CA4-1
area CA4-1
CA3 pyramidal cell
CAA
cerebral amyloid angiopathy
cabergoline
c. monotherapy
c. study
cabin
magnetic shielded c.
cable
braided Spectra UHMWPE surgical c.
braided titanium c.
coaxial c.
c. nerve graft
SecureStrand c.
Songer c.
titanium c.
UHMWPE c.
ultra-high molecular weight polyethylene fiber c.
cabling
percutaneous c.
cachectic
cachexia
diabetic neuropathic c.
hypophysial c.
c. hypophysiopriva
pituitary c.
cacosmia
CAD
coronary artery disease
CADASIL
cerebral autosomal dominant arteriopathy with subcortical infarcts and leukoencephalopathy
Ca^{2+}-dependent
cadherin
calcium-dependent c.
Cadwell
C. 5200A somatosensory evoked potential unit
C. 5200A somatosensory evoked potential unit device
CAE
childhood absence epilepsy
caecum (*var. of* cecum)
Caenorhabditis elegans
caeruleospinalis
tractus c.
caeruleus
locus c.
caerulospinal tract
café au lait spot
Cafergot
caffeine
ergotamine tartrate and c.
c. holiday
c. intoxication
c. metabolism
c. response
c. sequela
c. toxicity
c. use disorder
c. withdrawal
caffeine-containing medication
caffeine-induced
c.-i. anxiety disorder
c.-i. contracture
c.-i. sleep disorder
c.-i. vasoconstriction
caffeine-related sequela
Caffey hyperostosis
CagA
cytotoxin-associated gene A
cage
BAK c.
DePuy AcroMed Harms c.
Lumbar I/F C.
Ray threaded fusion c.
Rotafix lumbar c.
threaded fusion c. (TFC)
titanium mesh c.
trapezoidal metal c.
Caitlin agitation
Cajal
horizontal cell of C.
C. horizontal cell
interstitial nucleus of C.
nucleus of C.
Cajal-Retzius
C.-R. cell
C.-R. neuron
Calan
calbindin
calcaneal gait
calcar avis
Cal Carb-HD
calcareous granule

calcarina
arteria c.
fissura c.
calcarine
c. artery
c. complex
c. cortex
c. cortex infarction
c. fasciculus
c. fissure
c. spur
c. sulcus
calcarinus
sulcus c.
calcaroid
Calcibind
calcifediol
Calciferol
C. Injection
C. Oral
calcification
basal ganglia c.
c. of basal ganglion
cranial c.
dystrophic c.
gyriform intracranial c.
idiopathic c.
intracranial c.
Calcijex
Calcimar Injection
calcineurin inhibitor
calcinosis
cerebral c.
c. intervertebralis
c., Raynaud phenomenon, esophageal motility disorders, sclerodactyly, and telangiectasia (CREST)
tumoral c.
calcitonin
c. gene-related peptide (CGRP)
c. gene-related polypeptide
c. receptor-like receptor (CRLR)
calcitriol
calcium
c. bromide
c. carbonate
cerebrospinal fluid c.
c. channel antagonist
c. channel blocker
c. channel blocking agent
c. chloride
c. citrate
c. disodium edetate
c. disodium versenate
c. disorder
c. embolus
c. glubionate
c. gluceptate
c. gluconate
intracellular c.
c. ion
c. ionophore
c. lactate
low c.
c. metabolism imbalance
c. paradox
c. phosphatase bone paste
c. phosphate bioceramic
c. phosphate cement
c. pyrophosphate dihydrate (CPPD)
c. pyrophosphate dihydrate arthropathy
c. pyrophosphate dihydrate decomposition disease
serum c.
calcium-ATPase
calcium-calmodulin kinase II
calcium-dependent
c.-d. cadherin
c.-d. rhythmic cell
calcoaceticus
Acinetobacter c.
calculus, pl. **calculi**
cerebral c.
Caldwell
C. high-speed magnetic stimulator
C. projection
Caldwell-Luc
C.-L. incision
C.-L. procedure
calf compartment syndrome
caliber
bullet c.
calibration
automated test target c.
Boundary Shift Integral c.
low-voltage c.
caliciform ending
caliculus ophthalmicus
California encephalitis
calisthenics
Calleja
island of C.
C. islet
Call-Fleming syndrome
callosal
c. agenesis
c. apraxia
c. area
c. commissure
c. commissurotomy
c. convolution
c. gyrus
c. lesion
c. marginal branch
c. section

c. splenium
c. sulcus
callosi
genu corporis c.
pars frontalis corporis c.
pars occipitalis corporis c.
pedunculus corporis c.
radiatio corporis c.
raphe corporis c.
rostrum corporis c.
splenium corporis c.
stria longitudinalis lateralis corporis c.
stria longitudinalis medialis corporis c.
sulcus corporis c.
taeniola corporis c.
tapetum corporis c.
truncus corporis c.
tuber corporis c.
vena dorsalis corporis c.
vena posterior corporis c.
callosomarginal
c. artery
c. fissure
c. sulcus
callosomarginalis
sulcus c.
callosotomy
anterior c.
corpus c.
posterior c.
radiosurgical corpus c.
callosum
agenesis of corpus c.
body of corpus c.
corpus c.
dorsal vein of corpus c.
frontal part of corpus c.
genu of corpus c.
hypogenetic corpus c.
occipital part of corpus c.
peduncle of corpus c.
posterior vein of corpus c.
radiation of corpus c.
rostrum of corpus c.
splenium of corpus c.
sulcus of corpus c.
transverse stria of corpus c.
trunk of corpus c.
calm
c. hypotonic coma
c. wakefulness state
Calman carotid clamp
calming effect
calmodulin dysfunction
calmodulin-independent neuronal nitric oxide synthase activity
calmodulin-regulated event
caloric
c. intake
c. nystagmus
c. test
c. testing
calorifacient
calorigenic source
calorimetry
calpain inhibitor
calpainopathy
calvaria, pl. **calvariae**
calvarial
c. bone
c. hemangioma
c. hook
c. metastasis
c. tuberculosis
CAM
cell adhesion molecule
computer-assisted myelography
Cambridge Mental Disorders of the Elderly Examination
camera
AxioCam c.
CTI-Siemens 933/08-12 PET c.
GE Maxicamera gamma c.
Multispect 3 c.
scintillation c.
time-of-flight positron emission tomographic c.
6-camera Vicon motion capture system
Camino
C. fiberoptic ICP monitor
C. intracranial catheter
C. intracranial pressure monitoring system
C. intraparenchymal fiberoptic device
C. microventricular bolt
C. OLM ICP monitor
C. subdural screw
C. transducer catheter
C. ventricular bolt

NOTES

cAMP
adenosine 3′,5′-cyclic monophosphate
cAMP receptor protein
cAMP response element
cAMP response element binding protein
Campath
C. injection
C. IV
Campbell nerve root retractor
campotomy
camptocormia
camptospasm
Camptothecin
Campylobacter
C. jejuni
C. jejuni infection
Camurati-Engelmann
C.-E. disease
C.-E. syndrome
Canadian
C. Cognitive Abilities Test, Form 7
C. Neurological Scale (CNS)
C. Test of Cognitive Skills
canal
arachnoid c.
Arnold c.
auditory c.
Bichat c.
bony c.
caudal c.
central c.
Cotunnius c.
craniopharyngeal c.
Dorello c.
Guyon c.
haversian c.
Hensen c.
Hunter c.
infraorbital c.
internal auditory c.
c. knife
lateral semicircular c. (LSC)
limb of bony semicircular c.
Löwenberg c.
neural c.
optic c.
c. paresis
posterior semicircular c. (PSC)
semicircular c.
spinal c.
c. stenosis
superior semicircular c. (SSC)
uniting c.
c. of Vesalius
vidian c.
canaliculus, pl. **canaliculi**
c. reuniens
canalis, pl. **canales**
c. reuniens
canalium semicircularium
canarc-1 gene
Canavan
C. disease
C. leukodystrophy
C. sclerosis
Canavan-van Bogaert-Bertrand disease
cancellation
fat/water signal c.
phase c.
cancellous
c. bone
c. core
c. screw
cancer-associated myositis
Candida
C. albicans
C. infection
candidal
c. meningitis
c. microabscess
candidate
c. gene
c. gene strategy
C. Profile Record
candidiasis
cane
Thera C.
canine spasm
caninus
risus c.
spasmus c.
canis
Toxocara c.
cannabis-based medicine
cannabis intoxication
Cannon-Bard theory
Cannon theory
cannula
Adson brain-exploring c.
Adson brain-extracting c.
Bergstrom c.
Bucy-Frazier coagulation c.
Bucy-Frazier suction c.
Dorsey ventricular c.
Dyonics c.
Elsberg brain c.
Elsberg ventricular c.
Frazier brain-exploring c.
Frazier ventricular c.
Fujita suction c.
Haynes brain c.
introducer c.

large egress c.
McCain TMJ c.
Portnoy ventricular c.
Scott c.
Sedan c.
side-cutting c.
Sluijter-Mehta SMK-C10 c.
straightening c.

cannulated
c. drill bit
c. screw

cannulation
unilateral pedicle c.

canonical neuron

canopy ventilation monitor

Cantelli sign

CANVAS
Computer-Aided Neurovascular Analysis and Simulation
CANVAS protocol

canyon
Jamestown C. (JC)

CAO
carotid artery occlusion

cap
c. of ampullary crest
Bremer torque-limiting c.
c. myopathy
Navigus cranial base and c.
c. sign

capability
cognitive c.
metabolic c.

capacitance
membrane c.

capacity
cognitive c.
cranial c.
empathic c.
forced vital c. (FVC)
functional c.
intrinsic c.
metacognitive c.
neural c.
paranormal c.
vital c.
volitional c.
working c.

capelike sensory loss

capillariomotor

capillary
c. angioma
c. fracture
c. hemangioma
c. telangiectasia

capistratus
trismus c.

CAPIT
core assessment program for intracerebral transplantation

capita (*pl. of* caput)

capitis
dolor c.
semispinalis c.
splenius c.

caplet
Mytelase c.
Symax-SR c.

capnography

capnometer
MicroSpan C. 8800

Capozide

capreomycin

capsaicin

capsid protein

Capsin

capsula, pl. **capsulae**
crus anterius capsulae
crus posterius capsulae
c. externa
c. extrema
c. ganglii
c. interna
c. nuclei dentati
capsulae nuclei lentiformis

capsular infarction

capsulatum
Histoplasma c.
Histoplasmosis c.

capsule
anterior limb of internal c.
bromfenac sodium c.
c. cell
Depakote Sprinkle c.
Duradrin c.
Exelon c.
external c.
extreme c.
Fastlene c.
gabapentin c.
ganglion c.
genu of internal c.
Indochron E-R c.
internal c.

NOTES

C

capsule *(continued)*
Kadian sustained-release morphine c.
Keep Alert c.
Metadate CD extended-release c.
methylphenidate HCl extended-release c.
Nimotop c.
otic c.
posterior limb of internal c.
Pro-Fast HS c.
Pro-Fast SR c.
retrolenticular limb of internal c.
retrolenticular part of internal c.
retrolentiform limb of internal c.
Ritalin LA extended-release c.
sublenticular limb of internal c.
sublenticular part of internal c.
sublentiform limb of internal c.
suprasellar c.
Zonegran c.
zonisamide c.

capsulolabral complex

capsulotomy
gamma c.

captation

captopril

capture
IgM antibody c.

caput, pl. **capita**
c. cornus
c. nuclei caudati
c. succedaneum

CARASIL
cerebral autosomal recessive arteriopathy with subcortical infarcts and leukoencephalopathy

carbachol

carbamazepine

carbamylation

carbamylcholine chloride

carbamyl phosphate synthetase deficiency

carbapenem

Carbatrol

carbenicillin disodium

Carbex

Carb-HD
Cal C.-HD

carbidopa
levodopa and c.

carbidopa-levodopa

carbinol dehydratase deficiency

Carbocaine with Neo-Cobefrin

carbocyanine dye

carbohydrate
c. metabolic disorder
c. metabolism
c. metabolism disorder

carbohydrate-deficient
c.-d. glycoprotein
c.-d. glycoprotein syndrome
c.-d. transferrin

carbon
c. dioxide (CO_2)
c. dioxide arterial pressure
c. dioxide chemoreceptor
c. dioxide laser
c. dioxide tension
c. monoxide poisoning
c. tetrachloride poisoning

carbonate
calcium c.
lithium c.
magnesium c.

carbonic
c. acid
c. anhydrase
c. anhydrase inhibitor

carboxylase
acetyl coenzyme A c.
c. defect
3-methylcrotonyl-CoA c.
propionyl-CoA c.
pyruvate c.

carboxyl-terminal region

carboxypenicillin

carbromal

carcinoembryonic antigen (CEA)

carcinoma, pl. **carcinomata**
acinic cell c.
adenoid cystic c.
choroid plexus c.
embryonal cell c.
leptomeningeal c.
meningeal c.
neuroendocrine c. (NEC)
pancreatic c.
c. peripheral neuropathy
c. in situ
small cell c.
squamous cell c.

carcinomatosis
leptomeningeal c.
meningeal c.

carcinomatosum
coma c.

carcinomatous
c. encephalomyelopathy
c. meningitis
c. myelopathy
c. neuromyopathy
c. neuropathy
c. polyneuropathy

card
Boston Diagnostic Aphasia Exam-Cookie Theft C.
diary c.

cardiac
c. arrhythmia
c. catheterization
c. embolism
c. function test
c. ganglion
c. gating
c. glycoside
c. monitoring
c. nerve
c. pacemaker artifact
c. plexus
c. rhabdomyoma
c. rhythm
c. risk index
c. syncope
cardiaca
ganglia c.
cardiacus
plexus c.
cardinal
c. direction of gaze
c. sign
cardioaccelerating center
cardioballistic artifact
Cardiocap II pressure monitor
Cardio-Conray
cardioembolic stroke
cardiofacial syndrome
cardiogenic
c. embolism
c. shock
Cardiografin
cardioinhibitory center
Cardiolite
cardiomyopathy
cardioneural
Cardiopulmonary Paragon 8500 bed
CardioSearch sensor
cardiospasm
cardiovascular
c. control center
c. effect of sleep
carditis
rheumatic c.
care
collaborative c.
comprehensive c.
end-of-life c.
K+ C.
pattern of c.
postoperative c.
respite c.
standard of c.
standard c.
caregiver
c. burden
c. characteristic
c. depression
c. outcome
c. stress
carina, pl. **carinae**
c. fornicis
carinate abdomen
carinii
Pneumocystis c.
C-arm
C-a. fluoroscopic apparatus
C-a. fluoroscopy
reversible C-a.
carmine
indigo c.
carmustine
carnitine
c. muscle metabolism
c. palmitoyltransferase
c. palmitoyltransferase deficiency
c. serum level
c. transport defect
Carnitor Injection
carotici
ramus sinus c.
caroticocavernous fistula
caroticojugular spine
caroticooculomotor membrane
caroticotympanic
c. artery
c. nerve
caroticotympanici
nervi c.
caroticum
rete mirabile c.
carotid
aberrant c.
c. ablative procedure
c. Amytal procedure
c. angiogram
c. arteriography
c. artery
c. artery agenesis
c. artery aneurysm
c. artery angioplasty and stent placement
c. artery disease

C

NOTES

carotid *(continued)*
c. artery dissection
c. artery occlusion (CAO)
c. artery sacrifice
c. artery stenosis
C. Artery Stenosis with Asymptomatic Narrowing: Operation Versus Aspirin (CASANOVA)
C. Artery Stenosis with Asymptomatic Narrowing: Operation Versus Aspirin Study
c. artery stenting
c. atherosclerosis
c. baroceptor stimulation
c. bifurcation
c. body
c. body transplant
c. body tumor
c. branch of glossopharyngeal nerve [CN IX]
c. bruit
c. cave aneurysm
c. circulation
c. content
distal c.
c. endarterectomy
c. ganglion
c. occlusion
c. plaque hematoma
c. plexus
c. preservation
c. preservation technique
c. pulsation
c. rete
c. ring
c. sheath
c. sinus branch
c. sinus hypersensitivity
c. sinus hypersensitivity-induced syncope
c. sinus massage
c. sinus nerve
c. sinus reflex
c. sinus syndrome
c. vein

carotid-basilar anastomosis
carotid-cavernous sinus fistula
carotid-dural fistula
carotid-ophthalmic artery aneurysm
carotid-vertebral
c.-v. anastomosis
c.-v. vein bypass graft

carotodynia, carotidynia
carpal tunnel syndrome (CTS)
Carpenter syndrome
carpopedal
c. contraction
c. spasm

carpoptosis, carpoptosia
carposcope
carrageenan, carragheenin
carrier
DYT1 c.
parkin c.
Yasargil ligature c.

Carrow Auditory-Visual Abilities test
Carr-Purcell-Meiboom-Gill sequence
Carr-Purcell sequence
Carter immobilization cushion
Cartesian coordinate representation
cartilage
c. cranioplasty
c. inflammation
c. plate
thyroid c.
Tutoplast costal c.

cartilaginis thyroideae
cartilaginous
c. endplate
c. tumor

caryochrome
caryothecae
cisterna c.

CAS
computer-assisted surgery

Casal necklace appearance in pellagra
CASANOVA
Carotid Artery Stenosis with Asymptomatic Narrowing: Operation Versus Aspirin
CASANOVA Study

cascade
arachidonic acid c.
central injury c.
coagulation c.
immediate early gene c.
ischemic c.
pathophysiological c.

case
c. control experimental study design
c. formulation
C. IV System
Pyramesh c.
c. study

caseating granuloma
caseous necrosis
Caspar
C. anterior cervical plate
C. anterior plate fixation
C. cervical retractor
C. cervical screw
C. craniotome
C. disc space spreader
C. drill
C. headholder
C. plating

C. retraction post
C. trapezoidal plate
caspase-3 activation
caspase-activated DNAse
caspase-independent mechanism
caspase inhibitor
CASS
computer-assisted stereotactic surgery
CASS digital readout floorstand
CASS whole-brain mapping system
cassava plant tropical myeloneuropathy
cast
endocranial c.
hinged c.
Risser-Cotrel body c.
Castellani-Low sign
Castleman disease
Castroviejo eye suture forceps
CAT
chloramphenicol acetyl transferase
computed axial tomography
computerized axial tomography
CAT scan
CAT scanning
catabolic pathway
cataclysmic headache
catalase pathway
catalepsy
cataleptic attack
cataleptoid, cataleptiform
catamenial
c. epilepsy
c. migraine
c. migraine headache
c. seizure
c. seizure pattern
cataphasia
cataplectic
cataplexy, cataplexis
c. mechanism
Catapres
cataract-oligophrenia syndrome
catastrophic
c. effect
c. event
c. migraine
c. reaction
catatonia protracta
catatonic
c. motor behavior
c. patient
c. rigidity
c. stupor
catch-22 syndrome
catchment
CAT/CLAMS
Clinical Adaptive Test/Clinical Linguistic and Auditory Milestone Scale
catecholamine
c. lesion
peripheral c.
c. receptor
catecholamine-induced
c.-i. change
c.-i. thermogenesis
catecholaminergic
c. nucleus
c. pathway
catechol-*O*-methyltransferase (COMT)
c.-*O*-m. gene
c.-*O*-m. inhibitor
catechol-methyltransferase inhibitor
categorization
symptom c.
category
arousal c.
diagnostic c.
disorder c.
dysphoric c.
early-onset c.
c. fluency test
Functional Ambulation C. (FAC)
late-onset c.
somatic c.
category-specific
c.-s. naming
c.-s. semantic impairment
catelectrotonic state
catelectrotonus
cathepsin B, G
catheter
Abramson c.
Accu-Flo ventricular c.
afterloading c.
angiographic c.
Argyll trocar c.
balloon c.
Berenstein guiding c.
Camino intracranial c.
Camino transducer c.
cisterna magna c.
Codman ventricular silicone c.
c. coil

C

NOTES

catheter *(continued)*
Cook mini-compression balloon c.
Cordis Brite Tip guiding c.
cup c.
delivery c.
distal c.
double-lumen Swan-Ganz c.
dummy seed c.
DuPen epidural c.
Ekos ultrasound c.
Endeavor nondetachable silicone balloon c.
Envoy guide c.
ePTFE ventricular shunt c.
Fasguide c.
FasTracker-18 infusion c.
Fogarty embolectomy c.
guide c.
Heplock c.
Hickman c.
ICP c.
ICP-T fiberoptic ICP intracranial temperature c.
ICP-T fiberoptic ICP monitoring c.
intracranial pressure c.
intraventricular c.
ITC radiopaque balloon c.
Lapras c.
lumbar drainage c.
Micro-Soft Stream sidehole infusion c.
Micro-Vac suction c.
Mikaelsson c.
monorail aspiration c.
nondetachable silicone balloon c.
peripherally inserted central c. (PICC)
peritoneal c.
Phoenix Anti-Blok ventricular c.
polyethylene intravenous c.
Portnoy ventricular c.
Prowler Plus c.
Pudenz ventricular c.
Racz Tun-L-Kath c.
Raimondi peritoneal c.
Raimondi spring c.
Raimondi ventricular c.
Rapid Transit c.
rheolytic c.
Scott silicone ventricular c.
Shaw c.
Shiley c.
Silastic c.
SilverHawk c.
Simmons c.
Simpson c.
Soaker c.
spinal c.
Swan-Ganz c.
thin-wall introducer c.
toposcopic c.
Tracker-10, -18 c.
Tracker infusion c.
transducer-tipped c.
transfemoral c.
Tun-L-Kath epidural c.
tunnelable ventricular ICP c.
Turbo Tracker c.
ventriculostomy c.
Ventrix SD fiberoptic subdural ICP c.

catheter-induced subclavian vein thrombosis

catheterization
cardiac c.
superselective c.

catheter/pump

catochus

catscratch
c. disease (CSD)
c. fever

cat's-eye amaurosis

cauda, pl. **caudae**
c. equina
c. equina avulsion
c. equina compression
c. equina incarceration
c. equina syndrome
c. fasciae dentatae
c. nuclei caudati
c. striati

caudal
c. canal
c. cerebellar peduncle (CCP)
c. colliculus
c. colliculus commissure
c. hook
c. lamina resection
c. neuropore
c. olivary nucleus
c. peduncle of thalamus
c. pontine reticular nucleus
c. regression syndrome
c. to rostral
c. stroke
c. transtentorial herniation

caudalis
brachium colliculi c.
colliculus c.
hilum nuclei olivaris c.
lobulus semilunaris c.
nuclei colliculi c.
nucleus reticularis pontis c.
nucleus tegmenti pontis c.
nucleus vestibularis c.
pars c.
pedunculus cerebellaris c.

subnucleus c.
trigeminal nucleus c.
caudate
c. cell
c. nucleus
c. tissue
c. volume
caudati
caput nuclei c.
cauda nuclei c.
corpus nuclei c.
rami caudae nuclei c.
venae nuclei c.
caudatolenticular
caudatum
caudatus
colliculus c.
nucleus c.
caudolenticulares
pontes grisei c.
caudolenticular gray bridge
causal-attributional theory
causalgia
causalgic pain
causality
phenomenalistic c.
reverse c.
causal mechanism
causative
c. homozygous mutation
c. mechanism
c. organism
cause
contextual c.
neurobiological c.
cause-effect relationship
cautery
Aesculap bipolar c.
BICAP c.
bipolar c.
Concept hand-held c.
c. hook
Mira c.
monopolar c.
right-angle bipolar c.
suction c.
cava (*pl. of* cavum)
Cavalieri direct estimator method
cave
Meckel c.
septum pellucidum c.
trigeminal c.
caveolin-3 protein
cavernoma
cavernoma-related epilepsy
cavernosa
corpora c.
cavernosal nerve
cavernosus
sinus c.
cavernous
c. angioma
c. carotid aneurysm
c. hemangioma
c. malformation (CM)
c. nerve
c. plexus
c. sinus
c. sinus aneurysm
c. sinus fistula
c. sinus lesion
c. sinus meningioma
c. sinus syndrome
c. sinus thrombophlebitis
c. sinus thrombosis
c. sinus tumor
cavitas
c. epiduralis
c. septi pellucidi
c. subarachnoidea
c. trigeminalis
cavitation
spinal cord c.
Cavitron
C. dissector
C. laser
C. Ultrasonic Surgical Aspirator (CUSA)
cavity
epidural c.
head c.
nasal c.
oral c.
c. of septum pellucidum
sinonasal c.
subarachnoid c.
subdural c.
syringomyelic c.
syrinx c.
trigeminal c.
tympanic c.
cavum, pl. **cava**
c. epidurale
inferior vena cava

NOTES

cavum *(continued)*
c. meckelii
c. psalterii
c. septi pellucidi
c. septum pellucidum
c. subarachnoideum
c. subdurale
c. trigeminale
c. vergae
Cawthorne-Cooksey vestibular exercise
Cayler syndrome
CBC
complete blood count
CBF
cerebral blood flow
CBF reduction
CBF study
CBI
closed brain injury
CBI stereotactic headholder
CBV
cerebral blood volume
C1-C2
C1-C2 cable fixation
C1-C2 posterior arthrodesis
CCA
chimpanzee coryza agent
common carotid artery
CCA clamp
C_2-ceramide
CCI
chronic constrictive injury
ccipital bone malformation
CCK
cholecystokinin
CCK-4
cholecystokinin tetrapeptide
CCK-8
cholecystokinin octapeptide
CCM1
CCM1 gene
CCM1 gene mutation
CCM2 gene
CCM3 gene
CCP
caudal cerebellar peduncle
CCTV-EEG
continuous video-electroencephalogram monitoring
CD
combination drug
CD Horizon Eclipse spinal system
CD Horizon Sextant percutaneous screw-rod system
Metadate CD
C-D
Cotrel-Dubousset
C-D instrumentation
C-D instrumentation device
C-D instrumentation fixation strength
C-D instrumentation rigidity
C-D rod insertion
C-D screw modification
CD4
CD4 cell
CD4 lymphocyte
CD29+ memory cell
CD34 staining
CD44 antigen
CD4/CD8 ratio
CD68-positive macrophage
CDD
childhood disintegrative disorder
CDK2NA gene
cDNA
complementary deoxyribonucleic acid
CDNF
ciliary-deprived neurotropic factor
CDR
Clinical Dementia Rating
CDR Scale
CEA
carcinoembryonic antigen
CEA-Tc 99m
cebocephaly
cecocentral scotoma
cecum, caecum
Vicq d'Azyr foramen c.
CED
chondroectodermal dysplasia
CEEB
Center for Ecology, Evolution and Behavior
cefepime
cefuroxime
CEI
continuous extravascular infusion
converting enzyme inhibitor
Celexa
celiac
c. disease
c. ganglion
c. nerve
c. plexus
celiaca
ganglia c.
celiacus
plexus nervosus c.
cell
abnormal-shaped c.
adenohypophysial c.
c. adhesion molecule (CAM)
adrenal chromaffin c.
adult neural stem c.
agger nasi c.
air c.
Alzheimer c.

amacrine c.
ameboid c.
anterior horn c.
antigen-specific T-suppressor c.
Antoni A, B c.
apolar c.
APUD c.
arachnoid c.
astroglia c.
auditory receptor c.
B c.
balloon c.
basket c.
Bergmann glial c.
Betz c.
Bevan-Lewis c.
36B10 glioma c.
bipolar retinal c.
blob c.
blood c.
bone marrow stem c.
bone marrow stromal c.
border c.
Böttcher c.
bovine chromaffin c.
BrDu immunolabeling c.
BrDu-positive c.
bursting c.
Cajal horizontal c.
Cajal-Retzius c.
calcium-dependent rhythmic c.
capsule c.
CA3 pyramidal c.
caudate c.
CD4 c.
CD29+ memory c.
cerebellar granular c.
cerebellar granule c.
chandelier c.
chief c.
choroid plexus c.
chromaffin c.
Clarke c.
cochlear hair c.
color-opponent c.
column c.
commissural c.
compound granule c.
Corti c.
corticotroph c.
cuboidal c.
c. culture
c. cycle
cytotoxic T c.
dark c.
c. death
Deiters c.
c. division
Dogiel c.
dorsal horn c.
dorsal root ganglion c.
downgaze paralysis, ataxia/athetosis and foam c. (DAF)
effector c.
effector T c.
embryonic stem c.
ependymal c.
epithelioid c.
ethmoid air c.
excitable c.
external pillar c.
Fañanás c.
fatty granule c.
fibroblastic-like c.
foam c.
forebrain c.
ganglion c.
gemästete c.
gemistocytic c.
giant dopamine-containing c. (GDC)
giant pyramidal Betz c.
Gierke c.
gitter c.
glial c.
glitter c.
globoid c.
globose c.
Golgi epithelial c.
gonadotroph c.
grandmother c.
granule c.
gustatory c.
gyrochrome c.
hair c.
hamster c.
hecatomeral c.
hematopoietic dendritic c.
hemosiderin-laden c.
Hensen c.
heteromeric c.
hilar c.
HNK c.
horn c.
Hortega c.

NOTES

cell *(continued)*
human adult bone marrow mesenchymal stem c. (hMSCs)
human brain microvascular endothelial c. (HBMEC)
human neonatal kidney c.
human Purkinje c.
hypothalamic pacemaker c.
immune c.
immunocompetent c.
internal pillar c.
interstitial c.
intervertebral disc c.
intracarotid marrow c.
c. isolation
karyochrome c.
lactotroph c.
Langerhans c.
large polymorphic ganglion c.
Leydig tumor c.
c. line
lipid-laden stromal c.
c. loss
lupus erythematosus c.
lymphokine-activated killer c.
macroglia c.
macrophage-derived c.
mammalian c.
Martinotti c.
mastoid air c.
Mauthner c.
MBP-reactive T c.
c. membrane lipid
meningothelial arachnoid c.
meningothelial cap c.
Merkel tactile c.
mesoglial c.
Meynert solitary c.
microglia c.
midget bipolar c.
migratory c.
misshapen c.
mitral c.
mononuclear c. (MNC)
mossy c.
motor c.
Müller glial c.
Müller radial c.
multipolar c.
multipotential c.
myelin-damaging T c.
myelin-producing c.
myxomatous c.
Nageotte c.
natural killer c.
c. necrosis
neoplastic c.
nerve c.
neural crest c.
neural hamster c.
neural progenitor c.
neural stem c.
neural tube floor plate c.
neurilemma sheath c.
neuroendocrine transducer c.
neuroepithelial c.
neuroglia c.
neuroprogenitor c.
neurosecretory c.
nigral TH-positve c.
nonneural c.
normal c.
NT2 c.
olfactory ensheathing c.
olfactory receptor c.
olfactory sheathing c.
oligodendrocyte-like c. (OLC)
oligodendrocyte lineage c.
oligodendroglia c.
oligodendroglial lineage c.
Opalski c.
pancreatic beta c.
parafollicular c.
PC12 c.
perigemmal c.
periglomerular c.
peripheral blood mononuclear c. (PBMC)
peripheral nerve c.
perivascular mononuclear c.
phalangeal c.
physaliphorous c.
pia-arachnoid c.
Pick c.
pillar c.
pineal c.
porcine dopaminergic c.
primary neuronal c.
primitive neural c.
c. processing
progenitor c.
c. proliferation
proliferative malignant glial c.
pseudounipolar ganglion c.
Purkinje c.
PV-positive c.
pyramidal c.
radial glial c.
reactive c.
Renshaw c.
resting T c.
retinal ganglion c. (RGC)
Rolando c.
Sala c.
satellite c.
C. Saver
Schaffer collateral c.
Schultze c.

Schwann c.
sensory c.
Sertoli c.
SK-N-SH c.
small intensely fluorescent c.
somatotroph c.
S phase c.
spider c.
spindle c.
stem serotonergic c.
c. survival
syncytiotrophoblastic giant c. (STGC)
T c.
tactile c.
taste c.
tau-negative nerve c.
tautomeral c.
TH1 c.
TH2 c.
thymic myoid c.
thyrotroph c.
touch c.
transducer c.
T regulatory c.
tuberous sclerosis monster c.
tufted c.
tumor c.
TUNEL-positive c.
tunnel c.
unipolar c.
vector-producing c. (VPC)
ventral mesencephalic dopaminergic c.
vestibular hair c.
visual receptor c.
VZV-specific T c.
wandering c.
white blood c. (WBC)
xenogeneic chromaffin c.

cella, pl. **cellae**
c. media

cell-mediated immunity

cell-permeable

cellular
c. brain edema
c. component
c. immune function
c. immune response
c. ion homeostasis
c. kinetics
c. layers of cortex
c. lineage
c. macromolecule
c. migration disorder
c. organelle
c. prion protein (PrP^c)
c. respiratory function
c. store
c. system
c. therapy

cellulosa
vagina c.

cellulose
c. acetate polymer
oxidized regenerated c.

Celontin

cement
BoneSource hydroxyapatite c.
calcium phosphate c.

cenesthesia, coenesthesia

cenesthesic, cenesthetic

Cenestin

Cenolate

center
accelerating c.
Alzheimer Disease C. (ADC)
Alzheimer Disease Research C. (ADRC)
anospinal c.
apneustic c.
Association of Sleep Disorder C.
auditory word c.
C. for Brain Research and Holoprosencephaly and Related Malformations
Broca c.
Budge c.
cardioaccelerating c.
cardioinhibitory c.
cardiovascular control c.
ciliospinal c.
communal residential c.
coughing c.
defecation c.
deglutition c.
C. for Ecology, Evolution and Behavior (CEEB)
ejaculatory c.
eupraxic c.
expiratory c.
feeding c.
gaze pontine c.
genital c.

NOTES

center *(continued)*
genitospinal c.
glossokinesthetic c.
heat-regulating c.
higher c.
imprinting c. (IC)
inspiratory c.
Kronecker c.
Louisiana State University Medical C. (LSUMC)
medullary c.
micturition c.
Minnesota Regional Sleep Disorders C.
motor speech c.
nerve c.
panting c.
pneumotaxic c.
polypneic c.
pontine lateral gaze c.
regulatory c.
respiratory c.
retrovesical c.
satiety c.
semioval c.
sensory speech c.
sleep-generating c.
speech c.
sudorific c.
swallowing c.
sweat c.
thermoregulatory c.
thirst c.
UCLA Brain Mapping C.
vasoconstrictor c.
vasodilator c.
vasomotor c.
vesical c.
vesicospinal c.
vital c.
vomiting c.
Wernicke c.

centra (*pl. of* centrum)

central
c. alexia
c. alveolar hypoventilation syndrome
c. amaurosis
c. amygdaloid nucleus
c. anticholinergic syndrome
c. anticholinergic toxicity
c. auditory pathway
c. benzodiazepine receptor
c. canal
c. caudate nucleus
c. cerebral sulcus
c. chemosensitivity
c. cholinergic system
c. chromatolysis
c. cord injury syndrome
c. core disease
c. core myopathy
c. dazzle
c. deafness
c. direct-current bright spot
c. dopamine content
c. dopaminergic antagonism
C. European encephalitis
C. European tick-borne encephalitis virus
C. European tick-borne fever
c. excitatory state
c. facial paresis
c. ganglioneuroma
c. gelatinous substance of spinal cord
c. gray
c. gray matter region
c. gray substance
c. gyrus
c. hypoventilation syndrome
c. inflammatory demyelination
c. injury cascade
c. and lateral intermediate substance
c. lateral nucleus of thalamus
c. lesion
c. lobule
c. lobule of cerebellum
c. lobule wing
c. nervous system (CNS)
c. nervous system abnormality
c. nervous system dysfunction
c. nervous system hemorrhage
c. nervous system hypersomnolence
c. nervous system influenza virus infection
c. nervous system leukemia
c. nervous system lymphoma
c. nervous system malformation
c. nervous system myelination
c. nervous system neural crest
c. nervous system nocardiosis
c. nervous system ontogenesis
c. nervous system stimulant, nonamphetamine
c. nervous system tumor
c. neuritis
c. neurocytoma
c. nystagmus
c. paralysis
c. paraphasia
c. part of lateral ventricle
c. peduncle of thalamus
c. pontine myelinolysis
c. post-stroke pain
c. proprioception integration deficit
c. respiratory chemoreception

c. respiratory neuron
c. retinal fovea
c. role
c. sacral line
c. sensitization
c. sensory loss
c. sleep apnea (CSA)
c. sleep apnea syndrome
c. somatosensory conduction time
c. sulcus of insula
c. tegmental fasciculus
c. tegmental tract
c. thalamic radiation
c. timing process
c. transactional core
c. transtentorial herniation
c. venous channel
c. venous pressure
c. vertigo
c. vestibular system
c. vision acuity

centrale
systema nervosum c.

centralis
ala lobuli c.
ala lobulis c.
amaurosis c.
area c.
nucleus amygdalae c.
nucleus caudalis c.
nucleus cuneatus pars c.
pars inferior alae lobuli c.
pars superior ali lobuli c.
substantia gelatinosa c.
substantia grisea c.
substantia intermedia c.
sulcus c.
tractus tegmentalis c.

centralization phenomenon

central-type neurofibromatosis

centrencephalic
c. epilepsy
c. integrating system

centrifugal
c. current
c. nerve

centripetal
c. current
c. nerve
c. spread

centroblastic B-cell lymphoma

centrocecal visual field

centrofacial lentiginosis

centrokinesia

centrokinetic

centromedian thalamic nucleus

centromedianus
nucleus c.

centronuclear myopathy

centrophose

centrotemporal
c. paroxysmal focus
c. sharp wave

centrum, pl. **centra**
c. medianum
c. medullare
c. ovale
c. semiovale
Vieussens c.

cephalad

cephalalgia, cephalgia
benign coital c.
histamine c.
histaminic c.
Horton histamine c.
pharyngotympanic c.

cephalea
c. attonita
epileptic c.

cephaledema

cephalemia

cephalexin

cephalgia (*var. of* cephalalgia)

cephalgic attack

cephalhematocele
Stromeyer c.

cephalhematoma (*var. of* cephalohematoma)

cephalhydrocele traumatica

cephalic
c. angle
c. flexure
c. tetanus

cephalitis

cephalocele
orbital c.

cephalocentesis

cephalochordate

cephalodynia

cephalogyric

cephalohematocele

cephalohematoma, cephalhematoma
c. deformans

cephalohemometer

NOTES

cephalomedullary angle
cephalomeningitis
cephalometer
Bertillon c.
cephalometric
c. analysis
c. angle
c. measurement
c. radiograph
cephalometrography
cephalomotor
cephalooculocutaneous telangiectasia
cephalopalpebral reflex
cephalopathy
cephaloplegia
cephalopolysyndactyly
Greig c.
cephaloridine
cephalorrhachidian index
cephalosporin
fourth-generation c.
third-generation c.
cephalostat
cephalothin
cephalotrigeminal angiomatosis
cephapirin
cephradine
ceptor
chemical c.
contact c.
distance c.
ceramic vertebral spacer
ceramidase
ceramide
c. dihexoside
c. trihexoside
trihexosyl c.
Ceraxon
***c-erbB-2*-encoded oncoprotein**
cercopithecoid
cerea flexibilitas
cerebella (*pl. of* cerebellum)
cerebellae
ramus tonsillae c.
cerebellar
c. abscess
c. activation
c. aggregation culture
c. aggregation culture for teratogenicity testing
c. aplasia
c. apoplexy
c. arachnoid cyst
c. artery
c. artery infarction
c. astrocytoma
c. attachment
c. cerebral palsy
c. cognitive affective syndrome
c. cortex
c. cortical degeneration
c. degeneration ataxia
c. dysmetria
c. ectopia
c. encephalitis
c. ependymoma
c. fit
c. fit seizure
c. folium
c. fossa
c. frenulum
c. gait
c. gliosarcoma
c. granular cell
c. granule cell
c. granule neuron
c. hematoma
c. hemiataxia
c. hemisphere
c. hemisphere syndrome
c. hemorrhage
c. hemorrhage syndrome
c. hypoperfusion
c. malaria
c. mass
c. metabolism
c. mutism
c. nucleus
c. nystagmus
c. pathway
c. peduncle
c. pressure cone
c. pyramid
c. region
c. retraction
c. retractor
c. rigidity
c. speech
c. sulcus
c. tentorium
c. tonsil
c. tonsillar herniation
c. tremor
c. tumor
c. vein
c. vermal hypoplasia
c. vermian atrophy
c. vermis dysgenesis
c. volume
cerebellares
nuclei c.
cerebellaris
cortex c.
fossa c.
cerebelli
ala c.
alae lingulae c.
amygdala c.

arbor vitae c.
arteria inferior anterior c.
arteria inferior posterior c.
arteria superior c.
brachium conjunctivum c.
corpus medullare c.
cortex c.
culmen c.
facies inferior hemispherii c.
facies superior hemispherii c.
falx c.
fasciculus uncinatus c.
fissurae c.
fissura horizontalis c.
fissura intercruralis c.
fissura posterolateralis c.
fissura prima c.
fissura secunda c.
fissura transversa c.
folia c.
frenulum c.
incisura tentorii c.
laminae albae c.
laminae medullares c.
lingua c.
lingula c.
lobulus centralis corporis c.
lobulus paramedianus c.
lobulus quadrangularis anterior c.
lobulus quadrangularis posterior c.
lobulus simplex c.
lobus posterior c.
lobus rostralis c.
monticulus c.
nodulus c.
nuclei c.
nucleus dentatus c.
nucleus lateralis c.
nucleus medialis c.
pedunculi c.
pons c.
stratum gangliosum c.
stratum granulosum corticis c.
stratum moleculare corticis c.
stratum plexiforme c.
stratum purkinjense corticis c.
tentorium c.
tonsilla c.
uvula c.
vallecula c.
venae inferiores c.
venae superiores c.
vena precentralis c.
vermis c.
vincula lingulae c.

cerebellifugal

cerebellin

cerebellipetal

cerebellitis
postinfectious c.

cerebellohypothalamic fiber

cerebellolental

cerebellomedullaris
cisterna c.
c. posterior

cerebellomedullary
c. cistern
c. fissure
c. malformation syndrome

cerebellomesencephalic fissure

cerebellomesoencephalic fissure Perspex rod

cerebelloolivares
fibrae c.

cerebelloolivary
c. degeneration
c. fiber

cerebellopontine (CP)
c. angle (CPA)
c. angle approach
c. angle arachnoid cyst
c. angle cistern
c. angle schwannoma
c. angle surgery
c. angle syndrome
c. angle tumor
c. cisternography
c. recess

cerebellorubralis
tractus c.

cerebellorubral tract

cerebellorubrospinal tract

cerebellospinal
c. fiber
c. tract

cerebellotegmental tract

cerebellothalamic tract

cerebellothalamicus
tractus c.

cerebellovestibular dysfunction

cerebellum, pl. **cerebella**
anterior notch of c.
arborescent white substance of c.
body of c.

NOTES

cerebellum *(continued)*
central lobule of c.
cortical substance of c.
crescentic lobule of c.
dentate nucleus of c.
Flechsig bundle in c.
folia of c.
Gowers bundle in c.
granular layer of c.
hemisphere of c.
horizontal fissure of c.
incisure of tentorium of c.
inverse c.
lingula of c.
medullary body of c.
middle lobe of c.
molecular layer of c.
nuclear layer of c.
pons et c.
posterior lobe of c.
posterior notch of c.
primary fissure of c.
pyramis of c.
rostral lobe of c.
secondary fissure of c.
c. superior crus
tongue of c.
tonsil of c.
transverse fissure of c.
uncinate fasciculus of c.
uvula of c.
vallecula of c.
vein of c.
white laminae of c.
white layer of c.
white substance of c.
cerebra (*pl. of* cerebrum)
cerebral
c. abscess
c. acetylcholine nicotinic receptor
c. adiposity
c. agraphia
c. amaurosis
c. amebiasis
c. amyloid angiopathy (CAA)
c. anaplastic astrocytoma
c. angiography
c. angiomatosis
c. anoxia
c. anoxic-ischemic injury
c. anthrax
c. antioxidant activity
c. aplasia
c. apoplexy
c. apotentiality
c. aqueduct
c. aqueduct compression
c. aqueduct of Sylvius
c. arterial aneurysm
c. arterial circle
c. arteriography
c. arteriosclerosis
c. arteriovenous oxygen content difference
c. artery
c. artery aneurysm
c. artery dissection
c. artery fetal persistence
c. artery infarction
c. artery thrombosis
c. ataxia
c. atherosclerosis
c. autosomal dominant arteriopathy with subcortical infarcts and leukoencephalopathy (CADASIL)
c. autosomal recessive arteriopathy with subcortical infarcts and leukoencephalopathy (CARASIL)
c. axonopathy
c. beriberi
c. blindness
c. blood flow (CBF)
c. blood flow agent
c. blood flow rheology
c. blood flow study
c. blood vessel
c. blood volume (CBV)
c. brucellosis
c. calcinosis
c. calculus
c. cavernous angioma
c. circulation
c. cladosporiosis
c. commissure
c. contusion
c. convexity
c. cortex
c. cortex of Ateles
c. cysticercus granuloma
c. death
c. decompression
c. decortication
c. degenerative disorder
c. diataxia
c. digital angiogram
c. disease
c. dominance
c. dyschromatopsia
c. dysfunction
c. dysgenesis
c. dysplasia
c. dysrhythmia
c. edema
c. electrical measurement
c. embolus
c. fissure
c. flexure
c. fluid marker

c. folate deficiency
c. foreign body embolization
c. formed-element embolism
c. gaze paresis
c. gigantism
c. glioblastoma
c. glioma
c. gumma
c. gyrus
c. hemianesthesia
c. hemicorticectomy
c. hemidecortication
c. hemisphere
c. hemodynamics
c. hemodynamics and oxygenation
c. hemorrhage
c. hemosiderosis
c. hernia
c. herniation
c. hydatid
c. hyperesthesia
c. hypertension
c. hypomyelination
c. hypoperfusion
c. hypoxia
c. impairment
c. ischemia
c. ischemia steal
c. laceration
c. lacuna
c. layer of retina
c. lesion
c. lipidosis
c. lobe
c. localization
c. lymphoma
c. malaria
c. malaria infection
c. mantle
c. mapping of apraxia
c. metabolic rate
c. metabolic rate of glucose (CMRglc)
c. metabolic rate of oxygen ($CMRO_2$)
c. metastasis
c. microbleed
c. microembolism
c. nerve
c. neuroblastoma
c. nocardiosis
c. palsy
c. palsy infant stimulation program
c. peduncle
c. peduncular atrophy
c. perfusion
c. perfusion pressure
c. perinatal injury
c. poliodystrophy
c. poliomyelitis
c. porosis
c. potential
c. pressure autoregulation
progressive c.
c. protection
c. protective therapy
c. ptosis
c. radiation necrosis
c. region
c. revascularization
c. salt wasting
c. salt wasting syndrome
c. sclerosis
c. sensory input
c. sinus
c. sphingolipidosis
c. stalk
c. steal syndrome
c. structure
c. sulcus
c. tetanus
c. thermometry
c. tonsil
c. toxoplasmosis
c. trauma
c. tremor
c. trigone
c. tuberculosis
c. vasodilating agent
c. vasoreactivity
c. vasospasm
c. vein
c. vein angioma
c. vein thrombosis
c. venous malformation (CVM)
c. venous thrombosis
c. ventricle
c. ventriculography
c. vertigo
c. vesicle
c. vomiting

cerebrale
tache c.
trigonum c.

NOTES

cerebrales
sulci c.
cerebralgia
cerebralia
juga c.
cerebralis
adiposis c.
cortex c.
mycetism c.
pedunculus c.
cerebration
cerebri
aditus ad aqueductum c.
anus c.
apertura aqueductus c.
apophysis c.
aqueductus c.
astrocytosis c.
basis pedunculi c.
circulus arteriosus c.
cisterna fossae lateralis c.
cisterna venae magnae c.
commissura magna c.
commissura posterior c.
commotio c.
contusio c.
cortex c.
crus c.
epiphysis c.
facies inferior hemispherii c.
facies medialis et inferior hemispherii c.
facies superolateralis hemispherii c.
falx c.
familial gliomatosis c.
fibrae arcuatae c.
fissura longitudinalis c.
fissura transversa c.
formatio reticularis pedunculi c.
fossa lateralis c.
fungus c.
glioblastosis c.
gliomatosis c.
gyri c.
gyrus transitivi c.
hemiseptum c.
hemispherium c.
hypophysis c.
labium c.
lacuna c.
lamina molecularis corticis c.
lamina terminalis c.
lobi c.
lobus frontalis c.
lobus occipitalis c.
lobus parietalis c.
lymphomatosis c.
margo inferior c.
margo inferolateralis hemispherii c.
margo inferomedialis hemispherii c.
margo medialis c.
margo superomedialis c.
medial sulcus of crus c.
membrana c.
pars anterior pedunculi c.
pars dorsalis pedunculi c.
pars ventralis pedunculi c.
pedunculus c.
poliodystrophia c.
polus frontalis hemispherii c.
polus occipitalis hemispherii c.
polus temporalis c.
pseudomotor c.
pseudotumor c.
ramus anterior sulci lateralis c.
ramus ascendens sulci lateralis c.
ramus posterior sulci lateralis c.
sulci interlobares c.
sulcus centralis c.
sulcus lateralis pedunculi c.
sulcus lunatus c.
sulcus medialis cruris c.
tutamina c.
unguis ventriculi lateralis c.
venae anteriores c.
venae inferiores c.
venae internae c.
venae profundae c.
venae superficiales c.
venae superiores c.
vena magna c.
vena media profunda c.
vena media superficialis c.
ventriculus dexter c.
ventriculus lateralis c.
ventriculus quartus c.
ventriculus sinister c.
ventriculus tertius c.
zero cerebral pseudotumor c.
cerebrifugal
cerebripetal
cerebritis
lupus c.
suppurative c.
cerebroatrophic hyperammonemia
cerebrocerebellar projection
cerebrocortical nerve terminal
cerebrofaciothoracic dysplasia syndrome
cerebrohepatorenal syndrome
cerebrology
cerebroma
cerebromacular
c. degeneration
c. dystrophy
cerebromalacia
cerebromedullary cistern
cerebromeningeal
cerebromeningitis

cerebropathy
cerebrophysiology
cerebropontile
cerebroretinal
c. angiomatosis
c. degeneration
cerebrosclerosis
cerebroside
c. lipidosis
c. lipoidosis
c. reticulocytosis
c. sulfatase
cerebrosidosis
cerebrosis
cerebrospinal
c. axis
c. fever
c. fluid (CSF)
c. fluid absorption
c. fluid calcium
c. fluid ferritin level
c. fluid fistula
c. fluid formation
c. fluid glucose
c. fluid lactic acid
c. fluid leak
c. fluid leakage
c. fluid leukocyte
c. fluid otorrhea
c. fluid pathway
c. fluid pleocytosis
c. fluid pressure
c. fluid protein
c. fluid rhinorrhea
c. fluid shunt
c. fluid volume
c. index
c. meningitis
c. syphilis
c. system
cerebrospinalis
liquor c.
cerebrospinant
cerebrostomy
cerebrotendinous
c. cholesterolosis
c. xanthomatosis
cerebrotomy
cerebrovascular
c. accident (CVA)
c. accident dementia
c. amyloidosis
c. aneurysm
c. angiography
c. angioma
c. aphasia
c. arterial dissection
c. arterial thrombosis
c. computed tomography
c. disease
c. dysregulation
c. embolism
c. embryonic development
c. hemorrhage
c. infarction
c. ischemia
c. lesion
c. magnetic resonance imaging
c. malformation
c. morphology
c. neurosyphilis
c. pathology
c. regulation
c. resistance
c. syndrome
c. ulceration
c. venous thrombosis
cerebrum, pl. **cerebra**
anterior ramus of lateral sulcus of c.
aqueduct c.
arcuate fiber of c.
arterial circle of c.
ascending ramus of lateral sulcus of c.
cistern of great vein of c.
cistern of lateral fossa of c.
frontal lobe of c.
great transverse fissure of c.
gyri of c.
lamina terminalis of c.
lobe of c.
longitudinal fissure of c.
occipital lobe of c.
occipital pole of c.
parietal lobe of c.
superolateral surface of c.
temporal pole of c.
transverse fissure of c.
Cerebyx
Cereport
Ceresine
Ceretec imaging kit
cerium

NOTES

cerivastatin
ceroid lipofuscinosis
cerulean
locus c.
ceruloplasmin
c. deficiency
c. gene
serum c.
c. serum level
ceruminoma
cervical
c. aortic knuckle
c. arthrodesis
c. carotid bifurcation
c. collar
c. compression syndrome
c. cord lesion
c. corpectomy
c. curvature index
c. decompression surgery
c. discectomy
c. disc excision
c. disc herniation
c. disc syndrome
c. dumbbell tumor
c. dystonia
c. enlargement
c. enlargement of spinal cord
c. epidural abscess
c. epidural steroid injection
c. fibrositis
c. flexor synergy
c. flexure
c. fusion syndrome
c. immobilization device (CID)
c. intersegmental vein
c. interspace
c. intramedullary tumor
c. manipulation
c. muscle spasm
c. myelography
c. myospasm
c. nerve
c. nerve root injury
c. neural foramen
c. nucleus
c. part of spinal cord
c. pedicle screw
c. perivascular sympathectomy
c. plate
c. plexus
c. radiculopathy
c. resting posture
c. rib and band syndrome
c. root distribution
c. screw insertion technique
c. segment of spinal cord [C1–C8]
c. spinal column injury
c. spinal stenosis
c. spine
c. spine arthritis
c. spine atlantoaxial instability
c. spine basilar impression
c. spine decompression
c. spine injury
c. spine internal fixation
c. spine kyphotic deformity
c. spine laminectomy
c. spine posterior fusion
c. spine posterior ligament disruption
c. spine rheumatoid disease
c. spine screw-plate fixation
c. spine stabilization
c. spine stabilization procedure
c. spine trauma
c. spondylosis
c. spondylosis without myelopathy
c. spondylotic myelopathy
c. spondylotic myelopathy fusion technique
c. spondylotic myelopathy vertebrectomy
c. steroid epidural nerve block
c. subluxation
c. sympathetic chain location
c. syringomyelia
c. tension myositis
c. tension syndrome
c. vertebra
c. vertigo
c. vessel compression
c. whiplash
cervicales
nervi c.
cervicalia
segmenta c. 1–8
segmentum medullae spinalis c.
cervicalis
ansa c.
descendens c.
inferior root of ansa c.
intumescentia c.
nervus transversus c.
plexus c.
posterior root of ansa c.
radix anterior ansae c.
radix inferior ansae c.
radix posterior ansae c.
radix superior ansae c.
ramus lateralis rami posterioris nervi c.
ramus medialis rami posterioris nervi c.
ramus thyrohyoideus ansae c.
root of ansa c.
superior limb of ansa c.
superior root of ansa c.

cervicalium
rami anteriores nervorum c.
rami dorsales nervorum c.
rami posteriores nervorum c.
rami ventrales nervorum c.
cervices (*pl. of* cervix)
cervicis
descendens c.
c. muscle
splenius c.
cervicobrachialgia
cervicobrachial syndrome
cervicocephalic arterial dissection
cervicocollic reflex
cervicodynia
cervicogenic headache
cervicolumbar phenomenon
cervicomedullary
c. deformity
c. junction
c. junction compression
c. kink
c. tumor
cervicooccipital fusion
cervicothoracic
c. ganglion
c. junction
c. junction stabilization
c. junction surgery
c. orthosis
c. pedicle anatomy
c. pedicle angle
cervicothoracicum
ganglion c.
Cervive anterior cervical plating system
cervix, pl. **cervices**
c. of axon
c. columnae posterioris
c. cornus dorsalis medullae spinalis
c. cornus posterioris medullae spinalis
cesium fluoride scintillation detector
Cestan-Chenais syndrome
Cestan-Raymond syndrome
Cestan syndrome
cesticidal
cestode infection
CF
climbing fiber
C-factor
CFE
chronic focal encephalitis
CFI
cut-flow index
C-fiber
C-f. activity
C-f. evoked response
C-f. nociceptor
C-f. reflex
C-Flex
REMstar Plus with C-F.
REMstar Pro with C-F.
c-fos gene
CGRP
calcitonin gene-related peptide
CH
cluster headache
CH50 assay
Chaddock
C. reflex
C. sign
Chagas disease
chain
c. behavior
beta myosin heavy c.
electron transport c.
human neurofilament light c.
immunoglobulin kappa light c.
kappa light c.
lambda light c.
nuclear c.
oligosaccharide c.
c. reflex
respiratory c.
sympathetic c.
variable heavy c. (VH)
chaining technique
chair
Bárány c.
Combisit surgeon's c.
chalky white disc edema
chamber
anechoic c.
drip c.
flush c.
Monoplace hyperbaric c.
multiplace c.
Sechrist monoplace hyperbaric c.
Chamberlain palatooccipital line
chameleon tongue
chamomile
German c.
champagne-bottle leg
Champion Trauma Score

NOTES

Chance fracture
chancre
hard c.
chandelier cell
change
abulic mental c.
age-related brain c.
age-related pharmacodynamic c.
age-related pharmacokinetic c.
astrocytic c.
baseline-to-endpoint c.
binocular acuity c.
biochemical c.
blood flow c.
catecholamine-induced c.
chronic c.
circadian rhythm c.
circumscribed c.
Clinical Global Impression of C.
Clinician's Interview-Based Impression of C.
cognitive c.
Crooke hyaline c.
deep white matter hyperintensity c.
degenerative discogenic vertebral c.
degenerative spine c.
electrical c.
electrolyte c.
electrophysiologic c.
c. in energy
Fairbanks c.
Frisén-grade c.
global c.
hormonal c.
hyperintensity c.
interictal behavior c.
interictal personality c.
Interview-Based Impression of C.
intrapsychic c.
maturational c.
memory c.
mental status c.
metabolic c.
methylphenidate-induced c.
microvasculitic c.
morphologic c.
negative c.
neurochemical c.
neuropeptide c.
newly emergent categorical c.
nutritional c.
onion bulb c.
pathological c.
perivascular c.
personality c.
polyneuropathy, organomegaly, endocrinopathy, monoclonal gammopathy, skin c.'s (POEMS)
pressure-gradient c.
radiation-induced morphologic c.
reflex c.
c. in sleep pattern
stoichiometric c.
structural c.
subjective mood c.
taste c.
telangiectatic c.
trophic c.
vascular c.
vasomotor c.
visual c.
white matter c.
channel
adenosine triphosphate-dependent potassium c.
axolemmal ion c.
blob c.
central venous c.
chloride c.
grasp c.
ion c.
c. kinetic abnormality
ligand-gated ion c.
L-type calcium c.
membrane ion c.
potassium c.
transmitter-gated ion c.
T-type calcium c.
voltage-gated calcium c. (VGCC)
voltage-gated potassium c.
voltage-gated sodium c.
voltage-regulated calcium c.
4-channel
4-c. Aesculap ventriculoscope
4-c. transcranial Doppler monitor
8-channel
8-c. muscle stimulator
8-c. whole-head magnetometer
20-channel Beckman EEG instrument
37-channel biomagnetometer
channelopathy
epileptogenic c.
Chapman scale
characteristic
active sleep c.
aneurysmal c.
attack c.
caregiver c.
clinical c.
comorbid c.
confusional arousal c.
core c.
CSF c.
demographic c.
electrical c.
environment c.
graft-handling c.
human sleep c.

c. manifestation
narcolepsy c.
neuropsychologic c.
objective trauma c.
c. pattern of motivation
phenomenological c.
predictive c.
quiet sleep c.
receiver operating c. (ROC)
signal-noise c.
sleep c.
temporal c.
trait c.
trauma c.

CharcoAid

Charcot
C. artery
C. arthropathy
C. disease
C. gait
C. joint
C. sign
C. triad
C. vertigo

Charcot-Bouchard
C.-B. intracerebral aneurysm
C.-B. microaneurysm

Charcot-Marie syndrome

Charcot-Marie-Tooth
C.-M.-T. atrophy
C.-M.-T. disease
C.-M.-T. disease type 1, 2
C.-M.-T. phenotype

Charcot-Weiss-Baker syndrome

CHARGE
coloboma, heart disease, atresia choanae, retarded growth, genital anomalies, ear anomalies
CHARGE syndrome

charged particle radiosurgery

Charité disc prosthesis

Charles Bonnet syndrome

Charlevoix-Saguenay
C.-S. ataxia
C.-S. syndrome

charley horse

Charlie
The C. Foundation

Charlin syndrome

Charnley suction drain

CHASA
Children's Hemiplegia and Stroke Association

chasing spike

Chaslin gliosis

Chassaignac tubercle

CHAT
Checklist for Autism in Toddlers

Chatillon dolorimeter

Chealamide

checkerboard field

Checklist-90
Symptom C.-90

checklist
C. for Autism in Toddlers (CHAT)
symptom c.

Chediak-Higashi syndrome

cheek phenomenon

cheese reaction headache

cheilophagia

cheiloschisis

cheiralgia paresthetica

cheirobrachialgia, chirobrachialgia

cheirognostic

cheirokinesthesia, chirokinesthesia

cheirokinesthetic

cheirospasm, chirospasm

chelation therapy

chemical
c. aseptic meningitis
atomic, biologic, c. (ABC)
c. ceptor
c. denervation
c. hemostasis
c. injury
c. neurolysis
psychoactive c.
c. rhizotomy
c. shift
c. shift anisotropy
c. shift artifact
c. signaling
c. sympathectomy
c. toxin

chemically induced seizure

chemical-mechanical transduction

chemical-shift imaging

chemiluminescence

chemoattractant
c. axonal outgrowth
T-cell alpha c. (ITAC)

chemoceptor (*var. of* chemoreceptor)
chemodectoma
petrous ridge c.
chemodenervation
chemokine
c. CCL-20/CCR6 complex
CSF c.
chemoneurolysis
glycerol c.
percutaneous retrogasserian glycerol c.
chemonucleolysis
chemopallidectomy
chemopallidothalamectomy
chemopallidotomy
chemoperception
chemoreception
central respiratory c.
chemoreceptor, chemoceptor
carbon dioxide c.
medullary c.
peripheral c.
c. tumor
chemoreflex
chemosensitive zone
chemosensitivity
central c.
chemosensitivity-enhancing agent
chemosensory
c. receptor
c. stimulus
chemosis
orbital c.
chemothalamectomy
chemothalamotomy
chemotherapy
alkylating c.
c. antiviral
blood-brain barrier disruption c.
combination c.
cyclohexylchloroethylnitrosurea c.
glioma c.
high-dose systemic c.
intrathecal c.
intratumoral c.
PCV c.
salvage c.
systemic c.
chemotransmitter
chenodeoxycholic acid
Cherry
C. brain retractor
C. laminectomy retractor
C. osteotome
C. traction tongs
Cherry-Kerrison
C.-K. laminectomy forceps
C.-K. laminectomy rongeur
cherry-red
c.-r. spot
c.-r. spot myoclonus syndrome
chewer
sleep c.
chewing
c. automatism
c. behavior
Cheyne disease
Cheyne-Stokes
C.-S. breathing
C.-S. central apnea
C.-S. respiration
CHF
congestive heart failure
Chiari
C. deformity
C. formation
C. II syndrome
C. malformation dysraphism
C. malformation type I–IV
C. malformation with headache
chiaroscuro
chiasm
cistern of c.
glioma of optic c.
optic c.
prefixed c.
chiasma, pl. **chiasmata**
c. opticum
c. syndrome
chiasmal
c. apoplexy
c. arachnoiditis
c. compression
c. epidermoid
c. lesion
c. syndrome
chiasmapexy
transsphenoidal c.
chiasmata (*pl. of* chiasma)
chiasmatic
c. cistern
c. defect
c. glioma
c. lesion
c. recess
c. sulcus
c. syndrome
c. tumor
chiasmatic-hypothalamic pilocytic astrocytoma
chiasmaticus
ramus c.
sulcus c.
chiasmatis
cisterna c.
sulcus c.
chicken-wire vascular pattern

chief
c. cell
c. cell of corpus pineale
child
c. abuse with craniocerebral trauma
megacephalic c.
megacephalous c.
childhood
c. absence epilepsy (CAE)
c. absence epilepsy evolving to juvenile myoclonic epilepsy
c. absence epilepsy with generalized tonic-clonic seizure
alternating hemiplegia of c.
c. ataxia with cerebral hypomyelination
c. benign focal epilepsy
benign paroxysmal vertigo of c.
benign partial epilepsy of c.
C. Brain Tumor Consortium
C. Brain Tumor Consortium database
c. disintegrative disorder (CDD)
c. epilepsy with occipital paroxysm
c. moyamoya disease
c. muscular dystrophy
c. myositis
c. optic glioma
polymorphic epilepsy of c.
c. primitive neuroectodermal tumor
progressive bulbar palsy of c.
progressive bulbar paralysis of c.
c. schizophrenia
torsion disease of c.
transient tic disorder of c.
childhood-onset
c.-o. dystonia
c.-o. epilepsy
c.-o. Tourette syndrome
children
Apraxia Profile: A Descriptive Assessment Tool for C.
subclinical status epilepticus induced by sleep in c.
children's
C. Coma Score
C. Hemiplegia and Stroke Association (CHASA)
C. Hospital brain spatula
C. Hospital clip
C. Silapap
c. sleep habits questionnaire
chill
nervous c.
chimeric stimulant
chimpanzee coryza agent (CCA)
chin
c. jerk
c. reflex
Chinese
C. medicine
C. paralytic syndrome
Chippaux-Smirak arch index
chirobrachialgia (*var. of* cheirobrachialgia)
chirognostic
chirokinesthesia (*var. of* cheirokinesthesia)
chiropractic spinal manipulation
chirospasm (*var. of* cheirospasm)
chisel
Adson laminectomy c.
D'Errico lamina c.
Freer c.
Hajek c.
chloral
amylene c.
chlorambucil
chloramphenicol
c. acetyl transferase (CAT)
c. sodium succinate
chlordiazepoxide
amitriptyline hydrochloride and c.
c. hydrochloride
chlorhexidine
c. gluconate
c. shampoo
chloride
ammonium c.
butyl c.
calcium c.
carbamylcholine c.
c. channel
c. conductance
c. disorder
edrophonium c.
magnesium c.
manganese c.
oxybutynin c.
potassium c.
serum c.
sodium c.
^{201}Tl c.
chlorimipramine

C

NOTES

chlormethiazole
chloroethylnitrosourea
lipophilic c.
chloroform
chloroma
Chloromycetin
chloroquine
chlorothiazide
chlorpheniramine maleate
chlorphenoxamine
chlorproethazine
chlorpromazine
c. HCl
c. hydrochloride
chlorprothixene
chlorthalidone
Chlor-Trimeton
choanal atresia
Chodzko reflex
Choice
C. PT exchange wire
C. PT guidewire
choked disc
Cholebrine
cholecystokinin (CCK)
c. octapeptide (CCK-8)
c. tetrapeptide (CCK-4)
cholera
cholera-toxin-catalyzed densitometry
choleric constitutional type
choleromania
cholestanol
cholesteatoma
congenital c.
intracranial c.
cholesteatomatous
cholesterinosis (*var. of* cholesterolosis)
cholesterol
c. accumulation
c. crystal
c. cyst
c. embolism
c. ester storage disease
c. granuloma
c. metabolism
c. serum level
cholesterol-lowering therapy
cholesterolosis, cholesterinosis
cerebrotendinous c.
cholestyramine
choline acetyltransferase
choline/*N*-acetyl-aspartate (Cho/NAA)
choline/*N*-acetyl-aspartate ratio
cholinergic
c. activity
c. approach
c. crisis
c. deficit
c. dysfunction
c. effect
c. fiber
c. input
c. neuron
c. neurotransmission
c. system
c. therapy
c. transmission
cholinesterase
c. inhibitor
c. inhibitory poisoning
cholinoceptive
cholinomimetic therapy
Chlolografin
Cholovue
Cho/NAA
choline/*N*-acetyl-aspartate
Cho/NAA ratio
chondritis
nasal c.
chondroblastoma
chondrocalcinosis
chondrodystrophic myotonia
chondrodystrophy
chondroectodermal dysplasia (CED)
chondrohypoplasia
chondroitin-4-sulfate
chondroitin-6-sulfate
chondroitin sulfate proteoglycan
chondroma
juxtacortical c.
chondromatous tumor
chondromyxoid fibroma
chondroosteodystrophy
chondrosarcoma
chondroskeleton
Chopper-Dixon hybrid imaging
chorda, pl. **chordae**
c. magna
c. spinalis
c. tympani
c. tympani nerve
chordae willisii
chordoblastoma
chordocarcinoma
chordoid meningioma
chordoma
clival c.
chordosarcoma
chordotomy
chorea
acanthocytosis with c.
acute c.
autoimmune c.
automatic c.
benign familial c.
benign hereditary c.
Bergeron c.

chronic progressive hereditary c.
chronic progressive nonhereditary c.
c. cordis
c. corpuscle
dancing c.
degenerative c.
c. dimidiata
drug-induced c.
Dubini c.
electric c.
c. festinans
fibrillary c.
c. gravidarum
habit c.
hemilateral c.
Henoch c.
hereditary benign c.
hereditary nonprogressive c.
Huntington c.
hysterical c.
c. immune
infectious c.
c. insaniens
juvenile c.
kinesigenic c.
laryngeal c.
c. magna
c. major
methodical c.
mimetic c.
c. minor
c. mollis
Morvan c.
c. nocturna
nongenetic c.
c. nutans
oral contraceptive-induced c.
paralytic c.
c. paralytica
phenytoin-induced c.
posthemiplegic c.
prehemiplegic c.
procursive c.
rheumatic c.
rhythmic c.
c. rotatoria
saltatory c.
Schrötter c.
senile c.
1-sided c.
simple c.
sporadic c.
Sydenham c.
tetanoid c.
thyrotoxicosis-induced c.
unilateral c.
vascular c.

chorea-acanthocytosis

choreatic atonia

choreic
c. abasia
c. dyskinesia
c. gait
c. movement
c. syndrome

choreicus
status c.

choreiform
c. disorder
c. movement

choreoacanthocytosis

choreoathetoid
c. cerebral palsy
c. movement

choreoathetosis
benign infantile familial convulsions plus paroxysmal c.
congenital c.
dystonic c.
familial benign c.
familial paroxysmal c.
kinesigenic c.
paroxysmal kinesigenic c.
phenytoin-induced c.
psychotic c.
thyrotoxicosis-induced c.

choreoid

choreophrasia

choriocarcinoma
pineal regional c.

choriomeningitis
benign lymphocytic c.
lymphocytic c.

chorionic
c. gonadotropin
c. villus sampling (CVS)

chorioretinitis

choristoma nest

choroid
basal lamina of c.
basal layer of c.
c. branch
c. detachment
c. enlargement

NOTES

choroid *(continued)*
c. fissure
c. glomus
c. line
c. membrane
c. plexus
c. plexus ablation
c. plexus adenoma
c. plexus carcinoma
c. plexus cell
c. plexus extirpation
c. plexus of fourth ventricle
c. plexus hemangioma
c. plexus hemorrhage
c. plexus of lateral ventricle
c. plexus papilloma
c. plexus of third ventricle
c. plexus villus
c. plexus water hammer effect
c. skein
c. tela of fourth ventricle
c. tela of third ventricle
c. vein
choroidal
c. blush
c. detachment
c. fissure
c. fold
lateral posterior c.
medial posterior c.
c. metastasis
c. osteoma
c. pericallosal artery
c. xanthoma
choroidal-hippocampal
c.-h. fissure
c.-h. fissure complex
choroidea
arteria c.
fissura c.
lamina c.
plica c.
taenia c.
tela c.
tenia c.
choroideae
lamina basalis c.
choroidectomy
choroidei
rami c.
choroideremia
choroideum
glomus c.
choroideus
plexus c.
choroidopathy
Christensen-Krabbe disease
Christmas disease
CHRNA4 gene
CHRNA7 gene
chromaffin
c. cell
c. cell transplant
c. tumor
chromaffinoma
chromaffinopathy
chromatic
c. audition
c. granule
chromatin-negative
chromatin-positive
chromatolysis, chromatinolysis
central c.
retrograde c.
transsynaptic c.
chromatolytic
chromesthesia
chromium
chromogranin A
chromolysis
chromophil
c. adenoma
c. corpuscle
c. granule
c. substance
chromophobe
c. adenoma
c. cell of anterior lobe of hypophysis
chromophobic adenoma
chromophose
chromosomal
c. aberration
c. anomaly
c. banding technique
c. polysomy
chromosome
c. 4, 13, 14, 15, 17, 18, 21, 22
control c.
human c. 20
linear c.
loss of heterozygosity c. 10 (LOH10)
marker c.
c. (9_p) monosomy
c. 1p
c. 6p
c. 7p13-p15
c. 2q
c. 2q21-33
c. 2q24
c. 5q33-55
c. 6q
c. 6q24
c. 7q21.2
c. 8q
c. 8q13-21
c. 8q24

c. 10q22-24
c. 15q14
c. 15q24
c. 16q
c. 16q24.1
c. 19q11-13
c. 19q13.3
c. 20q
c. 20q13.2
c. 20q13.3
c. 21q22.1
c. 21q22.3
c. 3q25.2-q27
ring c.
c. study
c. walking
X c.

chronic
c. adhesive arachnoiditis
c. administration
c. African sleeping sickness
c. angle-closure glaucoma
c. anterior poliomyelitis
c. ataxia
c. basal meningitis with cranial nerve paralysis
c. change
c. cluster headache
c. communicating hydrocephalus
c. constrictive injury (CCI)
c. corticosteroid therapy
c. course
c. delirium
c. dysthymia
c. familial polyneuritis
c. fatigability
c. fatigue
c. fatigue and immune dysfunction syndrome
c. focal encephalitis (CFE)
c. hepatic failure peripheral neuropathy
c. hyperventilation syndrome
c. illness behavior
c. inflammatory demyelinating polyneuropathy (CIDP)
c. inflammatory demyelinating polyradiculoneuropathy (CIDP)
c. inflammatory demyelinating polyradiculopathy
c. inflammatory demyelinating sensorimotor neuropathy
c. insomnia
c. insomnia contributing factor
c. insomnia medical factor
c. insomnia medication effect
c. insomnia psychiatric factor
c. intractable pain
c. lung disease
c. migrainous neuralgia
c. motor tic disorder
c. myeloid leukemia
c. neurologic disorder
c. neuropsychologic disorder
c. nonprogressive headache
c. occlusion
c. ocular ischemia
c. paranoid reaction
c. paraparesis
c. paroxysmal hemicrania (CPH)
c. paroxysmal hemicrania headache
c. paroxysmal hemicrania-tic syndrome
c. partial epilepsy
c. pattern
c. plaque
c. progressive external ophthalmoplegia (CPEO)
c. progressive headache
c. progressive hereditary chorea
c. progressive myelopathy
c. progressive nonhereditary chorea
c. progressive syphilitic meningoencephalitis
c. relapsing polyneuropathy
c. relapsing polyradiculoneuropathy
c. response
c. sleep disorder
c. spinal epidural infection
c. spinal intradural infection
c. subdural hematoma
c. thrombus
c. tic
c. traumatic encephalopathy
c. trypanosomiasis
c. vertigo

chronica
encephalitis subcorticalis c.

chronobiology

chronometric and force generation task

chronotherapy

chuck
T-handle Jacob c.

C

NOTES

Churg-Strauss
C.-S. syndrome
C.-S. vasculitis
Chvostek sign
Chvostek-Weiss sign
chylous leakage
Chymodiactin
chymopapain
Cibacalcin Injection
Cibalith
Cibalith-S
cicatrix, pl. **cicatrices**
brain c.
meningocerebral c.
CID
cervical immobilization device
CID Picture Spine
CIDP
chronic inflammatory demyelinating polyneuropathy
chronic inflammatory demyelinating polyradiculoneuropathy
cigarette smoking
cigar-shaped diffusion ellipsoid
ciguatera
ciguatoxin
cilia (*pl. of* cilium)
ciliare
ganglion c.
ramus nervi oculomotorii ganglii ad c.
ciliari
ramus communicans nervi nasociliaris cum ganglio c.
ciliaris
radix brevis ganglii c.
radix longa ganglii c.
radix nasociliaris ganglii c.
radix oculomotoria ganglii c.
radix parasympathica ganglii c.
radix sympathica ganglii c.
ramus sympathicus ganglii c.
ciliary
c. ganglion
c. ganglionic plexus
c. migraine
c. migraine headache
c. nerve
c. neuralgia
c. neurotrophic factor (CNF)
ciliary-deprived neurotropic factor (CDNF)
ciliochoroidal detachment
ciliospinal
c. center
c. reflex
ciliotomy
cilium, pl. **cilia**
cilostazol
CIM
critical illness myopathy
cimetidine
cinanesthesia (*var. of* kinanesthesia)
Cincinnati Stroke Scale
cinclisis
cincture sensation
cinematic magnetic resonance imaging
cine phase contrast magnetic resonance imaging
cinerea
ala c.
commissura c.
fascia c.
fasciola c.
lamina c.
substantia c.
cinereae
nucleus alae c.
cinereal
cinerei
rami tuberis c.
cinereum
hamartoma of tuber c.
tuber c.
tuberculum c.
cinereus
locus c.
cineritious
cinesalgia
cineseismography
cingula (*pl. of* cingulum)
cingularis
ramus c.
cingulate
c. convolution
c. epilepsy
c. gyrus
c. gyrus dysgenesis
c. gyrus eversion
c. herniation
c. motor area (CMA)
c. operation
posterior c.
c. response
c. sulcus
c. tissue
cingulectomy
cinguli
fasciola cinerea c.
gyrus c.
isthmus gyri c.
isthmus of gyrus c.
sulcus c.
cingulothalamic artery
cingulotomy
rostral c.
stereotactic c.
cingulum, pl. **cingula**

c. bundle
sulcus of c.
cingulumotomy
circadian
c. clock
c. dysrhythmia
c. modulator
c. pacemaker
c. rhythm
c. rhythm change
c. rhythmicity
c. rhythm sleep disorder
c. system
c. timing
circannual
c. cycle
c. rhythm
circle
cerebral arterial c.
Haller c.
Papez c.
Ridley c.
c. of Willis
c. of Willis aneurysm
c. of Zinn-Haller
Zinn vascular c.
CircOlectric bed
circuit
basal ganglia-thalamocortical motor c.
cortex c.
cortical-striatal-pallidal-thalamic neural c.
dysfunctional neural c.
error detection c.
frontal subcortical brain c.
frontothalamic c.
lateral orbitofrontal c.
neuroanatomic c.
Papez c.
reflex c.
reverberating c.
traditional limbic c.
circuitry
amygdala fear c.
brain c.
cortical language c.
dysfunctional c.
frontal-cerebellar-thalamic c.
frontostriatal c.
limbic c.
normal c.
reciprocal c.
reward c.
striatofrontal c.
circular
c. fiber
c. laminar hook with offset top
c. nystagmus
c. sinus
c. sulcus of insula
c. sulcus of Reil
circulares
fibrae c.
circularis
sinus c.
circulating
c. androgen
c. leptin level
circulation
anterior c.
carotid c.
cerebral c.
collateral c.
cutaneous c.
intracranial c.
macro-eCVR-FV c.
micro-eCVR-FV c.
muscular c.
posterior c.
splanchnic c.
thalamic c.
vertebrobasilar c.
circulus, pl. **circuli**
c. arteriosus cerebri
c. arteriosus halleri
c. vasculosus nervi optici
c. venosus halleri
c. venosus ridleyi
circumcallosal
circumduction gait
circumference
head c.
circumferential branch
circumflex
c. nerve
c. nerve trauma
circumgemmal
circuminsular
circumlocution
circumscribed
c. amnesia
c. cerebral atrophy
c. change

NOTES

circumscribed *(continued)*
c. craniomalacia
c. edema
c. lesion
c. pyocephalus
c. region
circumscribing incision
circumscripta
meningitis serosa c.
osteoporosis c.
circumventricular organ
cirsoid aneurysm
cisapride
***cis*-parinaric acid**
13-*cis*-retinoic acid (13-CRA)
***cis*-retinoic acid (CRA)**
cistern
ambient c.
arachnoid c.
arachnoiditis of opticochiasmatic c.
basal c.
cerebellomedullary c.
cerebellopontine angle c.
cerebromedullary c.
c. of chiasm
chiasmatic c.
crural c.
fossa of Sylvius c.
great c.
c. of great cerebral vein
c. of great vein of cerebrum
insular c.
interpeduncular c.
c. of lamina terminalis
lateral cerebellomedullary c.
c. of lateral cerebral fossa
c. of lateral fossa of cerebrum
lumbar c.
mesencephalic c.
c. of nuclear envelope
obliterated basal c.
opticochiasmatic c.
parasellar c.
pericallosal c.
perimesencephalic c.
pontine c.
posterior cerebellomedullary c.
premedullary c.
prepontine c.
quadrigeminal c.
subarachnoid c.
subarachnoidal c.
superior c.
suprasellar c.
sylvian c.
c. sylvii
c. of Sylvius fossa
trigeminal c.
cisterna, pl. **cisternae**
c. ambiens
c. basalis
c. caryothecae
c. cerebellomedullaris
c. cerebellomedullaris lateralis
c. cerebellomedullaris posterior
c. chiasmatis
c. cruralis
c. fossae lateralis
c. fossae lateralis cerebri
c. fossae sylvii
c. intercruralis profunda
c. interpeduncularis
c. laminae terminalis
c. lumbalis
c. lumbar
c. magna
c. magna catheter
c. magna enlargement
c. pericallosa
c. pontis
c. pontocerebellaris
c. quadrigeminalis
cisternae subarachnoideae
cisternae subarachnoideales
c. sulci lateralis
c. superioris
c. venae magnae
c. venae magnae cerebri
cisternal
c. clot
c. puncture
cisternal-peritoneal shunt
cisternal-pleural shunt
cisternogram
indium c.
isotope c.
radioisotope c.
cisternography
cerebellopontine c.
computed tomographic c.
intraoperative c.
isotope c.
isotopic c.
perioperative c.
radioisotope c.
radionuclide c.
citalopram HBr
Citanest Plain
Citelli angle
Citracal
citrate
calcium c.
potassium acetate, potassium bicarbonate, and potassium c.
potassium bicarbonate, potassium chloride, and potassium c.
sufentanil c.
citric acid cycle

***Citrobacter* meningitis**
citrullinemia
citrullinuria
CIVRA
continuous intravenous regional anesthesia
CJD
Creutzfeldt-Jakob disease
c-jun gene
CK
creatine kinase
CK-MB
creatine kinase-MB fraction
cladiosic
cladosporiosis
cerebral c.
cladribine
clamp
adapted reference c.
Apofix interlaminar c.
Bigelow calvaria c.
Calman carotid c.
CCA c.
Crile c.
Crutchfield carotid artery c.
Dandy c.
Diethrich bulldog c.
Duvol lung c.
Gardner neurosurgical skull c.
Halifax interlaminar c.
head c.
interlaminar c.
Jacobson-Potts vascular c.
Javid carotid c.
Kindt carotid c.
Kocher c.
Kocher-Lovelace c.
Mayfield head c.
Mayfield neurosurgical skill c.
mosquito c.
Olivecrona aneurysm c.
Péan c.
3-point skull c.
Poppen-Blalock carotid c.
Roosen c.
Salibi carotid artery c.
Schnidt c.
Schwartz temporary intracranial artery c.
Selverstone c.
sizing c.
Sugita head c.
suture c.
Thompson carotid c.
Thumb-Saver introducer c.
Yasargil carotid c.
clamping mechanism
clang association
Clarke
C. cell
C. column
C. nucleus
nucleus dorsalis of C.
C. stereotactic instrument
Clark electrode
Clarus SpineScope
clasp-knife
c.-k. effect
c.-k. phenomenon
c.-k. reflex
c.-k. response
c.-k. rigidity
c.-k. spasticity
clasp knife
class
Gardner-Robertson c.
c. I–III evidence
pyranocarboxylic acid c.
classic
c. apraxia
c. brain tumor headache
c. cervical rib syndrome
c. conditioning
c. dissecting aneurysm
c. migraine
c. narcolepsy tetrad
classification
alcoholic c.
American Heart Association Stroke Outcome C. (AHA-SOC)
American Spinal Cord Injury Association c.
Antoni A neurinoma c.
basal ganglia c.
Brodmann c.
Eden c.
empirical c.
endplate damage c.
Engel postoperative seizure c.
Fränkel c.
Functional Ambulation C.
Hannover c.
headache c.
Hunt-Hess aneurysm c.

C

NOTES

classification *(continued)*
Hunt-Hess neurological c.
Hunt and Kosnik c.
International Working Formulation c.
Kernohan system of glioma c.
Kiel c.
Kistler subarachnoid hemorrhage c.
LeFort c.
Melmon and Rosen c.
modified Fischer c.
Newcastle c.
Nordstadt c.
Oxfordshire Community Stroke Project c.
Paykel c.
Ratliff avascular necrosis c.
Russell-Rubinstein cerebrovascular malformation c.
seizure c.
Spetzler-Martin c.
Sunderland c.
Sundt carotid ulceration c.
Suzuki c.
c. system
Toyama c.
Universal Spine C.
WHO astrocytoma c.

Claude-Bernard syndrome
Claude syndrome
claudication
disabling neurogenic c.
intermittent neurogenic c.
jaw c.
mental c.
neurogenic c. (NC)
visual c.

claustral layer
claustrum, pl. **claustra**
clava
claval
clavate papillae
clavi (*pl. of* clavus)
Claviceps purpurea
clavulanic acid
clavus, pl. **clavi**
c. clinical grouping
c. hystericus

clawed pedicle hook
clawhand deformity
clay shoveler's fracture
clear
c. cell ependymoma
c. cell meningioma

clearance
creatinine c.
dopamine c.
c. rate

clearing
artifactual c.

cleavage
symmetric c.

cleft
atypical c.
branchial c.
Lanterman c.
pharyngeal c.
primary synaptic c.
Schmidt-Lanterman c.
secondary synaptic c.
c. spine
subneural c.
synaptic c.

cleidocranial dysostosis
Cleocin
Clerambault syndrome
clericorum
dysphonia c.

Clevenger fissure
click
jaw c.
c. stimulation

click-evoked vestibular myogenic potential
climbing fiber (CF)
clinical
C. Adaptive Test/Clinical Linguistic and Auditory Milestone Scale (CAT/CLAMS)
c. armamentarium
c. characteristic
c. comparison study
c. conceptualization
c. condition
c. correlate
c. criterion
c. data
c. dementia
C. Dementia Rating (CDR)
C. Dementia Rating Scale
c. difference
c. effect
c. efficacy
c. electromagnetic flowmeter
c. electromagnetic flowmeter clip
c. formulation
C. Global Impression of Change
C. Global Improvement Scale
c. heterogeneity
c. ictal event
c. improvement
c. instability
c. intervention
c. intervention program
C. Linguistic Auditory Milestone Scale
c. manifestation

c. method
c. monitoring
c. monitoring technique
c. neurology
c. neuropsychology
c. neuroscientist
C. Observations of Motor and Postural Skills
c. phenomenology
c. phenomenon
c. phenotype
c. predictor
c. procedure
c. progression
c. relevance
c. response
c. seizure
c. sequela
c. sign
c. stability
c. subtype
c. symptom
c. syndrome
C. Test of Sensory Interaction and Balance (CTSIB)
c. theory
c. thinking
c. trial
c. variable
c. visit

clinically
c. adverse sequela
c. isolated syndrome
c. relevant classification system

clinician
C. Awareness Score
C. Global Rating Scale
C. Rated Overall Life Impairment
c. rating

clinician-rated
c.-r. cognitive symptom
c.-r. scale

Clinician's Interview-Based Impression of Change

clinicopathological

clinicopathologic study

Clinitron air bed

clinodactyly

clinoid
anterior c.
c. process

clinoidal
c. aneurysm
c. dura
c. meningioma
c. process
c. segment

clinoidectomy
anterior extradural c.
extradural c.

Clinoril

ClinSeg

clioquinol

clip
Acland c.
Adson scalp c.
aneurysm c.
angled aneurysm c.
c. application
c. applier
Backhaus towel c.
bayonet aneurysm c.
Beimer-Clip aneurysm c.
booster c.
Braun-Yasargil right-angle c.
Children's Hospital c.
clinical electromagnetic flowmeter c.
Codman aneurysm c.
Cologne-pattern scalp c.
crankshaft c.
cross-legged c.
Delrin plastic scalp c.
distal basilar temporary c.
Drake fenestrated c.
Drake-Kees c.
Elgiloy c.
fenestrated aneurysm c.
ferromagnetic intracerebral aneurysm c.
c. force meter
c. graft
heavy-duty straight c.
Heifetz c.
Heifetz-Weck c.
Kerr c.
LeRoy-Raney scalp c.
Ligaclip c.
c. ligation of aneurysm
L-shaped aneurysm c.
magnetic resonance-compatible c.
Mayfield aneurysm c.
McFadden-Kees c.

NOTES

clip *(continued)*
McKenzie hemostasis c.
McKenzie silver c.
Michel scalp c.
microvascular c.
mini-Sugita c.
nonferromagnetic c.
Olivecrona c.
c. placement
plastic scalp c.
primary c.
Raney scalp c.
right-angle booster c.
scalp c.
Schwartz aneurysm c.
Scoville c.
Slimline c.
Spetzler titanium aneurysm c.
straight aneurysm c.
Sugita aneurysm c.
Sugita cross-legged c.
Sugita-Ikakogyo c.
Sugita side-curved bayonet c.
Sugita temporary straight c.
Sundt booster c.
Sundt cross-legged c.
Sundt-Kees encircling patch c.
Sundt-Kees graft c.
Sundt-Kees Slimline c.
Sundt straddling c.
temporary c.
titanium aneurysm c.
Vari-Angle aneurysm c.
Weck c.
Yasargil-Aesculap spring c.
Yasargil cross-legged c.
Yasargil titanium aneurysm c.
Yasargil vessel c.
Zimmer c.
clip-induced stricture
clipped aneurysm
clipping
aneurysm c.
microsurgical neck c.
proximal c.
shank c.
surgical c.
clip-reinforced cotton sling
clip-type electrode
clitoridis
nervi cavernosi c.
nervus dorsalis c.
clival
c. chordoma
c. meningioma
c. mucocele
clivales
rami c.
clivus, pl. **clivi**
Blumenbach c.
c. canal line
lobulus clivi
lobus clivi
lower c.
c. meningioma
c. monticulus
mucopyocele of c.
CLN1 gene
CLN2 gene
CLN3 gene
CLN5 gene
CLN8 gene
cloaca therapy
clock
circadian c.
c. drawing test
internal circadian c.
clodanolene
clofazimine
clomethiazole
clomipramine
clonal
c. evolution hypothesis
c. expansion
clonazepam
clonic
c. block
c. contraction
c. convulsion
c. seizure
c. spasm
clonicity
clonicotonic seizure
clonidine
c. hydrochloride
topical c.
cloning
functional c.
clonogenic cell assay
clonospasm
clonus
ankle c.
foot c.
patellar c.
persistent c.
subsultus c.
sustained ankle c.
toe c.
wrist c.
clopenthixol
clopidogrel bisulfate
Cloquet
C. ganglion
C. pseudoganglion
clorazepate dipotassium
clorgyline
closed
c. angiography

c. brain injury (CBI)
c. Cotrel-Dubousset hook
c. disc space infection
c. galea
c. head injury
c. head injury screener
c. head syndrome
c. loop reflex
c. skull fracture
c. transverse process TSRH hook
closed-chain functional assessment
closed-circuit
c.-c. television electroencephalographic telemetry
c.-c. television monitoring
clostridial infection
Clostridium
C. botulinum
C. difficile
C. tetani
closure
approximating c.
neural tube c.
premature c.
c. pressure
scalp c.
vacuum-assisted c. (VAC)
watertight c.
clot
cisternal c.
cobweb-like c.
clotrimazole
clotting
c. disorder
c. factor deficiency
clouded-state epilepsy
clouding
corneal c.
cloudy cornea
cloverleaf
c. skull
c. skull syndrome
Cloward
C. back fusion
C. blade retractor
C. bone graft impactor
C. brain retractor
C. cautery hook
C. cervical arthrodesis
C. cervical disc approach
C. cervical dislocation reducer
C. cervical vertebra spreader
C. disc rongeur
C. double-hinge cervical retractor handle
C. dural hook
C. dural retractor
C. elevator
C. instrument
C. lamina spreader
C. lumbar lamina retractor
C. nerve root retractor
C. operation
C. procedure
C. skin retractor
C. small cervical retractor
C. spinal fusion osteotome
C. surgical saddle
C. technique
C. tissue retractor
Cloward-Cone ring curette
Cloward-Cushing vein retractor
Cloward-English laminectomy rongeur
Cloward-Hoen laminectomy retractor
clozapine therapy
Clozaril
cloze procedure
CLS
Coffin-Lowry syndrome
club ending of Bartelmez
clumsy
c. child syndrome
c. hand syndrome
cluneal nerve
cluster
c. A, B, C disorder
c. analysis
apolipoprotein gene c.
c. breathing
c. B trait
c. C, D symptom
diagnostic c.
dissociative symptom c.
DSM c.
eccentric A c.
emotional B c.
c. headache (CH)
microglial c.
c. period
c. of symptom
cluster-tic syndrome
cluttering
c. in speech
speech and language c.

NOTES

Clymer-Barrett Readiness Test, Revised
CM
cavernous malformation
CMA
cingulate motor area
CMA 600 neuromonitoring system
CMAP
compound motor action potential
compound muscle action potential
CMAP amplitude
CMD
congenital muscular dystrophy
merosin-deficient CMD
CMFTD
congenital muscle fiber-type disproportion
CMRglc
cerebral metabolic rate of glucose
$CMRO_2$
cerebral metabolic rate of oxygen
CMS
congenital myasthenic syndrome
CMS AccuProbe 450 system
CMV
controlled mechanical ventilation
cytomegalovirus
CMV encephalitis
CMV meningitis
CMV polyradiculomyelitis
CMV-PRAM
cytomegalovirus polyradiculomyelitis
CNAP
compound nerve action potential
CNCD
Consortium of Neurology Clerkship Directors
CNF
ciliary neurotrophic factor
C-nociceptor filter-evoked central abnormality
cnot gene
CNR
contrast-to-noise ratio
CNS
Canadian Neurological Scale
central nervous system
CNS abnormality
CNS insult
CNS involvement
CNS leukostasis
CNS lymphoma
CNS manifestation
CNS nocardiosis
CNS vasculature
CO_2
carbon dioxide
end-tidal CO_2
CO_2 inhalation
CO_2 narcosis
coactivation
coactive strategy
coagulase-negative staphylococcus
coagulation
c. cascade
c. defect
c. disorder
disseminated intravascular c. (DIC)
coagulative necrosis
coagulator
ASSI c.
bipolar c.
Concept bipolar c.
Fukushima monopolar malleable c.
Malis CMC-II bipolar c.
Malis solid-state c.
Polar-Mate c.
solid-state c.
coagulopathy
consumptive c.
coagulum
cryoprecipitate c.
coaptation
direct end-to-end c.
coarctation
aorta c.
coarse
c. nystagmus
c. tremor
coating of aneurysm
Coats disease
coaxial
c. cable
c. needle electrode
cobalamin
c. metabolism disorder
c. reductase deficiency
cobalt
c. Gray equivalent
c. samarium magnet
cobalt-60
collimated c.-60
Cobb
C. angle
C. angle determination
C. method
C. method of measuring kyphosis
C. periosteal elevator
C. syndrome
C. technique
cobblestone degeneration
Coblation-based spinal surgery system
cobweb-like clot
cocaine
c. intoxication
neonatal drug addiction with c.
c. withdrawal
cocaine-induced choreoathetoid movement

coccidioidal
c. complement fixation of cerebrospinal fluid
c. meningitis
Coccidioides
C. immitis
C. infection
coccidioidomycosis
coccygea
segmentum c. 1–3
segmentum medullae spinalis c.
coccygeal
c. ganglion
c. ligament
c. nerve
c. part of spinal cord
c. plexus
c. segment of spinal cord
c. vertebra
coccygei
ramus anterior nervi c.
ramus dorsalis nervi c.
ramus posterior nervi c.
ramus ventralis nervi c.
coccyges (*pl. of* coccyx)
coccygeus
nervi sacrales et nervus c.
nervus c.
plexus c.
coccygodynia
coccyx, pl. **coccyges**
posterior surgical exposure of sacrum and c.
cochlea, pl. **cochleae**
apical turn of c.
aqueductus c.
cupula c.
ganglion spirale c.
lamina basilaris c.
membranous c.
spiral ganglion of c.
vestibular fissure of c.
cochlear
c. aplasia
c. aqueduct
c. duct
c. ganglion
c. hair cell
c. implant
c. microphonic potential
c. nerve examination
c. nucleus
c. part of vestibulocochlear nerve
c. recess
c. response time
c. root of eighth nerve
c. root of vestibulocochlear nerve
c. vascular supply
cochleare
ganglion c.
cochleares
nuclei c.
cochlearis
crista basilaris ductus c.
ductus c.
nervus c.
nuclei nervi c.
paries vestibularis ductus c.
pars c.
radix c.
recessus c.
cochleogram
cochleopalpebral reflex
cochleopupillary reflex
cochleosacculotomy
cochleostapedial reflex
cochleovestibular compression syndrome
Cochrane Collaboration
Cockayne syndrome
cocktail chatter in hydrocephalus
coconut sound
code
gene c.
gustatory c.
multimodal c.
c. substitution-immediate recall-accuracy
codeine
Empracet with c.
c. neurotoxicity
Codman
C. aneurysm clip
C. anterior cervical plate system
C. Bactiseal antimicrobial impregnated catheter system
C. cranioblade
C. drill
C. Hakim programmable valve
C. IC
C. neurological headrest system
C. scissors
C. slit valve
C. ventricular silicone
C. ventricular silicone catheter

NOTES

Codman-Harper laminectomy rongeur
Codman-Kerrison laminectomy rongeur
Codman-Leksell laminectomy rongeur
Codman-Medos programmable valve
Codman-Schlesinger cervical laminectomy rongeur
coefficient
alpha c.
apparent diffusion c. (ADC)
contingency c.
familiar correlation c.
high alpha c.
low alpha c.
olfactory c.
scoring c.
Spearman correlation c.
c. of variation (COV)
coeliaca
ganglia c.
coeliaci
rami renales plexus c.
coeliacus
plexus c.
coenesthesia (*var. of* cenesthesia)
coenzyme
acetyl c. A
coercion program
coeruleus
locus c. (LC)
nucleus c.
coexisting
c. aneurysm
c. medical condition
Coffin-Lowry syndrome (CLS)
Coffin-Siris syndrome
COGA
Collaborative Study on the Genetics of Alcoholism
Cogan
C. lid twitch
C. oculomotor apraxia
C. syndrome
C. syndrome vasculitis
Cogentin
Cogent microillumination technology
Cognex
cognition
altered c.
Burns Brief Inventory of Communication and C.
constriction of c.
c. disorder
frontally based c.
impaired c.
premorbid c.
social c.
visuospatial constructive c.
cognitive
C. Abilities Screening Scale
C. Abilities Test, Form 5
C. Adaptive Computer Help
c. analytic therapy
c. behavioral group therapy
c. capability
c. capacity
c. change
c. decline
c. deficit
c. deterioration
c. difficulty
c. disorder
c. disturbance
c. domain
c. dysfunction
c. dysmetria
c. enhancement therapy
c. exercise
c. factor
C. Failures Questionnaire
c. fatigue
c. fluctuation
c. function
c. function assessment
c. function deficiency
c. function development
c. function immaturity
c. functioning
c. generation of affect
c. impairment
c. impairment of depression
c. impairment, no dementia
c. improvement
c. intervention
c. maturity
c. measure
c. mechanism
c. method
c. neuropsychology
c. neuroscience
c. pathology
c. performance
c. potential
c. profile
c. reserve
c. score
C. Skills Assessment Battery, Second Edition
c. slowing
c. state
c. status
c. subsystem
c. symptom
c. task
c. technique
c. tendency
c. test battery
c. testing
c. trajectory

cognitively intact
cognizance
CogScreen Aeromedical Edition
cogwheel
c. phenomenon
c. rigidity
c. sign
Cohen syndrome
coherence
phase c.
coherent
c. model
c. motion
c. negative picture-caption pair
c. positive picture-caption pair
coil
3-axis gradient c.
body c.
butterfly c.
catheter c.
crossed c.
Dacron-fibered platinum c.
detachable c.
Dixon radiofrequency c.
electrodetachable platinum c.
c. embolization
endovascular c.
figure-of-8 c.
Golay gradient c.
gradient c.
Guglielmi detachable c. (GDC)
head c.
Helmholtz c.
Hilal c.
Ivalon wire c.
occlusion c.
orthogonal square Helmholtz c.
phased-array c.
platinum c.
c. protrusion
quadrature head c.
radiofrequency head c.
receiver c.
RF c.
saddle c.
shim c.
solenoid c.
surface c.
thrombogenic c.
transverse gradient c.
Yasargil-Leyla brain retractor z-gradient c.
z-gradient c.
coiled spring
coiling
aneurysmal c.
intravascular c.
c. procedure
coital headache
colchicine
cold
c. acclimation
c. detection threshold
c. effector
c. injury
c. receptor
c. sensitivity
c. stimulus headache
cold-induced allodynia
cold-sensitive neuron
Coleman method
coli
Escherichia c.
colic lead
colla (*pl. of* collum)
collaboration
Cochrane C.
collaborative
c. care
C. Study on the Genetics of Alcoholism (COGA)
collagen
Avitene microfibrillar c.
intercellular c.
microfibrillar c.
c. vascular disease
c. vascular disease vasculitis
collagenase
c. inhibition
interstitial c.
collagenase-activating factor
collagen-impregnated Dacron
collapse
alar soft tissue c.
bone graft c.
c. delirium
disc space c.
graft c.
hemispheric c.
interspace c.
upper airway c.
vertebral c.

NOTES

collapsible tissue retractor
collar
Belmont c.
cervical c.
Exo-Static c.
hard c.
c. immobilization
Miami Acute Care cervical c.
Miami J c.
Newport c.
Philadelphia c.
Plastazote cervical c.
plastic c.
collateral
c. blood flow
c. blood supply
c. circulation
c. eminence
c. fiber
c. fissure
c. nerve sprouting
c. sulcus
c. trigone
c. vessel
collaterale
trigonum c.
collateralis
eminentia c.
fissura c.
sulcus c.
collector
common venous c.
Collet-Sicard syndrome
Collet syndrome
colli
nervus transversus c.
rami inferiores nervi transversi c.
rami superiores nervi transversi c.
collicular artery
colliculorum
commissura c.
colliculus, pl. **colliculi**
anterior c.
brachium of caudal c.
brachium of inferior c.
brachium of rostral c.
brachium of superior c.
caudal c.
c. caudalis
c. caudatus
commissure of inferior c.
commissure of superior c.
deep gray layer of superior c.
deep white layer of superior c.
facial c.
c. facialis
gray layer of superior c.
c. inferior
inferior nasal c.
intermediate white layer of superior c.
middle gray layer of superior c.
nuclei of caudal c.
nuclei of inferior c.
rostral c.
c. rostralis
superficial gray layer of superior c.
superior c.
zonal layer of superior c.
Collier
C. sign
C. tract
collimated cobalt-60
collimation
collimator
external c.
c. helmet
multileaf c.
stereoguide c.
Collins law of survival after brain tumor
collision
electron c.
c. tumor
collodion attachment
colloid
c. cyst
c. cyst of third ventricle
c. oncotic pressure
technetium albumin c.
technetium-99m sulfur c.
collum, pl. **colla**
coloboma, heart disease, atresia choanae, retarded growth, genital anomalies, ear anomalies (CHARGE)
Cologne-pattern scalp clip
Colonna shelf procedure
colony-forming efficiency
color
c. agnosia
c. anomia
c. flow duplex ultrasonography
c. taste
c. velocity imaging quantification
c. vision
c. vision disturbance
c. vision loss
c. visual loss
Colorado
C. microdissection needle
C. microneedle
C. tick fever viral encephalitis
3-color FACScan analysis
color-flow
c.-f. Doppler
c.-f. Doppler sonography
c.-f. imaging

color-opponent cell
colpocephaly
column
anterior gray c.
anterolateral c.
bony spinal c.
branchial efferent c.
Burdach c.
c. cell
Clarke c.
dorsal gray c.
forniceal c.
c. of fornix
fundamental c.
general somatic afferent c.
general somatic efferent c.
general visceral afferent c.
general visceral efferent c.
Goll c.
Gowers c.
gray c.
intermediate c.
intermediolateral cell c.
lateral c.
Lissauer c.
osteochondral spinal c.
Rolando c.
special somatic afferent c.
special visceral efferent c.
spinal c.
Spitzka-Lissauer c.
c. of Spitzka and Lissauer
Stilling c.
striomotor c.
thoracic c.
Türck c.
ventral white c.
vertebral c.
3-column
3-c. cervical spine injury
3-c. concept
columna, pl. **columnae**
c. anterior
c. anterior medullae spinalis
c. dorsalis medullae spinalis
c. fornicis
columnae griseae
columnae griseae medullae spinalis
c. intermedia
c. intermedia medullae spinalis
c. intermediolateralis medullae spinalis
c. lateralis
c. posterior
c. posterior medullae spinalis
c. thoracica
c. ventralis medullae spinalis
c. vertebralis
2-column cervical spine injury
coma
adrenocortical c.
agrypnodal c.
alcoholic c.
alpha frequency c.
apoplectic c.
calm hypotonic c.
c. carcinomatosum
diabetic c.
flaccid c.
hepatic c.
c. hepaticum
hyperosmolar nonketotic c.
hypoglycemic c.
hypopituitary c.
hypoventilation c.
Kussmaul c.
metabolic c.
myxedema c.
nonketotic hyperglycemic hyperosmolar c.
pentobarbital c.
postanoxic c.
c. scale
spindle c.
thyrotoxic c.
uremic c.
c. vigil
comatose
comb bundle
combination
c. chemotherapy
c. drug (CD)
c. headache
Isola spinal implant system plate-rod c.
muscle-fascia-Gelfoam c.
c. needle electrode
orthogonal c.
paradoxical c.
c. strategy
combined
c. anterior and posterior approach
c. aphasia

NOTES

combined *(continued)*
c. flexion-distraction injury and burst fracture
c. low cervical and transthoracic approach
c. predictive power
c. presigmoid-transtransversarium intradural approach
c. sclerosis
c. supra/infratentorial-transsinus approach
c. system disease
c. transsylvian and middle fossa approach
Combisit surgeon's chair
Combitrans transducer
Combivir
comedication
ComfortClassic nasal mask
ComfortFull nasal mask
ComfortGel nasal mask
comma
c. bundle of Schultze
c. tract of Schultze
command
verbal c.
commensalism
comminuted skull fracture
comminution
commissura, pl. **commissurae**
c. alba anterior
c. alba anterior medullae spinalis
c. alba posterior
c. alba posterior medullae spinalis
c. anterior grisea
c. cinerea
c. colliculi inferioris
c. colliculi rostralis
c. colliculi superioris
c. colliculorum
c. epithalamica
c. fornicis
c. grisea anterior
c. grisea anterior medullae spinalis
c. grisea anterior/posterior medullae spinalis
c. grisea posterior
c. grisea posterior medullae spinalis
c. habenularum
c. hippocampus
c. magna cerebri
c. olivarum
c. posterior cerebri
c. posterior grisea
c. supraoptica dorsalis
commissurae supraopticae
c. supraoptica ventralis
c. ventralis alba
commissural
c. aphasia
c. cell
c. fiber
c. myelotomy
c. neurofiber
c. plate
commissuralis
fibra c.
neurofibra c.
commissure
anterior commissure-posterior c. (AC-PC)
anterior gray c.
anterior white c.
callosal c.
caudal colliculus c.
cerebral c.
c. of cerebral hemisphere
dorsal supraoptic c.
epithalamus c.
c. of fornix
Ganser c.
gray c.
Gudden c.
habenular c.
hippocampal c.
c. of inferior colliculus
Meynert c.
nucleus of posterior c.
posterior cerebral c.
posterior gray c.
rostral colliculus c.
c. of superior colliculus
supraoptic c.
ventral white c.
Wernekinck c.
white c.
commissurotomy
callosal c.
percutaneous balloon c.
committee
AANS/CNS Outcomes C.
common
c. basal vein
c. carotid artery (CCA)
c. carotid nervous plexus
c. central process
c. crus
c. fibular nerve
c. iliac artery injury
c. membranous limb of membranous semicircular duct
c. migraine
c. peroneal nerve
c. sensibility
c. venous collector
c. venous confluence

commotio
c. cerebri
c. spinalis
communal residential center
commune
crus membranaceum c.
sensorium c.
communicans
macula c.
ramus c.
communicantes
gray rami c.
rami c.
white rami c.
communicating
c. branch
c. branch of auriculotemporal nerve with facial nerve
c. branch of chorda tympani with lingual nerve
c. branch of facial nerve with glossopharyngeal nerve
c. branch of facial nerve with tympanic plexus
c. branch of fibular artery
c. branch of intermediate nerve with tympanic plexus
c. branch of lacrimal nerve with zygomatic nerve
c. branch of lingual nerve with hypoglossal nerve
c. branch of median nerve with ulnar nerve
c. branch of nasociliary nerve with ciliary ganglion
c. branch of otic ganglion to auriculotemporal nerve
c. branch of otic ganglion to chorda tympani
c. branch of otic ganglion with chorda tympani
c. branch of otic ganglion with medial pterygoid nerve
c. branch of peroneal artery
c. branch of radial nerve with ulnar nerve
c. branch of spinal nerve
c. branch of superficial radial nerve with ulnar nerve
c. branch of sympathetic trunk
c. branch of tympanic plexus with auricular branch of vagus nerve
c. branch with nasociliary nerve
c. hydrocephalus
communication
c. difficulty
c. disorder
emotional c.
facilitation of c.
c. function
functional c. (FC)
gesture c.
c. impairment
mime c.
nonverbal c.
pathological c.
C.'s Profile Questionnaire
c. skill
C. Skills Profile
c. tool
verbal c.
Communicative Abilities in Daily Living
communis
nervus fibularis c.
plexus caroticus c.
ramus communicans fibularis nervi fibularis c.
ramus communicans peroneus nervi peronei c.
sacculus c.
community-acquired bacterial meningitis
Community-Oriented Programs Environment Scale
comorbid
c. characteristic
c. condition
c. dementia
c. disease
c. headache
c. illness
c. sleep disorder
c. syndrome
comorbidity
age-related c.
medical c.
compacta
pars c.
substantia nigra pars c. (SNc)
compact myelin
company
neurologic c.
compartment
extradural c.
infratentorial c.

NOTES

compartment *(continued)*
intracranial c.
lateral sellar c.
c. syndrome
Compass
C. arc-quadrant stereotactic system
C. frame-based stereotactic system
C. stereotactic phantom
compassionate-use basis
compassionate use of drugs
compatibility
ABO antigen c.
MRI c.
compensated hydrocephalus
compensation
gradient c.
load c.
compensatory
c. innervation
c. scoliosis
Comperm tubular elastic bandage
competency
c. assessment
high degree of c.
low threshold of c.
maternal c.
competent
mentally c.
competition
hemisphere c.
intermodal c.
complainant-listener relationship
complement
c. activation
c. fixation antibody test
c. fixation antibody titer
c. fixation inhibition
c. symptom-focused assessment
complementary
c. deoxyribonucleic acid (cDNA)
c. medicine
complete
c. blood count (CBC)
c. flaccid extremity paralysis
c. iridoplegia
c. lateral hemilaminectomy
c. tetanus
c. transverse myelitis
c. visual loss
completed stroke
completus
tetanus c.
complex
c. absence
acoustic nerve c.
acquired immunodeficiency syndrome dementia c.
adrenoleukodystrophy/adrenomyeloneuropathy c.
AIDS dementia c. (ADC)
ALD/AMN c.
ALS-PD c.
amygdaloid c.
amyotrophic lateral sclerosis-Parkinson dementia c.
antigen-antibody c.
aperiodic c.
avidin-biotin peroxidase c.
brain wave c.
calcarine c.
capsulolabral c.
chemokine CCL-20/CCR6 c.
choroidal-hippocampal fissure c.
Dandy-Walker c.
discoligamentous c.
c. disease
disorganized symptom c.
dynein-dynactin c.
c. febrile convulsion
c. febrile seizure
c. finger routine
c. fracture
c. fracture pattern
Guam parkinsonism-dementia c.
c. hand routine
hippocampal c.
hippocampal-amygdala c.
histocompatibility c.
immune c.
inferior olivary c.
inferior orbitofrontal c.
c. intellectual aura
interictal c.
K c.
major histocompatibility c. (MHC)
mastoid c.
membrane attack c.
c. meningioma
c. motor seizure
occipitoatlantoaxial c.
oculomotor nuclear c.
omphalocele-exstrophy-imperforate anus-spinal defects c.
c. paradigm
Parkinson disease and lateral sclerosis-dementia c.
c. partial nocturnal seizure
c. partial status
c. partial status epilepticus
PDH c.
perihypoglossal nuclear c.
periodic sharp-wave c.
plasmin-antiplasmin c.
polyspike-wave c.
posterior ligamentous c.
c. precipitated epilepsy
pyruvate dehydrogenase c.
c. regional pain syndrome

c. relationship
c. repetitive discharge (CRD)
respiratory c.
Rey-Osterrieth c.
Sakoda c.
c. segregation analysis
sharp-wave c.
slow-wave c.
Sokoda c.
spike-and-wave c.
spike-wave c.
superior olivary c.
symptom c.
syringomyelia-Chiari c.
Tag c.
c. task
troponin-tropomyosin c.
urethral c.
ventrobasal nucleus c.
ventrolateral nuclear c.
vertebrogenic symptom c.
c. visual perception

complexus olivaris inferior

compliance
intracranial c.
medication c.
c. rate
sustained c.
treatment c.

complicated
c. fracture
c. migraine

complication
adverse neurologic c.
drug-induced medical c.
c. following measles vaccination
c. following vaccination for mumps
halo c.
hardware c.
iatrogenic c.
immunization c.
infectious c.
Isola spinal implant system c.
liver transplant c.
lumbar puncture c.
mumps vaccination c.
neurologic c.
perioperative c.
rubella vaccination c.
screw-related c.
shunt-related c.
smallpox vaccination c.
transsphenoidal c.
treatment-related c.
ventilatory support neurologic c.

component
adrenomedullary c.
autonomous functional c.
bacterial cell wall c.
cellular c.
cross-sectional c.
endogenous electrophysiological c.
functional c.
genetic c.
hypermetabolic tumor c.
inotropic c.
Isola spinal implant system c.
physiological c.
Positive and Negative Syndrome Scale–Excitement C. (PANSS-EC)
prominent phobic anxiety c.
signal transducing receptor c.
c.'s of sleep
somatomotor c.
somatosensory c.
splanchnic motor c.
splanchnic sensory c.
sudomotor c.
thermogenic c.
true c.
vasomotor c.
visceral motor c.
visceral sensory c.

2-component microgrip precision control suction unit

composite
c. addition technique
c. disc prosthesis
c. index
Vineland Adaptive Behavior C.

compound
disease-modifying c.
c. granular corpuscle
c. granule cell
c. heterozygote
lipophilic c.
c. motor action potential (CMAP)
c. muscle action potential (CMAP)
c. muscle action potential amplitude
c. nerve action potential (CNAP)
porphyrin c.
primary active c.
c. skull fracture

NOTES

comprehensible speech
comprehensive
c. assessment
c. care
c. evaluation
C. Identification Process, Revised
C. Level of Consciousness Scale
C. Qualifying Examination
c. treatment planning
compressed
c. spectral analysis
c. spectral array
compressing neural element
compression
acute spinal cord c.
c. amplifier
c. anesthesia
ASIF broad dynamic c.
axial c.
balloon c.
brain c.
c. of brain
brainstem c.
cauda equina c.
cerebral aqueduct c.
cervical vessel c.
cervicomedullary junction c.
chiasmal c.
cranial nerve c.
epidural cord c.
extradural c.
c. fracture
Harrington rod instrumentation c.
c. instrumentation posterior construct
intervertebral disc c.
midbrain c.
nerve root c.
c. neuropathy
c. ophthalmodynamometer
optic chiasm c.
optic tract c.
c. paralysis
percutaneous trigeminal nerve c.
c. rod
c. rod treatment
spinal cord c.
c. spring
c. syndrome
thecal sac c.
c. U-rod
c. U-rod instrumentation
ventral medullary c.
ventral spinal cord c.
compression-rarefaction strain in craniocerebral trauma
compressive
c. mass lesion
c. myelopathy
c. neuropathy
c. rod
c. trigeminal nerve lesion
compromise
adenohypophysial c.
adrenocorticotropic c.
endocrinological c.
progressive neurologic c.
spinal canal c.
compromised
c. intellect
c. neurologic picture
Compton scattering
compulsive
c. drug administration
c. quality
c. reaction
c. spasms and tics
c. writing
computed
c. axial tomography (CAT)
c. tomographic cisternography
c. tomographic metrizamide myelography
c. tomography (CT)
computer
Brown-Roberts-Wells c.
c. navigation system
computer-aided
c.-a. image analysis
C.-A. Neurovascular Analysis and Simulation (CANVAS)
c.-a. sensory evaluator
c.-a. therapy
computer-assisted
c.-a. EEG signal analysis
c.-a. image-guided system
c.-a. myelography (CAM)
c.-a. neuroendoscopy
c.-a. placement
c.-a. stereotactic surgery (CASS)
c.-a. surgery (CAS)
c.-a. volumetric stereotactic approach
c.-a. volumetric stereotactic lesionectomy
computer-controlled
c.-c. neurological stimulation system
c.-c. neurological stimulation system cone
computer-guided therapy
computerized
c. axial tomography (CAT)
c. axial tomography scanning
c. EEG signal analysis
c. infrared telethermographic imaging
c. tomography scan

COMT
catechol-*O*-methyltransferase
COMT inhibitor
Comtan
conarium
concave
c. hyperdensity
c. hypodensity
concealed reflex
concentrate
factor IX complex c.
GABA c.
gamma-aminobutyric acid c.
concentrated anthrax
concentration
brain-derived HVA c.
elevated protein c.
glucose c.
hippocampal monoamine c.
homovanillic acid c.
HVA c.
hydrogen ion c.
impaired c.
interstitial serotonin c.
ligand c.
maximal plasma c.
minimal alveolar c. (MAC)
minimum effective c.
motion c.
plasma glutamate c.
protein c.
serum lipid c.
concentration-dependent abolition
concentric
c. fiber layer
c. herniation
c. needle electrode
c. sclerosis
c. visual field defect
concentrica
encephalitis periaxialis c.
leukoencephalitis periaxialis c.
concept
C. bipolar coagulator
body c.
3-column c.
C. hand-held cautery
Heidelberg c.
c. of spiritual coping
von Monakow diaschisis c.
c. of will
Winslow c.
conceptual
c. ability
c. limitation
c. planning
c. problem
c. system
conceptualization
clinical c.
Lindamood Auditory C.
spatial c.
conceptualizing
Concerta
concordant
c. interictal epileptiform abnormality
c. result
concrete
c. operation
c. operational development
c. operational stage
concupiscence
concurrent
c. headaches
c. video-EEG recording
concussion
c. amnesia
c. assessment
brain c.
c. myelitis
recurrent c.
repeat c.
c. severity
spinal cord c.
sports-related c.
Standardized Assessment of C.
condensation
mitochondrial c.
c. stimulation
condition
activating c.
amnesic disorder due to general medical c.
clinical c.
coexisting medical c.
comorbid c.
craniofacial c.
degenerative spine c.
dementia due to hepatic c.
disabling neurological c.
experimental c.
haloperidol c.
heterogeneous c.
hypomyelinating c.

NOTES

condition *(continued)*
neuromuscular c.
noise c.
nonprogressive myoclonus c.
proband c.
respondent c.
REST c.
sleep-related c.
stimulation c.
subcortical c.
treatment c.
underlying c.
conditioned
c. drug response
c. fear association
c. insomnia
c. reflex (CR)
c. stimulation
c. stimulus (CS)
conditioning
classic c.
conductance
chloride c.
voltage-activated c.
conduction
c. anesthesia
antidromic c.
c. aphasia
avalanche c.
axonal c.
c. block
bone c.
c. delay
ephaptic c.
motor c.
nerve signal c.
saltatorial c.
saltatory c.
speed of c.
synaptic c.
c. testing
c. time
c. velocity
conductor
Adson c.
Bailey c.
Davis c.
conduit
peripheral nerve regeneration c.
condylar
c. approach
c. hypoplasia
condyle
c. dissection
c. resection
condylectomy
mandibular c.
cone
bifurcation c.
c. cell of retina
cerebellar pressure c.
computer-controlled neurological stimulation system c.
c. fiber
growth c.
implantation c.
C. laminectomy retractor
layer of rods and c.'s
medullary c.
pressure c.
retinal c.
C. ring curette
C. scalp retractor
C. skull punch
C. skull punch forceps
C. skull traction tongs
spinal cord terminal c.
C. suction biopsy curette
C. suction tube
C. ventricular needle
C. wire-twisting forceps
Cone-Grant technique
confabulatory
c. amnesia
c. amnestic state
confetti skin lesion
configuration
Cotrel-Dubousset hook claw c.
dumbbell tumor c.
triangular base-transverse bar c.
venous lake c.
confirmed
angiographically c.
conflict
escalating c.
horizontal c.
neurovascular c.
vertical c.
visual-vestibular c.
confluence
common venous c.
c. of sinus
confluens sinuum
confluent central necrosis
confocal
c. laser scanning
c. laser scanning microscope
conformal radiotherapy
conformation
beta B-sheet c.
confrontation
premature c.
c. stage
c. testing
confusion
nocturnal c.
postictal c.
postoperative c.

right-left c.
sudden c.
confusional
c. arousal
c. arousal characteristic
c. migraine
c. state
congenita
amyoplasia c.
amyotonia c.
aplasia cutis c.
myotonia c.
paramyotonia c.
congenital
c. anomaly
c. aplastic anemia
c. arachnodactyly
c. atonic pseudoparalysis
c. bilateral perisylvian polymicrogyria
c. bilateral perisylvian syndrome
c. central hypoventilation syndrome
c. cerebellar atrophy
c. cerebral aneurysm
c. cerebral palsy
c. cholesteatoma
c. choreoathetosis
c. cytomegalovirus infection
c. defect of cranial bone
c. defect of cranial bones dysraphism
c. dilation
c. dysplastic angiomatosis
c. dysplastic angiopathy
c. facial diplegia
c. hamartomatosis
c. heart disease
c. hemolytic anemia
c. herpes simplex virus infection
c. hippocampal sclerosis
c. Horner syndrome
c. hydrocephalus
c. hypomyelination neuropathy
c. hypothesis
c. hypothyroidism
c. infratentorial disorder
c. insensitivity to pain
c. kyphosis
c. laxity of ligament
c. malformation
c. muscle fiber-type disproportion (CMFTD)
c. muscular dystrophy (CMD)
c. myasthenia
c. myasthenia gravis
c. myasthenic syndrome (CMS)
c. myopathy
c. neurosyphilis
c. nystagmus
c. ocular motor apraxia
c. pain c.
c. paramyotonia
c. porencephaly
c. rubella
c. scalp defect dysraphism
c. scoliosis
c. sensory neuropathy
c. spastic paraplegia
c. suprabulbar paresis
c. toxoplasmosis
c. tumor
c. varicella
c. virilizing adrenal hyperplasia
congenitalis
alopecia triangularis c.
congestion
brain c.
nasal c.
neurotonic c.
congestive heart failure (CHF)
congophilic
c. amyloid
c. amyloid angiopathy
Congress of Neurological Surgeons
congruence
congruous hemianopia
coni (*pl. of* conus)
conjoined
c. nerve roots
c. twins
conjugal
c. tension
c. visitation
conjugate
c. contraversive eye movement
c. downward deviation
c. eye deviation
c. fixed gaze
c. horizontal gaze
c. nystagmus
c. paralysis
conjugated eye movement
conjunctiva, pl. **conjunctivae**

NOTES

conjunctiva *(continued)*
decussation of brachia c.
fornix c.
conjunctival
c. cul-de-sac
c. injection
conjunctivi
decussatio brachii c.
conjunctivitis
connection
interbrain connection
intracortical c.
monosynaptic c.
neuroanatomic c.
patterning synaptic c.
reciprocal c.
synaptic c.
thalamocortical c.
therapeutic c.
connective
c. tissue
c. tissue disease
connectivity pattern
connector
adjustable pedicle c.
dual bypass c.
intrinsic transverse c.
longitudinal member to anchor c.
stepdown c.
straight c.
tandem c.
transverse c.
connexin
c. gene
c. 32 protein
connexus interthalamicus
Conradi-Hünermann syndrome
Conradi syndrome
consanguinity
parental c.
consciousness
altered level of c.
arousal component of c.
decreased c.
c. impaired
level of c.
loss of c.
c. stress reaction
threshold of c.
conscious simulation
consensual
c. gaze
c. response pupil
consequence
neurobehavioral c.
psychological c.
sleepiness c.
conservation
energy c.
conservative cutoff score
consideration
etiopathogenetic c.
consistent
c. aura
c. delivery
c. response
console
Dissectron ultrasonic neurosurgical aspirator c.
Marconi Medical Systems c.
consolidation
memory c.
Consortium
Childhood Brain Tumor C.
C. to Establish a Registry for Alzheimer Disease
European Brain Injury C.
C. of Neurology Clerkship Directors (CNCD)
North American Brain Tumor C. (NABTC)
Consta
Risperdal C.
constant
c. current stimulator
relaxation c.
T1 relaxation c.
T2 relaxation c.
time c.
constitutional medicine
constraint-induced therapy
constriction of cognition
construct
anterior c.
AO dynamic compression plate c.
compression instrumentation posterior c.
double-rod c.
Edwards modular system bridging sleeve c.
Edwards modular system compression c.
Edwards modular system distraction-lordosis c.
Edwards modular system kyphoreduction c.
Edwards modular system neutralization c.
Edwards modular system rod-sleeve c.
Edwards modular system scoliosis c.
Edwards modular system spondylo c.
Edwards modular system standard sleeve c.
Guiot-Talairach c.
hook-to-screw L4-S1 compression c.

iliosacral and iliac fixation c.
pedicle screw c.
posterior c.
psychological c.
c. research
rigid cantilever beam c.
rod-hook c.
screw-to-screw compression c.
segmental compression c.
single-rod c.
Texas Scottish Rite Hospital double-rod c.
titanium c.
TSRH double-rod c.
TSRH pedicle screw-laminar claw c.
upper cervical spine anterior c.
upper cervical spine posterior c.
Wiltse system double-rod c.
Wiltse system H c.
Wiltse system single-rod c.

construction
c. ability
c. apraxia
endocentric c.
visuospatial c.

constructional
c. ability
c. agraphia
c. impairment

Constulose

consumption
brain oxygen c.
dietary caffeine c.
medicinal caffeine c.
nervous c.

consumptive coagulopathy

contact
c. ceptor
c. compressive forceps
endplate-to-graft c.
linguadental c.
c. receptor
c. sense

contagion
primitive c.

contained disc

container exercise

contamination
bacterial wound c.

content
bone mineral c.
carotid c.
central dopamine c.

context
space c.
spatial-temporal c.
time c.

contextual
c. association
c. cause
C. Memory test

contiguity disorder aphasia

contiguous
c. gene syndrome
c. nonoverlapping axial CT
c. supramarginal gyrus
c. voxel

continence
fecal c.
urine c.

contingency coefficient

contingent negative variation

continua
aura c.
epilepsia partialis c.
hemicrania c.

continuous
c. amnesia
c. anatomical passive exerciser
c. approach
c. cognitive testing
c. daytime drowsiness
c. electromyographic recording
c. extravascular infusion (CEI)
c. inflammatory process
c. intrathecal baclofen infusion
c. intravenous infusion
c. intravenous regional anesthesia (CIVRA)
c. maintenance medication
c. muscle fiber activity syndrome
c. online recording
c. performance task-accuracy
c. performance task-efficiency
C. Performance test (CPT)
c. positive airway pressure (CPAP)
c. spike and wave during sleep
c. tremor
c. variable
c. venous oximetry
c. video-electroencephalogram monitoring (CCTV-EEG)

NOTES

continuous *(continued)*
C. Visual Memory Test, Revised
c. wave (CW)
continuous-wave
c.-w. Doppler
c.-w. Doppler imaging
c.-w. technique
contour
Cupid's bow c.
C. Emboli artificial embolization device
field c.
illusionary c. (IC)
pitch c.
real c. (RC)
contoured
c. anterior spinal plate
c. anterior spinal plate drill guide
c. anterior spinal plate technique
contraction
carpopedal c.
clonic c.
c. fasciculation
fibrillary c.
idiomuscular c.
maximal voluntary c.
maximum voluntary c. (MVC)
myotatic c.
nonepileptic myoclonic c.
paradoxical c.
Rossolimo c.
tetanic c.
tonic c.
twitch c.
contractual alliance
contracture
c. arachnodactyly
caffeine-induced c.
Dupuytren c.
fixed c.
functional c.
myotatic c.
organic c.
Skoog release of Dupuytren c.
Volkmann c.
contrafissura
contralateral
c. anesthesia
c. biopsy
c. conjugate gaze
c. eye
c. facial paralysis
c. hemiparesis
c. hemiplegia
c. homonymous hemianopia
c. loss
c. monocular nystagmus
c. reflex
c. routing of signal
c. routing of sound
c. sign
c. somatosensory cortex
c. straight leg raising test
c. tactical hypesthesia
c. temporary artery
c. transcallosal approach
contralesional
c. hand
c. hemifield
contrapulsion
ocular c.
c. of saccade
contrast
c. density
c. dye reaction
c. echocardiography magnetic resonance angiography
c. echocardiography magnetic resonance angiography
c. enhancement
c. enhancement imaging
gadolinium c.
inherent c.
iodinated radiographic c.
c. medium
c. opacification
paramagnetic c.
c. sensitivity reduction
soft tissue c.
spontaneous echo c.
contrast-enhanced
c.-e. CT
c.-e. CT scan
c.-e. magnetic resonance angiography
c.-e. MR angiography
c.-e. MRI
c.-e. MR image
c.-e. MR imaging
contrastimulus
contrast-to-noise ratio (CNR)
Contraves stand
Contraves-type floorstand
contrecoup
c. contusion
fracture by c.
c. injury
c. injury of brain
contribution
extracellular c.
intracellular c.
therapeutic c.
control
aberrant autocrine c.
Adcon-L adhesion c.
airway c.
breathing c.
c. chromosome

diffuse noxious inhibitory c. (DNIC)
double visual c.
3D positional c.
Engel classification system for postoperative seizure c. class I–IV
graphomotor c.
idiodynamic c.
immediate c.
impaired c.
inadequate impulse c.
motor c.
c. picture-caption pair
reflex c.
sense of c.
sphincter c.
synergic c.
televised radiofluoroscopic c.
tonic inhibitor c.
tumor c.
vestibuloequilibratory c.

controlled
c. hypothermia
c. mechanical ventilation (CMV)
c. medication trial
C. Oral Word Association (COWA)
C. Oral Word Association test

contusio cerebri

contusion
brain c.
cerebral c.
contrecoup c.
cortical c.
facial c.
gliding c.
hemorrhagic c.
scalp c.
spinal cord c.
wind c.

conus, pl. **coni**
c. medullaris
c. medullaris lesion
c. medullaris root avulsion
c. medullaris syndrome
c. perimedullary arteriovenous fistula
c. terminalis

convection-enhanced drug delivery

conventional
c. factor analysis
c. fractionated irradiation
c. neuroleptic
c. neuroleptic agent
c. neuroleptic drug
c. neuroleptic treatment
c. pharmacotherapy

convergence
c. abnormality
c. insufficiency
c. nucleus of Perlia
c. projection theory
c. spasm

convergence-divergence pattern

convergence-evoked nystagmus

convergence-retraction nystagmus

convergent
c. beam irradiation
c. strabismus

Conversational Skills Rating Scale

converse ocular dipping

conversion
c. disorder
metabolic c.
c. reaction
c. V profile

converter
analog-to-digital c.
digital-to-analog c.

converting enzyme inhibitor (CEI)

Convery polyarticular disability index

convexity
cerebral c.
cortical c.
c. meningioma
c. metastatic tumor

convexobasia

convolution
angular c.
anterior central c.
ascending frontal c.
ascending parietal c.
Broca c.
callosal c.
cingulate c.
first temporal c.
Heschl c.
hippocampal c.
inferior frontal c.
inferior temporal c.
middle frontal c.
middle temporal c.
occipitotemporal c.

NOTES

convolution *(continued)*
posterior central c.
second temporal c.
superior frontal c.
superior temporal c.
supramarginal c.
third temporal c.
transitional c.
transverse temporal c.
Zuckerkandl c.
convulsant threshold
convulsion
autosomal dominant febrile c.
benign familial infantile c.
benign familial neonatal c.
clonic c.
complex febrile c.
coordinate c.
eclamptic c.
epileptiform c.
ether c.
febrile c.
generalized tonic-clonic c.
GTC c.
hysterical c.
hysteroid c.
immediate posttraumatic c.
infantile c.
mimetic c.
mimic c.
paroxysmal c.
salaam c.
static c.
tetanic c.
tonic c.
uremic c.
convulsive
c. reflex
c. seizure
c. state
c. status epilepticus
c. syncope
c. therapy
c. tic
c. tic with coprolalia
convulsivus
status c.
Cook
C. mini-compression balloon catheter
C. stereotactic guide
cooling
autocerebral c.
brain c.
c. helmet
nasopharyngeal c.
c. technique
c. therapy
whole-body c.
Coombs test
cooperativity
criterion of c.
Cooper method
coordinate
c. convulsion
MEG sensorimotor mapping c.
Z c.
coordinated reflex
coordination
fluid c.
impaired c.
poor c.
sudden loss of c.
c. testing
coordinatus
spasmus c.
Copaxone
coping
concept of spiritual c.
maladaptive c.
c. response
c. strategy
copious salivation
copodyskinesia
copolymer
ethylene vinyl alcohol c.
copolymer-1
glatiramer c.-1
copper
c. deposition
serum c.
c. sulfate hydrogel
c. wire effect
Copper-Constantan thermocouple
copper-jacketed bullet
coprolalia
convulsive tic with c.
coprophemia
coproporphyria
hereditary c.
urine c.
copropraxia
copula
coracobrachialis
branch to c.
coral
madreporic c.
cord
accessory portion of spinal c.
anterior column of spinal c.
anterior median fissure of spinal c.
anterolateral column of spinal c.
apex of dorsal horn of spinal c.
apex of posterior horn of spinal c.
arachnoid of spinal c.
autonomic column of spinal c.
base of dorsal horn of spinal c.
base of posterior horn of spinal c.

Bergmann c.
c. bladder
central gelatinous substance of spinal c.
cervical enlargement of spinal c.
cervical part of spinal c.
cervical segment of spinal c. [C1–C8]
coccygeal part of spinal c.
coccygeal segment of spinal c.
cornu of spinal c.
dentate ligament of spinal c.
dorsal column of spinal c.
dorsal funicular column of spinal c.
dorsal median fissure of spinal c.
dura mater of spinal c.
c. embarrassment
fiber tract of spinal c.
gelatinous substance of posterior horn of spinal c.
glioma of spinal c.
gracile fasciculus of spinal c.
intermediate column of spinal c.
intermediate zone of spinal c.
intermediolateral cell column of spinal c.
lateral column of spinal c.
lateral funiculus of spinal c.
Lissauer tract of spinal c.
lumbar enlargement of spinal c.
lumbar part of spinal c.
lumbosacral enlargement of spinal c.
phrenic nucleus of anterior column of spinal c.
posterior column of spinal c.
posterior median fissure of spinal c.
posterior median sulcus of spinal c.
posteromedian column of spinal c.
postmortem spinal c.
segment of spinal c.
spinal c.
subacute combined degeneration of spinal c.
c. syndrome
tethered spinal c.
thoracic part of spinal c.
ventral column of spinal c.
ventral fasciculus proprius of spinal c.
ventral median fissure of spinal c.
vocal c.
Weitbrecht c.
white column of spinal c.
white commissure of spinal c.
white substance of spinal c.
Wilde c.
Willis c.

cordectomy

cordis

C. Brite Tip guiding catheter
chorea c.
C. implantable drug reservoir device
C. Secor implantable pump

Cordis-Hakim

C.-H. shunt system
C.-H. valve

cordopexy

cordotomy

anterolateral c.
c. hook holder
open c.
percutaneous c.
posterior column c.
spinothalamic c.
stereotactic c.

core

c. assessment program for intracerebral transplantation (CAPIT)
bone c.
cancellous c.
central transactional c.
c. characteristic
c. cognitive disturbance
c. pain
c. problem
c. sleep
c. temperature
c. temperature fluctuation

corectopia

coregistered image

coregistration

multimodality image c.

Corgard

Cori disease

corkscrew dural hook

cornea

cloudy c.

NOTES

corneal
c. anesthesia
c. anoxia
c. clouding
c. reflex
c. reflex testing
c. respiration
Cornelia de Lange syndrome
Cornell Scale for Depression in Dementia
corneomandibular reflex
corneomental reflex
corneopterygoid reflex
corn-picker's pupil
cornu, pl. **cornua**
c. ammonis
c. anterius
c. anterius medullae spinalis
c. anterius ventriculi lateralis
c. dorsalis medullae spinalis
c. frontale ventriculi lateralis
c. inferius
c. inferius cartilaginis thyroideae
c. inferius hiatus saphenus
c. inferius marginis
c. inferius ventriculi lateralis
c. laterale
c. laterale medullae spinalis
cornua of lateral ventricle
c. occipitale ventriculi lateralis
c. posterius
c. posterius medullae spinalis
c. posterius ventriculi lateralis
c. of spinal cord
c. temporale ventriculi lateralis
c. ventrale medullae spinalis
cornus
caput c.
corona, pl. **coronae**
c. radiata
Zinn c.
coronal
c. cleft vertebra
c. craniectomy
c. insonation plane
c. orientation
c. plane deformity
c. plane deformity sagittal translation
c. plumbline
c. scalp incision
c. section
c. suture
c. synostosis
coronary
c. artery bypass grafting
c. artery disease (CAD)
c. atherosclerosis
coronata
Cryptococcus c.
coronavirus
corpectomy
anterior c.
cervical c.
median c.
c. model
stackable cage c.
vertebral body c.
corpora (*pl. of* corpus)
corporal agnosia
corporation
Interventional Therapeutics C. (ITC)
corpulence
corpus, pl. **corpora**
c. amygdaloideum
c. aorticum
corpora arenacea
corpora bigemina
c. callosal impingement
c. callosotomy
c. callosum
c. callosum agenesis
c. callosum dysgenesis
corpora cavernosa
c. dentatum
c. fimbriatum
c. fimbriatum hippocampus
c. fornicis
c. geniculatum externum
c. geniculatum internum
c. geniculatum laterale
c. geniculatum mediale
c. juxtarestiforme
c. luteum
c. luysii
c. mamillare
c. medullare cerebelli
c. nuclei caudati
c. olivare
c. paraterminale
c. pineale
c. pontobulbare
corpora quadrigemina
c. quadrigeminum anterius
c. quadrigeminum posterius
c. restiforme
c. striatum
c. striatum syndrome
c. subthalamicum
c. trapezoideum
corpuscallostomy
corpuscle
articular c.
axile c.
axis c.
bulboid c.
chorea c.

chromophil c.
compound granular c.
Dogiel c.
genital c.
Gluge c.
Golgi c.
Golgi-Mazzoni c.
Herbst c.
Krause c.
lamellated c.
lingual c.
Mazzoni c.
Meissner c.
Merkel c.
oval c.
pacchionian c.
Pacini c.
pacinian c.
Purkinje c.
Ruffini c.
Schwalbe c.
tactile c.
taste c.
terminal nerve c.
Timofeew c.
touch c.
Valentin c.
Vater c.
Vater-Pacini c.

corpusculum, pl. **corpuscula**
c. articulare
corpuscula articularia
corpuscula bulboidea
c. genitale
corpuscula lamellosa
c. lamellosum
corpuscula nervosa terminalia
c. nervosum terminale
c. tactus
corpuscula tactus

correction
anterior c.
King type I–V curve posterior c.
kyphosis c.
mechanism of c.
rotational c.
small-volume c. (SVC)
surgical c.

correlate
anatomical c.
biologic c.
clinical c.
differential c.

correlation
image c.
intraclass c.
item-total c.
c. method
potential c.
c. time

corridor
transcallosal interforniceal c.

corroborative test

corrugator supercilii muscle

corset
lumbosacral c.
Warm 'n Form lumbosacral c.

Cortech guidance

Cortef

cortex, pl. **cortices**
adrenal c.
agranular c.
amorphous fraction of adrenal c.
anterior cingulate c.
articular c.
association c.
auditory association c.
calcarine c.
cellular layers of c.
cerebellar c.
c. cerebellaris
c. cerebelli
cerebral c.
c. cerebralis
c. cerebri
c. circuit
contralateral somatosensory c.
dispensable c.
dorsal premotor c.
dorsolateral prefrontal c.
double c.
dysgranular c.
eloquent c.
entorhinal c.
epileptogenic c.
excitomotor c.
extrastriate visual c.
extrastriate V5/MT c.
free functional c.
frontotemporal c.
fusiform cell of cerebral c.
ganglionic layer of cerebellar c.
ganglionic layer of cerebral c.

NOTES

cortex *(continued)*
granular layer of cerebellar c.
granular layer of cerebral c.
gustatory c.
hemispheric hippocampal c.
heteromodal association c.
heterotypic c.
homotypic c.
inferior prefrontal c.
inferior temporal c.
insular c.
ipsilateral somatosensory c.
ipsilateral temporal c.
lamina of the cerebral c.
laminated c.
language-associated c.
language-specific c.
lateral orbitofrontal c.
layer of cerebellar c.
layer of cerebral c.
limbic c.
medial frontal c.
medial orbitofrontal c.
medial prefrontal c. (mPFC)
medial temporal c.
mesial epileptogenic c.
mesial frontal c.
molecular layer of cerebellar c.
molecular layer of cerebral c.
motor c.
multiform layer of cerebral c.
multimodal association c.
nonolfactory c.
occipital c.
occipitotemporal c.
olfactory c.
opercular c.
orbital prefrontal c.
orbitofrontal c.
paralimbic c.
parastriate c.
parietal c.
periamygdaloid c.
perilesional inhibitory c.
perirolandic parietal c.
peristriate c.
perisylvian c.
piriform c.
plexiform layer of cerebral c.
polymicrogyric c.
posterior language c.
posterior parietal c. (PPC)
postinduction occipital c.
prefrontal c.
preinduction occipital c.
premotor c.
prepiriform c.
primary auditory c.
primary motor c.
primary sensorimotor c.
primary sensory c.
primary somatosensory c.
primary visual c.
right basilar mesial temporoparietal c.
rolandic c.
rostral medial prefrontal c.
secondary sensory c.
secondary somatosensory c.
secondary visual c.
sensory c.
somatosensory c.
somesthetic c.
stellate cell of cerebral c.
striate c.
subcortical band heterotopia/double c.
subcortical ectopic c.
sulcal prefrontal c.
supplementary motor c.
temporal c.
unimodal association c.
ventromedial prefrontal c.
vertebral body anterior c.
visual association c.
zonal layer of cerebral c.

Cortexplorer cerebral blood flow monitor

Corti
C. cell
C. ganglion
C. organ
C. pillar
pillar cell of C.
C. rod

cortical
c. achromia
c. activity
c. amygdaloid nucleus
c. aphasia
c. apraxia
c. area
c. arousal
c. atrophy
c. audiometry
c. basal ganglionic degeneration
c. blindness
c. contusion
c. convexity
c. deafness
c. dementia
c. development malformation
c. disconnection syndrome
c. dysgenesis
c. dysplasia
c. epilepsy
c. epileptogenic focus
c. fast wave

c. functional mapping
c. functioning
c. gray matter
c. gray matter deficit
c. gray region
c. hamartoma
c. incision coronary dilator
c. infarction
c. input
c. language circuitry
c. lesion
c. Lewy body
c. mapping of memory function
c. metabolism
c. microcirculatory flow
c. microdysgenesia
c. motor output
c. myoclonus
c. neuritic plaque
c. obliteration
c. organization
c. pathology
c. plasticity
c. plate
c. pyramidal neuron
c. reorganization
c. resection
c. screw
c. seizure focus
c. sensibility
c. sensory loss
c. somatosensory evoked potential
c. spreading depression (CSD)
c. stimulation
c. structure
c. substance of cerebellum
c. sulcus
c. tissue
c. transient ischemia
c. tuber
c. undercutting
c. vein
c. venous thrombosis
c. volume

corticalis
agenesia c.
nucleus amygdalae c.
pars c.

corticalization
cortical-striatal-pallidal-thalamic neural circuit
corticectomy
frontal c.
occipital c.
parietal c.

cortices (*pl. of* cortex)
corticifugal
corticipetal
corticoafferent
corticoautonomic
corticobulbar
c. deficit
c. fiber
c. motor neuron
c. pathway
c. tract

corticobulbaris
tractus c.

corticocancellous strut
corticocerebellum
corticodiencephalic
corticoefferent
corticofugal pathway
corticography
corticohypothalamic tract
corticomedial
corticomeningeal angiomatosis
corticomesencephalic
c. fiber
c. tract

corticomesencephalicae
fibrae c.

corticonucleares
fibrae c.

corticopeduncular
corticopontinae
fibrae c.

corticopontine
c. fiber
c. tract

corticopontini
tractus c.

corticopontocerebellar tract
corticoreticulares
fibrae c.

corticorubral
c. fiber
c. tract

corticorubrales
fibrae c.

corticospinal
c. atrophy
c. axon

NOTES

corticospinal *(continued)*
c. disease
c. fiber
c. motor neuron
c. motor pathway
c. motor system dysfunction
c. pathway lesion
c. tract
corticospinales
fibrae c.
corticospinalis
tractus c.
corticosteroid
oral c.
postoperative c.
c. therapy
corticostriatal slice
corticothalamicae
fibrae c.
corticothalamic fiber
corticotomy
Ilizarov c.
subperiosteal c.
corticotroph cell
corticotrophic axis
corticotropin
corticotropin-releasing
c.-r. factor
c.-r. hormone (CRH)
cortisol
c. level
c. and sodium succinate
cortisone acetate
cortistatin neuropeptide
cortone acetate
Corynebacterium diphtheriae
Cosman-Roberts-Wells (CRW)
CRW stereotactic head frame
CRW stereotactic ring
CRW stereotactic system
costal arch reflex
costaricensis
Angiostrongylus c.
Costen syndrome
costimulatory
c. molecule expression
c. signal
c. stimulus
costocervical artery
costoclavicular syndrome
cost-of-illness study
costopectoral reflex
costotransversectomy
c. approach
posterolateral c.
costotransverse ligament
costovertebral ligament
cosyntropin
cotinine
serum c.
cotransmitter
peptide c.
Cotrel
C. pedicle screw
C. pedicle screw fixation strength
C. pedicle screw rigidity
Cotrel-Dubousset (C-D)
C.-D. distraction system
C.-D. dynamic transverse traction device
C.-D. fixation
C.-D. hook claw configuration
C.-D. pedicle screw instrumentation
C.-D. rod
C.-D. rod flexibility
C.-D. screw-rod system
C.-D. spinal instrumentation
cotrimoxazole
Cotte
C. operation
C. presacral neurectomy
Cottle
C. elevator
C. knife
Cottle-Neivert retractor
cotton
oxidized c.
c. pad
c. pledget
c. wrap
cottonoid
c. covering
c. pledget
cotton-wool
c.-w. plaque
c.-w. sign
c.-w. spot
Cotugno disease
cotunnii
aqueductus c.
Cotunnius
C. aqueduct
C. canal
C. disease
C. nerve
couch
Boston neurosurgical c.
Siemens c.
couch-mounted head frame
cough
habit c.
c. headache
c. reflex
c. syncope
trigeminal c.

coughing
c. center
c. sign
council
Medical Research C. (MRC)
count
absolute neutrophil c. (ANC)
complete blood c. (CBC)
platelet c.
radioactive c.
white blood cell c.
counteracting impulsivity
countercurrent immunoelectrophoresis test
counterintuitive relationship
countermeasure
sleepiness c.
Counterpoint electromyograph
counterpulsion
enhanced external c. (EECP)
external c. (ECP)
countertransference
counting disruption
coup injury of brain
Couples BrainMap
coupling
excitation-contraction c.
G-protein c.
spin-spin c.
courage
Dutch C.
Cournand arteriogram needle
Cournand-Grino arteriogram needle
course
chronic c.
developmental c.
Functional Obstacle C.
c. of illness measure
long-term c.
rapid fluctuating c.
recurrent c.
temporal c.
Courtship Analysis
couvade crapulent
COV
coefficient of variation
covariation
intersegmental c.
cover
Accu-Flo polyethylene bur hole c.
Accu-Flo silicone rubber bur hole c.
bur hole c.
c. test
titanium mini bur hole c.
coverage
neocortical c.
whole-brain c.
covering
cottonoid c.
meningeal c.
meningothelial c.
titanium mini bur hole c.
covert face recognition
COWA
Controlled Oral Word Association
Cowden disease
Cowdry inclusion body type A, B
Cowdry-type intranuclear inclusion body
CO_2-withdrawal seizure test
COX
cyclooxygenase
COX-1
cyclooxygenase-1
COX-2
cyclooxygenase-2
COX-2 inhibitor
***Coxiella burnetii* infection**
Cox regression analysis
coxsackie encephalitis
coxsackievirus
c. A, B
c. infection paralytic syndrome
c. meningitis
CP
cerebellopontine
CPA
cerebellopontine angle
CPAP
continuous positive airway pressure
nasal CPAP
CPEO
chronic progressive external ophthalmoplegia
CPH
chronic paroxysmal hemicrania
CPH-tic syndrome
CPPD
calcium pyrophosphate dihydrate
CPT
Continuous Performance test
current perception threshold

C

NOTES

CR
conditioned reflex
Sinemet CR
CRA
cis-retinoic acid
13-CRA
13-*cis*-retinoic acid
cracked pot sign
crack-like vessel
crackling
parchment c.
craft palsy
Cragg thrombolytic brush
Craig vertebral body biopsy instrument
cramp
accessory c.
c. benign fasciculation
benign fasciculation with c.
intermittent c.
leg c.
miner's c.
muscle c.
musician's c.
nocturnal leg c.
pianist's c.
seamstress's c.
shaving c.
stoker's c.
tailor's c.
violinist's c.
waiter's c.
watchmaker's c.
writer's c.
crania (*pl. of* cranium)
cranial
c. access device
c. aneurysm
c. anomaly
c. arachnoid
c. arachnoid mater
c. arteritis
c. artery
c. autonomic ganglia
c. autonomic symptom
c. bifida
c. bone fixation plate
c. bone graft
c. calcification
c. capacity
c. cerebellar peduncle
c. computed tomography
c. cracked pot sign
c. cuff
c. dermal sinus
c. dysmorphism
c. epidural abscess
c. extension
c. flexure
c. fracture
c. insufflation
c. Jacobs hook
c. motor nucleus
c. muscle
c. nerve
c. nerve abnormality
c. nerve compression
c. nerve congenital disorder
c. nerve damage
c. nerve deficit
c. nerve dissection
c. nerve dysfunction
c. nerve examination
c. nerve heredodegenerative disease
c. nerve manipulation
c. nerve monitoring
c. nerve neoplasm
c. nerve palsy
c. nerve postinfectious disorder
c. nerve regeneration
c. nerve repair
c. nerve trauma
c. neuralgia
c. neuropathy
c. olivary nucleus
c. osteomyelitis
c. osteopetrosis
c. osteosynthesis
c. osteosynthesis system
c. perforator
c. perfusion pressure
c. pia mater
c. plating system
c. polyneuritis
c. polyneuropathy
c. puncture
c. radiosurgery
c. reflex
c. rongeur
c. rongeur forceps
c. root
c. settling
c. suture
c. synostosis
c. ultrasonography
c. ultrasound
c. vault
c. vault trephination
c. venous obstruction
craniales
nervi c.
radices c.
cranialis
arachnoidea mater c.
arachnoid mater c.
frenulum veli medullaris c.
ganglion sensorium nervi c.
nucleus nervi c.

nucleus olivaris c.
pia mater c.
cranialium
nuclei nervorum c.
cranialization
craniamphitomy
craniectomy
bilateral craniectomies
coronal c.
decompressive c.
linear c.
metopic c.
partial-thickness c.
retromastoid suboccipital c.
retrosigmoid c.
suboccipital c.
cranii
osteoporosis circumscripta c.
periostitis interna c.
pneumatocele c.
cranioblade
Acra-Cut c.
Codman c.
Spiral Flute c.
craniobuccal cyst
CranioCap custom-made cranial orthosis
craniocardiac reflex
craniocele
craniocephalic disproportion
craniocerebellocardiac syndrome
craniocerebral
c. drug trauma
c. missile injury
trauma c.
c. trauma hyperventilation
craniocervical
c. flexion test
c. junction
c. junction injury
c. plate
c. region
craniofacial
c. angle
c. condition
c. dysjunction
c. dysostosis
c. dysraphism
c. malformation
c. osteotomy
c. reconstruction
c. remodeling
c. resection
c. structure
c. surgery
craniofrontonasal dysplasia
craniognomy
craniolacunia
craniology
Gall c.
craniomalacia
circumscribed c.
craniomaxillofacial plating system
craniomeningocele
craniometaphysial dysplasia
craniometry
cranioorbital
c. deformity
c. zygomatic craniotomy
craniopathy
craniopharyngeal
c. canal
c. duct tumor
craniopharyngioma
adamantinomatous c.
ameloblastomatous c.
cystic papillomatous c.
intrasellar c.
monocystic c.
cranioplasty
acrylic c.
alloplastic c.
aluminum c.
cartilage c.
metallic c.
methylmethacrylate c.
c. plate
rib c.
tantalum c.
vascularized split calvarial c.
craniopuncture
craniorachischisis
craniosacral
c. nervous system
c. vault (CV)
c. vault 4 (CV4)
cranioschisis
craniosclerosis
cranioscopy
craniosinus fistula
craniospinal
c. irradiation
c. meningioma
c. MRI with gadolinium enhancement

NOTES

craniospinal *(continued)*
c. sensory ganglion
c. space
craniostenosis
craniosynostosis
lambdoid c.
sagittal c.
craniotabes
craniotome
Anspach c.
Caspar c.
Freiberg c.
Hall neurosurgical c.
Midas Rex c.
Mira Mark V c.
Smith air c.
craniotomy
attached c.
awake c.
bifrontal c.
cranioorbital zygomatic c.
CT-assisted stereotactic c.
c. cut
detached c.
endoscope-assisted c.
c. flap
frontal c.
frontotemporal c.
frontotemporoparietal c.
keyhole c.
open stereotactic c.
orbital zygomatic c.
osteoplastic c.
parietal c.
parietooccipital c.
posterior fossa c.
pterional c.
radical decompressive c.
retromastoid c.
retrosigmoid c.
right parietal occipital vertex c.
right temporoparietal c.
stereotactic-guided c.
stereotactic microsurgical c.
subfrontal c.
suboccipital c.
suprabrow transorbital roof c.
supratentorial c.
temporal c.
temporooccipital c.
trephine c.
Yasargil c.
craniotonoscopy
craniotopography
craniotrypesis
craniovertebral junction
cranium, pl. **crania**
beaten copper c.
bifid c.
c. bifidum
c. bifidum cysticum
c. bifidum occultum
pediatric c.
cranium-affixed fiducial
crankshaft
c. clip
c. phenomenon
crapulent
couvade c.
crapulous
crash induction of anesthesia
Crawford dural elevator
CRD
complex repetitive discharge
CRD on electromyogram
C-reactive
C-r. protein (CRP)
C-r. protein test
crease
hand palmar c.
palmar c.
simian c.
creatine
c. kinase (CK)
c. kinase equilibrium
c. kinase-MB fraction (CK-MB)
c. phosphokinase
c. transporter defect
creatinine
c. clearance
c. deficiency syndrome
c. kinase serum level
urinary c.
creation
kyphosis c.
lordosis c.
creative reasoning test
CREB binding protein
Cre + Cho ratio
Creed dissector
creeping palsy
Cree Questionnaire
cremasteric reflex
crepuscular state
crescendo
c. sleep
c. transient ischemic attack
crescentic lobule of cerebellum
CREST
calcinosis, Raynaud phenomenon, esophageal motility disorders, sclerodactyly, and telangiectasia
CREST syndrome
crest
acoustic c.
acousticofacial c.
ampullary c.
cap of ampullary c.

central nervous system neural c.
falciform c.
ganglionic c.
neural c.
neuroepithelium of ampullary c.
supramastoid c.
transverse c.
triangular c.
trigeminal c.
vestibular c.
c. of vestibule

Creutzfeldt-Jakob disease (CJD)

CRH
corticotropin-releasing hormone

criblé
état c.

cribriform plate

cribrosa
lamina c.
macula c.

cribrosae
maculae c.

cribrosus
status c.

Crichton-Browne sign

cricoarytenoid
c. ankylosis
c. muscle

cricoid ring

cricopharyngeal
c. achalasia
c. muscle

cricothyrotomy

cri du chat syndrome

Crigler-Najjar
C.-N. disease
C.-N. syndrome

Crile
C. artery forceps
C. clamp
C. gasserian ganglion knife
C. gasserian ganglion knife and dissector
C. head traction
C. hemostat
C. needle holder
C. nerve hook
C. nerve hook and dissector
C. retractor

crisis, pl. **crises**
adrenal c.
cholinergic c.
gastric c.
laryngeal c.
myasthenic c.
nephralgic c.
oculocephalogyric c.
oculogyric c.
parkinsonian c.
spondylolisthetic c.
tabetic c.
tyramine-induced hypertensive c.
visceral c.

crispation

crista, pl. **cristae**
c. ampullaris
c. basilaris ductus
c. basilaris ductus cochlearis
c. galli
c. quarta
c. transversa
c. transversalis
c. transversa meatus acustici interni
c. triangularis
c. vestibuli

criterion, pl. **criteria**
c. of associativity
Barkhof MRI criteria
Bartel criteria
clinical c.
c. of cooperativity
dependence c.
diagnostic c.
c. F
field-tested c.
Gordon criteria
Hunt and Hess criteria
c. level
level-of-care c.
MacNab criteria
McDonald criteria
Mulholland and Gunn criteria
Nyquist sampling criteria
Osserman criteria
patient placement c.
Poser criteria
a priori c.
criteria of Rechtschaffen and Kales
restrictive c.
criteria of Rowland
Schumacher criteria
c. of specificity
traditional circulatory criteria (TCC)

C

NOTES

criterion *(continued)*
Volpe criteria
White and Panjabi criteria
***Crithidia* IFA test**
critical
c. illness myopathy (CIM)
c. illness polyneuropathy
c. perfusion
criticus
status c.
Crixivan
CRLR
calcitonin receptor-like receptor
Crockard
C. retractor
C. transoral clip applier
Crock-Yamagishi system
crocodile tears syndrome
Crohn disease
Cronbach alpha
Crooke
C. granule
C. hyaline change
C. hyalinization
cross
Ranvier c.
cross-aggregation
cross-bracing
spinal rod c.-b.
Wiltse system c.-b.
Cross-Cultural Smell Identification Test
crossed
c. adductor jerk
c. adductor reflex
c. adductor sign
c. anesthesia
c. aphasia
c. coil
c. extension reflex
c. eye
c. hemianesthesia
c. hemiplegia
c. knee jerk
c. knee reflex
c. laterality
c. lens
c. paralysis
c. phrenic phenomenon
c. pyramidal tract
c. reflex of pelvis
c. spinoadductor reflex
crossed immunoelectrophoresis
crossed-screw fixation
cross-face
c.-f. anastomosis
c.-f. graft
cross-facial nerve graft anastomosis
cross-flow reserve
crossing
arteriovenous c.
Mistichelli c.
Crossing-Off Test
cross-legged
c.-l. clip
c.-l. progression
crosslink
Edwards modular system rod c.
Galveston fixation with TSRH c.
c. gamma
Texas Scottish Rite Hospital c.
crosslinking
crossover study
cross-reacting nerve glycoconjugate
cross-sectional
c.-s. area (CSA)
c.-s. assessment
c.-s. component
c.-s. evaluation
c.-s. experimental study design
c.-s. image
c.-s. research
c.-s. snapshot
c.-s. study
crossway
sensory c.
croup
postextubation c.
Crouzon
C. disease
C. syndrome
crowding theory
Crowe sign
Crow-Fukase syndrome
crown
Bremer halo c.
radiate c.
crown-heel length
crown-rump length
CRP
C-reactive protein
cruciata
hemianesthesia c.
hemiplegia c.
cruciate
c. eminence
c. ligament
cruciform
c. eminence
c. slit valve
cruciformis
eminentia c.
crura (*pl. of* crus)
crural
c. ataxia
c. cistern
c. interosseus nerve
c. monoplegia

c. paresis
c. plexus
cruralis
cisterna c.
cruris
nervus interosseus c.
tegmen c.
crus, pl. **crura**
c. anterius capsulae
c. anterius capsulae internae
cerebellum superior c.
c. cerebri
common c.
c. fornicis
c. of fornix
internal capsule anterior c.
internal capsule posterior c.
crura membranacea
crura membranacea ampullaria ductuum semicircularium
c. membranaceum commune
c. membranaceum commune ductuum semicircularium
c. membranaceum simplex
c. membranaceum simplex ductus semicircularis
crura ossea
crura ossea canalium semicircularium
c. posterius capsulae
c. posterius capsulae internae
crush injury
crusotomy
crutch
c. palsy
c. paralysis
Crutchfield
C. carotid artery clamp
C. drill point
C. hand drill
C. skeletal traction tongs
C. skull traction tongs
Crutchfield-Raney skull traction tongs
Cruveilhier
C. atrophy
C. disease
C. paralysis
C. plexus
cruzi
Trypanosoma c.
Cruz trypanosomiasis
CRW
Cosman-Roberts-Wells
CRW arc system
CRW base frame
CRW head frame
CRW stereotactic system
CRx Diamond valve
cry
epileptic c.
c. reflex
cryalgesia
cryanesthesia
cryesthesia
crying-cat syndrome
crymodynia
cryoanalgesia
cryocooler assembly
Cryocup ice massager
cryoglobulinemia
cryoglobulinemic vasculitis
cryohypophysectomy
transsphenoidal c.
cryolesion
brain c.
cryomagnet
Cryomedical Sciences, Inc.
cryomicrotome sectioning
cryopallidectomy
cryoprecipitate coagulum
cryopreserved tissue
cryoprobe
cryopulvinectomy
cryospasm
cryostat
cryosurgery
cryothalamectomy
cryothalamotomy
cryptic
c. arteriovenous malformation
c. cerebrovascular malformation
c. vascular malformation
cryptococcal
c. antigen
granuloma c.
c. infection
c. meningitis
c. organism
c. polysaccharide antigen test
c. spondylitis
cryptococcoma
cryptococcosis
intracranial c.

NOTES

Cryptococcus
- *C. albicans*
- *C. coronata*
- *C.* infection
- *C. neoformans*

cryptogenic
- c. drop attack
- c. epileptic encephalopathy
- c. hemifacial spasm
- c. infarction
- c. infection
- c. late-onset epilepsy
- c. myoclonic epilepsy
- c. neocortical epilepsy
- c. partial epilepsy
- c. stroke

cryptomerorachischisis
cryptotia
crystal
- cholesterol c.

crystallin
crystalline birefringence
crystallizable
- fragment c. (Fc)

crystallization
- symptom c.

CS
conditioned stimulus
CSA
central sleep apnea
cross-sectional area
CSD
catscratch disease
cortical spreading depression
CSF
cerebrospinal fluid
- CSF analysis
- CSF bacterial culture
- CSF characteristic
- CSF chemokine
- CSF Gram stain
- CSF marker
- CSF otorrhea
- CSF outflow pathway
- CSF pressure syndrome
- CSF rhinorrhea
- CSF to serum glucose ratio
- CSF shunt
- CSF tau protein abnormality

C-shaped
- C-s. incision
- C-s. microplate
- C-s. resistive magnet
- C-s. scalp flap

CT
computed tomography
- CT bone window
- contiguous nonoverlapping axial CT
- contrast-enhanced CT
- dynamic CT
- metrizamide-enhanced CT
- CT scan
- serial CT
- stable xenon CT
- xenon CT
- xenon-enhanced CT

CT-assisted stereotactic craniotomy
C-Tek anterior cervical plate system
C-terminal fragment
C-terminus
CT-guided
- CT-g. biopsy
- CT-g. stereotactic evacuation

CTI-Siemens
- CTI-S. 933/08-12 PET camera
- CTI-S. 933 tomograph

CTS
carpal tunnel syndrome
CTSIB
Clinical Test of Sensory Interaction and Balance
C-type natriuretic peptide
Cuban epidemic neuropathy
cubital
- c. nerve
- c. tunnel
- c. tunnel syndrome

cuboidal cell
cuboidodigital reflex
cue
- auditory c.
- c. effect
- environmental c.
- external c.
- interoceptive c.
- nonverbal c.
- response-produced c.
- semantic c.
- specific sensory c.
- trauma c.
- verbal c.

cue-induced subjective effect
cueing
- attentional c.
- semantic c.
- sensory c.

Cueva cranial nerve electrode
cuff
- cranial c.
- Finapres finger c.
- perivascular c.

cuffing
- perivascular c.

cuirass
- analgesic c.
- tabetic c.

cul-de-sac
- conjunctival c.-d.-s.

Culler hook
culmen, pl. **culmina**
c. cerebelli
culminis
lobulus c.
culture
blood c.
bullying c.
cell c.
cerebellar aggregation c.
CSF bacterial c.
C. Fair Intelligence Test
forebrain cell c.
fungal c.
immortalized primary cell c.
c. medium
tissue c.
culture-specific intervention
Cummins disc prosthesis
cumulative
c. dose
c. effect
c. medication reduction
c. stressor
c. trauma disorder
cuneate
c. fasciculus
c. funiculus
c. nucleus
c. tubercle
cuneati
nucleus funiculi c.
tuberculum nuclei c.
cuneatum
tuberculum c.
cuneatus
fasciculus c.
nucleus c.
cunei (*pl. of* cuneus)
cuneiform
c. lobe
c. nucleus
cuneiformis
lobulus c.
nucleus c.
cuneocerebellar
c. fiber
c. tract
cuneocerebellares
fibrae c.
cuneospinales
fibrae c.
cuneospinal fiber
cuneus, pl. **cunei**
cup
c. catheter
c. ear
c. forceps
ocular c.
optic c.
Cupid's
C. bow contour
C. bow sign
Cuprimine
cup-to-disc ratio
cupula, pl. **cupulae**
ampullary c.
c. cochlea
c. cristae ampullaris
cupular
c. part
c. part of epitympanic recess
cupularis
pars c.
cupulate part
cupulolithiasis
curare poisoning
curarization-induced flaccidity
curette, curet
blunt-ring c.
bone c.
Cloward-Cone ring c.
Cone ring c.
Cone suction biopsy c.
disc c.
downbiting Epstein c.
Epstein c.
flat back c.
Halle bone c.
Hardy c.
Hibbs spinal c.
Hibbs-Spratt spinal fusion c.
Howard spinal c.
Jansen bone c.
Malis c.
Marino transsphenoidal c.
Mayfield spinal c.
oval c.
pituitary c.
Raney stirrup-loop c.
Ray pituitary c.
reverse-angled c.
Rhoton blunt-ring c.
Rhoton loop c.

NOTES

curette *(continued)*
Rhoton spoon c.
Richards c.
ring c.
Scoville ruptured disc c.
Semmes c.
straight ring c.
transsphenoidal c.
vertical ring c.
current
alternating c. (AC)
ascending c.
audiofrequency eddy c.
centrifugal c.
centripetal c.
demarcation c.
c. depression
descending c.
direct c. (DC)
eddy c.
electrotonic c.
hyperpolarization-activated cationic c.
hyperpolarization-activated chloride c.
hyperpolarizing c.
inhibitory postsynaptic c.
c. of injury
nerve-action c.
c. perception threshold (CPT)
radiofrequency eddy c.
receptor-mediated c.
Curschmann-Steinert
C.-S. disease
C.-S. syndrome
curse
Ondine c.
cursiva
epilepsia c.
curtailed sleep
curvature
vertebral c.
curve
accommodation c.
area under c.
best-fit c.
developmental c.
double thoracic c.
frequency dispersion c.
isodose c.
Kaplan-Meier survival c.
King type I–V c.
low single thoracic c.
lumbar c.
nonlinear developmental c.
c. progression
right thoracic c.
rigid c.
severe rigid right thoracic c.
signal intensity c.
specific c.
strength-duration c.
survival c.
thoracolumbar c.
time-density c.
curved
c. cannula with locking dilator
c. conventional microscissors
c. electrode
c. incision
c. knot-tying forceps
c. microneedle holder
c. vertebral surface
curved-tipped spatula
CUSA
Cavitron Ultrasonic Surgical Aspirator
CUSA CEM system
CUSA electrosurgical module
CUSA system 200 straight autoclavable handpiece
CUSA tip
Cushing
C. basophilia
C. basophilism
C. bayonet forceps
C. bipolar forceps
C. bivalve retractor
C. brain forceps
C. brain spatula
C. brain spatula spoon
C. cranial bur
C. cranial perforator
C. cranial rongeur
C. decompressive retractor
C. disease
C. dressing forceps
C. dural hook
C. dural hook knife
C. effect
C. gasserian ganglion hook
C. intervertebral disc rongeur
C. Little Joker elevator
C. monopolar forceps
C. nerve hook
C. nerve retractor
C. periosteal elevator
C. phenomenon
C. pituitary elevator
C. pituitary scoop
C. pituitary spoon
C. reflex
C. response
C. saw
C. saw guide
C. staphylorrhaphy elevator
C. subtemporal retractor
C. syndrome
C. technique

C. tissue forceps
C. triad in brain tumor
C. ulcer
C. vein retractor
C. ventricular needle
Cushing-Landolt speculum
cushingoid
cushion
Carter immobilization c.
Vac-Lok c.
custom implant
customized jig
cut
craniotomy c.
Panama c.
visual field c.
cutaneomeningospinal angiomatosis
cutaneous
c. abnormality
c. adenoma
c. allodynia
c. angioma
c. anthrax
c. circulation
c. electrical stimulation
c. horn
c. mechanoreceptor
c. meningioma
c. nerve
c. neurofibromatosis
c. nociceptor
c. pupil reflex
c. receptor
c. sensation
cutaneus
nervus c.
ramus c.
cut-film angiography
cut-flow index (CFI)
cutis
neuroma c.
cutoff score
cutter
dowel c.
Howmedica microfixation system plate c.
Leibinger Micro System plate c.
CV
craniosacral vault
CV4
craniosacral vault 4
CVA
cerebrovascular accident
CVM
cerebral venous malformation
CVS
chorionic villus sampling
CW
continuous wave
cyanide poisoning
cyanoacrylate
N-butyl c.
c. glue
c. polymer sealant
cyanophilous
cyanopsia, cyanopia
cyanotic congenital heart disease
CyberKnife
Accuray C.
C. planning system
C. robotic radiosurgery system
C. stereotactic radiosurgery/radiotherapy system
C. technique
cybermedicine
cybernetics
Cyberonics vagus nerve stimulator electrode
Cyberware digitizer
Cybon surgical navigation tool
cyclase
adenyl c.
adenylate c.
adenylyl c.
guanylate c.
guanylyl c.
cycle
c.'s of afternystagmus
brain wave c.
cell c.
circannual c.
citric acid c.
disturbed sleep-wake c.
fusion-defusion c.
Hodgkin c.
introjective-projective c.
late luteal phase of menstrual c.
menstrual c.
normal sleep c.
sleep c.
sleep-awake c.
sleep-wake c.
urea c.

NOTES

cyclic
c. adenosine monophosphate
c. alteration
c. deoxyribonucleic acid
c. depression
c. endoperoxide
c. vomiting
c. vomiting syndrome
cyclicity
sleep-wake c.
cyclin box
cyclin-dependent kinase inhibitory protein
cycling
futile c.
phase c.
cyclizine
cyclobarbital
cyclobenzaprine hydrochloride
cyclohexylchloroethylnitrosurea chemotherapy
cyclooxygenase (COX)
c. enzyme
c. inhibitor
cyclooxygenase-1 (COX-1)
cyclooxygenase-2 (COX-2)
Cyclopan
cyclopentolate
cyclophosphamide
cyclopia
cycloplegia
cyclops lesion
cycloserine
cyclosporine, cyclosporin A
cyclothyme
cyclothymic PD
cyclotorsion
eye c.
Cygnus PFS Image-Guided system
cylinder
axis c.
pneumatic c.
Ruffini c.
terminal c.
cylindraxis
cylindrical spiral myopathy
cylindroma
Cymbalta
cynic spasm
Cyon nerve
cyproheptadine hydrochloride
cyst
aneurysmal bone c.
apoplectic c.
arachnoid c.
arachnoidal c.
bilateral arachnoid c.'s
bilateral choroid plexus c.'s
bone c.
brain c.
cerebellar arachnoid c.
cerebellopontine angle arachnoid c.
cholesterol c.
colloid c.
craniobuccal c.
Dandy-Walker c.
daughter c.
dentigerous c.
dermoid c.
endodermal c.
enteric c.
enterogenous c.
ependymal c.
epidermoid c.
extradural c.
extraforaminal synovial c.
c. fenestration
foramen magnum c.
foregut c.
frontoparietal convexity c.
giant sacral perineural c.
glial parenchymal c.
hydatid c.
interhemispheric c.
intracerebral hydatid c.
intracranial arachnoid c.
intradiploic epidermoid c.
intramedullary epidermoid c.
intraneural ganglion c.
intraparenchymal c.
intrapituitary c.
intrasellar Rathke cleft c.
intraspinal c.
juxtaarticular c.
leptomeningeal c.
lumbar synovial c.
middle cranial fossa c.
mucous retention c.
nasopharyngeal mucus retention c.
neural c.
neurenteric c.
neuroenteric c.
neuroepithelial c.
nonenteric c.
paraphysial c.
paraventricular c.
perineurial c.
pineal c.
pontine hydatid c.
pontomedullary epidermoid c.
porencephalic c.
posttraumatic leptomeningeal c.
primary epidural c.
quadrigeminal arachnoid c.
radicular c.
Rathke cleft c.
Rathke pouch c.
recurrent enteric c.

retinal c.
sacral nerve root c.
sellar c.
soapsuds c.
solitary hydatid c.
spinal canal hydatid c.
spinal cord arachnoid c.
spinal endodermal c.
spinal neurenteric c.
spinal synovial c.
spindle-shaped c.
subarachnoid ependymal c.
subperiosteal c.
suprasellar c.
synovial c.
Tarlov c.
temporal arachnoid c.
thyroglossal duct c.
Tornwaldt c.
unicameral bone c.
c. wall excision
xanthogranulomatous c.
xanthomatous Rathke cleft c.

cystadenoma
apocrine c.
cystine c.
eccrine c.
c. lymphomatosum

cystathionine synthetase deficiency
cystathioninuria aminoaciduria
cystatin B, C
cysteine
c. protease
c. protease inhibitor
c. proteinase
secreted protein acidic and rich in c.

cystic
c. astrocytoma
c. degenerative disorder
c. encephalomalacia
c. fibrosis
c. hydroma
c. intraparenchymal meningioma
c. lacunar infarction
c. mass
c. medial necrosis
c. microadenoma
c. myelomalacia
c. papillomatous craniopharyngioma
c. periventricular leukomalacia

cystica
hydronephrosis in spina bifida c.
spina bifida c.
urinary infection in spina bifida c.

cysticercal infection
cysticerci
subarachnoid c.

cysticercosis
intraventricular c.

cysticercus
migrating intraventricular c.

cysticum
cranium bifidum c.

cystine cystadenoma
cystoatrial shunt
Cystografin
cystoma
papilliferous c.

cystoscope
cytarabine liposome
cytoarchitectonic abnormality
cytoarchitectonics
cytoarchitectural asymmetry
cytoarchitecture
neural c.

cytochrome
c. *c*
c. *c* oxidase
c. *c* oxidase deficiency
c. oxidase defect
c. oxidase deficiency
c. P
c. P450 metabolism

cytodendrite
cytodistal
cytodomain
cytogenetic study
cytoid body
cytokeratin
low molecular weight c.

cytokine
c. bias
inflammatory c.
c. inhibitor
interacting c.
TH1 c.
TH2 c.

cytology
cytolysis

NOTES

cytomegalic
c. inclusion disease
c. inclusion virus
cytomegalovirus (CMV)
c. meningitis
c. polyradiculomyelitis (CMV-PRAM)
c. ventriculoencephalitis
Cytomel
cytometry
flow c.
cytopathy
mitochondrial c.
cytophotometry
Feulgen c.
cytoplasm
neuronal c.
cytoplasmic
c. body myopathy
c. desmin filament
c. dynein
c. inclusion
c. microtubule
c. organelle
cytoprotective
cytoproximal
cytoreduction
cytoreductive surgery
cytosine
c. arabinoside (ara-C)
c. arabinoside therapy
cytoskeletal
c. abnormality
c. degradation
c. protein
c. structure
cytoskeletal membrane event
cytoskeleton
axonal c.
cytosol fluid
cytotoxic
c. agent
c. drug
c. edema
c. lymphocyte
c. T cell
cytotoxin-associated gene A (CagA)
Cytoxan
C. Injection
C. Oral
Czarnecki sign
Czerny suture

2D
2-dimensional
2D graphic localization
2D multiplanar reconstructed image
D2
D2 blockade
D2 occupancy
D2 receptor
3D
3-dimensional
3D hexahedral element
3D positional adjustability
3D positional control
3D relationship analysis
3D titanium mini bone plate
D3 receptor
dab1 gene
daboia
dacarbazine
d'accoucheur
main d.
daclizumab
DaCosta syndrome
Dacron
collagen-impregnated D.
Dacron-fibered platinum coil
dacryoadenitis
dacryocystic epilepsy
dacryocystis
dacryocystitis
dacryocystocele
dactinomycin
dactylospasm
DAF
downgaze paralysis, ataxia/athetosis and foam cell
DAF syndrome
Dahlgren cranial rongeur
DAI
diffuse axonal injury
daily
d. living activities
d. living activities affecting sleep
D. Rating Scale
D. Record of Severity of Problems
Dalalone
daledalin tosylate
DAM-80 amplifier
damage
acute neuronal d.
amygdala d.
anoxic d.
anterior cervical surgery vocal cord d.
axonal d.
body ego d.
brain d. (BD)
cranial nerve d.
diencephalic d.
excitotoxic cell d.
free radical d.
frontal cortex d.
HI-induced brain d.
hypoxic brain d.
hypoxic-ischemic brain d.
iatrogenic d.
insult-induced neuronal d.
intrinsic d.
irreversible brain d.
ischemic brain d.
left hemisphere d. (LHD)
liver d.
nerve d.
neuronal d.
occipital cortex d.
oxidative d.
parietal cortex d.
retraction-induced cerebral d.
self-inflicted d.
temporal cortex d.
zygapophysial joint d.
Damasio and Damasio template
dampened waveform
Dana
D. operation
D. posterior rhizotomy
Dana-Farber Cancer Institute protocol
danaparoid sodium
danazol
dance
Saint Anthony d.
Saint Guy d.
Saint Vitus d.
dancing
d. chorea
d. disease
d. eye
d. spasm
Dandy
D. clamp
D. maneuver
D. myocutaneous scalp flap
D. nerve hook
D. neurological scissors
D. neurosurgical scissors
D. operation
D. probe
D. scalp hemostatic forceps
D. suction tube

Dandy *(continued)*
D. trigeminal nerve scissors
D. ventricular needle
Dandy-Walker
D.-W. complex
D.-W. cyst
D.-W. deformity
D.-W. malformation
D.-W. phenomenon
D.-W. syndrome
Danek
Medtronic Sofamor D.
danger
physical d.
danger-laden schema vulnerability
dangerous image
Danielssen-Boeck disease
Danielssen disease
Danocrine
Danon disease
Dantrium
dantrolene sodium
dapsone neuropathy
Daraprim
dark
d. cell
D. Warrior epilepsy
Darkschewitsch
nucleus of D.
dartos reflex
darwinian reflex
darwinism
neural d.
dashed gray velocity trace
Das-Naglieri Cognitive Assessment System
DAT
dementia Alzheimer type
dopamine transporter
DAT autoradiography
DAT gene
DAT for PCA
data, sing. **datum**
d. acquisition bandwidth
d. acquisition system
anecdotal d.
d. base
clinical d.
followup d.
functional imaging d.
interictal d.
longitudinal expert evaluation using all available d.
mental d.
narrative d.
nutraceutical d.
postmortem d.
quantitative d.
in vivo d.
databank
trauma coma d. (TCDB)
database
Childhood Brain Tumor Consortium d.
whole-brain mapping d.
DATATOP
deprenyl and tocopherol antioxidative therapy of parkinsonism
date rape drug
Datex infrared CO_2 monitor
datum (*sing. of* data)
Datura arborea
daughter
d. abscess
d. cyst
Daumas-Duport
D.-D. astrocytoma grading system
D.-D. tumor grading system
DAVF
dural arteriovenous fistula
Davidenkow syndrome
Davidoff age stratification
Davidoff-Dyke-Masson syndrome
Davis
D. brain retractor
D. brain spatula
D. coagulating forceps
D. conductor
D. dura dissector
D. dural separator
D. monopolar forceps
D. nerve separator
D. nerve separator-spatula
D. nerve spatula
D. percussion hammer
D. rib spreader
D. saw guide
D. scalp retractor
Dawson encephalitis
Daxolin
Daypro
daytime
d. consequences of sleeplessness
d. drowsiness
d. fatigability
d. fatigue
d. hallucination
d. sleep hangover
d. sleepiness
d. somnolence
d. stupor
dazzle
central d.
DBAS
Dysfunctional Beliefs and Attitudes about Sleep

DBD
dementia behavior disturbance
DBD Scale
DBF
distant brain failure
DBS
deep brain stimulation
DBS electrode
DBS electrode implantation
DC
direct current
DC SQUID sensor
DC SQUID sensor decompressive
3D-CTA
3-dimensional computed tomographic angiography
DCX gene
D-dimer
de
de Lange syndrome
De Mayo 2-point discrimination device
De Monte grading
de Morsier syndrome
de novo
de novo aneurysm
de novo appearance
de novo development
de novo metachronous neoplasm
de novo mutation
de novo nonconvulsive status epilepticus
de novo Parkinson disease
de novo synthesis
de pensós echo
de Quervain disease
De Sanctis-Cacchione syndrome
De Toni-Fanconi syndrome
dead
brain d. (BD)
d. hand
d. space
deafferentation
hemispherical d.
d. pain
d. pain syndrome
deafferented state
deafness
central d.
cortical d.
high-frequency d.
infantile X-linked d.
midbrain d.
nerve d.
neural d.
progressive hereditary nerve d.
pure word d.
retrocochlear d.
sensorineural d.
word d.
dealkylation
deaminase
myoadenylate d.
porphobilinogen d.
deamino-D-arginine vasopressin
death
apoptotic cell d.
brain d. (BD)
cell d.
cerebral d.
ischemic neuronal cell d.
living d.
neuronal cell d.
programmed cell d. (PCD)
Deaver
D. method
D. retractor
DeBakey
D. endarterectomy scissors
D. forceps
D. rib spreader
debarquement
mal de d.
DeBastiani
D. distractor
D. external fixator
D. frame
debilitating
d. dysphoric symptom
d. headache
d. illness
Debrancher enzyme deficiency
Debré-Sémélaigne pseudomyotonia
Debre-Sémélaigne syndrome
debridement
principle of d.
radical d.
debulking procedure
Decadron
decanoate
nandrolone d.
decarboxylase
amine precursor uptake d. (APUD)
aromatic amino acid d. (AADC)

NOTES

decarboxylase *(continued)*
glutamate d.
glutamic acid d.
glutamine d. (GAD)
ornithine d.
decarboxylation
decathexis
decay
free induction d. (FID)
decentration
decerebellation
decerebrate
decorticate and d.
d. posturing
d. rigidity
d. state
decerebration
bloodless d.
decerebrize
decision
Brawner d.
Decker
D. alligator forceps
D. alligator scissors
D. microsurgical forceps
D. microsurgical scissors
declarative
d. emotional memory processing
d. memory
d. memory process
decline
cognitive d.
functional d.
global cognitive d.
hippocampal d.
hormonal d.
inexorable d.
progressive cognitive d.
d. rate
subjective memory d.
terminal cognitive d.
declive, declivis
decompensation
hepatic d.
decomposition of movement
decompression
anterior d.
bone graft d.
cerebral d.
cervical spine d.
d. equipment
extensive posterior d.
foramen magnum d.
foraminal d.
hindbrain d.
interlaminar d.
internal d.
laser disc d. (LDD)
lumbar spine d.
microvascular d. (MVD)
nerve d.
d. operation
optic nerve sheath d. (ONSD)
orbital d.
posterior d.
sacral spine d.
d. sickness
simple d.
spinal d.
suboccipital d.
subtemporal d.
surgical d.
thoracic spine d.
thoracolumbar spine d.
timing of d.
transantral ethmoidal orbital d.
trigeminal d.
vascular d.
ventricular d.
vertebral body d.
decompressive
d. craniectomy
DC SQUID sensor d.
d. laminectomy
d. sickness
d. surgery
deconditioning
decorticate
d. and decerebrate
d. posturing
d. rigidity
d. state
decortication
cerebral d.
reversible d.
d. technique
decoy
myelin d.
decreased
d. consciousness
d. fine finger movement
d. interest in activity
d. need for sleep
d. oxygen level
d. respiratory drive
d. sleep efficiency
decremental
d. activity
d. response
decrescendo discharge
decubitus
d. paralysis
d. position
d. ulcer
decussate
decussatio, pl. **decussationes**
d. brachii conjunctivi
d. fibrarum nervorum trochlearium

d. fontinalis
d. lemnisci mediales
d. lemniscorum
d. motoria
d. pedunculorum cerebellarium superiorum
d. pyramidum
d. sensoria
d. tegmentalis anterior
d. tegmentalis posterior

decussation
anterior tegmental d.
d. of brachia conjunctiva
dorsal column d.
dorsal tegmental d.
d. of fillet
Forel d.
fountain d.
Held d.
impaired d.
d. of medial lemniscus
Meynert fountain d.
motor d.
optic d.
posterior tegmental d.
d. of pyramid
pyramidal d.
rubrospinal d.
d. of superior cerebellar peduncle
tectospinal d.
tegmental d.
d. of trochlear nerve
d. of trochlear nerve fiber
ventral tegmental d.
Wernekinck d.

dedifferentiation hypothesis

deductive reasoning test

deep
d. abdominal reflex
d. brain extension
d. brain lead
d. brain microelectrode recording
d. brain stimulation (DBS)
d. brain stimulation for mood disorder
d. cerebellar nucleus
d. gray layer of superior colliculus
d. hypothermic circulatory arrest
d. middle cerebral vein
d. nucleus
d. origin
d. retractor
d. sensibility
d. tendon reflex (DTR)
d. transitional gyrus
d. tumor
d. vein thrombosis
d. venous thrombosis
d. white layer of superior colliculus
d. white matter
d. white matter hyperintensity
d. white matter hyperintensity change
d. white matter lesion (DWML)
d. white matter pathology
d. white matter region

deer tick

defatigation

defecation center

defect
activation d.
afferent pupillary d.
altitudinal visual field d.
arcuate visual field d.
arousal d.
asymptomatic visual field d.
autosomal dominant genetic d.
carboxylase d.
carnitine transport d.
chiasmatic d.
coagulation d.
concentric visual field d.
creatine transporter d.
cytochrome oxidase d.
developmental d.
dural d.
extradural d.
field d.
focal plaquelike d.
galactosidase d.
glycosphingolipid metabolic d.
hematopoietic stem cell d.
imprinting d.
methylene tetrahydrofolate reductase d.
midline fusion d.
mitochondrial transport d.
multiple genetic d.'s
neural tube d. (NTD)
nonhomonymous field d.
partial homonymous field d.
pediatric stroke from septal d.
postoperative skull d.

NOTES

defect *(continued)*
protrusio d.
pursuit d.
relative afferent pupillary d. (RAPD)
residual dense nasal d.
smooth pursuit d.
sulfur metabolism d.
temporoparietal d.
visual field d.
defective glucose transport
defense
egomechanism of d.
endogenous antioxidative d.
heat d.
normal heat d.
d. reflex
deferens
plexus of ductus d.
deferentialis
plexus d.
deferoxamine
deferred shock
deficiency
N-acetylglutamate synthetase d.
acid lipase d.
acid maltase d.
acyl-CoA dehydrogenase d.
acyl-CoA oxidase d.
adenosine monophosphate deaminase d.
adenylosuccinate lyase d.
adult acid maltase d.
aldosterone d.
aminoaciduria d.
antithrombin III d.
aqueous humor d.
arginase d.
argininosuccinic acid synthase d.
arginosuccinate lyase d.
arylsulfatase A d.
aspartoacylase d.
AT III d.
beta-hexosaminidase A d.
bifunctional protein d.
bioenergetic d.
biopterin d.
biotin holocarboxylase synthetase d.
biotinidase d.
carbamyl phosphate synthetase d.
carbinol dehydratase d.
carnitine palmitoyltransferase d.
cerebral folate d.
ceruloplasmin d.
clotting factor d.
cobalamin reductase d.
cognitive function d.
cystathionine synthetase d.
cytochrome *c* oxidase d.
cytochrome oxidase d.
Debrancher enzyme d.
dementia due to vitamin d.
dihydrobiopterin synthetase d.
dihydropteridine reductase d.
dihydropyrimidinase d.
dihydropyrimidine dehydrogenase d.
endplate acetylcholinesterase d.
factor VII d.
factor VIII d.
factor IX d.
factor XII d.
folate d.
folic acid d.
fructose-1,6-diphosphatase d.
galactokinase d.
galactose-1-phosphate uridyltransferase d.
galactosylceramidase d.
glucuronidase d.
glutamyl cysteine synthetase d.
glutathione synthetase d.
glycerol kinase d.
glycogen debrancher d.
growth hormone d.
hereditary high-density lipoprotein d.
hexosaminidase d.
holocarboxylase synthetase d.
hypocretin d.
hypoxanthine guanine phosphoribosyltransferase d.
idiopathic growth hormone d.
infantile acid maltase d.
intellectual d.
intrinsic factor d.
iodine d.
iron d.
isoniazid-induced pyridoxine d.
LCHAD d.
literacy d.
merosin d.
mevalonate kinase d.
molybdenum cofactor d.
multiple carboxylase d.'s
muscle phosphorylase d.
myelin basic protein d.
myoadenylate deaminase d.
myopathic carnitine d.
myophosphorylase d.
neuraminidase d.
ornithine-ketoacid aminotransferase d.
ornithine transcarbamoylase d. (OTCD)
phenylalanine hydroxylase d.
phosphofructokinase transferase d.
phosphoglycerate kinase d.
phosphoglycerate mutase d.

phosphorylase d.
platelet glycoprotein Ia/IIa d.
protein C, S d.
6-PT d.
purine nucleotide phosphorylase d.
pyridoxine d.
pyruvate carboxylase d.
pyruvate kinase d.
quantal release d.
racemase d.
respiratory chain complex I d.
riboflavin d.
sarcoglycan d.
sepiapterin reductase d.
succinic semialdehyde dehydrogenase d.
sulfatase A d.
thiamine d.
thyroid d.
triosephosphate isomerase d.
uridine monophosphate synthase d.
vitamin B1 d.
vitamin B6 d.
vitamin B12 d.
vitamin D d.
vitamin E d.

deficient
d. social judgment
d. spinous process

deficit
auditory transfer d.
balance d.
behavior d.
bimanual coordination d.
central proprioception integration d.
cholinergic d.
cognitive d.
cortical gray matter d.
corticobulbar d.
cranial nerve d.
delayed ischemic neurological d. (DIND)
emotional memory d.
executive function d.
expressive language d.
expressive speech d.
focal neurologic d.
frontal lobe-related d.
functional d.
gaze d.
general temporal processing d.
iatrogenic d.
instrumental function d.
intellectual function d.
interlimb coordination d.
lexical-syntactic d.
magnocellular d.
memory function d.
motor d.
neurological d.
neuropsychologic d.
olfactory d.
perfusion d.
permanent cranial nerve d.
proprioceptive sensory d.
radicular motor d.
resolving ischemic neurologic d. (RIND)
d. reversal
reversible ischemic neurologic d. (RIND)
segmental sensory d.
sensory d.
sleep d.
subcortical d.
d. syndrome
tactile transfer d.
transfer d.
unilateral d.
upward gaze d.
verbal memory d.
verbal reasoning d.
vestibular d.
visual field d.
visuospatial d.
volitional d.

defined
d. aura
d. meningitis
d. neurulation
d. tremor

definition
arteriovenous malformation nidus d.
AVM nidus d.
diagnostic d.
3-dimensional target d.
nidus d.
pediatric respiratory d.

deflazacort

deflection
d. force
high-voltage d.
initial upward d.

NOTES

D

deflection *(continued)*
in-phase d.
out-of-phase d.
deformans
cephalohematoma d.
dystonia musculorum d. (DMD)
musculorum d.
osteitis d.
recessive dystonia musculorum d.
spondylitis d.
spondylosis d.
deformation
morphological d.
shear-strain d.
trefoil tendon d.
deformity
d. analysis
Arnold-Chiari d.
bull's-eye d.
cervical spine kyphotic d.
cervicomedullary d.
Chiari d.
clawhand d.
coronal plane d.
cranioorbital d.
Dandy-Walker d.
drop-finger d.
drop-thumb d.
fixed d.
flat back d.
hand d.
hindbrain d.
J-sella d.
Klippel-Feil d.
kyphotic d.
lateral compression d.
lumbar spine kyphotic d.
main en griffe d.
musculoskeletal d.
pes cavus d.
posttraumatic spinal d.
progressive d.
saddle nose d.
sagittal d.
scoliotic paralytic d.
skeletal d.
spinal coronal plane d.
swan-neck d.
thoracic spine scoliotic d.
thoracolumbar gibbus d.
vertebral compression d.
deformity/instability
spinal d./i.
deganglionate
degeneratio micans
degeneration
acquired hepatocerebral d.
adiposogenital d.
Alzheimer neurofibrillary d.
ascending d.
axon d.
axonal d.
axoplasm d.
cerebellar cortical d.
cerebelloolivary d.
cerebromacular d.
cerebroretinal d.
cobblestone d.
cortical basal ganglionic d.
dentatorubral d.
descending d.
disc d.
end-organ d.
fascicular d.
fibrinoid d.
frontal lobe d.
frontotemporal lobar d.
glistening d.
Gombault d.
granular d.
granulovacuolar d.
gray d.
hepatocerebral d.
hepatolenticular d.
Holmes cortical cerebellar d.
hyaline d.
hypertrophic olivary d.
infantile neuronal d.
lattice d.
lenticular progressive d.
Marchi d.
Menzel olivopontocerebellar d.
neurofibrillary d.
neuronal d.
Nissl d.
olivary d.
olivopontocerebellar d.
orthograde d.
oxidative d.
pallidal d.
paraneoplastic cerebellar d.
paraneoplastic cerebral d.
parenchymatous cerebellar d.
paving stone d.
pontosubicular d.
premature infant pontosubicular d.
primary neuronal d.
primary progressive cerebellar d.
pseudocystic d.
Purkinje cell d.
Ramsay Hunt type of inherited dentatorubral d.
reaction of d.
retinal d.
retrograde d.
rim d.
Rosenthal d.
secondary d.

spinal disc d.
spinocerebellar d. (SCD)
spinopontine d.
spongy d.
striatonigral d.
subacute cerebellar d.
subacute combined d.
synaptic d.
transneuronal d.
transsynaptic d.
traumatic d.
Türck d.
uratic d.
vacuolar d.
wallerian d.
white matter d.
Wilson hepatolenticular d.

degenerative
d. arthritis
d. brain disease
d. cervical disc disease
d. cervical spine disease
d. cervical spine disorder
d. chorea
d. dementia
d. discogenic endplate disease
d. discogenic vertebral change
d. hypothesis
d. lumbar scoliosis
d. lumbar spine fusion
d. lumbar spondylosis
d. narrowing
d. neuronal disorder
d. spine change
d. spine condition
d. spondylolisthesis
d. spondylosis
d. spondylosis decompression and fusion
d. subluxation

degloving
midface d.

deglutition
d. center
d. paralysis
d. reflex

Degos disease

degradable starch microsphere (DSM)

degradation
cytoskeletal d.
dopamine d.
elastin d.
leucine d.
myelin d.
NO-induced DNA d.

degustation

dehisced wound

7-dehydrocholesterol

dehydroepiandrosterone (DHEA)
d. sulfate (DHEA-S)

dehydrogenase
alcohol d.
aldehyde d.
dihydrolipoyl d.
flavoprotein d.
glutaryl-CoA d.
lactate d.
long-chain hydroxy Acyl-CoA d. (LCHAD, LCHD)
phosphogluconate d. (PGD)
pyruvate d. (PDH)

deiterospinal tract

Deiters
D. cell
D. nucleus
D. process

déjà
d. vu
d. vu aura

Dejerine
D. anterior bulb syndrome
D. disease
D. hand phenomenon
D. onion peel sensory loss
D. percussion hammer
D. peripheral neurotabes
D. reflex
D. sign

Dejerine-Davis percussion hammer

Dejerine-Klumpke
D.-K. palsy
D.-K. paralysis
D.-K. syndrome

Dejerine-Landouzy dystrophy

Dejerine-Lichtheim phenomenon

Dejerine-Roussy syndrome

Dejerine-Sottas
D.-S. atrophy
D.-S. disease
D.-S. peripheral neuropathy
D.-S. syndrome

Dejerine-Thomas
D.-T. atrophy
D.-T. syndrome

NOTES

delavirdine
delay
benign maturation d.
conduction d.
developmental d.
global developmental d. (GDD)
interpeak d.
d. of kindling
psychomotor d.
readout d.
transcallosal conduction d.
delayed
d. after depolarization
d. apoplexy
d. axotomy
d. cerebral vasospasm
d. coma after hypoxia
d. computed tomographic myelography
d. hydrocephalus
d. hypersensitivity reaction
d. ischemic deterioration
d. ischemic neurological deficit (DIND)
D. List Recall test
d. postischemic hypoperfusion
d. recall index
d. reflex
d. sensation
d. shock
d. sleep phase
d. sleep-phase syndrome
d. traumatic intracerebral hematoma (DTICH)
d. traumatic intracerebral hemorrhage
delayed-onset postherpetic neuralgia
deleterious effect
deletion
d. mutation
15q11-q13 d.
deliberate infliction of pain
deliria (*pl. of* delirium)
deliriant
delirifacient
delirious
d. patient
d. shock
delirium, pl. **deliria**
acute d.
ammonium chloride d.
anxious d.
chronic d.
collapse d.
d. ebriosorum
eclamptic d.
low d.
d. mussitans
muttering d.
d. palingnosticum
pathophysiology of d.
phencyclidine d.
d. phenomenology
posttraumatic d.
D. Rating Scale (DRS)
secondary d.
senile d.
substance-induced d.
toxic d.
d. tremens (DT)
d. unit
d. verborum
Delis-Kaplan Executive Function System
delivery
d. catheter
consistent d.
convection-enhanced drug d.
gene therapy d.
d. guidewire
intraarterial drug d.
intraparenchymal drug d.
intraventricular drug d.
polymer drug d.
viral d.
Delrin
D. plastic scalp clip
D. rod
delta
d. activity
d. activity stage
d. fornicis
d. gene
monorhythmic frontal d. (MFD)
d. rhythm
d. sleep
D. valve
D. valve in ventriculoperitoneal shunt
d. wave
delta-aminolevulinate dehydratase porphyria
delta-function arterial plasma
Deltasone
delta-9-tetrahydrocannabinol
deltoid-splitting incision
delusional
d. and hallucinatory syndrome
d. misidentification syndrome
Demadex
demand
biochemical oxygen d. (BOD)
functional d.
demarcation
d. current
d. potential
DeMartel
D. scalp flap forceps
D. wire saw

demeclocycline
demented patient
dementia
acquired d.
AD-related d.
AIDS d.
alcohol persisting d.
Alzheimer atrophic d.
Alzheimer disease-related d.
Alzheimer senile d. (ASD)
d. Alzheimer type (DAT)
d. of the Alzheimer type
Alzheimer-type senile d.
amyotrophic lateral sclerosis-Parkinson d. (ALS-PD)
D. Assessment Battery
d. behavior disturbance (DBD)
Binswanger d.
cerebrovascular accident d.
clinical d.
cognitive impairment, no d.
comorbid d.
Cornell Scale for Depression in D.
cortical d.
degenerative d.
depressed-type presenile d.
depression in d.
depressive d.
dialysis d.
diffuse Lewy body d. (DLBD)
d. due to hepatic condition
d. due to multiple etiologies
d. due to vitamin deficiency
epileptic d.
ethical aspects of d.
evolving d.
frontal lobe d.
d. frontal type
frontotemporal d. (FTD)
global d.
Gottfries-Brane-Steen Rating Scale for D.
hereditary dysphasic d.
HIV-associated d.
d. homozygous
hydrocephalic d.
hysterical d.
incident d.
infarction d.
d. insomnia
irreversible d.
ischemic vascular d.
late-life d.
Lewy body d.
Manchester and Oxford Universities Scale for the Psychopathological Assessment of D. (MOUSEPAD)
Mariana d. (MD)
mild d.
moderate d.
D. Mood Assessment Scale
multiinfarct d. (MID)
multiple sclerosis d.
neurodegenerative d.
non-Alzheimer frontal lobe-type d.
obstructive d.
occult presenile d.
paralytic d.
d. paralytica
d. paralytica juvenilis
paranoid-type arteriosclerotic d.
paranoid-type presenile d.
paranoid-type senile d.
d. paratonia progressiva
paretic d.
d. patient
pellagra d.
poststroke d.
posttraumatic d.
d. praecox
preexisting d.
premorbid d.
presenile d.
prestroke d.
primary senile d.
d. prodrome
d. progression
prominent d.
d. pugilistica
reversible d.
semantic d. (SD)
senile d.
severe d.
d. severity
subcortical ischemic vascular d.
d. syndrome
d. syndrome of depression
toxic d.
uncomplicated arteriosclerotic d.
uncomplicated presenile d.
uncomplicated senile d.
vascular d. (VaD)
vitamin B12 deficiency d.

NOTES

dementia *(continued)*
Wernicke d.
d. with Lewy body (DLB)
dementia-aphonia
dementia-related
d.-r. hypersomnia
d.-r. insomnia
dementing illness
Demianoff sign
demodulator
demographic
d. characteristic
d. feature
d. risk factor
d. variable
demonstration
Ames d.
demyelinate
demyelinated myelitis
demyelinating
d. encephalopathy
d. neuropathy
d. polyneuropathy
d. polyradiculoneuropathy
d. procedure
d. trigeminal nerve lesion
d. white matter disease
demyelination, demyelinization
central inflammatory d.
local d.
multifocal subcortical d.
osmotic d.
segmental d.
demyelinative
d. disorder
d. spinal fluid profile
dendriform
dendrite
apical d.
d. arborization
d. proliferation
d. synaptogenesis
dendritic
d. arbor
d. plasticity
d. process
d. shaft
d. shape
d. spine
d. spine density
d. thorn
d. tree
d. tuft
dendrodendritic synapse
dendroid
dendron
dendrophagocytosis
dendrophilia
dendrotomy
denervate
denervated
d. fiber
d. muscle atrophy
denervation
autonomic d.
chemical d.
Krause d.
law of d.
muscle d.
d. neuronal hypersensitivity
nigrostriatal d.
d. pain syndrome
dengue
d. fever
d. myelitis
d. viral encephalitis
d. virus
denial of illness
Denis
D. Browne syndrome
D. forceps
Denny-Brown
D.-B. sensory radicular neuropathy
D.-B. syndrome
dens, pl. **dentes**
d. anterior screw fixation
densa
macula d.
dense
d. amnesia
d. hemianopia
d. hemiparesis
d. hemiplegia
d. sensory loss
densitometric analysis
densitometry
cholera-toxin-catalyzed d.
optical d.
density
bone mineral d.
contrast d.
dendritic spine d.
fiber d.
GFAP fiber d.
intraepidermal nerve fiber d.
lumbosacral junction bone d.
proton d.
receptor d.
relative optical d. (ROD)
spectral d.
spin d.
striatal dopamine transporter d.
synaptic d.
density-modulated spectral array (DSA)
dental
d. nerve
d. pathology

dentata
fissura d.
hilus of fascia d.
dentatae
cauda fasciae d.
dentate
d. band
d. fascia
d. fissure
d. gyrus
d. ligament
d. ligament of spinal cord
d. nucleus
d. nucleus of cerebellum
dentatectomy
dentated serration
dentati
capsula nuclei d.
hilum nuclei d.
strata gyri d.
dentatorubral
d. atrophy
d. cerebellar atrophy with polymyoclonus
d. degeneration
d. fiber
dentatorubrales
fibrae d.
dentatorubropallidoluysian atrophy (DRPLA)
dentatothalamic
d. fiber
d. tract
dentatum
corpus d.
dentatus
gyrus d.
nucleus d.
dentes (*pl. of* dens)
denticola
Treponema d.
denticulate ligament
denticulatum
ligamentum d.
dentiform
dentigerous cyst
dentinogenesis imperfecta
Denver
D. hydrocephalus shunt
D. valve
Denver-II Developmental screening test
deontologic theory
deoxygenation
deoxyguanosine
d. kinase (DGUOK)
d. kinase gene
deoxyhemoglobin
intracellular d.
deoxynucleoside triphosphate
deoxyribonuclease (DNAse)
deoxyribonucleic acid (DNA)
Depacon
Depakene
Depakote
D. ER
D. Sprinkle capsule
depalatalization
dependence
d. criterion
substance d.
d. trait
dependency
wheelchair d.
dependent
blood oxygenation level d. (BOLD)
blood oxygen level d. (BOLD)
dose d.
shunt d.
depigmentation of noradrenergic brainstem nucleus
depMedalone Injection
DepoCyt
Depoject Injection
depolarization
d. block
delayed after d.
early after d.
late after d.
primary afferent d. (PAD)
depolarization-dependent synaptic transmission
depolarize
Depo-Medrol Injection
Depopred Injection
deposit
bulky leptomeningeal d.
extradural d.
intracellular insoluble protein d.
lipofuscinosis granular osmiophilic d.
vascular immune d.
deposition
amyloid plaque d.

NOTES

D

deposition *(continued)*
copper d.
hemosiderin d.
depot
Fluanxol D.
d. form
Depo-Testosterone
deprenyl and tocopherol antioxidative therapy of parkinsonism (DATATOP)
depressed
d. corneal reflex
d. gag reflex
d. migraineur
d. skull fracture
d. ventilatory response to hypercapnia
depressed-type presenile dementia
depression
agitated d.
alcohol-induced d.
anxious somatic d.
caregiver d.
cognitive impairment of d.
cortical spreading d. (CSD)
current d.
cyclic d.
d. in dementia
dementia syndrome of d.
drug-induced d.
drug-resistant d.
endplate d.
exaggerated d.
geriatric d.
headache, insomnia, and d. (HID)
hysterical d.
d. inventory
later-life d.
level of d.
major d.
manifestation of d.
myxedema d.
nuclear d.
paradoxical d.
paralyzing d.
postactivation d.
poststroke d.
post-TIA d.
pseudodementia of d.
pure d.
reversible cognitive impairment of d.
ruminative d.
d. severity
sleep disturbance in major d.
somatic d.
d. spectrum disease
sporadic d.
spreading d.
subjective d.
subsyndromal d.
symptomatic d.
syndromic d.
unspecified d.
visual field d.
depression-related chronic insomnia
depressive
d. auditory hallucination
d. breakthrough
d. dementia
d. disease
d. executive dysfunction
d. mixed state
d. olfactory hallucination
d. pseudodementia
d. psychoneurotic reaction
d. psychotic reaction
d. situational reaction
d. stupor
d. syndrome
d. visual hallucination
depressive-type
depressomotor
depressor
d. anguli oris muscle
d. fiber
d. nerve of Ludwig
d. reflex
deprivation
rapid eye movement d.
REM d.
sensory d.
sleep d. (SD)
volitional sleep d.
depth
d. electrode
d. guard
d. recording
skin d.
wire penetration d.
depth-recorded electroencephalogram
DePuy
D. AcroMed Harms cage
D. nerve hook
deramciclane
deranged neural development
derangement
metabolic d.
derby hat fracture
deregulation
emotional d.
derivation
neoplasm of lymphocytic d.
derivative
ergotamine d.
hematoporphyrin d.
valproic acid and d.
derived
endothelium d.

dermabrasion bur
dermal
d. meningioma
d. sinus
dermatan sulfate
DermaTemp infrared thermographic sensor
dermatica
zona d.
dermatitidis
Blastomyces d.
dermatofibrosarcoma protuberans
dermatogenic torticollis
dermatoglyphic pattern
dermatome
d. pain
thoracic d.
trigeminal d.
dermatomic area
dermatomyositis
juvenile d.
dermatomyotome
dermatoneurology
dermatoneurosis
dermatoplastic infantile ganglioglioma
dermatosensory evoked potential
dermohygrometer
dermoid
d. cyst
d. tumor
dermometer
dermometry
dermoneurosis
dermoneurotropic
Derogatis
D. Affects Balance Scale
D. Affects Balance Scale, Revised
D. Stress Profile
D'Errico
D. bayonet pituitary forceps
D. brain spatula
D. enlarging drill bur
D. hypophysial forceps
D. lamina chisel
D. nerve root retractor
D. perforating drill
D. perforating drill bur
D. periosteal elevator
D. skull trephine
D. tissue forceps
D. ventricular needle
D'Errico-Adson retractor
desacralize
desaturation
arterial oxygen d.
d. index (DI)
descendens
d. cervicalis
d. cervicis
d. hypoglossi
descending
d. branch
d. current
d. degeneration
d. motor pathway
d. neuritis
d. nucleus of trigeminus
d. tract of trigeminal nerve
desensitization
behavioral d.
eye movement d.
deserpidine
desferrioxamine
desflurane
design
case control experimental study d.
cross-sectional experimental study d.
hook hollow-ground connection d.
hook V-groove connection d.
Isola spinal implant system d.
longitudinal experimental study d.
mechanical plate d.
naturalistic d.
pedicle screw linkage d.
prospective experimental study d.
retrospective experimental study d.
spinal implant d.
transpedicular fixation system d.
d. for vision frame
d. for vision side shield
desipramine
desmethylclomipramine
desmin
d. storage myopathy
d. tumor marker
desminopathy
desmocytoma
desmodynia
desmoplastic
d. cerebral astrocytoma
d. infantile ganglioglioma
d. medulloblastoma
desmopressin acetate

NOTES

desmosterolosis
Desormaux endoscope
desoxycorticosterone acetate
desoxymorphine
desoxyphenobarbital
destruction
bony element d.
destructive
d. interference technique
d. stereotactic lesion
desynchronization
d. activity
event-related d.
postmovement beta d.
desynchronized
d. discharge pattern
d. sleep
desynchronous
Desyrel
DET
diethyltryptamine
detachable
d. coil
d. silicone balloon
detached
d. cranial section
d. craniotomy
detachment
choroid d.
choroidal d.
ciliochoroidal d.
dural d.
retinal d.
detail response to small white space
detection
mutation d.
odor d.
signal d.
spike d.
taurine d.
detector
body movement d.
cesium fluoride scintillation d.
phase-sensitive d.
quadrature d.
deterioration
cognitive d.
delayed ischemic d.
end-of-dose d.
functional d.
memory d.
neurologic d.
d. process
progressive neurologic d.
determinant
biologic d.
determination
Cobb angle d.
fusion limit d.
serum enzyme d.
determining sleepiness
detoxicate
detrusor
d. areflexia
d. hyperreflexia
d. reflex
detrusor-external sphincter dyssynergia
detrusor-sphincter dyssynergia
detrusor-striated sphincter dyssynergia
deutencephalon
devascularized
developing
D. Cognitive Abilities Test, Second Edition
d. spine
d. stroke
development
brain d.
cerebrovascular embryonic d.
cognitive function d.
concrete operational d.
de novo d.
deranged neural d.
dissociated motor d.
disturbance of intellectual d.
egocentric stage of d.
fine motor d.
focal malformation of cortical d.
d. malformation
neonatal language d.
neurobiology of early childhood d.
perinatal d.
postoperative intellectual d.
psychomotor d.
rhythm of lags and spurts in d.
spinal cord segmentation in embryonic d.
developmental
d. articulatory apraxia
D. Assessment of the Severely Handicapped
d. course
d. curve
d. defect
d. delay
d. disorder screening
d. effect
d. failure
d. history
d. language disorder (DLD)
d. malformation
D. Observation Checklist System
d. perspective
d. process
d. quotient in Down syndrome
d. root

d. surveillance
d. task

deviant stimulus

deviation

alternating skew d.
conjugate downward d.
conjugate eye d.
disconjugate eye d.
eye-gaze d.
head d.
ipsilateral tonic d.
nasal septal d.
ocular d.
vertical ocular d.
wrong-way d.

Devic disease

device

Angio-Seal closure d.
angle measurement d.
anterior internal fixation d.
antisiphon d.
assistive technology d.
Attractor retrieval d.
balloon occlusion-aspiration embolus entrapment d.
Bassett electrical stimulation d.
braided occlusion d.
Cadwell 5200A somatosensory evoked potential unit d.
Camino intraparenchymal fiberoptic d.
C-D instrumentation d.
cervical immobilization d. (CID)
Contour Emboli artificial embolization d.
Cordis implantable drug reservoir d.
Cotrel-Dubousset dynamic transverse traction d.
cranial access d.
De Mayo 2-point discrimination d.
DeWald spinal d.
Dunn d.
Dwyer d.
dynamic transverse traction d.
Edwards modular system sacral fixation d.
endoscope lens cleansing d.
ferromagnetic monitoring d.
Fischer-Leibinger bur hole-mounted fixation d.
fixation d.
flow-controlled d.
fracture fixation d.
frameless stereotactic d.
Galtac d.
GDC SynerG detachment d.
gravitational d.
Harrington rod instrumentation distraction outrigger d.
head fixation d.
Heyer-Schulte antisiphon d.
inanimate learning d.
In-Exsufflator respiratory d.
InterFix RP threaded spinal fusion cage d.
interspinous spacer d.
intraaortic balloon counterpulsation d.
intravascular d.
Kaneda anterior spine stabilizing d.
Kostuik-Harrington d.
Leksell adapter to Mayfield d.
malleable microsurgical suction d.
mandibular advancing d.
Mayfield/Acciss stereotactic d.
Medelec 5-channel neurophysiological d.
Microvena retrieval d.
MurphyScope neurologic d.
Neuromed Octrode implantable d.
newer generation d.
Nicolet Pathfinder I recording d.
noise-reduction d.
Novo-10a CBF measuring d.
optical d.
OssaTron d.
PDN d.
Perclose closure d.
Portnoy DPV d.
precalibrated pointing d.
prosthetic disc nucleus d.
Quartzo d.
Roeder manipulative aptitude test d.
roentgen knife stereotactic radiosurgical d.
sequential compression d.
Silastic d.
SilverHawk d.
Snore Guard mandibular repositioning d.
Sofamor spinal instrument d.

D

NOTES

device *(continued)*
Somanetics INVOS cerebral oximeter d.
SomaSensor d.
superconducting quantum interference d. (SQUID)
SynchroMed drug administration d.
Tacticon peripheral neuropathy screening d.
Taylor halter d.
Texas Scottish Rite Hospital corkscrew d.
Texas Scottish Rite Hospital mini-corkscrew d.
tongue-locking d.
tongue-retaining d.
d. for transverse traction (DTT)
ultrasonic aspirating d.
VasoSeal closure d.
Viking II nerve monitoring d.
z-touch laser d.
Device/M2
DeVilbiss
D. cranial rongeur
D. rongeur forceps
D. skull trephine
DeVivo disease
DeWald spinal device
Dewar posterior cervical fixation procedure
DEXA, DXA
dual-energy x-ray absorptiometry
dexamethasone suppression test
dexanabinol
dexclamol hydrochloride
Dexedrine
dexmedetomidine
dexmethylphenidate HCl
dexterity
manual d.
dextran
dextroamphetamine
amphetamine and d.
d. neurotoxicity
dextrocerebral
dextromanual
dextropedal
dextrorotoscoliosis
dextroscoliosis
dextrosinistral
Dextrostix Uristix
Deyerle sciatic tension test
DFF
DNA fragmentation factor
2DFT
2-dimensional Fourier transform
2DFT gradient-echo imaging
2DFT GRASS
2DFT time-of-flight MR angiography
3DFT
3-dimensional Fourier transform
anisotropic 3DFT
3DFT gradient-echo MR imaging
3DFT GRASS
isotropic 3DFT
DGUOK
deoxyguanosine kinase
DHA
docosahexaenoic acid
DHEA
dehydroepiandrosterone
DHEA-S
dehydroepiandrosterone sulfate
D.H.E. 45 Injection
DI
desaturation index
diabetes-related ataxia
diabetic
d. amyotrophy
d. arthropathy
d. coma
d. ketoacidosis (DKA)
d. lumbosacral radiculoplexus neuropathy (DLRPN)
d. mononeuritis multiplex
d. myelopathy
d. neuropathic cachexia
d. neuropathy neuralgia pain
d. oculomotor palsy
d. polyradiculopathy
d. pseudotabes
d. sensorimotor polyneuropathy
d. third nerve palsy
d. thoracic radiculopathy
diabetica
tabes d.
Diabinese
diagnosis, pl. **diagnoses**
autopsy-confirmed d.
2-dimensional d.
headache differential d.
narcolepsy d.
neurologic d.
pendulum of d.
diagnostic
d. ambiguity
d. anesthesia
d. apraxia
d. aspect
d. assessment
d. block
d. boundary
d. category
d. cluster
d. criterion
d. definition

d. impression
d. marker
d. measure
d. method
d. monitoring
d. noise
d. process
d. profile
d. template

diagonal
d. band
d. nystagmus

diagonalis
bandaletta d.
d. stria
stria d.

diagram
pulse timing d.
vector d.

Dial Away Pain 400 electrotherapy unit

dialing
random digital d.

dialysis
d. dementia
d. disequilibrium
d. disequilibrium syndrome
d. encephalopathy syndrome

diamagnetism

diameter
axonal d.
effective pedicle d.
effective thread d.
fiber d.
horizontal pedicle d.
lumbar spine pedicle d.
midsagittal d.
pedicle d.
sagittal pedicle d.
thoracic spine pedicle d.
transcerebellar d.
transpedicular fixation effective pedicle d.
transverse pedicle d.
vertical pedicle d.

diametral measurement

diamond
d. bit
d. bur
d. high-speed air drill
d. knife
D. valve flow-regulating shunt

Diamox challenge testing

diaphragm
lumbar part of d.
d. paralysis
d. of sella
sella turcica d.
d. of sella turcica

diaphragma, pl. **diaphragmata**
d. sellae

diaphragmatic
d. nerve
d. plexus
d. tic
d. weakness

diaphragmatis
pars anterior facies d.
pars lumbalis d.

diaplexus

diary
d. card
sleep d.

diaschisis

Diasonics magnetic resonance imaging

diastasis
suture d.

Diastat

diastatic skull fracture

diastematocrania

diastematomyelia dysraphism

diastole-phased pulsatile infusion

diastolic blood pressure

diataxia
cerebral d.
d. cerebralis infantilis

diathesis
bipolar d.
epileptic d.
spasmodic d.
spasmophilic d.

diatrizoate meglumine

diatrizoic acid

Diazemuls Injection

diazepam
D. Intensol
d. rectal gel

diazoxide

dibasic calcium phosphate

dibenzepin benzothiazine

dibenzodiazepine

Dibenzyline

dibromodulcitol

DIC
disseminated intravascular coagulation

NOTES

D

dicarboxylic aminoaciduria
dichloralphenazone
dichloroacetate
dichlorodifluoromethane and trichloromonofluoromethane
dichlorotetrafluoroethane
ethyl chloride and d.
dichlorphenamide
dichotomous parameter
Dick AO fixateur interne
Dickman
method of D.
Dickson method
DICOM
digital imaging and communication in medicine
DICOM format
dicoumarol
dicyclomine
didanosine
diencephala (*pl. of* diencephalon)
diencephalic
d. astrocytoma
d. damage
d. epilepsy
d. glioma
d. lesion
d. membrane
d. syndrome of infancy
d. transition area
d. vein
diencephalohypophysial
diencephalon, pl. **diencephala**
ventricle of d.
diet
d. adherence
Evers raw food d.
gluten-free d.
ketogenic d.
low-salt d.
MacDougall multiple sclerosis d.
phenylalanine-restricted d.
d. termination
d. therapy
dietary
d. caffeine consumption
d. neurotoxin
Diethrich bulldog clamp
diethylenetriamine pentaacetic acid (DTPA)
diethylstilbestrol
diethyltryptamine (DET)
diet-induced hyperketonemia
DIF
diffuse interstitial fibrosis
DiFerrante disease
difference
behavioral d.
cerebral arteriovenous oxygen content d.
clinical d.
dose-related d.
functional d.
genetic d.
gray/white matter d.
hormonal d.
mean consecutive d.
mean sorted d.
metabolic d.
morphological d.
pharmacological d.
religious d.
true d.
differential
D. Ability Scale
d. beneficial effect
d. correlate
d. display of messenger ribonucleic acid
d. increase
d. interaction
d. pressure shunt
d. pressure valve
d. threshold
differentiation
brain d.
neuronal d.
retrogressive d.
Schwann cell d.
difficile
Clostridium d.
difficulty
breathing d.
cognitive d.
communication d.
index of d. (ID)
sudden vision d.
word-finding d.
diffusa
encephalitis periaxialis d.
diffuse
d. axonal injury (DAI)
d. bilateral slowing
d. brain atrophy
d. brain injury
d. cellular astrocytoma
d. cerebral histiocytosis
d. cerebral sclerosis
d. disseminated atheroembolism
d. distribution of activity
d. fibrillary astrocytic tumor
d. gliosis
d. heteropsia
d. idiopathic skeletal hyperostosis (DISH)
d. infantile familial sclerosis
d. interstitial fibrosis (DIF)

d. intrinsic brainstem tumor
d. Lewy body dementia (DLBD)
d. Lewy body disease
d. necrotizing leukoencephalopathy
d. noxious inhibitory control (DNIC)
d. pontine glioma
d. pontine lesion
d. Rosenthal fiber formation
d. white matter disease
d. white matter shearing injury

diffused reflex

diffusion
anisotropic d.
identity d.
normoxic d.
d. respiration
d. tension imaging
d. tensor imaging (DTI)
d. tensor magnetic resonance imaging
d. tensor MRI
d. transmission

diffusion-perfusion magnetic resonance imaging

diffusion-weighted
d.-w. echo planar image (DW-EPI)
d.-w. imaging (DWI)
d.-w. magnetic resonance imaging
d.-w. scanning

diffusivity
transverse d.

diffusum
angiokeratoma corporis d.

diflavin free radical

diflunisal

difluoromethylornithine

digastric
d. line
d. muscle
d. nerve

DiGeorge syndrome

digit
d. span backward (DSB)
d. span forward (DSF)

digital
d. holography
d. imaging and communication in medicine (DICOM)
d. intravenous angiography
d. nerve
d. pinch
d. polysomnography
d. radiography (DR)
d. reflex
d. signal analysis
d. subtraction angiogram
d. subtraction angiography (DSA)
d. subtraction venography
d. subtraction venous angiography
d. subtraction venous angiography slice
d. syncope
d. temple massage
d. vascular imaging (DVI)
d. vernier scale

digital-to-analog converter

digitationes hippocampus

digitized
d. instrument
d. spinography

digitizer
Cyberware d.
3-dimensional sonic d.
infrared d.
optical d.

digressed speech

dihexoside
ceramide d.

dihomogammalinolenic acid

dihydrate
calcium pyrophosphate d. (CPPD)

dihydrobiopterin synthetase deficiency

dihydrochloride
pramipexole d.
triethylene tetramine d.

dihydroergotamine
d. mesylate
d. mesylate nasal spray

dihydroindolone

dihydrolipoamide acetyltransferase

dihydrolipoyl
d. dehydrogenase
d. transacetylase

dihydromorphinone hydrochloride

dihydropteridine
d. reductase
d. reductase deficiency

dihydropyrimidinase deficiency

dihydropyrimidine dehydrogenase deficiency

dihydrotachysterol

dihydroxyphenylalanine

3,4-dihydroxyphenylalanine

NOTES

D

5,7-dihydroxytryptamine
Dilantin Kapseals
dilatans
pneumosinus d.
dilated
d. intercavernous sinus
d. poorly reactive pupil
dilation, dilatation
aneurysmal d.
arachnoid nerve root sheath d.
bilateral pupil d.
congenital d.
episcleral vascular d.
hypertensive d.
infundibular d.
junctional d.
progressive ventricular d.
unilateral pupil d.
vascular d.
ventricular d.
dilator
cortical incision coronary d.
curved cannula with locking d.
Eder-Puestow metal olive d.
straight cannula with locking d.
tissue d.
dileptic seizure
dilute Russell viper venom time (DRVVT)
dimeglumine
gadopentetate d.
dimenhydrinate
dimension
abstract versus representational d.
disorganization d.
Isola spinal implant system d.
pedicle d.
personality d.
positive symptom d.
sensory d.
symptom d.
2-dimensional
2-d. diagnosis
2-d. electrophoresis
2-d. Fourier transform (2DFT)
2-d. Fourier transform gradient-echo imaging
2-d. mapping
2-d. proton echo planar spectroscopic imaging
3-dimensional (3D)
3-d. acquisition
3-d. computed tomographic angiography (3D-CTA)
3-d. digitizer neuronavigator
3-d. fast low-angle shot imaging
3-d. Fourier transform (3DFT)
3-d. Fourier transform gradient-echo imaging
3-d. neuroimaging
3-d. postprocessing software
3-d. reconstruction
3-d. reconstruction wand
3-d. slice
3-d. sonic digitizer
3-d. SPECT phantom
3-d. spoiled GRASS sequence
3-d. target definition
3-d. vector analysis
dimensional rating
dimercaprol
dimerization
receptor d.
2,5-dimethoxy-4-methylamphetamine
4-dimethoxyphenylethylamine
dimethoxyquinazoline
dimethylamine sulfate (DMAS)
dimethylaminoethyl methacrylate
dimethyl sulfoxide (DMSO)
dimethyltryptamine
dimidiata
chorea d.
dimness of vision
dimple
acromial d.
sacral d.
DIND
delayed ischemic neurological deficit
Dingman
D. mouth gag
D. oral retraction system
dinitrate
isosorbide d.
dinitrophenol peripheral neuropathy
dinoflagellate
dinucleotide
flavin adenine d. (FAD)
dioctyl sodium sulfosuccinate
diode
light-emitting d. (LED)
diodone
Diodrast
Dionosil
dioxide
carbon d. (CO_2)
partial arterial gas tension of carbon d.
thorium d.
diphasic
d. dyskinesia
d. milk fever
diphenhydramine hydrochloride
diphenoxylate neurotoxicity
diphenylbutylpiperidine
diphenylhydantoin
diphosphate
adenosine d. (ADP)
guanosine d.

diphtheria
d. peripheral neuropathy
d., tetanus toxoids, and pertussis vaccine
diphtheriae
Corynebacterium d.
diphtheric polyneuropathy
diphtheritic
d. neuropathy
d. paralysis
diplegia
atonic-astatic d.
brachial d.
congenital facial d.
facial d.
Förster d.
infantile d.
masticatory d.
spastic d.
diploë
diploic vein
diplomyelia
diplophonia
diplopia
acquired vertical d.
monocular d.
diploscope
dipole
equivalent current d.
d. field
d. localization
magnetic d.
d. tracing
dipole-dipole
d.-d. interaction
d.-d. relaxation
dipotassium
clorazepate d.
dipping
converse ocular d.
ocular d.
Diprivan
Diprotrizoate
direct
d. auditory compound actional potential
d. brain stimulation
d. cortical stimulation and somatosensory evoked potential (SSEP)
d. current (DC)
d. embolectomy
d. end-to-end coaptation
d. fracture
d. lateral vein
d. multiplanar imaging
d. pyramidal tract
d. screw fixation technique
d. thermogenic effect
d. vision surgery
direction
flow d.
phase-encoding d.
directive
advance d.
director
Consortium of Neurology Clerkship D.'s (CNCD)
disability
abstracting d.
overall d.
partial d.
perception of d.
reversible ischemic neurologic d. (RIND)
selective reading d.
disabling
d. headache
d. neurogenic claudication
d. neurological condition
d. positional vertigo (DPV)
disarray
myofibrillary d.
disaster-related
d.-r. avoidant symptom
d.-r. intrusive symptom
disc, disk
artificial intervertebral d.
artificial spinal d.
d. at risk
Bardeen d.
choked d.
contained d.
d. curette
d. degeneration
d. edema
embryonic d.
extruded d.
frayed d.
free fragment d.
herniated cervical d.
herniated intervertebral d.
d. herniation
immature intervertebral d.

NOTES

disc *(continued)*
injury of intervertebral d.
intervertebral d.
intraspinal herniated d.
Link SB Charité d.
magnetic d.
d. matrix proteoglycan
Merkel tactile d.
noncontained d.
optic d.
PDN prosthetic d.
plastic-covered hydrogel d.
d. prolapse
protruded d.
d. protrusion
d. punch
Ranvier tactile d.
d. replacement
d. rongeur
d. rupture
ruptured d.
sequestrated d.
slipped d.
d. space
d. space collapse
d. space infection
d. space narrowing
d. substitute
d. syndrome
synthetic intervertebral d.
tactile d.
vacuum d.
Z d.

discectomy, diskectomy
anterior d.
automated percutaneous lumbar d. (APLD)
cervical d.
lumbar d.
microlumbar d.
microsurgery d.
microsurgical d. (MSD)
Robinson anterior cervical d.
thoracic d.
thoracoscopic anterior d.
transthoracic d.

discharge
beta-alpha-theta-delta d.'s
bilateral independent periodic lateralized epileptiform d.'s (BIPLEDs)
bilaterally synchronous epileptic d.'s
bizarre high-frequency d.
bizarre repetitive d.'s
complex repetitive d. (CRD)
decrescendo d.
double d.
EEG anteromesial temporal d.
epileptic d.
epileptiform burst d.
exercise-induced sympathetic d.
focal epileptiform d.
grouped d.
hippocampal seizure d.
hypersynchronous d.
ictal focal epileptiform d.
interictal bisynchronous d.
interictal focal epileptiform d.
interictal generalized spike-and-wave d.
interictal spike d.
iterative d.
monosynaptic reflex d.
motor unit d.
multiple d.'s
myokymic d.
myotonic d.
nervous d.
neural d.
neuromyotonic d.
notched appearance of spike-wave d.
paroxysmal epileptiform d.
d. pattern
periodic lateralizing epileptiform d. (PLED)
polyspike-and-wave d.
polysynaptic d.
premature d.
pseudoperiodic d.
rate of recovery at d.
repetitive d.
rhythmic d.
rhythmical midtemporal d.
rolandic epileptiform d.
spike d.
spike-and-wave electroencephalographic d.
spike-wave d.
subclinical rhythmic EEG d.
sympathetic d.
synchronized neuronal d.
synchronous corticofugal epileptic d.
synchronous spike-and-wave d.
triple d.
unilateral interictal focal epileptic d.
waning d.

discharging lesion

disci (*pl. of* discus)

disciform, diskiform

discission knife

discitis, diskitis
iatrogenic d.
intervertebral d.
pyogenic d.

discogenic, diskogenic
d. sclerosis
discogram, diskogram
discography, diskography
discoid
d. marker
d. skin lesion
discoidectomy
discoligamentous
d. complex
d. injury
discomfiture
disconjugate eye deviation
disconnection
d. apraxia
d. syndrome
discontinuity
Bruch membrane d.
facial nerve d.
nerve d.
discopathy
traumatic cervical d.
discordance
d. of movement
d. of voice
discordant sibling
discoscope
percutaneous d.
discotomy, diskotomy
discountenance
Discourse Comprehension test
discrete
d. emotional response
d. locus stimulation
d. symptom
discriminant stimulus
discrimination
odor d.
pure-tone d.
Sweet 2-point d.
word d.
disc-shaped diffusion ellipsoid
discus, pl. **disci**
d. lentiformis
disease
acquired cardiac d.
acute Marchiafava-Bignami d.
Adamantiades-Behçet d.
Adams-Stokes d.
Addison d.
adjacent level d.
adult polyglucosan body d.
advanced cortical d.
Aicardi-Goutières d.
akinetic-rigid Huntington d.
Akureyri d.
Alexander d.
Alpers d.
Alzheimer d. (AD)
Andersen d.
anterior horn cell d.
antiepileptic drug-induced bone d.
Antopol d.
aortocranial d.
Aran-Duchenne d.
Armstrong d.
arterial occlusive d.
arteriosclerotic brain d.
arteritis cardiovascular d.
atheromatous d.
atherosclerotic cardiovascular d. (ASCVD)
Australian X d.
autoimmune d.
Ayala d.
Azorean d.
Azorean-Joseph-Machado d.
Ballet d.
Baló d.
Baltic myoclonus d.
Bamberger d.
Bannister d.
basilar-vertebral artery d.
Bassen-Kornzweig d.
Batten d.
Batten-Mayou d.
Baxter d.
Bayle d.
Bechterew d.
Becker d.
Begbie d.
Behçet d.
Behr d.
Bernard-Soulier d.
Bernhardt d.
Bielschowsky d.
Bielschowsky-Jansky d.
Biemond d.
Billroth d.
Binswanger d.
Blocq d.
Bloom d.
bone marrow transplantation graft-versus-host d.

D

NOTES

disease *(continued)*
Bornholm d.
Bosin d.
Bourneville d.
Bourneville-Pringle d.
brain d.
brancher enzyme deficiency d.
Brill-Zinsser d.
Briquet d.
Brissaud d.
Brodie d.
Brushfield-Wyatt d.
Buschke d.
Busse-Buschke d.
calcium pyrophosphate dihydrate decomposition d.
Camurati-Engelmann d.
Canavan d.
Canavan-van Bogaert-Bertrand d.
carotid artery d.
Castleman d.
catscratch d. (CSD)
celiac d.
central core d.
cerebral d.
cerebrovascular d.
cervical spine rheumatoid d.
Chagas d.
Charcot d.
Charcot-Marie-Tooth d. type 1, 2
Cheyne d.
childhood moyamoya d.
cholesterol ester storage d.
Christensen-Krabbe d.
Christmas d.
chronic lung d.
Coats d.
collagen vascular d.
combined system d.
comorbid d.
complex d.
congenital heart d.
connective tissue d.
Consortium to Establish a Registry for Alzheimer D.
Cori d.
coronary artery d. (CAD)
corticospinal d.
Cotugno d.
Cotunnius d.
Cowden d.
cranial nerve heredodegenerative d.
Creutzfeldt-Jakob d. (CJD)
Crigler-Najjar d.
Crohn d.
Crouzon d.
Cruveilhier d.
Curschmann-Steinert d.
Cushing d.
cyanotic congenital heart d.
cytomegalic inclusion d.
dancing d.
Danielssen d.
Danielssen-Boeck d.
Danon d.
degenerative brain d.
degenerative cervical disc d.
degenerative cervical spine d.
degenerative discogenic endplate d.
Degos d.
Dejerine d.
Dejerine-Sottas d.
demyelinating white matter d.
de novo Parkinson d.
depression spectrum d.
depressive d.
de Quervain d.
Devic d.
DeVivo d.
DiFerrante d.
diffuse Lewy body d.
diffuse white matter d.
disseminated d.
Dorfman-Chanarin d.
drug-induced white matter d.
Dubini d.
Duchenne d.
Duchenne-Aran d.
Duchenne-Griesinger d.
Eales d.
early-onset familial Alzheimer d.
early-onset Parkinson d.
Ehlers-Danlos d. type IV
Emery-Dreifuss d.
end-stage renal d.
Engelmann d.
enterococcal d.
epidural hemorrhage epidural metastatic d.
Erb d.
Erb-Charcot d.
Erb-Goldflam d.
Erdheim-Chester d.
Escobar d.
d. etiology
Eulenburg d.
d. exacerbation
exophytic joint d.
extracranial carotid occlusive d.
extracranial occlusive vascular d.
extrapyramidal motor system d.
Fabry d.
Fahr d.
familial Alzheimer d.
familial Creutzfeldt-Jakob d. (fCJD)
familial Parkinson d.
familial paroxysmal choreoathetosis d.

familial startle d.
Farber d.
fatal hereditary d.
Fazio-Londe d.
Feer d.
Flatau-Schilder d.
Foix-Alajouanine d.
Folling d.
foot-and-mouth d. (FMD)
Forbes d.
Forbes-Cori d.
Forestier d.
Fothergill d.
Freiberg-Kohler d.
Friedmann d.
Friedreich d.
Fuerstner d.
Fukuyama d.
fusion d.
Gaucher d.
Gerhardt d.
Gerlier d.
Gerstmann-Sträussler-Scheinker d.
Gilles de la Tourette d.
Glanzmann d.
glial d.
glutamyl ribose-5-phosphate storage d.
glycogen storage d.
Goldflam d.
Goldflam-Erb d.
Gowers d.
Graefe d.
graft-versus-host d. (GVHD)
Graves d.
Greenfield d.
Guinon d.
Haglund d.
Hallervorden-Spatz d.
Hammond d.
Hand-Schüller-Christian d.
Hansen d.
Hartnup d.
Heidenhain d.
Heine-Medin d.
hematologic d.
hemisphere d.
hemoglobin H, SC d.
hepatocerebral d.
hepatolenticular d.
hereditary neurodegenerative d.
hereditary striatopallidal d.
heredodegenerative d.
Hers d.
heterogeneous system d.
Heubner d.
Hirayama d.
Hirschsprung d.
Hodgkin d.
Hoehn and Yahr staging of Parkinson d.
Holmes cerebellar degeneration d.
Hoppe-Goldflam d.
Horton d.
Hunt d.
Hunter d.
Huntington d.
Hurler d.
Hurler-Scheie d.
Hurst d.
hyalin inclusion d.
hydatid d.
iatrogenic Creutzfeldt-Jakob d. (iCJD)
Iceland d.
I-cell d.
idiopathic Parkinson d.
inclusion cell d.
infantile Gaucher d.
infantile multisystem inflammatory d.
infantile Refsum d.
inflammatory demyelinating d.
intracranial d.
intradural inflammatory d.
intraneuronal inclusion d.
intrinsic d.
ischemic cerebrovascular d.
Jakob-Creutzfeldt d.
Jansky-Bielschowsky d.
Jeep driver's d.
Joseph d.
jumper d.
jumping Frenchmen of Maine d.
juvenile Huntington d.
juvenile nonneuropathic Niemann-Pick d.
Kawasaki d.
Kearns-Sayre d.
Kennedy d.
Kennedy-Fischbeck d.
kinky-hair d.
Kinnier-Wilson d.
Klippel d.

NOTES

disease *(continued)*
konzo d.
Krabbe d.
Krabbe-Weber-Dimitri d.
Kraepelin-Morel d.
Kufs d.
Kugelberg-Welander d.
Kumlinge d.
Kyasanur Forest d.
labyrinthine d.
Lafora body d.
Landouzy-Dejerine d.
Lasègue d.
late-onset Werdnig-Hoffmann d.
Leber d.
Legg d.
Leigh d.
leptomeningeal neoplastic d.
Lesch-Nyhan d.
Letterer-Siwe d.
Lewy body d.
Lhermitte-Duclos d.
Lichtheim d.
Lindau-von Hippel d.
Little d.
Lou Gehrig d.
lower motor neuron d.
Luft d.
lumbar disc d.
lumbar facet d.
Lyme d.
Lyodura-associated Creutzfeldt-Jakob d.
lysosomal storage d.
Lytico-Bodig d.
Machado-Joseph d.
mad cow d.
malignant lymphoproliferative d.
maple syrup urine d.
Marie-Foix-Alajouanine d.
Marie-Strümpell d.
Marie-Tooth d.
Maroteaux-Lamy d.
McArdle d.
Medin d.
medullary cystic d. (MCD)
Meige d.
Ménière d.
Menkes d.
Merzbacher-Pelizaeus d.
metastatic d.
Milton d.
Minamata d.
Minor d.
Mitchell d.
mitochondrial d. (MD)
mixed connective tissue d. (MCTD)
Möbius d.
Morel-Kraepelin d.
Morgagni d.
Morquio d.
Morton d.
Morvan d.
motor neuron d. (MND)
motor pathways d.
motor system d.
motor unit d.
moyamoya d.
multicore d.
Munchausen d.
Murray Valley d.
muscle-eye-brain d.
myelinoclastic d.
Nasu-Hakola d.
Neftel d.
neonatal hemorrhagic d.
neonatal Pelizaeus-Merzbacher d.
nerve root d.
neuro-Behçet d.
neurodegenerative d.
neuroendocrine d.
neurologic complication from cardiac d.
neuromuscular junction d.
new variant Creutzfeldt-Jakob d.
Niemann d.
Niemann-Pick d. (type A, B, C) (NPD)
nonneoplastic d.
nonviral infectious d.
Norrie d.
occlusive cerebrovascular d.
oculocraniosomatic d.
Ollier d.
Oppenheim d.
orbital d.
organic brain d. (OBD)
Paget d.
paraneoplastic neurologic d.
paraneoplastic neurological d.
parkin d.
parkin-related d.
Parkinson d.
Parrot d.
Parry-Romberg d.
Parsonage-Turner d.
pediatric moyamoya d.
pediatric stroke from rheumatic heart d.
Pelizaeus-Merzbacher d.
peripheral nerve d.
peripheral vascular d.
periventricular d.
peroxisomal d.
Pette-Döring d.
Peyronie d.
Pick d.

polyglucosan storage d.
polyglutamine d.
Pompe d., type 1, 2
Portuguese-Azorean d.
Pott d.
Pringle d.
prion d.
progressive brain d.
progressive neurological d.
progressive neuromuscular d.
pseudo-Hurler d.
pseudomyotonia d.
pulseless d.
pyramidal tract d.
Quincke d.
Rabot d.
Raynaud d.
Refsum d.
Rendu-Osler-Weber d.
restrictive lung d.
reversible motor neuron d.
rigid spine d.
rippling muscle d.
Romberg d.
Rosai-Dorfman d. (RDD)
Roth d.
Roussy-Lévy d.
Rust d.
Salla d.
sanatorium d.
Sandhoff d.
Sanfilippo d.
Santavuori d.
Santavuori-Haltia d.
Santavuori-Haltia-Hagberg d.
Schaumberg d.
Scheie d.
Scheuermann d.
Schilder d.
Schindler d.
Schmitt d.
Scholz d.
Seitelberger d.
self-induced artifactual skin d.
self-perpetuated d.
Selter d.
Shy-Drager d.
sialic acid storage d.
sickle cell d.
Siemerling-Creutzfeldt d.
Sly d.
small vessel d.
Spielmeyer-Sjögren d.
Spielmeyer-Vogt d.
Spielmeyer-Vogt-Sjögren d.
spinal cord d.
spinal metastatic d.
sporadic Creutzfeldt-Jakob d. (sCJD)
startle d.
Steele-Richardson-Olszewski d.
Steinert d.
St. Martin d.
Stokes-Adams d.
storage d.
structural intracranial d.
Strümpell d.
Strümpell-Leichtenstern d.
Strümpell-Lorrain d.
Strümpell-Marie d.
Strümpell-Westphal d.
Sturge d.
Sturge-Weber d.
subcortical cerebrovascular d.
subcortical small vessel d.
Swash-Schwartz d.
Sweet d.
swineherd d.
Sydenham d.
symptomatic extrapulmonary d.
systemic inflammatory d.
systemic neoplastic d.
Takayasu d.
Talma d.
Tangier d.
Tarui d.
Tay-Sachs d.
Thomsen d.
thoracolumbar degenerative d.
Thornton-Griggs-Moxley d.
thyroid d.
Tooth d.
Tourette d.
transient white matter d.
transmissible neurodegenerative d.
Trevor d.
triplet-repeat d.
Ullrich d.
Unverricht d.
Unverricht-Lafora d.
Unverricht-Lundborg d.
upper motor neuron d.
van Bogaert d.
van Bogaert-Canavan d.

NOTES

disease *(continued)*
vanishing white matter d.
variant Creutzfeldt-Jakob d. (vCJD)
vascular Parkinson d.
venous occlusive d.
venous thromboembolic d. (VTED)
vertebrobasilar d.
Virchow d.
Vogt d.
Vogt-Spielmeyer d.
von Economo d.
von Gierke d.
von Hippel d.
von Hippel-Lindau d.
von Recklinghausen d.
von Willebrand d.
Wartenberg d.
Weber-Christian d.
Welander d.
Werdnig-Hoffmann d.
Wernicke d.
Weston Hurst d.
Westphal d.
Whipple d.
white matter degenerative d.
Whytt d.
Wilson d.
Winkelman d.
Wohlfart-Kugelberg-Welander d.
Wolman d.
X-linked Charcot-Marie-Tooth d.
Ziehen-Oppenheim d.
disease-altering treatment
disease-associated antibody
disease-modifying
d.-m. agent (DMA)
d.-m. agent therapy
d.-m. compound
d.-m. drug (DMD)
disengagement mechanism
disequilibrium
dialysis d.
frontal d.
gait d.
neurochemical d.
subcortical d.
DISH
diffuse idiopathic skeletal hyperostosis
dishpan fracture
disialyl ganglioside
disimmune polyneuropathy
disinterest
social d.
disk (*var. of* disc)
diskectomy (*var. of* discectomy)
diskiform (*var. of* disciform)
diskitis (*var. of* discitis)
diskogenic (*var. of* discogenic)
diskogram (*var. of* discogram)
diskography (*var. of* discography)
diskotomy (*var. of* discotomy)
dislocation
atlantoaxial d.
fracture d.
rotatory d.
temporomandibular joint d.
dislodgment
hook d.
lead d.
dismutase
superoxide d. (SOD)
disodium
carbenicillin d.
d. etidronate
disofenin
technetium-99m d.
disomy
uniparental d.
disopyramide phosphate
disorder
abnormal sleep-wake schedule d.
accommodation d.
acoustic nerve d.
acute neuropsychologic d.
acute pain d.
adjustment sleep d.
adult-onset movement d.
alcohol-dependent sleep d.
aluminum toxic d.
amino acid metabolic d.
amnesic d.
aneurysm-associated d.
antibody-mediated d.
apperceptive d.
apraxic d.
arousal d.
arsenic toxic d.
articulation d.
Asperger d.
atypical gait d.
atypical somatoform d.
atypical stereotyped movement d.
atypical tic d.
auditory perceptual d.
autonomic arousal d.
autosomal dominant movement d.
balance d.
behavior d.
behavioral d.
biotin metabolic d.
bipolar I d.
bleeding d.
brain d.
caffeine-induced anxiety d.
caffeine-induced sleep d.
caffeine use d.
calcium d.
carbohydrate metabolic d.

carbohydrate metabolism d.
d. category
cellular migration d.
cerebral degenerative d.
childhood disintegrative d. (CDD)
chloride d.
choreiform d.
chronic motor tic d.
chronic neurologic d.
chronic neuropsychologic d.
chronic sleep d.
circadian rhythm sleep d.
clotting d.
cluster A, B, C d.
coagulation d.
cobalamin metabolism d.
cognition d.
cognitive d.
communication d.
comorbid sleep d.
congenital infratentorial d.
conversion d.
cranial nerve congenital d.
cranial nerve postinfectious d.
cumulative trauma d.
cystic degenerative d.
deep brain stimulation for mood d.
degenerative cervical spine d.
degenerative neuronal d.
demyelinative d.
developmental language d. (DLD)
drug-induced movement d.
drug-induced neuromuscular d.
dysmyelinating/hypomyelinating d.
electrolyte metabolism d.
endocrine d.
environmental sleep d.
d.'s of excessive somnolence (DOES)
extrapyramidal d.
extrinsic sleep d.
eye movement d.
facial neuromotor d.
fatty acid oxidation d.
free-running circadian sleep d.
frontal gait d.
functional voice d.
gait d.
generalized anxiety d. (GAD)
genetic d.
global amnestic d.
global anterograde memory d.
glucose homeostasis d.
glycoprotein degradation d.
glycoprotein storage d.
hereditary brachial plexus d.
hereditary sensory and autonomic d.
heterogenous d.
histidine metabolism d.
Huntington diseaselike d.
hyperkinetic conduct d.
hyperkinetic impulse d.
hyperkinetic motor d.
hyperkinetic movement d.
hypnotic-dependent sleep d.
hysterical gait d.
hysterical movement d.
inherited global neurodegenerative d.
d. of initiation and maintenance of sleep
insomnia-related panic d.
intermittent explosive d.
ion channel d.
irregular sleep-wake d.
jet lag sleep d.
labyrinthine d.
lead toxic d.
limb movement d.
limb psychogenic d.
limit-setting sleep d.
lipid-lipoprotein metabolism d.
lipid metabolism d.
lipid storage d.
lipoprotein metabolic d.
low back pain psychogenic d.
lymphoproliferative d.
lysine metabolism d.
lysosomal storage d.
magnesium d.
major depression d.
manganese toxic d.
mastication d.
medical/neurological d.
medication-induced movement d.
meningoradicular d.
mercury toxic d.
metabolic d.
metallic toxic d.
metal metabolic d.
metal metabolism d.
mitochondrial metabolic d.

NOTES

disorder *(continued)*
mixed receptive/expressive language d.
monogenetic d.
mood disorder associated with sleep d.
mood spectrum d.
motor neuron d.
motor psychogenic d.
motor retardation developmental delay d.
movement d.
multiple-tic d. (MTD)
multisystemic d.
muscle inflammatory d.
muscle myotonic d.
muscle psychogenic d.
musculoskeletal psychogenic d.
myeloproliferative d.
nervous system d.
neural migration d.
neural tube development d.
neurobehavioral d.
neurocirculatory d.
neurodegenerative movement d.
neurogenic d.
neurologic d.
neurometabolic d.
neuromuscular junction d.
neuronal lysosomal storage d.
neuronal migration d.
neuronal proliferation d.
neuroophthalmic d.
neuropsychologic d.
nonapneic sleep d.
nonentrained sleep-wake d.
non-24-hour sleep-wake d.
occupational neurotic d.
ophthalmic d.
optokinetic d.
organic anxiety d.
organic brain d.
organic delusional d.
organic mental d.
organic mood d.
organic personality d.
organic psychiatric d.
organic toxic d.
pachygyria-type cortical neuronal migration d.
pain d.
paralytic psychosomatic d.
paraneoplastic neurologic d.
paroxysmal sleep d.
periodic limb movement d. (PLMD)
peripheral nervous system d.
peroxisomal metabolic d.
peroxisome biogenesis d. (PBD)
pervasive development d. (PDD)
pervasive developmental d.
phosphate d.
physical comorbid d.
plant toxic d.
postsynaptic d.
potassium d.
potential cumulative trauma d.
presynaptic d.
primary thought d.
pronunciation d.
prothrombotic d.
psychoactive substance-induced organic mental d.
psychogenic learning d.
psychogenic limb d.
psychogenic motor d.
psychogenic muscle d.
psychogenic musculoskeletal d.
psychogenic neurocirculatory d.
psychogenic obsessional d.
psychogenic pain d.
psychogenic respiratory d.
psychogenic rheumatic d.
psychogenic skin d.
psychogenic sleep d.
psychogenic stomach d.
purine metabolic d.
pyrimidine metabolic d.
recurrent mood d.
reflex d.
REM sleep behavior d.
REM sleep-related d.
renal amino acid transport d.
rhythmic movement d.
seasonal affective d. (SAD)
secondary d.
self-perceived cognitive d.
senile gait d.
serotonin excess d.
serum lipoprotein d.
shift work-related sleep d.
shift work sleep d.
sleep disorder associated with mental d.
sleep-onset association d.
sleep psychogenic d.
sleep-related breathing d. (SRBD)
sleep-starts d.
sleeptalking d.
sleep terror d.
sleep-wake transition d.
smell d.
sodium channel d.
solitary aggressive-type conduct d.
somatization d.
somatoform d.
spectrum d.
speech developmental d.

sphingolipid metabolism d.
spinal cord d.
spoken language d.
startle d.
stereotyped movement d.
stereotypic movement d.
stimulant-dependent sleep d.
substance-induced organic mental d.
substantia nigra d.
swallowing d.
systemic giant cell d.
taste d.
temporary personality d.
thallium toxic d.
tic d.
tic-related obsessive-compulsive d.
toxic d.
toxin-induced sleep d.
transient d.
trauma spectrum d.
traumatic brachial plexus d.
triple repeat d.
tyrosine metabolism d.
urea cycle d.
vascular higher level gait d.
vestibular d.
violent conduct d.
visceral d.
visual field d.
visual image movement d.
vocal tic d.
wakefulness d.
X-linked cortical migration d.
Z-disc d.

disordered personality function

disorganization
background d.
d. dimension
EEG background d.
segmental arterial d.
d. symptom

disorganized
d. speech
d. symptom complex
d. thinking

disorientation
visuospatial d.

Disotate

disparity
pupil size d.

dispensable cortex

dispersion
intravoxel phase d.
nuclear magnetic relaxation d.
temporal d.

displacement
d. of interhemispheric fissure
significant d.
traumatic d.

disposable Doppler-constant thermocouple sensor

disproportion
congenital muscle fiber-type d. (CMFTD)
craniocephalic d.
muscle fiber-type d.

disrupted occipitocervical articulation

disruption
anterior column d.
autonomic d.
axonal transport d.
blood-brain barrier d. (BBBD)
brain function d.
cervical spine posterior ligament d.
counting d.
focal axonal d.
frank d.
incudostapedial d.
level of d.
d. of normal activity
pedicle cortex d.
sleep d.

disruptive
d. impact
d. psychotic patient

dissecting
d. aneurysm
d. forceps
d. hook

dissection
arterial d.
bone d.
bone/ligament d.
bony d.
carotid artery d.
cerebral artery d.
cerebrovascular arterial d.
cervicocephalic arterial d.
condyle d.
cranial nerve d.
extracranial vascular d.
familial cervicocephalic arterial d.
hard palate d.

NOTES

D

dissection *(continued)*
incisural d.
intracranial vascular d.
intradural d.
jugular vein d.
middle fossa floor/petrous d.
muscle d.
parotid d.
soft tissue d.
subperiosteal d.
subtemporal d.
suction d.
sylvian d.
thoracic outlet syndrome d.
vascular d.
vertebral d.
dissector
aneurysm neck d.
Angell James d.
Cavitron d.
Creed d.
Crile gasserian ganglion knife and d.
Crile nerve hook and d.
Davis dura d.
Effler-Groves d.
endarterectomy d.
Field suction d.
Freer d.
golf-stick d.
Hajek-Ballenger d.
Hardy d.
hockey-stick d.
Jannetta aneurysm neck d.
joker d.
Kocher d.
Malis d.
Marino transsphenoidal d.
Maroon-Jannetta d.
McDonald d.
Milligan d.
needle d.
neural d.
Oldberg d.
Olivecrona dura d.
Rayport dura and knife d.
Rhoton ball d.
Rochester lamina d.
Scoville d.
Smithwick d.
spatula d.
teardrop d.
tissue plane d.
Toennis-Adson d.
Toennis dura d.
ultrasonic d.
Dissectron ultrasonic neurosurgical aspirator console
disseminata
alopecia d.
disseminated
d. central nervous system histoplasmosis
d. CNS histoplasmosis
d. disease
d. encephalomyelitis
d. intravascular coagulation (DIC)
d. leiomyosarcoma
d. sclerosis
dissociable mechanism
dissociated
d. anesthesia
d. motor development
d. nystagmus
d. sensory loss
dissociation
albuminocytologic d.
d. level
d. measure
nonpathological d.
d. of numbers
d. of objects
occipitocervical d. (OCD)
pathological d.
pupil light-near d.
d. sensibility
sleep d.
d. symptom
syringomyelic d.
tabetic d.
visual-kinetic d.
dissociative
d. amnesia
d. anesthesia
d. anesthetic
d. patient
d. psychoneurotic reaction
d. response
d. symptom cluster
d. tendency
distal
d. anterior cerebral artery aneurysm
d. axonopathy
d. basilar temporary clip
d. carotid
d. catheter
d. catheter lengthening
d. lenticulostriate artery aneurysm
d. medial striate artery
d. motor latency
d. motor paresis
d. muscle
d. muscular dystrophy
d. myopathy
d. occlusion
d. part of anterior lobe of hypophysis

d. sensory polyneuropathy (DSP)
d. stimulation generator
d. symmetric axonal sensorimotor neuropathy
d. symmetric polyneuropathy
d. sympathetic stump
d. tingling on percussion (DTP)

distalis
pars d.

distance
d. ceptor
internodal d.
interpeduncular d.
interuncal d.
d. sense

distant
d. brain failure (DBF)
d. metastasis

distensae
striae d.

distensible tissue

distinction
primary/secondary d.
taste d.

distortion
body image d.
body schema d.
eddy current d.
local field d.
reality d.
significant subjective d.
subjective d.

distraction
anterior d.
apical d.
d. bar
d. force
Harrington d.
d. instrumentation
d. instrumentation biomechanics
d. laminoplasty
d. rod

distraction/compression scoliosis treatment

distractive flexion injury

distractor
asymmetric visual d.
DeBastiani d.

distribution
bimodal d.
Boltzmann d.
butterfly d.
cervical root d.
fixed d.
girdle-type pain d.
nervous d.
onion-skin d.
regional d.
sensory d.
stocking-glove d.
d. volume ratio (DVR)
von Mises stress d.

disturbance
acid-base d.
appetitive d.
balance d.
bladder d.
bowel d.
cognitive d.
color vision d.
core cognitive d.
dementia behavior d. (DBD)
electrolyte d.
endocrine d.
focal neurologic d.
gait d.
global assessment of sensory d.
hemisensory d.
hypomania associated with sleep d.
d. of intellectual development
language d.
memory d.
metabolic d.
mood d.
nocturnal sleep d.
oculomotor d.
perceptual d.
peripheral vasomotor d.
physical d.
posttraumatic mental d.
psychomotor behavioral d.
schizophrenia-related sleep d.
sleep d.
sleep-related respiratory d.
sleep-wake schedule d.
speech d.
sphincter d.
sphincteric d.
temporospatial orientation d.
transient emotional d.
visual d.

disturbed
emotionally d.

NOTES

disturbed *(continued)*
d. sleep
d. sleep-wake cycle
disulfiram
disuse
d. atrophy
d. osteoporosis
d. supersensitivity
diuretic
Diuril
diurnal
d. epilepsy
d. mood variation
d. nap
d. sleepiness
divalent cation transporter
divalproex sodium
divergence
d. insufficiency
synergistic d.
diverticularization
diverticulum, pl. **diverticula**
meningeal diverticula
diverting shunt tube
diving
d. reflex
d. spinal cord injury
divisio, pl. **divisiones**
divisiones anteriores plexus brachialis
d. autonomica systematis nervosi peripherici
divisiones posteriores plexus brachialis
division
anterior primary d.
cell d.
lobar d.
Divry-van
D.-v. Bogaert familial corticomeningeal angiomatosis
D.-v. Bogaert syndrome
Dix-Hallpike
D.-H. maneuver
D.-H. test
Dixon
D. method opposed imaging
D. radiofrequency coil
dizygotic twin
dizziness
sudden d.
DKA
diabetic ketoacidosis
olanzapine-associated DKA
DLB
dementia with Lewy body
DLBD
diffuse Lewy body dementia
DLD
developmental language disorder
DLRPN
diabetic lumbosacral radiculoplexus neuropathy
DMA
disease-modifying agent
DMA therapy
DMAS
dimethylamine sulfate
DMD
disease-modifying drug
Duchenne muscular dystrophy
dystonia musculorum deformans
DMD gene
DMD phenotype
D-Med Injection
DMSO
dimethyl sulfoxide
DNA
deoxyribonucleic acid
DNA analysis
double-stranded DNA
DNA fragmentation factor (DFF)
genomic DNA
DNA hybridization
DNA marker
mitochondrial DNA
DNA protein kinase
DNA repair enzyme
DNA repletion syndrome
viral DNA
DNA virus
DNAse
deoxyribonuclease
caspase-activated DNAse
DNIC
diffuse noxious inhibitory control
dobutamine
docetaxel
docking
neurotransmitter vessel d.
docosahexaenoic acid (DHA)
documented pseudarthrosis
Doc ventral cervical stabilization system
DOES
disorders of excessive somnolence
dog
seizure-alerting d.
Dogbone anterior cervical plate fixation system
Dogiel
D. cell
D. corpuscle
Dolenc technique
Dolgic
dolichocephaly
dolichoectasia
intracranial arterial d.

dolichoectatic
- d. aneurysm
- d. internal carotid artery

doll's
- d. eye maneuver
- d. eye phenomenon
- d. eye reaction
- d. eye reflex
- d. eye sign
- d. head anesthesia
- d. head phenomenon

Dolophine

dolor capitis

dolorific

dolorificus
- trismus d.

dolorimeter
- Chatillon d.

dolorimetry

dolorogenic zone

dolorology

dolorosa
- analgesia d.
- anesthesia d.
- hypalgesia d.
- paraplegia d.

dolorosum
- punctum d.

domain
- analog d.
- cognitive d.
- Fas-associated death d.
- d. of functioning
- microtubule-binding d.
- neuropsychologic d.
- N-terminal d.
- particle d.

dome
- d. of aneurysm
- aneurysmal d.
- double d.

dominance
- cerebral d.
- lack of clear-cut cerebral d.
- left hemisphere d.
- left/right hemisphere d.
- mixed cerebral d.
- right hemisphere d.

dominant
- autosomal d.
- d. frequency
- d. hemisphere
- d. hemisphere dysfunction
- d. hemisphere function
- d. hemisphere infarction
- d. hemisphere lesion
- d. hemisphere parietal area
- d. hemisphere temporal area

domperidone

Donaghy angled suture needle holder

Donaldson line

donepezil hydrochloride

donor
- beating-heart brain-dead d.
- blood d.

Doose syndrome

dopa
- d. decarboxylase inhibitor
- methyl d.

dopamine
- d. agonist
- d. beta hydrolase (DPH)
- brain d.
- d. clearance
- d. degradation
- d. D_2 receptor
- d. enhancement
- d. hydrochloride
- d. metabolism
- d. neurotoxicity
- d. neurotransmission
- d. pathway
- d. projection
- d. receptor blockade
- d. receptor blocker
- d. release
- d. stimulation
- striatal d.
- d. synthesis
- d. system
- d. transporter (DAT)
- d. transporter autoradiography
- d. uptake site

dopamine-acetylcholine imbalance

dopamine-innervated limbic region

dopamine-modulating transmitter system

dopaminergic
- d. activity
- d. antagonist
- d. antagonist-related exacerbation
- d. blocking drug
- d. effect
- d. inhibition
- d. medication

dopaminergic *(continued)*
d. modulation
d. neuron
d. projection
d. stimulant
d. system
d. therapy
d. tone
d. treatment
d. tuberoinfundibular pathway
dopaminergic-cholinergic balance
dopa-responsive dystonia
Doppler
color-flow D.
continuous-wave D.
D. effect
D. flowmetry
D. frequency spectrum
D. imaging
Mizuho surgical D.
multifrequency transcranial D.
Neuroguard transcranial D.
D. precordial end-tidal carbon dioxide monitoring
D. probe
D. pulsatility index
pulsed D.
pulse wave D.
D. sonography
transcranial D. (TCD)
D. ultrasonography
D. ultrasound
D. ultrasound monitor
Doral
Dorello canal
Dorfman-Chanarin disease
dormant basket cell hypothesis
Dormarex Oral
dorsal
d. accessory olivary nucleus
d. anterior cingulate region
d. aponeurotic expansion hood
d. callosal vein
d. central gray
d. cochlear nucleus
d. column decussation
d. column sensory pathway
d. column sensory tract
d. column of spinal cord
d. column stimulation
d. column stimulator
d. column syndrome
d. cord stimulation
d. enteric fistula
d. funicular column of spinal cord
d. funiculus
d. gray column
d. horn
d. horn cell
d. horn neuron
d. horn neuronal response
d. hypothalamic area
d. hypothalamic region
d. intermediate sulcus
d. lateral geniculate nucleus
d. limbic region
d. longitudinal fasciculus
d. median fissure of medulla oblongata
d. median fissure of spinal cord
d. median sulcus
d. mesencephalic syndrome
d. midbrain glioma
d. midbrain syndrome
d. motor nucleus of vagus
d. neocortical region
d. nucleus of thalamus
d. nucleus of trapezoid body
d. nucleus of vagus
d. pallidum
d. part of pons
d. plate of neural tube
d. premammillary nucleus
d. premotor cortex
d. ramus
d. raphe
d. raphe nucleus
d. reflex
d. rhizotomy
d. root entry zone (DREZ)
d. root entry zone lesion
d. root entry zone lesioning
d. root ganglion (DRG)
d. root ganglion cell
d. root of spinal nerve
d. scapular nerve
d. septal nucleus
d. spinal root
d. spine
d. spinocerebellar tract
d. spinocerebellar tract neuron
d. stream
d. stream dysfunction
d. stream structure
d. striatum
d. subcutaneous space
d. supraoptic commissure
d. tegmental decussation
d. thalamus
d. thoracic nucleus
d. trigeminothalamic tract
d. vagal nucleus
d. vein of corpus callosum
dorsale
pallidum d.
striatum d.
tuber d.

dorsalis
Abadie sign of tabes d.
area hypothalamica d.
commissura supraoptica d.
fasciculus longitudinalis d.
funiculus d.
hypertrophic pachymeningitis d.
lamina d.
nucleus campi d.
nucleus hypothalamicus d.
nucleus olivaris accessorius d.
nucleus paramedianus d.
nucleus premammillaris d.
nucleus thoracicus d.
nucleus vagalis d.
radix d.
ramus corporis callosi d.
regio hypothalamica d.
spina d.
tabes d.
tetanus d.
thalamus d.
tractus spinocerebellaris d.
Dorsey
D. dural separator
D. ventricular cannula
dorsiflex
dorsolateral
d. caudate nucleus
d. fasciculus
d. prefrontal cortex
d. prefrontal cortical area
d. prefrontal syndrome
d. region
d. resection
d. sulcus
d. tract
dorsolateralis
fasciculus d.
tractus d.
dorsomedial
d. hypothalamic nucleus
d. mesencephalic syndrome
d. nucleus of hypothalamus
d. thalamotomy
dorsomedialis
nucleus hypothalamicus d.
dorsum
d. pedis reflex
d. sellae atrophy
d. sellae erosion
dosage
medication d.
neuroleptic d.
radiosurgical d.
steroid d.
total neuroleptic d.
dose
anticholinergic d.
cumulative d.
d. dependent
effective d. (ED)
equivalent d.
d. escalation
full d.
improper d.
lithium d.
marginally therapeutic d.
maximum tolerated d.
minimal lethal d. (MLD)
modal d.
neuroleptic d.
nominal standard d.
oral d.
periphery d.
priming d.
radiation d.
d. range
d. reduction
d. reduction method
d. reduction strategy
sequential d.
standard d.
steady-state d.
subtherapeutic d.
dose-dependent neurotoxicity
dose-limiting toxicity
Dosepak
Medrol D.
dose-related difference
dose-response
d.-r. relation
d.-r. relationship
dosimeter
thermoluminescent d.
dosimetry
dosing
bolus d.
energy d.
fixed d.
flexible neuroleptic d.
neuroleptic d.
Dospan

NOTES

dot
line frequency noise d.
dothiepin hydrochloride
dot-probe task
double
d. antihelix
d. cortex
d. discharge
d. dome
d. elevator palsy
d. fishhook retractor
d. fragment sign
d. hemiplegia
d. major curve pattern
d. major curve scoliosis
d. spring ball valve
d. taper
d. thoracic curve
d. thoracic curve scoliosis
d. vision
d. visual control
d. yoke
d. Zielke instrumentation
double-action rongeur
double-blind
d.-b. drug study
d.-b. placebo-controlled trial
d.-b. placebo trial
double-compartment hydrocephalus
double-congenital athetosis
doublecortin gene
double-detector Vertex system
double-donut system
double-L spinal rod
double-lumen Swan-Ganz catheter
double-point threshold
double-pore vent system
double-rod
d.-r. construct
d.-r. technique
double-step
double-stranded
d.-s. deoxyribonucleic acid (dsDNA)
d.-s. DNA
d.-s. DNA virus
double-vector
d.-v. blade
d.-v. brain spatula
douloureux
tic d.
dowel cutter
down
d. gaze
D. syndrome
D. syndrome clinical feature
D. syndrome dermatoglyphic pattern
D. syndrome pathology
D. syndrome screening
downbeat nystagmus
downbiting Epstein curette
downgaze
d. paralysis, ataxia/athetosis and foam cell (DAF)
d. paresis
Downing retractor
down-moving optokinetic nystagmus
downsized circular laminar hook
downstream signaling
downturned corners of mouth
downward gaze paresis
doxazosin mesylate
doxepin hydrochloride
doxogenic
doxorubicin hydrochloride
Doyen
D. cylindrical bur
D. rib spreader
D. spherical bur
Doyère eminence
d-penicillamine
D-penicillamine treatment
DPH
dopamine beta hydrolase
DPV
disabling positional vertigo
DR
digital radiography
dracunculiasis
Drager MTC transducer
drain
Charnley suction d.
external ventricular d.
Hemovac Hydrocoat d.
Heyer-Schulte wound d.
Jackson-Pratt d.
lumbar d.
Shirley d.
subarachnoid d.
subgaleal d.
Surgivac d.
Wound-Evac d.
drainage
bur hole d.
epidural venous d.
external ventricular d.
infratentorial venous d.
lumbar d.
serial percutaneous needle d.
Spetzler-Martin grade III medium-size lesion with deep venous d.
Spetzler-Martin grade II small lesion with deep venous d.
spinal d.
stereotactic catheter d.
subarachnoid d.
syrinx d.
ventricular d.

draining vein
Drake
D. fenestrated clip
D. tandem clipping technique
D. tourniquet
Drake-Kees clip
Dramamine Less Drowsy Formula
drape
NeuroDrape surgical d.
OPMI microscopic d.
Dravet syndrome
DRD2 gene
dreaming sleep
dreamlike state
dreamy state
Dressinet netting bandage
dressing
Allevyn d.
d. apraxia
dry sterile d.
DuoDERM d.
Fabco gauze d.
Flexinet d.
d. forceps
hourglass d.
Inerpan flexible burn d.
Kaltostat d.
Kerlix d.
Mills d.
modified Robert Jones d.
Mother Jones d.
NeoDerm d.
OpSite d.
Owen gauze d.
Reston d.
Sof-Rol d.
Sof-Wick d.
Stimson d.
surgical d.
Surgicel Nu-Knit d.
Tubex gauze d.
DREZ
dorsal root entry zone
DREZ electrode
DREZ lesioning
DREZ procedure
DREZ surgery
DREZotomy
microsurgical DREZotomy
DRG
dorsal root ganglion
drift
EEG amplifier d.
genic d.
mesenchymal d.
drill
acorn d.
Acra-Cut wire pass d.
air d.
air-powered d.
Anspach 65K d.
Black Max high-speed d.
Caspar d.
Codman d.
Crutchfield hand d.
D'Errico perforating d.
diamond high-speed air d.
electric d.
Fisch d.
d. guide
d. guide with drill bit
Hall Surgairtome II d.
Hall UltraPower d.
Hall Versipower d.
high-speed air d.
Hudson d.
McKenzie perforating twist d.
MedNext high-speed d.
Midas Rex d.
Mira Mark III cranial d.
Phoenix cranial d.
power d.
powered automatic-stopping d.
Quick Connect twist d.
right-angle d.
Stryker d.
Xpress 100 disposable perforator bur hole d.
drilling technique
Drinker tank respirator
drinking
thymogenic d.
drip
d. chamber
perfusate d.
Drisdol Oral
drive
abnormal respiratory d.
acquired d.
affiliation d.
affiliative d.
d. behavior
decreased respiratory d.

NOTES

drive *(continued)*
kinetic d.
physiological d.
primary d.
secondary d.
sleep d.
stimulus d. (SD)
thermal d.
vestibulospinal d.
wakefulness d.
driver's thigh
driving
photic d.
d. risk
dromedary gait
dromica
epilepsia d.
dromotropic
dromotropism
negative d.
positive d.
dronabinol
Drooling
D. Rating Scale
D. Severity and Frequency Scale
droopy shoulder syndrome
drop
d. attack
d. foot
d. hand
d. metastasis
d. seizure
toe d.
wrist d.
droperidol
drop-finger deformity
dropfoot, drop foot
dropped foot
drop-thumb deformity
drowning
near d.
drowsiness
continuous daytime d.
daytime d.
incapacitating d.
pathological d.
rhythmic midtemporal burst of d.
rhythmic midtemporal theta of d. (RMTD)
DRPLA
dentatorubropallidoluysian atrophy
DRS
Delirium Rating Scale
DRSP
drug-resistant *Streptococcus pneumoniae*
drug
d. action
add-on d.
d. administration
antagonist d.
antiabsence antiepileptic d.
anticholinergic d.
antidote d.
antiepileptic d. (AED)
antimuscarinic d.
antiplatelet d.
anxiolytic d.
atypical antipsychotic d.
combination d. (CD)
compassionate use of d.'s
conventional neuroleptic d.
cytotoxic d.
date rape d.
disease-modifying d. (DMD)
dopaminergic blocking d.
d. efficacy
enzyme-inducing antiepileptic d.
d. fever
d. half-life
d. holiday
hypnotic d.
illicit d.
immunosuppressive d.
d. infusion pump
d. intervention
d. intoxication
intramuscular administered d.
d. metabolism
neuroleptic d.
oral administered d.
ototoxic d.
phenytoin interaction with other d.'s
platinum-based d.
psychedelic d.
d. reaction
d. regimen
d. reinforcement
d. risk analysis message system
sympathomimetic d.
d. tapering
d. tetanus
d. toxicity
d. transporter
tricyclic d.
d. war
d. washout
d. withdrawal seizure
drug-induced
d.-i. chorea
d.-i. depression
d.-i. dystonia
d.-i. encephalopathy
d.-i. hallucination
d.-i. hallucinatory state
d.-i. insomnia
d.-i. medical complication
d.-i. movement disorder

d.-i. myoglobinuria
d.-i. negative symptom
d.-i. neuromuscular disorder
d.-i. nystagmus
d.-i. organic personality syndrome
d.-i. paranoid state
d.-i. parkinsonism
d.-i. semihypnotic state
d.-i. status epilepticus
d.-i. tremor
d.-i. white matter disease
drug-like desire state
drug-naïve patient
drug-related dyskinesia
drug-resistant
d.-r. depression
d.-r. localization-related seizure
d.-r. *Streptococcus pneumoniae* (DRSP)
drug/toxin-induced tremor
Drummond
D. spinous wiring technique
D. wire
drunkenness
sleep d.
DRVVT
dilute Russell viper venom time
dry
d. beriberi
d. eye syndrome
d. leprosy
d. sterile dressing
DSA
density-modulated spectral array
digital subtraction angiography
DSB
digit span backward
dsDNA
double-stranded deoxyribonucleic acid
D2-selective dopamine agonist
DSF
digit span forward
DSM
degradable starch microsphere
DSM cluster
DSP
distal sensory polyneuropathy
DT
delirium tremens
DTI
diffusion tensor imaging
DTICH
delayed traumatic intracerebral hematoma
DTP
distal tingling on percussion
DTPA
diethylenetriamine pentaacetic acid
gadolinium DTPA
DTR
deep tendon reflex
DTT
device for transverse traction
DTT implant
dual
d. bypass connector
d. compression scoliosis treatment
d. mechanism of action
d. octapolar lead
d. pathology
d. quadrapolar lead
D. Quattrode spinal cord stimulation system
d. tasking
dual-energy x-ray absorptiometry (DEXA, DXA)
dualism
mind/body d.
molecular d.
dual-isotope SPECT
dual-photon absorptiometry
dual-switch valve
Duane retraction syndrome
Dubini
D. chorea
D. disease
Duchenne
D. disease
D. muscular dystrophy (DMD)
D. paralysis
D. sign
D. smile
D. syndrome
Duchenne-Aran
D.-A. disease
D.-A. spinal muscular atrophy
Duchenne-Davidoff-Masson syndrome
Duchenne-Erb
D.-E. paralysis
D.-E. syndrome
Duchenne-Griesinger disease
Duchenne-Landouzy dystrophy
duck-billed anodized spatula

D

NOTES

Duckworth
D. phenomenon
D. sign
duct
ampullary limb of semicircular d.
basal lamina of cochlear d.
basilar crest of cochlear d.
basilar membrane of cochlear d.
cochlear d.
common membranous limb of membranous semicircular d.
endolymphatic d.
Hensen d.
lacrimal d.
medullary collecting d. (MCD)
parotid d.
perilymphatic d.
semicircular d.
simple membranous limb of semicircular d.
Stensen d.
uniting d.
utriculosaccular d.
ductus
d. cochlearis
crista basilaris d.
d. endolymphaticus
d. perilymphaticus
d. reuniens
d. semicirculares
d. semicircularis
d. semicircularis anterior
d. semicircularis lateralis
d. semicircularis posterior
d. utriculosaccularis
ductuum
ampullaria d.
Duke Twins Study of Memory in Aging
Dulbecco modified Eagle medium
dull unremitting headache
duloxetine hydrochloride
Dumbach cranial titanium mesh
dumbbell
d. ganglioneuroma
d. lesion
d. neuroblastoma
d. neurofibroma
d. tumor
d. tumor configuration
dumbbell-shaped
d.-s. neurinoma
d.-s. spinal cavernous hemangioma
dumbbell-type neuroblastoma
dummy seed catheter
Duncan
D. syndrome
D. ventricle
Dunn device
Dunnett test
Duo-Cline bed wedge
DuoDERM dressing
DuPen epidural catheter
duplex
d. scanning
d. transmission
duplication
d. anomaly
d. mutation
Dupuytren contracture
dura
clinoidal d.
endosteal d.
freeze-dried cadaveric d.
d. hook
lyophilized cadaveric d.
d. mater
d. mater of brain
d. mater encephali
d. mater of spinal cord
d. mater spinalis
d. propria
scarred d.
supratentorial d.
Tisseel artificial d.
durabolin
Duradrin capsule
duraencephalosynangiosis
DuraGen dural graft matrix
Duragesic Transdermal
Dura-Guard dural repair patch
Dura-Kold ice wrap
dural
d. arteriovenous fistula (DAVF)
d. arteriovenous malformation
d. attachment
d. defect
d. detachment
d. ectasia
d. endothelioma
d. fibrosis
d. graft
d. grafting
d. hematoma
d. incision
d. margin
d. metastasis
d. part of filum terminale
d. penetration
d. punch
d. repair
d. retractor
d. ring
d. sac
d. sac effacement
d. scissors
d. separator
d. septum

d. sheath
d. sinus occlusion
d. tack-up suture
d. tail
d. tear
d. terminal filament
d. venous fistula
d. venous sinus
d. venous sinus thrombosis
duralis
sinus venosi d.
duraplasty
dura-protecting forceps
duration
minimum d.
movement d. (MD)
stimulus d.
d. tetany
Duret
D. hemorrhage
D. lesion
Durkan CTS gauge
duroarachnitis
durocutaneous fistula
durotomy
frontotemporal d.
incidental d.
paramedian d.
petty d.
Dutch Courage
duteplase
Duvol lung clamp
DVI
digital vascular imaging
DVR
distribution volume ratio
dwarf
bird-headed d.
dwarfism
hypothyroid d.
pituitary d.
DW-EPI
diffusion-weighted echo planar image
DWI
diffusion-weighted imaging
DWML
deep white matter lesion
Dwyer
D. device
D. instrument
D. instrumentation biomechanics
DXA (*var. of* DEXA)
Dyazide
dye
carbocyanine d.
dying-back
d.-b. neuropathy
d.-b. polyneuropathy
Dyke-Davidoff-Mason syndrome
Dyke-Davidoff syndrome
dynactin
mutant d.
dynamic
adaptation d.
d. ambulatory balance
d. aphasia
attachment d.
d. bed
d. block
d. compression plate instrumentation
d. CT
d. EMG-assisted biomechanical model
d. entrapment of vertebral artery
flow d.
d. formulation
d. gait index
hemispheric d.
intermediate hemispheric d.
lateral hemispheric d.
medial hemispheric d.
D. mesh pre-angled connecting bar
d. mutation
d. polarity
power d.
d. reference arc
d. referencing
religious d.
d. single-photon emission computed tomography
d. standing balance
temporal d.
d. transverse traction device
d. variable
dynamogenesis
dynamogenic
dynamogeny
dynamometer
bulb d.
dynein
cytoplasmic d.
d. protein
dynein-dynactin complex
dynorphin

NOTES

Dyonics
D. cannula
D. rod-lens endoscope
dysacusis
dysangiogenesis
hemorrhagic d.
dysantigraphia
dysaphia
dysaphic
dysarthria
apraxic d.
ataxic d.
athetoid d.
athetosic d.
flaccid d.
hyperkinetic d.
hypokinetic d.
labial d.
laryngeal d.
d. literalis
lower motor neuron d.
parkinsonian d.
peripheral d.
progressive d.
rigid d.
sensual d.
somesthetic d.
spastic d.
d. syllabaris spasmodica
dysarthria-clumsy hand syndrome
dysarthric
dysarthrosis
dysautonomia
familial d.
histamine test in familial d.
dysautonomic feature
dysbasia lordotica progressiva
dyscalculia
dyscheiral, dyschiral
dyscheiria, dyschiria
dyschromatopsia
cerebral d.
dyscinesia (*var. of* dyskinesia)
dysconjugate
d. gaze
d. movement
dyscontrol
dysdiadochokinesia, dysdiadochocinesia
dysdiadochokinesis
dysdiadochokinetic
dysembryoplastic neuroepithelial tumor
dyserethism
dysergia
dysesthesia
facial d.
dysexecutive
D. Questionnaire
d. syndrome
dysferlin band
dysferlinopathy
dysfibrous layer
dysfunction
autonomic d.
bilateral hemisphere d.
brain d.
bulbar d.
calmodulin d.
central nervous system d.
cerebellovestibular d.
cerebral d.
cholinergic d.
cognitive d.
corticospinal motor system d.
cranial nerve d.
depressive executive d.
dominant hemisphere d.
dorsal stream d.
emptying d.
executive d.
eye tracking d.
focal cortical d.
focal temporal lobe d.
frontal cortical d.
frontal lobe d.
global cognitive d.
higher cerebral d.
hypothalamic d.
hypothalamic-pituitary d.
immunologic d.
interictal physiologic d.
lacrimal gland d.
lingual airway d.
lobar d.
lower motor neuron d.
magnocellular d.
maternal d.
memory d.
minimal brain d.
mitochondrial d.
neurocognitive d.
nondominant hemisphere d.
ocular muscle d.
oculosympathetic d.
olfactory d.
optokinetic reflex d.
organic d.
pituitary d.
postictal cognitive d.
pyramidal tract d.
refractory erectile d.
renal d.
salivary gland d.
sensory integration d.
serotonergic d.
sexual d.
small-fiber d.
somatosensory d.
sphincter d.

striatofrontal d.
swallowing d.
temporal lobe d.
trigeminal motor d.
upper motor neuron d.
utriculosaccular d.

dysfunctional
D. Beliefs and Attitudes about Sleep (DBAS)
d. circuitry
d. dopamine system
d. neural circuit

dysgenesis
cerebellar vermis d.
cerebral d.
cingulate gyrus d.
corpus callosum d.
cortical d.
hemispheric cerebral d.
macroscopic d.

dysgenetic syndrome

dysgerminoma
parasellar d.

dysgeusia

dysgnosia

dysgranular cortex

dysgraphia

dysjunction
craniofacial d.

dysjunctive
d. gaze
d. nystagmus

dyskinesia, dyscinesia, dyskinesis
d. algera
anticonvulsant-induced d.
belly dancer d.
biliary d.
buccolingual d.
choreic d.
diphasic d.
drug-related d.
dystonic paroxysmal nonkinesigenic d.
extrapyramidal d.
faciobuccolingual d.
kinesigenic paroxysmal d.
levodopa-induced d.
ocular d.
oral d.
oral-buccal-lingual d.
orolingual-buccal d.
paroxysmal exertional d.
paroxysmal kinesigenic d.
paroxysmal nonkinesigenic d. (PNKD)
peak-dose d.
tardive oral d.
tardive orobuccal d.
withdrawal-emergent d.

dyskinetic

dyslexia
surface d.

dyslogia

dysmegalopsia

dysmetria
cerebellar d.
cognitive d.
lower limb d.
ocular d.
saccadic d.
truncal d.

dysmnesic syndrome

dysmorphic syndrome

dysmorphism, dysmorphia
cranial d.
facial d.

dysmyelinating/hypomyelinating disorder

dysmyelination

dysmyelinisatus

dysmyotonia

dysnomia
amnesic d.

dysnystaxis

dysorthographia

dysostosis
cleidocranial d.
craniofacial d.
mandibulofacial d.

dyspallia

dysphagia
D. Evaluation Protocol
neurogenic d.
receptive d.

dysphasia
Broca d.
hereditary d.
Wernicke d.

dysphasic

dysphonia
adductor d.
d. clericorum
d. spastica

NOTES

dysphoria
omnipresent d.
premenstrual d.
dysphoric
d. category
d. character structure
d. manic state
d. patient
dysphrasia
dysplasia
anhidrotic ectodermal d.
bony d.
brain d.
cerebral d.
chondroectodermal d. (CED)
cortical d.
craniofrontonasal d.
craniometaphysial d.
fibromuscular d. (FMD)
fibrous d.
focal cortical d.
müllerian duct aplasia, renal aplasia, cervicothoracic somite d.
odontoid d.
posterior quadrantic d.
septooptic d.
septooptic-pituitary d.
sphenoid wing d.
thanatophoric d.
dysplastic
d. gangliocytoma
d. spondylolisthesis
dyspnea
functional d.
nocturnal d.
sighing d.
dyspraxia
ideomotor d.
innervatory d.
limb-kinetic d.
oromotor d.
speech d.
dysprosium-DTPA
dysprosody
expressive d.
receptive d.
sensory d.
dysraphicus
status d.
dysraphism, dysraphia
anencephaly d.
Chiari malformation d.
congenital defect of cranial bones d.
congenital scalp defect d.
craniofacial d.
diastematomyelia d.
encephalocele d.
hydromyelia d.
meningomyelocele d.
neurodermal sinus d.
occult spinal d.
sacral agenesis d.
spina bifida d.
spinal d.
syringomyelia d.
tectocerebellar d.
dysreflexia
autonomic d. (AD)
dysregulated
d. neurotransmission
d. stress response
d. T-cell function
dysregulation
biologic d.
cerebrovascular d.
hypothalamic d.
immune d.
neurologic d.
sleep-related respiratory d.
dysrhythmia
cerebral d.
circadian d.
electroencephalographic d.
paroxysmal cerebral d.
dysrhythmic
dyssomnia
dysspondylism
dysstatic
dyssynergia
d. cerebellaris myoclonica
d. cerebellaris progressiva
detrusor-external sphincter d.
detrusor-sphincter d.
detrusor-striated sphincter d.
dystasia
hereditary areflexic d.
Roussy-Lévy hereditary areflexic d.
dystaxia
sensory d.
dysthymia
chronic d.
dystonia
d. 1 (DYT1)
action d.
adult-onset d.
anterocollis d.
arm d.
athetosic d.
breathy d.
cervical d.
childhood-onset d.
d. deformans progressiva
dopa-responsive d.
drug-induced d.
end-of-dose d.
d. examination
facial d.

focal hand d.
generalized d.
hereditary d.
hypnogenic paroxysmal d.
jerky primary d.
d. lenticularis
D. Movement Scale
d. musculorum
d. musculorum deformans (DMD)
musician's d.
myoclonic d.
nocturnal paroxysmal d.
nuchal d.
off-period d.
on-period d.
oromandibular d.
oropharyngeal d.
paradoxical phenomenon of d.
paroxysmal nocturnal d.
pathogenic d.
postanoxic d.
primary d.
psychogenic d.
secondary d.
segmental d.
spastic d.
symptomatic d.
tardive d.
torsion d.
transient d.
d. treatment
whispering d.

dystonic
d. amyotrophy
d. cerebral palsy
d. choreoathetosis
d. gait
d. movement
d. paroxysmal nonkinesigenic dyskinesia
d. reaction
d. spasm
d. torticollis
d. tremor

dystopia
orbital d.
pituitary d.

dystrophia
d. adiposogenitalis
d. musculorum progressiva
d. myotonica

dystrophic
d. calcification
d. neurite
d. neuron

dystrophica
myotonia d.

dystrophin

dystrophinopathy

dystrophoneurosis

dystrophy
adiposogenital d.
adult pseudohypertrophic muscular d.
Aran-Duchenne muscular d.
Barnes d.
Becker-Kiener d.
Becker-type tardive muscular d.
Becker variant of Duchenne d.
benign X-linked recessive muscular d.
Bogaert-Bertrand spongy d.
cerebromacular d.
childhood muscular d.
congenital muscular d. (CMD)
Dejerine-Landouzy d.
distal muscular d.
Duchenne-Landouzy d.
Duchenne muscular d. (DMD)
Emery-Dreifuss muscular d.
Erb muscular d.
facioscapulohumeral muscular d.
FSH d.
Fukuyama congenital muscular d.
Fukuyama-type congenital muscular d.
Gowers muscular d.
humeroperoneal muscular d.
infantile neuroaxonal d.
Kiloh-Nevin ocular form of progressive muscular d.
Landouzy d.
Landouzy-Dejerine muscular d.
Leyden-Möbius muscular d.
limb-girdle muscular d.
merosin-positive congenital muscular d.
muscular d.
myotonic muscular d.
neuroaxonal d.
oculogastrointestinal muscular d.
oculopharyngeal muscular d. (OPMD)

D

NOTES

dystrophy *(continued)*
pelvofemoral muscular d.
progressive muscular d.
pseudohypertrophic muscular d.
reflex sympathetic d. (RSD)
rigid spine muscular d.
scapulohumeral muscular d.
scapuloperoneal muscular d.
severe childhood autosomal recessive muscular d.
Simmerlin d.
Steinert myotonic d.
sympathetic reflex d.
Thomsen d.
Welander muscular d.
X-linked recessive muscular d.

dystropy

DYT1
dystonia 1
DYT1 carrier
DYT1 dystonia mutation
DYT1 gene

E1
ubiquitin-activating enzyme E1
E2
ubiquitin-conjugating enzyme E2
E3
ubiquitin-ligating enzyme E3
e4 allele
e4/e4 genotype
E9000 Power System
EA-2
episodic ataxia type 2
EAE
experimental allergic encephalitis
Eagle
E. minimum essential medium
E. rigid anterior cervical plate system
E. syndrome
Eales disease
ear
e. cartilage inflammation
cup e.
e. forceps
Earle salts
early
e. after depolarization
e. brain overgrowth
e. final awakening
e. life adversity
e. morning akinesia
e. mortality
e. pharmacological intervention
e. posttraumatic epilepsy
e. right anterior negativity
e. satiety
e. seizure
e. speech impairment
e. treatment diabetic retinopathy study
e. warning sign
early-onset
e.-o. ataxia
e.-o. category
e.-o. familial Alzheimer disease
e.-o. ischemic stroke
e.-o. Parkinson disease
e.-o. scoliosis
East
E. African sleeping sickness
E. African trypanosomiasis
eastern
e. equine encephalitis
e. equine encephalomyelitis (EEE)
easy
e. fatigability
e. fatigue
EasyGuide Neuro image-guided surgery system
eating
e. epilepsy
e. seizure
Eaton-Lambert syndrome
EB
ethidium bromide
Ebbinghaus test
EBI
EBI Array spinal system
EBI Omega21 spinal fixation system
EBI V-Force thread technology
ebriosorum
delirium e.
EBRT
external beam radiotherapy
EBV
Epstein-Barr virus
EBV encephalitis
ECA
extracranial carotid artery
ECA study
ECA-PCA bypass surgery
eccentric
e. A cluster
e. arteriosclerosis
e. growth
ecchondrosis
ecchymosis, pl. **ecchymoses**
bilateral medial orbital ecchymoses
mastoid e.
orbital e.
periorbital e.
posterior e.
eccrine
e. angiomatous hamartoma
e. cystadenoma
e. gland
echeosis
Echlin laminectomy rongeur
Echlin-Luer rongeur
ECHO
enteric cytopathic human orphan
ECHO virus
echo
de pensós e.
gradient e. (GRE)
gradient-recalled e.
Hahn e.

echo *(continued)*
e. planar diffusion- and perfusion-weighted imaging scan
e. planar image
e. planar imaging
radiofrequency-induced e.
rapid spin e. (RSE)
e. reaction
e. speech
spin e.
spoiled gradient e.
e. time (TE)
turbo-spin e.
T1-weighted spin e.
T2-weighted spin e.
echodensity
intraparenchymal periventricular e.
echoencephalography
echographia
echokinesis, echokinesia
echolalia
echomimia
echomotism
echopathy
echophrasia
echopraxia
echovirus
e. infection ataxia
e. meningitis
Echovist
ECI
electrocerebral inactivity
EC-IC
extracranial-intracranial
EC-IC arterial bypass
Ecker fissure
eclampsia
puerperal e.
eclamptic
e. amentia
e. convulsion
e. delirium
e. idiocy
e. seizure
e. symptom
eclamptogenic, eclamptogenous
Eclipse TENS unit
ECM
extracellular matrix
ECoG
electrocorticography
ECoG monitoring
ecologic framework
ecology
human e.
economic viewpoint
ECP
external counterpulsion
ECS
electrocerebral silence
ECST
European Carotid Surgery Trial
ectal origin
ectasia
basilar e.
dural e.
segmental e.
ectatic vessel
ectoderm
embryonic neural e.
neural e.
ectodermal implant
ectomorphic
ectopia
cerebellar e.
e. lentis
posterior pituitary gland e.
ectopic
e. ACTH syndrome
e. bone formation
e. hormone
e. intracranial retinoblastoma
e. neuron
e. pinealoma
e. pituitary adenoma (EPA)
e. pituitary gland
ectropion
ED
effective dose
EDAS
encephaloduroarteriosynangiosis
EDAS procedure
eddy
e. current
e. current distortion
e. current heating
EDE
effective dose equivalent
edema
airway e.
alimentary e.
angioneurotic e.
blue e.
brain e.
brainstem e.
cellular brain e.
cerebral e.
chalky white disc e.
circumscribed e.
cytotoxic e.
disc e.
extrapontine e.
focal e.
granulocytic brain e.
hereditary angioneurotic e. (HANE)
holohemispheric vasogenic e.
interstitial e.

interstitial hydrocephalic e.
intraneural e.
ipsilateral vasogenic e.
ischemic brain e.
malignant brain e.
meningioma-associated cerebral e.
nerve root e.
neurogenic pulmonary e. (NPE)
optic disc e.
orthostatic e.
pericephalic e.
perifocal e.
periodic e.
peritumoral brain e.
pulmonary e.
Quincke e.
retroauricular e.
temporary e.
vasogenic e.

Eden classification

Eder-Puestow metal olive dilator

edetate
calcium disodium e.

edge
e. artifact
e. enhancement
e. fracture

Edinburgh
E. 2 Coma Scale
E. Questionnaire

Edinger
E. fiber
E. nucleus

Edinger-Westphal nucleus

edition
Alcadd Test, Revised E.
Assessment of Aphasia and Related Disorders, Second E.
Bedside Evaluation Screening Test, Second E.
Cognitive Skills Assessment Battery, Second E.
CogScreen Aeromedical E.
Developing Cognitive Abilities Test, Second E.

Edmonton extension tongs

EDRF
endothelium-derived relaxing factor

edrophonium
e. chloride
e. chloride test

EDS
Ehlers-Danlos syndrome
excessive daytime sleepiness

EDSS
Expanded Disability Status Scale

education
American Council for Headache E.

Edwards
E. instrumentation
E. modular system
E. modular system bridging sleeve construct
E. modular system compression construct
E. modular system construct selection
E. modular system distraction-lordosis construct
E. modular system dynamic loading
E. modular system kyphoreduction construct
E. modular system load sharing
E. modular system neutralization construct
E. modular system rod crosslink
E. modular system rod-sleeve construct
E. modular system sacral fixation device
E. modular system scoliosis construct
E. modular system spinal rod-sleeve
E. modular system spondylo construct
E. modular system standard sleeve construct
E. modular system universal rod
E. sacral screw
E. syndrome

Edwards/Barbaro syringo-peritoneal shunt

Edwards-Levine rod

EECP
enhanced external counterpulsion

EEE
eastern equine encephalomyelitis

EEG
electroencephalogram
electroencephalography
EEG activating procedure

NOTES

EEG *(continued)*
EEG activation
EEG alpha blocking
EEG alpha pattern
EEG alpha rhythm
EEG alpha spindle
EEG alpha wave
EEG amplifier drift
EEG anachronism
EEG anteromesial temporal discharge
attenuation of alpha rhythm on EEG
EEG background disorganization
Bancaud phenomenon on EEG
baseline EEG
blunt spike-and-wave complex on EEG
frontal intermittent rhythmic delta activity on EEG
ictal pattern on EEG
ictal scalp EEG
interictal EEG
low-voltage EEG
mixed-frequency EEG
scattered dysrhythmic slow activity on EEG
sleep-deprived EEG
waking background EEG
EEG with NP lead

efavirenz

effacement
basal cistern e.
dural sac e.
nerve root sheath e.
sulcus e.
ventricle e.

effect
adverse negative immunosuppressive e.
adverse side e.
age e.
antagonistic e.
anticholinergic e.
anticonvulsant e.
antidopaminergic e.
antihistaminergic e.
antimuscarinic e.
antinociceptive e.
antioxidant e.
antiseizure e.
bandwagon e.
behavioral e.
blast e.
Bohr e.
Bohr-Haldane e.
boxcar e.
brain metabolic e.
bystander e.
calming e.
catastrophic e.
cholinergic e.
choroid plexus water hammer e.
chronic insomnia medication e.
clasp-knife e.
clinical e.
copper wire e.
cue e.
cue-induced subjective e.
cumulative e.
Cushing e.
deleterious e.
developmental e.
differential beneficial e.
direct thermogenic e.
dopaminergic e.
Doppler e.
enhanced e.
euphoric e.
extrapyramidal motor side e.
Féré e.
first-night e.
flow-induced influx e.
frontal cortex damage e.
gastrointestinal side e.
genetic e.
genomic e.
Hawthorn e.
head trauma e.
heat e.
hypermetabolic e.
iatrogenic e.
IC e.
immunosuppressive e.
inflow e.
inhibitory e.
insulin e.
interactive e.
Lazarus e.
limbic e.
limited e.
local mass e.
long-lasting drug e.
magnetohydrodynamic e.
main e.
mass e.
maximal e.
measurement e.
medical e.
medication-related side e.
medication side e.
metabolic e.
Mierzejewski e.
missile e.
modified Stroop e.
Mozart e.
muscarinic side e.
muscle-relaxing e.

negative immunosuppressive e.
negative priming e.
neurochemical e.
neuroprotective e.
neurotoxic e.
neurotropic e.
nonsignificant protective e.
noradrenergic e.
oral appliance side e.
Orbeli e.
panicogenic e.
paradoxical e.
peak behavioral e.
peripheral antimuscarinic side e.
phase-shift e.
phenothiazine toxic e.
positive e.
primary e.
proconvulsant e.
progesterone e.
protective e.
psychiatric e.
psychodynamic e.
psychological e.
psychotropic e.
putative e.
radiation e.
rebound e.
recency e.
reinforcing e.
salicylate toxic e.
secondary e.
serial position e.'s
serotonergic side e.
siphon e.
e. size
specific e.
stalk e.
steal e.
stimulation-related adverse e.
stimulatory e.
subjective e.
sundowner e.
susceptibility e.
sympathectomy e.
thermogenic e.
threshold e.
time-of-flight e.
time-on-task e.
toxic side e.
treatment-emergent extrapyramidal side e.
tricyclic e.
Tyndall e.
undifferentiated e.
Vulpian e.
washboard e.
Wedensky e.
withdrawal e.

effected pain

effective
e. dose (ED)
e. dose equivalent (EDE)
e. half time (Te)
e. level
e. pedicle diameter
e. technique
e. thread diameter

effectiveness
long-term e.
relative biologic e. (RBE)
relative biological e.
treatment e.

effector
e. cell
cold e.
heat e.
e. organ
e. T cell
warm e.

efferent
e. fiber
gamma e.
e. limb
e. motor unit
e. nerve
e. neurofiber
e. pathway
e. relation
e. sympathetic activity

efferentes
neurofibrae e.

Effer-K

effervescent
K+ Care E.
K-Electrolyte E.
Klorvess E.
K-Lyte E.
potassium bicarbonate and potassium chloride, e.
potassium bicarbonate and potassium citrate, e.

Effexor

NOTES

efficacy
clinical e.
drug e.
lack of e.
relational e.
e. scale
e. study
therapeutic e.
efficiency
colony-forming e.
decreased sleep e.
index of forecasting e.
sleep e.
Effler-Groves dissector
effort syndrome
effusion
subdural e.
EGF
epidermal growth factor
EGFR
epidermal growth factor receptor
eggcrate mattress
egg-shelling procedure
egocentric stage of development
egomechanism of defense
egosyntonic trait
EGR2 gene
Ehlers-Danlos
E.-D. disease
E.-D. disease type IV
E.-D. syndrome (EDS)
Ehrenritter ganglion
EIA
electroimmunoassay
MAC EIA
Eichhorst
E. atrophy
E. neuritis
eicosanoid production
eicosapentaenoic acid
eight-and-a-half syndrome
eighth
e. cranial nerve [CN VIII]
e. nerve herpetic neuritis
e. nerve tumor
Eisenlohr syndrome
ejaculatio retardata
ejaculatory
e. center
e. speech
ejection fraction
Ekbom syndrome
Ekos ultrasound catheter
ELANA
excimer laser-assisted nonocclusive anastomosis
Elan-E electronic motor system
elantrine
elastase
myeloid e.
plasma e.
Elastica-Masson stain
Elastica van Gieson stain
Elastica-Verhoeff stain
elasticity
infant spine e.
elastic-type
e.-t. disc prosthesis
e.-t. disc replacement
elasticum
pseudoxanthoma e.
elastin
e. degradation
e. gene
elastomeric balloon
Elavil
elbow
e. jerk
e. reflex
Eldepryl
elderly
Informant Questionnaire on Cognitive Decline in the E.
elective mutism
electric
e. chorea
e. differential therapy
e. drill
General E. (GE)
e. knife
electrical
e. activity
e. change
e. characteristic
e. cortical stimulation
e. evoked potential
e. injury
e. signal
e. silence
e. status epilepticus
e. status epilepticus during slow sleep
e. status epilepticus of sleep
e. stimulation of centromedian thalamic nucleus
e. stimulation mapping
electrically evoked pain
Electri-Cool cold therapy system
electroanalgesia
electroaxonography
electroblotting
electrocautery
Aspen e.
bipolar e.
Fox bipolar e.
monopolar e.

electrocerebral
  e. activity
  e. inactivator
  e. inactivity (ECI)
  e. silence (ECS)
electrocoagulation
  RF e.
electrocochleogram
electrocochleography
electrocontractility
electroconvulsive
  e. seizure
  e. therapy
electrocorticogram
electrocorticography (ECoG)
  intraoperative e.
electrode
  active surface e.
  Ad-Tech Spencer platinum depth e.
  A-frame e.
  anterior cheek e.
  Aspen laparoscopy e.
  bifilar needle e.
  bipolar needle e.
  bipolar stimulating e.
  Clark e.
  clip-type e.
  coaxial needle e.
  combination needle e.
  concentric needle e.
  Cueva cranial nerve e.
  curved e.
  Cyberonics vagus nerve stimulator e.
  DBS e.
  depth e.
  DREZ e.
  El-Naggar-Nashold right-angled nucleus caudalis DREZ e.
  epidural peg e.
  exploring e.
  external auditory meatus e.
  external canthus e.
  4F bipolar e.
  flexible wire e.
  foramen ovale e.
  ground e.
  helical e.
  e. impedance
  indifferent e.
  intracerebral depth e.
  Kanpolat CT e.
  Levin thermocouple cordotomy e.
  loose e.
  mandibular notch e.
  metal e.
  e. migration
  monopolar needle e.
  monopolar stimulating e.
  multilead e.
  Nashold TC e.
  nasopharyngeal e.
  needle e.
  Nichrome cylindrical e.
  peg e.
  percutaneous epidural e.
  Pisces e.
  Pisces-Quad e.
  platinum microwire e.
  Quad e.
  Ray RRE-TM thermistor e.
  record e.
  recording e.
  reference e.
  Resume e.
  scalp e.
  self-adhering e.
  self-attaching e.
  semiinvasive e.
  Silverman placement of e.
  silver-silver chloride e.
  Sluijter-Mehta thermocouple e.
  Somatics monitoring e.
  Spencer probe depth e.
  sphenoidal e.
  spring-loaded e.
  Stephenson-Gibbs reference e.
  stimulating e.
  straight needle e.
  subdural grid e.
  subdural strip e.
  surface e.
  temporary percutaneous SCS e.
  thermistor e.
  Thymapad stimulus e.
  trigeminal e.
  tripolar nerve cuff e.
  Wolfram needle e.
  Wyler cylindrical subdural e.
electrodecrement
electrode-pop artifact
electrode-popping artifact
electrodermal

NOTES

electrodetachable
e. balloon
e. platinum coil
electrodiagnosis
electrodiagnostic
e. medicine
e. study
e. testing
electroencephalogram (EEG)
e. activation
alerting maneuver on e.
alerting stimulus on e.
aliasing on e.
ambulatory e. (AEEG)
audiovisual e.
e. BEAM technique
e. brain electrical activity method technique
e. burst suppression pattern
depth-recorded e.
flat e.
HFF on e.
hippocampal e.
hypersynchronous e.
interictal e.
intracranial e. (ICEEG)
IRDA on e.
isoelectric e.
Janz response on e.
Laplacian montage on e.
LFF on e.
MFD wave on e.
normal e. (NEEG)
OIRDA on e.
PDA on e.
POSTS on e.
quantitative e. (QEEG)
e. rhythm
RMTD on e.
stereotactic depth e. (SDEEG)
e. study
surface scalp e.
electroencephalograph
electroencephalographer
electroencephalographic
e. burst suppression
e. dysrhythmia
e. pattern
e. wave
electroencephalography (EEG)
ambulatory e. (AEEG)
intracranial e.
scalp ictal e.
scalp-sphenoidal e.
single-fiber e. (SFEMG)
stereotactic depth e. (SDEEG)
subdural e.
electroencephalography-guided cortical resection
electroencephaloscope
electrogram
electrograph
electrographic
e. seizure
e. seizure activity
electrography
electrogustometry
electroimmunoassay (EIA)
electrolyte
e. change
e. disturbance
e. imbalance
e. metabolism disorder
electromagnetic
e. flowmeter
e. flow probe
e. focusing field
e. focusing field probe
e. interference (EMI)
e. radiation
electromicturation
electromuscular sensibility
electromyelogram
electromyelography
electromyogram (EMG)
CRD on e.
Erb point stimulation on e.
MUAP on e.
SNAP on e.
electromyogram-triggered neuromuscular stimulation
electromyograph
Counterpoint e.
Medelec MS91 e.
electromyographic (EMG)
e. artifact
e. feedback
e. incomplete interference pattern
e. potential
e. response
electromyography (EMG)
facial e.
needle e.
single-fiber e.
sphincter e.
electron
e. collision
e. micrograph
e. microscopy
e. transport chain
e. transport particle (ETP)
electron-coupled nuclear spin-spin interaction
electroneurogram (ENoG)
electroneurography (ENoG)
facial e.
electroneurolysis
electroneuromyography

electronic
e. monitor
e. monitoring
e. stimulator
electronystagmography (ENG)
electrooculogram
electrooculographic analysis
electrooculography (EOG)
electropathology
electrophoresis
agarose gel e.
2-dimensional e.
protein e.
pulsed-field gel e.
sodium dodecyl sulfate-polyacrylamide gel e.
thin-layer agarose gel e.
electrophrenic respiration
electrophysiologic
e. change
e. integrity
e. study
e. test
e. testing
electrophysiological
e. guidance
e. mapping
e. procedure
e. stimulation
electrophysiology test
electroretinogram
electroretinography (ERG)
electroshock seizure threshold
electrosleep
electrospectrogram
electrospectrography
electrospinogram
electrospinography
electrostimulation
electrotherapeutic
e. sleep
e. sleep therapy
electrotherapy
intradiscal e. (IDET)
electrothrombosis
electrotonic
e. current
e. junction
e. synapse
electrotonus
elegans
Caenorhabditis e.
Elekta
E. Leksell rongeur
E. robotic surgical microscope
E. stereotactic head frame
E. viewing wand
element
cAMP response e.
compressing neural e.
3D hexahedral e.
gestural e.
glioneuronal e.
identical e.'s
postural e.
truss e.
elephantiasis neuromatosa
eletriptan
Eleutherococcus senticosus
elevated
e. core temperature
e. protein concentration
e. score
elevation
flap e.
ischemia-induced e.
mood e.
nonfocal e.
e. paresis
prolactin e.
T-score e.
elevator
Adson e.
Cloward e.
Cobb periosteal e.
Cottle e.
Crawford dural e.
Cushing Little Joker e.
Cushing periosteal e.
Cushing pituitary e.
Cushing staphylorrhaphy e.
D'Errico periosteal e.
Frazier dural e.
Freer septal e.
Hajek-Ballenger septal e.
Jannetta duckbill e.
Jarit periosteal e.
Kennerdell-Maroon e.
Key e.
Langenbeck periosteal e.
Malis e.
periosteal e.
round-tipped periosteal e.
Yasargil e.

E

NOTES

elevatus
iatrogenic e.
eleventh cranial nerve [CN XI]
elfin
e. facies
e. facies syndrome
Elgiloy
E. clip
E. clip material
elicitation
affect e.
emotion e.
ELISA
enzyme-linked immunosorbent assay
ELISA Quantikine kit
ELISA test
ellipsis
ellipsoid
cigar-shaped diffusion e.
disc-shaped diffusion e.
elliptical
e. incision
e. nystagmus
El-Naggar-Nashold right-angled nucleus caudalis DREZ electrode
eloquent cortex
Elsberg
E. brain cannula
E. test
E. ventricular cannula
elusive illness state
E-M
erythema multiforme
E-M syndrome
EM
extraordinary meridian
emarginate
emargination
embarrassment
cord e.
nerve root e.
respiratory e.
embedding
paraffin e.
embolden
embolectomy
direct e.
emboli (*pl. of* embolus)
embolic
e. apoplexy
e. infarction
e. phenomenon
e. source
e. stroke
emboliformis
nucleus e.
emboliform nucleus
emboligenic
embolism
air e.
arterial gas e. (AGE)
artery-to-artery e.
cardiac e.
cardiogenic e.
cerebral formed-element e.
cerebrovascular e.
cholesterol e.
fat e.
paradoxical air e.
paradoxical cerebral e.
pulmonary e.
retinal e.
rheumatic fever cerebral e.
spinal e.
therapeutic e.
venous e.
embolization
cerebral foreign body e.
coil e.
flow-directed e.
Histoacryl e.
partial e.
particulate e.
percutaneous intraarterial e.
percutaneous transvenous coil e.
platinum coil e.
selective e.
staged e.
stent-supported coil e.
superselective e.
therapeutic e.
transarterial platinum coil e.
transtorcular e.
venous-side e.
embolophrasia
embolus, pl. **emboli**
air e.
artery-artery e.
calcium e.
cerebral e.
fat e.
fibrin-platelet-fibrin e.
Gelfoam powder e.
organism e.
platelet-fibrin e.
septic e.
embolus-to-blood ratio
embryologic zone
embryonal cell carcinoma
embryonic
e. cervical somite
e. disc
e. implant
e. isoform
e. neural ectoderm
e. stem cell
e. tail

EMC
encephalomyocarditis
EMC encephalitis
EMDR
eye movement desensitization and reprocessing
emergency
neurologic e.
emerinopathy
Emery-Dreifuss
E.-D. disease
E.-D. muscular dystrophy
emetine peripheral neuropathy
EMG
electromyogram
electromyographic
electromyography
automatic decompensation EMG
EMG biofeedback
EMG examination
needle EMG
Nomad-LE EMG
single-fiber EMG (SFEMG)
EMG stimulator
triggered EMG
EMG-triggered neuromuscular stimulation
EMI
electromagnetic interference
eminence
abducens e.
arcuate e.
collateral e.
cruciate e.
cruciform e.
Doyère e.
eminentia teres facial e.
facial e.
hypoglossal e.
malar e.
medial e.
median e.
olivary e.
postfundibular e.
pyramidal e.
restiform e.
round e.
terete e.
thenar e.
trigeminal e.
eminentia, pl. **eminentiae**
e. abducentis
e. collateralis
e. cruciformis
e. facialis
e. hypoglossi
e. medialis
e. medialis fossae rhomboideae
e. mediana
e. pyramidalis
e. restiformis
e. teres
e. teres facial eminence
vagi e.
emissary
e. foramen
e. vein
emission computed tomography
EMLA
eutectic mixture of local anesthetics
Emory Functional Ambulation Profile
emotion
e. elicitation
e. production
emotional
e. amnesia
e. B cluster
e. communication
e. control therapy
e. deregulation
e. excitability
e. expression
e. factor
e. functioning
e. incontinence
e. information processing
e. input
e. instability
e. lability
e. leukocytosis
e. mechanism
e. memory
e. memory deficit
e. memory process
e. memory processing
e. memory score
e. neglect
e. numbness
e. overlay
e. reactivity
e. regulation
e. release therapy
e. speech
e. stimulation

NOTES

E

emotional *(continued)*
e. stimulus
e. trajectory
emotionally disturbed
emotion-related activation
emotive
e. stimulus
e. theory
empathic
e. capacity
e. failure
emphasis
bilateral temporoparietal e.
emphysema
subgaleal e.
empirical
e. approach
e. basis
e. classification
e. finding
e. limitation
e. research
e. study
e. therapy
empiricism
scientific e.
Empracet with codeine
emprosthotonos position
empty
e. delta sign
e. sella
e. sella sign
e. sella syndrome
e. set
e. triangle sign
emptying dysfunction
empyema
spinal epidural e.
subdural e.
emulsion
polyvinyl acetate e.
EMV
eye-motor-verbal
en
en bloc
en bloc laminoplasty
en bloc resection
en bloc spondylectomy
En gene
en passage feeder artery
en plaque growth
en plaque meningioma
enanthate
testosterone e.
enantiomer
encapsulated
e. brain abscess
e. end organ
encapsulation
polymer e.
encephala (*pl. of* encephalon)
encephalalgia
encephalatrophic
encephalatrophy
encephalauxe
encephalemia
encephali
arachnoidea mater e.
arachnoid mater e.
arteriae e.
bulbus e.
dura mater e.
pia mater e.
truncus e.
encephalic
e. angioma
e. asymmetry
e. nerve
e. trunk
e. vertigo
e. vesicle
encephalitic
encephalitis, pl. **encephalitides**
acute disseminated e.
acute hemorrhagic e.
acute inclusion body e.
acute necrotizing e.
anti-Ma2-associated e.
arboviral e.
Australian X e.
bacterial e.
benign myalgic e.
brainstem e.
bunyavirus e.
California e.
Central European e.
cerebellar e.
chronic focal e. (CFE)
CMV e.
Colorado tick fever viral e.
coxsackie e.
Dawson e.
dengue viral e.
eastern equine e.
EBV e.
EMC e.
enteroviral e.
epidemic e.
equine e.
experimental allergic e. (EAE)
Far East Russian e.
fatal e.
focal suppurative e.
forest-spring e.
fulminant necrotizing e.
granulomatous e.
Hayem e.

e. hemorrhagica
herpes/herpetic e.
herpes simplex virus e. (HSVE)
herpesvirus e.
herpes zoster e.
HSV e.
hyperergic e.
Ilhéus e.
inclusion body e.
influenzal e.
Japanese B e.
e. japonica
La Crosse e.
lead e.
Leichtenstern e.
e. lethargica
limbic e.
lymphocytic choriomeningitis virus e.
lymphogranuloma venereum e.
Marie-Strümpell e.
measles e.
measles inclusion body e.
Mengo e.
metabolic e.
microglial nodular e.
mumps e.
Murray Valley e.
Mycoplasma pneumoniae e.
necrotizing e.
e. neonatorum
Nipah virus e.
e. periaxialis
e. periaxialis concentrica
e. periaxialis diffusa
postinfectious brainstem e.
postinfective e.
postvaccinal e.
Powassan e.
primary e.
psittacosis e.
purulent e.
e. pyogenica
Rasmussen chronic focal e.
rotavirus e.
Russian autumn e.
Russian autumnal e.
Russian endemic e.
Russian forest spring e.
Russian spring-summer e.
Russian tick-borne e.
Russian vernal e.
Schilder e.
secondary e.
Semliki Forest e.
septic e.
St. Louis e.
Strümpell-Leichtenstern e.
subacute inclusion body e.
subacute measles e.
e. subcorticalis chronica
subcorticalis chronica e.
summer e.
suppurative e.
tick-borne e. (Central European subtype)
toxoplasmic e. (TE)
van Bogaert e.
varicella e.
Venezuelan equine e.
vernal e.
vernoestival e.
Vienna e.
viral e.
von Economo e.
Western equine e.
West Nile e.
woodcutter's e.
yellow fever e.

encephalitogen

encephalitogenic protein

encephalization

encephalocele

anterior basal e.
basal e.
e. dysraphism
frontal e.
frontoethmoidal e.
frontosphenoidal e.
nasoethmoidal e.
nasofrontal e.
nasoorbital e.
occipital e.
orbital e.
parietal e.
sphenoethmoidal e.
sphenoid e.
sphenoidal e.
sphenomaxillary e.
sphenoorbital e.
suboccipital e.
transethmoidal e.
transsphenoidal e.

NOTES

encephaloclastic
e. microcephaly
e. porencephaly
encephalocystocele
encephalodialysis
encephaloduroarteriosynangiosis (EDAS)
encephalodynia
encephalodysplasia
encephalofacial angiomatosis
encephalogaleosynangiosis
encephalogram
isoelectric e.
encephalography
encephaloid
encephalolith
encephalology
encephaloma
encephalomalacia
cystic e.
end-stage ischemic e.
multicystic e.
subcortical e.
encephalomeningitis
encephalomeningocele
encephalomeningopathy
encephalometer
encephalomyelitis
acute demyelinating e.
acute disseminated e. (ADE)
acute disseminating e.
acute necrotizing hemorrhagic e.
allergic e.
benign myalgic e.
disseminated e.
eastern equine e. (EEE)
epidemic myalgic e.
experimental allergic e.
experimental autoimmune e.
granulomatous e.
Leigh subacute necrotizing e.
necrotizing e.
paraneoplastic e.
postinfectious disseminated e.
postparainfectious e.
postvaccinal e.
subacute necrotizing e.
Theiler murine e.
toxoplasmic e.
vaccination e.
varicella zoster e.
Venezuelan equine e. (VEE)
viral e.
virus e.
western equine e. (WEE)
zoster e.
encephalomyelocele
encephalomyeloneuropathy
nonspecific e.
encephalomyelonic axis
encephalomyelopathy
carcinomatous e.
epidemic myalgic e.
necrotizing e.
paracarcinomatous e.
paraneoplastic e.
postinfection e.
postvaccinal e.
subacute necrotizing e. (SNE)
encephalomyeloradiculitis
encephalomyeloradiculopathy
encephalomyocarditis (EMC)
encephalomyopathy
mitochondrial neurogastrointestinal e.
encephalomyosynangiosis
encephalon, pl. **encephala**
encephalonarcosis
encephalopathia addisonia
encephalopathic
encephalopathy
AIDS e.
alcoholic e.
amyotrophic type of spongiform e.
anoxic-ischemic e.
arteriosclerotic e.
autosomal recessive syndrome of e.
bilirubin e.
Binswanger e.
bovine spongiform e.
chronic traumatic e.
cryptogenic epileptic e.
demyelinating e.
drug-induced e.
epileptic e.
ethylmalonic e.
familial e.
fulminant hepatic e.
glycine e.
Heidenhain type of spongiform e.
hemorrhagic e.
hepatic e.
HIV e.
hyperkinetic e.
hypernatremic e.
hypertensive e.
hypoglycemic e.
hyponatremic e.
hypoparathyroid e.
hypoxic-hypercarbic e.
hypoxic-ischemic e. (HIE)
infantile subacute necrotizing e.
ischemic-hypoxic e.
lead e.
Leigh necrotizing e.
liver e.
Lyme e.
metabolic e.
methotrexate e.

mitochondrial neurogastrointestinal e. (MNGIE)
multicystic e.
myoclonic e.
myoneurogastrointestinal e.
necrotizing e.
Nevin-Jones subacute spongiform e.
palindromic e.
pancreatic e.
pertussis vaccination e.
portal systemic e.
postanoxic e.
postcontusion syndrome e.
post pertussis vaccination e.
post rabies vaccination e.
postvaccinal e.
progressive degenerative subcortical e.
progressive dialysis e.
progressive spongiform e.
progressive subcortical e.
progressive traumatic e.
pulmonary e.
recurrent e.
reversible e.
saturnine e.
septic e.
severe postanoxic e.
spongiform virus e.
subacute periventricular necrotizing e.
subacute spongiform e.
subcortical arteriosclerotic e.
subcortical vascular e.
thiamine deficiency e.
thyrotoxic e.
transmissible spongiform e. (TSE)
transmissible spongiform viral e.
traumatic progressive e.
uremic e.
vaccination e.
Wernicke e.
Wernicke-Korsakoff e.

encephalopsy
encephalopuncture
encephalopyosis
encephaloradiculitis
encephalorrhachidian
encephalorrhagia
pericapillary e.
encephaloschisis
encephalosclerosis
encephaloscope
encephaloscopy
encephalosepsis
encephalosis
encephalospinal
encephalotome
encephalotomy
encephalotrigeminal
e. angiomatosis
e. angiomatosis seizure
e. vascular syndrome
enclosed
e. macroadenoma
e. space
encoding
frequency e.
phase e.
velocity e.
encroachment
foraminal e.
spinal canal e.
end
e. bulb
e. organ
e. plate
endarterectomy
carotid e.
e. dissector
endarteritis
Heubner e.
endbrain
end-brush
end-bulb
Endeavor
E. balloon
E. Instructional Rating System
E. nondetachable silicone balloon catheter
endemic
e. hiccups
e. neuritis
e. paralytic vertigo
e. poliomyelitis
endemica
panneuritis e.
Endep
end-gaze physiologic nystagmus
ending
anulospiral e.
caliciform e.
epilemmal e.
flower-spray e.

NOTES

ending *(continued)*
free nerve e.
hederiform e.
nerve e.
nonencapsulated nerve e.
presynaptic nerve e.
primary e.
Ruffini e.
secondary e.
sole-plate e.
sympathetic nerve e.
synaptic e.
end-ischemic
end-labeling
terminal deoxynucleotide transferase-mediated nick e.-l.
endoaneurysmoplasty
endoaneurysmorrhaphy
endocarditis
pediatric stroke from Libman-Sacks e.
endoceliac
endocentric construction
endocept
endocranial cast
endocraniosis
endocranitis
endocranium
endocrine
e. axis
e. disorder
e. disturbance
e. function
e. gland
e. myopathy
e. secretion
e. system
endocrine-inactive pituitary adenoma
endocrinologic
endocrinological compromise
endocrinopathy
endodermal
e. cyst
e. sinus
e. sinus tumor
endoesophageal pressure measurement
end-of-dose
e.-o.-d. bradykinesia
e.-o.-d. deterioration
e.-o.-d. dystonia
end-of-life care
endogenous
e. abnormality
e. adenosine
e. antioxidant
e. antioxidative defense
e. benzodiazepine-like toxin
e. brain mechanism
e. chromosomal promoter
e. circadian rhythm
e. electrophysiological component
e. fiber
e. force
e. neuroprotective agent
e. oxidant
e. pyrogen (EP)
e. steroid hormone
e. thyrotoxicosis
e. transmitter
endoglycosidase
endolemniscalis
nucleus e.
endolemniscal nucleus
endolymphatic
e. duct
e. hydrops
e. sac
endolymphaticus
ductus e.
endolymph production
endomeninx
endomysium
endonasal skull-base endoscopy
endoneurial
e. fluid
e. tube
endoneuritis
endoneurium
endoneurolysis
endonuclease
restriction e.
endopeduncularis
nucleus e.
endopeduncular nucleus
endoperineuritis
endoperoxide
cyclic e.
endoplasmic reticulum
endoprosthesis
Wallgraft e.
end-organ degeneration
endorphin
endorphinergic
endorrhachis
endosaccular
e. coil placement
e. occlusion
e. packing
endoscope
angled-lens e.
angled-shaft e.
Desormaux e.
Dyonics rod-lens e.
flexible e.
Gaab e.
e. holder
Hopkins II e.
e. lens cleansing device

malleable e.
percutaneous spinal e.
Perneczky-designed microscope-assisting e.
rigid rod-lens e.
e. videocamera
Wolf e.
endoscope-assisted craniotomy
endoscope-controlled microsurgery
endoscopic
e. approach
e. endonasal transsphenoidal surgery
e. microneurosurgery
e. sinus surgery
e. skull-base surgery
e. sphenoidal biopsy
e. third ventriculostomy (ETV)
e. transpsoas fusion
e. visualization
endoscopic-assisted
endoscopy
endonasal skull-base e.
heads-up adjunctive e.
intraventricular e.
Karl Storz e.
laser-assisted spinal e.
transcranial skull-base e.
virtual e.
endostatin
endosteal dura
endothelial
e. adhesion molecule
e. cell-derived procoagulant
e. cell inhibitor
e. cell-stimulating angiogenesis factor
e. cell-stimulating glioma
e. injury
e. monolayer
e. nitric oxide synthase
endothelin (ET)
endothelin-1 (ET-1)
e.-1 platinum-Dacron microcoil
e.-1 platinum-Dacron microcoil endotracheal tube
endothelioma
dural e.
endotheliomatous meningioma
endothelium
e. derived
vascular e.
endothelium-derived relaxing factor (EDRF)
endotherm
endothermic
endothermy
endotoxin
gram-negative e.
meningococcal e.
endotracheal tube
endovascular
e. balloon occlusion
e. carotid sacrifice
e. coil
e. technique
e. therapy
endovasculoscopy
endplate, end-plate
e. acetylcholinesterase deficiency
e. activity
artificial e.
bony e.
cartilaginous e.
e. damage classification
e. depression
e. instability
lower bony e.
metallic e.
motor e.
muscle e.
e. potential (EPP)
soft/spongy e.
upper bony e.
endplate-to-graft contact
end-point
e.-p. CGI score
e.-p. nystagmus
end-product
advanced glycation e.-p. (AGE)
Endrate
end-stage
e.-s. ischemic encephalomalacia
e.-s. renal disease
end-state functioning
end-tidal
e.-t. carbon dioxide monitoring
e.-t. CO_2
e.-t. nitrogen monitoring
end-to-end anastomosis
Enduron

E

NOTES

endyma
end-zone pain
energy
change in e.
e. conservation
e. dosing
e. failure
intense e.
e. lack
Law of Specific Nerve E.
e. metabolism
e. requirement
enervation
enflurane
ENG
electronystagmography
Engel
E. classification system for postoperative seizure control class I–IV
E. postoperative seizure classification
E. Seizure Outcome Scale
Engelmann disease
engorgement
brain e.
engrailed gene
engram
engraphia
enhanced
e. effect
e. external counterpulsion (EECP)
e. physiologic tremor
e. sensitivity
enhancement
contrast e.
craniospinal MRI with gadolinium e.
dopamine e.
edge e.
flow-related e.
gadolinium e.
homogenous tumor e.
meningeal e.
MR imaging with gadolinium e.
nodular e.
paramagnetic contrast e.
postsynaptic e.
relaxation rate e.
selective relaxation e.
vertebral endplate e.
enhancing
e. exophytic tumor
e. lesion
e. ring
enkephalin
enkephalinergic
enlarged
e. brain
e. pupil
enlargement
biparietal e.
cervical e.
choroid e.
cisterna magna e.
head e.
lumbosacral e.
moyamoya collateral e.
sulcal e.
tympanic e.
ventricular e.
enlarging bur
Enlon Injection
ENoG
electroneurogram
electroneurography
enophthalmos
Enovil
enoxaparin
entacapone
Entamoeba
E. histolytica
E. histolytica cerebral amebiasis
entasia, entasis
entatic state
enteric
e. cyst
e. cytopathic human orphan (ECHO)
e. cytopathic human orphan virus
e. virus infection
entericus
plexus e.
entering root
Enterobacter
enterococcal disease
enterocolitica
Yersinia e.
enterogastric reflex
enterogenous cyst
enteropathic arthritis
enteroviral encephalitis
enterovirus
e. infection
e. meningitis
enthesitis
enthesopathy
enthlasis
entoptic pulse
entorbital fissure
entorhinal
e. area
e. cortex
e. cortex atrophy
entorhinal-hippocampal system

entrance
sellar e.
entrapment
foraminal e.
median nerve e.
e. mononeuropathy
nerve e.
e. neuropathy
PIN e.
suprascapular nerve e.
ulnar nerve e.
entropy
wavelet e.
entry
e. point
e. site
e. wound
e. zone
e. zone lesion
entubulation technique
enucleation
tumor e.
enucleator
Hardy microsurgical e.
Marino transsphenoidal e.
enuresis
functional e.
nocturnal primary e.
primary e.
enuretic absence
envelope
cistern of nuclear e.
nuclear e.
environmental
e. assessment
e. cue
e. factor
e. impediment
e. influence
e. neurology
e. press
e. process
e. sleep disorder
e. sound recognition
e. susceptibility
e. toxin
environment characteristic
Envision anterior cervical plate system
Envoy guide catheter
enzymatic binding site
enzyme
e. activation
e. autoinduction
cyclooxygenase e.
DNA repair e.
ET-converting e.
Fas-associated death domain-like interleukin-converting e.
hepatic e.
Hind III e.
interleukin-1 B-converting e.
lipolytic e.
neurotransmitter metabolic e.
porphyria synthesizing e.
rate-limiting e.
e. replacement therapy
enzyme-inducing
e.-i. antiepileptic
e.-i. antiepileptic drug
enzyme-linked immunosorbent assay (ELISA)
EOG
electrooculography
EOM
extraocular movement
eosinophil adenoma
eosinophilia-myalgia syndrome
eosinophilic
e. granuloma
e. granulomatosis
e. leukocyte
e. meningitis
e. meningoencephalitis
e. myeloencephalitis
e. myositis
eosin stain
EP
endogenous pyrogen
evoked potential
EPA
ectopic pituitary adenoma
EPAP
exhalation positive airway pressure
ependopathy
ependyma
fetal e.
ventricular e.
ependymal
e. cell
e. cyst
e. layer
e. tumor
e. zone

NOTES

ependymitis
granular e.
e. granularis
ependymoblastoma
ependymocyte
ependymocytoma
ependymoma
anaplastic e.
cerebellar e.
clear cell e.
exophytic e.
intracranial e.
intramedullary e.
myxopapillary e.
sacrococcygeal myxopapillary e.
spinal e.
subcutaneous sacrococcygeal myxopapillary e.
supratentorial lobar e.
ependymopathy
ephapse
ephaptic
e. conduction
e. transmission
ephebophilia
Ephedra sinica
ephedrine
e. sulfate
e., theophylline, phenobarbital
epicerebral space
epicondylectomy
medial e.
epicortical lesion
epicranium
epicritic
e. sensation
e. sensibility
epidemic
e. cerebrospinal meningitis
e. encephalitis
e. multiple sclerosis
e. myalgic encephalomyelitis
e. myalgic encephalomyelopathy
e. neuromyasthenia
e. poliomyelitis
e. tetany
e. typhus
e. vertigo
epidemica
myalgia cruris e.
tetania e.
epidemiological
E. Catchment Area Study
e. research
e. study
epidemiology
Multi-Institutional Research in Alzheimer Genetic E.
pandemic e.
epidermal
e. growth factor (EGF)
e. growth factor receptor (EGFR)
e. growth factor receptor gene
e. growth factor-tyrosine kinase inhibitor
e. necrolysis
e. nevus syndrome
epidermidis
Staphylococcus e.
epidermoid
chiasmal e.
e. cyst
e. lipoma
torcular e.
e. tumor
epidermoidoma
epidural
e. abscess
e. abscess evacuation
e. aerocele
e. angiolipoma
e. block
e. cavernous hemangioma
e. cavity
e. cord compression
e. fat
e. hematoma
e. hemorrhage
e. hemorrhage epidural metastatic disease
e. implant
e. infection
e. lipomatosis
e. meningioma
e. meningitis
e. needle
e. neuroplasty
e. peg electrode
e. pneumatosis
e. pneumocephalus
e. space
e. steroid injection
e. tumor
e. tumor evacuation
e. venography
e. venous drainage
e. venous plexus
epidurale
cavum e.
spatium e.
epiduralis
cavitas e.
epidurography
epifascicular epineurium
epigastric
e. aura
e. plexus
e. reflex

epilemma
epilemmal ending
epilepsia
e. arithmetica
e. cursiva
e. dromica
e. gravior
e. major
e. minor
e. nutans
e. partialis continua
e. tarda
epilepsy
abdominal e.
activated e.
adolescent-onset e.
adult-onset e.
affective prodrome of e.
age-dependent e.
akinetic e.
alcoholic e.
alcohol-precipitated e.
amygdalar e.
anosognosic e.
atonic e.
audiogenic e.
automatic e.
autonomic e.
autosomal dominant nocturnal frontal lobe e.
autosomal dominant temporal lobe e.
Baltic myoclonus e.
benign adult familial myoclonic e.
benign childhood partial e.
benign focal e.
benign occipital e.
benign rolandic e.
bilateral mesial temporal lobe e.
Bravais-jacksonian e.
catamenial e.
cavernoma-related e.
centrencephalic e.
childhood absence e. (CAE)
childhood absence epilepsy evolving to juvenile myoclonic e.
childhood benign focal e.
childhood-onset e.
chronic partial e.
cingulate e.
clouded-state e.
complex precipitated e.
cortical e.
cryptogenic late-onset e.
cryptogenic myoclonic e.
cryptogenic neocortical e.
cryptogenic partial e.
dacryocystic e.
Dark Warrior e.
diencephalic e.
diurnal e.
early posttraumatic e.
eating e.
e. etiology
extratemporal lobe e.
familial adult myoclonic e.
familial mesial temporal lobe e.
familial myoclonus e.
familial progressive myoclonic e.
febrile e.
fictitious e.
focal frontal lobe e.
E. Foundation
frontal lobe e.
gelastic e.
e. gene
generalized tonic-clonic e.
grand mal e.
haut mal e.
hemiconvulsion, hemiplegia, and e. (HHE)
hippocampal e.
hot water e.
idiopathic/cryptogenic e.
idiopathic generalized e.
idiopathic partial e.
e. implant
impulsive petit mal e.
infant-onset e.
e. insomnia
insular e.
intermittent myoclonus e.
International League Against E.
intractable grand mal e.
intractable psychomotor e.
Jackson e.
jacksonian e.
juvenile absence e.
juvenile myoclonic e.
Kojewnikoff e.
Lafora familial myoclonic e.
laryngeal e.
late e.
latent e.

E

NOTES

epilepsy *(continued)*
lateral-onset temporal lobe e.
local e.
localization-related e.
Lundborg myoclonic e.
major e.
malignant familial myoclonic e.
masked e.
matutinal e.
medial temporal lobe e.
medically intractable partial e.
menstrual e.
mixed-type e.
musicogenic e.
myoclonic astatic petit mal e.
myoclonus e.
National Society for E. (NSE)
neocortical e.
neocortical temporal lobe e.
Nintendo e.
nocturnal frontal lobe e.
occipital lobe e.
opercular e.
orbitofrontal e.
parietal lobe e.
partial complex e.
partial temporal lobe e.
pattern-induced e.
pattern-sensitive e.
pediatric and adolescent e. (PAE)
petit mal e.
pharmacoresistent e.
photogenic e.
physiologic e.
postapoplectic e.
poststroke e.
posttraumatic e.
e. prevalence
primary generalized e.
primary rhinencephalic psychomotor e.
procursive e.
progressive familial myoclonic e.
progressive myoclonus e. (PME)
psychogenic e.
psychomotor e.
pyridoxine-dependent e.
reflex e.
refractory partial e.
resistant e.
rolandic e.
rotatory e.
secondary generalized e.
self-induced e.
sensory-precipitated e.
situation-related e.
sleep e.
sleep-related e.
somnambulic e.
startle e.
sudden unexplained death in e. (SUDEP)
supplementary motor area e.
e. surgery
E. Surgery Inventory-55
surgical e.
symptomatic partial e.
e. syndrome
syndrome-related e.
tardy e.
television-induced e.
temporal lobe e.
temporolimbic e.
tonic e.
tornado e.
uncinate e.
Unverricht-Lundborg myoclonus e.
Unverricht myoclonus e.
vasomotor e.
vasovagal e.
vestibulogenic e.
video game e.
visceral e.
visual reflex e.

epileptic
e. absence
e. aura
e. automatism
e. cephalea
e. clouded state
e. cry
e. dementia
e. diathesis
e. discharge
e. drop attack
e. encephalopathy
e. event
e. fall
e. focus
e. migraineur
e. negative myoclonus
e. neuron
e. neuronal aggregate
e. prodrome
e. seizure
e. spasm
e. twilight state

epileptica absentia

epilepticus
absence status e.
complex partial status e.
convulsive status e.
de novo nonconvulsive status e.
drug-induced status e.
electrical status e.
focal status e.
furor e.
generalized convulsive status e.

globus e.
ictus e.
nonconvulsive status e.
pentobarbital in status e.
pseudo status e.
refractory status e.
status e. (SE)
tonic-clonic status e.
tonic status e.
epileptiform
e. activity
e. burst
e. burst discharge
e. bursting
e. convulsion
e. neuralgia
epileptogenesis
age-related e.
progressive e.
secondary e.
epileptogenic
e. brain injury
e. burst
e. channelopathy
e. cortex
e. focus
e. stimulation
e. structural lesion
e. temporal lesion
e. zone
epileptogenicity
intrinsic e.
epileptogenous
epileptoid
orthostatic e.
epileptologist
epileptology
epileptosis
epiloia
epimysium
epinephrine-anesthetic mixture
epinephrine toxicity
epineural
epineurectomy
epineurial neurorrhaphy
epineurium
epifascicular e.
epineurolysis
epiphenomenon
epiphora
epiphysis cerebri
epipial
episcleral vascular dilation
episcleritis
episode
habitual sleep e.
mitochondrial encephalomyopathy with lactic acidosis and strokelike e.'s (MELAS)
mitochondrial myopathy, encephalopathy, lactic acidosis, strokelike e.'s (MELAS)
nocturnal confusional e.
nocturnal hypotensive e.
pollakiuria e.
sleep bruxism e.
strokelike e.
episodic
e. amnesia
e. ataxia type 2 (EA-2)
e. cluster headache
e. dyscontrol syndrome
e. memory
e. memory function
e. nocturnal wandering
e. paroxysmal hemicrania
e. tension-type headache (ETTH)
e. vertigo
epispinal space
epistemic
epistemology
genetic e.
epistolary
epithalamic
epithalamica
commissura e.
epithalamus commissure
epithelial
e. choroid layer
e. hemangioendothelioma
e. lamina
e. membrane antigen tumor marker
epithelialis
lamina choroidea e.
epithelioid
e. cell
e. hemangioendothelioma
e. histiocyte
epithelioma
epitheliopathy
multifocal placoid pigment e.
placoid pigment e.
retinal pigment e.

E

NOTES

epithelioserosa
zona e.
epithelium
olfactory e.
retinal pigment e.
sense e.
sensory e.
subcapsular e.
epitope
beta-amyloid-related e.
brain e.'s
ganglioside e.
surface e.
epitympanici
pars cupularis recessus e.
epivaginal connective tissue
Epival
E-Plate
ABC E-P.
Epley procedure
EPM2 gene
EPO
evening primrose oil
epoch
Frequency Analysis of Consecutive E. (FACE)
epoxide hydrolase
epoxy-mounted preamplifier
EPP
endplate potential
EPS
exophthalmos-producing substance
extrapyramidal sign
extrapyramidal symptom
epsilon
apolipoprotein e. (ApoE)
apolipoprotein e. 4 (APOe4)
e. opiate receptor
epsilon-aminocaproic acid
epsilon-sarcoglycan gene
EPSP
excitatory postsynaptic potential
Epstein
E. curette
E. neurological hammer
E. staging system
E. symptom
Epstein-Barr virus (EBV)
ePTFE
expanded polytetrafluoroethylene
ePTFE ventricular shunt catheter
Epworth Sleepiness Scale (ESS)
equal potential
Equanil
equation
Bloch e.
Goldman constant field e.
Larmor e.
logistic regression e.
Nernst e.
Poiseuille e.
Solomon-Bloembergen e.
Equilet
equilibration
hanging-drop e.
equilibratory ataxia
equilibrium
creatine kinase e.
Hardy-Weinberg e.
sense of e.
equina
cauda e.
equine
e. encephalitis
e. gait
Equinox EEG neuromonitoring system
equinus position
equipment
adaptive e.
Baltimore Therapeutic E. (BTE)
decompression e.
insertion e.
stainless steel e.
Vitallium e.
equipotential
EquiTest
equivalent
cobalt Gray e.
e. current dipole
e. dose
effective dose e. (EDE)
migraine e.
equivocal finding
ER
extended release
Depakote ER
Erb
E. atrophy
E. disease
E. injury
E. muscular dystrophy
E. palsy
E. point
E. point stimulation on electromyogram
E. sclerosis
E. sign
E. spinal paralysis
E. syphilitic spastic paraplegia
Erb-Charcot disease
Erb-Duchenne
E.-D. palsy
E.-D. paralysis
E.-D. syndrome
Erb-Duchenne-Klumpke
E.-D.-K. injury
E.-D.-K. injury to brachial plexus

Erben
E. phenomenon
E. reflex
E. sign
Erb-Goldflam disease
Erb-Westphal sign
Erdheim-Chester disease
Erdheim tumor
erection
painful e.
sleep-related painful e.
erector-spinal reflex
erect torso posture
erethism mercurialis
ERG
electroretinography
ERG theory
ergocalciferol
ergoesthesiograph
ergogenic aid
Ergomar
ergonovine
Ergostat
ergot
ergotamine
e. derivative
e. tartrate
e. tartrate and caffeine
ergot-derivative dopamine agonist
ergot-derived medication
ergotica
tabes e.
ergotropic
erigentes
nervi e.
erlotinib
erosion
dorsum sellae e.
vascular e.
erosive sphenoid mucocele
erratic
e. absorption
e. sleep
error
e. detection circuit
frequency e.
gross medical e.
line bisection e. (LBE)
measurement e.
paraphasic e.
perceptual e.
registration e.
root mean square e.
target localization e.
target registration e. (TRE)
volume-averaging e.
error-free performance
ERS
extended, rotated, sidebent
ERSL
extended, rotated, sidebent left
ERSR
extended, rotated, sidebent right
ERT
estrogen replacement therapy
eruption
palatal mucosal e.
perioral e.
vesicular e.
erythema
e. chronicum migrans
e. multiforme (E-M)
e. multiforme-like
erythematosus
lupus e.
pediatric stroke from systemic lupus e.
systemic lupus e. (SLE)
erythredema polyneuritis
erythroblastosis fetalis
erythrocyte
e. protoporphyria
e. sedimentation rate (ESR)
erythromelalgia
head e.
erythroprosopalgia
escalating conflict
escalation
dose e.
escape phenomenon
Escherich
E. reflex
E. sign
Escherichia
E. coli
E. coli meningitis
escitalopram oxalate
Escobar
E. disease
E. syndrome
E-selectin level
esmolol
esodeviation
esodic nerve

E

NOTES

esoethmoiditis
esophageal
e. achalasia
e. airway
e. perforation
e. pH monitoring
e. plexus
e. pressure monitoring
esophagi
pars cervicalis e.
pars thoracica e.
esophagosalivary reflex
esophagus
thoracic part of e.
esotropia
Espocan combined spinal/epidural needle
ESR
erythrocyte sedimentation rate
ESRRL
extension, sidebent right, rotated left
ESS
Epworth Sleepiness Scale
European Stroke Scale
essential
e. anosmia
e. blepharospasm
e. headache
e. hypotonia
e. myoclonus
e. palatal tremor
e. thrombocytosis
Essex-Lopresti axial fixation
ESSF
external spinal skeletal fixation
Essick cell band
estazolam
esterase
acetylcholine e.
Esterom
esthematology
esthesia
esthesic
esthesiodic system
esthesiogenesis
esthesiogenic
esthesiography
esthesiology
esthesiometer
Semmes-Weinstein e.
Weber e.
esthesiometry
esthesioneuroblastoma
olfactory e.
esthesioneurocytoma
esthesioneurosis
esthesionosus
esthesiophysiology
esthesioscopy
estimated cerebrovascular resistance
estimation
suprathreshold taste intensity e.
estradiol
ethinyl e.
estradiol-17 B
estrogen
e. level
e. receptor
e. replacement therapy (ERT)
estrogen-related protein
estrogen-to-progesterone ratio
estrogen-withdrawal headache
estrous behavior
ET
endothelin
alpha ET
ET-1
endothelin-1
état
é. criblé
é. lacunaire
ET-converting enzyme
eterobarb
ethacrynic acid
ethambutol
ethanol
e. treatment
e. withdrawal
ethaverine hydrochloride
ETHE1 gene
ether convulsion
ethical aspects of dementia
Ethicon Ligaclip
ethidium bromide (EB)
ethinyl estradiol
ethiodized oil
ethionamide
ethmoid
e. air cell
e. sinus
ethmoidal
e. meningoencephalocele
e. nerve
e. osteotomy
ethopropazine
ethosuximide
ethotoin
ethyl
e. alcohol peripheral neuropathy
e. chloride and dichlorotetrafluoroethane
e. loflazepate
ethyl-eicosapentaenoic acid
ethylene
e. glycol poisoning
e. vinyl alcohol copolymer
e. vinyl alcohol copolymer liquid
ethylenediaminetetraacetic acid
ethylene-vinyl acetate (EVAc)

ethylester
levodopa e.
ethylmalonic
e. aciduria
e. encephalopathy
ethyltryptamine
alpha e.
etidocaine
etidronate
disodium e.
technetium e.
etifoxine
etiological heterogeneity
etiologic role
etiology
dementia due to multiple e.'s
disease e.
epilepsy e.
multifactorial e.
organic e.
e. theory
etiopathogenesis
MS e.
etiopathogenetic
e. consideration
e. mechanism
ETM1 gene
ETM2 gene
etodolac
etodroxizine
etomidate injection
etomidate-propylene glycol infusion
etoposide
ETP
electron transport particle
etretinate
etryptamine
ETTH
episodic tension-type headache
ETV
endoscopic third ventriculostomy
eukaryotic
e. homolog
e. messenger
Eulenburg disease
eumetria
euphoria
euphoric effect
eupractic
eupraxia
eupraxic center
European
E. Brain Injury Consortium
E. Carotid Surgery Trial (ECST)
E. Sleep Research Society
E. Society for Sleep Research
E. Stroke Scale (ESS)
EuroQol visual analog scale
eurycephalic, eurycephalous
eurythmic
eutectic mixture of local anesthetics (EMLA)
euthymic memory
EVAc
ethylene-vinyl acetate
evacuation
CT-guided stereotactic e.
epidural abscess e.
epidural tumor e.
hematoma e.
transsphenoidal e.
evaluating sleeplessness
evaluation
acute physiologic assessment and chronic health e. (APACHE)
bulbocavernosus reflex e.
comprehensive e.
cross-sectional e.
myasthenia gravis e.
neurologic e.
Neurometer CPT/C for nerve e.
neurophysiologic e.
pedicle e.
preoperative e.
seizure e.
serum lead level e.
surgery e.
evaluator
computer-aided sensory e.
Recovery Attitude and Treatment E. (RAATE)
Evans
E. index
E. ratio
E. syndrome
evasive movement
even-echo rephasing
evening
e. headache
e. primrose oil (EPO)
event
acoustic signature e.
acute life-threatening e. (ALTE)

NOTES

E

event *(continued)*
calmodulin-regulated e.
catastrophic e.
clinical ictal e.
cytoskeletal membrane e.
epileptic e.
genomic e.
ictal e.
ischemic e.
e. memory
multifactorial e.
neurologic e.
nocturnal e.
nonepileptic e.
partial arousal e.
psychogenic e.
e. recall
e. recall score
sequence of e.'s
teeth-grinding e.
transient focal neurologic e. (TFNE)
event-related
e.-r. brain potential study
e.-r. desynchronization
e.-r. innocuous somatosensory stimulation paradigm
e.-r. potential
Evershears surgical instrument
eversion
cingulate gyrus e.
Evers raw food diet
evidence
anatomical e.
anecdotal e.
bias-free e.
biologic e.
class I–III e.
evidence-based medicine
evisceroneurotomy
evoked
e. affect
e. cortical response
e. potential (EP)
e. potential trending
e. seizure
evolution
E. 1 precision robot
stroke in e.
evolving
e. dementia
e. hematoma
Ewald-Hudson forceps
Ewald second law
E wave
Ewing sarcoma
ex
ex vivo
ex vivo technique
exacerbation
disease e.
dopaminergic antagonist-related e.
headache e.
e. rate
seizure e.
spontaneous e.
symptom e.
exaggerated
e. depression
e. response
exam
examination
Boston Diagnostic Aphasia E.
Cambridge Mental Disorders of the Elderly E.
cochlear nerve e.
Comprehensive Qualifying E.
cranial nerve e.
dystonia e.
EMG e.
funduscopic e.
glossopharyngeal nerve e.
Hertel exophthalmometry e.
idiographic e.
lateral dominance e.
mental status e.
Mini-Mental State E. (MMSE)
motor development e.
muscle e.
Navy neurologic screening e.
needle electrode e. (NEE)
neurologic e. (NE)
neuropathologic e.
nystagmus e.
ocular motility e.
oculomotor nerve e.
olfactory nerve e.
ophthalmologic e.
optic nerve e.
posture e.
sensory perceptual e.
slit-lamp e.
soft sign in neurologic e.
sternocleidomastoid muscle testing in spinal accessory nerve e.
Stroke Data Bank Neurologic Rush Alzheimer Registry E.
tangent screen e.
vagus nerve e.
vestibular nerve e.
exanthem subitum
Excel double-tipped microcatheter
excessive
e. daytime sleepiness (EDS)
e. daytime somnolence
e. diffuse low- and medium-wave beta activity
e. exercise

e. fatigability
e. fatigue
e. lead exposure
e. salivation
e. sleep inertia
e. speech
excessively erect posture
exchange
blood-gas e.
blood-tissue e.
e. force
plasma e. (PE)
excimer laser-assisted nonocclusive anastomosis (ELANA)
excision
cervical disc e.
cyst wall e.
extratemporal e.
radical disc e.
retropulsed bone e.
total e.
excitability
altered axonal e.
emotional e.
membrane e.
neuronal e.
somatodendritic e.
e. test
thalamocortical e.
excitable
e. area
e. cell
excitation
glutamate e.
number of e.
postsynaptic e.
selective e.
excitation-contraction coupling
excitatory
e. afferent
e. amino acid
e. amino acid receptor
e. amino acid receptor inhibitor
e. irradiation
e. lesion
e. neurotransmitter
e. postsynaptic potential (EPSP)
e. pyramidal neuron
e. stimulus
excitomotor cortex
excitoreflex nerve
excitor nerve
excitotoxic
e. cell damage
e. neuronal cell injury
e. neurotransmitter antagonist
excitotoxicity
glutamate e.
glutamatergic e.
excitotoxin inhibitor
excyclotorsion
executive
e. deficit transient global amnesia
e. dysfunction
e. function
e. function deficit
e. process
Exelon capsule
exencephalic, exencephalous
exencephalocele
exencephaly
exercise
e. adherence
aerobic e.
Cawthorne-Cooksey vestibular e.
cognitive e.
container e.
excessive e.
intellectual e.
physical e.
PNF e.
e. protocol
verbal memory e.
exercise-induced
e.-i. myoglobinuria
e.-i. seizure
e.-i. sympathetic discharge
exerciser
continuous anatomical passive e.
exertional headache
exhalation positive airway pressure (EPAP)
exhaustion
heat e.
postactivation e.
posttetanic e.
existential-humanistic theory
exit
e. block
e. site
e. wound
exiting segment
Exner plexus
exodic nerve

NOTES

exogenous
e. fiber
e. force
e. nitric oxide
e. reaction
exon splicing
exophthalmometer
Hertel e.
exophthalmos
exophthalmos-producing substance (EPS)
exophytic
e. brainstem glioma
e. ependymoma
e. joint disease
exorbitance
Exo-Static collar
exotoxin
Pseudomonas e.
exotropia
paralytic pontine e.
expanded
E. Disability Status Scale (EDSS)
e. polytetrafluoroethylene (ePTFE)
expansion
clonal e.
field e.
maxillomandibular e. (MME)
trinucleotide repeat e.
volume e.
expectancy
life e.
quality-adjusted life e. (QALE)
e. wave
experience-induced cortical plasticity
experiential
e. aura
e. factor
experimental
e. allergic encephalitis (EAE)
e. allergic encephalomyelitis
e. autoimmune encephalomyelitis
e. condition
e. intervention
e. study
e. therapy
expiratory center
exploding head syndrome
exploration
brachial plexus e.
stereotactic biopsy e.
surgical e.
therapeutic e.
transcranial orbital e.
exploratory incision
exploring electrode
explosive
e. psychotic state
e. speech
exposure
anterior surgical e.
bony e.
bright light e.
excessive lead e.
extradural e.
fetal mercury e.
fetal phenytoin e.
half-and-half e.
e. keratopathy
light e.
membrane phosphatidylserine e.
middle fossa e.
midline e.
neuroleptic e.
occupational e.
organophosphate e.
pack-year e.
pesticide e.
prolonged e.
radiation e.
surgical e.
thoracolumbar junction surgical e.
thoracolumbar spine anterior e.
toxic e.
e. to trauma
upper cervical spine anterior e.
vertebral e.
in vivo situational e.
x-ray e.
exposure-based intervention
expressed skull fracture
expression
costimulatory molecule e.
emotional e.
facial e.
e. level
microarray gene e.
neurofilament e.
neuronal NADPH-diaphorase/NOS e.
neurotrophic factor e.
nontoxic gene e.
pattern of e.
phenotypic e.
RNA e.
expressive
e. aphasia
e. dysprosody
e. language
e. language deficit
e. speech deficit
expressive-receptive aphasia
Extencaps
Micro-K 10 E.
extended
e. ADL
e. phenytoin sodium
e. release (ER)
e., rotated, sidebent (ERS)

e., rotated, sidebent left (ERSL)
e., rotated, sidebent right (ERSR)
e. sector ultrasonic probe
e. subfrontal approach

extending axon

extension
brachioradialis transfer for wrist e.
cranial e.
deep brain e.
extrameatal tumor e.
e. injury
e. injury posterior atlantoaxial arthrodesis
intrasellar e.
neurite e.
Orascoptic loupe e.
paraplegia in e.
passive e.
radiolucent operating room table e.
e., sidebent right, rotated left (ESRRL)
e. stability
subependymal e.
suprasellar e.
tumor e.

extension-type cervical spine injury

extensive
e. neoplasm
e. posterior decompression
e. seizure focus

extensor
e. plantar response
e. tetanus
e. toe response

exterior band of Baillarger

externa
capsula e.
glia limitans e.
globus pallidus e.
hematorrhachis e.
lamina medullaris thalami e.
lamina pyramidalis e.
ophthalmoplegia e.
pachymeningitis e.

externae
fibrae arcuatae e.
stria laminae granularis e.

external
e. acoustic meatus
e. arcuate fiber
e. auditory canal mass
e. auditory meatus electrode
e. auditory meatus reflex
e. band of Baillarger
e. beam radiotherapy (EBRT)
e. bracing
e. canthus electrode
e. capsule
e. carotid artery
e. collimator
e. corticotectal tract
e. counterpulsion (ECP)
e. cue
e. cuneate nucleus
e. granular layer
e. hydrocephalus
e. immobilization
e. intercostal muscle
e. line of Baillarger
e. malleolar sign
e. maxillary plexus
e. medullary lamina
e. memory aid
e. meningitis
e. nuclear layer of retina
e. oblique reflex
e. pillar cell
e. popliteal nerve
e. pyocephalus
e. radiation
e. rhinoplasty
e. sheath of optic nerve
e. source
e. speech
e. speech stimulus
e. spinal skeletal fixation (ESSF)
e. spinal skeletal fixator
e. support system
e. terminal filament
e. ventricular drain
e. ventricular drainage
e. vertebral venous plexus

externi
nervi carotici e.
nervus meatus acustici e.

externum
corpus geniculatum e.
filum terminale e.
stratum limitans e.
stratum nucleare e.
stratum plexiforme e.

externus
nervus spermaticus e.
plexus caroticus e.

NOTES

exteroceptive nervous system
exteroceptor
exterofective system
extirpate
extirpation
choroid plexus e.
tumor e.
extorsion
extraaxial
e. cavernous hemangioma
e. lesion
extracanalicular acoustic neuroma
extracellular
e. acidosis
e. action potential
e. calcium activity
e. contribution
e. matrix (ECM)
e. matrix protein
e. matrix proteoglycan
e. proteosome
e. signal-regulated protein
e. space
extracerebral
e. activity
e. aneurysm
e. cavernous angioma
e. hematoma
extraconal lesion
extracorporeal
e. membrane oxygenation
e. membrane oxygenation affecting cognitive function
extracorticospinal
e. system
e. tract
extracranial
e. aneurysm
e. arteritis
e. carotid artery (ECA)
e. carotid occlusive disease
e. ganglion
e. mass lesion
e. meningioma
e. occlusive vascular disease
e. pneumatocele
e. pneumocele
e. radiosurgery
e. shunt
e. vascular dissection
extracraniale
ganglion e.
extracranial-intracranial (EC-IC)
e.-i. bypass
e.-i. bypass surgery
extracranial-to-intracranial bypass procedure
extract
kava e.
perchlorate e.
extradural
e. abscess
e. anastomosis
e. balloon
e. clinoidectomy
e. compartment
e. compression
e. cyst
e. defect
e. deposit
e. exposure
e. hemangioma
e. hematoma
e. hematorrhachis
e. hemorrhage
e. infection
e. injection
e. meningioma
e. phase
e. space
e. spinal metastasis
e. tumor
e. vertebral artery
extradurale
spatium e.
extraforaminal
e. lumbar disc herniation
e. synovial cyst
extrafusal fiber
extrageniculate
extrajunctional nucleus
extralemniscal
e. myelotomy
e. system
extraluminal
extrameatal
e. intracapsular tumor
e. tumor extension
extramedullary
e. hemangioma
e. spinal cord tumor
extrameningeal tuberculous infection
extramesial temporal lesion
extramuscular substrate
extraocular
e. motility
e. movement (EOM)
e. muscle
e. muscle involvement
e. muscle palsy
e. muscle paresis
e. paralysis
extraordinary meridian (EM)
extrapineal
e. pinealoma
e. pinealoma false neuroma

extrapolar region
extrapontine edema
extrapyramidal
e. cerebral palsy
e. disorder
e. dyskinesia
e. motor feature
e. motor side effect
e. motor system
e. motor system disease
e. nucleus
e. pathway
e. rigidity
e. sign (EPS)
e. symptom (EPS)
e. symptom potential
e. syndrome
e. syndrome symptom
extraspinal
e. leiomyoma
e. nerve stimulation
extrastriatal dopamine transmission
extrastriate
e. visual cortex
e. V5/MT cortex
extrasynaptic receptor
extratemporal
e. excision
e. lobectomy
e. lobe epilepsy
e. resection
e. seizure
extraterritorial spontaneous pain
extrathymic pathway
extrema
capsula e.
extreme
e. capsule
e. lateral inferior transcondylar approach
e. lateral transcondylar approach
e. narrowing limit
e. range
e. somatosensory evoked potential
extremely low-frequency magnetic field
extrinsic sleep disorder
extruded disc
extrusion
bone graft e.
wire e.
extubation
postoperative e.
eye
black e.
e. blink
e. blink artifact
e. blink conditioning test
e. blinking
contralateral e.
crossed e.
e. cyclotorsion
dancing e.
glassy e.
e. lead
lusterless e.
e. movement artifact
e. movement desensitization
e. movement desensitization and reprocessing (EMDR)
e. movement disorder
e. movement measurement
e. movement testing
e. muscle weakness
e. pain
paretic e.
raccoon e.
red e.
e. rolling
e. tracking
e. tracking dysfunction
eye-blink response
eyebrow
e. flash
e. incision
eye-closure reflex
eye-gaze deviation
eyelash sign
eyelid
e. myoclonia
e. myokymia
e. ptosis
e. retraction
eye-motor-verbal (EMV)
e.-m.-v. profile
eyes, motor, voice-verbal
eye-to-eye gaze
E-Z
E-Z Flap cranial bone plate
E-Z flap cranial flap fixation system
EZBrace orthosis

NOTES

FA
fractional anisotropy
Fabco gauze dressing
Fabry disease
FAC
Functional Ambulation Category
FACE
Frequency Analysis of Consecutive Epochs
face
anthropomorphic f.
immobile f.
masklike f.
Mooney f.
f. recognition
f. search
upside-down Mooney f.
face-dominant hemisphere
face-evoked magnetic field
face-nondominant hemisphere
facet, facette
bony f.
f. excision technique
f. fracture
f. fracture stabilization wiring
f. hypertrophy
f. injection
f. joint
f. joint preparation
f. joint splaying
f. joint syndrome
locked f.
f. replacement
f. rhizotomy
f. subluxation stabilization wiring
facetectomy
partial f.
facial
f. agnosia
f. anesthesia
f. apraxia
f. artery
f. asymmetry
f. colliculus
f. contusion
f. diplegia
F. Disability Index
f. dysesthesia
f. dysmorphism
f. dystonia
f. electromyography
f. electroneurography
f. eminence
f. expression
f. expression automatism
f. flushing
f. fracture
f. genu
f. grimace
f. grimacing
f. habit spasm
f. hematoma
f. hemiatrophy of Romberg
f. hemiplegia
f. hemispasm
f. hillock
f. migraine
f. motor nucleus
f. myokymia
f. nerve branch
f. nerve [CN VII]
f. nerve congenital anomaly
f. nerve discontinuity
f. nerve function
f. nerve injury
f. nerve paralysis
f. nerve perinatal trauma
f. neuralgia
f. neuroma
f. neuromotor disorder
f. neuropathy
f. nucleus
f. numbness
f. osteosynthesis
f. pain
f. palsy
f. plexus
f. profiling
f. progressive atrophy
f. progressive hemiatrophy
f. reanimation
f. recognition
f. reflex
f. root
f. sign
f. symmetry
f. tic
f. trophoneurosis
f. twitching
f. vision
f. weakness
faciali
rami communicantes nervi auriculotemporalis cum nervi f.
facialis
area nervi f.
colliculus f.
eminentia f.
ganglion geniculatum nervi f.
ganglion geniculi nervi f.

facialis *(continued)*
geniculum nervi f.
geniculum nervus f.
genu nervi f.
nervus f. [CN VII]
nucleus nervi f.
f. phenomenon
radix nervi f.
rami buccales nervi f.
rami zygomatici nervi f.
ramus cervicalis nervi f.
ramus colli nervi f.
ramus digastricus nervi f.
ramus lingualis nervi f.
ramus marginalis mandibularis nervi f.
ramus stylohyoideus nervi f.
facies
asymmetrical crying f. (ACF)
birdlike f.
elfin f.
hatchet f.
Hutchinson f.
f. inferior hemispherii cerebelli
f. inferior hemispherii cerebri
mask f.
masked f.
masklike f.
f. medialis et inferior hemispherii cerebri
moon f.
myasthenic f.
myopathic f.
myotonic f.
Parkinson f.
f. superior hemispherii cerebelli
f. superolateralis hemispherii cerebri
facilitation
f. of communication
intracortical inhibition and f.
postactivation f.
postspike f.
posttetanic f.
proprioceptive neuromuscular f. (PNF)
Wedensky f.
facility
sleep disorder f.
facioauricular vertebral (FAV)
faciobrachiocrural involvement
faciobuccolingual dyskinesia
faciocephalic pain
faciolingual
facioorbital penetration
facioplegia
facioplegic
f. migraine
f. migraine headache
facioscapulohumeral
f. atrophy
f. muscular dystrophy
faciostenosis
FACScan analysis
fact
anatomic f.
factitious attack
factor
age-specific risk f.
antihemophilic f. A, C
apoptosis-inducing f. (AIF)
assimilative f.
attitudinal risk f.
background f.
basal endothelium-derived relaxing f.
basic fibroblast growth f.
biologic risk f.
biomechanical f.
brain-derived neurotrophic f. (BDNF)
brain-derived neurotropic f.
chronic insomnia contributing f.
chronic insomnia medical f.
chronic insomnia psychiatric f.
ciliary-deprived neurotropic f. (CDNF)
ciliary neurotrophic f. (CNF)
cognitive f.
collagenase-activating f.
corticotropin-releasing f.
demographic risk f.
DNA fragmentation f. (DFF)
emotional f.
endothelial cell-stimulating angiogenesis f.
endothelium-derived relaxing f. (EDRF)
environmental f.
epidermal growth f. (EGF)
experiential f.
Fiblast trafermin growth f.
fibroblastic growth f. (FGF)
filling f.
fork head response f.
genetic f.
genetic risk f.
glial cell line-derived neurotrophic f.
glial-derived neurotrophic f. (GDNF)
glial line-derived neurotrophic f.
granulocyte-macrophage colony-stimulating f. (GM-CSF)
growth hormone-release inhibiting f. (GHRIF)
Hageman f.
helix-loop-helix response f.

hepatocyte growth f.
hepatocyte growth factor/scatter f. (HGF/SF)
HLH f.
homeodomain f.
human f.
hyperpolarizing f.
hypothalamic-releasing f.
insulin growth f.
insulinlike growth f. (IGF)
ischemia-modifying f.
f. IX complex concentrate
f. IX deficiency
leukemia inhibitory f. (LIF)
melanocyte-inhibiting f.
melanotropin-releasing f. (MRF)
middle glial cell line-derived neurotrophic f.
midlife cardiovascular risk f.
motivation f.
motivational/behavioral f.
nerve growth f. (NGF)
neural growth f.
neurobiological f.
neurophysiological phenotypic f.
neurotic f.
neurotrophic f.
nonspecific neurotic f.
obsessional Q f.
occupational risk f.
orthogonal depression f.
pathogenic f.
pathophysiologic f.
pharmacologic f.
phenotypic f.
phenylketonuria genetic f.
plasma f.
platelet-activating f. (PAF)
platelet-derived growth f. (PDGF)
potential predisposing f.
precipitating f.
predictive f.
pretraumatic risk f.
primary risk f.
prognostic f.
prolactin-inhibiting f. (PIF)
prolactin-releasing f. (PRF)
Q f.
quality f.
radiolabeled neurotrophic f.
rheumatoid f.
f. score
serum von Willebrand f.
state f.
Stuart-Power f.
susceptibility f.
synthetic corticotropin-releasing f.
transcription f.
transforming growth f. (TGF)
tumor necrosis f. (TNF)
vascular endothelial growth f. (VEGF)
vascular growth f.
f. VII deficiency
f. VIII antigen tumor marker
f. VIII deficiency
vitamin K-dependent clotting f. II, VII, IX, X
f. V Leiden
von Willebrand f. (vWF)
f. XII deficiency

factor-1
redox f.-1

factor-alpha
recombinant human tumor necrosis f.-a.
tumor necrosis f.-a. (TNF-alpha)

factual memory

FAD
flavin adenine dinucleotide

Fahn-Tolosa-Marin tremor rating scale

Fahr
F. disease
F. syndrome

failed
f. back surgery syndrome
f. back syndrome with documented pseudarthrosis
f. lumbar puncture

failure
age-associated memory f.
autonomic f.
brain functional f.
congestive heart f. (CHF)
developmental f.
distant brain f. (DBF)
empathic f.
energy f.
fatigue f.
functional f.
Harrington rod instrumentation f.
instrumentation f.
isolated gait ignition f.
metal f.

NOTES

failure *(continued)*
poliomyelitis-induced respiratory f.
pure autonomic f.
recall f.
spinal implant load to f.
visual f.
Fairbanks
F. change
F. method
Fajersztajn crossed sciatic sign
FAK
focal adhesion kinase
FAK protein
falcate
falces (*pl. of* falx)
falcial
falciform
f. crest
f. lobe
f. process
falciformis
f. hiatus sapheni
lobus f.
falcine
f. meningioma
falciparum
Plasmodium f.
Falconer lobectomy
falcotentorial meningioma
falcula
falcular
fall
epileptic f.
f. risk
fallopian neuritis
Fallopio foramen
FALS
familial amyotrophic lateral sclerosis
false
f. localizing sign
f. negative
f. neuroma
f. neurotransmitter
f. positive
false-negative PCR
false-positive rate
falx, pl. **falces**
f. cerebelli
f. cerebri
f. hypoplasia
f. meningioma
parasagittal f.
F. sign
famciclovir
familial
f. adult myoclonic epilepsy
f. Alzheimer disease
f. amyloid neuropathy
f. amyloidosis
f. amyloidotic polyneuropathy
F. Amyloid Polyneuropathy World Transplant Registry
f. amyotrophic lateral sclerosis (FALS)
f. arteriovenous malformation
f. autosomal recessive idiopathic myoclonic epilepsy of infancy
f. benign choreoathetosis
f. centrolobar sclerosis
f. cervicocephalic arterial dissection
f. cortical tremor
f. Creutzfeldt-Jakob disease (fCJD)
f. dysautonomia
f. dysautonomia syndrome
f. dyskalemic periodic paralysis
f. encephalopathy
f. episodic ataxia
f. fatal insomnia
f. form of amyotrophic lateral sclerosis
f. glioma
f. gliomatosis cerebri
f. glycosuria
f. hemiplegic migraine (FHM)
f. hypercholesterolemia
f. hypokalemic periodic paralysis
f. infantile bilateral striatal necrosis
f. infantile myasthenia
f. intracranial aneurysm (FIA)
f. Mediterranean fever (FMF)
f. medulloblastoma
f. mesial temporal lobe epilepsy
f. myoclonus epilepsy
f. neurovisceral lipidosis
f. neuroviscerolipidosis
f. Parkinson disease
f. paroxysmal choreoathetosis
f. paroxysmal choreoathetosis disease
f. paroxysmal kinesigenic ataxia
f. partial epilepsy with variable foci
f. progressive myoclonic epilepsy
f. restless leg syndrome
f. schwannomatosis
f. spastic ataxia
f. spastic paraplegia
f. spinal muscular atrophy
f. startle disease
f. transmission
familiar correlation coefficient
family
leucine zipper f.
zinc-finger f.
fan
f. retractor
f. sign
Fañanás cell

Fanconi
F. anemia
F. syndrome
far
F. East Russian encephalitis
f. lateral inferior suboccipital approach
Faraday shield
Farber
F. disease
F. lipogranulomatosis
farcinica
Nocardia f.
Farley retractor
farnesyl transferase inhibitor
FAS
fetal alcohol syndrome
Fas-associated
F.-a. death domain
F.-a. death domain-like interleukin-converting enzyme
fascia, pl. **fasciae**
f. cinerea
f. dentata hippocampus
dentate f.
infraspinous f.
f. lata sling
lumbodorsal f. (LDF)
vertebral f.
fascia-muscle-fascia sandwich
fascicle
medial longitudinal f.
muscle f.
nerve f.
peripheral nerve f.
fascicular
f. adaptation
f. degeneration
f. graft
f. ophthalmoplegia
fasciculation
contraction f.
cramp benign f.
muscle f.
f. potential
fasciculitis
thalamic f.
fasciculus, pl. **fasciculi**
f. aberrans of Monakow
alvear f.
f. anterior proprius
anterior pyramidal f.
arcuate f.
Burdach cuneate f.
calcarine f.
central tegmental f.
f. circumolivaris pyramidis
f. corticospinalis anterior
f. corticospinalis lateralis
cuneate f.
f. cuneatus
dorsal longitudinal f.
dorsolateral f.
f. dorsolateralis
fasciculus subcallosus for superior occipitofrontal f.
Flechsig f.
Foville f.
frontooccipital f.
Gowers f.
gracile f.
f. gracilis
f. gracilis medullae oblongatae
f. gracilis medullae spinalis
hooked f.
inferior longitudinal f.
inferior occipitofrontal f.
interfascicular f.
f. interfascicularis (FI)
intersegmental f.
interstitial nucleus of medial longitudinal f.
f. lateralis plexus brachialis
f. lateralis proprius
lateral pyramidal f.
lenticular f.
f. lenticularis
Lissauer f.
fasciculi longitudinales pontis
f. longitudinalis dorsalis
f. longitudinalis inferior
f. longitudinalis medialis
f. longitudinalis posterior
f. longitudinalis superior
longitudinal pontine f.
macular f.
f. macularis
f. mamillotegmentalis
f. mamillothalamicus
mammillotegmental f.
mammillothalamic f.
marginal f.
f. marginalis
f. medialis telencephali

NOTES

fasciculus *(continued)*
medial longitudinal f. (MLF)
median longitudinal f.
f. of Meynert
Meynert f.
nucleus of cuneate f.
oblique pontine f.
f. obliquus pontis
occipitofrontal f.
f. occipitofrontalis
f. occipitofrontalis inferior
f. occipitofrontalis superior
oval f.
f. pedunculomamillaris
pedunculomammillary f.
perpendicular f.
proper f.
fasciculi proprii
f. proprius anterior
f. proprius anterior medullae spinalis
f. proprius dorsalis medullae spinalis
f. proprius lateralis
f. proprius lateralis medullae spinalis
f. proprius posterior medullae spinalis
f. pyramidalis anterior
f. pyramidalis lateralis
retroflex f.
f. retroflexus
f. rotundus
round f.
rubroreticular f.
fasciculi rubroreticulares
Schütz f.
semilunar f.
f. semilunaris
septomarginal f.
f. septomarginalis
slender f.
f. solitarius
solitary f.
subcallosal f.
f. subcallosus
subthalamic f.
f. subthalamicus
f. sulcomarginalis
superior longitudinal f.
superior occipitofrontal f.
thalamic f.
f. thalamicus
f. thalamomamillaris
f. thalamomammillaris
transverse f.
fasciculi transversi
Türck f.
unciform f.
f. uncinatus
f. uncinatus cerebelli
Vicq d'Azyr f.
wedge-shaped f.

fasciola, pl. **fasciolae**
f. cinerea
f. cinerea cinguli

fasciolar gyrus

fasciolaris
gyrus f.

Fasguide catheter

fast
f. axonal transport
f. channel syndrome
F. Dasher 14 wire
f. field-potential rhythm
f. Fourier transform (FFT)
f. Fourier transformation spectrum analyzer
f. gradient recalled spectroscopic imaging technique
F. Health Knowledge Test, 1986 Revision
f. imaging
f. imaging with steady precession (FISP)
f. low-angle shot (FLASH)
f. low-angle shot sequence
f. motor unit
f. saccadic eye movement
f. spin-echo inversion recovery sequence
f. spin-echo scan

fast-acting agent

fast-frequency repetitive transcranial magnetic stimulation

fastigatum

fastigial
f. nucleus
f. pressor response

fastigii
nucleus f.

fastigiobulbar
f. fiber
f. tract

fastigiobulbaris
tractus f.

fastigiospinal
f. fiber
f. tract

fastigiospinalis
tractus f.

fastigium

Fastlene capsule

FasTracker-18 infusion catheter

fast-scan magnetic resonance

fat
f. embolism
f. embolus

epidural f.
f. malabsorption
vertebral marrow f.

fatal
f. arrhythmia
f. encephalitis
f. familial insomnia (FFI)
f. hemorrhage
f. hereditary disease
f. hypothermia

fat-free mass

fatigability
auditory f.
chronic f.
daytime f.
easy f.
excessive f.
nervous f.
psychogenic f.
stimulation f.
sustained f.

fatigue
chronic f.
cognitive f.
daytime f.
easy f.
excessive f.
f. failure
f. failure response
implant f.
metal f.
sense of f.
stapedius muscle f.
f. of systemic illness

fat-patch graft

fat-suppression
f.-s. MR imaging
f.-s. technique

fatty
f. acid oxidation
f. acid oxidation disorder
f. acid transport into mitochondria
f. degeneration in Reye syndrome
f. granule cell
f. streak

fat/water
f./w. chemical shift
f./w. signal cancellation

fauces
branch of lingual nerve to isthmus of f.

faucial
f. paralysis
f. reflex

FAV
facioauricular vertebral
FAV syndrome

Favaloro-Morse sternal spreader

Fazio-Londe
F.-L. atrophy
F.-L. disease
F.-L. syndrome

FBS
feedback signal

FC
functional communication

Fc
fragment crystallizable
Fc fragment

fCJD
familial Creutzfeldt-Jakob disease

FCR
flexor carpi radialis

FDG
fluorodeoxyglucose
FDG method

FDG-PET
fluorodeoxyglucose positron emission tomography

fear
f. association
ictal f.
lingering f.

feature
demographic f.
Down syndrome clinical f.
dysautonomic f.
extrapyramidal motor f.
gross pathological f.
hemodynamic f.
histological f.
junctural f.
leonine facial f.
morphologic f.
myopathic f.
neurobehavioral f.
neurologic f.
paralinguistic f.
pathological f.
sleep f.

featureless headache

febarbamate

F

NOTES

febrile
f. convulsion
f. epilepsy
f. seizure
fecal
f. continence
f. soiling
feedback
electromyographic f.
f. mechanism
molecular f.
negative f.
positive f.
f. projection
f. sensitivity
f. signal (FBS)
f. system
feedforward projection
feeding
f. artery
f. artery of aneurysm
f. center
f. difficulties in cerebral palsy
f. mean arterial pressure (FMAP)
feel-good molecule
Feer disease
FEF
forced expiratory flow
Fehling TOP ejector punch
felbamate
Felbatol
feltwork
Kaes f.
Felty syndrome
FemBack
Femcet
femoral
f. cutaneous nerve
f. introducer sheath
f. nerve stretch test
f. neuropathy
f. reflex
femoralis
nervus f.
plexus f.
rami cutanei anteriores nervi f.
rami musculares nervi f.
femoris
nervus quadratus f.
femoroabdominal reflex
fenestra
fenestrated
f. aneurysm clip
f. oculomotor nerve
fenestration
bur hole neuroendoscopic f.
cyst f.
fenisorex
fenobam
Fenton reaction
Féré effect
Féréol-Graux palsy
Ferguson
F. brain suction tip
F. brain suction tube
F. suction
Ferguson-Critchley ataxia
ferpentetate
technetium-99m f.
Ferrein foramen
Ferris
F. Smith-Kerrison laminectomy rongeur
F. Smith-Kerrison punch
ferrite
barium f.
ferritin
serum f.
f. test
ferromagnetic
f. artifact
f. bullet
f. implant
f. intracerebral aneurysm clip
f. monitoring device
ferrous sulfate neurotoxicity
ferroxidase
multicopper f.
ferruginea
substantia f.
ferrugineus
locus f.
ferumoxide injectable solution
festinans
chorea f.
festinating gait
fetal
f. adenoma
f. AIDS transmission
f. alcohol syndrome (FAS)
f. brain
f. brain transitory neuron
f. cell transplantation
f. cerebrovascular system
f. dopaminergic tissue implant
f. ependyma
f. growth retardation
f. heart rate monitoring
f. hydrocephalus
f. mercury exposure
f. mesencephalic grafting
f. mesencephalic tissue
f. neural implant
f. neural transplant
f. phenytoin exposure
f. planum
f. planum temporal lateralization
f. position

f. response
f. shunt procedure
f. substantia nigra
f. tau
f. tissue transplant
f. transfusion
f. valproic acid syndrome

fetalis
erythroblastosis f.

fetoprotein
alpha f. (AFP)

feud
blood f.

Feulgen cytophotometry

fever
acute rheumatic f.
Argentinian hemorrhigic f.
Bolivian hemorrhagic f.
catscratch f.
f. caused by infection (FI)
Central European tick-borne f.
cerebrospinal f.
dengue f.
diphasic milk f.
drug f.
familial Mediterranean f. (FMF)
hemorrhagic f.
Jarisch-Herxheimer f.
Katayama f.
meningotyphoid f.
Q f.
relapsing f.
rheumatic f.
Rift Valley f.
Rocky Mountain spotted f.
saddleback f.
South African tick-bite f.
spotted f.
tick-borne relapsing f.
trypanosome f.
typhus f.
undulant f.
West Nile f.
yellow f.
Zika f.

FFA
fusiform face area

FFbH-R
Hannover Functional Ability Questionnaire for measuring back pain-related functional limitations

FFI
fatal familial insomnia

FFM
free-fat mass

FFT
fast Fourier transform

FGF
fibroblastic growth factor

FGFR
fibroblast growth factor receptor

FGFR2
fibroblast growth factor receptor 2

FGFR1 gene

FHM
familial hemiplegic migraine

FI
fasciculus interfascicularis
fever caused by infection

FIA
familial intracranial aneurysm

fiber
A f.
accelerator f.
A-delta f.
adrenergic f.
afferent nerve f.
alpha f.
amygdalofugal f.
anastomosing f.
anastomotic f.
anterior external arcuate f.
anulospiral f.
anulus fibrosus f.
arcuate f.
association f.
augmentor f.
autonomic nerve f.
B f.
Bergmann f.
beta f.
bulbar corticonuclear f.
Burdach f.
C f.
cerebellohypothalamic f.
cerebelloolivary f.
cerebellospinal f.
cholinergic f.
circular f.
climbing f. (CF)
collateral f.
commissural f.
cone f.

fiber *(continued)*
corticobulbar f.
corticomesencephalic f.
corticopontine f.
corticorubral f.
corticospinal f.
corticothalamic f.
cuneocerebellar f.
cuneospinal f.
decussation of trochlear nerve f.
denervated f.
f. density
dentatorubral f.
dentatothalamic f.
depressor f.
f. diameter
f. dissection technique
Edinger f.
efferent f.
endogenous f.
exogenous f.
external arcuate f.
extrafusal f.
fastigiobulbar f.
fastigiospinal f.
frontopontine f.
gamma f.
geniculostriate f.
Goll f.
gracile spinal f.
Gratiolet radiating f.
gray f.
heterodesmotic f.
homodesmotic f.
hypoglossal nerve f.
hypothalamocerebellar f.
hypothalamospinal f.
inhibitory f.
inner cone f.
intergemmal nerve f.
internal arcuate f.
internuncial f.
intersegmental f.
intraaxial f.
intracortical transverse f.
intraepidermal nerve f. (IENF)
intrafusal f.
intragemmal nerve f.
intrasegmental f.
intrathalamic f.
intrinsic f.
layer of nerve f.'s
lemniscal f.
long association f.
longitudinal pontine f.
Mauthner f.
mechanoreceptor f.
medullated nerve f.
mesencephalic corticonuclear f.
microthin plastic f.
Monakow f.
monoaminergic f.
mossy f.
motor f.
Müller f.
muscle f.
myelinated nerve f.
Myer f.
myoclonic epilepsy with ragged red f.'s (MERRF)
nerve f.
neuroglial f.
nigrostriate f.
nociceptive C f.
nonmedullated f.
nuclear bag f.
nuclear chain f.
nucleocortical f.
oblique gastric f.
occipitopontine f.
occipitotectal f.
olivocerebellar f.
olivospinal f.
outer cone f.
pain f.
pain-transmitting nerve f.
parallel f.
paraventricular f.
parietopontine f.
peptidergic f.
periventricular f.
pilomotor f.
pontine corticonuclear f.
pontocerebellar f.
postcommissural f.
posterior external arcuate f.
postganglionic nerve f.
preganglionic autonomic f.
preganglionic nerve f.
pressor f.
pretectoolivary f.
projection f.
pyramidal f.
radicular f.
ragged red f. (RRF)
raphespinal f.
Rasmussen nerve f.
reinnervated f.
Reissner f.
Remak f.
Retzius f.
rod f.
Rosenthal f.
rubroolivary f.
rubrothalamic f.
sensory myelinated f.
f. sensory tract
short association f.

f. size
somatic afferent f.
somatic efferent f.
somatic nerve f.
spinocuneate f.
spinogracile f.
spinohypothalamic f.
spinomesencephalic f.
spinoolivary f.
spinoperiaqueductal f.
spinoreticular f.
spinotectal f.
spinothalamic f.
Stilling f.
stria terminalis f.
striatonigral f.
subcortical U f.
sudomotor f.
supraoptic f.
T f.
tangential nerve f.
tautomeric f.
tectoolivary f.
tectopontine f.
tectoreticular f.
temporopontine f.
tendril f.
thalamocortical f.
f. tract of spinal cord
f. tract transection
transverse pontine f.
trigeminothalamic f.
ultra-high molecular weight polyethylene f.
ultraterminal f.
unmyelinated f.
varicose f.
vasomotor f.
visceral afferent f.
visceral efferent f.
visceral nerve f.
von Monakow f.

fiberoptic
f. illuminator
f. nasopharyngolaryngoscopy

fiberoptics

fiberscope
superfine f.

Fiblast trafermin growth factor

fibra, pl. **fibrae**
fibrae arcuatae cerebri
fibrae arcuatae externae
fibrae arcuatae externae anteriores
fibrae arcuatae externae posteriores
fibrae arcuatae internae
fibrae associationes brevis
fibrae associationes longae
fibrae cerebelloolivares
fibrae circulares
fibrae commissurales telencephali
f. commissuralis
fibrae corticomesencephalicae
fibrae corticonucleares
fibrae corticonucleares bulbus
fibrae corticonucleares mesencephali
fibrae corticonucleares pontis
fibrae corticopontinae
fibrae corticoreticulares
fibrae corticorubrales
fibrae corticospinales
fibrae corticothalamicae
fibrae cuneocerebellares
fibrae cuneospinales
fibrae frontopontinae
fibrae gracilispinales
f. hypothalamospinales
f. intrathalamicae
f. occipitopontinae
f. occipitotectales
f. olivospinales
f. paraventriculares
f. parietopontinae
f. periventriculares
f. pontis longitudinales
f. pontis profundae
f. pontis superficialis
f. pontis transversae
f. pontocerebellares
f. postcommissurales
f. precommissurales
f. pretectoolivares
f. pyramidales
f. rubroolivares
f. spinocuneatae
f. spinograciles
f. spinohypothalamicae
f. spinomesencephalicae
f. spinoolivares
f. spinoperiaqueductales
f. spinoreticulares
f. spinotectales
f. striae terminalis
f. supraopticae
f. supraopticohypophysiales

F

NOTES

fibra *(continued)*
f. tectoolivares
f. tectopontinae
f. tectoreticulares
f. temporopontinae
fibrae dentatorubrales
fibril
Abeta f.
beta-amyloid f.
bundle of f.'s
Golgi side f.
nerve f.
thioflavin-positive f.
fibrillar basket
fibrillary
f. aggregate
f. astrocyte
f. astrocytoma
f. chorea
f. contraction
f. glia
f. myoclonia
f. neuroma
f. tremor
fibrillation
atrial f.
nonrheumatic atrial f.
paroxysmal atrial f.
f. potential
ventricular f.
fibrillinopathy
fibrillogenesis
fibrin
f. adhesive sealant
f. bandage
f. film
f. glue
f. glue-soaked Gelfoam
f. thrombus
fibrinogen
fibrinoid degeneration
fibrinolysin
fibrinolysis
intracisternal f.
fibrinolytic agent
fibrin-platelet-fibrin embolus
fibroblast
f. growth factor receptor (FGFR)
f. growth factor receptor 2 (FGFR2)
senescent f.
transfected f.
fibroblastic
f. growth factor (FGF)
f. meningioma
f. proliferation
fibroblastic-like cell
fibroblastoma
perineural f.
fibrodysplasia ossificans
fibrogliosis
fibrohistiocytoma
malignant f.
fibrolipoma
fibroma
chondromyxoid f.
gingival f.
ossifying f.
periungual f.
psammomatoid ossifying f.
sinonasal psammomatoid ossifying f.
subungual f.
ungual f.
fibromatosis
juvenile f.
fibromuscular
f. dysplasia (FMD)
f. hyperplasia
fibromyalgia
fibromyelinic plaque
fibronectin synthesis
fibroneuroma
fibroplasia
retrolental f.
fibropsammoma
fibrosa
meninx f.
fibrosarcoma
fibrosclerosis
multifocal f.
systemic multifocal f.
fibrosing arachnoiditis
fibrosis
arachnoid f.
cystic f.
diffuse interstitial f. (DIF)
dural f.
leptomeningeal f.
meningeal f.
muscle f.
postradiation f.
progressive leptomeningeal f.
f. radiation
retroperitoneal f.
root sleeve f.
fibrositic headache
fibrositis
cervical f.
fibrosum
molluscum f.
fibrous
f. astrocyte
f. dysplasia
f. mesothelioma
f. plaque
f. sarcoma
f. sheath of optic nerve

fibroxanthoma
fibroxanthosarcoma
fibular
f. allograft
f. grafting
f. nerve
f. peg
fictitious
f. epilepsy
f. seizure
FID
free induction decay
repeated FID
fiducial
cranium-affixed f.
inexact f.
f. marker
MKM f.
radiopaque f.
field
abuse f.
barrel f.
Broca f.
Brodmann cytoarchitectonic f.
centrocecal visual f.
checkerboard f.
f. contour
f. defect
dipole f.
electromagnetic focusing f.
f. expansion
extremely low-frequency magnetic f.
face-evoked magnetic f.
f. of Forel
fringing f.
frontal eye f.
f. of gaze
Goldmann visual f.
f. gradient
gradient magnetic f.
H f.
harmonic error f.
f. homogeneity
Humphrey visual f.
f. independence-dependence
f. inhomogeneity
lateral central tegmental f.
lattice f.
f. magnet
magnetic f.
main f.
medial central tegmental f.
nerve f.
nucleus of dorsal f.
nucleus of medial f.
nucleus of perizonal f.
nucleus of prerubral f.
nucleus of ventral f.
occipital eye f.
parietal eye f.
f. pattern
prerubral f.
pulsating electromagnetic f.
pulsed electromagnetic f. (PEMF)
radiation f.
radiofrequency electromagnetic f.
f. shift
static magnetic f.
f. strength
F. suction dissector
supplementary eye f. (SEF)
vector f.
f. of view
Wernicke f.
z-gradient f.
Fielding
F. and Hawkins classification system
F. membrane
field-tested criterion
FIENS
Foundation for International Education in Neurological Surgery
fifth
f. cranial nerve [CN V]
f. ventricle
fight-or-flight mechanism
Figueira syndrome
figure
fortification f.
myelin f.
figure-ground perception
figure-of-8 coil
fila (*pl. of* filum)
filament
actin f.
cytoplasmic desmin f.
dural terminal f.
external terminal f.
filum terminale pial f.
glial f.
helical-like f.
internal terminal f.

NOTES

filament *(continued)*
meningeal f.
myosin f.
paired helical f.
pial terminal f.
f. protein
root f.
spinal ater f.
spinal nerve root f.
straight f.
terminal f.
filamin
f. A mutation
f. 1 gene
FilaminA gene (*FLNA*)
filiformis
nucleus f.
filiform nucleus
fillet
decussation of f.
lateral f.
f. layer
medial f.
triangle of f.
trigone of f.
filling factor
film
absorbable gelatin f.
Accu-Flo dura f.
fibrin f.
Instat fibrin f.
orthogonal f.
filovaricosis
filter
analog f.
high-frequency f. (HFF)
high linear f.
low-frequency f. (LFF)
low-pass f.
Millipore f.
muscle f.
notch f.
roll-off f.
shunt f.
filtered-back projection
filter-evoked central abnormality
filtering
antialias f.
perceptual f.
signal f.
filum, pl. **fila**
f. durae matris spinalis
fila olfactoria
olfactory f.
radicular f.
fila radicularia
fila radicularia nervi spinalis
f. spinale
terminal f.
f. terminale
f. terminale externum
f. terminale internum
f. terminale lesion
f. terminale pial filament
f. terminale syndrome
fimbria, pl. **fimbriae**
f. of hippocampus
tenia fibriae
fimbria-fornix lesion
fimbriatum
corpus f.
fimbriodentate sulcus
fimbriodentatus
sulcus f.
final common pathway
Finapres finger cuff
finding
angiographic f.
bipolar polysomnographic f.
empirical f.
equivocal f.
motor f.
obtained f.
pathological f.
postmortem f.
spurious f.
fine
f. motor development
f. motor function
f. rapid nystagmus
f. touch microsurgery
f. touch sensation
f. tremor
fine-cup forceps
fine-tipped up-angled and down-angled bipolar forceps
finger
f. agnosia
f. anomia
f. fracture technique
f. indicator
jerk f.
lock f.
f. phenomenon
f. response
snap f.
spring f.
trigger f.
finger-nose test
fingerprint body myopathy
finger-tapping task
finger tapping test
finger-thumb reflex
finger-to-finger test
finger-to-nose test
finish bur

finite
f. element analysis
f. element model
Finnish-type familial amyloid polyneuropathy
Finnish variant of neuronal ceroid lipofuscinosis
Finochietto
F. retractor
F. rib spreader
Fiorinal
FIRDA
frontal intermittent rhythmic delta activity
firing
neuronal element f.
sustained high-frequency repetitive f. (SRF)
firma
terra f.
FIR.S.T.
first seizure study
first
f. cranial nerve [CN I]
f. seizure study (FIR.S.T.)
f. somatosensory area
f. temporal convolution
f. temporal gyrus
f. visual area
first-degree
f.-d. nystagmus
f.-d. relative
first-episode patient
first-line therapy
first-night effect
first-order
f.-o. elimination kinetics
f.-o. neuron
first-rank symptom
first-trimester maternal seizure
Fisch
F. drill
F. dural hook
F. micro hook
Fischer
F. grade
F. stereotaxy system
F. syndrome
Fischer-Leibinger bur hole-mounted fixation device
FISH
fluorescence in situ hybridization
fish
puffer f.
f. vertebra
Fisher
F. exact test
F. grading
F. syndrome
Fishgold line
FISP
fast imaging with steady precession
fissura, pl. **fissurae**
f. calcarina
fissurae cerebelli
f. cerebri lateralis
f. choroidea
f. collateralis
f. dentata
f. hippocampus
f. horizontalis
f. horizontalis cerebelli
f. intercruralis cerebelli
f. intersemilunaris
f. intraculminalis
f. longitudinalis cerebri
f. mediana anterior medullae oblongatae
f. mediana anterior medullae spinalis
f. mediana ventralis medullae oblongatae
f. mediana ventralis medullae spinalis
f. parietooccipitalis
f. petrooccipitalis
f. posterior superior
f. posterolateralis
f. posterolateralis cerebelli
f. precentralis
f. preculminalis
f. prepyramidalis
f. prima cerebelli
f. secunda cerebelli
f. sphenooccipitalis
f. transversa cerebelli
f. transversa cerebri
fissure
ansoparamedian f.
f. of anulus
ape f.
Bichat f.
Broca f.
Burdach f.

NOTES

F

fissure *(continued)*
calcarine f.
callosomarginal f.
cerebellomedullary f.
cerebellomesencephalic f.
cerebral f.
choroid f.
choroidal f.
choroidal-hippocampal f.
Clevenger f.
collateral f.
dentate f.
displacement of interhemispheric f.
Ecker f.
entorbital f.
great horizontal f.
great longitudinal f.
hippocampal f.
inferior orbital f.
inferofrontal f.
intercrural f.
interhemispheric f.
intersemilunar f.
intraculminate f.
lateral cerebral f.
longitudinal cerebral f.
lunate f.
Monro f.
optic f.
Pansch f.
paracentral f.
parietooccipital f.
postcentral f.
postclival f.
posterior median f.
posterior superior f.
posterolateral f.
posthippocampal f.
postlingual f.
postlunate f.
postpyramidal f.
postrhinal f.
precentral f.
preclival f.
preculminate f.
precuneal f.
prenodular f.
prepyramidal f.
presylvian f.
retrotonsillar f.
rhinal f.
f. of Rolando
Schwalbe f.
simian f.
subfrontal f.
subtemporal f.
superfrontal f.
superior orbital f. (SOF)
superior temporal f.
sylvian f.
f. of Sylvius
transtemporal f.
transverse cerebral f.
zygal f.

fistula, pl. **fistulae**
arteriovenous f.
Brescia-Cimino f.
caroticocavernous f.
carotid-cavernous sinus f.
carotid-dural f.
cavernous sinus f.
cerebrospinal fluid f.
conus perimedullary arteriovenous f.
craniosinus f.
dorsal enteric f.
dural arteriovenous f. (DAVF)
dural venous f.
durocutaneous f.
iatrogenic carotid-cavernous f.
intradural retromedullary arteriovenous f.
perilymph f. (PLF)
perilymphatic f.
posterior fossa dural arteriovenous f.
pulmonary arteriovenous f.
radiculomedullary f.
spinal dural arteriovenous f. (SDAVF)
trauma-induced f.
wall f.

fistula-induced sinus thrombosis

fistular
premedullary arteriovenous f.

fit
cerebellar f.
uncinate f.

Fite stain

fixateur interne

fixation
adjunctive screw f.
anterior metallic f.
anterior plate f.
anterior screw f.
anterior spinal f.
Arbeitsgemeinschaft für Osteosynthesefragen-Association for the Study of Internal F. (AO-ASIF)
Association for the Study of Internal F. (ASIF)
atlantoaxial f.
Caspar anterior plate f.
C1-C2 cable f.
cervical spine internal f.
cervical spine screw-plate f.
Cotrel-Dubousset f.
crossed-screw f.

dens anterior screw f.
f. device
Essex-Lopresti axial f.
external spinal skeletal f. (ESSF)
Galveston f.
Halifax clamp posterior cervical f.
Harrington rod f.
hook-plate f.
iliac f.
f. instability
intermaxillary f.
internal spinal f.
lumbar pedicle f.
lumbar spine segmental f.
lumbar spine transpedicular f.
Luque-Galveston f.
Luque loop f.
Magerl posterior C1-C2 screw f.
mandibular f.
Manual of Internal F.
Modulock posterior spinal f.
multiple-point sacral f.
f. nystagmus
occipitocervical f.
odontoid fracture internal f.
pedicle screw-rod f.
pedicular f.
pelvic f.
plate f.
plate-screw f.
posterior cervical f.
posterior segmental f.
reduction f.
ReFix noninvasive f.
rigid internal f.
rod f.
Roy-Camille posterior screw plate f.
sacral pedicle screw f.
sacral spine f.
sacrum fusion screw f.
scoliotic curve f.
screw f.
segmental f.
semirigid pedicle screw-plate f.
Sofwire spinal f.
spinal f.
spinopelvic transiliac f. (STIF)
spondylolisthesis reduction f.
sublaminar f.
f. technique
Texas Scottish Rite Hospital rod f.
transarticular screw f.
transpedicular screw-rod f.
transverse f.
TSRH rod f.
visual f.

fixative
Bouin-Hollande f.

fixator
AO internal f.
DeBastiani external f.
external spinal skeletal f.
intermediate head f.
ReFix stereotactic head f.
Vermont spinal f.

fixed
f. contracture
f. deformity
f. distribution
f. dosing
f. dosing arm
f. gaze
f. lumbar kyphosis
f. pupil
f. spasm
f. torticollis

fixed-action pattern

fixed-dose stimulation

fixed-head screw

fixedness
functional f.

FK506 neurotoxicity

F-labeled fluoromisonidazole positron emission tomography

flaccid
f. coma
f. dysarthria
f. paralysis
f. paraparesis
f. paresis

flaccida
pars f.

flaccidity
curarization-induced f.

FLAIR
fluid-attenuated inversion recovery
FLAIR sequence magnetic resonance imaging

flame-shaped hemorrhage

flame-tip bur

Flanagan spinal fusion gouge

flap
axial pattern scalp f.

NOTES

flap *(continued)*
bicoronal scalp f.
bone f.
craniotomy f.
C-shaped scalp f.
Dandy myocutaneous scalp f.
f. elevation
free bone f.
horseshoe-shaped f.
I-shaped scalp f.
island pedicle scalp f.
liver f.
lumbar periosteal turnover f.
myocutaneous f.
neurovascular f.
osteoplastic bone f.
palatopharyngeal f.
pedicled pericranial f.
pericranial temporalis f.
reversible uvulopalatal f.
scalp f.
sickle f.
skin f.
supraorbital pericranial f.
trapdoor-type f.
U-shaped scalp f.
uvulopalatal f. (UPF)
flapping tremor
flare
axon f.
FLASH
fast low-angle shot
flash
eyebrow f.
flash-frozen tumor specimen
flashing pain syndrome
flat
f. back curette
f. back deformity
f. back syndrome
f. electroencephalogram
f. occiput
f. tire sign
f. top wave
Flatau law
Flatau-Schilder disease
flattening
f. of gyrus
occiput f.
flavin
f. adenine dinucleotide (FAD)
f. mononucleotide (FMN)
flavin-containing mono-oxygenase metabolic system
Flavivirus
flavoprotein dehydrogenase
flavum
ligamentum f.
flecainide
Flechsig
F. area
F. bundle in cerebellum
F. fasciculus
F. ground bundle
oval area of F.
F. primordial zone
semilunar nucleus of F.
F. tract
fleece
Stilling f.
fleeting
f. auditory hallucination
f. visual hallucination
flexed posture
Flexeril
Flex Foam orthosis
flexibilitas
cerea f.
flexibility
Cotrel-Dubousset rod f.
mental f.
flexible
f. arm microretractor
f. arm retractor
f. endoscope
f. neuroleptic dosing
f. wire electrode
Flexicair bed
Flexinet dressing
flexion
f. burst fracture
flicker thumb f.
forceful forward f.
forceful sidewise f.
forelimb f.
forward f.
full f.
f. injury
f. injury posterior atlantoaxial arthrodesis
paraplegia in f.
passive f.
f. reflex testing
sidewise f.
spontaneous f.
f. stability
flexion-compression spine injury stabilization
flexion-distraction injury
flexion-extension injury
flexion-extension-mediated injury
flexor
f. carpi radialis (FCR)
f. carpi radialis muscle
f. reflex
f. tetanus
flexura, pl. **flexurae**

flexure
basicranial f.
cephalic f.
cerebral f.
cervical f.
cranial f.
mesencephalic f.
pontine f.
telencephalic f.
transverse rhombencephalic f.
flicker
f. frequency grating
f. thumb flexion
Flickinger
formula of F.
flip angle
flittering scotoma
FLNA
FilaminA gene
floating-forehead operation
floccule
flocculi (*pl. of* flocculus)
flocculonodular
f. arteriovenous malformation
f. lobe
f. lobule
f. node
flocculonodularis
lobus f.
flocculus, pl. **flocculi**
accessory f.
peduncle of f.
pedunculus f.
flomoxef
floor
fourth ventricle f.
lateral ventricle f.
f. plate
temporal fossa f.
third ventricle f.
floorstand
CASS digital readout f.
Contraves-type f.
floppy
f. head syndrome
f. infant syndrome
FloSeal
F. hemostatic agent
F. Matrix hemostatic sealant
Flouren law
flow
absolute f.
anterior cingulate f.
autoregulation of cerebral blood f.
axoplasmic f.
f. birefringence
blood f.
brain blood f.
cerebral blood f. (CBF)
collateral blood f.
cortical microcirculatory f.
f. cytometry
f. detection technique
f. direction
f. dynamic
forced expiratory f. (FEF)
global cerebral blood f. (gCBF)
hemispheric blood f.
hemispheric cross f.
hypothalamic blood f.
intraarterial f.
local cerebral blood f. (LCBF)
f. misregistration
orbital blood f.
prefrontal f.
regional cerebral blood f. (rCBF)
f. regulated suction tube
resting anterior cingulate f.
retrograde blood f.
spinal cord blood f.
spinal cord white matter blood f.
f. theory
f. tracer
f. velocity
whole-brain blood f.
xenon CT cerebral blood f.
flow-controlled device
flow-directed embolization
flower basket of Bochdalek
flower-spray
f.-s. ending
f.-s. organ of Ruffini
flow-induced influx effect
flow-limitation arousal
flowmeter
clinical electromagnetic f.
electromagnetic f.
laser Doppler f. (LDF)
flowmetry
Doppler f.
laser Doppler f.
flow-related enhancement

NOTES

flow-sensitive
f.-s. magnetic resonance imaging
f.-s. MR imaging
FLP
Functional Limitation Profile
Fluanxol Depot
fluconazole
fluctuation
cognitive f.
core temperature f.
motor f.
on-off motor f.
orthostatic f.
temperature f.
5-flucytosine
flucytosine blood level
fludrocortisone
fluency
abnormal f.
fluent
f. aphasia
f. speech
Fluftex gauze roll
fluid
f. ability
f. balance
cerebrospinal f. (CSF)
coccidioidal complement fixation of cerebrospinal f.
f. coordination
cytosol f.
endoneurial f.
limulus lysate assay of cerebrospinal f.
mononuclear pleocytosis of cerebrospinal f.
f. percussion head injury
pleocytosis of cerebrospinal f.
f. retention
spinal f.
subgaleal cerebrospinal f.
Traube-Hering-Mayer wave in cerebrospinal f.
ventricular f.
xanthochromia of cerebrospinal f.
fluid-attenuated
f.-a. inversion recovery (FLAIR)
f.-a. inversion recovery sequence magnetic resonance imaging
fluidity
increased platelet membrane f.
f. of movement
flu-like syndrome
flumazenil
flumezapine
flunarizine
fluorescein
intrathecal f.
fluorescence
autofluorescence focal f.
f. in situ hybridization (FISH)
fluorescent treponemal antibody absorption test
fluorocytosine
fluorodeoxyglucose (FDG)
f. PET study
f. positron emission tomography (FDG-PET)
positron emission tomography-f. (PET-FDG)
fluorodopa
f. positron emission tomographic scan
f. positron emission tomography
fluorography
pulsed f.
fluorometer
FluoroNav
F. virtual fluoroscopic system
F. virtual fluoroscopy system
fluorophore
fluoroptic
f. thermometry probe
f. thermometry system
fluoroscopic
f. image guidance
f. imaging
fluoroscopically guided injection
fluoroscopy
C-arm f.
intraoperative lateral f.
fluorosis
5-fluorouracil
fluorouracil therapy
fluoxetine
f. intoxication
f. treatment
fluoxymesterone
fluphenazine hydrochloride
flurazepam
flurry of myoclonic jerks
flush
f. chamber
perilimbal f.
flushing
facial f.
hemifacial f.
flutamide
fluticasone
flutter
ocular f.
fluvoxamine maleate
flux
ion f.
magnetic f.
microcirculatory red cell f.
Flynn-Aird syndrome

FMAP
feeding mean arterial pressure
FMD
fibromuscular dysplasia
foot-and-mouth disease
FMF
familial Mediterranean fever
FMN
flavin mononucleotide
f-MRI
functional magnetic resonance imaging
BOLD f-MRI
foam
f. cell
gelatin f.
Ivalon f.
polyvinyl alcohol f.
PV f.
focal
f. acute headache
f. adhesion kinase (FAK)
f. akathisia
f. artery ischemia
f. axonal disruption
f. brain syndrome
f. cerebral head injury
f. cerebral ischemia
f. cortical architecture
f. cortical dysfunction
f. cortical dysplasia
f. delta slow-wave activity
f. edema
f. epileptiform activity
f. epileptiform discharge
f. frontal lobe epilepsy
f. hand dystonia
f. infection
f. jerking
f. lesion
f. malformation of cortical development
f. motor seizure
f. muscular atrophy
f. neonatal hypotonia
f. neurological sign
f. neurologic deficit
f. neurologic disturbance
f. neurologic sign
f. neuropathy
f. nodular heterotopia
f. plaquelike defect
f. pontine leukoencephaly
f. radiation
f. resection
f. sclerosis
f. sensorimotor sign
f. slowing
f. slowing of background rhythm
f. slow-wave abnormality
f. status epilepticus
f. stereotactic injection
f. suppurative encephalitis
f. temporal lobe dysfunction
FocalSeal-S surgical sealant
focus, pl. **foci**
anaplastic f.
benign epilepsy with occipital f.
centrotemporal paroxysmal f.
cortical epileptogenic f.
cortical seizure f.
epileptic f.
epileptogenic f.
extensive seizure f.
familial partial epilepsy with variable foci
f. of hemorrhage
inward f.
occult frontal f.
outward f.
restricted f.
rolandic paroxysmal f.
secondary epileptogenic f.
tuberculous f.
focused radiation therapy
FOG
freezing of gait
Fogarty embolectomy catheter
Foix-Alajouanine
F.-A. disease
F.-A. myelitis
F.-A. syndrome
Foix-Cavany-Marie syndrome
Foix syndrome
folate
f. deficiency
serum f.
fold
choroidal f.
interclinoid f.
medullary f.
neural f.
petroclinoid f.
postsynaptic f.
retrotarsal f.

foldover
image f.
folia (*pl. of* folium)
folic
f. acid
f. acid deficiency
folii
lobulus f.
folinic acid
folium, pl. **folia**
cerebellar f.
folia cerebelli
folia of cerebellum
f. of vermis
follicle
hair f.
follicle-stimulating hormone (FSH)
follicle-stimulating/luteinizing hormone adenoma
follicularis
alopecia f.
Folling disease
following gaze
followup, follow-up
f. data
systematic f.
f. visit
Fonar Upright MRI
fontanelle
fonticulus nasofrontalis
fontinalis
decussatio f.
food
f. allergy insomnia
mercury-contaminated f.
food-borne botulism
foot
astrocytic end f.
f. clonus
dropped f.
Friedreich f.
f. of hippocampus
Morton f.
perineuronal end f.
perivascular end f.
precapillary end f.
f. reflex
f. slap
spastic equinus f.
sucker f.
f. tapping
foot-and-mouth disease (FMD)
footdrop
footplate of stapes
foramen, pl. **foramina**
arachnoid f.
Bichat f.
f. caecum medullae oblongatae
f. caecum posterius
cervical neural f.
emissary f.
Fallopio f.
Ferrein f.
f. of Froesch
great f.
greater sciatic f.
Hyrtl f.
interventricular f.
f. interventriculare
intervertebral f.
jugular f.
f. jugulare
f. jugulare tumor
f. of Key and Retzius
f. of Key-Retzius
f. lacerum
f. lateralis ventriculi quarti
f. of Luschka
f. of Magendie
f. magnum
f. magnum cyst
f. magnum decompression
f. magnum herniation
f. magnum line
f. of Monro
foramina nervosa
neural f.
open exit f.
f. ovale
f. ovale electrode
f. ovale tumor
Pacchioni f.
pacchionian f.
parietal f.
posterior lacerate f.
Retzius f.
f. rotundum
f. rotundum tumor
Schwalbe f.
skull base foramina
f. spinosum (FS)
stylomastoid f.
f. of Vesalius
Vicq d'Azyr f.
foraminal
f. approach
f. decompression
f. encroachment
f. entrapment
f. herniation
f. stenosis
foraminosus
foraminotomy
microendoscopic f.
microscopic f.
foraminulum, pl. **foraminula**
Forbes-Cori disease
Forbes disease

force
- f. application
- F. 2 CEM generator
- deflection f.
- distraction f.
- endogenous f.
- exchange f.
- exogenous f.
- fraction maximal voluntary contraction f.
- f. nucleus
- shearing f.
- societal f.
- f. transducer

forced
- f. choice of recognition test
- f. expiratory flow (FEF)
- f. grasping reflex
- f. impulse
- f. medication
- f. relationship
- f. vital capacity (FVC)

forceful
- f. flexion injury
- f. forward flexion
- f. sidewise flexion

forceps
- Adson bipolar f.
- Adson-Brown f.
- Adson clip-introducing f.
- Adson cup f.
- Adson dressing f.
- Adson hemostatic f.
- Adson hypophysial f.
- Adson-Mixter neurosurgical f.
- Adson tissue f.
- alligator cup f.
- f. anterior
- Babcock f.
- bayonet f.
- bipolar bayonet f.
- bipolar coagulating f.
- bipolar electrocautery f.
- bipolar long-shaft f.
- brain clip f.
- brain spatula f.
- brain tumor f.
- Brown-Adson f.
- Castroviejo eye suture f.
- Cherry-Kerrison laminectomy f.
- Cone skull punch f.
- Cone wire-twisting f.
- contact compressive f.
- cranial rongeur f.
- Crile artery f.
- cup f.
- curved knot-tying f.
- Cushing bayonet f.
- Cushing bipolar f.
- Cushing brain f.
- Cushing dressing f.
- Cushing monopolar f.
- Cushing tissue f.
- Dandy scalp hemostatic f.
- Davis coagulating f.
- Davis monopolar f.
- DeBakey f.
- Decker alligator f.
- Decker microsurgical f.
- DeMartel scalp flap f.
- Denis f.
- D'Errico bayonet pituitary f.
- D'Errico hypophysial f.
- D'Errico tissue f.
- DeVilbiss rongeur f.
- dissecting f.
- dressing f.
- dura-protecting f.
- ear f.
- Ewald-Hudson f.
- fine-cup f.
- fine-tipped up-angled and down-angled bipolar f.
- Fox bipolar electrocautery f.
- f. fracture
- frontal f.
- f. frontalis
- Gerald f.
- Greenwood bipolar and suction f.
- Grünwald ear f.
- Hajek-Koffler bone punch f.
- Halsted artery f.
- Halsted mosquito f.
- Hardy bayonet dressing f.
- Hardy microsurgical bayonet bipolar f.
- Hardy sella punch f.
- Heifetz cup serrated ring f.
- hemostatic f.
- Hirsch hypophysis punch f.
- Howmedica microfixation system plate-holding f.
- Hudson f.
- Hunt angled serrated ring f.

NOTES

forceps *(continued)*
Hunt angled-tip f.
Hunt grasping f.
Hunt-Yasargil pituitary f.
Hurd bone-cutting f.
hypophysectomy f.
hypophysial f.
hypophysis punch f.
Jacobson mosquito f.
Jannetta alligator f.
Jannetta bayonet f.
Jansen-Middleton f.
Jansen monopolar f.
Jarell f.
Jarit brain f.
Jarit tendon-pulling f.
Jerald f.
jeweler's bipolar f.
Johnson brain tumor f.
Knight f.
laminectomy punch f.
Leibinger Micro System plate-holding f.
LeRoy scalp clip-applying f.
Love-Gruenwald intervertebral disc f.
Love-Gruenwald pituitary f.
Love-Kerrison rongeur f.
Luc ethmoid f.
MacCarty f.
major f.
Malis angled bayonet f.
Malis irrigation f.
Malis-Jensen microbipolar f.
Malis jeweler's bipolar f.
Maryland tissue-grasping f.
McGill f.
McKenzie brain clip f.
McKenzie clip-applying f.
McKenzie clip-bending f.
McKenzie clip-introducing f.
microartery f.
microbipolar f.
microcup f.
microsurgery f.
microvascular f.
Miles punch biopsy f.
minor f.
monopolar tissue f.
mosquito f.
Moynihan f.
Nicola f.
occipital f.
f. occipitalis
Oldberg pituitary f.
Olivecrona-Toennis clip-applying f.
Péan f.
peapod intervertebral disc f.
pituitary f.
plain f.
f. posterior
Preston ligamentum flavum f.
Raimondi infant scalp hemostatic f.
Raney coagulating f.
Raney rongeur f.
Raney scalp clip-applying f.
Rhoton-Cushing f.
Rhoton dissecting f.
Rhoton-Tew bipolar f.
Richter laminectomy punch f.
ringed formed f.
round-handled f.
scalp clip f.
scalp flap f.
Scharff microbipolar and suction f.
Scoville brain clip-applying f.
Scoville brain spatula f.
sella punch f.
Spencer biopsy f.
spinal perforating f.
sponge-holding f.
straight knot-tying f.
straight-line bayonet f.
f. tip
tissue f.
Toennis tumor f.
transsphenoidal bipolar f.
tying f.
Yasargil artery f.
Yasargil bayonet f.
Yasargil clip-applying f.
Yasargil flat serrated ring f.
Yasargil hypophysial f.
Yasargil knotting f.
Yasargil micro f.
Yasargil tumor f.

forearm
f. jerk
f. sign

forebrain
f. activity
f. cell
f. cell culture
magnocellular basal f.
f. vesicle

foregut cyst

forehead
remodeled f.

foreign
f. body
f. body granuloma
f. body migration

Forel
area of F.
F. decussation
field of F.
tegmental field of F.

forelimb
f. flexion
f. kinematics
f. motor
Forestier disease
forest-spring encephalitis
forgetfulness
benign senescent f.
senescent f.
fork
Hardy 3-prong f.
f. head gene
f. head response factor
Jannetta f.
Sugita f.
forking of sylvian aqueduct
form
f. birefringence
depot f.
major f.
minor f.
scrapie f.
trimeric f.
wave f.
formal dose-escalation protocol
format
DICOM f.
formate
butyl f.
formatio, pl. **formationes**
f. hippocampalis
f. reticularis
f. reticularis medullae oblongatae
f. reticularis medullae spinalis
f. reticularis pedunculi cerebri
f. reticularis tegmenti mesencephali
f. reticularis tegmenti pontis
formation
abscess f.
aneurysm f.
bone matrix f.
brainstem reticular f.
cerebrospinal fluid f.
Chiari f.
diffuse Rosenthal fiber f.
ectopic bone f.
free radical f.
granuloma f.
hemostatic plug f.
hippocampal f.
medulla oblongata reticular f.
meningioma f.
mesencephalic reticular f.
mesencephalon reticular f.
midbrain reticular f.
mucocele f.
neural plate f.
onion bulb f.
osteophyte f.
paramedian pontine reticular f. (PPRF)
pons reticular f.
pontine paramedian reticular f.
pontine parareticular f.
posttraumatic symptom f.
reticular f.
Rosenthal fiber f.
rouleaux f.
spinal cord reticular f.
syrinx f.
tegmental reticular f.
formed visual hallucination
forme fruste
former smoker
formication sign
formula, pl. **formulae**
Abercrombie neuronal cell count f.
Dramamine Less Drowsy F.
F. EM oral solution
f. of Flickinger
parenteral f.
Penn cube function f.
formulation
case f.
clinical f.
dynamic f.
fornicate gyrus
fornicati
uncus gyri f.
fornicatus
gyrus f.
isthmus of gyrus f.
forniceal column
fornicis
carina f.
columna f.
commissura f.
corpus f.
crus f.
delta f.
stria f.
tenia f.
fornix, pl. **fornices**
anterior pillar of f.

NOTES

fornix *(continued)*
body of f.
column of f.
commissure of f.
f. conjunctiva
crus of f.
pillar of f.
posterior pillar of f.
transverse f.
Förster
F. diplegia
F. syndrome
fortification
f. figure
f. spectrum
forward
digit span f. (DSF)
f. flexion
f. modeling
spatial span f. (SSF)
fosazepam
fosphenytoin
FOS protein
FOSQ
Functional Outcomes of Sleep Questionnaire
fossa, pl. **fossae**
anterior cranial f.
anterior recess of interpeduncular f.
cerebellar f.
f. cerebellaris
cistern of lateral cerebral f.
cistern of Sylvius f.
hypophysial f.
f. incudis
inferior aperture of axillary f.
infratemporal f. (ITF)
interpeduncular f.
f. interpeduncularis
lateral cerebral f.
f. lateralis cerebri
limiting sulcus of rhomboid f.
middle cranial f.
f. ovalis
posterior cranial f.
posterior pituitary f.
posterior recess of interpeduncular f.
pterygoid f.
pterygopalatine f.
rhomboid f.
f. rhomboidea
f. of Rosenmüller
rostral posterior f.
sphenoidal f.
superior aperture of axillary f.
sylvian f.
f. of Sylvius
f. of Sylvius cistern
temporal f.
fossula, pl. **fossulae**
Foster
F. frame
F. Kennedy syndrome
FOT
functional occupational therapy
Fothergill
F. disease
F. neuralgia
Foundation
Epilepsy F.
F. for International Education in Neurological Surgery (FIENS)
International Tremor F.
National Brain Tumor F.
The Charlie F.
fountain decussation
FOUR
Full Outline of Unresponsiveness
FOUR coma score
Fourier
F. analysis
F. pulsatility index
F. spectroscopy
F. synthesis
F. transform
F. transform algorithm
F. transformation zeugmatography
F. transform technique
fourth
f. cervical nerve (C4)
f. cranial nerve [CN IV]
f. nerve palsy
f. ventricle
f. ventricle floor
f. ventricle fovea
fourth-generation cephalosporin
fovea, pl. **foveae**
anterior f.
f. centralis maculae luteae
f. centralis retinae
central retinal f.
fourth ventricle f.
inferior f.
superior f.
foveal vision
foveola, pl. **foveolae**
Foville
F. fasciculus
F. syndrome
fowleri
Naegleria f.
Fox
F. bipolar electrocautery
F. bipolar electrocautery forceps
FPA
frontopolar artery

fraction
creatine kinase-MB f. (CK-MB)
ejection f.
growth f.
f. maximal voluntary contraction force
oxygen extraction f. (OEF)
regional oxygen extraction f.
S-phase f.
fractional anisotropy (FA)
fractionated
f. radiation therapy
f. radiotherapy
fractionation protocol
fracture
anterior column f.
anteroposterior f.
articular mass separation f.
atlantal f.
atlas-axis combination f.
atlas burst f.
axial burst f.
axial loading f.
axis-atlas combination f.
basal skull f.
basilar skull f.
blow-out f.
burst f.
capillary f.
Chance f.
clay shoveler's f.
closed skull f.
combined flexion-distraction injury and burst f.
comminuted skull f.
complex f.
complicated f.
compound skull f.
compression f.
f. by contrecoup
cranial f.
depressed skull f.
derby hat f.
diastatic skull f.
direct f.
dishpan f.
f. dislocation
edge f.
expressed skull f.
facet f.
facial f.
f. fixation device
flexion burst f.
forceps f.
growing skull f.
growth plate f.
gutter f.
hairline f.
hangman's f.
indirect f.
Jefferson f.
lateral f.
LeFort f.
linear skull f.
low lumbar spine f.
lumbar spine burst f.
lumbosacral junction f.
maxillofacial f.
neural arch f.
neurogenic f.
nondepressed skull f.
odontoid f.
open skull f.
orbital floor f.
perinatal clavicle f.
perinatal humerus f.
ping-pong f.
pond f.
f. reduction
rib f.
ring f.
sacral insufficiency f.
sacral stress f.
sagittal slice f.
seatbelt f.
sentinel spinous process f.
shear f.
simple skull f.
skull f.
slice f.
slot f.
spinous process f.
f. stabilization
stable f.
stellate endplate f.
stellate skull f.
step f.
teardrop f.
thoracic spine f.
thoracolumbar burst f.
translational f.
transverse vertebral body f.
type II odontoid f.
unstable f.

NOTES

fracture *(continued)*
vertebral f.
wedge-compression f.
f. with scoliosis
zygomatic f.
fracture-dislocation
f.-d. reduction
thoracolumbar spine f.-d.
fragile X syndrome
fragilis
Bacteroides f.
fragility
nuclear f.
vascular f.
fragmatome
fragment
bone f.
f. crystallizable (Fc)
C-terminal f.
Fc f.
free f.
intracranial f.
missed f.
missile f.
proteolytic f.
retained bullet f.
tangle f.
fragmentary myoclonus
fragmentation
internucleosomal DNA f.
f. of nocturnal sleep
sleep f.
fragmented syndrome
frame
Andrews f.
Brown-Roberts-Wells head f.
Budde-Greenberg-Sugita stereotactic head f.
Cosman-Roberts-Wells stereotactic head f.
couch-mounted head f.
CRW base f.
CRW head f.
DeBastiani f.
design for vision f.
Elekta stereotactic head f.
f. fixation scanner-assisted target localization
Foster f.
Gill-Thomas-Cosman f.
Greenberg retractor f.
head f.
Horsley-Clarke stereotactic f.
Komai stereotactic head f.
Laitinen stereoguide 2000 arc-centered stereotactic f.
Leksell-Elekta stereotactic f.
Leksell G stereotactic head f.
Lex-Ton spinal f.
Mayfield fixation f.
Mussen f.
OBT stereotactic f.
Olivier-Bertrand-Tipal f.
operative wedge f.
Patil stereotactic head f.
Pelorus stereotactic f.
3-point fixation f.
4-poster f.
Radionics CRW stereotactic head f.
Reichert-Mundinger-Fischer stereotactic head f.
Reichert-Mundinger stereotactic head f.
Relton-Hall f.
rigid f.
servohydraulic test f.
stereotactic f.
f. stereotaxy
Stryker f.
Sugita multipurpose head f.
Talairach stereotactic f.
Tarbell-Loeffler-Cosman f.
Todd-Wells stereotactic f.
Wilson f.
ZD f.
frame-based radiosurgical system
frameless
f. and armless stereotactic neuronavigation
f. stereotactic device
f. stereotactic microsurgery
f. stereotactic technique
f. stereotaxy
f. stereotaxy system
framework
ecologic f.
multidimensional f.
Framingham
F. Eye Study
F. Heart Study
franca
lingua f.
frank
f. catatonic stupor
f. disc herniation
f. disruption
f. lesion
Fränkel
F. classification
F. classification of spinal cord injury
F. grading system
F. scale
F. sign
Frankenhäuser ganglion
Frankfurt Complaint Questionnaire
franklinic taste
frataxin gene PCR

frayed disc
Frazier
F. brain-exploring cannula
F. brain trocar
F. cordotomy knife
F. dural elevator
F. dural guide
F. dural hook
F. dural scissors
F. dural separator
F. laminectomy retractor
F. lighted brain retractor
F. nerve hook
F. pituitary knife
F. stylet
F. suction
F. suction tip
F. suction tube
F. ventricular cannula
F. ventricular needle
Frazier-Spiller
F.-S. operation
F.-S. rhizotomy
freckling
inguinal f.
free
f. bone flap
f. fragment
f. fragment disc
f. functional cortex
f. induction decay (FID)
f. induction signal
f. nerve ending
f. radical
f. radical damage
f. radical formation
f. radical homeostasis
f. radical hypothesis
f. radical scavenger
f. radical scavenging mechanism
seizure f.
free-fat mass (FFM)
freehand
f. injection
F. neuroprosthetic system
f. ultrasound-guided intervention
Freeman-Sheldon syndrome
Freer
F. chisel
F. dissector
F. septal elevator
Freer-Swanson ganglion knife
free-running circadian sleep disorder
freeze-dried cadaveric dura
freezing
f. of gait (FOG)
f. phenomenon
Fregoli phenomenon/syndrome
Freiberg
F. craniotome
F. so-called infarction
Freiberg-Kohler disease
French
F. brain retractor
F. polio
F. rod bender
F. rod bender frontal
Frenchay Aphasia Screening test
Frenkel symptom
frenulum, pl. **frenula**
buccal f.
cerebellar f.
f. cerebelli
f. of Giacomini
multiple buccal frenula
rostral medullary vellum f.
f. of superior medullary velum
f. veli medullaris cranialis
f. veli medullaris rostralis
f. veli medullaris superioris
f. veli medullaris superius
frenzied psychomotor activity
frequency
alpha rhythm f.
F. Analysis of Consecutive Epochs (FACE)
angular f.
background alpha f.
f. dispersion curve
dominant f.
f. encoding
f. error
haplotype f.
high-filter f.
Larmor f.
low-filter f.
low linear f.
mean alpha f.
Nyquist f.
offset f.
precessional f.
f. range
resonant f.
seizure f.

NOTES

frequency *(continued)*
f. shift
spatial f.
spectral edge f. (SEF)
spike f.
theta peak f.
frequency-encoding gradient
frequent headaches
Fresnel paste-on prism
Frey
F. irritation hair
F. syndrome
friable artery
Friderichsen-Waterhouse syndrome
fried egg artifact
Friedmann
F. disease
F. vasomotor syndrome
Friedreich
F. disease
F. foot
F. hereditary ataxia
F. tabes
fringe
radical f.
fringing field
Frisén-grade change
Froesch
foramen of F.
Frohse
arcade of F.
Froin syndrome
Froment
F. paper sign
F. prehensile thumb sign
frontal
f. abasia
anterior f.
f. artery
f. ataxia
f. brain perfusion
f. brain region
f. branch neurectomy
f. convexity meningioma
f. cortex damage
f. cortex damage effect
f. cortical dysfunction
f. cortical function
f. corticectomy
f. craniotomy
f. disequilibrium
f. encephalocele
f. eye field
f. forceps
French rod bender f.
f. gait disorder
f. groove
f. gyrectomy
f. gyrus
f. headache
f. horn
f. hypoperfusion
f. interhemispheric space
f. intermittent rhythmic delta activity (FIRDA)
f. intermittent rhythmic delta activity on EEG
f. lobe
f. lobe abscess
f. lobe abstraction/problem solving
f. lobe of cerebrum
f. lobe degeneration
f. lobe dementia
f. lobe dysfunction
f. lobe epilepsy
f. lobe function
f. lobe impairment
f. lobe infarction
f. lobe lesion
f. lobe-related deficit
f. lobe seizure
f. lobe seizure with complex behavior
f. lobe syndrome
f. lobe tumor
f. lobe volume
f. lobotomy
f. metabolism
f. neoplasm
f. nerve
f. operculum
f. part of corpus callosum
f. plane
f. plane growth abnormality
f. polar branch
f. pole
f. subcortical brain circuit
f. temporal atrophy
f. tuber
f. white matter lesion
frontal-cerebellar-thalamic circuitry
frontale
operculum f.
frontalis
alopecia liminaris f.
forceps f.
lobus f.
nervus f.
pars orbitalis ossis f.
polus f.
sulci orbitales lobi f.
sulcus olfactorius lobi f.
frontally based cognition
frontocortical
f. aphasia
f. area

frontoethmoidal
f. encephalocele
f. recess
frontolenticular aphasia
frontomarginalis
sulcus f.
frontonasomaxillary osteotomy
frontooccipital fasciculus
frontoorbital
f. advancement
f. area
f. osteotomy
frontoparallel plane
frontoparietal
ascending f. (ASFP)
f. convexity cyst
f. operculum
frontoparietale
operculum f.
frontopolar
f. artery (FPA)
f. lead
frontopontinae
fibrae f.
frontopontine
f. fiber
f. tract
frontopontinus
tractus f.
frontopontocerebellar pathway
frontosphenoidal encephalocele
frontostriatal
f. circuitry
f. pathway
frontotemporal
f. approach
f. cortex
f. craniotomy
f. dementia (FTD)
f. durotomy
f. lobar degeneration
f. slowing
f. tract
frontotemporoparietal craniotomy
frontothalamic circuit
front tap
front-tap reflex
Froriep ganglion
frost
uremic f.
frovatriptan succinate
fructose-1,6-diphosphatase deficiency
fructose intolerance
fruste, pl. **frustes**
forme f.
Fryns syndrome
FS
foramen spinosum
FS MRI
FSH
follicle-stimulating hormone
FSH dystrophy
FTD
frontotemporal dementia
fucosidosis
Fuerstner disease
fugax
amaurosis f.
proctalgia f.
Fugl-Meyer assessment
Fujita
F. method
F. suction cannula
Fukuhara syndrome
Fukushima
F. cavernous bypass
F. monopolar malleable coagulator
F. retractor
fukutin
f. allele
f. gene
f. mutation
f. protein
Fukuyama
F. congenital muscular dystrophy
F. disease
F. syndrome
Fukuyama-type congenital muscular dystrophy
fulgurating migraine
full
f. dose
f. flexion
F. Outline of Unresponsiveness (FOUR)
f. remission
f. syndrome
f. width at half maximum (FWHM)
full-blown syndrome
full-dose-treated patient
fullness
aural f.
full-night polysomnography

F

NOTES

full-thickness necrosis
fulminant
f. hepatic encephalopathy
f. hydrocephalus
f. necrotizing encephalitis
f. neuroleptic malignant syndrome
Fulton laminectomy rongeur
fumarate
quetiapine f.
fumigatus
Aspergillus f.
function
allomeric f.
altered cognitive f.
anorectal f.
autonomic f.
autonomous f.
axis f.
behavioral f.
biologic window on CNS f.
cellular immune f.
cellular respiratory f.
cognitive f.
communication f.
cortical mapping of memory f.
disordered personality f.
dominant hemisphere f.
dysregulated T-cell f.
endocrine f.
episodic memory f.
executive f.
extracorporeal membrane oxygenation affecting cognitive f.
facial nerve f.
fine motor f.
frontal cortical f.
frontal lobe f.
GABA inhibitory f.
gastric f.
genital f.
global f.
gustatory f.
harmonic f.
higher cognitive f.
higher neural f.
impaired cerebral f.
impaired limbic-diencephalic f.
indolamine f.
intellectual f.
ipsilateral motor f.
isomeric f.
left ventricular f.
Legendre f.
leukemia therapy affecting cognitive f.
level of cognitive f.
linear rate-response f.
LSUMC classification of motor and sensory f.
memory f.
motor f.
motoric f.
myelinated nerve fiber f.
neural f.
neurologic f.
neuronal f.
nondominant hemisphere f.
nonlinear rate-response f.
noradrenergic system f.
olfactory f.
ovarian f.
psychosocial f.
renal f.
residual language f.
reverse learning f.
secretory f.
semantic memory f.
sensory f.
f. of sleep
spectral density f.
spinal cord f.
T-cell f.
thermoeffector f.
thermoregulatory f.
f. type
urinary tract f.
vestibular f.
visuospatial f.
working memory f.
functional
f. activation
f. activation PET scanning
F. Ambulation Category (FAC)
F. Ambulation Classification
f. analysis
f. anatomical perspective
f. anosmia
f. aphasia
f. aphonia
f. apoplexy
f. approach
f. assessment
f. brain imaging
f. brain imaging study
f. capacity
f. cloning
f. communication (FC)
f. component
f. contracture
f. decline
f. deficit
f. demand
f. deterioration
f. difference
f. dyspnea
f. electrical stimulation
f. enuresis
F. Ergonomic Prolo Scale

f. failure
F. Fitness Assessment for Adults over 60 Years
f. fixedness
f. funnel
f. hearing impairment
f. hippocampal inactivation
f. imaging data
f. imaging technique
F. Independence Measure
f. language recovery
f. limitation
F. Limitation Profile (FLP)
f. loss
f. magnetic resonance imaging (f-MRI)
f. MRI study
f. neuroimaging
f. neuromuscular stimulation
f. neuropharmacology
f. neurosurgery
f. object
F. Obstacle Course
f. occupational therapy (FOT)
F. Outcomes of Sleep Questionnaire (FOSQ)
f. pain
f. psychiatric syndrome
f. rehabilitation
f. retrograde amnesia
f. spasm
f. status
F. Status Index
f. stereotaxy
f. terminal innervation ratio
f. vaginismus
f. vertebral spinal unit
f. voice disorder

functional/cognitive impairment
functionalism
functioning
adaptive f.
baseline cognitive f.
brain f.
cognitive f.
cortical f.
domain of f.
emotional f.
end-state f.
general verbal intellectual f.
global f.
impaired attentional f.
intellectual f.
level of f.
f. measure
measure of general cognitive f.
neuropsychologic f.
overall cognitive f.
physical f.
premorbid f.
verbal intellectual f.
visuospatial f.
in vivo brain f.

fundamental
f. cognitive process
f. column
f. conceptual problem
f. neural mechanism
f. predisposition

fundus of aneurysm
funduscopic examination
fungal
f. culture
f. infection
f. meningitis
f. smear

fungiform papillae
fungus, pl. **fungi**
f. cerebri
f. isolation

funicular
f. graft
f. myelitis
f. myelosis

funiculitis
funiculus, pl. **funiculi**
anterior f.
cuneate f.
dorsal f.
f. dorsalis
f. gracilis
lateral f.
f. lateralis
f. lateralis medullae oblongatae
funiculi medullae spinalis
medulla oblongata lateral f.
posterior f.
f. posterior medullae oblongatae
f. separans
f. solitarius
spinal cord ventricular f.
f. teres
ventral f.
f. ventralis medullae spinalis

NOTES

F

funnel
functional f.
pial f.
f. plot
f. vision
furcal nerve
furegrelate
furifosmin
technetium-99m f.
furor epilepticus
furosemide
furrowed band
fused spine
fusiform
f. aneurysm
f. aneurysm neck
f. cell of cerebral cortex
f. face area (FFA)
f. gyrus
f. layer
fusiformis
gyrus f.
lobulus f.
fusimotor
f. axon
f. nerve
fusion
Adkins spinal f.
Albee lumbar spinal f.
anterior cervical discectomy and f.
anterior lumbar interbody f. (ALIF)
anterior lumbar spine interbody f.
atlantoaxial f.
Bailey-Badgley cervical spine f.
Bosworth spinal f.
Brooks cervical f.
Brooks-Jenkins atlantoaxial f.
cervical spine posterior f.
cervicooccipital f.
Cloward back f.
degenerative lumbar spine f.
degenerative spondylosis decompression and f.
f. disease
endoscopic transpsoas f.
Gallie cervical f.
Gallie spinal f.
Goldstein spinal f.
Harris-Smith cervical f.
Henry-Geist spinal f.
Hibbs-Jones spinal f.
interbody f.
interfacet wiring and f.
intertransverse process f.
f. limit determination
f. line
long segment spinal f.
lower cervical spine f.
lumbar interbody f.
lumbosacral f.
f. nonunion rate
occipitoatlantoaxial f.
occipitocervical f.
posterior lumbar interbody f. (PLIF)
posterior spinal f.
posterolateral lumbar spinal f.
posterolateral lumbosacral f.
posterolateral spinal f.
Robinson anterior cervical f.
sacral spine f.
selective thoracic spine f.
short segment spinal f.
Simmons cervical spine f.
single-level spinal f.
in situ spinal f.
solid f.
spinal f.
f. stiffness
f. technique
thoracic spinal f.
transforaminal lumbar interbody f. (TLIF)
upper cervical spine f.
variable stereotactic image f.
vertebral f.
Wiltberger f.
fusion-defusion cycle
futile cycling
FVC
forced vital capacity
F-wave
F-w. monitoring
F-w. test
FWHM
full width at half maximum

Gaab endoscope
GABA
gamma-aminobutyric acid
GABA agonist
GABA concentrate
GABA inhibitory function
GABA receptor
GABA transaminase
$GABA_B$
$GABA_B$ receptor
$GABA_B$ receptor-mediated inhibition
GABA-A
gamma-aminobutyric acid type A
GABAergic
G. cortical interneuron
G. inhibition
G. neuron
GABA-mediated inhibitory synaptic transmission
gabapentin capsule
GABAR
$GABA_A$ receptor
$GABA_A$ receptor (GABAR)
GABAR-mediated inhibition
Gabitril
GAD
generalized anxiety disorder
glutamine decarboxylase
gadodiamide
gadolinium
g. contrast
g. diethylenetriamine pentaacetic acid (Gd-DTPA)
g. diethylenetriamine pentaacetic acid-enhanced MR
g. DTPA
g. enhancement
gadolinium-enhanced
g.-e. MR angiography (Gd-MRA)
g.-e. MRI
g.-e. MR imaging
gadolinium-enhancing lesion
gadopentetate dimeglumine
gadoteridol
GAD-specific intervention
Gaenslen test
GAG
glycosaminoglycan
gag
Dingman mouth g.
g. reflex
g. reflex loss
g. reflex test
Gagel granuloma
gain-of-function abnormality
gait
g. abnormality
G. Abnormality Rating Scale
g. apraxia
g. ataxia
ataxic g.
broad-based g.
calcaneal g.
cerebellar g.
Charcot g.
choreic g.
circumduction g.
g. disequilibrium
g. disorder
g. disorder, autoantibody, late-age onset polyneuropathy
g. disturbance
dromedary g.
dystonic g.
equine g.
festinating g.
freezing of g. (FOG)
gluteal g.
gluteus maximus g.
gluteus medius g.
helicopod g.
hemiparetic g.
hemiplegic g.
high steppage g.
hip extensor g.
hysterical g.
g. impairment
intermittent double-step g.
maximus g.
myopathic g.
paraparetic g.
paraplegic spastic g.
parkinsonian g.
posterior column dysfunction g.
propulsive g.
quadriceps g.
scissors g.
shuffling g.
small-step g.
spastic g.
g. speed
staggering g.
steppage g.
tabetic g.
teddy bear g.
toppling g.
Trendelenburg g.
waddling g.
galactokinase deficiency
galactose-6-sulfate sulfatase

G

galactosemia
galactose-1-phosphate
g.-p. accumulation
g.-p. uridyltransferase deficiency
galactosialidosis
galactosidase
beta g.
g. defect
galactoside
alpha g. A, B
galactosylceramidase deficiency
galactosylceramide lipidosis
galactosylsphingosine accumulation
galantamine
g. HBr
g. hydrobromide
Galante disc degeneration score
Galant reflex
Galassi
G. classification system
G. pupillary phenomenon
galea
g. aponeurotica
closed g.
galeatomy
Galen
G. anastomosis
great cerebral vein of G.
G. nerve
vein of G.
G. vein malformation
galenic draining group
gallamine triethiodide
Gall craniology
galli
crista g.
wing of crista g.
Gallie
G. cervical fusion
G. spinal fusion
G. wiring technique
Gallie-Rodgers technique
gallium
g. nitrate
g. scan
gallium-67
galloping tongue
Galtac device
Galt skull trephine
galvanic
g. skin reaction
g. skin reflex (GSR)
g. skin resistance (GSR)
g. skin response (GSR)
g. vertigo
g. vestibular stimulation
galvanogustometer
galvanometer
galvanopalpation
Galveston
G. fixation
G. fixation with TSRH
G. fixation with TSRH crosslink
G. Orientation and Awareness test
GAMA
General Ability Measure for Adults
Gambian trypanosomiasis
Gambierdiscus toxicus
gamete
gamma
g. aminobutyric acid agonist
g. capsulotomy
g. carboxylated protein
crosslink g.
g. efferent
g. efferent system
g. fiber
g. globulin
g. hydroxybutyrate and amphetamine
g. irradiation
g. knife
G. knife instrument
g. knife radiosurgery (GKRS)
g. loop
G. Maxicamera
g. motoneuron
g. motor neuron
g. motor system
g. ray
g. rhythm
g. rigidity
g. secretase
g. thalamotomy
g. wave
gamma-acetylenic-GABA
gamma-aminobutyric
g.-a. acid (GABA)
g.-a. acid concentrate
g.-a. acid type A (GABA-A)
gamma-aminolevulinic
g.-a. acid
g.-a. acid dehydratase activity
gamma-glutamyl transferase
gamma-glutamyl transpeptidase
gamma-interferon treatment
gamma-linolenic acid
gamma-vinyl-GABA
gammopathy
benign monoclonal g.
IgM monoclonal g.
monoclonal g.
GAN
giant axonal neuropathy gene
ganaxolone
ganciclovir
GAN gene
ganglia (*pl. of* ganglion)

ganglial
gangliated nerve
gangliectomy
gangliform
ganglii
capsula g.
stroma g.
gangliitis
gangliocyte
gangliocytoma
dysplastic g.
sellar g.
ganglioformis
intumescentia g.
ganglioglioma
dermatoplastic infantile g.
desmoplastic infantile g.
infantile g.
ganglioglioneurocytoma
ganglioglioneuroma
gangliolysis
percutaneous radiofrequency g.
ganglioma
intracerebral g.
ganglion, pl. **ganglia**
aberrant g.
acousticofacial g.
Andersch g.
aorticorenal g.
ganglia aorticorenalia
Arnold g.
auditory g.
Auerbach g.
auricular g.
autonomic g.
g. of autonomic plexus
basal g.
Bezold g.
Blandin g.
Bochdalek g.
Bock g.
Böttcher g.
branch of internal carotid artery to trigeminal g.
branch of oculomotor nerve to ciliary g.
calcification of basal g.
g. capsule
cardiac g.
ganglia cardiaca
carotid g.
celiac g.
ganglia celiaca
g. cell
g. cell of dorsal spinal root
g. cell of retina
g. cervicale inferius
g. cervicale medium
g. cervicale superius
cervicothoracic g.
g. cervicothoracicum
g. ciliare
ciliary g.
Cloquet g.
coccygeal g.
cochlear g.
g. cochleare
ganglia coeliaca
communicating branch of nasociliary nerve with ciliary g.
Corti g.
cranial autonomic ganglia
ganglia craniospinalia sensoria
craniospinal sensory g.
dorsal root g. (DRG)
Ehrenritter g.
extracranial g.
g. extracraniale
g. of facial nerve
Frankenhäuser g.
Froriep g.
gasserian g.
geniculate g. (GG)
g. geniculatum nervi facialis
g. geniculi
g. geniculi nervi facialis
glossopharyngeal nerve jugular g.
glossopharyngeal nerve lower g.
glossopharyngeal nerve rostral g.
Gudden g.
g. habenula
g. hook
hypogastric g.
g. impar
inferior cervical g.
inferior mesenteric g.
inferior petrosal g.
g. inferius nervi glossopharyngei
g. inferius nervi vagus
inhibitory g.
intercrural g.
ganglia intermedia
intermediate g.
g. of intermediate nerve

G

NOTES

ganglion *(continued)*
interpeduncular g.
intervertebral g.
intracranial g.
g. isthmus
jugular g.
Laumonier g.
Lee g.
lenticular g.
Lobstein g.
long root of ciliary g.
Ludwig g.
ganglia lumbalia
lumbar g.
marbled appearance of basal g.
Meckel lesser g.
Meissner g.
g. mesentericum inferius
g. mesentericum superius
middle cervical g.
motor root of ciliary g.
Müller g.
nasal g.
nerve g.
neural g.
g. nevi splanchnici
nodose g.
oculomotor root of ciliary g.
otic g.
g. oticum
parasympathetic root of ciliary g.
parasympathetic root of otic g.
parasympathetic root of pterygopalatine g.
parasympathetic root of sublingual g.
parasympathetic root of submandibular g.
paravertebral g.
pelvic g.
ganglia pelvica
ganglia pelvina
petrosal g.
petrous g.
phrenic g.
ganglia phrenica
ganglia plexuum autonomicorum
ganglia plexuum visceralium
posterior root g.
prevertebral g.
pterygopalatine g.
g. pterygopalatinum
radiocapitellar joint g.
Remak g.
renal g.
ganglia renalia
Ribes g.
root of otic g.
g. rostralis nervi glossopharyngei
g. rostralis nervi vagus
sacral g.
ganglia sacralia
Scarpa g.
Schacher g.
semilunar g.
g. sensorium nervi cranialis
g. sensorium nervi spinalis
sensory root of ciliary g.
sensory root of otic g.
sensory root of submandibular g.
short root of ciliary g.
Soemmerring g.
solar g.
sphenomaxillary g.
sphenopalatine g.
spiral cochlear g.
g. spirale cochlea
splanchnic g.
stellate g.
g. stellatum
sublingual g.
g. sublinguale
submandibular g.
g. submandibulare
submaxillary g.
superior cervical g. (SCG)
superior mesenteric g.
g. superius nervi glossopharyngei
g. superius nervi vagus
suprarenal g.
sympathetic g.
ganglia of sympathetic trunk
g. of sympathetic trunk
g. sympatheticum
g. sympathicum
terminal g.
g. terminale
ganglia thoracica
thoracic splanchnic g.
g. thoracicum splanchnicum
trigeminal g.
g. trigeminale
ganglia trunci sympathici
g. of trunk of vagus
tympanic g.
g. tympanicum
vagus nerve jugular g.
vagus nerve rostral g.
Valentin tympanic g.
ventricular g.
vertebral g.
g. vertebrale
vestibular g.
g. vestibulare
Vieussens g.
g. viscerale
visceral plexus g.

Walther g.
Wrisberg g.
ganglionaris
lamina pyramidalis g.
ganglionated
ganglionectomy
Meckel sphenopalatine g.
sphenopalatine g.
superior cervical g.
ganglioneuritis
ganglioneuroblastoma
ganglioneurocytoma
ganglioneurofibroma
ganglioneuroma
central g.
dumbbell g.
ganglioneuromatosis
ganglionic
g. blocking agent
g. cell layer of retina
g. crest
g. cyst in synovial tendon sheath
g. glioma
g. layer
g. layer of cerebellar cortex
g. layer of cerebral cortex
g. layer of optic nerve
g. motor neuron
g. stratum of optic nerve
ganglionicum
stratum g.
stroma g.
ganglionitis
gasserian g.
ganglionostomy
ganglioplegic
gangliosialidosis
ganglioside
disialyl g.
g. epitope
GM1 g.
g. lipidosis
g. monosialic acid
gangliosidosis
generalized g.
GM2 g.
infantile GM2 g.
type 1 GM1 g.
gangliosympathectomy
gangrene
trophic g.
Ganser
basal nucleus of G.
G. commissure
nucleus basalis of G.
gantry rotation
Gantzer muscle
gap
air-bone g.
g. junction
g. paradigm
treatment g.
widened interspinous g.
Garcin syndrome
Gardner
G. angle
G. headholder
G. meningocele repair
G. neurosurgical skull clamp
G. operation
G. and Robertson classification system
G. syndrome
Gardner-Robertson
G.-R. class
G.-R. hearing grade
Gardner-Wells
G.-W. headrest
G.-W. tongs
Garrett orientation line
gas
arterial blood g. (ABG)
g. chromatography mass spectrometry
Ga scintigraphy
Gaskell nerve
gasping
g. for breath
inspiratory g.
gasserian
g. ganglion
g. ganglion area
g. ganglionitis
g. ganglion neuroma
Gass syndrome
gastric
g. bypass surgery
g. coronary plexus
g. crisis
g. function
g. nerve
g. neurasthenia

NOTES

G

gastric *(continued)*
g. tetany
g. vertigo
gastrica
tetania g.
gastrici
plexus g.
gastrocolic reflex
gastroenteritis
gastroepiploic plexus
Gastrografin
gastroileac reflex
gastrointestinal
g. bleeding
g. secretion
g. side effect
g. symptom grouping
gastrulation
gate
g. control hypothesis
g. control theory
g. control theory of pain
gating
cardiac g.
g. mechanism
sensory g.
Gaucher disease
gauge
Durkan CTS g.
Padgett baseline pinch g.
pressure g.
strain g.
gauntlet anesthesia
gaussian noise
gaze
blank g.
cardinal direction of g.
conjugate fixed g.
conjugate horizontal g.
consensual g.
contralateral conjugate g.
g. deficit
down g.
dysconjugate g.
dysjunctive g.
eye-to-eye g.
field of g.
fixed g.
following g.
horizontal g.
g. impairment
ipsilateral tonic conjugate g.
lateral g.
g. palsy
g. paralysis
g. paresis
periodic alternating g.
ping-pong g.
g. pontine center
g. preference
g. refixational shift
restriction of inward g.
vertical g.
gaze-coordinating aggregate
gaze-evoked
g.-e. amaurosis
g.-e. blindness
g.-e. nystagmus
g.-e. visual loss
gaze-paretic nystagmus
gB
glycoprotein B
GBM
glioblastoma multiforme
GCA
giant cell arteritis
gCBF
global cerebral blood flow
GCS
Glasgow Coma Score
GDC
giant dopamine-containing cell
Guglielmi detachable coil
GDC SynerG detachment device
GDD
global developmental delay
Gd-DTPA
gadolinium diethylenetriamine pentaacetic acid
Gd-DTPA-enhanced cranial MR imaging
Gd-MRA
gadolinium-enhanced MR angiography
GDNF
glial-derived neurotrophic factor
GDS
Global Deterioration Scale
GE
General Electric
GE 9800 CT system
GE Maxicamera gamma camera
GE Signa scanning
GE Vector scanning
gearshift probe
GEFS+
generalized epilepsy with febrile seizures plus
Geigel reflex
gel
diazepam rectal g.
H.P. Acthar G.
gelastic
g. epilepsy
g. seizure
gelatin
g. foam
g. phantom
g. sponge

gelatinosa
substantia g.
gelatinosus
nucleus g.
gelatinous
g. hematoma
g. nucleus
g. substance
g. substance of posterior horn of spinal cord
Gelfoam
fibrin glue-soaked G.
G. pad
papaverine-soaked G.
G. pledget
G. powder embolus
thrombin-soaked G.
Gélineau syndrome
Gellman instrumentation
gelotripsy
Gelpi retractor
Gelusil
gemästete cell
gemistocyte
gemistocytic
g. astrocyte
g. astrocytoma
g. cell
g. reaction
gemistocytoma
gemma gustatoria
Gemnisyn
Gemonil
gender-specific analysis
gene
achaete-scute g.
alpha-synuclein g.
amyloid precursor protein g.
ataxia g.
bcl-2 g.
Bcl-xL g.
canarc-1 g.
candidate g.
catechol-*O*-methyltransferase g.
CCM1 g.
CCM2 g.
CCM3 g.
CDK2NA g.
ceruloplasmin g.
c-fos g.
CHRNA4 g.
CHRNA7 g.
c-jun g.
CLN1 g.
CLN2 g.
CLN3 g.
CLN5 g.
CLN8 g.
cnot g.
g. code
connexin g.
g. conservation in patterning
cytotoxin-associated g. A (CagA)
dab1 g.
DAT g.
DCX g.
delta g.
deoxyguanosine kinase g.
DMD g.
doublecortin g.
DRD2 g.
DYT1 g.
EGR2 g.
elastin g.
En g.
engrailed g.
epidermal growth factor receptor g.
epilepsy g.
EPM2A g.
epsilon-sarcoglycan g.
ERG2 g.
ETHE1 g.
ETM1 g.
ETM2 g.
g. families in patterning
FGFR3 g.
filamin 1 g.
FilaminA g. (*FLNA*)
fork head g.
fukutin g.
GAN g.
giant axonal neuropathy g. (*GAN*)
gooseberry g.
gox g.
GRIK1 g.
growth arrest-specific g.
gsc g.
hepatic apoprotein g.
homeodomain g.
homologous g.
housekeeping g.
Hox g.
human doublecortin g.
immediate early g.

G

NOTES

gene *(continued)*
inverse polymerase chain reaction-based detection of frataxin g.
ion-channel g.
IT-15 g.
kallikrein g.
KCNQ2 g.
KCNQ3 g.
KIAA g.
krox g.
lamin a/c g. (*LMNA*)
leucine zipper g.
LIM g.
LIM-kinase g.
LIS1 g.
low-penetrance/high-frequency g.
LRRK2 g.
math g.
MDM2 g.
MeCP2 g.
MGC4607 g.
MLC1 g.
myotonic dystrophy g.
neuropeptide g.
NF-1 g.
NF-2 g.
nkx g.
noggin g.
notch g.
null g.
numb g.
organizer g.
otx g.
p53 g.
paired g.
parkin g.
patched g.
pax g.
phosphate-regulating g.
pigment g.
pigmentation-related g.
pitx g.
PMP-22 g.
PnP g.
polypeptide hormone g.
polyQ g.
potassium channel g.
prion protein g.
g. product
ptc g.
rapsyn g.
reelin g.
regulator g.
reln g.
retinoblastoma g.
SCA g.
SCN1B g.
seipin g.
shh g.
sialidase g.
slug g.
SMN g.
sporadic fatal insomnia prion protein g.
structural g.
suppressor g.
survival motor neuron g.
g. synergy
tau g.
TCOF1 g.
g. therapy
g. therapy delivery
g. therapy vector
thymidine kinase g. (TK2)
TOAD-64 g.
triple A syndrome g.
TSC1 g.
TSC2 g.
tumor suppressor g.
UBE3A g.
ubiquitin-ligase g.
unc-33 g.
wingless g.
wnt g.
zic g.
zinc-finger g.

GenePD study

genera (*pl. of* genus)

general
G. Ability Measure for Adults (GAMA)
g. cognitive status
G. Electric (GE)
G. Electric CT 9800 scanner
G. Electric Hi-Speed Advantage helical scanner
G. Electric Hi-Speed Spiral CT Scanner
G. Electric Signa 1.5-Tesla magnetic resonance scanner
g. endotracheal anesthesia
g. knowledge score
g. medical impairment
g. memory index
g. mood state
g. orotracheal anesthesia
g. paresis
g. paresis of insane
g. sensation
g. somatic afferent (GSA)
g. somatic afferent column
g. somatic efferent column
g. temporal processing deficit
g. verbal intellectual functioning
g. visceral afferent (GVA)
g. visceral afferent column
g. visceral efferent column

generalized
g. amnesia
g. anxiety disorder (GAD)
g. atypical absence seizure
g. auditory agnosia
g. convulsive status epilepticus
g. dystonia
g. epilepsy plus febrile seizure
g. epilepsy with febrile seizures plus (GEFS+)
g. gangliosidosis
g. headache
g. myasthenia gravis
g. myokymia
g. paralysis
g. periodic sharp wave
g. polyneuropathy
g. slowing
g. tetanus
g. tonic-clonic (GTC)
g. tonic-clonic convulsion
g. tonic-clonic epilepsy
g. tonic-clonic seizure (GTCS)

generation
g. of affect
lesion g.
mitochondrial free radical g.
pericyte edema g.
slow-wave g.
word g.

generator
alpha rhythm g.
distal stimulation g.
Force 2 CEM g.
high-frequency g.
implantable pulse g.
Itrel pulse g.
Medtronic 3470 pulse g.
model 100 pulse g.
model 101 pulse g.
Neuro N-50 lesion g.
pain g.
pattern g.
g. potential
programmable pulse g.
pulse g.
radiofrequency g.
Radionics RF lesion g.

generic negative symptom

genetic
g. alteration
g. alternation
g. basis
biochemical g.'s
g. component
g. difference
g. disorder
g. effect
g. epistemology
g. factor
g.'s of headache
g. heterogeneity
g. link
g. linkage analysis
g. locus
g. mapping
molecular g.'s
g. mutation
g. predisposition
g. programming
g. relationship
reverse g.'s
g. risk factor
g. screening
g. strategy
g. susceptibility
g. testing
g. tool
g. transmission
g. typing
g. variation
g. viewpoint

genic
g. balance
g. drift

genicula (*pl. of* geniculum)

geniculate
g. body
g. ganglion (GG)
g. herpes
g. neuralgia
g. nucleus
g. otalgia

geniculati
nucleus medialis magnocellularis corporis g.

geniculatus lateralis nucleus

geniculi
ganglion g.
gyrus g.

geniculocalcarine
g. radiation
g. tract

geniculocalvarium

NOTES

geniculocortical pathway
geniculostriate
g. fiber
g. pathway
g. tract
geniculum, pl. **genicula**
g. of facial nerve
g. nervi facialis
g. nervus facialis
genioglossus
g. advancement
g. advancement-hyoid myotomy
g. advancement procedure
g. muscle
geniohyoid muscle
genioplasty
genital
g. center
g. corpuscle
g. function
g. response
g. ulceration
genitale
corpusculum g.
genitofemoralis
ramus femoralis nervi g.
ramus genitalis nervi g.
genitofemoral nerve
genitospinal center
Gennari
G. band
line of G.
G. line
G. stria
stripe of G.
genome
herpes simplex virus g.
g. hybridization
genome-wide admixture scan
genomic
g. alteration
g. DNA
g. effect
g. event
g. imprinting
g. mechanism
genotype
ApoE g.
apolipoprotein E g.
Asp/Asp g.
e4/e4 g.
tryptophan hydroxylase allelic g.
genotypic
genotyping
gentamicin
intratympanic g.
genu, pl. **genua**
branch to internal capsule, g.
g. capsulae internae
g. corporis callosi
g. of corpus callosum
facial g.
g. of facial nerve
g. of internal capsule
g. nervi facialis
genus, pl. **genera**
Geodon
Gerald forceps
Gerbode-Burford rib spreader
Gerhardt disease
Gerhardt-Semon law
geriatric
g. depression
G. Depression Scale
g. neurology
g. rehabilitation
Gerlier disease
germ
g. cell tumor
g. cell tumor with synchronous lesions in pineal and suprasellar regions
German chamomile
germinal
g. matrix
g. matrix hemorrhage
germinoma
pineal g.
pure g.
tectal g.
germline mosaicism
geromorphism
Gerson therapy
Gerstmann-Sträussler-Scheinker
G.-S.-S. disease
G.-S.-S. syndrome
Gerstmann-Sträussler syndrome
Gerstmann syndrome
Geschwind syndrome
Gesell Developmental Scale
gestational polyneuropathy
gestural
g. automatism
g. element
gesture
g. communication
limb transitive g.
GFAP
glial fibrillary acidic protein
GFAP fiber density
GFAP gene activation
GFAP-stained process
GFP
global field power
GG
geniculate ganglion
Ghajar guide
ghost image

GHRH
growth hormone-releasing hormone
GHRIF
growth hormone-release inhibiting factor
Giacomini
band of G.
frenulum of G.
uncus band of G.
giant
g. axon
g. axonal neuropathy
g. axonal neuropathy gene (*GAN*)
g. basilar aneurysm
g. cell arteritis (GCA)
g. cell astrocytoma
g. cell glioblastoma
g. cell glioblastoma multiforme
g. cell granuloma
g. cell granulomatous hypophysitis
g. cell monstrocellular sarcoma of Zülch
g. cell tumor
g. cervical carotid artery aneurysm
g. dopamine-containing cell (GDC)
g. glomus tumor
g. intracranial aneurysm
g. motor unit action potential
g. neuron
g. petroclival hemangiopericytoma
g. pituitary adenoma
g. pituitary tumor
g. pyramidal Betz cell
g. saccular aneurysm
g. sacral perineural cyst
g. tortuous basilar artery
g. urticaria
Gianturco-Roubin II stent
gibberish aphasia
Gibbs
G. artifact
G. phenomenon
G. ring
giddy headache
Giemsa banding
Gierke
G. cell
G. respiratory bundle
Gifford reflex
gigans
urticaria g.
gigantea
urticaria g.
gigantism
cerebral g.
gigantocellular
g. glioma
g. nucleus of medulla oblongata
gigantocellularis
nucleus reticularis intermedius g.
Gigli
G. guide
G. saw
Gill
G. laminectomy
G. procedure
G. Thomas locator
Gilles
G. de la Tourette
G. de la Tourette disease
G. de la Tourette syndrome
Gilliatt-Sumner hand
Gill-Thomas-Cosman frame
ginger paralysis
gingival
g. fibroma
g. hyperplasia
gingko biloba
girdle
Ace halo pelvic g.
g. anesthesia
Hitzig g.
g. pain
g. sensation
Girdlestone laminectomy
girdle-type pain distribution
githagism
gitter cell, gitterzelle
GKRS
gamma knife radiosurgery
glabella
glabella-inion
g.-i. line
g.-i. line landmark
glabellar
g. approach
g. exposure osteotomy
g. reflex
g. tap
glabrous skin
gland
adrenal g.
apocrine g.
Bartholin g.
basal g.

NOTES

gland *(continued)*
eccrine g.
ectopic pituitary g.
endocrine g.
hemal g.
lacrimal g.
master g.
neural lobe of pituitary g.
pacchionian g.
parathyroid g.
pineal g.
pituitary g.
posterior lobe of pituitary g.
salivary g.
thyroid g.
von Ebner g.
glandula, pl. **glandulae**
g. basilaris
g. pinealis
g. pituitaria
glandular lobe of hypophysis
Glanzmann disease
Glaser automatic laminectomy retractor
Glasflex material
Glasgow
G. Assessment Schedule
G. Coma Score (GCS)
G. Outcome Scale
G. Outcome Score (GOS)
Glasscock triangle
glassy eye
glatiramer
g. acetate
g. copolymer-1
glaucoma
chronic angle-closure g.
low-tension g.
subacute angle-closure g.
glaucus
Aspergillus g.
Glees
method of G.
Gleevec
glia
fibrillary g.
g. limitans
g. limitans externa
radial g.
g. scar
gliacyte
Gliadel
G. implant
G. wafer
G. wafer treatment protocol
gliae
membrana limitans g.
glial
g. cell
g. cell line-derived
g. cell line-derived neurotrophic factor
g. cell maturation
g. cytoplasmic inclusion
g. disease
g. fibrillary acidic protein (GFAP)
g. fibrillary acidic protein activation
g. filament
g. limiting membrane
g. line-derived neurotrophic factor
g. metabolism
g. neuronal interaction
g. nodule
g. parenchymal cyst
g. reaction
g. scarring
g. tumor
g. tumorigenesis
glial-derived neurotrophic factor (GDNF)
glial-specific marker
GliaSite radiation therapy system
gliding contusion
glioblast
glioblastoma
cerebral g.
giant cell g.
g. multiforme (GBM)
occipital g.
g. xenograft
glioblastosis cerebri
gliocyte
gliocytoma
gliofibrillary
glioma
anaplastic mixed g.
g. angiogenesis
36B10 g. cell
biologically quiescent g.
brainstem g.
butterfly-type g.
cerebral g.
g. chemotherapy
chiasmatic g.
childhood optic g.
diencephalic g.
diffuse pontine g.
dorsal midbrain g.
endothelial cell-stimulating g.
exophytic brainstem g.
familial g.
ganglionic g.
gigantocellular g.
high-grade g.
hypothalamic g.
hypothalamic/chiasmatic g.
intracranial g.
low-grade g. (LGG)

malignant g.
medullary g.
mixed g.
multifocal g.
nasal g.
nonaplastic g.
optic g.
g. of optic chiasm
optic nerve g.
optic pathway g.
pediatric brainstem g.
periaqueductal g.
peripheral g.
pontine g.
radiation-induced g.
rolandoparietal g.
spinal cord g.
g. of spinal cord
subependymal mixed g.
supratentorial g.
tectal g.
tegmental g.
telangiectatic g.
g. telangiectodes
thalamic g.
uncommon g.

glioma-polyposis syndrome

gliomatosis

arachnoidal g.
g. cerebri
leptomeningeal g.
meningeal g.

gliomatous

gliomyxoma

glioneuroma

glioneuronal element

gliophagia

gliopil

gliosarcoma

cerebellar g.

gliosis

g. of aqueduct
aqueductal g.
astrocytic g.
Chaslin g.
diffuse g.
hemispheric g.
hemosiderin reactional g.
hypertrophic nodular g.
isomorphous g.
perivascular g.
piloid g.
progressive subcortical g.
reactive g.
unilateral g.

gliosome

gliotic white matter

glistening degeneration

glitter cell

global

g. AIMS score
g. amnesia
g. amnestic disorder
g. ANOVA
g. anterograde memory disorder
g. aphasia
g. assessment of sensory disturbance
g. brain lactate
G. Burden of Disease Study
g. cerebral blood flow (gCBF)
g. cerebral ischemia
g. change
g. clinical impression score
g. clinician-rated scale
g. cognitive decline
g. cognitive dysfunction
g. cognitive impairment
g. dementia
g. dementia rating scale
G. Deterioration Scale (GDS)
g. developmental delay (GDD)
g. distress index
g. field power (GFP)
g. function
g. functioning
g. gene replacement therapy
g. ischemic neuronal injury
g. measure
g. measure of impairment
g. metabolism
g. outcome
g. paralysis
G. Tic Rating Score
G. Utilization of Streptokinase and t-PA for Occluded Coronary Arteries (GUSTO-1)
g. well-being

globi (*pl. of* globus)

globoid

g. cell
g. cell leukodystrophy

NOTES

globose
g. cell
g. nucleus
globosus
nucleus g.
globule
Marchi g.
globulin
alpha-2 g.
gamma g.
homologous tetanus immune g. (HTIG)
human tetanus immune g.
intravenous gamma g.
intravenous immune g.
sex hormone-binding g. (SHBG)
testosterone-estradiol-binding g.
zoster immune g.
globus, pl. **globi**
g. epilepticus
g. hystericus
g. pallidus
g. pallidus externa
g. pallidus external segment
g. pallidus interna
g. pallidus internal segment
g. pallidus internus (GPi)
g. pallidus lateralis
g. pallidus medialis
glome
glomectomy
glomera (*pl. of* glomus)
glomerular layer of olfactory bulb
glomerule
glomerulus, pl. **glomeruli**
nonencapsulated nerve g.
olfactory g.
stereoselective g.
synaptic g.
glomus, pl. **glomera**
g. aorticum
g. arteriovenous malformation
g. body
choroid g.
g. choroideum
intravagal g.
g. intravagale
jugular g.
g. jugulare
g. jugulare tumor
g. jugulotympanicum
g. pulmonale
pulmonary g.
g. tympanicum
g. vagale
g. vagale tumor
glossectomy
reduction g.
glossokinesthetic, glossocinesthetic
g. center
glossokinetic
g. artifact
g. potential
glossolabiolaryngeal paralysis
glossolabiopharyngeal paralysis
glossolysis
glossopalatolabial paralysis
glossopharyngeal
g. cranial nerve [CN IX]
g. nerve examination
g. nerve jugular ganglion
g. nerve lower ganglion
g. nerve paralysis
g. nerve rootlet
g. nerve rostral ganglion
g. neuralgia (GPN)
g. neuropathy
g. tic
glossopharyngei
ganglion inferius nervi g.
ganglion rostralis nervi g.
ganglion superius nervi g.
nucleus nervi g.
rami linguales nervi g.
rami pharyngeal nervi g.
rami tonsillares nervi g.
ramus musculi stylopharyngei nervi g.
ramus sinus carotici nervi g.
glossopharyngeo
ramus communicans cum nervo g.
ramus communicans nervi facialis cum nervo g.
ramus communicans nervi vagi cum nervo g.
glossopharyngeolabial paralysis
glossopharyngeus
nervus g. [CN IX]
glossoplegia
glossospasm
glossotomy
labiomandibular g.
glossy skin
glottis
glove
g. anesthesia
Biogel Sensor surgical g.
mesh g.
glubionate
calcium g.
glucagon
gluceptate
calcium g.
technetium-99m g.
gluciphore
glucocerebrosidase

glucocorticoid
hypothalamic g.
glucocorticoid-induced
g.-i. bone loss
g.-i. osteoporosis
glucogenesis
glucomineralocorticoid
gluconate
calcium g.
chlorhexidine g.
magnesium g.
potassium chloride and potassium g.
potassium citrate and potassium g.
gluconeogenesis
glucophore
glucose
g. blood level
cerebral metabolic rate of g. (CMRglc)
cerebrospinal fluid g.
g. concentration
g. homeostasis disorder
g. hypermetabolism
g. metabolism
g. metabolism in brain
preischemic blood g.
g. tolerance
g. transport
g. transporter molecule
glucose-6-phosphate transport system
glucose-6-phosphatase
glucosephosphate isomerase
glucose transporter 1 (GLUT 1)
glucosidase
glucosylsphingosine accumulation
glucuroconjugation
glucuronic acid
glucuronidase
beta g.
g. deficiency
glucuronidation
glucuronide
glue
acrylic g.
autologous fibrin sealant g.
cyanoacrylate g.
fibrin g.
Histoacryl g.
Gluge corpuscle
GluR1
glutamate receptor 1
Glu-receptor antagonist
GLUT 1
glucose transporter 1
glutamate
g. decarboxylase
g. excitation
g. excitotoxicity
g. metabolism
metabotropic g.
monosodium g.
g. neurotoxicity
g. plus glutamine
g. receptor 1 (GluR1)
g. receptor antagonist
g. receptor-mediated neurodegeneration
g. receptor subtype
g. toxicity
g. transporter
g. transport velocity
glutamate-containing neuron
glutamate-mediated excitatory synaptic transmission
glutamatergic
g. excitotoxicity
g. hypoactivity
g. neuron
g. neurotransmission
g. pathway
g. response
g. synaptic transmission
glutamic acid decarboxylase
glutamide receptor subunit
glutamine
g. decarboxylase (GAD)
glutamate plus g.
glutamyl
g. cysteine synthetase deficiency
g. ribose-5-phosphate storage disease
g. transaminase
glutaraldehyde
glutaric
g. acid
g. aciduria type I-III
glutaryl-CoA dehydrogenase
glutathione (GSH)
g. peroxidase
g. persuades (GSHPx)
g. synthetase
g. synthetase deficiency

G

NOTES

gluteal
g. gait
g. nerve
g. reflex
gluten
g. ataxia
g. sensitivity
gluten-free diet
glutethimide group
gluteus
g. maximus gait
g. medius gait
glycan
O-linked g.
glycerol
g. chemoneurolysis
g. kinase deficiency
g. rhizotomy
g. test
glyceryl trinitrate
glycinate
aluminum g.
glycine
g. encephalopathy
ketotic g.
nonketotic g.
g. supplementation
glycoconjugate
cross-reacting nerve g.
glycogen
g. debrancher deficiency
g. storage disease
glycogen-derived pyruvate
glycogenosis (type I–VII)
glycogeusia
glycolipid
glycolysis
glycoprotein
g. B (gB)
carbohydrate-deficient g.
g. degradation disorder
integral membrane g.
membrane-bound g.
myelin-associated g. (MAG)
myelin oligodendrocyte g. (MOG)
myelin/oligodendrocyte g.
p170 g.
platelet g. IIb/IIIa
g. storage disorder
variant surface g. (VSG)
glycoproteinosis
glycoprotein-secreting adenoma
glycopyrrolate
glycorrhachia
glycosaminoglycan (GAG)
glycoside
cardiac g.
glycosphingolipid metabolic defect
glycosuria
familial g.
glycosylase
glycosylation pattern
glycyl
GM2 gangliosidosis
GM-CSF
granulocyte-macrophage colony-stimulating factor
GMFM
Gross Motor Function Measure
GM1 ganglioside
gnathic index
gnathostomiasis
gnosia
GnRH
gonadotropin-releasing hormone
Godtfredsen syndrome
Goebel syndrome
Golay gradient coil
gold
7C G. test
g. intoxication
g. peripheral neuropathy
g. weight implant
Golda reflex
Goldberg-Shprintzen syndrome
Goldenhar-Gorlin syndrome
Goldenhar syndrome
Goldflam disease
Goldflam-Erb disease
Goldman
G. constant field equation
G. perimetry
Goldmann visual field
Goldscheider test
Goldstein
G. spinal fusion
G. toe sign
Goldthwait sign
golf-stick dissector
Golgi
G. body
G. corpuscle
G. epithelial cell
G. reflex
G. side fibril
G. staining
G. system
G. tendon organ (GTO)
G. theory
G. type I, II neuron
vesiculation of the G.
Golgi-Mazzoni corpuscle
Goliath syndrome
Goll
G. column
G. column nucleus
G. fiber

nucleus of G.
tract of G.
Gombault
G. degeneration
G. neuritis
G. triangle
Gombault-Philippe triangle
Gomori
G. trichrome
G. trichrome stain
gonadotroph cell
gonadotropin
beta human chorionic g.
beta subunit of human chorionic g. (beta HCG)
chorionic g.
human chorionic g. (hCG)
gonadotropin-producing adenoma
gonadotropin-releasing hormone (GnRH, GRH)
gondii
Toxoplasma g.
gonioscopy
gonyalgia paresthetica
GoodKnight 420G Nasal CPAP System
Goody's Body Pain
gooseberry gene
gooseneck rongeur
Gordon
G. criteria
G. Diagnostic System
G. reflex
G. sign
G. and Sweet silver reticulin stain
G. symptom
Gore method
Gorlin
G. sign
G. syndrome
GOS
Glasgow Outcome Score
Gosling
G. pulsatility
G. pulsatility index
Gottfries-Brane-Steen Rating Scale for Dementia
Gottron sign
gouge
AO g.
Flanagan spinal fusion g.
Hibbs spinal fusion g.
Hoen lamina g.
Killian g.
spinal fusion g.
gout
tophaceous g.
gouty arthritis
Gowers
G. bundle
G. bundle in cerebellum
G. column
G. disease
G. fasciculus
G. maneuver
G. muscular dystrophy
G. phenomenon
G. sign
G. syndrome
G. tract
gown restriction
gox gene
GPCR
G-protein-coupled receptor
GPi
globus pallidus internus
GPN
glossopharyngeal neuralgia
G protein
G-protein
G-p. abnormality
G-p. coupling
G-protein-coupled receptor (GPCR)
gracile
g. fasciculus
g. fasciculus of medulla oblongata
g. fasciculus of spinal cord
g. lobule
g. nucleus
g. spinal fiber
g. tubercle
tuberculum g.
gracilis
fasciculus g.
funiculus g.
lobulus g.
nucleus fasciculi g.
nucleus funiculi g.
tubercle of nucleus g.
tuberculum nuclei g.
gracilispinales
fibrae g.
grade
Fischer g.
Gardner-Robertson hearing g.

NOTES

grade *(continued)*
Hughes disability g.
Hunt and Hess g. I–III
g. I–IV astrocytoma
g. I–IV spondylolisthesis
MRI g.
Simpson g.
Spetzler-Martin g.
Gradenigo syndrome
gradient
g. amplifier
bipolar g.
g. coil
g. compensation
g. echo (GRE)
g. echo imaging
g. echo MRI
field g.
frequency-encoding g.
magnetic field g.
g. magnetic field
g. moment
g. moment nulling
net electrochemical potential g.
phase-encoding g.
pulsed g.
readout g.
rephasing g.
rewinder g.
Ribot g.
slice-select encoding g.
g. slope
steep-dose g.
transmantle pressure g.
x g.
y g.
gradient-echo
g.-e. MR image
g.-e. MR imaging
gradient-echo echo planar image
gradient-echo magnetic resonance image
gradient-recalled
g.-r. acquisition in steady state (GRASS)
g.-r. echo
g.-r. echo image
g.-r. echo technique
gradient-refocused
g.-r. imaging
g.-r. sequence
grading
De Monte g.
Fisher g.
Hirsch g.
Kernohan g.
NPH g.
Simpson g.
tumor g.
gradiometer
axial g.
Graefe
G. disease
G. sign
G. spot
graft
acellular human dermal g.
adipose g.
adrenal medulla g.
aortobifemoral bypass g.
autochthonous g.
autogenous bone g.
autologous fat g.
barrel staved g.
bone g.
bovine pericardium for dural g.
bypass g.
cable nerve g.
carotid-vertebral vein bypass g.
clip g.
g. collapse
cranial bone g.
cross-face g.
dural g.
fascicular g.
fat-patch g.
funicular g.
greater auricular nerve g.
Hemashield enhanced g.
human dural substitute g.
hydroxyapatite g.
iliac bone g.
interbody g.
interfascicular g.
intracranial-extracranial nerve g.
intracranial-intratemporal nerve g.
Keystone g.
g. material alternative
g. migration
nerve g.
onlay dural g.
petrous carotid-to-intradural carotid saphenous vein g.
posterior bone g.
posterolateral bone g.
radial artery g.
rib g.
roof-patch g.
saphenous vein bypass g.
saphenous vein patch g.
g. site
in situ tricortical iliac crest block bone g.
skull bone g.
sleeve g.
split calvarial g.
split-thickness calvarial g.
strut g.

sural nerve bridge g.
sural nerve cable g.
sutureless onlay g.
Teflon tube g.
temporosuboccipital bone g.
tricortical iliac crest bone g.
Unilab Surgibone bovine bone g.
vascular patch g.
xenogeneic g.

graft-handling characteristic

grafting
allograft bone g.
g. anastomosis
autograft bone g.
bone g.
coronary artery bypass g.
dural g.
fetal mesencephalic g.
fibular g.
hypophysial g.
posterolateral bone g.
strut g.

Grafton demineralized bone matrix

graft-related problem

graft-versus-host disease (GVHD)

gram-negative
g.-n. bacillary meningitis
g.-n. bacillus
g.-n. endotoxin

Gram stain

grand
g. mal
g. mal epilepsy
g. mal seizure

grandmother cell

Granit loop

granular
g. cell myoblastoma
g. cell tumor
g. degeneration
g. ependymitis
g. layer
g. layer of cerebellar cortex
g. layer of cerebellum
g. layer of cerebral cortex
g. layer of retina
g. neuron

granulare
stratum g.

granularis
ependymitis g.

granulation
arachnoid g.
arachnoidal g.
pacchionian g.
g. tissue
Virchow g.

granule
azurophilic g.
Birbeck g.
calcareous g.
g. cell
g. cell axon
g. cell proliferation
chromatic g.
chromophil g.
Crooke g.
lipofuscin g.
meningeal g.
Nissl g.

granulocyte

granulocyte-macrophage colony-stimulating factor (GM-CSF)

granulocytic
g. brain edema
g. sarcoma

granuloma
caseating g.
cerebral cysticercus g.
cholesterol g.
g. cryptococcal
eosinophilic g.
foreign body g.
g. formation
Gagel g.
giant cell g.
intrasellar g.
lethal midline g.
parenchymal g.
petroclival cholesterol g.

granulomatosis
eosinophilic g.
Langerhans cell g.
lymphomatoid g.
Wegener g. (WG)

granulomatous
g. angiitis
g. arteritis
g. encephalitis
g. encephalomyelitis
g. hypophysitis

granulovacuolar degeneration

grapelike lesion

G

NOTES

graphanesthesia
graphesthesia
graphia
lexical g.
graphic
g. aphasia
g. impairment
graphomotor
g. aphasia
g. control
g. skill
graphospasm
Grashey aphasia
grasp
g. channel
g. reflex
grasper
lion's paw g.
grasping reflex
GRASS
gradient-recalled acquisition in steady state
2DFT GRASS
3DFT GRASS
sequential GRASS
Grasset
G. law
G. phenomenon
G. sign
Grasset-Bychowski sign
Grasset-Gaussel-Hoover sign
Grasset-Gaussel phenomenon
Grass stimulator S44
grating
flicker frequency g.
sensorimotor g.
spatial frequency g.
Gratiolet
G. radiating fiber
G. radiation
Graves
G. disease
G. ophthalmopathy
graviceptive
g. brainstem lesion
g. brainstem syndrome
g. pathway
gravidarum
chorea g.
tetania g.
gravior
epilepsia g.
gravireceptor
gravis
adult-onset myasthenia g.
congenital myasthenia g.
generalized myasthenia g.
juvenile myasthenia g.
myasthenia g. (MG)
neonatal myasthenia g.
neurasthenia g.
ocular myasthenia g.
penicillamine-induced myasthenia g.
seronegative myasthenia g.
transient neonatal myasthenia g.
gravitational device
gray (Gy)
g. baby syndrome
central g.
g. column
g. commissure
g. degeneration
dorsal central g.
g. fiber
g. layer of superior colliculus
g. matter
g. matter area
g. matter atrophy
g. matter lactate
g. matter lactate level
g. matter necrosis
g. matter region
g. matter tissue
periaqueductal central g.
periventricular g. (PVG)
g. rami communicantes
g. ramus
g. substance
g. tuber
g. tubercle
G. type I, II synapse
g. wing
gray/white
g./w. matter difference
g./w. matter junction
GRE
gradient echo
great
g. anterior medullary artery
g. cerebral vein
g. cerebral vein of Galen
g. cerebral vein of Galen aneurysm
g. cistern
g. foramen
g. horizontal fissure
g. longitudinal fissure
g. toe reflex
g. transverse fissure of cerebrum
greater
g. auricular nerve graft
g. occipital nerve
g. rhomboid muscle
g. sciatic foramen
g. superficial petrosal nerve (GSPN)
Greenberg
G. retracting system

G. retractor
G. retractor frame
G. retractor set
Greenberg-Sugita
G.-S. retractor
G.-S. retractor grid
Greenberg-type bar
Greenfield
G. classification of spinocerebellar ataxia
G. disease
Greenwood bipolar and suction forceps
Greig
G. cephalopolysyndactyly
G. cephalopolysyndactyly syndrome
Greitz-Bergstrom method
Grenoble stereotactic robot
GRH
gonadotropin-releasing hormone
grid
Greenberg-Sugita retractor g.
subdural g.
Griesinger sign
GRIK1 gene
grimace
facial g.
grimacing
facial g.
grinding
rhythmic teeth g.
teeth g.
tooth g.
grip
milkmaid's g.
pincer g.
syringe g.
grippe aurique
grip-strength test
grisea
commissura anterior g.
commissura posterior g.
griseae
columnae g.
griseofulvin peripheral neuropathy
griseum
indusium g.
groaning
nocturnal g.
Grocott stain
groove
anterior intermediate g.
anterolateral g.
anteromedian g.
arterial g.
frontal g.
meningioma of olfactory g.
neural g.
occipital g.
olfactory g.
parasagittal g.
pontomedullary g.
posterior intermediate g.
posterolateral g.
retroolivary g.
sagittal g.
vascular g.
gross
g. medical error
G. Motor Function Measure (GMFM)
g. pathological feature
g. total resection
ground
g. bundle
g. electrode
group
g. A beta-hemolytic streptococcus
amygdala nucleus g.
g. analysis
AO g.
Brain Tumor Study G. (BTSG)
g. B streptococcus
buzz g.
galenic draining g.
glutethimide g.
neurogenic fiber-type g.
osmophore g.
Parkinson Study G. (PSG)
pedunculopontine cholinergic g.
petrosal draining g.
Pittsburgh gamma knife g.
polyarteritis nodosa g.
primary g.
sapophore g.
Surgical Interbody Research G.
Swedish gamma knife g.
tentorial draining g.
transversospinalis muscle g.
ventral respiratory g.
grouped discharge
grouping
clavus clinical g.
gastrointestinal symptom g.
pseudoneurological symptom g.

G

NOTES

growing skull fracture
growth
g. arrest-specific gene
axonal g.
g. cone
eccentric g.
en plaque g.
g. factor inhibitor
g. fraction
g. hormone deficiency
g. hormone-producing adenoma
g. hormone-release inhibiting factor (GHRIF)
g. hormone-releasing hormone (GHRH)
meningioma g.
neurite g.
olfactory axonal g.
g. plate fracture
g. plate separation
spinal g.
vertebral body g.
growth-associated protein
growth-hormone-secreting adenoma
growth-inhibiting molecule
growth-plate
growth-promoting molecule
Gruber ligament
Gruca-Weiss spring
Grünwald
G. ear forceps
G. neurosurgical rongeur
gryochrome
GSA
general somatic afferent
gsc gene
GSH
glutathione
GSHPx
glutathione persuades
GSNO
nitrosoglutathione
GSPN
greater superficial petrosal nerve
GSR
galvanic skin reflex
galvanic skin resistance
galvanic skin response
GTC
generalized tonic-clonic
GTC convulsion
GTCS
generalized tonic-clonic seizure
GTO
Golgi tendon organ
GTP
guanosine triphosphate
Guamanian ALS
Guam parkinsonism-dementia complex
guanethidine sulfate
guanfacine
guanidine
guanine/cytosine ratio
guanine nucleotide
guanophore
guanosine
g. diphosphate
g. monophosphate
g. triphosphate (GTP)
guanylate cyclase
guanylyl cyclase
guard
depth g.
Midas Rex bur g.
snore g.
UltraPower bur g.
guarded tripole
Gubler
G. hemiplegia
G. line
G. paralysis
G. syndrome
Gudden
G. atrophy
G. commissure
G. ganglion
G. tegmental nucleus
Guglielmi
G. detachable coil (GDC)
G. detachable coil system
guidance
axon g.
Brown-Roberts-Wells computerized tomography stereotactic g.
Cortech g.
electrophysiological g.
fluoroscopic image g.
image g.
real-time g.
StealthStation system real-time g.
stereotactic g.
ultrasonographic g.
guide
Adson dural protector g.
Ad-Tech electrode g.
AO stopped-drill g.
g. catheter
contoured anterior spinal plate drill g.
Cook stereotactic g.
Cushing saw g.
Davis saw g.
drill g.
Frazier dural g.
Ghajar g.
Gigli g.
Hall-Dundar drill g.
hydrophilic g.

medication g.
Navigus trajectory g.
NeuraGen nerve g.
nut alignment g.
stereotactic g.
transpedicular drill g.
Yasargil ligature g.

guideline
oral appliance g.

guidepin, guide pin

guidewire, guide wire
Choice PT g.
delivery g.
J-tipped g.
Platinum Plus g.
Radifocus g.

Guillain-Barré
G.-B. polyneuritis
G.-B. postinfection peripheral neuropathy
G.-B. reflex
G.-B. syndrome

Guillain-Barré-Strohl syndrome

Guillain-Garcin syndrome

Guillain-Mollaret triangle

Guilland sign

Guinon disease

Guiot scheme

Guiot-Talairach construct

Gulf War syndrome

gullwing pattern

gumma
cerebral g.

gun
Omni clip g.

Gunn
Marcus G.
G. phenomenon
G. sign
G. syndrome

gunshot wound

gustation

gustatoria
anosmia g.
gemma g.

gustatorium
organum g.

gustatorius
porus g.

gustatory
g. agnosia
g. anesthesia
g. anomia
g. audition
g. aura
g. bud
g. cell
g. code
g. cortex
g. function
g. hallucination
g. hyperesthesia
g. lemniscus
g. nucleus
g. organ
g. pathway
g. pore
g. receiving area
g. receptor
g. sweating syndrome

gustatory-sudorific reflex

GUSTO-1
Global Utilization of Streptokinase and t-PA for Occluded Coronary Arteries

gustolacrimal reflex

gustometer

gustometry

gustus
organum g.

Guthrie test

gutter fracture

gutturotetany

Guy Neurological Disability Scale

Guyon canal

GVA
general visceral afferent

GVHD
graft-versus-host disease

Gy
gray

gyral
g. atrophy
g. infarction

gyrectomy
frontal g.

gyrencephalic

gyri (*pl. of* gyrus)

gyriform intracranial calcification

gyrochrome cell

gyromagnetic ratio

gyrometer

Gyroscan
Philips G. S5, S15

gyrose

G

NOTES

gyrospasm
gyrus, pl. **gyri**
angular g.
g. angularis
annectent g.
anterior central g.
anterior cingulate g.
anterior paracentral g.
anterior piriform g.
anterior transverse temporal g.
ascending frontal g.
ascending parietal g.
gyri breves insula
Broca g.
callosal g.
central g.
cerebral g.
gyri cerebri
gyri of cerebrum
cingulate g.
g. cinguli
contiguous supramarginal g.
deep transitional g.
dentate g.
g. dentatus
fasciolar g.
g. fasciolaris
first temporal g.
flattening of g.
fornicate g.
g. fornicatus
frontal g.
g. frontalis inferior
g. frontalis medialis
g. frontalis medius
g. frontalis superior
fusiform g.
g. fusiformis
g. geniculi
Heschl g.
hippocampal dentate g.
g. hippocampus
inferior frontal g.
inferior occipital g.
inferior parietal g.
inferior temporal g.
infracalcarine g.
insular g.
interlocking g.
intralimbic g.
isthmus of cingulate g.
lamination of g.
lateral occipitotemporal g.
lateral olfactory g.
layer of dentate g.
lingual g.
g. lingualis
g. longus insula
marginal g.
medial frontal g.
medial occipitotemporal g.
medial olfactory g.
middle frontal g.
middle occipital g.
middle temporal g.
occipital g.
g. occipitotemporalis lateralis
g. occipitotemporalis medialis
g. olfactorius lateralis
g. olfactorius medialis
olfactory g.
gyri orbitales
orbital part of inferior frontal g.
paracentral g.
g. paracentralis
g. paracentralis anterior
g. paracentralis posterior
parahippocampal g.
g. parahippocampalis
paraterminal g.
g. paraterminalis
parietal g.
postcentral g.
g. postcentralis
posterior central g.
posterior cingulate g.
posterior fusiform g.
posterior paracentral g.
posterior transverse temporal g.
precentral g.
g. precentralis
preinsular g.
prepiriform g.
quadrate g.
g. rectus
Retzius g.
short insular g.
splenial g.
straight g.
subcallosal g.
g. subcallosus
subcollateral g.
superior frontal g.
superior occipital g.
superior parietal g.
superior temporal lobe g.
supracallosal g.
supramarginal g.
g. supramarginalis
tail of dentate g.
temporal g.
gyri temporales transversi
g. temporalis inferior
g. temporalis medius
g. temporalis superior
g. temporalis transversalis posterior
g. temporalis transversus anterior

g. temporalis transversus posterior habena
transitional g.
g. transitivi cerebri
transverse temporal g.
Turner marginal g.
uncal g.
uncinate g.
vein of olfactory g.

NOTES

H
H field
H reflex
H response
H wave
H zone
H1 receptor
HAART
highly active antiretroviral therapy
habena, pl. **habenae**
gyrus temporalis transversus posterior h.
habenula, pl. **habenulae**
ganglion h.
nuclei habenulae
nucleus h.
habenulae perforatae
pineal h.
sulcus h.
trigone of h.
trigonum h.
habenular
h. body
h. commissure
h. nucleus
h. sulcus
h. trigone
habenularis
sulcus h.
habenularum
commissura h.
habenulointerpeduncularis
tractus h.
habenulointerpeduncular tract
habenulopeduncularis
tractus h.
habenulopeduncular tract
habit
h. chorea
h. cough
h. reversal training
smoking h.
h. spasm
h. tic
habitual
h. finger movement
h. posture
h. seizure
h. sleep episode
habitus
h. apoplecticus
marfanoid h.
Hachinski
H. ischemic scale
H. ischemic score
Hacker procedure
Haddad syndrome
Haeckel law
Haemophilus
H. aerophilus
H. influenzae
H. influenzae b
H. influenzae type B meningitis
H. parainfluenzae
Haenel symptom
Hageman factor
Hagen-Poiseuille law
Haglund disease
Hague Seizure Severity Scale
Hahn
H. echo
H. sign
Haid universal bone plate system
Haight-Finochietto rib spreader
Haight rib spreader
hair
auditory h.
h. cell
h. follicle
h. follicle receptor
Frey irritation h.
h. lead level
h. loss
olfactory h.
sensory h.
taste h.
von Frey h.
h. whorl pattern
hairline fracture
Hajdu-Cheney syndrome
Hajek
H. chisel
H. laminectomy punch
H. mallet
Hajek-Ballenger
H.-B. dissector
H.-B. septal elevator
Hajek-Koffler
H.-K. bone punch forceps
H.-K. laminectomy rongeur
H.-K. punch
Håkanson technique
Hakim
H. high-pressure valve
H. precision valve
H. programmable valve system
H. syndrome
Hakim-Cordis ventriculoperitoneal shunt
Hakuba
medial triangle of H.

Halcion
Haldol
half-and-half exposure
half base syndrome
half-Fourier imaging
half-life
drug h.-l.
half-NEX imaging
Halifax
H. clamp posterior cervical fixation
H. interlaminar clamp
H. interlaminar clamp system
Hall
H. neurosurgical craniotome
H. Osteon drill system kit
H. Osteon irrigation kit
H. Surgairtome II drill
H. UltraPower drill
H. Versipower drill
Hall-Dundar drill guide
Halle
H. bone curette
H. dura knife
H. nasal speculum
Haller
H. ansa
H. circle
H. line
H. unguis
halleri
circulus arteriosus h.
circulus venosus h.
Hallermann-Streiff syndrome
Hallervorden-Spatz
H.-S. disease
H.-S. syndrome
Hallervorden syndrome
Hallpike
H. maneuver
H. test
Hallpike-Bárány positioning maneuver
hallucal abnormality
hallucinated voice
hallucination
auditory h.
daytime h.
depressive auditory h.
depressive olfactory h.
depressive visual h.
drug-induced h.
fleeting auditory h.
fleeting visual h.
formed visual h.
gustatory h.
haptic h.
hypnagogic h.
hypnopompic h.
kaleidoscope h.
kinesthesia h.
lilliputian h.
nocturnal h.
nonpsychotic h.
olfactory h.
overt h.
palinoptic h.
running commentary h.
simple h.
sleep h.
speech h.
stump h.
tactile h.
third-person auditory h.
visual h.
vivid h.
hallucinative
hallucinatory
h. neuralgia
h. transient organic syndrome
halo
Ace low-profile MR h.
Ace Mark III h.
h. apparatus
h. application
h. brace
Bremer h.
Brown-Roberts-Wells head ring h.
h. complication
Houston h.
hyperechoic h.
hypoechogenic peritumoral h.
h. immobilization
h. orthosis
h. phenomenon
Philadelphia h.
h. pin
pulsating visual h.
h. retractor system
h. ring
h. ring adapter
Surgairtome II drill h.
h. vest
h. vest immobilization
haloperidol condition
Halotestin
halothane anesthesia
Halperon
Halstead modified technique
Halstead-Wepman Aphasia Screening test
Halsted
H. artery forceps
H. mosquito forceps
Halter traction
HAMA
human antimouse antibody
hamartoma
cortical h.
eccrine angiomatous h.

hypothalamic h.
subependymal h.
h. of tuber cinereum
vascular h.
ventromedial hypothalamic h.

hamartomatosis
congenital h.

hamartomatous lipoma

hammer
Babinski percussion h.
Berliner percussion h.
Buck neurological h.
Buck percussion h.
Davis percussion h.
Dejerine-Davis percussion h.
Dejerine percussion h.
Epstein neurological h.
Küntscher h.
Monreal reflex h.
neurological h.
percussion h.
Rabiner neurological h.
slotted h.
Taylor percussion h.
Trömner percussion h.

Hammill Multiability Achievement test

hammock bandage

Hammond disease

hamster cell

HAM/TSP
human T-cell lymphotropic virus type 1-associated myelopathy/tropical spastic paraparesis

hand
accoucheur's h.
all-median nerve h.
all-ulnar nerve h.
ape h.
h. ataxia
benediction h.
contralesional h.
dead h.
h. deformity
drop h.
H. Dynamometer test
Gilliatt-Sumner h.
h. grasp reflex
Marinesco succulent h.
mechanic's h.
h. nondominant
obstetric h.
obstetrical h.
h. palmar crease
phantom h.
preacher's h.
simian h.
striatal h.
H. Test, Revised 1983
upper h.
writing h.

handcuff neuropathy

handedness

handgrip task

handicap
International Classification of Impairments, Disabilities and H.'s (ICIDH)

handicapped
Developmental Assessment of the Severely H.

handle
bayonet h.
Cloward double-hinge cervical retractor h.
Hardy lateral knife h.

handpiece
CUSA system 200 straight autoclavable h.

Hand-Schüller-Christian disease

hand-shoulder syndrome

HANE
hereditary angioneurotic edema

hanging-drop equilibration

hangman's fracture

hangover
daytime sleep h.

Hanks buffered saline solution

Hannover
H. classification
H. Functional Ability Questionnaire for measuring back pain-related functional limitations (FFbH-R)
H. system

Hansen disease

haphalgesia

haplotype
alpha-synuclein h.
h. analysis
h. association
h. frequency
4-loci h.
6-loci h.
h. mapping
multiple-loci h.

NOTES

haptic hallucination
haptometer
hard
h. chancre
h. collar
h. disc herniation
h. palate dissection
h. tissue replacement (HTR)
h. tissue replacement-malleable facial implant (HTR-MFI)
h. tissue replacement-patient-matched
h. tissue replacement-patient-matched implant (HTR-PMI)
Harding W87 test
hardware
h. complication
TiMesh h.
Hardy
H. approach
H. attachment
H. bayonet dressing forceps
H. bivalve speculum
H. curette
H. dissector
H. lateral knife handle
H. lip retractor
H. microsurgical bayonet bipolar forceps
H. microsurgical enucleator
H. pituitary spoon
H. 3-prong fork
H. sella punch forceps
H. sellar punch
H. suction tube
Hardy-Rand-Rittler plate
Hardy-Weinberg equilibrium
Hare Psychopathy Checklist: Screening Version
Harken rib spreader
harkoseride
Harmon cervical approach
harmonic
h. error field
h. function
harmonious interaction
Harm posterior cervical plate
Harms technique
HAROLD
hemispheric asymmetry reduction in older adults
HARP
Harvard Atherosclerosis Reversibility Project
Harriluque
H. sublaminar wiring modification
H. technique
Harrington
H. distraction
H. pedicle hook
H. rod
H. rod fixation
H. rod and hook system
H. rod instrumentation
H. rod instrumentation compression
H. rod instrumentation distraction outrigger device
H. rod instrumentation failure
H. rod instrumentation force application
H. scissors
H. spreader
Harris
H. migraine
H. syndrome
Harris-Smith cervical fusion
Hartel
H. technique
H. treatment
Harting body
Hartley-Krause operation
Hartnup disease
Hartshill
H. Ransford loop
H. rectangle
H. rectangle rod
Harvard Atherosclerosis Reversibility Project (HARP)
harvesting
radial artery h. (RAH)
Hasegawa
H. Dementia Scale
H. Dementia Scale-Revised
hatchet facies
Hausa Speaking test
Hauser ambulation index
haut mal epilepsy
haversian canal
Hawthorn effect
Hayem encephalitis
Haynes brain cannula
HBMEC
human brain microvascular endothelial cell
HBO
hyperbaric oxygen
HBO therapy
HBr
hydrobromide
citalopram HBr
galantamine HBr
hCG
human chorionic gonadotropin
hCG-secreting suprasellar immature teratoma
HCHWA-D
hereditary cerebral hemorrhage with amyloidosis-Dutch type

HCl
hydrochloride
buprenorphine HCl
chlorpromazine HCl
dexmethylphenidate HCl
imipramine HCl
lazabemide HCl
maprotiline HCl
memantine HCl
methadone HCl
methamphetamine HCl
methylphenidate HCl
molindone HCl
naltrexone HCl
naratriptan HCl
nortriptyline HCl
selegiline HCl
tacrine HCl
tiagabine HCl
ziprasidone HCl
HCN-1 cell line
HCP
hypertrophic chromic pachymeningitis
HCT, Hct
hematocrit
HCVR
hypercapnic ventilatory response
HDL
high-density lipoprotein
HDSA
Huntington Disease Society of America
HDT
head-down tilt
head
h. area
h. banging
h. bobbing
h. of caudate nucleus
h. cavity
h. circumference
h. circumference measurement
h. clamp
h. coil
h. computed tomography
h. deviation
h. enlargement
h. erythromelalgia
h. fixation device
h. frame
h. impulse sign
h. impulse test
h. injury
h. jerking
h. line
h. movement
h. nodding in spasmus nutans
h. position in intracranial pressure increase
h. ring
h. spasm
h. tetanus
h. tilt
h. trauma
h. trauma effect
h. zone
headache
acute generalized h.
acute localized h.
acute recurrent h.
alarm clock h.
analgesic rebound h.
basilar artery migraine h.
benign exertional h.
Bickerstaff migraine h.
bifrontal h.
bilious h.
bioccipital h.
bitemporal h.
blind h.
brain abscess with h.
brain tumor with h.
cataclysmic h.
catamenial migraine h.
cervicogenic h.
cheese reaction h.
Chiari malformation with h.
chronic cluster h.
chronic nonprogressive h.
chronic paroxysmal hemicrania h.
chronic progressive h.
ciliary migraine h.
classic brain tumor h.
h. classification
cluster h. (CH)
coital h.
cold stimulus h.
combination h.
comorbid h.
concurrent h.'s
cough h.
debilitating h.
h. differential diagnosis
disabling h.
dull unremitting h.

NOTES

H

headache *(continued)*
episodic cluster h.
episodic tension-type h. (ETTH)
essential h.
estrogen-withdrawal h.
evening h.
h. exacerbation
exertional h.
facioplegic migraine h.
featureless h.
fibrositic h.
focal acute h.
frequent h.'s
frontal h.
generalized h.
genetics of h.
giddy h.
helmet h.
hemicrania continua h.
high-altitude h.
histaminic h.
Horton h.
hot dog h.
hyperemic h.
hypertension-related h.
hyperventilation h.
hypnic h.
hypoxia-related h.
ice cream h.
ice pick h.
idiopathic stabbing h.
indomethacin-sensitive h.
h., insomnia, and depression (HID)
intraventricular h. (IVH)
ipsilateral h.
jabs-and-jolts h.
leakage h.
lower-half h.
matutinal h.
medication-induced h.
medication overuse h.
metabolic h.
migraine h.
migraine-like h.
mixed h.
monosodium glutamate-induced h.
morning h.
muscle contraction h.
neuralgiform h.
nitrite h.
nodular h.
nonmigrainous vascular h.
nonpulsating h.
occasional h.
occipital h.
organic h.
orgasmic h.
otitis with h.
paroxysmal migraine h.
pathophysiology of h.
pectoralgic migraine h.
persistent daily h.
h. phenotype
phobia-induced migraine h.
postconcussion h.
postictal migrainous h.
postlumbar puncture h.
posttraumatic h.
preictal h.
premonitory h.
preorgasmic h.
primary cough h.
primary stabbing h.
primary thunderclap h.
progressive h.
psychogenic h.
pulsating h.
pyrexial h.
radiation injury h.
rapid eye movement sleep-locked h.
h. recurrence
recurrent h.
recurring h.
reflex h.
h. relief
REM sleep-locked h.
retinal migraine h.
seasonal migraine h.
secondary h.
severe h.
sex h.
sick h.
sinus h.
sinusitis with h.
sleep-related h.
spinal puncture h.
spondylotic h.
suboccipital h.
sudden-onset h.
sudden severe h.
swim goggle h.
Symonds h.
symptomatic h.
syncopal migraine h.
h. syndrome
temporal h.
tension-type h.
tension vascular h.
thunderclap h.
TMJ dysfunction with h.
toxic h.
traumatic h.
h. trigger
triptan rebound h.
trochlear h.
unilateral migraine h.
vacuum h.

vascular h.
vasodilator h.
vasomotor h.
vestibular migraine h.
violent onset h.
vomiting with h.
weekend h.
whole cranial h.
Willis h.
withdrawal h.
h. with hematoma
h. with vasculitis
Wolff h.

headache-free migraine
head-bobbing doll syndrome
head-down tilt (HDT)
head-dropping test
headframe
headholder, head holder
Caspar h.
CBI stereotactic h.
Gardner h.
integrated h.
Malcolm-Rand carbon-composite h.
Mayfield-Kees h.
Mayfield radiolucent h.
Mayfield skull-pin h.
Patil stereotactic h.
pin h.
pinion h.
3-point h.
radiolucent cranial pin h.
ReFix stereotactic h.
Sugita h.

headlamp
Keeler video h.

headlight
high-beam fiberoptic h.
LightWear h.
Orascoptic fiberoptic h.
Quadrilite 6000 fiberoptic h.

headrest
Brown-Roberts-Wells h.
Gardner-Wells h.
horseshoe h.
Light-Veley h.
Mayfield horseshoe h.
Mayfield-Kees h.
Mayfield radiolucent h.
multipurpose h.
pediatric h.
pin fixation h.
3-point h.
Reston foam-padded h.
Timo h.
Veley h.

headset
InstaTrak h.

heads-up
h.-u. adjunctive endoscopy
h.-u. imaging system

head-thrust test
head-to-head clinical trial
head-up tilt testing
HealosMP52 implant
HealosMP52-treated fusion site
health
bone h.
National Institute for Occupational Safety and h.'s (NIOSH)

hearing loss
heart
irritable h.
h. murmur
h. reflex
h. rhythm

heartbeat potential
heat
h. defense
h. defense response
h. effect
h. effector
h. exhaustion
h. hyperplasia
h. loss
h. pain threshold
h. shock protein
h. stress

heating
eddy current h.
radiofrequency h.

heat-loss
h.-l. apparatus
h.-l. mechanism
h.-l. pathway

heat-regulating center
heatstroke
heavy
h. meromyosin
h. metal intoxication
h. metal neuritis
h. metal neuropathy
h. particle radiotherapy

heavy-duty straight clip

NOTES

H

hebbian potentiation of synapse
hecatomeral cell
hecatomeric, hecateromeric
hederiform ending
heel
h. tap
h. walking
heel-knee-shin test
heel-knee test
heel-tap
h.-t. reaction
h.-t. test
heel-toe walking
heel-to-knee-to-toe test
heel-to-shin test
Heidelberg concept
Heidenhain
H. disease
H. syndrome
H. type of spongiform encephalopathy
Heifetz
H. carotid occluder
H. clip
H. cranial perforator
H. cup serrated ring forceps
H. procedure
H. skull perforator
Heifetz-Weck clip
heightened sensory perception
height vertigo
Heilbronner
H. sign
H. thigh
Heine-Medin disease
Held
H. bundle
H. decussation
H. end bulb
helical
h. CT angiography
h. electrode
helical-like filament
helices (*pl. of* helix)
helicoidal computerized tomography
helicopod gait
helicopodia
heliencephalitis
heliotrope rash
helix, pl. **helices**
helix-loop-helix (HLH)
h.-l.-h. response factor
helmet
collimator h.
cooling h.
h. headache
Sheffield collimator h.
Helmholtz coil
helminthic infection
Helweg bundle
hemal gland
hemangioblastoma
benign capillary h.
spinal h.
third ventricular h.
hemangioendothelioma
epithelial h.
epithelioid h.
kaposiform h.
Masson vegetant intravascular h.
vertebral h.
hemangioma
h. of brain
calvarial h.
capillary h.
cavernous h.
choroid plexus h.
dumbbell-shaped spinal cavernous h.
epidural cavernous h.
extraaxial cavernous h.
extradural h.
extramedullary h.
histiocytoid h.
infantile hemangioblastic h.
laryngeal h.
oral h.
pontomesencephalic cavernous h.
retropharyngeal h.
sacral h.
spinal h.
vertebral h.
hemangiomatosis
hemangiopericytic meningioma
hemangiopericytoma
giant petroclival h.
meningeal h.
Hemashield enhanced graft
hematencephalon
hematocephaly
hematocrit (HCT, Hct)
hematoencephalic barrier
hematogenous cell infiltration
hematologic disease
hematoma
acute subdural h.
balancing subdural h.
carotid plaque h.
cerebellar h.
chronic subdural h.
delayed traumatic intracerebral h. (DTICH)
dural h.
epidural h.
h. evacuation
evolving h.
extracerebral h.
extradural h.

facial h.
gelatinous h.
headache with h.
hemispheral h.
hypertensive h.
iatrogenic h.
infratemporal h.
interhemispheric h.
intracephalic h.
intracerebellar h.
intracerebral h.
intracranial h.
intramedullary h.
intramural h.
intraparenchymal h.
intraventricular h.
isodense subdural h.
nasal septum h.
occipital h.
optic nerve sheath h.
parenchymatous h.
posterior fossa extradural h.
retromembranous h.
retropharyngeal h.
scalp h.
spinal epidural h. (SEH)
spontaneous spinal epidural h. (SSEH)
subdural h.
subgaleal h.
subperiosteal h.
sylvian h.
traumatic h.

Hematome system
hematomyelia
hematomyelopore
hematopoietic
h. dendritic cell
h. stem cell defect
hematoporphyrin derivative
hematorrhachis, hemorrhachis
h. externa
extradural h.
h. interna
subdural h.
hematoxylin
acid h.
Mayer h.
phosphotungstic acid h. (PTAH)
hematoxylin-eosin stain
heme
h. biosynthesis
h. synthesis
hemeralopia
hemiacrosomia
hemiageusia, hemiageustia, hemigeusia
hemialgia
hemiamyosthenia
hemianalgesia
hemianesthesia
alternate h.
cerebral h.
crossed h.
h. cruciata
mesocephalic h.
pontine h.
spinal h.
hemianopia, hemianopsia, hemiopia
altitudinal h.
bilateral homonymous h.
bitemporal h.
congruous h.
contralateral homonymous h.
dense h.
heteronymous h.
homonymous h.
ipsilateral h.
macular h.
macular-sparing h.
paracentral h.
partial h.
quadrantic h.
hemianopic scotoma
hemianosmia
hemiapraxia
hemiasomatognosia
hemiasynergia
hemiataxia
cerebellar h.
hemiathetosis
hemiatrophy
facial progressive h.
lingual h.
progressive lingual h.
hemiballismus, hemiballism
hemibasal syndrome
hemicephalalgia
hemicerebrum
hemichorea
hemichorea-hemiballism syndrome
hemiconvulsion, hemiplegia, and epilepsy (HHE)

NOTES

H

hemiconvulsion-hemiplegia-epilepsy syndrome (HHES)
hemicord
hemicorporectomy
hemicorticectomy
cerebral h.
hemicrania
chronic paroxysmal h. (CPH)
h. continua
h. continua headache
episodic paroxysmal h.
paroxysmal h.
hemicranial pain
hemicranicus
status h.
hemicraniectomy
hemicraniosis
hemicraniotomy
hemidecortication
cerebral h.
hemideficit
motor h.
sensible h.
hemidepersonalization
hemidysergia
hemidysesthesia
hemidystonia
hemiepilepsy
hemifacial
h. flushing
h. microsomia
h. spasm (HFS)
h. weakness
hemifield
contralesional h.
ipsilesional h.
h. loss
nasal h.
h. slide phenomenon
hemigeusia (*var. of* hemiageusia)
hemi-hemimegalencephaly
hemihydranencephaly
hemihypalgesia
hemihyperesthesia
hemihyperkinesis
hemihypertonia
hemihypertrophy
hemihypesthesia, hemihypoesthesia
hemihypometria
hemihypotonia
hemilaminectomy
complete lateral h.
lumbar h.
partial h.
unilateral h.
hemilateral chorea
hemimegalencephaly
hemimicropsia
hemimyelomeningocele
hemineglect
h. syndrome
visuospatial h.
hemiopalgia
hemiopia (*var. of* hemianopia)
hemiparaplegia
hemiparesis
amobarbital-induced h.
ataxic h.
brain abscess with h.
contralateral h.
dense h.
hemiparetic h.
herald h.
hypesthetic ataxic h.
ipsilateral h.
paradoxical ipsilateral h.
premature infant spastic h.
pure motor h.
residual h.
spastic h.
transient h.
unilateral h.
hemiparesthesia
hemiparetic
h. gait
h. hemiparesis
hemiparkinsonian stiffness
hemiplegia
acute acquired h.
acutely acquired h.
h. alternans
alternating hypoglossal h.
bilateral spastic h.
contralateral h.
crossed h.
h. cruciata
dense h.
double h.
facial h.
Gubler h.
hysterical h.
infantile h.
left h.
h. migraine
motor h.
pure motor h.
right h.
spastic h.
spinal h.
superior alternating h.
Wernicke-Mann spastic h.
hemiplegic
h. amyotrophy
h. gait
h. idiocy
h. migraine
h. rigidity
hemirachischisis

hemisection
spinal cord h.
hemisensory
h. disturbance
h. loss
h. syndrome
hemiseptum cerebri
hemisoma
hemisomatognosia
hemispasm
facial h.
hemispatial neglect
hemispheral
h. hematoma
h. mass
hemisphere
cerebellar h.
h. of cerebellum
cerebral h.
commissure of cerebral h.
h. competition
h. disease
dominant h.
face-dominant h.
face-nondominant h.
inferior surface of cerebellar h.
inferior vein of cerebellar h.
ipsilateral h.
medial surface of cerebral h.
mesial h.
nondominant h.
quadrate lobe of cerebral h.
h. sequence
h. stroke
superior surface of cerebellar h.
superior vein of cerebellar h.
superolateral face of cerebral h.
ventricle of cerebral h.
hemispherectomy
anatomical h.
hemispheric
h. asymmetry reduction in older adults (HAROLD)
h. blood flow
h. cerebral dysgenesis
h. collapse
h. cross flow
h. disconnection syndrome
h. dynamic
h. gliosis
h. hippocampal cortex
h. infarction
h. stroke
hemispherical
h. contact probe
h. deafferentation
hemispherii
polus temporalis h.
hemispherium cerebri
hemispherotomy
hemitetany
hemithermoanesthesia
hemitongue
hemitonia
hemitransfixion incision
hemitremor
hemivagotony
hemivertebra
hemizygosity
hemochromatosis
hemoclip
Samuels-Weck h.
hemodilution
isovolemic h.
prophylactic hypertensive hypervolemic h.
hemodynamic
h. feature
h. resuscitation
h. system
hemodynamics
cerebral h.
hemoflagellate
hemoglobin
h. glutamer-250[bovine] oxygen-based therapeutic system
h. H, SC disease
hemoglobinopathy
sickle h.
hemoglobinuria
paroxysmal nocturnal h.
hemolysis
hemolytic uremia syndrome
hemolytic-uremic syndrome
hemoperfusion
hemophilia
Hemopure oxygen-based therapeutic system
hemorrhachis (*var. of* hematorrhachis)
hemorrhage
aneurysmal subarachnoid h.
apoplectic h.
arterial h.

NOTES

H

hemorrhage *(continued)*
artery of cerebral h.
8-ball h.
brainstem h.
central nervous system h.
cerebellar h.
cerebral h.
cerebrovascular h.
choroid plexus h.
delayed traumatic intracerebral h.
Duret h.
epidural h.
extradural h.
fatal h.
flame-shaped h.
focus of h.
germinal matrix h.
Hunt and Hess grading scale for aneurysmal subarachnoid h.
hypertensive basal ganglia h.
hypotensive h.
Icelandic form of intracranial h.
intertrabecular h.
intracapsular h.
intracerebral leukostatic h.
intracranial h.
intraocular h.
intraparenchymal h.
intraplaque h.
intratumor h.
intratumoral h.
intraventricular h.
Kistler classification of subarachnoid h.
lobar h.
mesencephalic h.
neonatal cerebral h.
neonatal intraventricular h.
nerve fiber layer h.
nonaneurysmal perimesencephalic subarachnoid h.
nondominant putaminal h.
nontraumatic subarachnoid h.
parenchymal cerebral h.
parenchymatous h.
perianeurysmal h.
periaqueductal h.
perimesencephalic nonaneurysmal subarachnoid h.
periventricular-intraventricular h. (PIH)
petechial h.
pontine h.
premature infant subarachnoid h.
primary pontine h.
primary subarachnoid supratentorial h.
putaminal h.
remote cerebellar h.
retinal h.
retrobulbar h.
severity grading for h.
silent intracerebral h.
slit h.
spinal cord h.
spinal epidural h.
spinal subarachnoid h.
spinal subdural h.
splinter h.
striate h.
subacute h.
subarachnoid h. (SAH)
subconjunctival h.
subcortical h.
subdural h.
subependymal h.
subgaleal h.
subhyaloid h.
subintimal h.
supratentorial subdural h.
syringomyelic h.
thalamic h.
thalamic-subthalamic h.
traumatic intracranial h.
traumatic meningeal h.
traumatic subarachnoid h. (TSAH)
vitreous h.

hemorrhagic
h. contusion
h. disease of newborn
h. dysangiogenesis
h. encephalopathy
h. fever
h. infarction
h. lesion
h. metastasis
h. necrosis
h. pachymeningitis
h. shearing injury
h. shock
h. softening
h. stroke
H. Stroke-Specific Quality of Life Instrument (HSQuale)
h. transformation (HT)

hemorrhagica
encephalitis h.

hemorrheology

hemosiderin
h. deposition
h. reactional gliosis
h. ring
h. scar

hemosiderin-laden cell

hemosiderin-stained brain

hemosiderosis
cerebral h.

hemostasis
absolute h.
chemical h.
hemostasis-related protein
hemostat
Avitene microfibrillar collagen h.
h. awl
Crile h.
Surgicel fibrillar absorbable h.
hemostatic
h. forceps
h. plug formation
hemotympanum
Hemovac Hydrocoat drain
Hendler test
Henle
H. fiber layer
ligament of H.
H. membrane
H. nervous layer
H. rhomboid sinus
H. sheath
H. spine
Hennebert sign
Henoch chorea
Henoch-Schönlein purpura
Henry-Geist spinal fusion
henselae
Bartonella h.
Rochalimaea h.
Hensen
H. canal
H. cell
H. duct
H. node
heparin
low molecular weight h.
h. sulfate
heparinization
heparinized
hepatic
h. apoprotein gene
h. coma
h. decompensation
h. disease-associated neuropathy
h. encephalopathy
h. encephalopathy treatment
h. enzyme
h. injury
h. oxidative metabolism
h. porphyria
hepaticum
coma h.
hepatis
pars anterior faciei diaphragmatis h.
pars posterior facies diaphragmatis h.
hepatocerebral
h. degeneration
h. disease
hepatocyte
h. growth factor
h. growth factor/scatter factor (HGF/SF)
hepatoiminodiacetic acid (HIDA)
hepatolenticular
h. degeneration
h. disease
hepatomegaly
hepatotoxicity
hepatropic virus
Heplock catheter
Heptalac
herald hemiparesis
herbal medicine
Herbst
H. appliance
H. corpuscle
hereditaria
adynamia episodica h.
hereditary
h. angioneurotic edema (HANE)
h. areflexic dystasia
h. ataxic syndrome
h. benign chorea
h. brachial plexus disorder
h. brachial plexus neuropathy
h. branchial myoclonus
h. cerebellar ataxia
h. cerebellar ataxia of Marie
h. cerebellar atrophy
h. cerebral hemorrhage with amyloidosis-Dutch type (HCHWA-D)
h. chin trembling
h. coproporphyria
h. dysphasia
h. dysphasic dementia
h. dystonia
h. essential tremor
h. hemorrhagic telangiectasia

NOTES

H

hereditary *(continued)*
h. high-density lipoprotein deficiency
h. hypertrophic neuropathy
h. motor-sensory neuropathy (HMSN)
h. myokymia
h. neuralgic amyotrophy
h. neurodegenerative disease
h. neuropathic amyloidosis
h. neuropathy with liability to pressure palsy (HNPP)
h. neuropathy with susceptibility to pressure palsy
h. nonprogressive chorea
h. photomyoclonus
h. posterior column ataxia
h. radicular sensory neuropathy
h. sensory and autonomic disorder
h. sensory autonomic neuropathy, type 1–4 (HSAN-1–4)
h. sensory motor neuropathy (HSMN)
h. sensory neuropathy (HSN)
h. sensory radicular neuropathy
h. sensory radiculopathy
h. spastic paraparesis (HSP)
h. spastic paraplegia
h. spinal ataxia
h. spinocerebellar ataxia syndrome
h. striatopallidal disease

heredoataxia

heredodegenerative disease

heredofamilial
h. amyloidosis
h. tremor

heredopathia atactica polyneuritiformis

heredotaxia

heregulin

Hering
sinus nerve of H.
H. sinus nerve

Hering-Breuer reflex

Hering-Traube wave

heritable neuropathy

Hermann Brain Dominance Instrument

Hermetian symmetry

Hermetic
H. external ventricular drainage system
H. II drainage management system
H. lumbar drainage system

hermsii
Borrelia h.

hernia
cerebral h.
meningeal h.

herniated
h. cervical disc
h. intervertebral disc
h. nucleus pulposus

herniation
brain h.
caudal transtentorial h.
central transtentorial h.
h. of cerebellar tonsil
cerebellar tonsillar h.
cerebral h.
cervical disc h.
cingulate h.
concentric h.
disc h.
extraforaminal lumbar disc h.
foramen magnum h.
foraminal h.
frank disc h.
hard disc h.
hippocampal h.
impending h.
incipient downward central brain h.
internal disc h.
intervertebral disc h.
intraspongy nuclear disc h.
lumbar disc h.
rostral transtentorial h.
soft disc h.
sphenoidal h.
spinal h.
subfalcial h.
subfalcine h.
subligamentous disc h.
h. syndrome
temporal lobe h.
tentorial h.
thoracic disc h.
tonsillar h.
transforaminal h.
transtentorial uncal h.
traumatic cervical disc h.
uncal transtentorial h.

herophili
torcular h.

herpes
geniculate h.
h. simplex
h. simplex virus (HSV)
h. simplex virus encephalitis (HSVE)
h. simplex virus genome
h. simplex virus type 1 (HSV-1)
h. simplex virus type 2 (HSV-2)
toxoplasmosis, other infections, rubella, cytomegalovirus infection, h.
h. zoster
h. zoster encephalitis
h. zoster neuritis
h. zoster ophthalmicus

h. zoster oticus
h. zoster virus (HZV)
h. zoster virus infection
herpes/herpetic encephalitis
herpesvirus
h. encephalitis
Herpesvirus simiae
human h. 6 (HHV6)
human herpesvirus 8/Kaposi sarcoma-associated h. (HHV8/KSHV)
h. infection type 6, 7
herpete
zoster sine h.
herpetic
h. meningoencephalitis
h. neuritis
Herring body
Herrmann
H. Brain Dominance Instrument, Revised
H. syndrome
Hers disease
Hertel
H. exophthalmometer
H. exophthalmometry examination
6-hertz spike
Heschl
H. convolution
H. gyrus
transverse temporal gyri of H.
Hess
H. screen test
trophotropic zone of H.
hetacillin
heteresthesia
heterochromatin
heterocyclic
heterodesmotic fiber
heterodimeric receptor
heteroganglionic
heterogeneity
allelic h.
clinical h.
etiological h.
genetic h.
locus h.
plaque h.
heterogeneous
h. condition
h. system disease
heterogenicity
phenotypic h.
heterogenous disorder
heterogeusia
heterokinesia, heterokinesis
heterolalia
heterologous stimulus
heteromeric cell
heteromodal association cortex
heteronuclear ribonucleic acid (hnRNA)
heteronymous
h. hemianopia
h. motoneuron
heteropathy
heterophasia
heterophemia, heterophemy
heteroplasm
heteropodal
heteropsia
diffuse h.
heteroreceptor
heterosexuality
heterosmia
heterotonia
heterotonic
heterotopia
h. agglomerate
band h.
bilateral periventricular nodular h.
focal nodular h.
incomplete band h.
isolated periventricular nodular h.
neuronal h.
nodular h.
periventricular nodular h.
subcortical band h.
subcortical laminar h.
subependymal diffuse h.
heterotopic
h. gray matter
h. interstitial neuropathy of infancy
h. ossification
h. pain
heterotrimeric
heterotropic neuron
heterotypic cortex
heterozygosity
heterozygote
compound h.
heterozygous factor V Leiden mutation
Heubner
H. arteritis

NOTES

H

Heubner *(continued)*
artery of H.
H. disease
H. endarteritis
recurrent artery of H.
heutoscopy
Hewlett-Packard pressure monitor
hexachlorophene toxicity
Hexadrol Phosphate
hexamethylmelamine
hexamethylpropyleneamine oxime (HMPAO)
hexapropymate
hexosaminidase
h. A, B
h. deficiency
hexose
Heyer-Pudenz valve
Heyer-Schulte
H.-S. antisiphon device
H.-S. bur hole valve
H.-S. neurosurgical shunt
H.-S. wound drain
HFF
high-frequency filter
HFF on electroencephalogram
HFPV
high-frequency percussive ventilation
HFS
hemifacial spasm
HGF/SF
hepatocyte growth factor/scatter factor
HHE
hemiconvulsion, hemiplegia, and epilepsy
HHE syndrome
HHES
hemiconvulsion-hemiplegia-epilepsy syndrome
HHF35 muscle-specific actin tumor marker
HHV6
human herpesvirus 6
HHV7
human herpesvirus 7
HHV8/KSHV
human herpesvirus 8/Kaposi sarcoma-associated herpesvirus
HHV6-MS
human herpesvirus 6/multiple sclerosis
hiatus
h. semilunaris
tentorial h.
Hibbs
H. spinal curette
H. spinal fusion gouge
Hibbs-Jones spinal fusion
Hibbs-Spratt spinal fusion curette
hiccup
endemic h.'s
idiopathic chronic h.'s
Hickman catheter
Hick syndrome
HID
headache, insomnia, and depression
HID syndrome
HIDA
hepatoiminodiacetic acid
technetium-99m HIDA
hidden observer phenomenon
hidradenoma
hidrocystoma
HIE
hypoxic-ischemic encephalopathy
high
h. air loss bed
h. alpha coefficient
h. amplitude
h. animal protein
h. arousal threshold
h. cervical cord injury
h. cervical spinal cord lesion
h. degree of competency
h. linear filter
h. molecular weight cytokeratin tumor marker
h. muscular resistance bed
h. osmolar contrast medium
h. pontine lesion
h. sensitivity
h. sodium
h. steppage gait
h. thoracic cord lesion
high-affinity binding site
high-altitude
h.-a. headache
h.-a. illness
high-beam fiberoptic headlight
high-density
h.-d. area
h.-d. lipoprotein (HDL)
h.-d. transient signal
high-dose
h.-d. dopaminergic agonist
h.-d. systemic chemotherapy
high-energy
h.-e. brachytherapy
h.-e. cellular store
h.-e. X-ray beam
higher
h. center
h. cerebral dysfunction
h. cognitive function
h. neural function
h. order motion
high-filter frequency
high-force Sundt clip system

high-frequency
h.-f. activity
h.-f. deafness
h.-f. filter (HFF)
h.-f. generator
h.-f. hearing impairment
h.-f. hearing loss
h.-f. oscillation
h.-f. percussive ventilation (HFPV)
high-functioning
h.-f. autistic individual
h.-f. patient
high-gain instability
high-grade
h.-g. glioma
h.-g. spondylolisthesis
h.-g. stenosis
h.-g. tumor
high-intensity
h.-i. click stimulation
h.-i. lesion
h.-i. signal
high-lesion load
highly
h. active antiretroviral therapy (HAART)
h. selective vagotomy
h. unsaturated fatty acid (HUFA)
high-potency neuroleptic
high-resolution
h.-r. brain SPECT
h.-r. brain SPECT system
h.-r. chromosome analysis
h.-r. contiguous T1-weighted gradient-echo MRI
h.-r. 3DFT MR imaging
h.-r. image
h.-r. MRI
high-risk
h.-r. lesion
h.-r. population
high-signal lesion
high-speed
h.-s. air drill
h.-s. microdrill
high-threshold mechanoreceptor
high-torque bur
High-Vision surgical telescope
high-voltage
h.-v. centrotemporal spike
h.-v. deflection
h.-v. slow and sharp activity
HI-induced brain damage
hila (*pl. of* hilum)
Hilal
H. coil
H. microcoil
hilar
h. adenopathy
h. cell
h. lymph node
Hilger facial nerve stimulator
hillock
axon h.
facial h.
Hilton
H. law
H. method
hilum, pl. **hila**
h. of dentate nucleus
h. of inferior olivary nucleus
h. nuclei dentati
h. nuclei olivaris
h. nuclei olivaris caudalis
h. nuclei olivaris inferioris
h. of olivary nucleus
hilus of fascia dentata
H-imipramine binding
hindbrain
h. decompression
h. deformity
h. ischemia
h. malformation
h. vesicle
Hind III enzyme
hinged cast
hip
h. axis
h. extensor gait
h. phenomenon
hip-flexion phenomenon
Hippel-Lindau
von H.-L. (VHL)
hippocampal
h. activation
h. amnesia
h. commissure
h. complex
h. convolution
h. decline
h. dentate gyrus
h. electroencephalogram
h. epilepsy
h. fissure

NOTES

hippocampal *(continued)*
h. formation
h. formation atrophy
h. formation subdivision
h. herniation
h. infarction
h. monoamine concentration
h. neuronal loss
h. oligemia
h. pattern
h. pyramidal cell loss
h. pyramidal neuron
h. raw volume
h. resection
h. sclerosis
h. seizure discharge
h. slice
h. slice model of seizure
h. sprouting
h. sulcus
h. volume loss
h. volumetric loss
h. volumetry
h. vulnerability
hippocampal-amygdala complex
hippocampalis
formatio h.
sulcus h.
hippocampectomy
hippocampus, pl. **hippocampi**
alveus of h.
commissura h.
corpus fimbriatum h.
digitationes h.
fascia dentata h.
fimbria of h.
fissura h.
foot of h.
gyrus h.
layer of h.
h. major
mammalian h.
h. minor
minor h.
oriens layer of h.
pes h.
radiate layer of h.
rudimentum h.
strata hippocampi
stratum lucidum h.
stratum moleculare h.
stratum oriens h.
stratum pyramidale h.
stratum radiatum h.
subiculum h.
sulcus h.
tenia hippocampi
uncus gyri h.
hippocratic aphorism
Hirano body
Hirayama disease
Hirsch
H. endonasal technique
H. grading
H. hypophysis punch forceps
Hirschberg
H. reflex
H. sign
H. test
Hirschsprung disease
hirsutism
hirundinis
nidus h.
His
isthmus of H.
H. perivascular space
histamine
h. antagonist
h. cephalalgia
h. test in familial dysautonomia
histamine-2 antagonist
histaminergic neuron
histaminic
h. cephalalgia
h. headache
histidine metabolism disorder
histidinemia aminoaciduria
histine
beta h.
histiocyte
epithelioid h.
histiocytoid hemangioma
histiocytoma
histiocytosis
diffuse cerebral h.
kerasin h.
sinus h.
histiocytosis X
Histoacryl
H. blue
H. embolization
H. glue
histochemical study
histocompatibility
h. antigen
h. complex
histogram
histologic
h. appearance
h. atypia
h. section
histological feature
histologically benign
histology
posttraumatic brain h.
tumor h.
histolytica
Entamoeba h.

histomorphometric
histonectomy
histoneurology
histopathologic
histopathology
Histoplasma
H. capsulatum
H. infection
H. meningitis
H. polysaccharide antigen
histoplasma
histoplasmosis
disseminated central nervous system h.
disseminated CNS h.
medullar h.
historrhexis
history
developmental h.
neurologic h.
neurologic-ophthalmologic h.
perinatal event in h.
sleep h.
histotoxic hypoxia
Hitachi
H. scanning electron microscope
H. spectrophotometer
Hitch model
Hitselberger sign
Hitzig girdle
HIV
human immunodeficiency virus
HIV encephalopathy
HIV myelopathy
HIV myopathy
HIV-1-envelope protein
HIV-associated
HIV-a. dementia
HIV-a. nemaline myopathy
HIV-a. vasculitic vasculopathy
Hivid
HIV-related
HIV-r. neuropathy
HIV-r. seizure
HIV-sensory neuropathy (HIV-SN)
HIV-SN
HIV-sensory neuropathy
HLA
human lymphocyte antigen
HLA typing
HLA-CW2 antigen
HLA-DR15 typing
HLA-DR2 antigen
HLH
helix-loop-helix
HLH factor
HMPAO
hexamethylpropyleneamine oxime
hMSCs
human adult bone marrow mesenchymal stem cell
HMSN
hereditary motor-sensory neuropathy
HNK
human neonatal kidney
HNK cell
HNPP
hereditary neuropathy with liability to pressure palsy
hnRNA
heteronuclear ribonucleic acid
hNT neuron
Hoche
H. bundle
H. tract
Hochsinger
H. phenomenon
H. sign
HOCl
hypochlorous acid
hockey-stick dissector
Hodgkin
H. cycle
H. disease
H. lymphoma
Hodgkin-Huxley assumption
Hoehn
H. and Yahr Disability Scale
H. and Yahr Parkinson staging
H. and Yahr staging of Parkinson disease
H. and Yahr staging system
Hoen
H. dural separator
H. intervertebral disc rongeur
H. lamina gouge
H. nerve hook
H. pituitary rongeur
H. ventricular needle
Hoffmann
H. and Mohr procedure
H. muscular atrophy
H. phenomenon

NOTES

Hoffmann *(continued)*
H. reflex
H. sign
Hoffmann-Werdnig syndrome
holder
Adson dural needle h.
Ayers needle h.
cordotomy hook h.
Crile needle h.
curved microneedle h.
Donaghy angled suture needle h.
endoscope h.
Holinger endarterectomy dissector h.
Jacobson needle h.
Malis needle h.
Micro-One needle h.
microsurgery needle h.
needle h.
neurosurgical needle h.
Texas Scottish Rite Hospital hook h.
Vari-Angle clip h.
Wangensteen needle h.
Webster needle h.
Yasargil needle h.
hole
black h.
bur h.
precoronal bur h.
h. preparation method
holiday
caffeine h.
drug h.
Holinger endarterectomy dissector holder
holistic
h. approach
h. medicine
h. regimen
Hollander test
Hollenhorst plaque
Hollingshead Index of Social Position
Hollingshead-Redlich scale
hollow stainless-steel trocar
Holmes
H. cerebellar degeneration disease
H. cortical cerebellar degeneration
H. phenomenon
H. sign
H. tremor
Holmes-Adie
H.-A. pupil
H.-A. syndrome
Holmes-Stewart phenomenon
holmium YAG laser
holoacrania
holocarboxylase
h. synthetase
h. synthetase deficiency
holocord hydromyelia
holography
digital h.
volumetric multiple-exposure transmission h. (VMETH)
holohemispheric vasogenic edema
holoprosencephaly
alobar h.
lobar h.
semilobar h.
holorachischisis
holotelencephaly
Holscher nerve root retractor
Holter
H. high-pressure valve
H. medium-pressure valve
H. monitor
H. monitor test
Holter-Hausner valve
Homans sign
homeoboxes in patterning
homeodomain
h. factor
h. gene
h. protein
homeostasis
cellular ion h.
free radical h.
homeostatic balance
homeostenosis
Homer Wright rosette
home safety risk
HomeTrac
Saunders cervical H.
homochronous
homocitrullinuria
homocysteine
h. acid
h. level
homocystinuria
adult-onset combined methylmalonic aciduria and h.
homodesmotic fiber
homodimer
homofenazine
homogenate
buffy coat h.
h. technique
homogeneity
field h.
spatial h.
homogeneous lesion
homogenous
h. reinforcement
h. tumor enhancement
homolateral

homolog, homologue
eukaryotic h.
homologous
h. gene
h. stimulus
h. tetanus immune globulin (HTIG)
homonomy
analysis of h.
homonymous
h. hemianopia
h. motoneuron
h. muscle
h. scintillating scotoma
homophone
homoplasmy
homotopic pain
homotypic cortex
homovanillic
h. acid (HVA)
h. acid concentration
h. acid test
homozygosity
homozygote
homozygous
dementia h.
h. state
homuncular organization phase reversal
homunculus
human h.
somatosensory h.
Honig working memory and brain activation model
hood
dorsal aponeurotic expansion h.
H. masking technique
hook
Adson dissecting h.
Adson dural h.
Adson nerve h.
anatomic h.
André anatomical h.
ball-tip nerve h.
bifid h.
blunt nerve h.
Bobechko sliding barrel h.
calvarial h.
caudal h.
cautery h.
clawed pedicle h.
closed Cotrel-Dubousset h.
closed transverse process TSRH h.
Cloward cautery h.
Cloward dural h.
corkscrew dural h.
cranial Jacobs h.
Crile nerve h.
Culler h.
Cushing dural h.
Cushing gasserian ganglion h.
Cushing nerve h.
Dandy nerve h.
DePuy nerve h.
h. dislodgment
dissecting h.
downsized circular laminar h.
dura h.
Fisch dural h.
Fisch micro h.
Frazier dural h.
Frazier nerve h.
ganglion h.
Harrington pedicle h.
Hoen nerve h.
h. hollow-ground connection design
intermediate C-D h.
Isola spinal implant system h.
Jannetta h.
Kennerdell-Maroon h.
Kilner h.
Krayenbuehl nerve h.
Lahey Clinic dural h.
Lahey Clinic nerve h.
laminar C-D h.
large ball nerve h.
Leatherman h.
Love nerve root h.
Lucae nerve h.
Malis nerve h.
Marino transsphenoidal h.
microball h.
modified right-angled h.
Moe alar h.
Moe spinal h.
Moe square-ended h.
multispan fracture h.
Murphy ball h.
narrow-blade laminar h.
nerve h.
open C-D h.
pear-shaped nerve h.
pediatric C-D h.
pediatric TSRH h.
pedicle C-D h.
retractor handle Cloward dural h.

NOTES

hook *(continued)*
- ribbed h.
- Rosser crypt h.
- Sachs dural h.
- Scoville nerve root h.
- Selverstone cordotomy h.
- side-opening laminar h.
- h. site
- Smithwick button h.
- Smithwick ganglion h.
- Smithwick sympathectomy h.
- square-ended h.
- straight nerve h.
- Texas Scottish Rite Hospital buttressed laminar h.
- Texas Scottish Rite Hospital circular laminar h.
- Texas Scottish Rite Hospital pedicle h.
- Texas Scottish Rite Hospital trial h.
- Toennis dural h.
- transection h.
- transsphenoidal h.
- TSRH buttressed laminar h.
- TSRH circular laminar h.
- TSRH pedicle h.
- h. V-groove connection design
- von Graefe strabismus h.
- Weary nerve h.
- wide-blade laminar h.
- Yasargil spring h.
- Zielke bifid h.
- Zimmer caudal h.

hooked
- h. bundle of Russell
- h. fasciculus

hook-plate fixation

hook-to-screw L4-S1 compression construct

Hoover sign

Hopkins
- H. II endoscope
- H. syndrome
- H. Verbal Learning test

Hoppe-Goldflam disease

horizontal
- h. axis
- h. cell of Cajal
- h. cell of retina
- h. conflict
- h. eye movement
- h. fissure of cerebellum
- h. gaze
- h. gaze palsy
- h. gaze paresis
- h. inhibition
- h. pedicle diameter
- h. pendular nystagmus
- h. vertigo

horizontalis
- fissura h.

hormonal
- h. change
- h. decline
- h. difference
- h. maturation
- h. receptor
- h. therapy

hormone
- adrenocorticotropic h. (ACTH)
- anterior pituitary h.
- antidiuretic h. (ADH)
- corticotropin-releasing h. (CRH)
- ectopic h.
- endogenous steroid h.
- follicle-stimulating h. (FSH)
- gonadotropin-releasing h. (GnRH, GRH)
- growth hormone-releasing h. (GHRH)
- hypothalamic regulating h.
- luteinizing h. (LH)
- luteinizing hormone-releasing h.
- maternal thyroid h.
- natriuretic h.
- parathyroid h. (PTH)
- peripheral steroid h.
- prolactin-inhibiting h.
- prolactin-releasing h. (PRH)
- h. replacement
- h. replacement therapy (HRT)
- sex h.
- steroid h.
- supplemental steroid h.
- syndrome of inappropriate secretion of antidiuretic h. (SIADH)
- thyroid-stimulating h. (TSH)
- thyrotropin-releasing h. (TRH)

horn
- Ammon h.
- anterior h.
- apex of posterior h.
- bulb of occipital h.
- h. cell
- cutaneous h.
- dorsal h.
- frontal h.
- inferior h.
- lateral ventricle occipital h.
- lateral ventricle posterior h.
- lateral ventricle temporal h.
- occipital h.
- posterior h.
- spinal cord lateral h.
- spinal cord ventral h.
- temporal h.

tip of posterior h.
vein of posterior h.
ventral h.
Horne-Ostberg questionnaire
Horner
H. ptosis
H. syndrome
Horner-Bernard syndrome
horse
charley h.
horseshoe
h. headrest
h. incision
horseshoe-shaped flap
Horsley
H. bone wax
H. dural separator
H. operation
H. rongeur
H. sign
Horsley-Clarke
H.-C. stereotactic apparatus
H.-C. stereotactic frame
Hortega
H. cell
H. neuroglia stain
Horton
H. disease
H. giant cell arteritis
H. headache
H. histamine cephalalgia
H. syndrome
hospital
Texas Scottish Rite H. (TSRH)
VA H.
hospital-acquired
h.-a. meningitis
h.-a. pneumonia
host
h. immune response
immunocompromised h.
hot
h. dog headache
h. knife
h. spot
h. water epilepsy
hot-spot phantom
Hounsfield unit (HU)
24-hour ambulatory monitoring
12-hour fasting lipid panel
hourglass
h. dressing
h. tumor
House-Brackmann
H.-B. Facial Nerve Function Grading Scale
H.-B. Score
House-Fisch
H.-F. dural retractor
H.-F. dural spatula
housekeeping gene
Houston halo
Howard spinal curette
Howmedica
H. microfixation cranial plate
H. microfixation system drill bit
H. microfixation system plate cutter
H. microfixation system plate-holding forceps
H. microfixation system pliers
Hox gene
Ho:YAG laser
Hoyt-Spencer sign
H.P. Acthar Gel
hPVR
human poliovirus receptor
H-reflex
357HR Magnum tablet
HRT
hormone replacement therapy
HSAN-1–4
hereditary sensory autonomic neuropathy, type 1–4
H-shaped microplate
HSMN
hereditary sensory motor neuropathy
HSN
hereditary sensory neuropathy
HSP
hereditary spastic paraparesis
HSQuale
Hemorrhagic Stroke-Specific Quality of Life Instrument
HSV
herpes simplex virus
HSV encephalitis
HSV-1
herpes simplex virus type 1
HSV-2
herpes simplex virus type 2

NOTES

HSVE
herpes simplex virus encephalitis
HT
hemorrhagic transformation
5-HT
5-hydroxytryptamine
5-HT agonist
5-HT receptor assay
5-HT releasing agent
5-HT reuptake inhibitor
5-HT1
5-HT1 receptor
serotonin 5-HT1
5-HT3 receptor
5-HT_2-D_2-antagonist
HTIG
homologous tetanus immune globulin
HTLV
human T-cell leukemia virus
HTLV-associated myelopathy/tropical spastic paraparesis
HTLV-I-associated myelopathy
5-HTP
5-hydroxytryptophan
HTR
hard tissue replacement
HTR polymer
HTR-MFI
hard tissue replacement-malleable facial implant
HTR-MFI chin implant
HTR-MFI curved implant
HTR-MFI malar implant
HTR-MFI paranasal implant
HTR-MFI premaxillary implant
HTR-MFI ramus implant
HTR-MFI straight implant
HTR-PMI
hard tissue replacement-patient-matched implant
HTR-PMI implant
HU
Hounsfield unit
Hu-Ab titer
Hu antibody
Hudson
H. brace
H. brace bur
H. cerebellar attachment
H. cranial drill set
H. cranial rongeur
H. drill
H. forceps
H. perforator
HUFA
highly unsaturated fatty acid
huffer's neuropathy
Hughes
H. disability grade
H. reflex
Hulka instrument
human
h. adult bone marrow mesenchymal stem cell (hMSCs)
h. antimouse antibody (HAMA)
h. botulism
h. brain microvascular endothelial cell (HBMEC)
h. cadaveric spine
h. chorionic gonadotropin (hCG)
h. chromosome 20
h. doublecortin gene
h. dural substitute
h. dural substitute graft
h. ecology
h. factor
h. herpesvirus 6 (HHV6)
h. herpesvirus 7 (HHV7)
h. herpesvirus 8/Kaposi sarcoma-associated herpesvirus (HHV8/KSHV)
h. herpesvirus 6/multiple sclerosis (HHV6-MS)
h. homunculus
h. immunodeficiency virus (HIV)
h. immunodeficiency virus infection
h. lymphocyte antigen (HLA)
h. neonatal kidney (HNK)
h. neonatal kidney cell
h. neurofilament light chain
h. poliovirus receptor (hPVR)
h. prion protein
h. Purkinje cell
h. relationship
h. sleep characteristic
h. strength
h. T-cell leukemia virus (HTLV)
h. T-cell lymphoma virus
h. T-cell lymphotropic virus
h. T-cell lymphotropic virus-associated myeloneuropathy
h. T-cell lymphotropic virus-associated myelopathy
h. T-cell lymphotropic virus type 1-associated myelopathy/tropical spastic paraparesis (HAM/TSP)
h. tetanus immune globulin
h. T-lymphotrophic virus-associated myelopathy
humeroperoneal muscular dystrophy
humidification
BiPAP Pro II with heated h.
REMstar Auto with heated h.
REMstar Plus with C-Flex and heated h.

REMstar Pro with C-Flex and heated h.
humoral
h. immune response
h. immune system
h. phototransduction
Humphrey visual field
Hunstad infusion needle
Hunt
H. angled serrated ring forceps
H. angled-tip forceps
H. atrophy
H. disease
H. grasping forceps
H. and Hess criteria
H. and Hess grade I–III
H. and Hess grading scale for aneurysmal subarachnoid hemorrhage
H. and Hess Stroke Scale
H. juvenile paralysis agitans
H. and Kosnik classification
H. neuralgia
H. paradoxic phenomenon
H. syndrome
Hunt-Early technique
Hunter
H. canal
H. disease
H. dural separator
H. open cord tendon implant
H. operation
H. syndrome
hunterian
h. ligation
h. ligation of aneurysm
Hunter-McAlpine syndrome
Hunt-Hess
H.-H. aneurysm classification
H.-H. aneurysm grading system
H.-H. neurological classification
H.-H. subarachnoid hemorrhage scale
huntingtin protein
Huntington
H. chorea
H. disease
H. diseaselike disorder
H. Disease Society of America (HDSA)
H. sign
Hunt-Kosnik classification of aneurysm
Hunt-Yasargil pituitary forceps
Hurd bone-cutting forceps
Hurler
H. disease
H. syndrome
Hurler-Scheie
H.-S. disease
H.-S. syndrome
Hurst disease
Husk bone rongeur
Hutchinson
H. facies
H. mask
H. pupil
H. sign
H. triad
Hutchinson-Gilford progeria syndrome
Hutchison
H. syndrome
H. triad in syphilis
HVA
homovanillic acid
HVA concentration
H-wave test
hyaline
h. arteriosclerosis
h. body myopathy
h. body of pituitary
h. degeneration
h. thickening
hyalin inclusion disease
hyalinization
Crooke h.
hyalophagia
hyaluronan
hyaluronic acid
hyaluronidase
hybridization
DNA h.
fluorescence in situ h. (FISH)
genome h.
Northern h.
in situ h.
suppression subtractive h. (SSH)
hybridoma
hydatid
cerebral h.
h. cyst
h. disease
Hydergine LC

NOTES

H

hydralazine
h. hydrochloride
h. and hydrochlorothiazide
hydranencephaly
Hydrap-ES
hydrate
amyl h.
amylene h.
hydraulic-type
h.-t. disc prosthesis
h.-t. disc replacement
hydrazine toxicity
hydrencephalocele
hydrencephalomeningocele
hydrencephalus
hydrencephaly macrocephaly
hydride
butyl h.
hydroadipsia
hydrobromide (HBr)
galantamine h.
hydrobulbia
hydrocarbon
aromatic h.
volatile h.
hydrocele spinalis
hydrocephalic
h. dementia
h. idiocy
h. infant
h. periventricular radiolucency
hydrocephalocele
hydrocephaloid
hydrocephalus, hydrocephaly
acquired h.
acute h.
aqueductal gliosis with h.'s
arrested h.
asymptomatic h.
bilateral h.
chronic communicating h.
cocktail chatter in h.
communicating h.
compensated h.
congenital h.
delayed h.
double-compartment h.
external h.
h. ex vacuo
fetal h.
fulminant h.
idiopathic normal-pressure h. (INPH)
infantile h.
internal h.
kaolin-induced h.
maximal h.
meningitic h.
multiloculated h.
neonatal h.
noncommunicating h.
normal-pressure h. (NPH)
normotensive h.
obstructing h.
obstructive h.
occult h.
otic h.
h. oversecretion
posthemorrhagic h.
postinfectious h.
postmeningitic h.
postoperative h.
posttraumatic h.
premature infant h.
primary h.
progressive h.
secondary h.
shunted h.
h. shunt procedure
subdural effusion with h.
symptomatic h.
tension h.
thrombotic h.
toxic h.
triventricular h.
uncompensated h.
unilateral h.
unshunted h.
vasospasm-related h.
X-linked h.
hydrochloride (HCl)
alfentanil h.
alphaprodine h.
amantadine h.
amitriptyline h.
aptiganel h.
azacyclonol h.
butaclamol h.
chlordiazepoxide h.
chlorpromazine h.
clonidine h.
cyclobenzaprine h.
cyproheptadine h.
dexclamol h.
dihydromorphinone h.
diphenhydramine h.
donepezil h.
dopamine h.
dothiepin h.
doxepin h.
doxorubicin h.
duloxetine h.
ethaverine h.
fluphenazine h.
hydralazine h.
hydromorphone h.
hydroxyzine h.
imafen h.

imipramine h.
isoetharine h.
meperidine h.
methadone h.
methylamphetamine h.
midodrine h.
naratriptan h.
nitrosourea h.
oxyphencyclimine h.
papaverine h.
pargyline h.
perphenazine and amitriptyline h.
phencyclidine h.
procarbazine h.
promethazine h.
proparacaine h.
propranolol h.
remifentanil h.
ropinirole h.
sertraline h.
tiagabine h.
tizanidine h.
trifluoperazine h.
trihexyphenidyl h.
trimethobenzamide h.
tryptizol h.
venlafaxine h.
ziprasidone h.
hydrochlorothiazide
benazepril and h.
hydralazine and h.
lisinopril and h.
methyldopa and h.
propranolol and h.
h. and spironolactone
h. and triamterene
hydrocortisone
Hydrocortone
H. Acetate
H. Phosphate
hydrodipsia
hydrodipsomania
HydroDIURIL
hydrodynamic theory
hydroencephalocele
hydrogel
copper sulfate h.
h. disc replacement
hydrogen ion concentration
hydrolase
dopamine beta h. (DPH)
epoxide h.
terminal h.
Hydrolene polymer
Hydroloid-G
hydroma
cystic h.
hydromeningitis
hydromeningocele
hydromeningoencephalocele
hydromicrocephaly
hydromorphone hydrochloride
hydromyelia
h. dysraphism
holocord h.
hydromyelocele
hydromyelomeningocele
hydronephrosis in spina bifida cystica
Hydro-Par
hydroperoxide
phospholipid h.
4-hydroperoxycyclophosphamide
hydrophilic guide
hydrophilicity
hydrophobia
hydrophobic
h. ligand
h. tetanus
hydrophobicity algorithm
hydrophorograph
hydropneumatic massage
hydropneumogony
hydrops
endolymphatic h.
hypertensive meningeal h.
labyrinthine h.
hydrorachis
hydrostatic valve
hydrosyringomyelia
hydroxide
magnesium aluminum h.
hydroxocobalamin
3-hydroxy-3-methylglutaric aciduria
hydroxyapatite
APS h.
h. block
h. graft
Interpore porous h.
hydroxybutyrate
beta h.
4-hydroxybutyric aciduria
hydroxychloroquine

NOTES

H

17-hydroxycorticosteroid
6-hydroxydopamine (6-OHDA)
hydroxyethylmethacrylate
2-hydroxyethylmethacrylate
hydroxyethyl methacrylate polymerizing solution
2-hydroxyglutaric aciduria
5-hydroxyindoleacetic acid
3-hydroxyisobutyric aciduria
hydroxyisovaleric aminoaciduria
hydroxylase
  beta h.
  plasma dopamine beta h.
  tryptophan h.
  tyrosine h.
hydroxylase-positive
  tyrosine h.-p.
hydroxylation
hydroxyl radical
hydroxyproline
hydroxyquinoline neurotoxicity
5-hydroxytryptamine (5-HT)
  5-h. receptor assay
5-hydroxytryptophan (5-HTP)
hydroxyurea
hydroxyzine
  h. hydrochloride
  h. pamoate
hygiene
  sleep h.
hygroma
  subdural h.
hyla
hyoglossus muscle
hyoid
  h. advancement
  h. bone
  h. muscle
  h. suspension
hypalgesia, hypoalgesia
  h. dolorosa
hypalgesic, hypalgetic
Hypaque
hypaxial
hyperabduction syndrome
hyperactive
  h. affect
  h. sympathetic response
  h. tendon reflex
hyperacusis, hyperacusia
hyperadrenalism
hyperadrenergic
  h. response
  h. state
hyperaesthetic (*var. of* hyperesthetic)
hyperageusia
hyperaldosteronism
hyperalgesia, hyperalgia
  auditory h.
  muscular h.
hyperalgesic zone
hyperalgetic
hyperalgia (*var. of* hyperalgesia)
hyperalimentation
hyperammonemia
  cerebroatrophic h.
  valproate-associated h.
hyperamylasemia
hyperaphia
hyperaphic
hyperargininemia
hyperarousal
  physiological h.
  h. symptom
hyperbaric
  h. oxygen (HBO)
  h. oxygen therapy
hyperbetaalaninemia-aminoaciduria
hyperbilirubinemia
  nonhemolytic h.
hypercalcemia
  neonatal h.
hypercalciuria
hypercapnia, hypercarbia
  depressed ventilatory response to h.
  profound h.
hypercapnic
  h. responsiveness
  h. ventilatory response (HCVR)
hypercatabolism
hypercellularity
hypercholesterolemia
  familial h.
hypercinesia (*var. of* hyperkinesis)
hypercinesis (*var. of* hyperkinesis)
hyper-CKemia
  idiopathic h.-C.
hypercoagulability
hypercoagulable state
hypercoagulation
hypercompensatory type
hypercortisolemia
hypercortisolism
hypercryalgesia
hypercryesthesia
hyperdense lesion
hyperdensity
  concave h.
hyperdopaminergic state
hyperdynamia
hyperdynamic
hyperechoic halo
hyperekplexia
hyperemia
  occlusive h.
  relative h.

hyperemic
h. headache
h. response
hyperenergetic behavior
hypereosinophilic syndrome
hyperequilibrium
hyperergasia
hyperergia, hypergia
hyperergic encephalitis
hyperesthesia
auditory h.
cerebral h.
gustatory h.
muscular h.
h. olfactoria
olfactory h.
oneiric h.
h. optica
tactile h.
vaginal h.
hyperesthetic, hyperaesthetic
hyperestrogenemia
hyperevolutism
hyperexcitability
neuronal h.
self-sustaining h.
hyperexcitable neuron
hyperextension
intraoperative neck h.
hyperextension-hyperflexion injury
hyperfibrinolysis
hyperflexion
hyperfractionated
h. irradiation
h. radiotherapy
hyperfractionation
hyperfrontality
hyperfunction
adrenocortical h.
hyperfusion
hypergammaglobulinemia
hypergamy
hyperganglionosis
hypergeusia
hypergia (*var. of* hyperergia)
hyperglycemia
ketotic h.
nonketotic h.
hyperglycemia-induced neuronal injury
hyperglycinemia
nonketotic h.
hyperglycorrhachia
hypergraphia
hyperhidrosis
palmar h.
sleep h.
hyperhomocystinemia
hypericum perforatum
hyperinsulinism, hyperinsulinemia
hyperintense
h. hyperosmolality
h. lesion
hyperintensity
h. change
deep white matter h.
incidental punctate white matter h.
MRI signal h.
periventricular h.
punctate white matter h.
h. rating
h. severity
signal h.
subcortical gray matter h.
white matter h.
hyperisotonic
hyperkalemia
hyperkalemic periodic paralysis
hyperkeratosis
hyperketonemia
diet-induced h.
hyperkinesis, hypercinesia, hypercinesis, hyperkinesia
h. sign
hyperkinetic
h. conduct disorder
h. dysarthria
h. encephalopathy
h. impulse disorder
h. motor disorder
h. movement disorder
h. reaction
h. syndrome
hyperkyphoscoliosis
neuropathic h.
hyperlaxity
joint h.
hyperlexia
hyperlipidemia
hyperlysinemia aminoaciduria
hyperlysinuria
hypermagnesemia
hypermetabolic
h. effect
h. tumor component

NOTES

H

hypermetabolism
glucose h.
hypermetamorphosis
hypermethioninemia-hyperornithinemia
hypermethylation
hypermetria
hypermimia
hypermotor seizure
hypermyelination
hypermyesthesia
hypermyotonia
hypernatremia
hypodipsic h.
hypernatremic encephalopathy
hypernephroma
hypernomic
hypernychthemeral syndrome
hyperorality
hyperornithinemia
hyperosmia
hyperosmolality
hyperintense h.
hyperosmolar
h. hyperglycemic nonketotic syndrome
h. nonketotic coma
hyperosmolarity
hyperosmotic agent
hyperostosis
Caffey h.
diffuse idiopathic skeletal h. (DISH)
h. frontalis interna
idiopathic skeletal h.
hyperostotic
h. lesion
h. spondylosis
hyperoxaluria
primary h.
hyperoxia
hyperpallesthesia
hyperparathyroidism
maternal h.
hyperpathia
hyperperfusion
h. syndrome
tissue h.
hyperphagia
hyperphenylalaninemia
hyperphosphatasia
hyperphosphorylated tau
hyperphrenic
hyperpipecolatemia
hyperpituitarism
hyperplasia
arachnoidal h.
congenital virilizing adrenal h.
fibromuscular h.
gingival h.
heat h.
multiglandular h.
papillary mucosal h.
somatotroph h.
static h.
vessel h.
hyperplastic-hypertrophic obesity
hyperpolarization
hyperpolarization-activated
h.-a. cationic current
h.-a. chloride current
hyperpolarizing
h. current
h. factor
hyperponesis
hyperponetic
hyperpragic
hyperpraxia
hyperprolactinemia
hyperprolinemia aminoaciduria
hyperpronation
hyperpselaphesia
hyperpyrexia
hyperreactive
hyperreflexia
asymmetric h.
autonomic h. (AH)
bilateral h.
detrusor h.
pathologic h.
spastic h.
unilateral h.
hyperresponsive
hypersalivation
hypersarcosinemia
hypersecretion
hypersecretory adenoma
hypersensitivity
carotid sinus h.
denervation neuronal h.
h. vasculitis
hypersomnia
dementia-related h.
idiopathic h.
h. parkinsonism
hypersomnolence
central nervous system h.
idiopathic CNS h.
hypersomnolent
hyperstimulation
adrenergic h.
hypersympathicotonus
hypersynchronous
h. activity
h. discharge
h. electroencephalogram
hypersynchrony
hypnagogic h.
hypnopompic h.

hypertarachia
hypertelorism
orbital h.
hypertension
benign intracranial h.
cerebral h.
idiopathic intracranial h. (IIH)
intracranial h.
malignant h.
neonatal h.
orthostatic h.
paroxysmal h.
postural h.
venous h.
h. with insomnia
hypertension-related headache
hypertensive
h. basal ganglia hemorrhage
h. dilation
h. encephalopathy
h. hematoma
h., hypervolemic, hemodilutional therapy
h. meningeal hydrops
h. pontine microhemorrhage
hyperthermalgesia
hyperthermesthesia
hyperthermia
malignant h.
microwave h.
rebound h.
hyperthermoesthesia
hyperthyroidism
apathetic h.
hyperthyroid neuropathy
hypertonia, hypertonicity, hypertonus
sympathetic h.
treatment-emergent h.
hypertonic
h. absence
h. cerebral palsy
hypertrichosis
hypertriglyceridemia
hypertrophic
h. arthritis
h. cervical pachymeningitis
h. chromic pachymeningitis (HCP)
h. cranial pachymeningitis
h. interstitial neuropathy
h. nodular gliosis
h. obesity
h. olivary degeneration
h. pachymeningitis dorsalis
hypertrophica
pachymeningitis cranialis h.
hypertrophied frenulum syndrome
hypertrophy
facet h.
muscle h.
muscular h.
pons h.
pontine h.
pseudomuscular h.
uncovertebral joint h.
hypertropia
over-right h.
hypertryptophanemia
hyperuricemia
hypervalinemia
hypervascularity
intratumoral h.
hypervascularization
hyperventilation
h. activating technique
autonomic h.
craniocerebral trauma h.
h. headache
precipitation by h.
h. seizure
h. test
h. tetany
hypervigilance
hyperviscosity syndrome
hypervitaminosis A
hypervolemia
hypervolemic treatment
hypesthesia, hypoesthesia
brachiofacial cortical h.
contralateral tactical h.
olfactory h.
trigeminal h.
hypesthetic ataxic hemiparesis
hyphema
hypnagogic
h. hallucination
h. hypersynchrony
h. image
h. state
hypnalgia
hypnapagogic
hypnic
h. headache
h. jerk

NOTES

H

hypnoanalytic
hypnocinematograph
hypnogenesis
hypnogenic
h. paroxysmal dystonia
h. spot
hypnogram
hypnoid
hypnoidal state
hypnolepsy
Hypnomidate
hypnopedia
hypnopompic
h. hallucination
h. hypersynchrony
h. image
hypnosis
hypnotic
h. action
h. activity
h. agent
h. drug
h. intoxication
h. medication
h. sedative
h. withdrawal
hypnotic-dependent
h.-d. insomnia
h.-d. sleep disorder
hypnotic-induced
hypnoticus
status h.
hypnotist
hypoactive
h. affect
h. limbic structure
hypoactivity
glutamatergic h.
hypoacusis
hypoadrenalism
hypoalgesia (*var. of* hypalgesia)
hypobetalipoproteinemia
hypoblast
hypobulia
hypocalcemia
neonatal h.
premature infant h.
hypocapnia
hypocapnic ventilatory response
hypochloremia
hypochlorous acid (HOCI)
hypochondria
hypochondriac
h. neurosis
h. paranoia
h. psychoneurotic reaction
hypochondriacal reaction
hypochondrial reflex
hypochondroplasia
hypocomplementemic urticarial vasculitis
hypocortisolemia
hypocretin
h. deficiency
h. neuron
h. system
hypocretin-1
hypocrisy
hypocrite
hypocupremia
hypodensity
concave h.
white matter h.
hypodipsic hypernatremia
hypoechogenic peritumoral halo
hypoequilibrium
hypoergic
hypoesthesia (*var. of* hypesthesia)
hypofibrinogenemia
hypofolatemia
hypofractionated radiosurgery
hypofrontality
hypofunction
hypoganglionosis
hypogastric
h. ganglion
h. nerve
h. reflex
hypogastricus
nervus h.
plexus h.
hypogenetic corpus callosum
hypogeusesthesia
hypogeusia
hypoglossal
h. canal lesion
h. cranial nerve
h. eminence
h. foramen tumor
h. nerve [CN XII]
h. nerve fiber
h. nerve palsy
h. nerve paresis
h. nerve testing
h. neuralgia
h. neuropathy
h. nucleus
h. triangle
h. trigone
hypoglossale
trigonum h.
hypoglossal-facial nerve anastomosis
hypoglossalis
nucleus h.
hypoglossi
ansa h.
descendens h.
eminentia h.
nucleus nervi h.

nucleus prepositus h.
rami linguales nervi h.
trigonum nervi h.
tuberculum h.
hypoglosso
rami communicantes nervi lingualis cum nervo h.
hypoglycemia
hypoglycemic
h. coma
h. encephalopathy
h. peripheral neuropathy
h. seizure
hypoglycorrhachia
hypogonadism with anosmia
hypohypnotic
hypointensity
hypokalemia
thiazide-induced h.
hypokalemic
h. metabolic acidosis
h. periodic paralysis
hypokinetic
h. dysarthria
h. syndrome
hypokyphosis
right thoracic curve with h.
thoracic h.
hypolemmal nerve terminal
hypolipidemic
hypologia
hypomagnesemia
neonatal h.
hypomania
h. associated with sleep disturbance
treatment-emergent h.
hypomanic quality
hypomelanosis of Ito
hypometabolism
interictal h.
parietooccipitotemporal h.
prefrontal h.
hypometamorphosis
hypometria
hypometric saccade
hypomotor seizure
hypomyelinating condition
hypomyelination
cerebral h.
childhood ataxia with cerebral h.
hypomyelinogenesis
hyponatremia
hyponatremic encephalopathy
hypopallesthesia
hypoparathyroid
h. encephalopathy
h. tetany
hypoparathyroidism
hypoperfusion
biparietal h.
bitemporal h.
cerebellar h.
cerebral h.
delayed postischemic h.
frontal h.
mesial temporal h.
parietal h.
parietooccipital h.
h. syndrome
temporoparietal h.
hypophonia
hypophonic aphasia
hypophosphatemia
hypophrasia
hypophyseal (*var. of* hypophysial)
hypophysectomize
hypophysectomy
h. forceps
partial central h.
total h.
transethmosphenoidal h.
transsphenoidal h.
unilateral h.
hypophyseoportal system
hypophyseopriva (*var. of* hypophysiopriva)
hypophyseoprivic (*var. of* hypophysioprivic)
hypophyseos
infundibulum lobi posterioris h.
lobus anterior h.
lobus glandularis h.
lobus posterior h.
pars intermedia lobi anterioris h.
pars nervosa h.
pars pharyngea h.
hypophyseotropic (*var. of* hypophysiotropic)
hypophysial, hypophyseal
h. aneurysm
h. cachexia
h. forceps
h. fossa
h. grafting

NOTES

H

hypophysial *(continued)*
h. portal system
h. stalk
h. syndrome
hypophysiopriva, hypophyseopriva
cachexia h.
hypophysioprivic, hypophyseoprivic
hypophysiosphenoidal syndrome
hypophysiotropic, hypophyseotropic
hypophysis
alpha cell of anterior lobe of h.
anterior lobe of h.
h. cerebri
chromophobe cell of anterior lobe of h.
distal part of anterior lobe of h.
glandular lobe of h.
infundibular part of anterior lobe of h.
neural lobe of h.
neural part of h.
pharyngeal h.
posterior lobe of h.
h. punch forceps
h. sicca
tentorium of h.
hypophysitis
giant cell granulomatous h.
granulomatous h.
lymphocytic h.
lymphoid h.
pseudotumoral lymphocytic h.
hypopituitarism
hypopituitary coma
hypoplasia
cerebellar vermal h.
condylar h.
falx h.
optic nerve h.
pituitary h.
hypopnea
hypoponesis
hypopotentia
hypopraxia
hyporeactive
hyporeflexia
multisegmental h.
radicular h.
hyposensitivity
hyposmia
hyposomnia
hyposomniac
hyposthenia
hypostheniant
hyposympathicotonus
hypotaxia
hypotelorism
hypotense lesion
hypotension
acute severe h.
idiopathic orthostatic h.
intracranial h. (IH)
neurogenic orthostatic h.
orthostatic h.
spontaneous intracranial h.
sympathotonic orthostatic h.
hypotensive
h. hemorrhage
h. retinopathy
h. surgery
hypothalami
infundibulum h.
lamina terminalis h.
nucleus anterior h.
nucleus arcuatus h.
nucleus dorsalis h.
nucleus dorsomedialis h.
nucleus paraventricularis h.
nucleus posterior h.
nucleus supraopticus h.
nucleus ventrolateralis h.
nucleus ventromedialis h.
hypothalamic
h. acromegaly
h. amenorrhea
h. area
h. astrocytoma
h. blood flow
h. dysfunction
h. dysregulation
h. glioma
h. glucocorticoid
h. hamartoma
h. infundibulum
h. lesion
h. nucleus
h. obesity
h. pacemaker cell
h. regulating hormone
h. regulatory input
h. savage syndrome
h. sulcus
h. thermostat
hypothalamicae
zona h.
hypothalamic/chiasmatic glioma
hypothalamic-hypophysial-gonadal axis
hypothalamicorum
rami nucleorum h.
hypothalamic-pituitary
h.-p. axis
h.-p. dysfunction
h.-p. system
hypothalamic-pituitary-adrenal axis
hypothalamic-pituitary-adrenocortical system
hypothalamic-releasing factor

hypothalamicus
ramus h.
sulcus h.
hypothalamocerebellar fiber
hypothalamohypophysial
h. portal system
h. tract
hypothalamohypophysialis
tractus h.
hypothalamospinal
h. fiber
h. tract
hypothalamospinales
fibrae h.
hypothalamotomy
hypothalamus
anterior h.
dorsomedial nucleus of h.
interstitial nucleus of anterior h.
lateral zone of h.
medial zone of h.
paraventricular nucleus of h.
posterior nucleus of h.
preoptic h.
supraoptic nucleus of h.
ventromedial nucleus of h.
zone of h.
hypothermia
controlled h.
fatal h.
h. I-bolt
regional h.
hypothermic metabolic index
hypothesis, pl. **hypotheses**
alpha, beta, gamma h.
clonal evolution h.
congenital h.
dedifferentiation h.
degenerative h.
dormant basket cell h.
free radical h.
gate control h.
jelly roll h.
lipid h.
mnemic h.
Penfield h.
upregulation/downregulation h.
hypothesis-driven
hypothymic
hypothyroid
h. dwarfism
h. neuropathy
hypothyroidism
congenital h.
neonatal h.
premature infant h.
hypotonia, hypotonus, hypotony
benign congenital h.
essential h.
focal neonatal h.
muscular h.
neonatal h.
nitrazepam-induced h.
ocular h.
hypotonic cerebral palsy
hypotonicity
hypotonus (*var. of* hypotonia)
hypotony (*var. of* hypotonia)
hypotropia
hypoventilation
h. coma
primary alveolar h.
hypovolemia
hypovolemic shock
hypoxanthine
h. guanine phosphoribosyltransferase
h. guanine phosphoribosyltransferase deficiency
hypoxemia
nocturnal h.
hypoxia
anemic h.
anoxic h.
cerebral h.
delayed coma after h.
histotoxic h.
hypoxic h.
ischemic h.
isocapnic h.
relative h.
short-term h.
stagnant h.
toxic h.
hypoxia-related headache
hypoxia-susceptible sector of Sommer
hypoxic
h. brain damage
h. cerebral vasodilatation
h. hypoxia
h. ischemia
h. ventilatory response
hypoxic-hypercarbic encephalopathy
hypoxic-ischemic
h.-i. brain

NOTES

H

hypoxic-ischemic *(continued)*
- h.-i. brain damage
- h.-i. encephalopathy (HIE)
- h.-i. fetal lesion
- h.-i. injury
- h.-i. insult

hypsarhythmia, hypsarrhythmia
hypsarrhythmic electroencephalographic pattern
hypsicephalic
hypsicephaly, hypsocephaly
hypsokinesis
Hyrtl
- H. anastomosis
- H. foramen
- H. loop

hysteresis
hysterica
- megalopia h.
- suffocation h.

hysterical
- h. amnesia
- h. anesthesia
- h. aphonia
- h. ataxia
- h. blindness
- h. chorea
- h. convulsion
- h. dementia
- h. depression
- h. fugue state
- h. gait
- h. gait disorder
- h. hearing impairment
- h. hemiplegia
- h. movement disorder
- h. mutism
- h. paralysis
- h. polydipsia
- h. pseudodementia
- h. seizure
- h. syncope
- h. torticollis
- h. tremor
- h. visual loss

hysteric coma-like state
hystericoneuralgic
hystericus
- clavus h.
- globus h.

hysterocatalepsy
hysteroepilepsy
hysteroepileptogenous point
hysterogenic, hysterogenous
hysteroid convulsion
Hytrast
HZV
- herpes zoster virus
  - HZV vasculitis-vasculopathy

I
I band
I substance
IADL
instrumental activities of daily living
IADSA
intraarterial digital subtraction angiography
IAP
intermittent acute porphyria
iatrogenic
i. carotid-cavernous fistula
i. complication
i. Creutzfeldt-Jakob disease (iCJD)
i. damage
i. deficit
i. discitis
i. effect
i. elevatus
i. hematoma
i. instability
i. lumbar kyphosis
IBBB
intrablood-brain barrier
I-bolt
hypothermia I-b.
Texas Scottish Rite Hospital I-b.
Ibuprohm
IC
illusionary contour
imprinting center
Codman IC
IC effect
ICA
internal carotid artery
ICA-occluded stable Xe/CT CBF study
ice
i. cream headache
i. pick headache
i. pick-like pain
i. pick pain
ICEEG
intracranial electroencephalogram
Iceland disease
Icelandic form of intracranial hemorrhage
I-cell disease
ichthyosis
ichthyotoxism
IC-IC
intracranial-intracranial
IC-IC bypass
ICIDH
International Classification of Impairments, Disabilities and Handicaps
iCJD
iatrogenic Creutzfeldt-Jakob disease
ICP
intracranial pressure
ICP Camino bolt
ICP catheter
ICP microsensor
ICP monitor
ICP waveform
ICP-T
intracranial pressure-temperature
ICP-T fiberoptic ICP intracranial temperature catheter
ICP-T fiberoptic ICP monitoring catheter
ictal
i. amnesia
i. automatism
i. cerebral perfusion pattern
i. confusional seizure
i. EEG pattern
i. epileptiform abnormality
i. epileptiform activity
i. epileptiform pattern
i. event
i. fear
i. focal epileptiform discharge
i. localization
i. onset zone
i. pattern on EEG
i. period
i. polygram
i. propagation
i. scalp EEG
i. semiology
i. single-photon emission computed tomography
i. speech
i. vomiting
ictus
i. epilepticus
i. paralyticus
i. sanguinis
ICU
intensive care unit
ICU myopathy
ICVM
intracranial vascular malformation
ID
index of difficulty

IDEA
Individuals with Disabilities Education Act
idealizing transference
ideal spinal implant
ideational
i. agnosia
i. apraxia
ideatory apraxia
idebenone
identical elements
identification
i. process
smell i.
identified trait
identity diffusion
ideokinetic apraxia
ideological orientation
ideomotion
ideomotor
i. apraxia
i. dyspraxia
ideoplastic stage
IDET
intradiscal electrotherapy
intradiscal electrothermal therapy
IDET procedure
idiocy
amaurotic i.
athetosic i.
eclamptic i.
hemiplegic i.
hydrocephalic i.
juvenile amaurotic i.
late infantile amaurotic i.
mongolian i.
paraplegic i.
idiodynamic control
idiogenic osmole
idioglossia
idiographic examination
idiojunctional rhythm
idiomuscular contraction
idiopathic
i. ataxic syndrome
i. bilateral vestibulopathy
i. calcification
i. central sleep apnea
i. chronic hiccups
i. CNS hypersomnolence
i. facial nerve palsy
i. generalized epilepsy
i. generalized epilepsy syndrome
i. growth hormone deficiency
i. hyper-CKemia
i. hypersomnia
i. hypertrophic cranial pachymeningitis
i. inflammatory myopathy (IIM)
i. insomnia
i. intracranial hypertension (IIH)
i. intracranial pachymeningitis
i. meningitis
i. muscular atrophy
i. myelofibrosis (IMF)
i. narcolepsy
i. normal-pressure hydrocephalus (INPH)
i. orbital pseudotumor
i. orthostatic hypotension
i. Parkinson disease
i. Parsonage-Turner syndrome
i. partial epilepsy
i. peripheral neuropathy
i. polyneuropathy
i. recurring stupor
i. seizure
i. skeletal hyperostosis
i. stabbing headache
i. syncope
i. thoracic scoliosis
i. thrombocytopenic purpura (ITP)
i. torticollis
i. trigeminal neuralgia (ITN)
idiopathic/cryptogenic epilepsy
idiopathy
idiophrenic
idioreflex
idiospasm
idiosyncrasia olfactoria
idiosyncratic
i. basis
i. intoxication
i. reaction
IDP
inflammatory demyelinating polyneuropathy
IDPL
injected dose per liter
iduronate sulfatase
IENF
intraepidermal nerve fiber
IFET
ischemic forearm exercise test
IFN
interferon
IFN-G
interferon gamma
IgA
immunoglobulin A
anti-GT1a IgA
IGF
insulinlike growth factor
IgG
immunoglobulin G
Iggo receptor
IgM
immunoglobulin M

IgM antibody capture
IgM monoclonal gammopathy
IgM paraproteinemic neuropathy
IGMIT
image-guided minimally invasive therapy
IgM-lambda paraprotein
IH
intracranial hypotension
IHS
International Headache Society
IHWOP
intracranial hypertension without papilledema
IIH
idiopathic intracranial hypertension
IIM
idiopathic inflammatory myopathy
IL
interleukin
I-labeled cocaine analog
ileocolic plexus
Iletin
Ilhéus encephalitis
iliac
i. artery injury
i. bone graft
i. crest bone graft stabilization
i. crest resection
i. crest syndrome
i. fixation
i. post
i. screw
iliacus
plexus i.
iliocostal muscle
iliofemoral thrombosis
iliohypogastrici
ramus cutaneus anterior nervi i.
ramus cutaneus lateralis nervi i.
iliohypogastric nerve
iliohypogastricus
nervus i.
ilioinguinalis
nervus i.
ilioinguinal nerve
iliopsoas muscle
iliopubic nerve
iliopubicus
nervus i.
iliosacral
i. and iliac fixation construct
i. region
i. screw
Ilizarov corticotomy
ill-defined
i.-d. aneurysm neck
i.-d. symptom
illegal drug synthesis
illicit drug
illness
autoimmune i.
brain i.
comorbid i.
debilitating i.
dementing i.
denial of i.
fatigue of systemic i.
high-altitude i.
long-term i.
mercury-induced i.
monophasic neurologic i.
neurological i.
objective severity of i.
outcome of i.
viral-mediated i.
illumination
Luxtec coaxial i.
illuminator
fiberoptic i.
XL i.
illusion
auditory i.
illusionary contour (IC)
illusory memory
imafen hydrochloride
image
accidental i.
i. acquisition time
autoradiographic i.
axial magnetic resonance i.
axial spin-echo i.
B-mode i.
body i.
contrast-enhanced MR i.
coregistered i.
i. correlation
cross-sectional i.
dangerous i.
diffusion-weighted echo planar i. (DW-EPI)
2D multiplanar reconstructed i.
echo planar i.
i. foldover

NOTES

image *(continued)*
i. formation principle
ghost i.
gradient-echo echo planar i.
gradient-echo magnetic resonance i.
gradient-echo MR i.
gradient-recalled echo i.
i. guidance
high-resolution i.
hypnagogic i.
hypnopompic i.
imperfect i.
incidental i.
in-phase i.
i. intensification
i. intensifier
Iso-C i.
long pulse repetition time/echo time i.
magnetic resonance i. (MRI)
magnetization transfer i.
midsagittal i.
motor i.
negative i.
i. neurosurgery
neutral i.
out-of-phase i.
PET i.
phantom i.
positive i.
proton-weighted i.
i. quality
raw speckled i.
reformatted i.
i. registration
sagittal spin-echo i.
sagittal T1-weighted SE i.
sagittal T1-weighted spin echo i.
sensory i.
short pulse repetition time/echo time i.
source i.
SPECT i.
spin-echo T1-weighted plan i.
stereotactic PET i.
tactile i.
thin-section i.
tilting of visual i.
T1-weighted magnetic resonance i.
T2-weighted magnetic resonance i.
T1-weighted MR i.
T2-weighted MR i.
T1-weighted spin-echo i.
T2-weighted spin-echo i.
T2-weighted turbo-gradient i.

image-complete resection

image-guided
i.-g. minimally invasive therapy (IGMIT)
i.-g. robotic radiosurgery
i.-g. solution
i.-g. stereotactic brain biopsy
i.-g. stereotaxis

image-integrated surgery treatment planning

Imagent BP

imager
Magnes 2500 WH i.
1.5-T i.

imagery training for persistent primary insomnia

imaging
i. artifact
blood oxygen level-dependent functional magnetic resonance i.
blood pool i.
brain i.
cerebrovascular magnetic resonance i.
chemical-shift i.
Chopper-Dixon hybrid i.
cinematic magnetic resonance i.
cine phase contrast magnetic resonance i.
color-flow i.
computerized infrared telethermographic i.
continuous-wave Doppler i.
contrast-enhanced MR i.
contrast enhancement i.
2DFT gradient-echo i.
3DFT gradient-echo MR i.
Diasonics magnetic resonance i.
diffusion-perfusion magnetic resonance i.
diffusion tension i.
diffusion tensor i. (DTI)
diffusion tensor magnetic resonance i.
diffusion-weighted i. (DWI)
diffusion-weighted magnetic resonance i.
digital vascular i. (DVI)
3-dimensional fast low-angle shot i.
2-dimensional Fourier transform gradient-echo i.
3-dimensional Fourier transform gradient-echo i.
2-dimensional proton echo planar spectroscopic i.
direct multiplanar i.
Dixon method opposed i.
Doppler i.
echo planar i.
fast i.
fat-suppression MR i.
FLAIR sequence magnetic resonance i.

flow-sensitive magnetic resonance i.
flow-sensitive MR i.
fluid-attenuated inversion recovery sequence magnetic resonance i.
fluoroscopic i.
functional brain i.
functional magnetic resonance i. (f-MRI)
gadolinium-enhanced MR i.
Gd-DTPA-enhanced cranial MR i.
gradient echo i.
gradient-echo MR i.
gradient-refocused i.
half-Fourier i.
half-NEX i.
high-resolution 3DFT MR i.
interventional magnetic resonance i. (iMRI)
intrinsic i.
line i.
Magnes magnetic source i.
magnetic resonance i. (MRI)
magnetic resonance perfusion i.
magnetic source i. (MSI)
i. method
i. modality
MR volumetry i.
multiplanar i.
multiple line-scan i.
multiple-plane i.
neurodiagnostic i.
neuroreceptor i.
neurovascular i.
nonproton magnetic resonance i.
nuclear i.
oblique sagittal gradient-echo MR i.
orthogonal polarized spectral i. (OPSI)
partial flip-angle i.
partial Fourier i.
perfusion-weighted i.
phase-sensitive gradient-echo MR i.
planar spin i.
point i.
i. protocol
proton i.
pulsed Doppler i.
quantitative i.
radionuclide i.
rapid acquisition radiofrequency-echo steady-state i.
real-time color Doppler i.
reproducible target i.
second harmonic i. (SHI)
sequential plane i.
sequential point i.
serial i.
short inversion recovery i.
simultaneous volume i.
spin-echo i.
spin-warp i.
structural magnetic resonance i.
i. study
suboptimal i.
subtraction i.
surface coil spectroscopic i.
surveillance i.
^{99m}Tc HMPAO SPECT i.
Tc-99m HMPAO cerebral perfusion SPECT i.
time-variance i. (TVI)
transcranial real-time color Doppler i.
in vivo i.

imatinib

imbalance
acid-base i.
autonomic i.
calcium metabolism i.
dopamine-acetylcholine i.
electrolyte i.
magnesium i.
metabolic i.
potassium i.
sodium i.
sympathetic i.
vasomotor i.

IMF
idiopathic myelofibrosis

imidazopyridine

iminoglycinuria

imipenem-cilastatin injection

imipramine
i. HCl
i. hydrochloride
i. neurotoxicity

imitative tetanus

Imitrex

immature
i. intervertebral disc
i. teratoma

immaturity
cognitive function i.

NOTES

immediate
i. control
i. early gene
i. early gene cascade
i. posttraumatic automatism
i. posttraumatic convulsion
immigration
macrophage i.
immitis
Coccidioides i.
immobile face
immobilization
collar i.
external i.
halo i.
halo vest i.
i. method
postoperative i.
spinal i.
sternooccipital-mandibular i. (SOMI)
Treponema pallidum i.
immobilizer
Vac-Lok bag i.
immortalized primary cell culture
immune
i. cell
chorea i.
i. complex
i. dysregulation
i. response
i. system
i. thrombocytopenic purpura (ITP)
immune-mediated
i.-m. mechanism
i.-m. neuropathy
immunity
cell-mediated i.
immunization complication
immunocompetent
i. cell
i. macrophage
immunocompromised host
immunocytochemical
i. analysis
i. assay
immunoelectrotransfer blot technique
immunofluorescence assay
immunoglobulin
i. A (IgA)
i. G (IgG)
i. kappa light chain
i. M (IgM)
i. treatment
immunohistochemical
i. study
i. technique
immunohistochemistry
BrDu i.
Southwestern i.
immunologic
i. abnormality
i. aspect
i. dysfunction
i. nitric oxide synthase
immunological paralysis
immunology
multiple sclerosis i.
immunomodulator
immunoperoxidase
i. method
i. procedure
i. staining
immunoreactive
plasma i. (PI-R)
immunostimulatory gene transfer
immunosuppressive
i. drug
i. effect
i. medication
i. therapy
immunotherapeutic agent
immunotoxin
immunoturbidimetry analyzer
impact
disruptive i.
pharmacologic i.
systemic i.
impactor
Cloward bone graft i.
vertebral body i.
impaired
Assessment for Persons Profoundly or Severely I.
i. attentional functioning
i. cerebral function
i. cognition
i. concentration
consciousness i.
i. control
i. coordination
i. decussation
i. drug metabolism
i. face recognition
i. limbic-diencephalic function
i. memory
i. migration of brain neuron
motorically i.
i. neuromuscular transmission
i. object recognition
i. vision
impairment
age-associated memory i.
age-related memory i.
anterior horn cell motor i.
autonomic i.
balance i.
basic i.
category-specific semantic i.

cerebral i.
Clinician Rated Overall Life I.
cognitive i.
communication i.
constructional i.
early speech i.
frontal lobe i.
functional/cognitive i.
functional hearing i.
gait i.
gaze i.
general medical i.
global cognitive i.
global measure of i.
graphic i.
high-frequency hearing i.
hysterical hearing i.
initial spoken language i.
intellectual i.
IQ-adjusted memory i.
late-life cognitive i.
level of i.
life i.
medical i.
memory i.
mental i.
mild cognitive i. (MCI)
motivation i.
motor i.
narrative speech perception i.
neurocognitive i.
nonlanguage cognitive i.
perceptual-motor ability i.
peripheral nerve level motor i.
phonologic assembly i.
postictal i.
preexisting cognitive i.
psychogenic hearing i.
psychomotor i.
i. rating score
root level motor i.
saccade i.
semantic memory i.
sensory i.
severe i.
social i.
speech processing i.
spinal nerve level motor i.
spoken language i.
supranuclear vertical gaze i.
temporal lobe i.
transient cognitive i. (TCI)
upper motor neuron i.
vascular cognitive i.
verbal memory i.
visual memory i.
volitional i.

impar
ganglion i.
nervus i.

impedance
i. artifact
i. audiometry
electrode i.
i. measurement
i. method
middle ear i.
static acoustic i.
i. value

impediment
environmental i.

impending herniation

imperfect
i. image
i. image registration

imperfecta
dentinogenesis i.
osteogenesis i. (OI)

impersistence
motor i.

impingement
anterior cord i.
corpus callosal i.

implant
Activa tremor control system i.
Arenberg-Denver inner ear valve i.
auditory brainstem i. (ABI)
broken existing i.
cochlear i.
custom i.
DTT i.
ectodermal i.
embryonic i.
epidural i.
epilepsy i.
i. fatigue
ferromagnetic i.
fetal dopaminergic tissue i.
fetal neural i.
Gliadel i.
gold weight i.
hard tissue replacement-malleable facial i. (HTR-MFI)

NOTES

implant *(continued)*
hard tissue replacement-patient-matched i. (HTR-PMI)
HealosMP52 i.
HTR-MFI chin i.
HTR-MFI curved i.
HTR-MFI malar i.
HTR-MFI paranasal i.
HTR-MFI premaxillary i.
HTR-MFI ramus i.
HTR-MFI straight i.
HTR-PMI i.
Hunter open cord tendon i.
ideal spinal i.
iodine-125 i.
KLS-Martin i.
lumbar anterior root stimulator i.
MacroSorb absorbable plate i.
metallic otologic i.
i. migration
NeuroControl Freehand i.
nicardipine prolonged-release i.
Nucleus 24 multichannel auditory brainstem i.
otologic i.
patient-matched i.
Polaris adjustable spinal cage i.
i. removal
Schwann cell i.
silicone i.
stainless steel i.
i. survival rate
tissue i.
TSRH i.
vagal nerve i.
vagus stimulator i.
Zielke VDS i.

implantable pulse generator

implantation
brachytherapy seed i.
i. cone
DBS electrode i.
nerve i.
screw i.
stereotactic i.
subdural grid i.
i. technique

implanted
i. infusion pump
i. polymer

implicit process

implosion therapy

impregnation
Bodian silver i.

impressio
i. petrosa pallii
i. petrosa pallii incisura
i. trigeminalis ossis temporalis

impression
basilar i.
cervical spine basilar i.
diagnostic i.

impressive aphasia

imprinting
i. center (IC)
i. center mutation analysis
i. defect
genomic i.

improper dose

improved
i. communication skill
Isollyl I.

improvement
behavioral i.
clinical i.
cognitive i.
life-changing i.
neurologic i.
spontaneous i.

impulse
i. asynchrony
forced i.
nerve i.
neural i.
i. neurosis
nociceptive i.

impulsive
i. petit mal epilepsy
i. spectrum

impulsive-aggressive trait

impulsivity
counteracting i.
lifetime i.

iMRI
interventional magnetic resonance imaging
PoleStar N-10 iMRI

Imuran

imus
nervus splanchnicus thoracicus i.

in
in situ hybridization
in situ photocoagulation
in situ spinal fusion
in situ tricortical iliac crest block bone graft
in toto
in utero teratologic agent
in vitro molecular study
in vitro spectra
in vivo benzodiazepine receptor binding
in vivo brain functioning
in vivo data
in vivo 1H magnetic resonance spectroscopy
in vivo imaging

in vivo optical spectroscopy (INVOS)
in vivo situational exposure
in vivo stereological assessment
in vivo technique
inability to function independently
inactivation
functional hippocampal i.
X i.
inactivator
electrocerebral i.
inactivity
behavioral i.
electrocerebral i. (ECI)
inadequate
i. impulse control
i. stimulus
i. therapy
inanimate learning device
inappropriate verbalizing
inattention
sensory i.
visual i.
inborn
i. error of metabolism
i. reflex
Inc.
Orthopedic Systems, I. (OSI)
incapacitating drowsiness
incarceration
cauda equina i.
incentive system
incerta
zona i.
incidence
age-specific cumulative i.
aneurysm i.
myelopathy i.
nonunion i.
incidental
i. aneurysm
i. dual pathology
i. durotomy
i. image
i. punctate white matter hyperintensity
incident dementia
incipient downward central brain herniation
incision
battledore i.
bifrontal i.
Brunner modified i.
Caldwell-Luc i.
circumscribing i.
coronal scalp i.
C-shaped i.
curved i.
deltoid-splitting i.
dural i.
elliptical i.
exploratory i.
eyebrow i.
hemitransfixion i.
horseshoe i.
Kocher collar i.
laterally convex dural i.
lateral rhinotomy i.
Lynch i.
Mayfield i.
midline i.
muscle-splitting i.
Naffziger straight midline i.
palatal mucosal i.
posterolateral costotransversectomy i.
question mark-shaped i.
right-sided submandibular transverse i.
S i.
scalp i.
skin i.
standard retroperitoneal flank i.
straight i.
tangential i.
transcortical i.
transverse i.
T-shaped i.
vertical midline i.
V-shaped i.
Weber-Fergusson i.
webspace i.
Y i.
incisional neuroma
incisive plexus
incisura, pl. **incisurae**
i. cerebelli anterior
i. cerebelli posterior
impressio petrosa pallii i.
i. jugularis ossis occipitalis
i. jugularis ossis temporalis
i. preoccipitalis
tentorial i.
i. tentorii
i. tentorii cerebelli

NOTES

incisural
i. dissection
i. space
incisure
Lanterman i.
Lanterman-Schmidt i.
occipital bone-jugular i.
preoccipital i.
Schmidt-Lanterman i.
temporal bone-jugular i.
tentorial i.
i. of tentorium of cerebellum
inclusion
i. body
i. body encephalitis
i. body myopathy
i. body myositis
i. cell disease
cytoplasmic i.
glial cytoplasmic i.
intracellular lipid i.
intraneuronal i.
i. lipoma
Pick i.
i. tumor
incomplete
i. alexia
i. band heterotopia
i. neurofibromatosis
i. neurologic injury
i. spinal cord injury
i. upper airway obstruction
incomplete-sentence test
inconsistent response
incontinence
emotional i.
urinary i.
incontinentia
i. pigmenti
i. pigmenti achromians
increase
differential i.
head position in intracranial pressure i.
intracranial pressure i.
mannitol in intracranial pressure i.
metabolic i.
increased
i. intracranial pressure
i. platelet membrane fluidity
i. rapid eye movement latency
i. signal
i. speech
i. Wormian bone
incremental response
incudis
fossa i.
incudostapedial
i. disruption
i. joint
indapamide
independence
loss of i.
independence-dependence
field i.-d.
independently
inability to function i.
Inderal LA
Inderide
index, pl. **indices, indexes**
ADL i.
alpha i.
ankle-brachial i.
anterior horn i.
apnea i. (AI)
apnea-hypopnea i. (AHI)
Ayala i.
Barthel I.
body mass i. (BMI)
brain perfusion i. (BPI)
breath-holding i. (BHI)
cardiac risk i.
cephalorrhachidian i.
cerebrospinal i.
cervical curvature i.
Chippaux-Smirak arch i.
composite i.
Convery polyarticular disability i.
cut-flow i. (CFI)
delayed recall i.
desaturation i. (DI)
i. of difficulty (ID)
Doppler pulsatility i.
dynamic gait i.
Evans i.
Facial Disability I.
i. of forecasting efficiency
Fourier pulsatility i.
Functional Status I.
general memory i.
global distress i.
gnathic i.
Gosling pulsatility i.
Hauser ambulation i.
hypothermic metabolic i.
K i.
Katz ADL I.
Keitel i.
Kenny ADL i.
Klaus height i.
labeling i.
lateralization i.
Life Satisfaction I.
Life Skills Profile i.
Lucas and Drucker Motor I.
lumbar spine i. (LSI)

McDowell Impairment I.
Mean Ambulation I.
memory i.
modified Barthel I.
Motricity I.
National Death I.
neurocognitive i.
neuroendocrine i.
Northwick Park Index of Independence in ADL i.
organism-specific antibody i.
overall risk i.
oxygen desaturation i. (ODI)
PICA i.
pipe stemming of ankle-brachial i.
Pittsburgh Sleep Quality I.
PLMS i.
poststress ankle/arm Doppler i.
pressure-volume i.
pulsatility i.
radiological pressure-volume i.
Rankin Disability I.
Reintegration to Normal Living I.
respiratory arousal i. (RAI)
respiratory disturbance i. (RDI)
resting ankle/arm Doppler i.
Ritchie i.
Rivermead ADL i.
Rivermead Mobility I.
RNL i.
Spinal Cord Motor Index and Sensory Indices
steal i.
Symptom Checklist 90-Revised Global Severity I.
TCD pulsatility i.

India ink
Indiana tome carpal tunnel release system
Indiana-type familial amyloid polyneuropathy
Indian variant lipofuscinosis
indicator
finger i.
sensor position i.
sleep position i. (SPI)

indices (*pl. of* index)
indifference to pain syndrome
indifferent electrode
indigo carmine
indigotin disulfonate sodium
indinavir
indirect
i. fracture
i. genetic transmission
i. mechanism
i. probe
i. reflex
i. striatopallidal pathway

indiscriminate lesion
indium cisternogram
indium-diethylene triamine pentaacetic acid study
indium-111 octreotide scintigraphy
individual
high-functioning autistic i.
I.'s with Disabilities Education Act (IDEA)

Indochron E-R capsule
indolamine function
indomethacin-responsive headache syndrome
indomethacin-sensitive headache
induced
i. aphasia
i. factitious symptom
i. hypocapnic central apnea

inducer
angiogenic i.

induction
neural i.

InDura intrathecal catheter and pump
indusium griseum
ineffective communication pattern
inequality
ventilation/perfusion i.

Inerpan flexible burn dressing
inertia
excessive sleep i.
sleep i.
i. time

inescapable pain
inexact fiducial
inexorable decline
In-Exsufflator respiratory device
infancy
diencephalic syndrome of i.
familial autosomal recessive idiopathic myoclonic epilepsy of i.
heterotopic interstitial neuropathy of i.
melanotic neuroectodermal tumor of i. (MNTI)

NOTES

infancy *(continued)*
myoclonic epilepsy of i.
spongy degeneration of i.
infant
hydrocephalic i.
i. muscle tone
i. REM sleep
i. sleep staging
i. spine elasticity
i. spine mobility
traction response of i.
infantile
i. acid maltase deficiency
i. amnesia
i. autism
i. beriberi
i. bilateral striatal necrosis
i. botulism
i. convulsion
i. diplegia
i. ganglioglioma
i. Gaucher disease
i. GM2 gangliosidosis
i. hemangioblastic hemangioma
i. hemiplegia
i. hydrocephalus
i. jerk myoclonus
i. lipofuscinosis
i. multisystem inflammatory disease
i. myofibrillar myopathy
i. myofibromatosis
i. neuroaxonal dystrophy
i. neuronal ceroid lipofuscinosis
i. neuronal degeneration
i. neuropathy
i. progressive spinal muscular atrophy
i. Refsum disease
i. spasm
i. spastic paraplegia
i. subacute necrotizing encephalopathy
i. tetany
i. tremor syndrome
i. X-linked ataxia
i. X-linked deafness
infantile-onset spinocerebellar ataxia
infantilis
diataxia cerebralis i.
poliodystrophia cerebri progressiva i.
progressiva i.
infant-onset epilepsy
infantum
roseola i.
infarction
acute cerebral i.
anterior communicating artery distribution i.
arteriolar i.
atherosclerotic i.
bicerebral i.
bilateral occipital i.'s
bilateral upper brainstem i.'s
borderzone i.
brain i.
brainstem i.
calcarine cortex i.
capsular i.
cerebellar artery i.
cerebral artery i.
cerebrovascular i.
cortical i.
cryptogenic i.
cystic lacunar i.
i. dementia
dominant hemisphere i.
embolic i.
Freiberg so-called i.
frontal lobe i.
gyral i.
hemispheric i.
hemorrhagic i.
hippocampal i.
inferolateral i.
ischemic brainstem i.
ischemic cerebral i.
labyrinthine i.
lacunar brain i.
large artery i.
large vessel i.
medium vessel i.
medullary i.
mesencephalic i.
midbrain i.
migraine-induced i.
migrainous i.
multiple cortical i.'s
myocardial i.
neonatal cerebral i.
nonembolic i.
nonseptic embolic brain i.
occipital lobe i.
optic nerve i.
paramedian i.
parietooccipital i.
perinatal trauma i.
photochemically induced graded spinal cord i.
photothrombotic i.
pituitary i.
pontine i.
posterior cerebral territory i.
putaminal i.
retinal i.
right frontoparietal i.
silent i.
small centrum ovale i.

small deep recent i.
small lacunar i.
small penetrator i. (SPI)
small vessel i.
spinal cord i.
striatocapsular i.
subacute cerebral i.
subcortical i.
subendocardial myocardial i.
temporal lobe i.
thalamic i.
thalamopeduncular i.
tuberothalamic i.
uncal i.
ventral pontine i.
vertebrobasilar i.
i. volume
watershed zone i.
white matter i.

infarct-like lesion

infection

Acanthamoeba i.
acute purulent meningitis i.
amebic i.
arenavirus i.
bacterial i.
baculovirus i.
Campylobacter jejuni i.
Candida i.
central nervous system influenza virus i.
cerebral malaria i.
cestode i.
chronic spinal epidural i.
chronic spinal intradural i.
closed disc space i.
clostridial i.
Coccidioides i.
congenital cytomegalovirus i.
congenital herpes simplex virus i.
Coxiella burnetii i.
cryptococcal i.
Cryptococcus i.
cryptogenic i.
cysticercal i.
disc space i.
enteric virus i.
enterovirus i.
epidural i.
extradural i.
extrameningeal tuberculous i.
fever caused by i. (FI)
focal i.
fungal i.
helminthic i.
herpesvirus i. type 6, 7
herpes zoster virus i.
Histoplasma i.
human immunodeficiency virus i.
intervertebral disc space i.
latent i.
Legionella pneumophila i.
leprosy i.
Lyssavirus i.
lytic i.
meningeal i.
mosquito bite i.
Mucor i.
Mycobacterium tuberculosis i.
Mycoplasma i.
mycotic i.
myxovirus i.
Naegleria i.
nematode i.
neonatal enterovirus i.
neonatal herpes simplex virus i.
nervous system i.
nosocomial i.
odontogenic i.
ophthalmic zoster i.
opportunistic CNS i.
orthomyxovirus i.
parainfluenza virus i.
paramyxovirus i.
parasitic i.
paraspinal i.
Phycomycetes rhizopus i.
pneumococcal i.
poliomyelitis i.
poliovirus i.
postoperative i.
i. prevention
protozoan i.
Q fever i.
retrovirus i.
rhabdovirus i.
Rhizopus i.
rickettsial i.
roseola i.
rubella i.
scalp i.
Shigella dysenteriae i.
slow virus i.
spinal cord i.

NOTES

infection *(continued)*
spirochetal i.
staphylococcal i.
streptococcal i.
syphilis i.
togavirus i.
toxocariasis i.
trematode i.
trichinosis i.
trypanosomiasis i.
tuberculosis i.
valve i.
varicella zoster virus i.
ventriculostomy-related i.
viral i.
Western equine encephalitis virus i.
zoster virus i.

infection-related neuropathy

infectious
i. aneurysm
i. chorea
i. complication
i. hepatitis peripheral neuropathy
i. meningitis
i. mononucleosis
i. ophthalmoplegia
i. polyneuritis
i. polyneuritis syndrome
i. retinopathy

infectiva
polioencephalitis i.

inferior
i. anastomotic vein
i. aperture of axillary fossa
area vestibularis i.
i. basal vein
i. cerebellar artery
i. cerebellar peduncle
i. cerebral surface
i. cerebral vein
i. cervical ganglion
i. choroid plexus
i. choroid vein
colliculus i.
complexus olivaris i.
i. dental nerve
i. extradural approach
fasciculus longitudinalis i.
fasciculus occipitofrontalis i.
i. fovea
i. frontal convolution
i. frontal gyrus
i. frontal sulcus
i. ganglion of glossopharyngeal nerve
i. ganglion of vagus nerve
gyrus frontalis i.
gyrus temporalis i.
i. horn
i. horn of lateral ventricle
i. laryngeal nerve
lobulus parietalis i.
lobulus semilunaris i.
i. longitudinal fasciculus
i. longitudinal sinus
macula cribrosa i.
i. medullary velum
i. mesenteric ganglion
i. nasal colliculus
nervus cardiacus cervicalis i.
nervus cutaneous brachii lateralis i.
nervus gluteus i.
nevus alveolus i.
nucleus olivaris i.
nucleus salivarius i.
nucleus salivatorius i.
nucleus vestibularis i.
i. occipital gyrus
i. occipitofrontal fasciculus
oliva i.
i. olivary complex
i. olivary nucleus
i. olive
i. orbital fissure
i. orbitofrontal complex
i. parietal gyrus
i. parietal lobule
i. parietal region
i. part of vestibulocochlear nerve
pedunculus cerebellaris i.
pedunculus thalami i.
i. periventricular white matter
i. petrosal ganglion
i. petrosal sinus
plexus dentalis i.
plexus hypogastricus i.
plexus mesentericus i.
plexus rectalis i.
i. polioencephalitis
i. pontine syndrome
i. prefrontal cortex
i. quadrigeminal brachium
i. rectus muscle
i. root of ansa cervicalis
i. root of cervical loop
i. root of vestibulocochlear nerve
i. sagittal sinus
i. salivary nucleus
i. semilunar lobule
sinus petrosus i.
sinus sagittalis i.
sulcus frontalis i.
sulcus temporalis i.
i. surface of cerebellar hemisphere
i. syndrome of red nucleus
tela choroidea i.
i. temporal convolution
i. temporal cortex

i. temporal gyrus
i. temporal sulcus
i. thalamic peduncle
i. thalamic radiation
i. thalamostriate vein
i. thyroid plexus
i. transvermian approach
i. vein of cerebellar hemisphere
i. vein of vermis
vena anastomotica i.
i. vena cava
vena choroidea i.
vena ventricularis i.
vena vermis i.
ventral posterior i. (VPI)
i. ventricular vein
i. vertebra
i. vestibular area
i. vestibular nucleus

inferiore
ramus communicans nervi laryngei superioris cum nervo laryngeo i.

inferiores
nervi anales i.
nervi clunium i.
nervi rectales i.
nuclei olivares i.
rami clunium i.
rami gluteales i.
venae cerebri i.
venae hemispherii cerebelli i.
venae thalamostriatae i.

inferioris
brachium colliculi i.
commissura colliculi i.
hilum nuclei olivaris i.
nuclei colliculi i.
nucleus linearis i.
nucleus reticularis intermedius pontis i.
pars opercularis gyri frontalis i.
pars orbitalis gyri frontalis i.
pars triangularis gyri frontalis i.
rami dentales inferiores plexus dentalis i.
rami gingivales inferiores plexus dentalis i.
vellus olivae i.

inferius
brachium quadrigeminum i.
cornu i.
ganglion cervicale i.
ganglion mesentericum i.
velum medullare i.

inferofrontal fissure

inferolateral
i. endonasal transsphenoidal approach
i. infarction
i. pontine artery

inferolateralis
margo i.

infiltrating
i. spinal angiolipoma
i. tumor

infiltration
hematogenous cell i.
perineural i.

InFix interbody fusion system

inflammation
arterial i.
cartilage i.
ear cartilage i.
ischemic ocular i.
lipopolysaccharide-induced i.
neurogenic i. (NI)
perivenular i.
spinal cord i.

inflammation-induced cell injury

inflammatory
i. cytokine
i. demyelinating disease
i. demyelinating neuropathy
i. demyelinating optic neuritis
i. demyelinating polyneuropathy (IDP)
i. demyelinating polyradiculoneuropathy
i. diabetic vasculopathy
i. lesion
i. myopathy
i. response

inflexibility
postural i.

infliximab-treated patient

inflow effect

influence
environmental i.
vestibulospinal i.

influenza
i. A antibody
i. A pandemic
i. virus myositis

NOTES

influenzae
Haemophilus i.
Haemophilus i. b
influenzal encephalitis
infolding
Informant
I. Awareness Score
I. Questionnaire on Cognitive Decline in the Elderly
information
afferent thermosensory i.
biochemical i.
i. processing
release of i.
sensory i.
i. technology
thermosensory i.
verbal i.
infracalcarine gyrus
infraclinoid aneurysm
infradian rhythm
infragranular
i. layer
i. region
infranuclear
i. lesion
i. paralysis
i. weakness
infraorbital
i. canal
i. injection
i. nerve
i. plexus
infraorbitalis
nervus i.
rami labiales superiores nervi i.
rami nasales externi nervi i.
rami nasales interni nervi i.
rami palpebrales inferiores nervi i.
infrared
i. digitizer
i. light-reflecting sphere
i. reflection oculography
i. thermography (IRT)
i. videosomnography
infraspinatus reflex
infraspinous fascia
infrastriate layer
infratemporal
i. approach
i. fossa (ITF)
i. fossa tumor
i. hematoma
infratentorial
i. arteriovenous malformation
i. compartment
i. lateral supracellular approach
i. lesion
i. Lindau tumor
i. neoplastic syndrome
i. neurological tumor
i. region
i. structural syndrome
i. supracerebellar
i. venous drainage
infratrochlearis
nervus i.
rami palpebrales nervi i.
infratrochlear nerve
infundibula (*pl. of* infundibulum)
infundibular
i. body
i. dilation
i. part
i. part of anterior lobe of hypophysis
i. recess
i. stalk
i. stem
infundibularis
nucleus i.
pars i.
recessus i.
infundibuli
recessus i.
infundibuloma
infundibulotubular region
infundibulum, pl. **infundibula**
aditus ad i.
i. hypothalami
hypothalamic i.
iter ad i.
i. lobi posterioris hypophyseos
i. neurohypophyseos
Infusaid M400 constant-flow pump
infusion
brain i.
brain-heart i. (BHI)
i. computed tomography
continuous extravascular i. (CEI)
continuous intrathecal baclofen i.
continuous intravenous i.
diastole-phased pulsatile i.
etomidate-propylene glycol i.
intraparenchymal i.
intraventricular i.
propofol i.
i. pump
Inge
I. cervical lamina spreader
I. laminectomy retractor
I. laminectomy spreader
ingestion
buckthorn i.
ingravescent apoplexy
ingrowth
neuronal i.

inguinal
  i. freckling
  i. reflex
inhalation
  i. anthrax
  CO_2 i.
  oxygen i.
  xenon i.
inherent contrast
inheritance
  autosomal dominant i.
  autosomal recessive i.
  maternal i.
  mendelian i.
inherited
  i. ataxia
  i. global neurodegenerative disorder
  i. neuropathy
inhibited response
inhibition
  collagenase i.
  complement fixation i.
  dopaminergic i.
  GABAergic i.
  $GABA_B$ receptor-mediated i.
  GABAR-mediated i.
  horizontal i.
  mediated neuronal i.
  paired-pulse i.
  pervasive i.
  reflexive saccade i.
  saccade i.
  short-interval intracortical i. (SICI)
  Wedensky i.
inhibitor
  acetyl cholinesterase i.
  angiogenic i.
  batimastat protease i.
  calcineurin i.
  calpain i.
  carbonic anhydrase i.
  caspase i.
  catechol-methyltransferase i.
  catechol-*O*-methyltransferase i.
  cholinesterase i.
  COMT i.
  converting enzyme i. (CEI)
  COX-2 i.
  cyclooxygenase i.
  cysteine protease i.
  cytokine i.
  dopa decarboxylase i.
  endothelial cell i.
  epidermal growth factor-tyrosine kinase i.
  excitatory amino acid receptor i.
  excitotoxin i.
  farnesyl transferase i.
  growth factor i.
  5-HT reuptake i.
  marimastat protease i.
  matrix metalloproteinase i.
  metalloprotease i.
  monoamine oxidase i. (MAOI)
  monoamine oxidase-B i.
  NOS i.
  peptide i.
  plasminogen activator i.
  polyamine biosynthesis i.
  protease i.
  protein kinase C i.
  reductase i.
  SAM i.
  selective norepinephrine reuptake i.
  selective phosphodiesterase i.
  selective serotonin reuptake i. (SSRI)
  serotonin norepinephrine reuptake i.
  signal transduction i.
  Src i.
  thromboxane synthase i.
  tissue factor pathway i.
  xanthine oxidase i.
inhibitory
  i. amino acid
  i. effect
  i. fiber
  i. ganglion
  i. loop
  i. nerve
  i. neurotransmitter
  i. postsynaptic current
  i. postsynaptic potential (IPSP)
  i. protein
  i. regulatory input
  i. synapse
  i. transmitter
  i. virus
inhomogeneity
  field i.
iniencephaly
inion
initial
  i. segment

NOTES

initial *(continued)*
i. spoken language impairment
i. stage
i. stress reaction
i. upward deflection
initiative
Parkinson Research The Organized Genetic I. (PROGENI)
injected dose per liter (IDPL)
injection
Adlone I.
A-methaPred I.
AquaMEPHYTON I.
botulinum toxin i.
Calciferol I.
Calcimar I.
Campath i.
Carnitor I.
cervical epidural steroid i.
Cibacalcin I.
conjunctival i.
Cytoxan I.
depMedalone I.
Depoject I.
Depo-Medrol I.
Depopred I.
D.H.E. 45 I.
Diazemuls I.
D-Med I.
Enlon I.
epidural steroid i.
etomidate i.
extradural i.
facet i.
fluoroscopically guided i.
focal stereotactic i.
freehand i.
imipenem-cilastatin i.
infraorbital i.
i. injury
intraarterial i.
intrahippocampal i.
intraneural phenol i.
intratumoral i.
intraventricular i.
Konakion I.
long-acting i.
Mestinon I.
Metastron I.
Miacalcin I.
M-Prednisol I.
Neosar I.
nerve root i.
Osteocalcin I.
paramagnetic contrast i.
prolotherapy i.
Regonol I.
Relefact TRH i.
retrobulbar i.
retrogasserian i.
Reversol I.
saline i.
Salmonine I.
stereotactic intracystic i.
sumatriptan succinate i.
Tensilon I.
THAM I.
THAM-E I.
Ureaphil I.
injured brain
injury
acceleration extension i.
accidental i.
acquired brain i. (ABI)
acute burst i.
acute central cervical spinal cord i.
anoxic i.
avulsion i.
axonal i.
axonal shearing i.
axonotmetic i.
birth i.
birth-related spinal cord i.
brachial plexus avulsion i.
brain i.
brainstem i. (BSI)
Brief Test of Head I.
burner i.
burst i.
cerebral anoxic-ischemic i.
cerebral perinatal i.
cervical nerve root i.
cervical spinal column i.
cervical spine i.
chemical i.
chronic constrictive i. (CCI)
closed brain i. (CBI)
closed head i.
cold i.
2-column cervical spine i.
3-column cervical spine i.
common iliac artery i.
contrecoup i.
craniocerebral missile i.
craniocervical junction i.
crush i.
current of i.
diffuse axonal i. (DAI)
diffuse brain i.
diffuse white matter shearing i.
discoligamentous i.
distractive flexion i.
diving spinal cord i.
electrical i.
endothelial i.
epileptogenic brain i.
Erb i.
Erb-Duchenne-Klumpke i.

excitotoxic neuronal cell i.
extension i.
extension-type cervical spine i.
facial nerve i.
flexion i.
flexion-distraction i.
flexion-extension i.
flexion-extension-mediated i.
fluid percussion head i.
focal cerebral head i.
forceful flexion i.
Fränkel classification of spinal cord i.
global ischemic neuronal i.
head i.
hemorrhagic shearing i.
hepatic i.
high cervical cord i.
hyperextension-hyperflexion i.
hyperglycemia-induced neuronal i.
hypoxic-ischemic i.
iliac artery i.
incomplete neurologic i.
incomplete spinal cord i.
inflammation-induced cell i.
injection i.
i. of intervertebral disc
ischemic i.
kainic acid-induced focal i.
laryngeal nerve i.
lightning i.
LSUMC classification of nerve i.
lumbar spine i.
lumbosacral spine plexus i.
mechanism of i.
middle column i.
mild head i.
minor head i. (MHI)
missile i.
i. morphology
multilobar i.
multiple impact i.'s
neonatal i.
nerve root i.
neural i.
neurologic i.
neuronal i.
old nerve i.
open head i.
optic nerve i.
oxidative cellular i.
oxygen radical-induced cellular i.
parasagittal cerebral i.
parasympathetic nerve i.
past head i.
pediatric spinal column i.
pediatric spinal cord i.
penetrating brain i.
penetrating spinal i.
perinatal obturator nerve i.
peripheral nerve i.
permanent i.
phrenic nerve i.
physical i.
postnatal i.
i. potential
quadriplegic i.
radiation i.
radical induced brain i.
repetitive motion i. (RMI)
retraction i.
rotational i.
rotationally induced shear-strain i.
secondary brain i.
seventh nerve i.
severe head i.
i. severity assessment
i. severity scale
i. severity score
shearing i.
skeletal muscle i.
soft tissue i.
i. spike
spinal cord i. (SCI)
sports-related spinal i.
stable cervical spine i.
stinger i.
suction i.
thoracic duct i.
thoracic spine i.
thoracolumbar spine flexion-distraction i.
tracheal i.
traction-type i.
transient plexus i.
transventricular i.
traumatic brain i. (TBI)
ureter i.
vascular i.
vena cava i.
vertebral artery i.
vertebral column i.
i. of war

NOTES

injury *(continued)*
whiplash i.
Wilbrand knee i.
ink
India i.
inlet
thoracic i.
in-line telesensor
innate reflex
inner
i. band of Baillarger
i. cone fiber
i. limiting layer
i. line of Baillarger
i. nuclear layer
i. plexiform layer
i. sheath of optic nerve
i. world
innervate
innervation
adrenergic i.
anomalous i.
i. apraxia
compensatory i.
median nerve i.
reciprocal i.
rudimentary sympathetic i.
innervatory
i. apraxia
i. dyspraxia
innominata
substantia i.
innominate
i. angiogram
i. artery
i. substance
i. vein
Innovative Magnetic Resonance Imaging System
INO
internuclear ophthalmoplegia
inoculation
intracerebral i.
inoperable tumor
iNOS
isoform of NO synthase
stressed-induced iNOS
inositol
i. triphosphate
i. 1,4,5-triphosphate (IP_3)
inotropic component
INPH
idiopathic normal-pressure hydrocephalus
in-phase
i.-p. deflection
i.-p. image
input
afferent i.
arterial plasma i.
behavioral i.
cerebral sensory i.
cholinergic i.
cortical i.
emotional i.
hypothalamic regulatory i.
inhibitory regulatory i.
phonetic i.
regulatory i.
vestibulospinal i.
INR
international normalized ratio
insane
general paresis of i.
insaniens
chorea i.
insecticide peripheral neuropathy
inserter
Texas Scottish Rite Hospital hook i.
insertion
C-D rod i.
i. equipment
oblique screw i.
pedicle screw i.
screw i.
sphenoidal electrode i.
Syracuse anterior I-plate i.
insertional activity
insertion/deletion polymorphism
inside-out signaling
insomnia
alcohol-induced i.
altitude i.
i. assessment tool
i. categories of subtypes
chronic i.
conditioned i.
dementia i.
dementia-related i.
depression-related chronic i.
drug-induced i.
epilepsy i.
familial fatal i.
fatal familial i. (FFI)
food allergy i.
hypertension with i.
hypnotic-dependent i.
idiopathic i.
imagery training for persistent primary i.
long-term i.
medication-induced i.
meditation for i.
mood disorder with chronic i.
neurologic illness i.
nicotine-induced i.
nocturnal i.
persistent primary i.

posttraumatic i.
primary i.
psychophysiologic i.
psychophysiological i.
rebound i.
recurrent i.
secondary i.
short-term i.
sleep initiation i.
sleep maintenance i.
subjective i.
terminal i.
transient i.
i. treatment
i. with steroids

insomnia-related panic disorder

inspiratory
i. center
i. gasping
i. positive airway pressure (IPAP)

instability
adjacent i.
atlantoaxial i.
autonomic i.
cervical spine atlantoaxial i.
clinical i.
emotional i.
endplate i.
fixation i.
high-gain i.
iatrogenic i.
lumbar spine i.
occipitoatlantoaxial i.
occipitocervical i.
phase i.
postural i.
sagittal plane i.
single-level ligamentous i.
spinal i.
vasomotor i.
vertebral cervical i.

instantaneous axotomy

instant scan

Instat fibrin film

InstaTrak
I. guidance system
I. headset

instillation procedure

instrument
Accurate Surgical and Scientific I.'s (ASSI)
Backlund stereotactic i.
i. calibration matrix
20-channel Beckman EEG i.
Clarke stereotactic i.
Cloward i.
Craig vertebral body biopsy i.
digitized i.
Dwyer i.
Evershears surgical i.
Gamma knife i.
Hemorrhagic Stroke-Specific Quality of Life I. (HSQuale)
Hermann Brain Dominance I.
Hulka i.
interspinous segmental spinal i.
Kloehn craniofacial i.
Malis bipolar i.
micro-Doppler i.
Micro-Three microsurgery i.
i. migration
Millet neurological test i.
model TC2-64B pulsed-range gated Doppler i.
Nicolet Compass EMG i.
pencil-grip i.
personality disorder i.
pistol-grip i.
primer i.
pulsed-range gated Doppler i.
Radionics bipolar i.
rating i.
Richmond subarachnoid screw i.
Ruggles Surgical I.
solid-state i.
spark-gap i.
SpeedReducer i.
spinal distraction i.
stereotactic i.
Ware i.
WHO i.
Yasargil i.
Yasargil-Aesculap i.
Zielke i.

instrumental
i. act
i. activities of daily living (IADL)
i. ADL
i. amusia
i. function deficit

instrumentalism

instrumentation
anterior distraction i.

NOTES

instrumentation *(continued)*
anterior-posterior fusion with segmental spinal i.
AO fixateur interne i.
AO notched i.
C-D i.
compression U-rod i.
Cotrel-Dubousset pedicle screw i.
Cotrel-Dubousset spinal i.
distraction i.
double Zielke i.
dynamic compression plate i.
Edwards i.
i. failure
Gellman i.
Harrington rod i.
interspinous segmental spinal i.
Isola i.
Jacobs locking hook spinal rod i.
Kambin i.
Kaneda anterior spinal i.
Louis i.
lumbar spine i.
lumbosacral spine transpedicular i.
Luque II segmental spinal i.
Luque semirigid segmental spinal i.
modular i.
Moss-Miami spinal i.
posterior cervical spinal i.
posterior distraction i.
posterior hook-rod spinal i.
rod-sleeve i.
sacral spine modular i.
sacral spine Universal i.
segmental spinal i. (SSI)
spinal i.
Steffee i.
stereotactic i.
Texas Scottish Rite Hospital i.
transpedicular spinal i.
TSRH i.
universal i.
variable screw placement system i.
VSP plate i.
Zielke i.
Z-plate anterior thoracolumbar i.

insufficiency
adrenal i.
adrenocortical i.
anterior pituitary i.
aortic i.
convergence i.
divergence i.
mechanical i.
muscular i.
parathyroid i.
renal i.
respiratory i.
testicular i.
vertebrobasilar i.

insufficient
i. sleep
i. sleep syndrome

insufflation
cranial i.

insula, pl. **insulae**
central sulcus of i.
circular sulcus of i.
gyri breves i.
gyrus longus i.
limen i.
lobus i.
long gyrus of i.
i. operculum
i. of Reil
short gyrus of i.
sulcus centralis i.
sulcus circularis i.
sulcus limitans of i.

insular
i. area
i. cistern
i. cortex
i. cortex tissue
i. epilepsy
i. gyrus
i. lobe
i. sclerosis
i. threshold
i. vein

insulares
venae i.

insularis
lobus i.
pars i.

insulated electrode needle

insulin
i. coma treatment
i. effect
i. growth factor
i. hypoglycemia test
i. shock treatment

insulinlike growth factor (IGF)

insult
brain i.
brief ischemic i.
CNS i.
hypoxic-ischemic i.
intraoperative neural i.
ischemic i.
perinatal unilateral cerebral ischemic i.
putative i.

insult-induced neuronal damage

intact
cognitively i.
i. reading skill

i. spinous lamina
i. spinous process
intake
caloric i.
integral
Boundary Shift I. (BSI)
i. membrane glycoprotein
i. role
Integra Selector ultrasonic aspiration
integrated
i. ECT system
i. headholder
i. sideport access portal
integration
Beery developmental test of visuomotor i.
integrative
i. approach
i. problem
integrity
electrophysiologic i.
ligamentous i.
motor neuron i.
physical i.
intellect
compromised i.
intellectual
i. ability
i. aphasia
i. aura
i. deficiency
i. exercise
i. function
i. function deficit
i. functioning
i. impairment
intelligence
i. quotient (IQ)
social i.
intense
i. energy
i. vascularity
intensification
image i.
intensifier
image i.
OEC-Diasonics mobile C-arm image i.
intensity
pairwise i.
i. of trauma
intensity-modulated radiation therapy
intensive
i. care unit (ICU)
i. motor activity
Intensol
Diazepam I.
intention
motor i.
i. myoclonus
i. spasm
i. tremor
intentional visually guided saccade
intent rating
intent-to-treat analysis
interacting cytokine
interaction
amygdala-prefrontal cortex-locus ceruleus i.
differential i.
dipole-dipole i.
electron-coupled nuclear spin-spin i.
glial neuronal i.
harmonious i.
neurochemical i.
pharmacodynamic i.
pharmacokinetic i.
physicochemical i.
posture i.
i. process analysis
protein binding i.
proton-electron dipole-dipole i.
social i.
state-trait i.
interactive
i. effect
i. voice response system
interannular segment
interarticularis
pars i.
interbody
i. fusion
i. graft
intercalary neuron
intercalated nucleus
intercalation
intercalatus
nucleus i.
intercavernous sinus
intercellular
i. collagen
i. matrix
intercerebral

NOTES

interclinoid
i. fold
i. ligament
intercolumnar tubercle
interconnected cerebral region
intercostal
i. artery
i. artery angiogram
i. muscle weakness
i. nerve
i. nerve nucleus
i. neuralgia
intercostales
nervi i.
intercostalis
rami mammarii laterales rami cutanei lateralis pectoralis nervi i.
rami mammarii mediales rami cutanei anterioris pectoralis nervi i.
ramus cutaneus anterior abdominalis nervi i.
ramus cutaneus anterior pectoralis nervi i.
ramus cutaneus lateralis abdominalis nervi i.
ramus cutaneus lateralis pectoralis nervi i.
intercostalium
rami musculares nervi nervorum i.
intercostobrachiales
nervi i.
intercostobrachial nerve
intercrural
i. fissure
i. ganglion
i. space
interdigital
i. neuritis
i. transfer
interdural tumor
interelectrode
interest
region of i. (ROI)
restricted i.
volume of i.
voxel of i. (VOI)
interface
air-brain i.
long-term bone-instrumentation i.
motor i.
sensory i.
interfacet wiring and fusion
interfascial approach
interfascicular
i. fasciculus
i. graft
i. neuroglia
interfascicularis
fasciculus i. (FI)
interference
electromagnetic i. (EMI)
ipsilateral visuospatial i.
interferon (IFN)
alpha i.
i. beta-1a
i. beta-1b
interferon-B
interferon gamma (IFN-G)
interfibrillary migration
InterFix RP threaded spinal fusion cage device
interforniceal approach
interganglionic
intergemmal nerve fiber
intergyral
interhemicerebral
interhemispheric
i. cyst
i. fissure
i. hematoma
i. propagation time
i. synchrony
interictal
i. behavior
i. behavior change
i. behavior syndrome
i. bisynchronous discharge
i. complex
i. data
i. EEG
i. EEG activity
i. electroencephalogram
i. epileptic personality
i. epileptiform abnormality
i. epileptiform activity
i. epileptiform spike
i. focal epileptiform discharge
i. generalized spike-and-wave discharge
i. hypometabolism
i. pattern
i. period
i. personality change
i. phenomenon
i. physiologic dysfunction
i. sharp wave
i. spike discharge
interior band of Baillarger
interlaminar
i. clamp
i. decompression
interleukin (IL)
i. beta
interleukin-1–15
interlimb coordination deficit
interlocking gyrus

intermaxillary fixation
intermedia
i. adenohypophyseos
area hypothalamica i.
columna i.
ganglia i.
massa i.
pars i.
regio hypothalamica i.
stria cochlearis i.
intermediae
nucleus dorsomedialis hypothalamicae i.
intermediary nerve
intermediate
i. acoustic stria
i. brain syndrome due to alcohol
i. C-D hook
i. cervical septum
i. column
i. column of spinal cord
i. ganglion
i. gray zone
i. head fixator
i. hemispheric dynamic
i. hypothalamic area
i. hypothalamic region
i. layer
i. mass
i. nerve
i. part
i. part of adenohypophysis
i. spinal muscular atrophy
i. white layer of superior colliculus
i. zone of spinal cord
intermedii
nervi supraclaviculares i.
rami temporales i.
intermediolateral
i. cell column
i. cell column of spinal cord
i. mesencephalic syndrome
i. nucleus
i. tract
intermediolateralis
nucleus i.
intermediomedialis
nucleus i.
ramus frontalis i.
intermediomedial nucleus
intermedium
septum cervicale i.
stratum griseum i.
stratum medullare i.
intermedius
nervus cutaneous dorsalis i.
nucleus linearis i.
nucleus ventralis i.
ventralis i.
intermeningeal space
intermesentericus
plexus i.
intermittent
i. acute porphyria (IAP)
i. cramp
i. double-step gait
i. explosive disorder
i. focal slowing
i. myoclonus epilepsy
i. neurogenic claudication
i. photic stimulation
i. rhythmic delta activity (IRDA)
i. tetanus
i. torticollis
intermodal competition
interna
capsula i.
globus pallidus i.
hematorrhachis i.
hyperostosis frontalis i.
lamina pyramidalis i.
mediodorsal globus pallidus i.
ophthalmoplegia i.
pachymeningitis i.
protuberantia occipitalis i.
tabula i.
internae
crus anterius capsulae i.
crus posterius capsulae i.
fibrae arcuatae i.
genu capsulae i.
pars cervicalis arteriae carotidis i.
pars retrolentiformis capsulae i.
pars sublentiformis capsulae i.
pars thalamolenticularis capsulae i.
rami cruris posterioris capsulae i.
rami genus capsulae i.
rami partis retrolentiformis capsulae i.
stria laminae granularis i.
stria laminae pyramidalis i.
venae cerebri i.

NOTES

internal
i. acoustic meatus
i. architecture neuronal size
i. arcuate fiber
i. auditory canal
i. band of Baillarger
i. capsule
i. capsule anterior crus
i. capsule posterior crus
i. capsule syndrome
i. carotid angiogram
i. carotid artery (ICA)
i. carotid artery aneurysm
i. carotid artery balloon test occlusion
i. carotid balloon test
i. cerebral vein
i. circadian clock
i. corticotectal tract
i. decompression
i. disc herniation
i. fixation plate-screw system
i. fixation of spine
i. fixation spring
i. hydrocephalus
i. jugular vein
i. line of Baillarger
i. medullary lamina
i. meningitis
i. model
i. neurolysis
i. ophthalmoplegia
i. pillar cell
i. popliteal nerve
i. pulse generating unit
i. pyocephalus
i. representation
i. respiration
i. selection
i. sense
i. sheath of optic nerve
i. spinal fixation
I. State Scale
i. terminal filament
i. vertebral venous plexus

international
I. Classification of Epilepsies and Epileptic Syndromes
I. Classification of Impairments, Disabilities and Handicaps (ICIDH)
I. Classification of Seizures
I. Cooperative Ataxia Rating Scale
I. Cooperative Study on the Timing of Aneurysm Surgery
I. Headache Society (IHS)
Interpore Cross I.
I. League Against Epilepsy
i. normalized ratio (INR)
I. Rett Syndrome Association (IRSA)
I. Study of Unruptured Intracranial Aneurysm (ISUIA)
I. 10–20 system of electrode placement
I. Tremor Foundation
I. Working Formulation classification

interne
AO-ASIF fixateur i.
AO fixateur i.
Dick AO fixateur i.
fixateur i.

interneuron
GABAergic cortical i.

interneuronal calcium modulation

interni
crista transversa meatus acustici i.
nervus musculi obturatorii i.

interno
ramus communicans nervi laryngei inferioris cum ramo laryngeo i.

internodal
i. distance
i. length
i. segment

internodale
segmentum i.

internode

internorum
stratum segmentorum externorum et i.

internuclearis
ophthalmoplegia i.

internuclear ophthalmoplegia (INO)

internucleosomal DNA fragmentation

internum
corpus geniculatum i.
filum terminale i.
stratum limitans i.
stratum nucleare i.
stratum plexiforme i.

internuncial
i. fiber
i. neuron
i. pathway

internus
globus pallidus i. (GPi)
nervus caroticus i.
nervus obturatorius i.
plexus caroticus i.

interoceptive
i. cue
i. nervous system

interoceptor

interofective system

interolivary region

interoreceptive

interosseous branch of medial terminal branch of deep fibular nerve
interparietal sulcus
interpeak
i. delay
i. latency
interpeduncular
i. cistern
i. distance
i. fossa
i. fossa lesion
i. ganglion
i. nucleus
i. space
i. trigone
interpeduncularis
cisterna i.
fossa i.
nucleus i.
substantia perforata i.
interpleural analgesia (IPA)
interpolation algorithm
Interpore
I. Cross International
I. porous hydroxyapatite
interposed nucleus
interpositospinalis
tractus i.
interpositospinal tract
interpositum
velum i.
interpositus
nucleus i.
interpulse time
interradial plexus
interscalene triangle
interscapular reflex
intersegmental
i. aberration
i. covariation
i. fasciculus
i. fiber
i. reflex
intersemilunar fissure
intersemilunaris
fissura i.
interspace
ballooning of vertebral i.
cervical i.
i. collapse
lumbar i.
thoracic i.
interspike interval
interspinous
i. ligamentum
i. segmental spinal instrument
i. segmental spinal instrumentation
i. segmental spinal instrumentation technique
i. spacer device
interstimulus interval
interstitial
i. amygdaloid nucleus
i. brachytherapy
i. cell
i. collagenase
i. edema
i. hydrocephalic edema
i. neuritis
i. nucleus of anterior hypothalamus
i. nucleus of Cajal
i. nucleus of medial longitudinal fasciculus
i. polymyositis
i. radiation source
i. radiation therapy
i. radiotherapy
i. serotonin concentration
interstitialis
nucleus amygdalae i.
interstitiospinalis
tractus i.
interstitiospinal tract
interstriate layer
interthalamica
adhesio i.
interthalamic adhesion
interthalamicus
connexus i.
intertrabecular hemorrhage
intertransverse process fusion
interuncal distance
intervaginal space of optic nerve
interval
atlantoaxial i.
interspike i.
interstimulus i.
mean interpotential i. (MIPI)
time i.
intervention
biologic i.
clinical i.
cognitive i.
culture-specific i.

NOTES

intervention *(continued)*
drug i.
early pharmacological i.
experimental i.
exposure-based i.
freehand ultrasound-guided i.
GAD-specific i.
neurosurgical i.
pharmacologic i.
pharmacological i.
static i.
targeted i.
therapeutic i.
verbal i.
interventional
i. magnetic resonance imaging (iMRI)
i. neuroradiology
i. radiology (IR)
I. Therapeutics Corporation (ITC)
interventriculare
foramen i.
interventricular foramen
intervertebral
i. disc
i. disc cell
i. disc compression
i. disc herniation
i. discitis
i. disc rupture
i. disc space infection
i. foramen
i. ganglion
i. osteochondrosis
i. punch
intervertebralis
anulus fibrous disci i.
calcinosis i.
nucleus pulposus disci i.
interview
Autism Diagnostic I.
research i.
Zarit burden i.
Interview-Based Impression of Change
intestinal
polyneuropathy, ophthalmoplegia, leukoencephalopathy, and i.
i. trauma
intolerance
fructose i.
intonation
voice i.
intoxication
aluminum i.
ammonia i.
amphetamine i.
anticonvulsant i.
bromide i.
Burundanga i.
caffeine i.
cannabis i.
cocaine i.
drug i.
fluoxetine i.
gold i.
heavy metal i.
hypnotic i.
idiosyncratic i.
lead i.
manganese i.
marijuana i.
mercury i.
narcotic i.
opioid i.
pathologic i.
pathological i.
phencyclidine i.
reversible i.
sedative i.
serum heavy metal i.
substance i.
thallium i.
water i.
intraabdominal
i. bleeding
i. neuroblastoma
intraaortic
i. balloon counterpulsation device
i. balloon pump
intraarachnoid
i. leptomeningeal malformation
i. neurovascular structure
intraarterial
i. Amytal testing
i. catheter angiography
i. catheterization angiography
i. digital subtraction angiogram
i. digital subtraction angiography (IADSA)
i. drug delivery
i. flow
i. injection
intraaural attenuation
intraaxial
i. brain lesion
i. fiber
i. neoplasm
intrablood-brain barrier (IBBB)
intracanalicular
i. lesion
i. segment
intracapsular hemorrhage
intracarotid
i. amobarbital testing
i. marrow cell
i. sodium Amytal memory testing

intracavernous
i. carotid aneurysm
i. tumor
intracavitary irradiation
intracellular
i. calcium
i. calcium block
i. contribution
i. deoxyhemoglobin
i. energy metabolism
i. insoluble protein deposit
i. ion
i. lipid inclusion
i. metabolic pathway
i. metabolic process
i. protein
i. second messenger
i. signal
intracephalic hematoma
intracerebellar
i. hematoma
i. nucleus
intracerebral
i. aneurysm
i. arteriovenous malformation
i. depth electrode
i. depth electrode monitoring
i. ganglioma
i. hematoma
i. Hodgkin lymphoma
i. hydatid cyst
i. inoculation
i. lesion
i. leukostatic hemorrhage
i. microdialysis
i. steal
i. water
intracerebroventricular administration of morphine
intracisternal
i. administration
i. fibrinolysis
i. puncture
i. thrombolysis
intraclass correlation
intraconal mass
intracortical
i. axon
i. connection
i. facilitatory pathway
i. inhibition and facilitation
i. transverse fiber

intracranial
i. aerocele
i. air
i. aneurysm
i. arachnoid cyst
i. arterial dolichoectasia
i. artery
i. astrocytoma
i. bifurcation
i. bleeding
i. brain volume
i. bruit
i. calcification
i. cavernous angioma
i. cholesteatoma
i. circulation
i. compartment
i. compliance
i. cryptococcosis
i. disease
i. electroencephalogram (ICEEG)
i. electroencephalography
i. ependymoma
i. epidural abscess
i. epidural pressure
i. fragment
i. ganglion
i. glioma
i. granulomatous arteritis
i. hematoma
i. hemorrhage
i. Hodgkin lymphoma
i. hypertension
i. hypertension without papilledema (IHWOP)
i. hypotension (IH)
intracranial to i.
i. mass lesion
i. meningioma
i. meningioma resection
i. MR angiography
i. navigation
i. neoplasm
i. neuroblastoma
i. neuronavigation
i. occlusion
i. pachymeningitis
i. part of optic nerve
i. plasmacytoma
i. pneumatocele
i. pneumocele
i. prechiasmatic segment

NOTES

intracranial *(continued)*
i. pressure (ICP)
i. pressure catheter
i. pressure Express digital monitor
i. pressure increase
i. pressure microsensor
i. pressure-temperature (ICP-T)
i. raw volume
i. recording
i. rhizotomy
i. sarcoidosis
i. schwannoma
i. seminoma
i. sinus thrombosis
i. steal phenomenon
i. steal syndrome
i. stenting
i. tuberculoma
i. tumor
i. vascular dissection
i. vascular malformation (ICVM, IVM)
i. venous malformation
i. venous sinus
intracranial-extracranial
i.-e. nerve graft
i.-e. transplantation
intracranial-intracranial (IC-IC)
i.-i. bypass
intracranial-intratemporal nerve graft
intracrine mechanism
intractable
i. chronic pain
i. grand mal epilepsy
i. paroxysmal spell
i. partial seizure
i. psychomotor epilepsy
i. somatic pain
i. unilateral pain
i. vertigo
intraculminalis
fissura i.
intraculminate fissure
intracutaneous reaction
intradermal angioma
intradiploic epidermoid cyst
intradiscal
i. electrotherapy (IDET)
i. electrothermal procedure
i. electrothermal therapy (IDET)
intradural
i. abscess
i. anastomosis
i. aneurysm
i. approach
i. dissection
i. draining vein
i. extramedullary mass lesion
i. inflammatory disease
i. lipoma
i. metastasis
i. phase
i. retractor
i. retromedullary arteriovenous fistula
i. segment
i. tumor
i. tumor surgery
intradural-extradural meningioma
intraepidermal
i. nerve fiber (IENF)
i. nerve fiber density
intrafascicular migration
intraforaminal approach
intrafusal fiber
intragemmal nerve fiber
intragracile sulcus
intragracilis
sulcus i.
intragyral
intrahippocampal
i. injection
i. microdialysis
intralabyrinthine schwannoma
intralamellaris
pachymeningitis i.
intralaminar nucleus
intralimbic gyrus
intraluminal thrombolysis
Intramedic PE-50 polyethylene tubing
intramedullary
i. ependymoma
i. epidermoid cyst
i. hematoma
i. lymphoma
i. nail
i. spinal cord tumor
i. spinal lesion
i. toxoplasmosis
i. tractotomy
intrameningeal
intramolecular
i. dipole-dipole mechanism
i. relaxation
intramural
i. hematoma
i. plexus
intramuscular
i. absorption
i. administered drug
i. administration
i. neurolysis
intranasal sumatriptan
intraneural
i. edema
i. ganglion cyst
i. neurofibrillary tangle
i. phenol injection

I

intraneuronal
- i. fibrillary tangle
- i. inclusion
- i. inclusion disease

intranidal aneurysm
intransigent
intransitive limb
intranuclear
- i. ophthalmoplegia
- i. receptor

intraocular
- i. hemorrhage
- i. neuritis
- i. pressure

intraocularis
- pars intralaminaris nervi optici i.
- pars prelaminaris nervi optici i.

intraoperative
- i. angiography
- i. balloon occlusion
- i. B-mode ultrasound
- i. cell saver
- i. cisternography
- i. dural tear
- i. electrical cortical stimulation (IOECS)
- i. electrocorticography
- i. facial nerve monitoring
- i. lateral fluoroscopy
- i. microendoscopy
- i. MRI
- i. neck hyperextension
- i. neural insult
- i. neuroinvestigational system
- i. neuromonitoring
- i. neurophysiological monitoring
- i. rupture
- i. stereotactic spatial localization
- i. ultrasonic probe
- i. x-ray

intraorbital
- i. arteriovenous malformation
- i. granular cell tumor
- i. lesion
- i. meningioma
- i. surgery

intraosseous
- i. meningioma
- i. schwannoma

intraparenchymal
- i. cyst
- i. drug delivery
- i. hematoma
- i. hemorrhage
- i. infusion
- i. mass
- i. meningioma
- i. periventricular echodensity

intraparietal
- i. sulcus
- i. sulcus of Turner

intraparietalis
- sulcus i.

intraparotideus
- plexus i.

intrapartum asphyxia
intraperitoneal (IP)
- i. receptor

intrapial
intrapituitary cyst
intraplaque hemorrhage
intrapontine
intrapsychic
- i. change
- i. origin
- i. world

intrarachidian
Intrascan ultrasound
intrasegmental
- i. fiber
- i. reflex

intrasellar
- i. craniopharyngioma
- i. extension
- i. granuloma
- i. growth hormone-secreting pituitary tumor
- i. lesion
- i. paraganglioma
- i. Rathke cleft cyst
- i. rhabdomyosarcoma

intrasinus transducer
intraspinal
- i. adenoma
- i. cyst
- i. drug infusion system
- i. epidermoid tumor
- i. epidural pressure
- i. herniated disc
- i. lesion
- i. meningioma
- i. vascular malformation

intraspinous muscle
intraspongy nuclear disc herniation

NOTES

intrasynaptic
intratentorial
i. atrophy
i. malformation
i. supracerebellar approach
intraterritorial anastomosis
intrathalamicae
fibrae i.
intrathalamic fiber
intrathecal
i. antibiotic
i. chemotherapy
i. contrast-enhanced CAT scan
i. drug therapy
i. fluorescein
i. IgG synthetic rate
i. immunoglobulin synthesis
i. infusion test
i. morphine analgesia
i. morphinotherapy
i. neurolysis
i. octreotide
i. pain management
intrathoracic bleeding
intratumoral
i. arteriovenous shunt
i. chemotherapy
i. hemorrhage
i. hypervascularity
i. injection
intratumor hemorrhage
intratympanic
i. aminoglycoside
i. gentamicin
intrauterine shunt procedure
intravagal
i. glomus
i. paraganglioma
intravagale
glomus i.
intravascular
i. balloon occlusion
i. coiling
i. device
i. ligature
i. lymphoma
i. pressure
i. streaming
intravenous (IV, I.V.)
i. gamma globulin
i. immune globulin
i. immune globulin humoral therapy
i. immunoglobulin treatment
i. medication
i. oxygen-15 water bolus technique
i. regional anesthesia (IVRA)
i. regional sympathetic blockade
intraventricular (I-V)
i. catheter
i. cysticercosis
i. drug delivery
i. endoscopy
i. headache (IVH)
i. hematoma
i. hemorrhage
i. infusion
i. injection
i. meningioma
i. septation
i. tumor
intravertebral
intravoxel phase dispersion
Intrel
I. II spinal cord stimulation system
I. II spinal cord stimulator
intrinsic
i. birefringence
i. brainstem tumor
i. capacity
i. cell suicide mechanism
i. damage
i. disease
i. epileptogenicity
i. factor deficiency
i. fiber
i. imaging
i. reflex
i. relationship
i. transverse connector
i. transverse connector role
intrinsic-negative runner
intrinsic-positive runner
introducer cannula
introjective-projective cycle
intromittent organ
intron
Intropaque
Intropin
intrusion in verbal learning
intrusive
i. memory
i. symptom
intubation
aqueductal i.
nasogastric i.
oral i.
intumescence
tympanic i.
intumescent
intumescentia
i. cervicalis
i. ganglioformis
i. lumbalis
i. lumbosacralis
i. tympanica
intussusception

invagination
basilar i.
invasive
i. electroencephalographic monitoring
i. pituitary adenoma
i. tumor
inventory
Beck Depression I. (BDI)
Bell Object Relations and Reality Testing I.
Brief Pain I.
Brief Symptom I.
depression i.
Epilepsy Surgery I.-55
Johns Hopkins Functioning I.
Minnesota Multiphasic Personality I. (MMPI)
Multidimensional Pain I.
Quality of Life in Epilepsy-89 I.
sleep-awake activity i.
Sleep-Wake Activity I. (SWAI)
i. of symptoms
inverse
i. Anton syndrome
i. Argyll Robertson pupil
i. cerebellum
i. ocular bobbing
i. polymerase chain reaction-based detection of frataxin gene
i. treatment planning
inversed jaw-winking syndrome
inversion
i. recovery
i. time
inverted radial reflex
investigation
neurodiagnostic i.
presurgical i.
investigatory reflex
inveterate
involuntary
i. medication
i. movement
i. nervous system
i. time-out
i. trembling
involution
thymic i.
involutional
i. paranoid reaction
i. psychotic reaction
involvement
brachiocrural i.
brain i.
bulbar i.
CNS i.
extraocular muscle i.
faciobrachiocrural i.
mononeuric i.
nervous system i.
sarcoidosis neuromuscular i.
sporadic nerve root i.
tumorous i.
INVOS
in vivo optical spectroscopy
INVOS 3100 cerebral oximeter monitoring system
INVOS transcranial cerebral oximeter
inward focus
iobenzamic acid
iobutoic acid
iocarmate meglumine
iocarmic acid
iodamide
Iodamoeba buetschlii **cerebral amebiasis**
iodide
metocurine i.
radioactive i.
iodinated radiographic contrast
iodine
i. deficiency
isotopic i.
protein-bound i. (PBI)
iodine-125 implant
iodipamide
i. meglumine
i. methylglucamine
iodized oil
iodoalphionic acid
iodopyracet
iodoxamate
iodoxamic acid
IOECS
intraoperative electrical cortical stimulation
ioglicate
ioglicic acid
ioglunide
ioglycamic acid
ioglycamide
iogulamide

NOTES

iohexol
i. CT ventriculogram
i. myelography
ion
argon i.
calcium i.
i. channel
i. channel disorder
i. flux
intracellular i.
positive i.
ion-channel gene
ionic
I. spine spacer system
i. stimulus
ionophore
calcium i.
iopamidol contrast medium
iopanoic acid
iophendylate
iophenoxic acid
iopromide
iopronic acid
iopydol
iopydone
iosefamate
iosefamic acid
ioseric acid
iosulamide
iosumetic acid
ioteric acid
iothalamate
meglumine i.
iothalamic acid
iotrol
iotroxamide
iotroxic acid
ioversol
Iowa Conners scale
ioxaglate
i. meglumine
i. sodium
ioxaglic acid
ioxithalamate
ioxithalamic acid
IP
intraperitoneal
IP_3
inositol 1,4,5-triphosphate
IPA
interpleural analgesia
IPAP
inspiratory positive airway pressure
I-plate
Syracuse anterior I-p.
ipodate acid
ipratropium bromide
ipsilateral
i. anosmia
i. approach
i. bleed
i. cerebellar ataxia
i. cerebellar sign
i. cortical activation
i. corticospinal tract sign
i. facial palsy
i. facial paralysis
i. facial paresis
i. fastigial nucleus
i. gaze palsy
i. headache
i. hemianopia
i. hemiparesis
i. hemisphere
i. loss
i. mesial temporal sclerosis
i. mesial temporal structure
i. middle cerebral artery
i. monocular blindness
i. motor function
i. neglect
i. projection
i. reflex
i. somatosensory cortex
i. stroke
i. temporal cortex
i. tonic conjugate gaze
i. tonic deviation
i. tragus
i. transcallosal technique
i. vasogenic edema
i. visuospatial interference
ipsilaterally blind
ipsilesional hemifield
ipsipulsion
ocular i.
IPSP
inhibitory postsynaptic potential
IQ
intelligence quotient
IQ-adjusted memory impairment
IR
interventional radiology
IRDA
intermittent rhythmic delta activity
IRDA on electroencephalogram
Iressa
iridis
rubeosis i.
iridium
iridium-192
iridocyclitis
iridoparalysis
iridoplegia
complete i.
reflex i.
sympathetic i.

iridotomy
argon laser i. (ALI)
iris
i. Lisch nodule
i. neovascularization
i. stellate pattern
iritis
white i.
iron
i. deficiency
i. ferrous sulfate
i. lung
i. metabolism
i. poisoning
i. replacement therapy
iron-ascorbate-DTPA
technetium-99m i.-a.-DTPA
iron-containing lesion
irradiation
conventional fractionated i.
convergent beam i.
craniospinal i.
excitatory i.
gamma i.
hyperfractionated i.
intracavitary i.
prophylactic craniospinal i.
selective i.
stereotactic i.
whole-brain i. (WBI)
x-ray i.
irreducible subluxation
irregular
i. nystagmus
i. sleep-wake disorder
i. sleep-wake pattern
irrelevant stimulus
irreversible
i. brain damage
i. dementia
i. limitation
irrigant
Neosporin GU I.
irrigation bipolar system
irrigator
Brackmann suction s.-i.
Kurze suction s.-i.
irritability
mechanical i.
nervous i.
specific i.
irritable
i. heart
i. nociceptor
i. syndrome
irritation
meningeal i.
nerve root i.
temperature i.
irritative
i. lesion
i. zone
IRSA
International Rett Syndrome Association
IRT
infrared thermography
Isaacs-Mertens syndrome
Isaac syndrome
ischemia
anoxic i.
brain i.
brainstem i.
cerebral i.
cerebrovascular i.
chronic ocular i.
cortical transient i.
focal artery i.
focal cerebral i.
global cerebral i.
hindbrain i.
hypoxic i.
ischemic i.
myoneural i.
nocturnal cardiac i.
posterior circulation i.
reversible i.
rostral brainstem i.
tourniquet i.
transient brainstem i.
vasomotor i.
vertebrobasilar i.
white matter i.
ischemia-induced elevation
ischemia-modifying factor
ischemic
i. anterior optic neuropathy
i. brain damage
i. brain edema
i. brainstem infarction
i. cascade
i. cerebral infarction
i. cerebrovascular disease
i. event

NOTES

ischemic *(continued)*
i. forearm exercise test (IFET)
i. hemispheric swelling
i. hypoxia
i. injury
i. insult
i. ischemia
i. lesion volume
i. lumbago
i. muscular atrophy
i. neuritis
i. neuron
i. neuronal cell death
i. ocular inflammation
i. pathology
i. penumbra
i. phenomenon
i. posterior optic neuropathy
i. preconditioning
i. stress
i. stroke
i. stroke pathophysiology
i. vascular dementia
i. white matter lesion
ischemic-hypoxic
i.-h. encephalopathy
i.-h. lesion
ischiadic
i. nerve
i. plexus
ischiadici
rami musculares nervi i.
ischiadicus
nervus i.
ischialgia
ischiodynia
ischioneuralgia
ischogyria
^{125}I seed
ISG
ISG viewing wand
ISG Wand navigation system
I-shaped scalp flap
Ishihara plate
island
i. of Calleja
neuroectodermal tumor pale i.
i. pedicle scalp flap
i. of Reil
syncytial i.
islet
Calleja i.
i. cell adenoma
Isle of Wight Study
isobutyl
isobutyl-2-cyanoacrylate
Iso-C
Iso-C image
Iso-C scan
Iso-C spin
isocapnic hypoxia
isocentric
i. linear accelerator
i. linear accelerator x-ray
isochromosome
isochronism
law of i.
isocoric pupil
isocortex
isodense
i. lesion
i. mass
i. subdural hematoma
isodisomy
isodose
i. curve
i. line
isoelectric
i. electroencephalogram
i. encephalogram
isoenergetic
isoenzyme
isoetharine hydrochloride
isoflavone
isoflurane anesthesia
isoform
brain i.
embryonic i.
i. of NO synthase (iNOS)
recombinant tau i.
3-repeat i.
4-repeat i.
isointense lesion
isokinetic dynamometric testing
Isola
I. instrumentation
I. spinal implant system
I. spinal implant system accessory
I. spinal implant system anchor
I. spinal implant system application
I. spinal implant system complication
I. spinal implant system component
I. spinal implant system design
I. spinal implant system dimension
I. spinal implant system eye rod
I. spinal implant system hook
I. spinal implant system iliac post
I. spinal implant system iliac screw
I. spinal implant system plate-rod combination
isolated
i. angiitis
i. angiitis of central nervous system
i. body lateropulsion

i. gait ignition failure
i. periventricular nodular heterotopia
i. phobia
i. radial nerve palsy
isolation
anterior horn cell i.
cell i.
fungus i.
mononuclear leukocyte i.
isolé
Isollyl Improved
isomerase
glucosephosphate i.
isomeric function
isometheptene mucate
isometric tremor
isomorphous gliosis
isoniazid
i. neuropathy
i. polyneuropathy
i. therapy
isoniazid-induced pyridoxine deficiency
isonicotinic acid peripheral neuropathy
Isopap
Isopaque
isopotential
isoproterenol tilt table test
isosorbide dinitrate
isothiocyanate
allyl i.
isotope
i. cisternogram
i. cisternography
isotopic
i. cisternography
i. iodine
isotretinoin
isotropic
i. band
i. 3DFT
i. 3-dimensional Fourier transform
i. linear material
isovaleric
i. acidemia aminoaciduria
i. aciduria
isovolemic hemodilution
isozyme
isthmi (*pl. of* isthmus)
isthmic spondylolisthesis
isthmoparalysis
isthmoplegia
isthmus, pl. **isthmi**
i. of cingulate gyrus
ganglion i.
i. gyri cinguli
i. of gyrus cinguli
i. of gyrus fornicatus
i. of His
i. of limbic lobe
i. rhombencephali
rhombencephalic i.
ISUIA
International Study of Unruptured Intracranial Aneurysm
IT-15 gene
ITAC
T-cell alpha chemoattractant
ITC
Interventional Therapeutics Corporation
ITC radiopaque balloon catheter
itch-specific central neuron
3-Item Delirium Scale
item-total correlation
iter
i. ad infundibulum
i. of Sylvius
i. a tertio ad quartum ventriculum
iterative discharge
ITF
infratemporal fossa
IT-MS infusion therapy
ITN
idiopathic trigeminal neuralgia
Ito
hypomelanosis of I.
ITP
idiopathic thrombocytopenic purpura
immune thrombocytopenic purpura
itraconazole
Itrel
I. pulse generator
I. 3 Spinal Cord Stimulation System
IV, I.V.
intravenous
Campath IV
I-V
intraventricular
Ivalon
I. embolic sponge
I. foam
I. particle
I. wire coil

NOTES

IVH
intraventricular headache
IVM
intracranial vascular malformation
IVRA
intravenous regional anesthesia
Iwamoto
method of Suzuki and I.
Ixodes
I. pacificus
I. scapularis
ixomyelitis

jabs-and-jolts
j.-a.-j. headache
j.-a.-j. syndrome
jacket
Minerva j.
jackknife
j. attack
j. seizure
j. spasm
Jackson
J. epilepsy
J. law
J. rule
J. sign
J. spine table
J. vagoaccessory hypoglossal paralysis
jacksonian
j. epilepsy
j. march
j. seizure
Jackson-Pratt drain
Jackson-Weiss syndrome
Jacobs
J. locking hook spinal rod
J. locking hook spinal rod instrumentation
J. locking hook spinal rod instrumentation modification
J. locking hook spinal rod technique
Jacobson
J. endarterectomy spatula
J. microneurosurgical scissors
J. microprobe
J. microvascular knife
J. mosquito forceps
J. needle holder
J. nerve
J. plexus
J. probe
J. reflex
J. suture pusher
J. vessel knife
Jacobson-Potts vascular clamp
Jacod
J. syndrome
J. triad
Jaeger-Hamby procedure
Jahnke syndrome
jake paralysis
Jakob-Creutzfeldt disease
Jamaica
J. ginger poisoning
J. ginger polyneuritis
Jamaican
J. neuropathy
J. vomiting sickness
Jamestown
J. Canyon (JC)
J. Canyon virus (JCV)
Janet test
Jannetta
J. alligator forceps
J. aneurysm neck dissector
J. bayonet forceps
J. duckbill elevator
J. fork
J. hook
J. knife
J. microvascular decompression procedure
J. posterior fossa retractor
J. probe
Jannetta-Kurze dissecting scissors
Jansen
J. bone curette
J. mastoid retractor
J. monopolar forceps
J. rasp
J. rongeur
J. scalp retractor
Jansen-Middleton
J.-M. forceps
J.-M. rongeur
J.-M. scissors
Jansen-Wagner retractor
Jansky-Bielschowsky disease
Janz
J. juvenile myoclonic seizure
J. response
J. response on electroencephalogram
syndrome of J.
J. syndrome
Japanese
J. B encephalitis
J. encephalitis virus
J. Society of Sleep Research
J. suction tip
Japanese-type familial amyloid polyneuropathy
japonica
encephalitis j.
Jarcho-Levin syndrome
Jarell forceps
jargon
j. aphasia
organ j.

Jarisch-Herxheimer
J.-H. fever
J.-H. fever reaction
Jarit
J. brain forceps
J. periosteal elevator
J. rotator
J. tendon-pulling forceps
Jarit-Kerrison laminectomy rongeur
Jarit-Liston bone rongeur
Jarit-Ruskin bone rongeur
Jasco spectropolarimeter
jaundice
nuclear j.
Java arthrodesis system
Javid
J. carotid clamp
J. shunt
jaw
j. claudication
j. click
j. jerk
j. stiffness
j. winking
jaw-jerk reflex
jaw-winking
j.-w. phenomenon
j.-w. reflex
j.-w. syndrome
jaw-working reflex
JB
jugular bulb
JC
Jamestown Canyon
JC virus
JCV
Jamestown Canyon virus
Jeep driver's disease
Jefferson
J. fracture
J. syndrome
jejuni
Campylobacter j.
jelly
j. nystagmus
j. roll hypothesis
Jendrassik maneuver
Jerald forceps
jerk
ankle j.
biceps j.
body j.
brisk jaw j.
chin j.
crossed adductor j.
crossed knee j.
elbow j.
j. finger
flurry of myoclonic j.'s
forearm j.
hypnic j.
jaw j.
knee j.
leg j.
macro square-wave j.
myoclonic j.
nocturnal leg j.
nystagmoid j.
paretic j.
photomyoclonic j.
quadriceps j.
square-wave j.
supinator j.
tendon j.
triceps surae j.
jerking
focal j.
head j.
shoulder j.
j. stiff-person syndrome
jerk-locked back-averaged recording
jerky
j. primary dystonia
j. seesaw nystagmus
Jervell-Lange-Nielsen syndrome
jet
j. lag phenomenon/syndrome
j. lag sleep disorder
jeweler's bipolar forceps
Jewett wave
jig
Ace Hershey halo j.
customized j.
loading j.
Joffroy
J. reflex
J. sign
Johanson-Blizzard syndrome
Johns
J. Hopkins Functioning Inventory
J. Hopkins Severity Scale
Johnson brain tumor forceps
Johnston alopecia
joint
apophysial j.
atlantoaxial j.
atlantooccipital j.
Charcot j.
facet j.
j. hyperlaxity
incudostapedial j.
neuropathic j.
j. position
radiohumeral j.
j. receptor
j. replacement
sacroiliac j.
j. sense

temporomandibular j. (TMJ)
zygapophysial j.
joker dissector
Jolly
J. reaction
J. test
jolt
lancinating electric shocklike j.
Joplin neuroma
Joseph disease
Jostent graft stent
Joubert syndrome
JPA
juvenile pilocytic astrocytoma
J receptor
J-sella deformity
J-tipped guidewire
judgment
deficient social j.
juga cerebralia
jugular
j. bulb (JB)
j. bulb oxyhemoglobin saturation monitoring (SjO_2)
j. bulb venous oxygen saturation
j. chain lymph node
j. foramen
j. foramen mass
j. foramen muscle
j. foramen schwannoma
j. foramen syndrome
j. ganglion
j. glomus
j. nerve
j. sign
j. vein
j. vein dissection
jugulare
foramen j.
glomus j.
jugularis
nervus j.
jugulocephalic vein
jugulosubclavian junction
jugulotympanicum
glomus j.
jumper
j. disease
j. disease of Maine
jump-graft hypoglossal-facial nerve anastomosis
jumping Frenchmen of Maine disease
junction
anterior cervical approach to cervicothoracic j.
cervicomedullary j.
cervicothoracic j.
craniocervical j.
craniovertebral j.
electrotonic j.
gap j.
gray/white matter j.
jugulosubclavian j.
liponeural j.
motor unit neuromuscular j.
myoneural j.
neuromuscular j.
pontomedullary j.
pontomesencephalic j.
posterior craniocervical j.
postsynaptic neuromuscular j.
sylvian/rolandic j.
temporoparietal j. (TPJ)
thoracolumbar j.
junctional
j. dilation
j. kyphosis
j. scotoma of Traquair
junctural feature
Junin virus
jurisprudential teaching model
Juster reflex
justification
neurobiological j.
juvenile
j. absence epilepsy
j. absence seizure
j. amaurotic idiocy
j. amyotrophy
j. angiofibroma
j. arteriovenous malformation
j. cerebellar astrocytoma
j. chorea
j. dermatomyositis
j. fibromatosis
j. Huntington disease
j. justice system
j. myasthenia gravis
j. myoclonic epilepsy
j. myxedema
j. neuronal ceroid lipofuscinosis
j. nonneuropathic Niemann-Pick disease
j. papillomatosis

NOTES

juvenile *(continued)*
  j. parkinsonism
  j. pilocytic astrocytoma (JPA)
  j. rheumatoid arthritis
  j. rheumatoid arthritis vasculitis
  j. spinal muscular atrophy
juvenilis
  dementia paralytica j.
juxtaarticular cyst
juxtacortical
  j. chondroma
  j. sarcoma
juxtallocortex
juxtapapillary uveitis
juxtapulmonary receptor
juxtarestiform body
juxtarestiforme
  corpus j.

K
potassium
K complex
K index
K+
K+ Care
K+ Care Effervescent
K-2000 surgical saw blade
Kabuki syndrome
Kadian sustained-release morphine capsule
Kaes
K. feltwork
line of K.
K. line
K. stria
Kaes-Bechterew
band of K.-B.
K.-B. layer
K.-B. stria
Kahn syndrome
kainate receptor
kainic
k. acid
k. acid-induced focal injury
kaleidoscope hallucination
Kales
criteria of Rechtschaffen and K.
kallikrein gene
Kallmann syndrome
Kaltostat dressing
Kambin instrumentation
Kanavel approach
Kandel stereotactic apparatus
Kaneda
K. anterior spinal instrumentation
K. anterior spinal/scoliosis system
K. anterior spinal system
K. anterior spine stabilizing device
K. SR spinal system
Kanpolat
K. CT electrode
K. electrode kit
Kaochlor SF
kaolin clotting time
kaolin-induced hydrocephalus
Kaon
Kaplan-Meier
K.-M. survival analysis
K.-M. survival curve
kaposiform hemangioendothelioma
Kaposi sarcoma
kappa
k. light chain
k. opiate receptor
k. score
k. wave
Kapseals
Dilantin K.
Karlin microknife
Karl Storz endoscopy
Karnofsky
K. performance scale
K. performance score (KPS)
K. rating scale
Karolinska Sleepiness Scale
Kartagener syndrome
karyochrome cell
karyotype
XYY k.
Kasabach-Merritt syndrome
Katayama fever
Kato
technique of Miyazaki and K.
Katz ADL Index
Katzman test
kava
k. extract
kava k.
Kawasaki
K. disease
K. disease vasculitis
Kayser-Fleischer corneal ring
K-Centrum anterior spinal fixation system
KCNQ3 gene
KCNq2 gene
33-kDa antigen
56kD protein
Keane Mobility bed
Kearns-Sayre
K.-S. disease
K.-S. syndrome
Keeler
K. Galilean loupe
K. panoramic loupe
K. video headlamp
Keen
K. operation
K. point
Keep Alert capsule
Kehrer reflex
Keitel index
K-Electrolyte Effervescent
Kelly-Goerss Compass stereotactic system
Kelly stereotactic system
Kelvin body
Kennedy
K. disease

Kennedy *(continued)*
K. disease test
K. syndrome
Kennedy-Fischbeck disease
Kennerdell-Maroon
K.-M. elevator
K.-M. hook
K.-M. orbital retractor
K.-M. technique
Kenney Self-Care Questionnaire
Kenny ADL index
Keppra
Kerandel symptom
kerasin histiocytosis
keratan sulfate
keratitis
neuroparalytic k.
neurotrophic k.
k. paralytica
keratoacanthoma
keratoconjunctivitis sicca
keratocyst
keratoderma blennorrhagicum
keratopathy
band k.
exposure k.
keratosis
k. obturans
seborrheic k.
keratotic lesion
keraunoneurosis
Kerlix dressing
kernicterus
neonatal k.
premature infant k.
Kernig
K. sign
K. test
Kernohan
K. classification of brain tumor
K. grading
K. notch
K. notch phenomenon
K. notch syndrome
K. sign
K. system
K. system of glioma classification
Kerr
K. clip
K. sign
Kerrison
K. bone punch
K. bone punch kinesthesiometer
K. microronguer
K. rongeur
Kestenbaum procedure
Ketalar
ketamine
NMDA antagonist k.
ketanserin
ketoacid accumulation
ketoacidosis
diabetic k. (DKA)
ketoaciduria
branched-chain k.
ketogenic diet
ketorolac tromethamine
ketotic
k. glycine
k. hyperglycemia
Kety-Schmidt method
Key elevator
keyhole
k. craniotomy
k. laminectomy
k. surgery
transsylvian k.
Key-Retzius
foramen of K.-R.
Keystone graft
KIAA gene
kidney
human neonatal k. (HNK)
Kiel classification
Kienböck phenomenon
killer
natural k. (NK)
Killian
K. gouge
K. operation
K. septum speculum
Kilner hook
Kiloh-Nevin
K.-N. ocular form of progressive muscular dystrophy
K.-N. ocular myopathy
K.-N. syndrome
KinAir bed
kinanesthesia, cinanesthesia
kinase
calcium-calmodulin k. II
creatine k. (CK)
deoxyguanosine k. (DGUOK)
DNA protein k.
focal adhesion k. (FAK)
mitogen-activated protein k.
phosphoglycerate k.
phosphorylase k.
protein k.
protein k. C (PKC)
serum creatinine k.
tyrosine k.
kindled seizure
kindling
amygdala k.
delay of k.
k. process
Kindt carotid clamp

kinematic
forelimb k.'s
kinematograph
kinesia paradoxica
kinesigenic
k. ataxia
k. attack
k. chorea
k. choreoathetosis
k. paroxysmal dyskinesia
k. trigger
kinesioneurosis
kinesipathy
kinesthesia hallucination
kinesthesiometer
Kerrison bone punch k.
kinesthesis
kinesthetic
k. aura
k. sense
kinetic
k. ataxia
k. cervical spine
k. drive
k. microplate reader
k. model
k. modeling
k. perimetry
k. strabismus
k. tremor
kinetics
cellular k.
first-order elimination k.
mode-switching k.
zero-order elimination k.
King
K. type I–V curve
K. type I–V curve posterior correction
K. type I–V scoliosis
kink
cervicomedullary k.
kinky-hair disease
Kinnier-Wilson disease
kinocilium
Kinsbourne syndrome
Kirby-Bauer disc diffusion method
Kirschner
K. pin
K. wire
K. wire placement
Kisch reflex
Kistler
K. classification of subarachnoid hemorrhage
K. subarachnoid hemorrhage classification
kit
Ceretec imaging k.
ELISA Quantikine k.
Hall Osteon drill system k.
Hall Osteon irrigation k.
Kanpolat electrode k.
KLS-Martin modular neuro k.
Laitinen high-precision stereotactic-assisted radiation therapy k.
Laitinen percutaneous tumor biopsy k.
Laserscope discography k.
Micro E irrigation k.
Micro 100 irrigation k.
Ototome irrigation k.
PainBuster infusion pump management k.
Radifocus introducer B k.
Shiley distention k.
stereotactic-assisted radiation therapy k.
Vectastain ABC k.
Kjellin syndrome
Klaus height index
Klearway oral appliance
Klebsiella pneumoniae **meningitis**
kleeblattschädel
Kleine-Levin
K.-L. syndrome
K.-L. syndrome prognosis
K.-L. syndrome treatment
Kleist sign
Klinefelter syndrome
Klippel disease
Klippel-Feil
K.-F. anomaly
K.-F. deformity
K.-F. syndrome
Klippel-Trenaunay syndrome
Klippel-Trenaunay-Weber syndrome
Klippel-Weil sign
Kloehn craniofacial instrument
Klonopin
Klorvess Effervescent
Klotrix
KLS-Martin
KLS-M. center drive screw

K

NOTES

KLS-Martin *(continued)*
KLS-M. implant
KLS-M. modular neuro kit
Klumpke
K. palsy
K. paralysis
Klumpke-Dejerine
K.-D. paralysis
K.-D. syndrome
Klüver
method of K.
Klüver-Barrera Luxol fast blue stain
Klüver-Bucy syndrome
K-Lyte/Cl
K-Lyte Effervescent
knee
k. jerk
k. phenomenon
k. reflex
Wilbrand k.
knee-chest position
knee-jerk reflex
knife
Adson dural k.
Adson right-angle k.
angular k.
arachnoid k.
Bucy cordotomy k.
canal k.
clasp k.
cobalt-60 gamma k.
Cottle k.
Crile gasserian ganglion k.
Cushing dural hook k.
diamond k.
discission k.
electric k.
Frazier cordotomy k.
Frazier pituitary k.
Freer-Swanson ganglion k.
gamma k.
Halle dura k.
hot k.
Jacobson microvascular k.
Jacobson vessel k.
Jannetta k.
Leksell Model C gamma k.
model U gamma k.
Olivecrona trigeminal k.
photon k.
platelet-shaped k.
Rayport dural dissector and k.
Stecher arachnoid k.
Toennis dura k.
Weary cordotomy k.
X K.
Yasargil arachnoid k.
Yasargil microvascular k.
Knight forceps
knismogenic
knob
olfactory k.
synaptic k.
Knodt rod
knuckle
cervical aortic k.
Koala Pad graphics tablet
Kobayashi retractor
Kocher
K. clamp
K. collar incision
K. dissector
K. point
K. reflex
Kocher-Debré-Semelaigne syndrome
Kocher-Lovelace clamp
Koenen tumor
Koerber-Salus-Elschnig syndrome
Koerte-Ballance operation
Koerte procedure
Kohlmeier-Degos syndrome
Kohnstamm phenomenon
Kojewnikoff epilepsy
Kölliker-Fuse nucleus
Kölliker reticulum
Komai stereotactic head frame
Komet
K. K-2000 surgical saw blade
K. K-wire/Steinman pin and delivery tray system
K. medical battery tester
K. Medical/Brasseler USA XK-95 high-speed drill system
Konakion Injection
koniocortex
auditory k.
konzo disease
Korsakoff
K. amnesia
K. syndrome
korsakoffian amnesia
Kostuik
K. rod
K. screw
Kostuik-Harrington
K.-H. device
K.-H. distraction system
KPS
Karnofsky performance score
Krabbe
K. diffuse sclerosis
K. disease
K. leukodystrophy
K. syndrome
Krabbe-Weber-Dimitri disease
Kraepelina paranoia
Kraepelin-Morel disease
Kraepelin schema

Krause
K. corpuscle
K. denervation
K. end bulb
K. operation
K. respiratory bundle
K. terminal bulb
Krayenbuehl nerve hook
Krimsky test
Kronecker
K. aneurysm needle
K. center
krox gene
Kruskal-Wallis
K.-W. H test
K.-W. test
k-space reordered by inversion time at each slice position
KTP/532 surgical laser
kubisagari, kubisagaru
Kufs disease
Kugelberg-Welander
K.-W. disease
K.-W. distal muscular atrophy
K.-W. distal myopathy
K.-W. juvenile spinal muscle atrophy
K.-W. syndrome
Kühne
K. phenomenon
K. spindle
K. terminal plate
Kuhnt intermediary tissue
Kumlinge disease
Kümmell spondylitis
Küntscher
K. hammer
K. nail
Kurtzke
K. Expanded Disability Status Scale
K. multiple sclerosis disability scale
K. score
Kurze
K. dissection scissors
K. suction irrigator
Kussmaul
K. aphasia
K. coma
K. paralysis
Kussmaul-Landry paralysis
Kveim test
kwashiorkor
K-wire
blunt K-w.
K-w. placement
Kyasanur Forest disease
kymoparalytica
myohypertrophia k.
kynurenic acid
kynurenine aminotransferase
Kyoto Multi-Institutional Study Group Pediatric Neurology
kyphoplasty
balloon k.
kyphoscoliosis
neurofibromatosis k.
k. secondary to neurofibromatosis
severe k.
thoracolumbar k.
kyphosis
acute angular k.
k. brace
Cobb method of measuring k.
congenital k.
k. correction
k. creation
fixed lumbar k.
iatrogenic lumbar k.
junctional k.
lumbar k.
postlaminectomy k.
posttraumatic k.
progressive k.
right thoracic curve with junctional k.
Scheuermann k.
thoracic k.
thoracolumbar k.
kyphotic
k. deformity
k. deformity pathomechanics
k. pelvis
KyphX Xpander inflatable bone tamp

NOTES

LA
long-acting
Inderal LA
Labbé
L. neurocirculatory syndrome
vein of L.
L. vein
labeling
l. index
photoaffinity l.
labia (*pl. of* labium)
labial
l. dysarthria
l. nerve
l. paralysis
lability
emotional l.
labiochorea
labioglossolaryngeal
l. palsy
l. paralysis
labioglossomandibular approach
labioglossopharyngeal paralysis
labiomandibular
l. approach
l. glossotomy
labium, pl. **labia**
l. cerebri
laboratory
basement l.
l. study
Venereal Disease Research L. (VDRL)
labyrinth
membranous l.
vestibular l.
labyrinthectomy
unit l. (UL)
labyrinthine
l. aplasia
l. apoplexy
l. concussion syndrome
l. disease
l. disorder
l. fistula test
l. hydrops
l. infarction
l. righting reflex
l. torticollis
l. vertigo
labyrinthitis
laceration
brain l.
cerebral l.
scalp l.
lacerum
foramen l.
L-acetylcarnitine
lack
l. of clear-cut cerebral dominance
l. of efficacy
energy l.
lacrimal
l. duct
l. gland
l. gland dysfunction
l. nerve
l. reflex
lacrimalis
nervus l.
pars orbitalis glandulae l.
lacrimogustatory reflex
La Crosse encephalitis
lactate
brain l.
calcium l.
l. dehydrogenase
global brain l.
gray matter l.
regional brain l.
Ringer l.
sodium l.
white matter l.
lactic
l. acidosis
l. acid production in perinatal asphyxia
l. acid serum level
lactoferrin
lactose metabolism
lactosuria
lactotroph cell
lactotrophic
Lactrodectus mactans
lacuna, pl. **lacunae**
cerebral l.
l. cerebri
lateral l.
lacunae laterales
lacunae lateralis
perisinusoidal l.
lacunaire
état l.
lacunar
l. amnesia
l. brain infarction
l. molecular layer
l. skull
l. state
l. stroke

L

lacunar *(continued)*
l. stroke manifestation
l. syndrome
lacunaris
status l.
lacunosum
stratum moleculare et substratum l.
lacunosus
status l.
Ladd fiberoptic system
laeso
vertigo ab stomacho l.
Lafora
L. body
L. body disease
L. familial myoclonic epilepsy
laforin
lag
bright light exposure for jet l.
lagophthalmos
Lahey
L. Clinic dural hook
L. Clinic nerve hook
L. score
Laitinen
L. high-precision stereotactic-assisted radiation therapy kit
L. percutaneous tumor biopsy kit
L. stereoadapter
L. stereoguide 2000 arc-centered stereotactic frame
L. stereotactic system
lake
lateral l.
venous l.
L-alanine acid
lalognosis
laloplegia
Lamaze technique
lambda
l. light chain
l. wave
lambdoid
l. activity
l. craniosynostosis
l. plagiocephaly
l. synostosis
lambdoidal suture
Lambert-Eaton
L.-E. myasthenic syndrome (LEMS)
L.-E. syndrome (LES)
Lambert syndrome
lamella, pl. **lamellae**
basal l.
triangular l.
vitreous l.
lamellar sheath
lamellated corpuscle
lamellosa
corpuscula l.
lamellosum
corpusculum l.
Lamictal
lamina, pl. **laminae**
l. affixa
l. alaris
laminae albae cerebelli
l. arcus vertebrae
basal l.
l. basalis
l. basalis choroideae
basilar l.
l. basilaris cochlea
l. of the cerebral cortex
l. choroidea
l. choroidea epithelialis
l. cinerea
l. cribrosa
l. dorsalis
epithelial l.
external medullary l.
intact spinous l.
internal medullary l.
laminae medullares cerebelli
laminae medullares thalami
l. medullaris
l. medullaris lateralis
l. medullaris lateralis corporis striati
l. medullaris medialis
l. medullaris medialis corporis striati
l. medullaris medialis nuclei lentiformis
l. medullaris thalami externa
l. of mesencephalic tectum
l. molecularis
l. molecularis corticis cerebri
l. multiformis
periclaustral l.
l. pyramidalis externa
l. pyramidalis ganglionaris
l. pyramidalis interna
l. quadrigemina
quadrigeminal l.
l. of Rexed
Rexed l.
rostral l.
l. rostralis
l. septi pellucidi
l. of septum pellucidum
spinal l. II
l. spinalis II
l. spreader
l. supraneuroporica
l. tecti
l. tecti mesencephali

l. terminalis (LT)
l. terminalis cerebri
l. terminalis of cerebrum
l. terminalis hypothalami
trapdoor l.
l. ventralis
l. of vertebral arch
l. vitrea
lamina-associated protein
lamin a/c gene (*LMNA*)
laminae (*pl. of* lamina)
laminaplasty (*var. of* laminoplasty)
laminar
l. C-D hook
l. cortex posterior aspect
l. cortical necrosis
l. cortical sclerosis
laminated cortex
lamination of gyrus
laminectomized spine
laminectomy
Beckman-Eaton l.
Beckman-Weitlaner l.
cervical spine l.
decompressive l.
Gill l.
Girdlestone l.
keyhole l.
multilevel l.
osteoplastic l.
4-place l.
l. punch forceps
l. roll
single-level decompressive l.
laminin
laminoforaminotomy
laminopathy
laminoplasty, laminaplasty
distraction l.
en bloc l.
open-door l.
spinous process-splitting l.
Tsuji l.
laminotomy
microendoscopic l.
microscopic l. (ML)
unilateral l.
Lamitrode lead
lamivudine
zidovudine and l.
lamprey spinal axon
Lance-Adams syndrome
lancinating
l. electric shocklike jolt
l. pain
lancisi
L. longitudinal nerve
striae l.
Landau
L. reflex
L. syndrome
Landau-Kleffner syndrome
landmark
bony l.
glabella-inion line l.
pedicle l.
surface l.
Landolt
L. pituitary speculum
L. spreader
Landouzy-Dejerine
L.-D. atrophy
L.-D. disease
L.-D. muscular dystrophy
Landouzy dystrophy
Landouzy-Grasset law
Landry
L. paralysis
L. syndrome
Landry-Guillain-Barré-Strohl syndrome
Landry-Guillain-Barré syndrome
Langenbeck periosteal elevator
Langer-Giedion syndrome
Langerhans
L. cell
L. cell granulomatosis
Langley nerve
language
l. alteration
l. area
l. disturbance
expressive l.
l. lateralization
l. manipulation
l. therapy
l. zone
language-associated cortex
language-induced seizure
language-specific
l.-s. brain activity
l.-s. cortex
lanreotide
Lanterman
L. cleft

NOTES

Lanterman *(continued)*
L. incisure
L. segment
Lanterman-Schmidt incisure
laparoscopic transperitoneal approach
Lapidus bed
Laplacian montage on electroencephalogram
Lapras catheter
lapse
memory l.
LAPSS
Los Angeles Prehospital Stroke Screen
lapsus lingua
large
l. artery infarction
l. ball nerve hook
l. egress cannula
l. polymorphic ganglion cell
l. vessel infarction
l. vessel vasculitis
large-scale neural system
Larmor
L. equation
L. frequency
L. precession
Larodopa
laryngeal
l. atresia
l. chorea
l. crisis
l. dysarthria
l. epilepsy
l. hemangioma
l. nerve
l. nerve injury
l. syncope
l. vertigo
laryngectomy
laryngismus
laryngoparalysis
laryngoplegia
laryngospasm
laryngospastic reflex
Lasègue
L. disease
L. sign
L. syndrome I, II
L. test
laser
argon l.
l. beam
carbon dioxide l.
Cavitron l.
l. disc decompression (LDD)
l. Doppler flowmeter (LDF)
l. Doppler flowmetry
l. Doppler spectroscopy
l. Doppler velocimetry
holmium YAG l.
Ho:YAG l.
KTP/532 surgical l.
Nd:YAG l.
l. nucleotomy
orthogonal l.
l. photocoagulation (LPC)
l. scanning microscope (LSM)
Sharplan l.
l. speckle
l. speckle pattern
l. surgery
l. tissue welding
l. uvulopalatoplasty (LUPP)
VersaPulse holmium l.
laser-assisted
l.-a. palatoplasty
l.-a. spinal endoscopy
l.-a. uvulopalatoplasty (LAUP)
Laserflo Doppler probe
Laserflow
L. blood perfusion monitor
L. BPM^2 real-time cerebral perfusion monitor
Laserscope discography kit
Lassa fever virus
lata
Tutoplast fascia l.
Latarjet nerve
late
l. after depolarization
l. distal hereditary myopathy
l. endosomal protein
l. epilepsy
l. infantile amaurotic idiocy
l. infantile neuronal ceroid lipofuscinosis
l. luteal phase of menstrual cycle
l. Lyme neuroborreliosis
l. seizure
l. whiplash syndrome
late-life
l.-l. cognitive impairment
l.-l. dementia
l.-l. migraine accompaniment
latency
blink reflex l.
distal motor l.
increased rapid eye movement l.
interpeak l.
mean sleep l.
REM l.
residual l.
sensory l.
sleep l.
terminal l.
l. of tibialis anterior activation
latency-evoked potential

latent
l. epilepsy
l. infection
l. ophthalmoplegia
l. period
l. reflex
l. tetany
l. zone
late-onset
l.-o. ataxia
l.-o. category
l.-o. ischemic stroke
l.-o. rod myopathy
l.-o. Werdnig-Hoffmann disease
late-phase long-term potentiation (L-LTP)
lateral
l. amygdaloid nucleus
l. aperture
l. aperture of fourth ventricle
l. atrial vein
l. bending stability
l. central tegmental field
l. cephalometric radiography
l. cerebellar region
l. cerebellomedullary cistern
l. cerebral fissure
l. cerebral fossa
l. cerebral sulcus
l. cervical nucleus
l. column
l. column of spinal cord
l. compression deformity
l. corticospinal tract
l. cuneate nucleus
l. direct vein
l. dominance examination
l. dorsal tegmentum
l. dorsal tegmentum nucleus
l. extracavitary approach
l. fasciculus proprius
l. femoral cutaneous nerve
l. fillet
l. foramina of Luschka
l. fossa of brain
l. fracture
l. funiculus
l. funiculus of spinal cord
l. gaze
l. gaze nystagmus
l. gaze palsy
l. geniculate body
l. geniculate nucleus (LGN)
l. ground bundle
l. habenular nucleus
l. hemispheric dynamic
l. hypothalamic area
l. hypothalamic region
l. inferior pontine syndrome
l. intermediate substance
l. intradural approach
l. lacuna
l. lake
l. lemniscus
l. lemniscus trigone
l. line organ
l. listhesis
l. longitudinal stria
l. mass screw
l. medullary lamina of corpus striatum
l. medullary lamina of lentiform nucleus
l. medullary lumina
l. medullary syndrome
l. midpontine syndrome
l. neocortex
l. nucleus of mammillary body
l. nucleus of medulla oblongata
l. nucleus of thalamus
l. nucleus of trapezoid body
l. occipital artery
l. occipital sulcus
l. occipitotemporal gyrus
l. olfactory gyrus
l. olfactory stria
l. olfactory tract
l. orbitofrontal circuit
l. orbitofrontal cortex
l. parabrachial nucleus
l. pericuneate nucleus
l. periventricular white matter
l. posterior choroidal
l. posterior choroidal artery
l. posterior nucleus
l. preoptic nucleus
l. projection
l. proprius bundle
l. pterygoid nerve
l. pulvinar nucleus
l. pyramidal fasciculus
l. pyramidal tract
l. rachiotomy
l. raphespinal tract

NOTES

lateral *(continued)*
l. recess of fourth ventricle
l. recess stenosis
l. rectus muscle
l. rectus palsy
l. recumbent position
l. reticular nucleus
l. reticulospinal tract
l. rhinotomy
l. rhinotomy incision
l. roentgenogram
l. root of median nerve
l. root of optic tract
l. rostral supplementary motor area
l. rotation
l. sellar compartment
l. semicircular canal (LSC)
l. septal nucleus
l. sinus
l. sinus thrombosis
l. skull base
l. spinal sclerosis
l. spinothalamic tract
l. superior olivary nucleus
l. superior pontine syndrome
l. tarsorrhaphy
l. temporal epileptogenic lesion
l. temporal resection
l. terminal branch of deep fibular nerve
l. thalamic peduncle
l. thoracic meningocele
l. tuberal nucleus
l. vein of lateral ventricle
ventral posterior l. (VPL)
l. ventricle floor
l. ventricle occipital horn
l. ventricle posterior horn
l. ventricle temporal horn
l. vertigo
l. vestibular nucleus
l. vestibulospinal tract
l. zone
l. zone of hypothalamus

laterale
cornu l.
corpus geniculatum l.

laterales
lacunae l.
nervi supraclaviculares l.
nuclei tuberales l.
rami medullares l.
ramus choroidei posteriores l.
venae directae l.

lateralis
area hypothalamica l.
arteria occipitalis l.
arteria orbitofrontalis l.
bulbus cornus occipitalis ventriculi l.
bulbus cornus posterioris ventriculi l.
cisterna cerebellomedullaris l.
cisterna fossae l.
cisterna sulci l.
columna l.
cornu anterius ventriculi l.
cornu frontale ventriculi l.
cornu inferius ventriculi l.
cornu occipitale ventriculi l.
cornu posterius ventriculi l.
cornu temporale ventriculi l.
ductus semicircularis l.
fasciculus corticospinalis l.
fasciculus proprius l.
fasciculus pyramidalis l.
fissura cerebri l.
funiculus l.
globus pallidus l.
gyrus occipitotemporalis l.
gyrus olfactorius l.
lacunae l.
lamina medullaris l.
lemniscus l.
nervi digitales plantares communes nervi plantaris l.
nervi digitales plantares proprii nervi plantaris l.
nervus ampullaris l.
nervus cutaneous dorsalis l.
nervus cutaneous surae l.
nervus cutaneus antebrachii l.
nervus pectoralis l.
nervus plantaris l.
nervus pterygoideus l.
nuclei lemnisci l.
nucleus amygdalae l.
nucleus centralis l.
nucleus cervicalis l.
nucleus corporis mammillaris l.
nucleus dorsalis corporis geniculati l.
nucleus geniculatus l.
nucleus habenularis l.
nucleus lemnisci l.
nucleus olivaris superior l.
nucleus parabrachialis l.
nucleus paragigantocellular l.
nucleus pericuneatus l.
nucleus preopticus l.
nucleus septalis l.
nucleus tractus olfactorii l.
nucleus ventralis l.
nucleus ventralis corporis geniculi l.
nucleus vestibularis l.
pars centralis ventriculi l.

pars dorsalis corporis geniculati l.
pars ventralis corporis geniculati l.
pedunculus thalami l.
plexus choroideus ventriculi l.
rami corporis geniculati l.
ramus choroidei ventriculi l.
ramus profundus nervi plantaris l.
ramus superficialis nervi plantaris l.
regio hypothalamica l.
stria longitudinalis l.
stria olfactoria l.
substantia intermedia centralis et l.
sulcus occipitalis l.
tela choroidea ventriculi l.
tractus corticospinalis l.
tractus pyramidalis l.
tractus raphespinalis l.
tractus spinothalamicus l.
tractus vestibulospinalis l.
trigonum collaterale ventriculi l.
trigonum lemnisci l.
vena atrii l.
vena lateralis ventriculi l.
vena medialis ventriculi l.
vena recessus l.
ventralis posterior l.
ventriculus l.
zona l.

laterality
crossed l.

lateralization
fetal planum temporal l.
l. index
language l.

lateralized
l. activity
l. artifact
l. brain language system

laterally convex dural incision

lateral-onset temporal lobe epilepsy

later-life depression

lateropulsion
body l.
l. of body movement
l. of eye movement
isolated body l.
ocular l.

latex
l. agglutination
l. balloon
l. particle agglutination test

latex-covered pledget

lathosterol

lathosterolosis

lathyrism

Latin American Sleep Society

latissimus dorsi muscle

latrotoxin
alpha l.
beta l.

lattice
l. degeneration
l. field

latticed layer

laughing
l. seizure
l. sickness

laughter reflex

Laumonier ganglion

LAUP
laser-assisted uvulopalatoplasty

Laurence-Biedl syndrome

Laurence-Moon-Bardet-Biedl syndrome

Laurence-Moon-Biedl syndrome

Laurence-Moon syndrome

Lausanne stereotactic robot

law
l.'s of association
autonomic affective l.
l. of average localization
Bastian l.
Bastian-Bruns l.
Bell l.
Bell-Magendie l.
Bernoulli l.
Boltzmann distribution l.
Bowditch l.
Broadbent l.
l. of denervation
Ewald second l.
Flatau l.
Flouren l.
Gerhardt-Semon l.
Grasset l.
Haeckel l.
Hagen-Poiseuille l.
Hilton l.
l. of isochronism
Jackson l.
Landouzy-Grasset l.
Leyden l.
Magendie l.
Müller l.
Pascal l.

NOTES

law *(continued)*
Poiseuille l.
l. of referred pain
restraint l.
Ribot l.
Ritter l.
Rosenbach l.
Semon l.
Sherrington l.
L. of Specific Nerve Energy
Stokes l.
3 strikes l.
l. of thirds
van der Kolk l.
wallerian l.
Lawford syndrome
laxity
zygapophysial joint l.
layer
bacillary l.
l. of Bechterew
Bechterew l.
l. of cerebellar cortex
l. of cerebral cortex
claustral l.
concentric fiber l.
l. of dentate gyrus
dysfibrous l.
ependymal l.
epithelial choroid l.
external granular l.
fillet l.
fusiform l.
ganglionic l.
granular l.
Henle fiber l.
Henle nervous l.
l. of hippocampus
infragranular l.
infrastriate l.
inner limiting l.
inner nuclear l.
inner plexiform l.
intermediate l.
interstriate l.
Kaes-Bechterew l.
lacunar molecular l.
latticed l.
magnocellular l.
mantle l.
marginal l.
Meynert l.
mitral cell l.
molecular l.
multiform l.
l. of nerve fibers
neuroepithelial l.
olfactory nerve l.
optic l.
oriens l.
outer limiting l.
outer nuclear l. (ONL)
outer plexiform l.
peripapillary nerve fiber l.
piriform neuron l.
l. of piriform neuron
plexiform l.
polymorphous l.
Purkinje cell l.
pyramidal cell l.
radiant l.
l. of rods and cones
rostral l.
stria of internal granular l.
stria of internal pyramidal l.
stria of molecular l.
subarachnoid blood l.
subcallosal l.
superior colliculus l.
suprastriate l.
ventricular l.
Waldeyer zonal l.
zonular l.
lazabemide HCl
Lazarus effect
L-baclofen
LBE
line bisection error
LBP
low back pain
LC
locus coeruleus
Hydergine LC
LCBF
local cerebral blood flow
LCHAD
long-chain hydroxy Acyl-CoA dehydrogenase
LCHAD deficiency
LCHD
long-chain hydroxy Acyl-CoA dehydrogenase
LCMV
lymphocytic choriomeningitis virus
LDA
low-density area
LDD
laser disc decompression
LDD delivery system
LDD procedure
LDF
laser Doppler flowmeter
lumbodorsal fascia
LDL
low-density lipoprotein
L-dopa/benserazide
L-dopa stimulation test
Leach-Nyhan syndrome

lead
colic l.
deep brain l.
l. dislodgment
dual octapolar l.
dual quadrapolar l.
EEG with NP l.
l. encephalitis
l. encephalopathy
eye l.
frontopolar l.
l. intoxication
Lamitrode l.
model 300 NCP bipolar l.
NCP l.
l. neuropathy
octapolar l.
l. palsy
l. paralysis
l. poisoning
l. toxic disorder
l. toxicity
lead-pipe rigidity
leak
anastomotic l.
cerebrospinal fluid l.
sentinel l.
leakage
cerebrospinal fluid l.
chylous l.
l. headache
learning
intrusion in verbal l.
word list l.
learning-based rehabilitation
Leatherman hook
Leber
L. congenital amaurosis
L. disease
L. hereditary optic atrophy
L. hereditary optic neuropathy
LED
light-emitting diode
LED probe
Lee
L. disc prosthesis
L. ganglion
Leeds
L. Anxiety Scale
L. Sleep Evaluation Questionnaire (LSEQ)
LeFort
L. classification
L. fracture
L. osteotomy
left
l. atrial myxoma
l. common carotid artery
extension, sidebent right, rotated l. (ESRRL)
l. frontal lobe
l. hemiplegia
l. hemisphere damage (LHD)
l. hemisphere dominance
l. hemisphere mechanism
l. planum temporal
l. thoracolumbar major curve pattern
l. ventricle
l. ventricular function
l. visuospatial neglect
left-bearing nystagmus
left/right
l./r. asymmetry
l./r. hemisphere dominance
left-sided
l.-s. apraxia
l.-s. thoracotomy
left-to-right shunt
leftward saccade
leg
champagne-bottle l.
l. cramp
l. cramp treatment
l. jerk
l. movement
l. movement monitoring
l. pain
l. phenomenon
restless l.'s
l. sign
Legend high-speed pneumatic system
Legendre
L. function
L. sign
Legg disease
***Legionella pneumophila* infection**
leg-raising test
Leibinger
L. 3D plate
L. Micro Imlants drill bit
L. microplate
L. Micro Plus plate

NOTES

Leibinger *(continued)*
L. Micro Plus screw
L. Micro System cranial fixation plate
L. Micro System plate cutter
L. Micro System plate-holding forceps
L. Micro System pliers
L. titanium mini-Würzburg implant system
Leica vibrating knife microtome
Leichtenstern
L. encephalitis
L. phenomenon
L. sign
Leiden
factor V L.
Leigh
L. disease
L. necrotizing encephalopathy
L. subacute necrotizing encephalomyelitis
L. syndrome
leiodystonia
leiomyoma
extraspinal l.
leiomyosarcoma
disseminated l.
Leksell
L. adapter to Mayfield device
L. apparatus
L. arc
L. gamma knife target series
L. GammaPlan computerized program
L. G stereotactic head frame
L. Micro-Stereotactic system
L. Model C gamma knife
L. posteroventral pallidotomy
L. rongeur
L. selector
L. stereotactic gamma unit
L. stereotactic gamma unit lens
L. SurgiPlan computerized program
L. technique
Leksell-Elekta stereotactic frame
Lemieux-Neemeh syndrome
Lemmon sternal spreader
lemniscal
l. fiber
l. pathway
l. system
l. trigone
lemniscorum
decussatio l.
lemniscus, pl. **lemnisci**
acoustic l.
auditory l.
decussation of medial l.
gustatory l.
lateral l.
l. lateralis
medial l.
l. medialis
nucleus of lateral l.
spinal l.
l. spinalis
stratum interolivare l.
trigeminal l.
l. trigeminalis
trigone of lateral l.
trigonum l.
LEMS
Lambert-Eaton myasthenic syndrome
length
age-dependent l.
crown-heel l.
crown-rump l.
internodal l.
pedicle screw chord l.
pedicle screw path l.
pulse l.
lengthening
distal catheter l.
l. reaction
Lenke
L. classification of adolescent idiopathic scoliosis
L. scoring system
Lennert lymphoma
Lennox-Gastaut
L.-G. pattern
L.-G. syndrome
Lennox syndrome
lens
crossed l.
Leksell stereotactic gamma unit l.
nucleus of l.
lenticula, pl. **lenticulae**
lenticular
l. ansa
l. aphasia
l. fasciculus
l. ganglion
l. loop
l. nucleus
l. progressive degeneration
lenticularis
ansa l.
dystonia l.
fasciculus l.
nucleus of ansa l.
nucleus ansae l.
lenticulooptic
lenticulostriate artery (LSA)
lenticulothalamic
lentiformis
capsulae nuclei l.

discus l.
lamina medullaris medialis nuclei l.
nucleus l.
lentiform nucleus
lentiginosis
centrofacial l.
lentis
ectopia l.
nucleus l.
lentiviral vector
leonine facial feature
leontiasis ossea
Leopard syndrome
leprae
Mycobacterium l.
leprechaunism
leprosy
anesthetic l.
articular l.
dry l.
l. infection
mutilating l.
l. peripheral neuropathy
trophoneurotic l.
leprous
l. neuropathy
l. polyneuritis
leptin
l. level
l. secretion
l. signal
leptomeningeal
l. anastomosis
l. capillary-venous angiomatosis
l. carcinoma
l. carcinomatosis
l. cyst
l. enhancement postcontrast administration
l. fibrosis
l. gliomatosis
l. metastasis
l. neoplastic disease
l. tumor
l. venous angioma
leptomeningeal/wedge cortical biopsy
leptomeninges (*pl. of* leptomeninx)
leptomeningeum
spatium l.
leptomeningioma
leptomeningitis
basilar l.
sarcomatous l.
leptomeningopathy
leptomeninx, pl. **leptomeninges**
leptomyelolipoma
leptospirosis lymphocytic meningitis
Leriche
L. operation
L. sympathectomy
L. syndrome
Leri sign
LeRoy-Raney scalp clip
LeRoy scalp clip-applying forceps
LES
Lambert-Eaton syndrome
Lesch-Nyhan
L.-N. disease
L.-N. syndrome
Leser-Trélat sign
lesion
acute cerebellar hemispheric l.
afferent digital l.
afferent nerve l.
angiocentric immunoproliferative l.
anterior parietal l.
anterochiasmatic l.
atrophic l.
auricular l.
axonal l.
basal ganglionic l.
biparietal l.
brachial plexus l.
brain l.
brainstem l.
bubbly bone l.
callosal l.
catecholamine l.
cavernous sinus l.
central l.
cerebral l.
cerebrovascular l.
cervical cord l.
chiasmal l.
chiasmatic l.
circumscribed l.
compressive mass l.
compressive trigeminal nerve l.
confetti skin l.
conus medullaris l.
cortical l.
corticospinal pathway l.

NOTES

lesion *(continued)*
cyclops l.
deep white matter l. (DWML)
demyelinating trigeminal nerve l.
destructive stereotactic l.
diencephalic l.
diffuse pontine l.
discharging l.
discoid skin l.
dominant hemisphere l.
dorsal root entry zone l.
dumbbell l.
Duret l.
enhancing l.
entry zone l.
epicortical l.
epileptogenic structural l.
epileptogenic temporal l.
excitatory l.
extraaxial l.
extraconal l.
extracranial mass l.
extramesial temporal l.
filum terminale l.
fimbria-fornix l.
focal l.
frank l.
frontal lobe l.
frontal white matter l.
gadolinium-enhancing l.
l. generation
grapelike l.
graviceptive brainstem l.
hemorrhagic l.
high cervical spinal cord l.
high-intensity l.
high pontine l.
high-risk l.
high-signal l.
high thoracic cord l.
homogeneous l.
hyperdense l.
hyperintense l.
hyperostotic l.
hypoglossal canal l.
hypotense l.
hypothalamic l.
hypoxic-ischemic fetal l.
indiscriminate l.
infarct-like l.
inflammatory l.
infranuclear l.
infratentorial l.
interpeduncular fossa l.
intraaxial brain l.
intracanalicular l.
intracerebral l.
intracranial mass l.
intradural extramedullary mass l.
intramedullary spinal l.
intraorbital l.
intrasellar l.
intraspinal l.
iron-containing l.
irritative l.
ischemic-hypoxic l.
ischemic white matter l.
isodense l.
isointense l.
keratotic l.
lateral temporal epileptogenic l.
leukoencephalopathic l.
l. load
low-density l.
lower motor neuron l.
low-grade l.
l. map
mass l.
Meckel cave l.
median nerve l.
mesial temporal epileptogenic l.
metabolic l.
metameric l.
microscopic l.
midbrain l.
midline developmental l.
mononeural l.
mucous membrane l.
multiple focal l.'s
multiple ring-enhancing l.'s
myelic l.
myelitic l.
nail l.
nasal l.
neoplastic l.
neurofibrillary l.
neurogenic l.
nondominant hemisphere l.
nonmeningiomatous malignant l.
nucleus basalis l.
obturator nerve l.
occipital l.
ocular l.
optic nerve l.
oral herpes l.
orbitomedial/cingulate l.
pallidal l.
paraorbital l.
parasagittal l.
parasellar l.
parietal cortex l.
parietal lobe l.
parietooccipital l.
peripheral nerve l.
peripheral oculomotor l.
periventricular hyperintense l.
periventricular white matter l.
peroneal nerve l.

Perthes-Bankart l.
petroclival l.
phrenic nerve l.
pigment epithelial l.
pineal l.
pituitary stalk l.
pontine l.
posterior column l.
posterior compartment l.
posterior fossa mass l.
posterior language area l.
posttraumatic frontal l.
potentially curable l.
prepontine l.
pretectal l.
pseudocystic hypodense l.
pseudomedial longitudinal fasciculus l.
pyramidal tract l.
radiofrequency l.
regurgitant l.
retrobulbar l.
retrochiasmal l.
retrochiasmatic l.
retrocochlear l.
ring-wall l.
root entry zone l.
rotationally induced shear-strain l.
sciatic nerve l.
senile leukoencephalopathic l.
single enhancing CT l.
skip l.
space-occupying brain l.
spinal cord l.
spinal mass l.
striatal l.
structural brain l.
subcortical l.
subtentorial l.
supranuclear l.
suprasellar l.
supratentorial structural l.
synchronous l.
tectal l.
tertiary neuron l.
thalamic l.
thoracic cord l.
T2 hyperintense l.
T1 hypointense l.
transverse cord l.
traumatic intracranial l.
T2-weighted MRI l.
ulnar nerve l.
underlying mass l.
underlying structural l.
unstable l.
upper motor neuron l.
well-circumscribed l.
well-defined focal brain l.
white matter l. (WML)

lesionectomy
computer-assisted volumetric stereotactic l.
stereotactic l.

lesion-induced cortical plasticity

lesioning
dorsal root entry zone l.
DREZ l.
nucleus caudalis-nucleus solitarius DREZ l.
radiofrequency l.
thermal l.
trigeminal l.
trigeminal nucleus caudalis l.

lesser superficial petrosal nerve (LSPN)

LET
linear energy transfer

lethal midline granuloma

lethargica
encephalitis l.

lethica
aphasia l.

letter
l. blindness
l. fluency test

Letterer-Siwe disease

leucine
l. degradation
l. serum level
l. zipper family
l. zipper gene

leucotome (*var. of* leukotome)

leucotomy (*var. of* leukotomy)

leucovorin

leukemia
central nervous system l.
chronic myeloid l.
l. inhibitory factor (LIF)
pediatric stroke from l.
periventricular l.
l. therapy affecting cognitive function

Leukeran

L

NOTES

leukoaraiosis
l. score
leukocyte
l. antigen typing
cerebrospinal fluid l.
eosinophilic l.
polymorphonuclear l. (PML)
l. scintigraphy
tumor-infiltrating l. (TIL)
leukocytoclastic vasculitis
leukocytosis
emotional l.
leukodystrophia cerebri progressiva
leukodystrophy
adrenal l.
Canavan l.
globoid cell l.
Krabbe l.
megalencephalic l.
metachromatic l.
Pelizaeus-Merzbacher l.
spongiform l.
spongy degeneration l.
sudanophilic l.
leukoencephalitis
acute epidemic l.
acute necrotizing hemorrhagic l.
necrotizing hemorrhagic l.
l. periaxialis concentrica
postinfectious l.
postvaccinal l.
sclerosing l.
subacute sclerosing l.
van Bogaert sclerosing l.
viral l.
leukoencephalopathic lesion
leukoencephalopathy
cerebral autosomal dominant arteriopathy with subcortical infarcts and l. (CADASIL)
cerebral autosomal recessive arteriopathy with subcortical infarcts and l. (CARASIL)
diffuse necrotizing l.
metachromatic l.
mitochondrial l.
multifocal l.
necrotizing l.
polycystic lipomembranous osteodysplasia with sclerosing l. (PLOSL)
progressive multifocal l. (PML)
l. radiation
subacute sclerosing l.
subcortical l.
leukoencephaly
focal pontine l.
progressive necrotizing l.
leukokoria
leukomalacia
cystic periventricular l.
periventricular l. (PVL)
premature infant periventricular l.
leukomyelitis
necrotizing hemorrhage l.
leukomyelopathy
leukopenia
transient l.
leukopoiesis
leukostasis
CNS l.
leukotome, leucotome
leukotomy, leucotomy
bimedial frontal l.
limbic l.
prefrontal l.
transorbital l.
ventromedial frontal l.
leukotriene modifier
leuprolide acetate
LEV
levetiracetam
levallorphan tartrate
levator
l. ani nerve
l. palatini
l. palpebrae muscle
l. scapulae
level
l. of abstraction
l. of activity
agitation l.
air-fluid l.
l. of alertness
ammonia blood l.
bilirubin serum l.
carnitine serum l.
cerebrospinal fluid ferritin l.
ceruloplasmin serum l.
cholesterol serum l.
circulating leptin l.
l. of cognitive function
l. of consciousness
cortisol l.
creatinine kinase serum l.
criterion l.
decreased oxygen l.
l. of depression
l. of disruption
dissociation l.
effective l.
E-selectin l.
estrogen l.
expression l.
flucytosine blood l.
l. of functioning
L. of Functioning Scale
glucose blood l.

gray matter lactate l.
hair lead l.
homocysteine l.
l. of impairment
lactic acid serum l.
leptin l.
leucine serum l.
linear interpolation l.
lipid serum l.
liver enzyme serum l.
low energy l.
lower circulating estrogen l.
meningioma prostaglandin l.
mental l.
molecular l.
muscle enzyme serum l.
neural noise l.
neural pathway l.
neurosegmental l.
nocturnal melatonin l.
orotic acid urine l.
oxalic acid urine l.
pathological l.
perceptual l.
performance l.
phenylalanine serum l.
phytanic acid l.
pipecolic acid l.
plasma homocysteine l.
plasma leptin l.
posttest l.
primitive emotional l.
progesterone l.
proline urine l.
l. of psychological pain
red cell folic acid l.
serum ammonia l.
serum androgen l.
serum caffeine l.
serum folic acid l.
spinal l.
symptom l.
synaptic protein l.
thyroid-stimulating hormone l.
urea blood l.
uric acid l.
vertebral l.
vitamin B12 l.
white matter lactate l.
zinc protoporphyrin l.

level-dependent
level-of-care criterion
levetiracetam (LEV)
Levine-Critchley syndrome
Levin thermocouple cordotomy electrode
Lev-Lenègre syndrome
levocarnitine
levodopa
l. and carbidopa
l. ethylester
levodopa/carbidopa
levodopa-induced dyskinesia
levonorgestrel
levopromazine
Lévy-Roussy syndrome
Lewis blood group activity
Lewy
L. body
L. body dementia
L. body disease
Lexapro
lexical
l. access
l. agraphia
l. graphia
l. process
l. word production
lexical-syntactic deficit
lexicon
orthographic l.
lexipafant
Lex-Ton spinal frame
Leyden
L. ataxia
L. law
L. neuritis
Leyden-Möbius
L.-M. muscular dystrophy
L.-M. syndrome
Leydig
L. neuron
L. tumor cell
Leyla
L. brain retractor
L. self-retaining tractor bar
L. self-retaining tractor bar lift
LFF
low-frequency filter
LFF on electroencephalogram
LGG
low-grade glioma
L-glutamate
L-glutamic acid

NOTES

LGMD2B
limb-girdle muscular dystrophy type 2B
LGN
lateral geniculate nucleus
LH
luteinizing hormone
LHD
left hemisphere damage
Lhermitte
L. phenomenon
L. sign
Lhermitte-Duclos disease
liberae
terminationes nervorum l.
liberatory maneuver
Librium
Lichtheim
L. aphasia
L. disease
L. plaque
L. sign
L. syndrome
licostinel
Liddell-Sherrington reflex
Liddle
L. dexamethasone suppression test
L. psychomotor poverty
lid nystagmus
lidocaine
l. test
l. transdermal patch
Lidoderm
lidofenin
technetium-99m l.
lienalis
plexus l.
lienal plexus
Liepmann apraxia
LIF
leukemia inhibitory factor
life
l. expectancy
l. impairment
L. Satisfaction Index
L. Skills Profile
L. Skills Profile index
l. span
L. Span Study
life-changing improvement
lifelong therapy
lifestyle modification
lifetime impulsivity
life-year
quality-adjusted l.-y. (QUALY)
Li-Fraumeni syndrome
lift
Leyla self-retaining tractor bar l.
pneumatic chair l.
lifter
Yasargil tissue l.
Ligaclip
L. applier
L. clip
Ethicon L.
ligament
alar l.
anterior longitudinal l.
atlantoepistrophic l.
axial-occipital l.
coccygeal l.
congenital laxity of l.
costotransverse l.
costovertebral l.
cruciate l.
dentate l.
denticulate l.
Gruber l.
l. of Henle
interclinoid l.
longitudinal l.
mamilloaccessory l. (MAL)
occipital-atlas-axis l.
ossification of posterior longitudinal l. (OPLL)
petrosphenoidal l.
posterior longitudinal l.
Struthers l.
transverse atlantal l.
yellow l.
ligamenta (*pl. of* ligamentum)
ligamentectomy
bilateral l.'s
ligamentous integrity
ligamentum, pl. **ligamenta**
l. denticulatum
l. flavum
interspinous l.
ligand
bidentate l.
l. concentration
hydrophobic l.
l. occupation
putative endogenous l.
receptor l.
l. selection
ligand-gated ion channel
ligase
ubiquitin protein l.
ligation
hunterian l.
ligature
intravascular l.
light
birefringence in polarized l.
l. chain paraprotein
l. effect on circadian rhythm
l. exposure

l. meromyosin
l. microscopy study
seizure induced by flickering l.
l. sleep
l. touch response
light-emitting diode (LED)
lightheaded
lightning
l. attacks in infantile spasm
l. injury
light-prompted button task
Light-Veley headrest
LightWare micro retractor
LightWear headlight
Lilienthal rib spreader
Liliequist
membrane of L.
lilliputian hallucination
limb
afferent l.
l. of bony semicircular canal
branch to internal capsule, posterior l.
branch to internal capsule, retrolentiform l.
efferent l.
intransitive l.
l. movement disorder
l. muscle
l. myokymia
paralyzed l.
phantom l.
l. psychogenic disorder
l. transitive gesture
l. tremor
l. weakness
limb-girdle
l.-g. muscular dystrophy
l.-g. muscular dystrophy type 2B (LGMD2B)
limb-girdle-trunk paresis
limbic
l. activation
l. brain region
l. circuitry
l. cortex
l. dopamine receptor
l. effect
l. encephalitis
l. leukotomy
l. lobe
l. neuronal firing rate
l. system
l. system pathway
l. system structure
limbic-related region
limbicus
lobus l.
Limbitrol
limb-kinetic
l.-k. apraxia
l.-k. dyspraxia
limbus vertebra
limen, pl. **limina**
l. insula
l. to twoness
LIM gene
liminal stimulus
liminometer
limit
extreme narrowing l.
l. setting
limitans
glia l.
sulcus l.
limitation
conceptual l.
empirical l.
functional l.
Hannover Functional Ability Questionnaire for measuring back pain-related functional l.'s (FFbH-R)
irreversible l.
receiver l.
vertical gaze l.
limited
l. effect
l. symptom attack
limiting
l. sulcus
l. sulcus of fourth ventricle
l. sulcus of Reil
l. sulcus of rhomboid fossa
limit-setting sleep disorder
***LIM*-kinase gene**
limp
antalgic l.
limulus
l. amebocyte lysate assay
l. lysate assay of cerebrospinal fluid
LINAC
linear accelerator

NOTES

LINAC *(continued)*
Boston LINAC
LINAC radiosurgery
LINAC radiosurgery system
LINAC-based radiosurgical system
lincomycin
Lindamood Auditory Conceptualization
Lindau tumor
Lindau-von Hippel disease
Lindegaard hemispheric ratio
Linder
L. sign
L. test
Lindermann bur
line
AC-PC l.
anterior commissure-posterior commissure l.
l. artifact
Baillarger l.
basal l.
l. of Bechterew
bimastoid l.
l. bisection error (LBE)
cell l.
central sacral l.
Chamberlain palatooccipital l.
choroid l.
clivus canal l.
digastric l.
Donaldson l.
Fishgold l.
foramen magnum l.
l. frequency noise dot
fusion l.
Garrett orientation l.
Gennari l.
l. of Gennari
glabella-inion l.
Gubler l.
Haller l.
HCN-1 cell l.
head l.
l. imaging
isodose l.
l. of Kaes
Kaes l.
linear regression l.
logarithmic regression l.
Lorentzian l.
M l.
major dense l.
major period l.
McGregor basal l.
McRae foramen magnum l.
Mees l.
midpoint to meatal l.
neural cell l.
Obersteiner-Redlich l.
occipital l.
palatooccipital l.
period l.
posterior canal l.
radiosignal l.
recruitment l.
rolandic l.
l. scanning
simian l.
soft l.
spinolamellar l.
spinous interlaminar l.
Swischuk l.
sylvian l.
tender l.
Ullmann l.
Voigt l.
Wackenheim clivus canal l.
l. width
lineage
cellular l.
linear
l. accelerator (LINAC)
l. accelerator radiosurgery
l. accelerator system
l. chromosome
l. craniectomy
l. energy transfer (LET)
l. interpolation level
l. least-square regression analysis
l. nevus sebaceus
l. nucleus
l. perspective
l. rate-response function
l. regression line
l. scale
l. skull fracture
line-derived
glial cell l.-d.
lingering fear
lingua, pl. **linguae**
l. cerebelli
l. franca
lapsus l.
nucleus fibrosus l.
septum l.
tremor l.
linguadental contact
lingual
l. airway dysfunction
l. branch
l. corpuscle
l. gyrus
l. hemiatrophy
l. muscle
l. nerve
l. paralysis
l. plexus
l. septum

l. trophoneurosis
l. vein
lingualis
gyrus l.
nervus l.
rami fauciales nervi l.
rami isthmi faucium nervi l.
rami linguales nervi l.
lingualplasty
lingula, pl. **lingulae**
l. cerebelli
l. of cerebellum
vincula l.
linguofacial vein
link
genetic l.
L. SB Charité disc
L. SB Charité disc prosthesis
linkage
l. analysis
l. object
rod l.
lion's paw grasper
Lioresal
liothyronine sodium
lip
l. reflex
rhombic l.
l. smacking automatism
lipase
acid l.
lipectomy
lipedematous alopecia
lipid
l. bilayer
cell membrane l.
l. hypothesis
l. metabolism disorder
l. peroxidation
l. recycling
serum l.
l. serum level
l. storage disorder
l. storage myopathy
lipid-containing vesicle
lipid-laden stromal cell
lipid-lipoprotein metabolism disorder
lipid-lowering agent
lipidosis, pl. **lipidoses**
cerebral l.
cerebroside l.
familial neurovisceral l.
galactosylceramide l.
ganglioside l.
neuronal l.
sphingomyelin l.
sulfatide l.
lipid-protein bilayer
lipiodol
lipodystrophy
lipofuscin granule
lipofuscinoses
lipofuscinosis
adult l.
ceroid l.
Finnish variant of neuronal ceroid l.
l. granular osmiophilic deposit
Indian variant l.
infantile l.
infantile neuronal ceroid l.
juvenile neuronal ceroid l.
late infantile neuronal ceroid l.
neuronal ceroid l. (NCL)
lipogranulomatosis
Farber l.
lipohyalinosis
lipoid
l. metabolism
l. proteinosis
lipoidosis
cerebroside l.
lipolysis
membrane l.
lipolytic enzyme
lipoma
epidermoid l.
hamartomatous l.
inclusion l.
intradural l.
quadrigeminal cistern l.
spinal l.
subarachnoid l.
subcutaneous l.
tectal l.
lipomatosis
epidural l.
lipomeningocele
lipomeningomyelocele
lipomyelocele
lipomyelomeningocele
lipomyeloschisis
liponeural junction

NOTES

lipophilic
l. chloroethylnitrosourea
l. compound
l. sodium
lipopolysaccharide
lipopolysaccharide-induced inflammation
lipoprotein
high-density l. (HDL)
low-density l. (LDL)
l. metabolic disorder
l. receptor-related protein
liposarcoma
liposome
cytarabine l.
lipoxygenase pathway
liquid
L. Embolic System
ethylene vinyl alcohol copolymer l.
liquor cerebrospinalis
Lisch nodule
LIS1 gene
lisinopril and hydrochlorothiazide
Lissauer
L. bundle
L. column
column of Spitzka and L.
L. fasciculus
L. marginal zone
L. paralysis
L. tract
L. tract of spinal cord
lissencephalic syndrome
lissencephaly, lissencephalia
l. syndrome
Walker l.
X-linked l.
list
recall of word l.
Listeria
L. monocytogenes
L. monocytogenes meningitis
Lister strain
listhesis
lateral l.
lisuride
Lite
Profile L.
Spinal-Stim L.
liter
injected dose per l. (IDPL)
literacy deficiency
literal
l. agraphia
l. paraphasia
literalis
dysarthria l.
lithium
l. carbonate
l. dose
l. treatment
Little disease
livedo reticularis
liver
l. damage
l. encephalopathy
l. enzyme serum level
l. flap
l. function test
l. phosphorylase
l. span
l. transplantation
l. transplant complication
Livierato sign
living
activities of daily l. (ADL)
Communicative Abilities in Daily L.
l. death
instrumental activities of daily l. (IADL)
Reintegration to Normal L. (RNL)
tasks of independent l.
L-LTP
late-phase long-term potentiation
L-lysine acid
LM
lower motor
LMN
lower motor neuron
LMNA
lamin a/c gene
load
axial l.
l. compensation
high-lesion l.
lesion l.
sensory l.
spine l.
torso flexion l.
loading
axial l.
Edwards modular system dynamic l.
l. jig
salient l.
spinal l.
l. strategy
lobar
l. atrophy
l. division
l. dysfunction
l. hemorrhage
l. holoprosencephaly
l. resection
l. sclerosis
lobe
burst temporal l.

cerebral l.
l. of cerebrum
cuneiform l.
falciform l.
flocculonodular l.
frontal l.
insular l.
isthmus of limbic l.
left frontal l.
limbic l.
medial temporal l.
mesial aspect of temporal l.
mesial part of frontal l.
mesiobasal temporal l.
mesiotemporal l.
neural l.
occipital l.
olfactory l.
optic l.
parietal l.
piriform l.
prefrontal l.
quadrate l.
right frontal l.
semilunar l.
Spigelius l.
temporal l.
uncus of temporal l.
vagal l.
visceral l.

lobectomy
anterior temporal l.
anteromesial temporal l.
extratemporal l.
Falconer l.
nondominant temporal l.
occipital l.
temporal l.

lobi (*pl. of* lobus)

lobotomy
frontal l.
prefrontal l.
radical prefrontal l.
transorbital l.

Lobstein ganglion

lobule
ala of central l.
ansiform l.
anterior lunate l.
anterior paracentral l.
biventer l.
biventral l.
central l.
flocculonodular l.
gracile l.
inferior parietal l.
inferior semilunar l.
myxoid l.
paracentral l.
paramedian l.
parietal l.
posterior lunate l.
quadrangular l.
quadrate l.
semilunar l.
simple l.
slender l.
superior parietal l. (SPL)
superior semilunar l.
wing of central l.

lobulet, lobulette

lobulus, pl. **lobuli**
l. biventer
l. biventralis
l. centralis corporis cerebelli
l. clivi
l. culminis
l. cuneiformis
l. folii
l. fusiformis
l. gracilis
l. paracentralis
l. paramedianus
l. paramedianus cerebelli
l. parietalis inferior
l. parietalis superior
l. quadrangularis
l. quadrangularis anterior cerebelli
l. quadrangularis posterior cerebelli
l. quadratus
lobuli semilunares
l. semilunaris caudalis
l. semilunaris inferior
l. semilunaris rostralis
l. semilunaris superior
l. simplex
l. simplex cerebelli

lobus, pl. **lobi**
l. anterior hypophyseos
lobi cerebri
l. clivi
l. falciformis
l. flocculonodularis
l. frontalis

NOTES

lobus *(continued)*
l. frontalis cerebri
l. glandularis hypophyseos
l. insula
l. insularis
l. limbicus
l. nervosus
l. nervosus neurohypophyseos
l. occipitalis
l. occipitalis cerebri
l. parietalis
l. parietalis cerebri
l. posterior cerebelli
l. posterior hypophyseos
l. rostralis cerebelli
l. temporalis
l. vagus
local
l. anesthesia
l. cerebral blood flow (LCBF)
l. circuit theory
l. demyelination
l. diagnostic block
l. epilepsy
l. excitatory state
l. field distortion
l. lymph node
l. mass effect
l. reduction in amplitude
l. reflex
l. sign
l. syncope
l. tetanus
l. tic
l. vasoconstrictive action
localization
l. agnosia
anatomic l.
autoradiographic l.
cerebral l.
2D graphic l.
dipole l.
frame fixation scanner-assisted target l.
ictal l.
intraoperative stereotactic spatial l.
law of average l.
manual target l.
pedicle l.
pneumotaxic l.
scanner-assisted target l.
spatial l.
stereotactic anatomic target l.
subcellular l.
target l.
ultrasonographic l.
x-ray l.
localization-related
l.-r. epilepsy
l.-r. seizure
l.-r. therapy
localized
l. amnesia
l. electroencephalographic seizure pattern
l. evoked potential
l. magnetic resonance
l. pruritus
l. restorative central nervous system gene therapy
localizer
Mayfield fiducial l.
Risser l.
Suetens-Gybels-Vandermeulen angiographic l.
ultrasonic l.
location
aneurysm l.
brain l.
cervical sympathetic chain l.
pedicle l.
locative
locator
Gill Thomas l.
loci (*pl. of* locus)
4-loci haplotype
6-loci haplotype
lock
l. finger
l. spasm
locked facet
locked-in syndrome
locoism
locomotion
brachial l.
locomotor ataxia
loculation syndrome
loculus, pl. **loculi**
meningeal l.
locus, pl. **loci**
l. caeruleus
l. cerulean
l. cinereus
l. coeruleus (LC)
l. coeruleus region
l. ferrugineus
genetic l.
l. heterogeneity
l. niger
l. of onset
l. perforatus anticus
l. perforatus posticus
quantitative trait l. (QTL)
Loewenthal
L. bundle
L. tract
loflazepate
ethyl l.

log
sleep l.
sleeplessness l.
logagraphia
logamnesia
logaphasia
logarithmic regression line
logarithm of odds score
logasthenia
logical memory subtest score
logistic
l. regression analysis
l. regression equation
logopathy
logoplegia
logospasm
LOH10
loss of heterozygosity chromosome 10
Lombard voice-reflex test
lomustine
long
l. association fiber
L. Beach stereotactic robot
l. gyrus of insula
l. pulse repetition time/echo time image
l. pulse repetition time/long echo time
l. pulse repetition time/long echo time spin-echo
l. root of ciliary ganglion
l. segment spinal fusion
l. sleep (LS)
l. sleeper
l. thoracic nerve
l. thoracic palsy
long-acting (LA)
l.-a. injectable medication
l.-a. injection
longae
fibrae associationes l.
long-chain
l.-c. fatty acid
l.-c. hydroxy Acyl-CoA dehydrogenase (LCHAD, LCHD)
longi
nervi ciliares l.
longitudinal
l. assessment
l. axis
l. cerebral fissure
l. experimental study design
l. expert evaluation using all available data
l. fissure of cerebrum
l. ligament
l. ligament rupture
l. magnetization
l. medial bundle
l. member to anchor connector
l. pontine bundle
l. pontine fasciculus
l. pontine fiber
l. relaxation
l. scan
l. sinus thrombus
l. spinal bar
longitudinales
fibrae pontis l.
long-lasting drug effect
longstanding
l. corticosteroid administration
l. symptom
long-stay ward
long-term
l.-t. associative memory
l.-t. bone-instrumentation interface
l.-t. course
l.-t. declarative memory
l.-t. disability assessment
l.-t. effectiveness
l.-t. effects of trauma
l.-t. illness
l.-t. insomnia
l.-t. naturalistic study
l.-t. outcome
l.-t. result
l.-t. stability
l.-t. storage of memory
l.-t. vasomotor tone renin
longus
l. capitis muscle
l. cervicis colli muscle
nervus thoracicus l.
loop
Blair-Ivy l.
gamma l.
Granit l.
Hartshill Ransford l.
l. of hypoglossal nerve
Hyrtl l.
inferior root of cervical l.
inhibitory l.
lenticular l.

NOTES

loop *(continued)*
Meyer l.
Meyer-Archambault l.
neuronal feedback l.
neuronal feed-forward l.
pallidostriatal feedback l.
peduncular l.
Ransford l.
l. of spinal nerve
subclavian l.
superior root of cervical l.
l. synapse
unipolar cutting l.
vascular l.
Vieussens l.
loose
l. belt artifact
l. electrode
loosening
pin l.
Lopressor
lorazepam
lordosis
l. creation
lumbar spine l.
l. preservation
thoracic spine l.
Lorentzian line
Lorenz
L. cranial plate
L. cranial screw
L. Neuro/skull base titanium osteosynthesis system
L. titanium screws and plate
Lorenzo oil
Los Angeles Prehospital Stroke Screen (LAPSS)
losigamone
loss
allelic l.
amygdala volumetric l.
axonal l.
blood l.
bone l.
capelike sensory l.
cell l.
central sensory l.
color vision l.
color visual l.
complete visual l.
l. of consciousness
contralateral l.
cortical sensory l.
Dejerine onion peel sensory l.
dense sensory l.
dissociated sensory l.
l. of energy metabolism
functional l.
gag reflex l.
gaze-evoked visual l.
glucocorticoid-induced bone l.
hair l.
hearing l.
heat l.
hemifield l.
hemisensory l.
l. of heterozygosity chromosome 10 (LOH10)
high-frequency hearing l.
hippocampal neuronal l.
hippocampal pyramidal cell l.
hippocampal volume l.
hippocampal volumetric l.
hysterical visual l.
l. of independence
ipsilateral l.
mechanical visual l.
l. of memory
natural hearing l.
neuronal l.
nonspecific neuronal l.
painless vision l.
partial visual l.
peripheral sensory l.
permanent visual l.
position l.
primary afferent l.
progressive visual l.
pure-tone hearing l.
l. of response
retrocochlear hearing l.
saddle-area sensory l.
l. of sensitivity
sensory l.
signal l.
stocking-glove sensory l.
surgical hearing l.
synapse l.
synaptic l.
topographic memory l.
transient monocular visual l.
unilateral hearing l.
unilateral visual l.
vibration l.
vision l.
visual acuity l.
volumetric l.
weight l.
loss-of-resistance technique
lotus neuropathy
Lou Gehrig disease
Louis-Bar syndrome
Louisiana State University Medical Center (LSUMC)
Louis instrumentation
lounging position
loupe
binocular l.

Keeler Galilean l.
Keeler panoramic l.
l. magnification

Love
L. nerve root hook
L. nerve root retractor
L. pituitary rongeur

Love-Adson wire tightener

Love-Gruenwald
L.-G. cranial rongeur
L.-G. disc rongeur
L.-G. intervertebral disc forceps
L.-G. pituitary forceps
L.-G. pituitary rongeur

Love-Kerrison
L.-K. laminectomy rongeur
L.-K. rongeur forceps

Lovén reflex

low
l. air loss bed
l. alpha coefficient
l. anger threshold
l. back pain (LBP)
l. back pain psychogenic disorder
l. back syndrome
l. blood gas partition
l. bone mass
l. calcium
l. cervical approach
l. delirium
l. EMG tone
l. energy level
l. linear frequency
l. lumbar spine fracture
l. molecular weight cytokeratin
l. molecular weight heparin
l. physical activity
l. potassium
L. Profile valve
l. serum albumin
l. single thoracic curve
l. threshold of competency

low-amplitude
l.-a. activity
l.-a. circadian rhythm

low-degree astrocytoma

low-density
l.-d. area (LDA)
l.-d. lesion
l.-d. lipoprotein (LDL)
l.-d. lipoprotein receptor

low-dose
l.-d. dopaminergic agonist
l.-d. estrogen replacement
l.-d. strategy

Löwenberg canal

low-energy gamma radiation

lower
l. abdominal periosteal reflex
l. basilar aneurysm
l. bony endplate
l. cervical spine
l. cervical spine fusion
l. cervical spine posterior stabilization
l. cervical spine procedure
l. circulating estrogen level
l. clivus
l. hook trial
l. limb dysmetria
l. lumbar spine
l. mortality
l. motor (LM)
l. motor neuron (LMN)
l. motor neuron disease
l. motor neuron dysarthria
l. motor neuron dysfunction
l. motor neuron lesion
l. motor neuron paralysis
l. motor neuron syndrome
l. pons
l. posterior lumbar spine and sacrum surgery
l. radicular syndrome
l. thoracic pedicle
l. thoracic spine

lower-half headache

lowest saturation of oxygen

Lowe syndrome

low-filter frequency

low-frequency
l.-f. activity
l.-f. filter (LFF)

low-grade
l.-g. diffuse astrocytoma
l.-g. glioma (LGG)
l.-g. lesion
l.-g. tumor

low-key response

low-melt temperature agarose

low-pass filter

low-penetrance/high-frequency gene

Lowry-MacLean syndrome

NOTES

L

low-salt diet
low-tension glaucoma
low-threshold mechanoreceptor (LTM)
low-voltage
l.-v. activity
l.-v. calibration
l.-v. EEG
loxapine
Loxitane C
Lozol
LP
lumbar puncture
LPC
laser photocoagulation
LRRK2
LRRK2 gene
LRRK2 mutation
LS
long sleep
Micro-K LS
LSA
lenticulostriate artery
LSC
lateral semicircular canal
LSEQ
Leeds Sleep Evaluation Questionnaire
L-shaped
L-s. aneurysm clip
L-s. microplate
LSI
lumbar spine index
LSM
laser scanning microscope
LSPN
lesser superficial petrosal nerve
LSUMC
Louisiana State University Medical Center
LSUMC classification of motor and sensory function
LSUMC classification of nerve injury
LT
lamina terminalis
LTM
low-threshold mechanoreceptor
L-triiodothyronine
L-tryptophan
L-type calcium channel
L-tyrosine acid
lubeluzole
Lucae
L. bone mallet
L. nerve hook
Lucas and Drucker Motor Index
lucent mass
Luc ethmoid forceps
Luciani triad
lucidum
septum l.
Ludwig
depressor nerve of L.
L. ganglion
L. nerve
Luer-Lok stopcock
luetic
l. aneurysm
l. meningitis
Luft disease
Luhr
L. microfixation cranial plate
L. microfixation system drill bit
L. microfixation system pliers
L. microplate
L. miniplate
L. pan plate
lumbago
ischemic l.
lumbales
nervi splanchnici l.
lumbalia
ganglia l.
segmentum l. 1–5
lumbalis
cisterna l.
intumescentia l.
plexus l.
rami musculares plexus l.
ramus lateralis rami posterioris nervi l.
ramus medialis rami posterioris nervi l.
segmentum medullae spinalis l.
lumbalium
rami anteriores nervorum l.
rami dorsales nervorum l.
rami posteriores nervorum l.
rami ventrales nervorum l.
lumbar
l. anterior root stimulator implant
l. arachnoid peritoneal shunt
l. artery
l. cistern
cisterna l.
l. curve
l. disc disease
l. discectomy
l. disc herniation
l. disc rupture
l. drain
l. drainage
l. drainage catheter
l. enlargement of spinal cord
l. epidural steroid
l. facet disease
l. flat back syndrome
l. ganglion

l. hemilaminectomy
L. I/F Cage
l. interbody arthrodesis
l. interbody fusion
l. interspace
l. kyphosis
l. lordosis preservation
l. meningocele
l. myelography
l. nerve
l. part of diaphragm
l. part of spinal cord
l. pedicle fixation
l. pedicle marker
l. pedicle screw
l. periosteal turnover flap
l. plexopathy
l. plexus
l. port
l. puncture (LP)
l. puncture complication
l. puncture needle
l. puncture pain
l. reflex
l. rheumatism
l. scoliosis
l. spinal stenosis
l. spine biopsy
l. spine burst fracture
l. spine decompression
l. spine index (LSI)
l. spine injury
l. spine instability
l. spine instrumentation
l. spine kyphotic deformity
l. spine lordosis
l. spine model
l. spine pedicle diameter
l. spine rotational stability
l. spine segmental fixation
l. spine stabilization
l. spine transpedicular fixation
l. spine trauma
l. spine vertebral osteosynthesis
l. spondylosis
l. sympathectomy
l. synovial cyst
l. tumor
l. vertebra

lumbares
nervi splanchnici l.

lumbaria
segmentum l.

lumbaris
plexus l.

lumbarization

lumbar-peritoneal shunting

lumboaortic intermesenteric plexus

lumboatrial shunt

lumbodorsal fascia (LDF)

lumboinguinalis
nervus l.

lumboinguinal nerve

lumboperitoneal shunt

lumbosacral
l. corset
l. enlargement
l. enlargement of spinal cord
l. fusion
l. junction bone density
l. junction cortical thickness
l. junction fracture
l. meningocele
l. myelomeningocele
l. plexus neuritis
l. radiculopathy
l. spine plexus injury
l. spine transpedicular instrumentation
l. trunk
l. vertebra

lumbosacralis
intumescentia l.
plexus l.
truncus l.

lumina
lateral medullary l.

luminal
l. occlusion
l. perfusate

Lumsden
pneumotaxic center of L.

lunate
l. fissure
l. sulcus

lunatus
sulcus l.

Lundborg myoclonic epilepsy

Lunesta

lung
iron l.
trench l.

NOTES

LUPP
laser uvulopalatoplasty
Lupron
lupus
l. anticoagulant
l. cerebritis
l. erythematosus
l. erythematosus cell
l. erythematosus peripheral neuropathy
Luque
L. II segmental spinal instrumentation
L. instrumentation concave technique
L. instrumentation convex technique
L. loop fixation
L. rectangle
L. ring
L. rod
L. rod migration
L. semirigid segmental spinal instrumentation
L. sublaminar wiring technique
L. wire
Luque-Galveston
L.-G. fixation
L.-G. post
Luschka
foramen of L.
lateral foramina of L.
L. nerve
neurocentral joint of L.
Lust
L. phenomenon
L. reflex
L. sign
lusterless eye
lutea
macula l.
luteae
fovea centralis maculae l.
luteal phase progesterone
luteinizing
l. hormone (LH)
l. hormone-releasing hormone
luteum
corpus l.
punctum l.
Luvox
luxation
rotary atlantoaxial l.
rotatory l.
Luxtec
L. coaxial illumination
L. illuminated surgical telescope
luxury
l. perfusion
l. perfusion syndrome
Luys
L. body
nucleus of L.
luysii
corpus l.
Lyell syndrome
Lyme
L. borreliosis
L. disease
L. encephalopathy
L. neuroborreliosis
L. neuropathy
lymphadenopathy
lymphangioma
lymphoblastoid
lymphocyte
CD4 l.
cytotoxic l.
peripheral blood l.
tumor-infiltrating l. (TIL)
lymphocytic
l. adenohypophysitis
l. choriomeningitis
l. choriomeningitis virus (LCMV)
l. choriomeningitis virus encephalitis
l. hypophysitis
l. meningitis
l. pleocytosis
lymphocytopenia
lymphocytosis
atypical l.
lymphoepithelial parotid tumor
lymphoepithelioma
lymphogranuloma venereum encephalitis
lymphoid hypophysitis
lymphoinvasion
lymphokine
lymphokine-activated killer cell
lymphoma
angiotropic l.
central nervous system l.
centroblastic B-cell l.
cerebral l.
CNS l.
Hodgkin l.
intracerebral Hodgkin l.
intracranial Hodgkin l.
intramedullary l.
intravascular l.
Lennert l.
malignant l.
meningeal l.
non-Hodgkin l. (NHL)
primary brain l.
primary central nervous system l. (PCNSL)
primary CNS l.
primary intramedullary l.

primary leptomeningeal l.
solitary extranodal l.
spinal cord tumor with l.
lymphomagenesis
lymphomatoid granulomatosis
lymphomatosis cerebri
lymphomatosum
cystadenoma l.
lymphomatous
l. meningitis
l. tumor
lymphopathy
ataxic l.
lymphoplasmacyte-rich meningioma
lymphoproliferative disorder
lymphotoxin
Lynch incision
Lyodura
Lyodura-associated Creutzfeldt-Jakob disease
Lyon data set
lyophilized cadaveric dura
Lyrica
lysergic acid diethylamide and strychnine
lysine metabolism disorder
lysolecithin patching
lysosomal
l. enzymatic activity
l. storage disease
l. storage disorder
***Lyssavirus* infection**
lytic infection
Lytico-Bodig disease

NOTES

M
M line
M response
M segment
M vector
M wave
M1
M1 agonist
M1 segment aneurysm
M2
M2 artery segment
M2 branch
M2 segment of right middle cerebral artery
99m
CEA-Tc 99m
Pertscan 99m
M-2 anterior plate system
MAC
minimal alveolar concentration
MAC EIA
MacCarty forceps
MacDougall multiple sclerosis diet
Macewen
M. sign
M. symptom
Machado-Joseph disease
machine
Accuray Neurotron 1000 m.
m. artifact
Burdick Eclipse ECG m.
Teca Sapphire EMG m.
mAChR
muscarinic acetylcholine receptor
Machupo virus
Mackenzie syndrome
MacNab criteria
macrencephaly, macrencephalia
macro
m. square-wave jerk
m. stimulation
macroadenoma
enclosed m.
pituitary m.
macroaneurysm
macrocephalic, macrocephalous
macrocephaly, macrocephalia
hydrencephaly m.
macrocheilia, macrochilia
macrocranium
macrocryoglobulinemia peripheral neuropathy
macro-eCVR-FV circulation
macroelectrical stimulation
macroelectrode technique
macroencephalon
macroglia cell
macroglobulinemia
m. peripheral neuropathy
Waldenstrom m.
m. of Waldenstrom
macroglossia
macrognathia
macrogyria
macroinstrument
macromolecule
cellular m.
myelin m.
macrophage
activated m.
CD68-positive m.
m. immigration
immunocompetent m.
perivascular m.
macrophage-derived cell
macrophthalmos
MacroPore sheet
macropsia
macroscopic
m. dysgenesis
m. magnetization moment
m. magnetization vector
MacroSorb absorbable plate implant
macrostereognosia
mactans
Lactrodectus m.
macula, pl. **maculae**
m. communicans
m. cribrosa
maculae cribrosae
m. cribrosa inferior
m. cribrosa media
m. cribrosa quarta
m. cribrosa superior
m. densa
m. lutea
neuroepithelium of m.
m. retinae
m. sacculi
m. utriculi
macular
m. fasciculus
m. hemianopia
m. sparing
macularis
fasciculus m.
macular-sparing hemianopia
maculoneural bundle
maculopapular rash

mad
m. cow disease
M. Hatter syndrome
M-ADL
morphine-Adcon-L
M-ADL paste
madness
myxedema m.
madreporic coral
MADRS
Montgomery and Asberg Depression Rating Scale
madurae
Actinomadura m.
Maffucci syndrome
MAG
myelin-associated glycoprotein
magaldrate
Magellan electromagnetic navigation system
Magendie
foramen of M.
M. law
median foramen of M.
M. space
Magendie-Hertwig
M.-H. sign
M.-H. syndrome
Magerl
M. hook-plate system
method of M.
M. plate-screw system
M. posterior C1-C2 screw fixation
magic
M. B1 balloon
m. bone
M. microcatheter
m. thinking
M. Wallstent
magna
arteria radicularis m.
chorda m.
chorea m.
cisterna m.
mega cisterna m.
radicularis m.
vena cerebri m.
magnae
cisterna venae m.
Magnan
M. sign
M. trombone movement
Magnes
M. magnetic source imaging
M. MEG system
M. 2500 WH imager
magnesium
m. aluminum hydroxide
m. balance
m. carbonate
m. chloride
m. deficiency infantile tremor syndrome
m. disorder
m. gluconate
m. hydroxide suspension
m. imbalance
m. oxide
m. salicylate
m. sulfate
magnet
Alnico Magneprobe m.
cobalt samarium m.
C-shaped resistive m.
field m.
main field m.
m. mode
open m.
permanent m.
PoleStar m.
m. quench
m. reaction
m. reflex
resistive m.
m. shielding
superconducting m.
0.5-T superconducting m.
magnetic
m. apraxia
m. dipole
m. disc
m. field
m. field gradient
m. field vector
m. flux
m. moment
m. resonance (MR)
m. resonance angiogram
m. resonance angiography (MRA)
m. resonance-compatible clip
m. resonance image (MRI)
m. resonance imaging (MRI)
m. resonance marker
m. resonance neurography (MRN)
m. resonance perfusion imaging
m. resonance signal
m. resonance spectroscopy (MRS)
m. resonance tomography (MRT)
m. resonance venography (MRV)
m. search coil recording
m. seizure therapy
m. shielded cabin
somatosensory evoked m.
m. source imaging (MSI)
m. stimulator
m. susceptibility
m. susceptibility artifact
m. transfer ratio

magnetization
longitudinal m.
spatial modulation of m. (SPAMM)
spin m.
m. transfer image
m. transfer ratio
transverse m.
magnetization-prepared rapid acquisition gradient echo sequence (MPRAGE)
magnetoelectric stimulation
magnetoelectrophysiology
magnetoencephalogram (M-EEG, MEG)
magnetoencephalograph
magnetoencephalography (MEG)
magnetohydrodynamic effect
Magnetom
M. Open scanner
M. SP 4000 1.5-Tesla system
M. Vision scanner
magnetometer
8-channel whole-head m.
magnetometry
synthetic aperture m. (SAM)
Magnevist
magni
ramus posterior nervi auricularis m.
magnification
loupe m.
magnitude
perturbation m.
magnocellular
m. basal forebrain
m. deficit
m. dysfunction
m. layer
m. neuron
m. pathway
m. reticular nucleus
m. visual system
magnocellularia
strata m.
magnocellularis
nucleus medialis m.
nucleus reticularis m.
magnum
M. 800 bed
foramen m.
magnus
M. and de Kleijn neck reflex
nervus auricularis m.
nucleus raphes m.
m. raphe nucleus
Magonate
Magstim
M. 200
M. Rapid magnetic stimulator
M. 200 stimulator
maidenhair tree
main
m. cuneate nucleus
m. d'accoucheur
m. effect
m. en griffe deformity
m. en singe
m. field
m. field magnet
m. sensory nucleus of trigeminus
m. succulente
Maine
jumper disease of M.
maintaining sleep
maintenance
m. medication
M. of Wakefulness Test (MWT)
major
m. break
chorea m.
m. dense line
m. depression
m. depression disorder
epilepsia m.
m. epilepsy
m. forceps
m. form
hippocampus m.
m. histocompatibility complex (MHC)
m. life stress
m. motor aphasia
m. motor seizure
nervus occipitalis m.
nervus palatinus m.
nervus petrosus m.
nervus splanchnicus thoracicus m.
m. period line
m. psychiatric syndrome
m. risk period
m. solution
majoris
rami nasales posteriores inferiores nervi palatini m.
sulcus nervi petrosi m.
MAL
mamilloaccessory ligament

NOTES

mal
m. de debarquement
grand m.
petit m.
pyknoleptic petit m.
malabsorption
fat m.
m. syndrome peripheral neuropathy
vitamin D m.
Malacarne
M. pyramid
M. space
malacia traumatica
maladaptive
m. coping
m. mechanism
m. pattern
m. pattern of motivation
maladie des tic
malaise
postexertional m.
malalignment
ocular m.
malar eminence
malaria
cerebellar m.
cerebral m.
therapeutic m.
malate
almotriptan m.
Malcolm-Rand carbon-composite headholder
maldevelopment
neural m.
maleate
chlorpheniramine m.
fluvoxamine m.
methysergide m.
perhexiline m.
prochlorperazine m.
timolol m.
trimipramine m.
malevolent thought system
malformation
angiographically occult intracranial vascular m. (AOIVM)
angiographically visualized vascular m. (AVVM)
Arnold-Chiari m.
arteriovenous m. (AVM)
auditory arteriovenous m.
brain arteriovenous m. (BAVM)
brainstem cavernous m.
cavernous m. (CM)
Center for Brain Research and Holoprosencephaly and Related M.'s
central nervous system m.
cerebral venous m. (CVM)
cerebrovascular m.
Chiari m. type I–IV
congenital m.
cortical development m.
craniofacial m.
cryptic arteriovenous m.
cryptic cerebrovascular m.
cryptic vascular m.
Dandy-Walker m.
development m.
developmental m.
dural arteriovenous m.
familial arteriovenous m.
flocculonodular arteriovenous m.
Galen vein m.
glomus arteriovenous m.
hindbrain m.
infratentorial arteriovenous m.
intraarachnoid leptomeningeal m.
intracerebral arteriovenous m.
intracranial vascular m. (ICVM, IVM)
intracranial venous m.
intraorbital arteriovenous m.
intraspinal vascular m.
intratentorial m.
juvenile arteriovenous m.
medial hemispheric arteriovenous m.
obliterated arteriovenous m.
occipital bone m.
occult cerebrovascular m. (OCVM)
occult vascular m. (OVM)
Osler-Weber-Rendu arteriovenous m.
pedicle screw m.
pial arteriovenous m.
punctate cavernous m.
radiculomeningeal spinal vascular m.
Spetzler-Martin classification of arteriovenous m.
spinal cord arteriovenous m.
split-cord m.
structural m.
supratentorial arteriovenous m.
thalamocaudate arteriovenous m.
vascular m.
vein of Galen m.
venous m.
Wyburn-Mason arteriovenous m.
malfunction
shunt m.
Malibu orthosis
malignancy
anterior skull base m.
nasopharyngeal m.
skull base m.
malignant
m. astrocytoma

m. atrophic papulosis
m. brain edema
m. brain tumor
m. eccrine poroma
m. endovascular papillary angioendothelioma
m. external otitis
m. familial myoclonic epilepsy
m. fibrohistiocytoma
m. germ cell tumor
m. glioma
m. hypertension
m. hyperthermia
m. lymphoma
m. lymphoproliferative disease
m. meningioma
m. neuroleptic syndrome
m. phenotype
m. purpura
m. stupor
m. teratoma

malingering

Malis
M. angled bayonet forceps
M. bipolar cautery scissors
M. bipolar instrument
M. bipolar microcoagulator
M. brain retractor
M. CMC-II bipolar coagulator
M. CMC-III electrosurgical system
M. curette
M. dissector
M. electrocoagulation unit
M. elevator
M. irrigating bipolar CMC-III
M. irrigation forceps
M. jeweler's bipolar forceps
M. ligature passer
M. needle holder
M. nerve hook
M. neurological scissors
M. solid-state coagulator
M. vessel supporter

Malis-Jensen microbipolar forceps

malleable
m. endoscope
m. microsurgical suction device
m. multipore suction tube

malleatory spasm

mallet
Hajek m.
Lucae bone m.

malnutrition
m. infantile tremor syndrome
protein-energy m.

malocclusion

malposition
screw m.

malum vertebrale suboccipitale

mamillare
corpus m.

mamillaris
nuclei corporis m.
pedunculus corporis m.

mamillary, mammillary
m. body
m. body volume
m. region

mamilloaccessory
m. ligament (MAL)
m. notch
m. ridge

mamillopeduncular tract

mamillotegmentalis
fasciculus m.

mamillotegmental tract

mamillothalamic tract

mamillothalamicus
fasciculus m.

mammalian
m. cell
m. hippocampus
m. olfactory system
m. vomeronasal system

mammary
m. body
m. neuralgia

mammillary (*var. of* mamillary)

mammillotegmental fasciculus

mammillothalamic fasciculus

mammosomatotroph cell adenoma

management
intrathecal pain m.
nonpharmacologic behavior m.
radiosurgical m.
seizure m.

Manchester and Oxford Universities Scale for the Psychopathological Assessment of Dementia (MOUSEPAD)

mandibular
m. advancing device
m. advancing oral appliance
m. condylectomy

mandibular *(continued)*
m. fixation
m. nerve
m. notch electrode
m. osteotomy
m. reflex
m. repositioner
m. retraction
m. swing technique
mandibularis
nervus m.
ramus meningeus nervi m.
mandibulofacial dysostosis
mandibulotomy
mandrel, mandril
steam-shaping m.
threaded m.
maneuver
Adson modified m.
Allen m.
Bárány m.
Bielschowsky m.
Buzzard m.
Dandy m.
Dix-Hallpike m.
doll's eye m.
Gowers m.
Hallpike m.
Hallpike-Bárány positioning m.
Jendrassik m.
liberatory m.
nasal airflow-inducing m. (NAIM)
Phalen m.
Schreiber m.
Spurling m.
Valsalva m.
manganese
m. chloride
m. intoxication
m. toxic disorder
m. toxicity
m. toxin
mania
sleep disturbance associated with m.
manic
m. patient
m. stare
m. syndrome
manie
m. de perfection
m. de rumination
manifest
m. symptom
m. tetany
manifesta
spina bifida m.
manifestation
behavioral m.
characteristic m.
clinical m.
CNS m.
m. of depression
lacunar stroke m.
neurobehavioral m.
neuroimaging m.
neurologic m.
neurotic m.
psychophysiologic m.
m. of resistance
somatic neurologic m.
man-in-a-barrel syndrome
manipulation
cervical m.
chiropractic spinal m.
cranial nerve m.
language m.
osteopathic spinal m.
m. stage
syntactic m.
manipulator
Mehrkoordinaten m. (MKM)
manner
allosteric m.
psychical m.
mannitol
m. in intracranial pressure increase
mannitol-induced cerebral vasodilatation
Mannkopf sign
mannose in mucolipidosis
mannosidase
alpha m.
beta m.
mannosidosis
alpha m.
beta m.
Mann-Whitney
M.-W. test
M.-W. U test
MANOVA
multivariate analysis of variance
mansoni
Schistosoma m.
mantle
brain m.
cerebral m.
m. layer
m. sclerosis
Mantoux interdermal tuberculin skin test
manual
m. dexterity
M. of Internal Fixation
m. target localization
m. vernier scale
manubrium

MAO
monoamine oxidase
MAO spectrophotometric assay
MAO-A gene polymorphism
MAOI
monoamine oxidase inhibitor
MAP
mitogen-activated protein
map
brain electrical activity m.
lesion m.
phase-contrast m.
retinotopic m.
somatosensory m.
statistical parametric m. (SPM)
Z-score m.
Mapap
maple syrup urine disease
maplike skull
mapped epilepsy syndrome
mapping
behavior m.
brain electrical activity m.
brainstem diencephalic m.
cortical functional m.
2-dimensional m.
electrical stimulation m.
electrophysiological m.
genetic m.
haplotype m.
parametric m.
phase m.
radiotherapy brain m.
somatosensory m.
spatiotemporal brain m.
speech and motor m.
stimulation m.
Talairach whole-brain m.
maprotiline HCl
MAR
melanoma-associated retinopathy
marasmic, marantic
m. thrombosis
m. thrombus
marasmus
marbled appearance of basal ganglion
Marcaine
Marcé study
march
jacksonian m.
Marchac forehead template
Marchant zone
Marchi
M. ball
M. degeneration
M. globule
M. reaction
M. tract
Marchiafava-Bignami syndrome
Marconi Medical Systems console
Marcus
M. grading scale for avascular necrosis
M. Gunn
M. Gunn phenomenon
M. Gunn pupil
M. Gunn sign
M. Gunn syndrome
marfanoid
m. craniosynostosis syndrome
m. habitus
Marfan syndrome
margaroid tumor
margin
dural m.
marginal
m. branch of cingulate sulcus
m. fasciculus
m. gyrus
m. layer
m. sinus
m. zone
marginalis
fasciculus m.
ramus m.
sinus m.
sulcus m.
marginally therapeutic dose
marginis
cornu inferius m.
margo
m. inferior cerebri
m. inferolateralis
m. inferolateralis hemispherii cerebri
m. inferomedialis hemispherii cerebri
m. medialis cerebri
m. superomedialis
m. superomedialis cerebri
Mariana dementia (MD)
Marie
M. ataxia
hereditary cerebellar ataxia of M.

NOTES

Marie *(continued)*
M. quadrilateral sign
M. quadrilateral space
Marie-Foix-Alajouanine
M.-F.-A. cerebellar atrophy
M.-F.-A. disease
Marie-Foix sign
Marie-Strümpell
M.-S. disease
M.-S. encephalitis
Marie-Tooth disease
marijuana intoxication
marimastat protease inhibitor
Marin Amat syndrome
Marinesco
M. sign
M. succulent hand
Marinesco-Garland syndrome
Marinesco-Radovici reflex
Marinesco-Sjögren syndrome
marine toxin
Marino
M. transsphenoidal curette
M. transsphenoidal dissector
M. transsphenoidal enucleator
M. transsphenoidal hook
marked motor agitation
marker
biochemical phenotypic m.
biochemical tumor m.
biologic m.
cerebral fluid m.
m. chromosome
CSF m.
desmin tumor m.
diagnostic m.
discoid m.
DNA m.
epithelial membrane antigen tumor m.
factor VIII antigen tumor m.
fiducial m.
glial-specific m.
HHF35 muscle-specific actin tumor m.
high molecular weight cytokeratin tumor m.
lumbar pedicle m.
magnetic resonance m.
metallic skin m.
pedicle m.
phenotypic m.
roentgenographic opaque m.
Schwann cell m.
serum m.
S-100 tumor m.
surface fiducial m.
thoracic pedicle m.
tumor m.
vimentin tumor m.
m. X syndrome
Markesbery-Griggs distal myopathy
Markham-Meyerding hemilaminectomy retractor
Markov
M. analysis methodology
M. decision analysis model
M. transition state
Marlex mesh
marmoratus
status m.
Maroon-Jannetta dissector
Maroteaux-Lamy
M.-L. disease
M.-L. syndrome
marrow
bone m.
vertebral m.
marsupial notch
Martin-Bell syndrome
Martin-Gruber anastomosis
Martin nerve root retractor
Martinotti cell
Maryland
M. coma scale
M. tissue-grasping forceps
Maryland-type familial amyloid polyneuropathy
Masini sign
mask
Aquaplast m.
ComfortClassic nasal m.
ComfortFull nasal m.
ComfortGel nasal m.
m. facies
Hutchinson m.
Parkinson m.
Parrot m.
tabetic m.
masked
m. epilepsy
m. facies
masking
metacontrast m.
m. pain
white noise m.
masklike
m. face
m. facies
mass
m. action theory
black m.
cerebellar m.
cystic m.
m. doubling time
m. effect
external auditory canal m.
fat-free m.

free-fat m. (FFM)
hemispheral m.
intermediate m.
intraconal m.
intraparenchymal m.
isodense m.
jugular foramen m.
m. lesion
low bone m.
lucent m.
m. media
muscle m.
parameningeal m.
parasagittal intracranial m.
parasellar m.
peak bone m.
petrous apex m.
pineal region m.
polyganglionic m.
posterior fossa m.
m. protrusion
pulsatile m.
red/blue pulsatile m.
m. reflex
serpiginous m.
smooth-bordered cystic m.
m. spectrometer
suprasellar m.
supratentorial m.
thermogenic tissue m.
tigroid m.
vascular intratympanic m.

massage
carotid sinus m.
digital temple m.
hydropneumatic m.
nerve-point m.
m. therapy
m. treatment

massager
Cryocup ice m.

massa intermedia

masseter
m. muscle
m. reflex
m. strength

masseteric nerve

massetericus
nervus m.

massive spasm

Masson
M. trichrome stain
M. vegetant intravascular hemangioendothelioma

Masson-Fontana stain

MAST
minimal access spinal technology

master gland

mastication disorder

masticatoria
monoplegia m.

masticatorius
nucleus m.

masticatory
m. attack
m. diplegia
m. muscle activity
m. nucleus
m. spasm

mastocytosis
systemic m.

mastoid
m. air cell
m. antrum
m. complex
m. ecchymosis
m. process
m. retractor

Matas
M. operation
M. test
M. treatment

matchbox sign

matching
prototype m.
M. to Simple test
surface m.
m. and tuning network

mater
cranial arachnoid m.
cranial pia m.
dura m.
pia m.
sinus of dura m.
spinal arachnoid m.
spinal pia m.
transverse sinus of dura m.
venous sinus of dura m.

material
alloplastic m.
ballistic m.
Biocoral graft m.
Elgiloy clip m.
Glasflex m.

NOTES

M

material *(continued)*
isotropic linear m.
MP-35 clip m.
necrotic m.
NeuroCell-HD porcine fetal neural m.
NeuroCell-PD porcine fetal neural m.
neutral m.
nonferrous m.
Phynox cobalt alloy clip m.
precollagenous filamentous m.
verbal m.

maternal
m. competency
m. deprivation syndrome
m. dysfunction
m. hyperparathyroidism
m. inheritance
m. seizure
m. thyroid hormone

mathematical optimization and logical dimensioning for radiotherapy

Mathew Stroke Scale

math gene

Matricaria recutita

matris
sinus transversus durae m.

matrix
Accell Total Bone M.
m. adhesion
AlloDerm acellular dermal m.
DuraGen dural graft m.
extracellular m. (ECM)
germinal m.
Grafton demineralized bone m.
instrument calibration m.
intercellular m.
m. metalloproteinase (MMP)
m. metalloproteinase inhibitor
m. metalloproteinase type 1
m. molecule
onlay collagen m.
parenchymal m.
m. protein
rigid body transformation m.
Surgiflo hemostatic m.

matter
anisotropy of white m.
cortical gray m.
deep white m.
gliotic white m.
gray m.
heterotopic gray m.
inferior periventricular white m.
lateral periventricular white m.
medial periventricular white m.
occipital gray m.
occipital white m.
parahippocampal white m.
periaqueductal gray m.
periventricular gray m.
periventricular white m.
pontine gray m.
sclerosis of white m.
spinal cord gray m.
spongy degeneration of cerebral white m.
subcortical gray m.
superior periventricular white m.
vanishing white m.
white m.

Mattis Dementia Rating Scale

mattress
Akros extended-care m.
Akros pressure m.
eggcrate m.

maturation
age-related m.
glial cell m.
hormonal m.
neocortex m.
neuroblast m.
Pandy m.
skeletal m.
spinal m.

maturational change

mature teratoma

maturity
cognitive m.
motor m.

matutinal
m. epilepsy
m. headache

Mauthner
M. cell
M. fiber
M. membrane
M. sheath

Maxalt

Maxenon 300-watt xenon light source

Maxicamera
Gamma M.

Maxidone

maxillaris
nervus m.
rami alveolares superiores anteriores nervi m.
rami alveolares superiores posteriores nervi m.
rami nasales posteriores superiores laterales nervi m.
rami nasales posteriores superiores mediales nervi m.
rami orbitales nervi m.
ramus alveolaris superiores medius nervi m.
ramus meningeus nervi m.

maxillary
m. antrum
m. artery
m. nerve
m. osteotomy
m. plexus
m. sinus
m. vein
maxillofacial
m. fracture
m. plating system
m. trauma
maxillomandibular
m. advancement (MMA)
m. artery
m. expansion (MME)
Maxillume 250-watt quartz halogen light source
Maxima II TENS unit
maximal
m. effect
m. electroshock-induced seizure
m. electroshock seizure (MES)
m. hydrocephalus
m. plasma concentration
m. stimulus
m. voluntary contraction
maximum
full width at half m. (FWHM)
m. intensity pixel reconstruction
m. intensity projection
m. intent rating
m. lethality rating
m. saccade peak velocity
m. tolerable amount
m. tolerated dose
m. voluntary contraction (MVC)
maximus gait
Maxwell pair
Mayberg limbic-cortical dysregulation model
Mayer
M. hematoxylin
M. reflex
Mayer-Gross closing-in phenomenon
Mayerson sign
Mayfield
M. aneurysm clip
M. brain spatula
M. disposable skull pin
M. fiducial localizer
M. fixation frame
M. head clamp
M. headrest system
M. horseshoe headrest
M. incision
M. miniature clip applier
M. neurosurgical skill clamp
M. pinion
M. radiolucent base unit
M. radiolucent headholder
M. radiolucent headrest
M. rongeur
M. skull cap pin
M. skull-pin headholder
M. spinal curette
M. surgical system
M. temporary aneurysm clip applier
M. tongs
Mayfield/Acciss stereotactic device
Mayfield-Kees
M.-K. headholder
M.-K. headrest
M.-K. skull fixation apparatus
M.-K. table attachment
Mayo
M. Alzheimer Disease Center/Alzheimer Disease Patient Registry
M. Asymptomatic Carotid Endarterectomy Study
M. block anesthesia
M. Clinic stereotactic robot
M. scissors
M. stand
May-White syndrome
Maze test
Mazzoni corpuscle
MBP
myelin basic protein
MBP-reactive T cell
MCA
middle cerebral artery
McArdle disease
MCAT
middle cerebral artery thrombosis
McCain
M. TMJ cannula
M. TMJ trocar
McCarthy reflex
McCormac reflex

M

NOTES

MCD
medullary collecting duct
medullary cystic disease
McDonald
M. criteria
M. dissector
McDowell Impairment Index
McFadden-Kees clip
McGill
M. forceps
M. Pain Questionnaire
McGregor basal line
McGuire screw system
M-channel
M-CHAT
Modified Checklist for Autism in Toddlers
MCI
mild cognitive impairment
McKenzie
M. brain clip forceps
M. clip-applying forceps
M. clip-bending forceps
M. clip-introducing forceps
M. enlarging bur
M. hemostasis clip
M. perforating twist drill
M. reservoir
M. silver clip
McLain-Weinstein classification of spinal tumors
McLeod syndrome
McLone and Knepper etiological theory
McRae foramen magnum line
MCTD
mixed connective tissue disease
M-current
MCV
motor conduction velocity
MD
Mariana dementia
mitochondrial disease
movement duration
MDAS
Memorial Delirium Assessment Scale
MDM2
murine double minute 2
MDM2 gene
MDMA
methylenedioxymethamphetamine
mean
m. alpha frequency
M. Ambulation Index
m. arterial blood pressure
m. consecutive difference
m. corpuscular volume
m. interpotential interval (MIPI)
m. intracranial raw volume
m. normalized whole brain volume
m. sleep latency
m. sorted difference
standard error of m. (SEM)
m. total weighted sum score
m. weighted score
measles
m. encephalitis
m. inclusion body encephalitis
m. panencephalitis
m. peripheral neuropathy
m., rubella and zoster (MRZ)
m. virus
measure
m. of balance
baseline m.
behavioral assessment m.
benchmark m.
cognitive m.
course of illness m.
diagnostic m.
dissociation m.
Functional Independence M.
functioning m.
m. of general cognitive functioning
global m.
Gross Motor Function M. (GMFM)
neglect m.
neurocognitive m.
neuropsychologic m.
number-recency m.
objective m.
outcome m.
overall cognitive m.
phenomenological m.
pretreatment m.
quality of life m.
quantitative m.
repeated m. (rm)
sensitive m.
state-dependent m.
Stroke Specific Quality of Life M. (SS-QOL)
Surrogate Outcome M.
symptom m.
therapeutic m.
measured stress
measurement
ankle reflex m.
blood flow m.
cephalometric m.
cerebral electrical m.
diametral m.
m. effect
endoesophageal pressure m.
m. error
eye movement m.
head circumference m.
impedance m.
M-mode electrocardiographic m.

premature infant head circumference m.
quality-of-life m.
reference m.
Schober m.
tremor m.
xenon CT m.

measurement/monitoring
nasal pressure m./m.

measuring
m. sensor
m. sleepiness

meatus
external acoustic m.
internal acoustic m.

mechanical
m. anosmia
m. insufficiency
m. irritability
m. nociceptor
m. plate design
m. receptor
m. sensory threshold
m. stability
m. ventilation
m. vertigo
m. visual loss

mechanical-type disc prosthesis

mechanics
quantum m.
spinal m.

mechanic's hand

mechanism
airstream m.
analogous brain m.
arousal m.
association m.
axonal m.
basic brain m.
brain metabolic m.
caspase-independent m.
cataplexy m.
causal m.
causative m.
clamping m.
cognitive m.
m. of correction
disengagement m.
dissociable m.
emotional m.
endogenous brain m.
etiopathogenetic m.
feedback m.
fight-or-flight m.
free radical scavenging m.
fundamental neural m.
gating m.
genomic m.
heat-loss m.
immune-mediated m.
indirect m.
m. of injury
intracrine m.
intramolecular dipole-dipole m.
intrinsic cell suicide m.
left hemisphere m.
maladaptive m.
metabolic m.
mote-beam m.
myoinositol transport m.
neural m.
neurobiological m.
neuronal m.
osmotic m.
paracrine m.
perceptual/cognitive m.
pharmacological m.
plastic compensatory m.
pneumatic splint m.
postsynaptic compensatory m.
primary m.
putative m.
relapse m.
right hemisphere m.
rotating m.
spring m.
sunburst m.
synaptic m.
thermogenic m.
vasculitic m.
1-way flow m.

mechanoreceptor
cutaneous m.
m. fiber
high-threshold m.
low-threshold m. (LTM)
pacinian m.
Ruffini m.

mechanoreflex

mechanosensory

Meckel
M. cave
M. cave lesion
M. lesser ganglion

NOTES

Meckel *(continued)*
M. space
M. sphenopalatine ganglionectomy
Meckel-Gruber syndrome
meckelii
cavum m.
MeCP2 gene
Medelec
M. 5-channel neurophysiological device
M. MS91 electromyograph
media (*pl. of* medium)
mediae
pars sphenoidalis arteriae cerebralis m.
medial
m. accessory olivary nucleus
m. amygdaloid nucleus
m. atrial vein
m. branch C2
m. central nucleus of thalamus
m. central tegmental field
m. cerebral surface
m. dorsal nucleus of thalamus
m. eminence
m. eminence of rhomboid
m. epicondylectomy
m. extradural approach
m. fillet
m. forebrain bundle
m. frontal cortex
m. frontal gyrus
m. frontal lobe syndrome
m. geniculate body
m. geniculate nucleus (MGN)
m. habenular nucleus
m. hemispheric arteriovenous malformation
m. hemispheric dynamic
m. inferior pontine syndrome
m. lemniscus
m. longitudinal bundle
m. longitudinal fascicle
m. longitudinal fasciculus (MLF)
m. longitudinal stria
m. magnocellular nucleus
m. medullary lamina of corpus striatum
m. medullary lamina of lentiform nucleus
m. medullary syndrome
m. nucleus of trapezoid body
m. occipital artery
m. occipitotemporal gyrus
m. olfactory gyrus
m. olfactory stria
m. operculum
m. orbitofrontal cortex
m. parabrachial nucleus
m. pericuneate nucleus
m. periventricular white matter
m. plantar nerve
m. posterior choroidal
m. prefrontal cortex (mPFC)
m. preoptic area
m. preoptic nucleus
m. rectus muscle
m. reticulospinal tract
m. root of median nerve
root of olfactory tract, lateral and m.
m. root of optic tract
m. rostral supplementary motor area
m. septal nucleus
m. striate artery
m. sulcus of crus cerebri
m. superior olivary nucleus
m. superior temporal
m. surface of cerebral hemisphere
m. temporal cortex
m. temporal lobe
m. temporal lobe epilepsy
m. temporal memory system
m. temporal structure
m. terminal branch of deep fibular nerve
m. terminal nucleus (MTN)
m. triangle of Hakuba
m. vein of lateral ventricle
m. ventral nucleus
ventral posterior m. (VPM)
m. vestibular nucleus
m. vestibulospinal tract
m. zone
m. zone of hypothalamus
mediale
corpus geniculatum m.
mediales
decussatio lemnisci m.
nervi supraclaviculares m.
nuclei geniculati m.
rami clunium m.
rami gluteales m.
rami medullares m.
ramus choroidei posteriores m.
medialis
arteria occipitalis m.
arteria orbitofrontalis m.
eminentia m.
fasciculus longitudinalis m.
globus pallidus m.
gyrus frontalis m.
gyrus occipitotemporalis m.
gyrus olfactorius m.
lamina medullaris m.
lemniscus m.

nervi digitales plantares communes nervi plantaris m.
nervi digitales plantares proprii nervi plantaris m.
nervus cutaneous antebrachii m.
nervus cutaneous brachii m.
nervus cutaneous dorsalis m.
nervus cutaneous surae m.
nervus pectoralis m.
nervus plantaris m.
nervus pterygoideus m.
nuclei corporis geniculati m.
nucleus amygdalae basalis m.
nucleus campi m.
nucleus corporis geniculati m.
nucleus corporis mammillaris m.
nucleus dorsalis corporis geniculati m.
nucleus habenularis m.
nucleus interstitiales fasciculi longitudinalis m.
nucleus mamillaris m.
nucleus olivaris accessorius m.
nucleus olivaris superior m.
nucleus parabrachialis m.
nucleus pericuneatus m.
nucleus preopticus m.
nucleus septalis m.
nucleus vestibularis m.
pars dorsalis corporis geniculati m.
pars ventralis corporis geniculati m.
ramus anterior nervi cutanei antebrachii m.
ramus posterior nervi cutanei antebrachii m.
stria longitudinalis m.
stria olfactoria m.
tractus vestibulospinalis m.
vena atrii m.
zona m.

median
m. aperture
m. aperture of fourth ventricle
m. cleft face syndrome
m. corpectomy
m. eminence
m. face syndrome
m. foramen of Magendie
m. frontal sulcus
m. longitudinal fasciculus
m. mixed nerve action potential
m. nerve
m. nerve entrapment
m. nerve innervation
m. nerve lesion
m. nerve trauma
m. preoptic nucleus
m. raphe of medulla oblongata
m. raphe nucleus
m. raphe of pons
m. sternotomy brachial plexopathy
m. sulcus of fourth ventricle

mediana
eminentia m.

mediani
nervi digitales palmares communes nervi m.
nervi digitales palmares proprii nervi m.
radix lateralis nervi m.
radix medialis nervi m.
rami musculares nervi m.
ramus palmaris nervi m.

medianum
centrum m.

medianus
nervus m.
nucleus preopticus m.
nucleus raphes m.

mediated neuronal inhibition

medical
m. comorbidity
m. effect
m. impairment
M. Outcomes Study Short Form Health Survey
m. parameter monitoring (MPM)
M. Research Council (MRC)
M. Research Council scale for strength testing
m. taper schedule
m. value system

medically
m. intractable partial epilepsy
m. refractory partial seizure
m. unexplained physical symptoms (MUPS)

medical/neurological disorder

medication
adjunctive m.
anticholinergic m.
antiretroviral m.
antiseizure m.
antiviral m.

NOTES

medication *(continued)*
caffeine-containing m.
m. compliance
continuous maintenance m.
dopaminergic m.
m. dosage
m. effect on sleep
ergot-derived m.
forced m.
m. guide
hypnotic m.
immunosuppressive m.
intravenous m.
involuntary m.
long-acting injectable m.
maintenance m.
neuroleptic m.
m. overuse headache
peripherally acting anticholinergic m.
prophylactic m.
psychiatric m.
psychotropic m.
pulmonary m.
m. reduction
m. refractoriness
m. regimen
rescue m.
m. side effect
m. stigma
m. tapering
m. taper schedule
vasodilating antihypertensive m.
weight-neutral psychotic m.
medication-induced
m.-i. depressive syndrome
m.-i. headache
m.-i. insomnia
m.-i. movement disorder
m.-i. REM sleep suppression
m.-i. seizure
m.-i. tremor
medication-related
m.-r. side effect
m.-r. sleepiness
medicinal caffeine consumption
medicine
American Academy of Sleep M.
cannabis-based m.
Chinese m.
complementary m.
constitutional m.
digital imaging and communication in m. (DICOM)
electrodiagnostic m.
evidence-based m.
herbal m.
holistic m.
western m.
Medicus bed
Mediflow pillow
medii
nervi clunium m.
Medin disease
mediodorsal
m. globus pallidus interna
m. nucleus
mediodorsalis
nucleus m.
mediopubic reflex
medioventralis
nucleus m.
Medisorb drug delivery system
MediSpacer
meditation-based stress reduction
meditation for insomnia
Mediterranean myoclonus
medium, pl. **media**
AngioConray contrast m.
arteria cerebri media
cella media
contrast m.
culture m.
Dulbecco modified Eagle m.
Eagle minimum essential m.
ganglion cervicale m.
high osmolar contrast m.
iopamidol contrast m.
macula cribrosa media
mass media
otitis media
scala media
stratum griseum m.
m. vessel infarction
^{133}XeSPECT contrast m.
medius
gyrus frontalis m.
gyrus temporalis m.
nervus cardiacus cervicalis m.
nervus meningeus m.
pedunculus cerebellaris m.
plexus rectalis m.
sulcus frontalis m.
sulcus temporalis m.
MedNext
M. bone dissecting system
M. high-speed drill
Medos-Hakim valve
Medos valve
Medpacific LD 5000 Laser-Doppler perfusion monitor
Medrad infusion pump
Medrol Dosepak
medronate
technetium-99m m.
medroxyprogesterone acetate
Medtronic
M. Itrel II neurostimulator

M. Midas Rex Legend system
M. Pisces Quad Plus
M. 3470 pulse generator
M. Sofamor Danek
M. SynchroMed implantable pump
M. Xtrel neurostimulator

medulla, pl. **medullae**
m. oblongata
m. oblongata lateral funiculus
m. oblongata reticular formation
posterior pyramid of m.
pyramid of m.
rostral ventrolateral m.
m. spinalis
ventrolateral surface of m.

medullare
centrum m.

medullares
striae m.

medullar histoplasmosis

medullaris
conus m.
lamina m.
stria m.
substantia m.
tethered conus m.
tubus m.

medullary
m. artery
m. artery of brain
m. body of cerebellum
m. body of vermis
m. center
m. chemoreceptor
m. collecting duct (MCD)
m. cone
m. cystic disease (MCD)
m. fold
m. glioma
m. infarction
m. inhibitory region
m. inhibitory zone
m. lamina of thalamus
m. layer of thalamus
m. plate
m. protrusion
m. pyramidotomy
m. raphe
m. raphe nucleus
m. reticulospinal tract
m. segment
m. sheath
m. sign
m. solitary tract
m. stria of fourth ventricle
m. stria of thalamus
m. substance
m. syndrome
m. teniae
m. tenia of thalamus
m. tractotomy
m. tube
m. tumor

medullated nerve fiber

medullation

medullectomy

medullitis

medulloblastoma
desmoplastic m.
familial m.
melanotic m.
vermian m.

medullocell

medulloepithelioma

medullomyoblastoma

medullopontine sulcus

medullovasculosa
area m.
zona m.

M-EEG
magnetoencephalogram

Mees line

mefenamic acid

Mefoxin

MEG
magnetoencephalogram
magnetoencephalography
MEG head-based coordinate system
MEG sensor
MEG sensorimotor mapping coordinate

mega
m. cisterna magna
M. Tilt and Turn bed

Mega-Air bed

megacephalia (*var. of* megacephaly)

megacephalic child

megacephalous child

megacephaly, megacephalia

megadolichobasilar anomaly

megadolichovertebrobasilar anomaly

megalencephalic leukodystrophy

megalencephalon

NOTES

M

megalencephaly
unilateral m.
megalgia
megalocephaly, megalocephalia
megaloencephalon
megaloencephaly
megalopapilla
megalopia hysterica
meglumine
diatrizoate m.
iocarmate m.
iodipamide m.
m. iothalamate
ioxaglate m.
m. metrizoate
Mehrkoordinaten manipulator (MKM)
Meige
M. disease
M. syndrome
Meissner
M. corpuscle
M. ganglion
M. plexus
melancholic type
melancholium
melanin pigment
melanocyte
melanocyte-inhibiting factor
melanocytoma
meningeal m.
melanoma-associated retinopathy (MAR)
melanophore
melanophorin
melanosis
neurocutaneous m.
melanotic
m. medulloblastoma
m. neuroectodermal tumor
m. neuroectodermal tumor of infancy (MNTI)
melanotropin-releasing factor (MRF)
MELAS
mitochondrial encephalomyopathy with lactic acidosis and strokelike episodes
mitochondrial myopathy, encephalopathy, lactic acidosis, strokelike episodes
MELAS syndrome
melatonin-replacement therapy
melatonin test
melitensis
Brucella m.
Melkersson-Rosenthal syndrome
Melkersson syndrome
Mellaril
Melmon and Rosen classification
Melnick-Fraser syndrome
melphalan
Melzack and Wall gate theory
memantine HCl
membrana, pl. **membranae**
m. basilaris
m. cerebri
m. limitans gliae
m. versicolor
membranacea
crura m.
membrane
arachnoid m.
m. attack complex
basement m.
basilar m.
brain synaptic m.
branch of auriculotemporal nerve to tympanic m.
m. capacitance
caroticooculomotor m.
choroid m.
diencephalic m.
m. excitability
Fielding m.
glial limiting m.
Henle m.
m. ion channel
m. of Liliequist
m. lipolysis
Mauthner m.
mesencephalic m.
middle m.
neuronal m.
nitrocellulose m.
m. phenotype
m. phosphatidylserine exposure
m. phospholipid
pial-glial m.
postsynaptic neuronal m.
m. potential
Preclude spinal m.
presynaptic m.
sarcolemma m.
Schwann m.
spiral m.
synaptic m.
m. valve
vestibular m.
vitreous m.
membrane-anchored aspartyl protease
membrane-associated protein
membrane-bound
m.-b. glycoprotein
m.-b. organelle
membranectomy
membranous
m. cochlea
m. labyrinth
m. labyrinth rupture
memoration
amnesic m.

memorial
M. Delirium Assessment Scale (MDAS)
M. Symptom Assessment Scale
memory
accuracy of m.
anterograde m.
auditory m.
Bower model of mood-congruent m.
m. change
m. consolidation
declarative m.
m. deterioration
m. disturbance
m. dysfunction
emotional m.
episodic m.
euthymic m.
event m.
factual m.
m. function
m. function deficit
illusory m.
impaired m.
m. impairment
m. index
intrusive m.
m. lapse
long-term associative m.
long-term declarative m.
long-term storage of m.
loss of m.
new m.
nondeclarative m.
nonverbal m.
old m.
m. organization
m. paradigm
m. performance
photographic m.
procedural m.
m. process
m. processing
prospective m.
recall m.
recent m.
recognition m.
recovered m.
m. reinforcement theory
remote m.
m. retrieval strategy
retrograde m.
Ribot law of m.
secondary verbal m.
selective m.
semantic m.
senile m.
short-term declarative m.
short-term visual m.
sound m.
spatial m.
superior long-term m.
m. system
tapping m.
m. task
top-down organization of m.
m. trace
verbal episodic m.
verbal working m.
veridical m.
visual episodic m.
visuospatial m.
working m.
memory-continuous performance
memory-guided saccade
Memotherm stent
MEMS
microelectromechanical system
MEN 1–3
multiple endocrine neoplasia, type 1–3
Mendel
M. dorsal foot reflex
M. instep reflex
Mendel-Bechterew
M.-B. reflex
M.-B. sign
mendelian
m. inheritance
m. pattern
mendicancy
pathological m.
Menezes
method of M.
Mengo encephalitis
Ménière
M. disease
M. syndrome
meningeal
m. angiomatosis
m. anthrax
m. artery
m. biopsy
m. carcinoma

NOTES

meningeal *(continued)*
m. carcinomatosis
m. covering
m. diverticula
m. enhancement
m. fibrosis
m. filament
m. gliomatosis
m. granule
m. hemangiopericytoma
m. hernia
m. infection
m. irritation
m. loculus
m. lymphoma
m. melanocytoma
m. nerve
m. neurosarcoidosis
m. neurosyphilis
m. pachymeningitis
m. pathogen
m. plexus
m. seeding
m. sign
m. syphilis
m. tumor
m. vein
meningematoma
meningeocortical (*var. of* meningocortical)
meningeorrhaphy
meninges (*pl. of* meninx)
meningeus
plexus m.
meninghematoma
meningioangiomatosis
meningioma
anaplastic m.
angioblastic m.
angiomatous m.
angioplastic m.
angle m.
atypical m.
benign m.
bifrontal malignant m.
cavernous sinus m.
chordoid m.
clear cell m.
clinoidal m.
clival m.
clivus m.
complex m.
convexity m.
craniospinal m.
cutaneous m.
cystic intraparenchymal m.
dermal m.
endotheliomatous m.
en plaque m.
epidural m.
extracranial m.
extradural m.
falcine m.
falcotentorial m.
falx m.
fibroblastic m.
m. formation
frontal convexity m.
m. growth
hemangiopericytic m.
intracranial m.
intradural-extradural m.
intraorbital m.
intraosseous m.
intraparenchymal m.
intraspinal m.
intraventricular m.
lymphoplasmacyte-rich m.
malignant m.
meningothelial m.
metaplastic m.
metastasizing m.
microcystic m.
multiple m.'s
olfactory groove m.
m. of olfactory groove
optic nerve sheath m.
outer sphenoid ridge m.
papillary m.
parasagittal m.
parasellar tentorial m.
parietal m.
perioptic m.
peritorcular m.
petroclinoclival m.
petroclival m.
petroclivotentorial m.
pineal m.
posterior fossa m.
m. prostaglandin level
psammomatous m.
m. resection
rhabdoid m.
secretory m.
sphenoid ridge m.
sphenoid wing m.
sphenoorbital m.
spinocranial m.
subdural m.
subfrontal m.
suprasellar m.
supratentorial m. (STM)
syncytial m.
tentorial apex m.
tentorial leaf m.
thoracic m.
torcular m.

transitional m.
tuberculum sellae m.
meningioma-associated cerebral edema
meningiomatosis
meningism
meningitic
m. hydrocephalus
m. neurosyphilis
m. streak
meningitidis
Neisseria m.
meningitis, pl. **meningitides**
Acanthamoeba m.
actinomycosis lymphocytic m.
acute cerebrospinal m. (ACM)
acute purulent m.
aseptic uremic m.
Bacilles anthracis m.
bacterial m.
basilar m.
benign lymphocytic m.
beta hemolytic streptococcus m.
blastomycotic m.
Brucella m.
candidal m.
carcinomatous m.
cerebrospinal m.
chemical aseptic m.
Citrobacter m.
CMV m.
coccidioidal m.
community-acquired bacterial m.
coxsackievirus m.
cryptococcal m.
cytomegalovirus m.
defined m.
echovirus m.
enterovirus m.
eosinophilic m.
epidemic cerebrospinal m.
epidural m.
Escherichia coli m.
external m.
fungal m.
gram-negative bacillary m.
Haemophilus influenzae type B m.
Histoplasma m.
hospital-acquired m.
idiopathic m.
infectious m.
m. inflammatory response
internal m.
Klebsiella pneumoniae m.
leptospirosis lymphocytic m.
Listeria monocytogenes m.
luetic m.
lymphocytic m.
lymphomatous m.
meningococcal m.
Mollaret m.
mumps m.
Naegleria m.
Neisseria meningitidis m.
neonatal m.
neoplastic m.
noninfectious m.
occlusive m.
ornithosis lymphocytic m.
m. ossificans
otic m.
paragonimiasis lymphocytic m.
parasitic m.
Pasteurella ureae m.
pneumococcal m.
postoperative aseptic m.
premature infant m.
Proteus m.
Pseudomonas aeruginosa m.
purulent m.
pyogenic m.
Salmonella m.
septic m.
serosa m.
m. serosa circumscripta
serous m.
m. serous spinalis
sinogenic m.
spinal m.
staphylococcal m.
sterile m.
streptococcal m.
Streptococcus agalactiae m.
Streptococcus aureus m.
Streptococcus pneumoniae m.
subacute m.
sympathetic m.
m. sympathica
tubercular m.
tuberculosis m.
tuberculous m.
viral m.
meningoarteritis
meningocele
lateral thoracic m.

NOTES

meningocele *(continued)*
lumbar m.
lumbosacral m.
sacral m.
spinal m.
spurious m.
traumatic m.
meningocerebral cicatrix
meningocerebritis
meningococcal
m. endotoxin
m. meningitis
meningococcemia
acute fulminating m.
meningocortical, meningeocortical
meningocyte
meningoencephalitis
acute primary hemorrhagic m.
amebic m.
anthrax m.
arbovirus m.
aseptic m.
bacterial m.
biundulant m.
chronic progressive syphilitic m.
eosinophilic m.
herpetic m.
mumps m.
murine typhus m.
nonvasculitic autoimmune inflammatory m.
primary amebic m.
Rocky Mountain spotted fever m.
sterile m.
syphilitic m.
toxoplasmic m.
meningoencephalocele
basal m.
ethmoidal m.
sphenoethmoidal m.
sphenoorbital m.
sphenopharyngeal m.
transsphenoidal m.
meningoencephalomyelitis
meningoencephalomyelopathy
meningoencephalopathy
meningofibroblastoma
meningogenic
meningohypophysial
m. branch
m. trunk
meningomyelitis
syphilitic m.
meningomyelocele dysraphism
meningomyeloencephalitis
meningopathy
meningopolyneuritis
tick-borne m.
meningorachidian vein
meningoradicular disorder
meningoradiculitis
meningorrhagia
meningorrhea
meningothelial
m. appearance
m. arachnoid cell
m. cap cell
m. covering
m. meningioma
meningothelioma
meningotyphoid fever
meningovascular
m. neurosyphilis
m. syphilis
meningovasculitis
syphilitic m.
meninigitis
Pasteurella m.
meninx, pl. **meninges**
basilar m.
m. fibrosa
m. primitiva
primitive m.
m. serosa
m. tenuis
vascular m.
m. vasculosa
meniscus, pl. **menisci**
tactile m.
m. tactus
Menkes
M. disease
M. kinky hair syndrome
menstrual
m. cycle
m. epilepsy
m. migraine
mental
m. agraphia
m. alertness
m. alternation test
m. arousal
m. claudication
m. data
m. flexibility
m. impairment
m. level
m. model
m. nerve
m. phenomenon
m. retardation
m. speed
m. status change
m. status examination
m. workload
mentalis
nervus m.
rami gingivales nervi m.

rami labiales nervi m.
rami mentales nervi m.
mentally competent
mentation
slowed m.
Menzel
M. ataxia
M. olivopontocerebellar atrophy
M. olivopontocerebellar degeneration
MEP
motor evoked potential
multimodality evoked potential
meperidine
m. analog
m. hydrochloride
m. and promethazine
Mephyton Oral
mepivacaine
MEPP
miniature endplate potential
meprobamate
meralgia paresthetica
mercurialis
erethism m.
mercurial tremor
mercury
m. intoxication
m. peripheral neuropathy
m. toxic disorder
m. toxicity
m. toxin
m. vapor poisoning
mercury-contaminated food
mercury-induced illness
Meretoja syndrome
Meretoja-type familial amyloid polyneuropathy
meridian
extraordinary m. (EM)
Merkel
M. corpuscle
M. tactile cell
M. tactile disc
Merocel tampon
merocoxalgia
meromyosin
heavy m.
light m.
merorachischisis, merorrhachischisis
merosin deficiency
merosin-deficient CMD
merosin-positive congenital muscular dystrophy
merosmia
MERRF
myoclonic epilepsy with ragged red fibers
MERRF syndrome
MERRLA
myoclonus epilepsy with ragged red fibers-lactic acidosis
MERRLA syndrome
Mersiline tape
Mersilk black silk suture
mertiatide
technetium-99m m.
Merzbacher-Pelizaeus disease
MES
maximal electroshock seizure
MES test
mesaxon
mesencephali
apertura aqueductus m.
aqueductus m.
fibrae corticonucleares m.
formatio reticularis tegmenti m.
lamina tecti m.
nuclei reticulares m.
sulcus lateralis m.
tectum m.
tegmentum m.
mesencephalic
m. cistern
m. corticonuclear fiber
m. flexure
m. hemorrhage
m. infarction
m. membrane
m. neuron
m. nucleus
m. nucleus of trigeminal nerve
m. nucleus of trigeminus
m. premotor structure
m. reticular formation
m. sign
m. tegmentum
m. tissue
m. tractotomy
m. tract of trigeminal nerve
m. transition area
m. transplant
m. vein

NOTES

mesencephalicae
venae m.
mesencephalicus
nucleus cuneiformis m.
mesencephalitis
mesencephalohypophysial
mesencephalon
m. aqueduct
oculomotor sulcus of m.
m. reticular formation
reticular nucleus of m.
ventral m.
mesencephalooculofacial angiomatosis
mesencephalotomy
mesenchymal drift
mesenchyme
paraxial m.
mesenteric vasculitis
mesh
Dumbach cranial titanium m.
m. glove
m. glove stimulation
Marlex m.
polylactic acid m.
tantalum m.
Teflon m.
mesial
m. aspect of temporal lobe
m. cerebral structure
m. epileptogenic cortex
m. frontal cortex
m. hemisphere
m. part of frontal lobe
m. prefrontal cortical area
m. surface
m. temporal epileptogenic lesion
m. temporal hypoperfusion
m. temporal sclerosis (MTS)
mesiobasal temporal lobe
mesiotemporal lobe
mesoblastic sensibility
mesocephalic hemianesthesia
mesocortex
mesocortical
m. dopamine pathway
m. dopaminergic system
mesocorticolimbic dopaminergic abnormality
mesoderm
mesoglia
mesoglial cell
mesolimbic
m. dopamine pathway
m. dopamine system
m. selectivity
mesolobus
mesomorphic
mesoneuritis
nodular m.
mesoridazine
mesothelioma
fibrous m.
messenger
eukaryotic m.
intracellular second m.
m. ribonucleic acid
Mestinon
M. Injection
M. Syrup
mesulergine
mesylate
benztropine m.
bromocriptine m.
dihydroergotamine m.
doxazosin m.
pergolide m.
rasagiline m.
reboxetine m.
traxoprodil m.
ziprasidone m.
metabolic
m. abnormality
m. acidosis
m. activation
m. activity
m. alkalosis
m. alteration
m. capability
m. change
m. coma
m. conversion
m. derangement
m. difference
m. disorder
m. disorder screening
m. disturbance
m. effect
m. encephalitis
m. encephalopathy
m. headache
m. imbalance
m. increase
m. lesion
m. mechanism
m. myopathy
m. pathway
m. process
m. rate
m. response
m. testing
metabolism
abnormal m.
albumin m.
alcohol m.
arachidonic acid m.
m. at rest
brain glucose m.
caffeine m.

carbohydrate m.
carnitine muscle m.
cerebellar m.
cholesterol m.
cortical m.
cytochrome P450 m.
dopamine m.
drug m.
energy m.
frontal m.
glial m.
global m.
glucose m.
glutamate m.
hepatic oxidative m.
impaired drug m.
inborn error of m.
intracellular energy m.
iron m.
lactose m.
lipoid m.
loss of energy m.
metal m.
methadone m.
neuronal m.
nitrogen m.
nucleic acid m.
parallel pathways of m.
phosphate m.
phytol m.
porphyrin m.
prefrontal m.
psychotropic m.
purine m.
regional glucose m.
striatal m.
striatus-orbitofrontal m.
temporal lobe m.
tetrahydrobiopterin m.

metabolite
active m.
bupropion m.
phosphoinositol m.
toxic m.

metabotropic
m. glutamate
m. glutamate receptor

metacarpohypothenar reflex

metacarpothenar reflex

metachromatic
m. leukodystrophy
m. leukodystrophy neuropathy
m. leukoencephalopathy

metachronous neoplasm

metacognitive capacity

metacontrast masking

Metadate
M. CD
M. CD extended-release capsule

metadrenaline

metaiodobenzyl-guanidine (MIBG)

metal
m. electrode
m. failure
m. fatigue
m. metabolic disorder
m. metabolism
m. metabolism disorder
m. neuropathy
m. object
m. plate

metallic
m. cranioplasty
m. endplate
m. foreign body
m. otologic implant
m. skin marker
m. toxic disorder
m. toxin
m. tremor

metalloendoprotease

metalloprotease inhibitor

metalloproteinase
matrix m. (MMP)
matrix m. type 1
tissue inhibitor of m. (TIMP)

metal-produced neuropathy

metameric
m. lesion
m. nervous system
m. syndrome

metamorphopsia

metaplastic meningioma

metaraminol bitartrate

metastasis, pl. **metastases**
brain m.
calvarial m.
cerebral m.
choroidal m.
distant m.
drop m.
dural m.
extradural spinal m.

NOTES

metastasis *(continued)*
hemorrhagic m.
intradural m.
leptomeningeal m.
miliary brain m.
ocular m.
retrobulbar orbital m.
spinal m.
subarachnoid space m.
metastasizing meningioma
metastatic
m. brain tumor
m. disease
m. tumor removal
Metastron Injection
metatarsalgia
Morton m.
metatarsal reflex
metathalamus
metaxalone
metencephalic
metencephalon
metencephalospinal
metenkephalin
meter
BioTrainer exercise m.
clip force m.
methacrylate
dimethylaminoethyl m.
methadone
m. HCl
m. hydrochloride
m. metabolism
methamphetamine HCl
methanol poisoning
methantheline
methazolamide
methcathinone
methemoglobin
methexenyl
methicillin-resistant staphylococcus
methiodal
methionine
methocarbamol
method
Anel m.
Antyllus m.
assessment m.
avidin-biotin-complex-peroxidase m.
Boundary Shift Integral m.
brain electrical activity m. (BEAM)
brain imaging m.
Brasdor m.
bundle nailing m.
Cavalieri direct estimator m.
clinical m.
Cobb m.
cognitive m.
Coleman m.
Cooper m.
correlation m.
Deaver m.
diagnostic m.
m. of Dickman
Dickson m.
dose reduction m.
Fairbanks m.
FDG m.
Fujita m.
m. of Glees
Gore m.
Greitz-Bergstrom m.
Hilton m.
hole preparation m.
imaging m.
immobilization m.
immunoperoxidase m.
impedance m.
Kety-Schmidt m.
Kirby-Bauer disc diffusion m.
m. of Klüver
m. of Magerl
m. of Menezes
Monte Carlo permutation m.
Moore m.
Pavlov m.
phase-contrast m.
Purmann m.
Q-sort m.
rating m.
reduction m.
Scarpa m.
Seldinger m.
Simmons m.
steady-state m.
m. of successive approximation
m. of Suzuki and Iwamoto
Taylor series linearization m.
Thane m.
Turnbull m.
Wardrop m.
Westergren m.
Winston-Lutz m.
Wintrobe m.
Xe clearance m.
xenon m.
zeta m.
methodical chorea
methodology
Markov analysis m.
methotrexate
m. encephalopathy
m. poisoning
m. sodium
methsuximide
methyl
m. alcohol peripheral neuropathy
m. alcohol poisoning

m. alcohol toxicity
m. alcohol toxin
m. dopa
methylamphetamine hydrochloride
methylcarbamic
methyl-CpG-binding protein
3-methylcrotonyl-CoA carboxylase
methylcrotonylglycinuria
beta m.
***N*-methyl-D-aspartate (NMDA)**
***N*-methyl-D-aspartate (NMDA)**
N-m.-D.-a. receptor
N-m.-D.-a. receptor antagonist
methyldopa and hydrochlorothiazide
methylene
m. blue
m. tetrahydrofolate reductase defect
methylenedioxymethamphetamine (MDMA)
m. and phencyclidine
methylglucamine
iodipamide m.
3-methylglutaconic aciduria
methylglyoxal bis(guanylhydrazone)
methylmalonic
m. acidemia
m. aciduria
m. aminoaciduria
methylmalonyl-CoA mutase
methylmethacrylate
m. block
m. cranioplastic plug
m. cranioplasty
m. spacer
methylphenidate
m. administration
m. HCl
m. HCl extended-release capsule
methylphenidate-induced change
methylphenobarbital
1-methyl-4-phenyl-1,2,3,6-tetrahydropyridine
***N*-methyl-4-phenyl-1,2,3,6-tetrahydropyridine**
methylprednisolone
m. acetate
m. and sodium succinate
methyltetrahydrofolate reductase mutation
methylxanthine-induced postural tremor
MethyPatch
methysergide maleate
metocurine iodide
metolazone
metopic
m. craniectomy
m. suture
m. synostosis
metopoplasty
metoprolol tartrate
metrizamide
m. contrast study
m. myelography
metrizamide-enhanced CT
metrizamide-filled balloon
metrizoate
meglumine m.
metrizoic acid
metronidazole
METRx
METRx system
METRx X-Tube retractor
metyrapone test
Metzenbaum scissors
mevalonate kinase deficiency
mevalonic aciduria
mevinolin
Mexate-AQ
mexiletine
Meyer
M. loop
M. sublaminar wiring technique
Meyer-Archambault loop
Meyerding
M. laminectomy blade
M. laminectomy retractor
Meyerding-Scoville blade
Meynert
basal nucleus of M.
M. commissure
M. fasciculus
fasciculus of M.
M. fountain decussation
M. layer
nucleus basalis of M.
retroflex bundle of M.
M. retroflex bundle
M. solitary cell
M. tract
MFD
monorhythmic frontal delta
MFD activity
MFD test

NOTES

M

MFD *(continued)*
MFD wave on electroencephalogram
MFMN
multifocal motor neuropathy
Mfn1-deficient mitochondria
Mfn2-deficient mitochondria
MFS
Miller-Fisher syndrome
MG
myasthenia gravis
MGBG
mitoguazone
MGC4607
MGC4607 gene
MGC4607 gene mutation
MGN
medial geniculate nucleus
MHC
major histocompatibility complex
MHI
minor head injury
Miacalcin
M. Injection
M. Nasal Spray
Miami
M. Acute Care cervical collar
M. J collar
MIBG
metaiodobenzyl-guanidine
micans
degeneratio m.
mication
Michele vertebral body trephine
Michel scalp clip
Michotte visual stimulus
micrencephalous
micrencephaly, micrencephalia, microencephaly
Micrins microsurgical suture
Micro
M. E irrigation kit
M. 100 irrigation kit
M. Plus screw
microabscess
candidal m.
microadenoma
cystic m.
pituitary m.
microadenomectomy
selective m.
microaerophilic streptococcus
Micro-Aire blade
microaneurysm
Charcot-Bouchard m.
microangiopathy
mineralizing m.
microarray gene expression
microartery forceps
microball hook
microbipolar forceps
microbleed
cerebral m.
microbore Tygon tube
microcatheter
Excel double-tipped m.
Magic m.
Prowler-14 m.
Prowler double-tipped m.
Rapid Transit m.
m. system
Tracker Excel m.
variable stiffness m.
microcephaly
encephaloclastic m.
schizencephalic m.
MicroChoice electric-powered surgical system
microcirculation
nerve root m.
microcirculatory
m. perfusion
m. red cell flux
microclip
Yasargil m.
microcoagulator
Malis bipolar m.
microcoil
endothelin-1 platinum-Dacron m.
Hilal m.
platinum Dacron m.
microconnector
microcoulomb
microcrania
microcup forceps
microcurette
Rhoton m.
Yasargil m.
microcyst
microcystic meningioma
microdactyly
microdeletion syndrome
microdialysis
intracerebral m.
intrahippocampal m.
microdiscectomy, microdiskectomy
microdissector
Rhoton m.
Yasargil m.
micro-Doppler instrument
microdrill
high-speed m.
system high-speed m.
microdysgenesia
cortical m.
microdysgenesis
micro-eCVR-FV circulation
microelectrode recording

microelectroencephalography
microelectromechanical system (MEMS)
microembolic signal
microembolism
cerebral m.
silent m.
microencephaly (*var. of* micrencephaly)
microendoscopic
m. discectomy system
m. foraminotomy
m. laminotomy
microendoscopy
intraoperative m.
microfibrillar collagen
microfilament
microforceps
Yasargil m.
microglia cell
microgliacyte
microglial
m. cluster
m. nodular encephalitis
microglioma
microgliomatosis
microgliosis
microglobulin
$beta_2$ m.
micrognathia
Robin sequence m.
micrograph
electron m.
micrography, micrographia
MicroGuide microelectrode recording system
microguidewire
microgyria
perisylvian m.
microgyrus
microhemagglutination-*Treponema pallidum* test
microhemorrhage
hypertensive pontine m.
microhook
Rhoton m.
microinfarction
microinjection
Micro-K
M.-K 10 Extencaps
M.-K LS
microknife
Karlin m.
microlumbar discectomy
micromesh
titanium m.
microneedle
Colorado m.
microneurography
microneurosurgery
endoscopic m.
microneurovascular anastomosis
Micro-One needle holder
microoperative
m. procedure
m. treatment
Micropaque
microphthalmos
micropituicyte
micropituitary rongeur
microplate
C-shaped m.
H-shaped m.
Leibinger m.
L-shaped m.
Luhr m.
Storz Microsystem m.
Synthes Microsystem m.
Micro-Plus titanium plating system
microporosity
microprobe
Jacobson m.
microprolactinoma
micropsia
microptic
microrasp
Yasargil m.
microretractor
flexible arm m.
microronguer
Kerrison m.
microsatellite marker analysis
microsaw
oscillating m.
Zimmer m.
microscissors
curved conventional m.
straight m.
Yasargil m.
microscope
confocal laser scanning m.
Elekta robotic surgical m.
Hitachi scanning electron m.
laser scanning m. (LSM)
MKM m.
Omni 2 m.

NOTES

microscope *(continued)*
operating m. VM 900
operative m.
OPMI surgical m.
Philips 400 transmission electron m.
pneumatic m.
robotic m.
surgical m.
SurgiScope robotic m.
Vario m.
Zeiss Axiovert m.
Zeiss-Contraves operating m.
Zeiss MKM m.
Zeiss operating m.
Zeiss OPMI Neuro/NC4 surgical m.
zoom m.
microscopic
m. endoscopy surgery
m. foraminotomy
m. laminotomy (ML)
m. lesion
m. neurosurgery
m. polyangiitis
microscopy
electron m.
scanning electron m.
transillumination m.
microseme
microsensor
ICP m.
intracranial pressure m.
microsleep
microsmatic
microsmic
Micro-Softplate
Micro-Soft Stream sidehole infusion catheter
microsomal isoenzyme metabolism profile
microsomia
hemifacial m.
MicroSpan Capnometer 8800
microsphere
degradable starch m. (DSM)
microstaple
Barouk m.
microstomia
Microsulfon
microsurgery
m. discectomy
endoscope-controlled m.
fine touch m.
m. forceps
frameless stereotactic m.
m. needle holder
microsurgical
m. discectomy (MSD)
m. DREZotomy
m. neck clipping
m. procedure
m. resection
m. technique
m. thoracoscopic vertebrectomy
microsuture
microsystem
microthin plastic fiber
Micro-Three microsurgery instrument
microtome
Leica vibrating knife m.
microtubule
cytoplasmic m.
microtubule-associated protein
microtubule-binding
m.-b. domain
m.-b. repeat
Micro-Vac suction catheter
microvascular
m. anastomosis
m. clip
m. compression syndrome
m. decompression (MVD)
m. forceps
m. pressure (MVP)
microvasculitic change
Microvena retrieval device
microvesicular steatosis
microvolt
microwave hyperthermia
Microzide
Micro-Z neuromuscular stimulator
micturition
m. center
m. reflex
m. syncope
MID
multiinfarct dementia
Midas
M. Rex bur guard
M. Rex craniotome
M. Rex craniotomy saw
M. Rex drill
M. Rex instrumentation system
M. Rex Legend System
M. Rex power system
midazolam
midbrain
aqueduct of m.
m. compression
m. deafness
m. infarction
m. lesion
opening of aqueduct of m.
m. perforating artery
m. reticular formation
rostral m.
tectum of m.

tegmentum of m.
m. tegmentum
m. vesicle
midcervical flexion myelopathy
middle
m. cerebellar peduncle
m. cerebral artery (MCA)
m. cerebral artery occlusion
m. cerebral artery thrombosis (MCAT)
m. cervical ganglion
m. column injury
m. cranial fossa
m. cranial fossa approach
m. cranial fossa cyst
m. ear impedance
m. fossa craniotomy approach
m. fossa exposure
m. fossa floor/petrous dissection
m. fossa transtentorial translabyrinthine approach
m. frontal convolution
m. frontal gyrus
m. frontal sulcus
m. glial cell line-derived neurotrophic factor
m. gray layer of superior colliculus
m. hemorrhoidal plexus
m. lobe of cerebellum
m. membrane
m. meningeal artery (MMA)
m. occipital gyrus
m. radicular syndrome
m. temporal convolution
m. temporal focal spike
m. temporal gyrus
m. temporal sulcus
midface
m. degloving
m. degloving technique
m. hypoplasia syndrome
m. retrusion
midget bipolar cell
midlife cardiovascular risk factor
midline
m. brain tumor
m. cervical tenderness
m. developmental lesion
m. exposure
m. fusion defect
m. incision
m. myelotomy
m. shift
m. spinal approach
m. syndrome
midodrine hydrochloride
midpoint to meatal line
midpontine syndrome
Midrin
midsagittal
m. diameter
m. image
m. section
midtegmentum
midtemporal seizure
Mierzejewski effect
Miethke dual-switch valve
miglustat
migraine
abdominal m.
acephalgic m.
acute confusional m.
affective prodrome of m.
autosomal dominant m.
basilar artery m.
basilar-type m.
Bickerstaff m.
catamenial m.
catastrophic m.
ciliary m.
classic m.
common m.
complicated m.
confusional m.
m. equivalent
facial m.
facioplegic m.
familial hemiplegic m. (FHM)
fulgurating m.
Harris m.
m. headache
headache-free m.
hemiplegia m.
hemiplegic m.
menstrual m.
migraine sans m.
m. neuralgia analgesic
neurologic m.
ophthalmic m.
ophthalmoplegic m.
paroxysmal m.
pectoralgic m.
refractory m.

NOTES

M

migraine *(continued)*
retinal m.
seasonal m.
status m.
syncopal m.
unilateral m.
m. variant
m. vasospasm
vestibular m.
m. with aura
m. without aura (MwoA)
migraine-associated stroke
migraine-free state
migraine-induced
m.-i. infarction
m.-i. stroke
migraine-like headache
migraineur
depressed m.
epileptic m.
migrainosus
status m.
migrainous
m. aura
m. cranial neuralgia
m. infarction
m. symptom
migralepsy
Migranal
migrans
erythema chronicum m.
visceral larva m.
migrating intraventricular cysticercus
migration
m. abnormality
electrode m.
foreign body m.
graft m.
implant m.
instrument m.
interfibrillary m.
intrafascicular m.
Luque rod m.
neuroblast m.
neuroepithelial cell m.
neuronal m.
perifascicular m.
rod m.
transendothelial m.
vertical m.
migratory
m. arthralgia
m. cell
m. pain
m. pathway
Mikaelsson catheter
Mikulicz operation
mild
m. cognitive impairment (MCI)
m. dementia
m. head injury
m. mental retardation
m. subsyndromal symptom
Miles punch biopsy forceps
miliary
m. aneurysm
m. brain metastasis
m. pulmonary tuberculosis
military neurosurgery
milk-ejection reflex
milkmaid's grip
Millard-Gubler syndrome
Mille
M. Pattes screw
M. Pattes technique
Miller-Dieker syndrome
Miller-Fisher
M.-F. syndrome (MFS)
M.-F. test
M.-F. variant of Guillain-Barré syndrome
Milles syndrome
Millet neurological test instrument
Milligan dissector
Millipore
M. filter
M. suture
Mills dressing
milrinone
Miltex rib spreader
Milton disease
Milwaukee brace
mime communication
mimetic
m. chorea
m. convulsion
m. muscle
m. paralysis
mimic
m. convulsion
m. spasm
m. tic
mimicry
molecular m.
Minamata disease
mind
m. blindness
m. power
mind/body dualism
mineralizing microangiopathy
miner's
m. cramp
m. nystagmus
Minerva
M. jacket
M. vest
mini
m. applier

M. Orbita plate
M. Würzburg screw
miniature
m. endplate potential (MEPP)
m. ultrasound transmitter
minicore-multicore myopathy
minicore myopathy
minimal
m. access spinal technology (MAST)
m. alveolar concentration (MAC)
m. brain dysfunction
m. lethal dose (MLD)
minimalist surgical strategy
minimally conscious state
Minimax 200-watt light source
Mini-Mental State Examination (MMSE)
minimizing stimulation
minimum
m. duration
m. effective concentration
m. incision surgery
m. intensity projection
mini-open
m.-o. approach
m.-o. technique
miniosmotic infusion pump
miniplate
Luhr m.
m. strut
titanium m.
mini-Sugita clip
mini-Würzburg implant system
Minnesota
M. Multiphasic Personality Inventory (MMPI)
M. Regional Sleep Disorders Center
minocycline
minor
chorea m.
M. disease
epilepsia m.
m. forceps
m. form
m. head injury (MHI)
hippocampus m.
m. hippocampus
m. motor seizure
nervus occipitalis m.
nervus petrosus m.
nervus splanchnicus thoracicus m.
M. sign
minores
nervi palatini m.
minoris
ramus renalis nervi splanchnici m.
sulcus nervi petrosi m.
minorum
rami tonsillares nervorum palatinorum m.
minute
murine double m. 2 (MDM2)
m. object
3-minute rule
miosis
paralytic m.
spastic m.
MIPI
mean interpotential interval
Mira
M. cautery
M. Mark III cranial drill
M. Mark III cranial drill set
M. Mark V craniotome
M. Mark V craniotome set
mirabile
rete m.
Mirapex
mirror
m. system
m. of Wernicke
mirrorlike property
mirror-writing
misconception
sleep-state m.
misdirection phenomenon
misery perfusion
Mishler valve
Miskimon cerebellar retractor
mismatch negativity
misonidazole
misoprostol
misperception
sleep state m.
misplaced thermocouple artifact
misregistration
flow m.
oblique flow m.
missed fragment
missense mutation
misshapen cell

NOTES

M

missile
m. effect
m. fragment
m. injury
Mistichelli crossing
Mitchell disease
mitochondria, sing. **mitochondrion**
fatty acid transport into m.
Mfn1-deficient m.
Mfn2-deficient m.
mitochondrial
m. condensation
m. cytopathy
m. deoxyribonucleic acid (mtDNA)
m. deoxyribonucleic acid analysis
m. depletion syndrome
m. disease (MD)
m. DNA
m. dysfunction
m. encephalomyopathy with lactic acidosis and strokelike episodes (MELAS)
m. encephalomyopathy with sensorimotor polyneuropathy
m. free radical generation
m. GTPase mitofusin 2 mutation
m. leukoencephalopathy
m. metabolic disorder
m. morphology
m. myopathy
m. myopathy, encephalopathy, lactic acidosis, strokelike episodes (MELAS)
m. neurogastrointestinal encephalomyopathy
m. neurogastrointestinal encephalopathy (MNGIE)
m. neuropathy
m. transport defect
Mitofsky-Aaksberg random digit dialing procedure
mitogen
mitogen-activated
m.-a. protein (MAP)
m.-a. protein kinase
mitoguazone (MGBG)
mitosis
neural tube formation m.
mitotane
mitotic
m. segregation
m. spindle apparatus
mitoxantrone
mitral
m. cell
m. cell layer
m. valve prolapse
mixed
m. aphasia
m. apnea
m. bipolar state
m. cerebral dominance
m. connective tissue disease (MCTD)
m. form cerebral palsy
m. germ cell tumor
m. glioma
m. growth hormone-prolactin cell adenoma
m. headache
m. headache syndrome
m. nerve
m. oligoastrocytoma
m. paralysis
m. pineal tumor
m. receptive/expressive language disorder
m. spasm
mixed-frequency EEG
mixed-type
m.-t. epilepsy
m.-t. psychopathic personality
Mixter ventricular needle
mixture
epinephrine-anesthetic m.
thrombogenic ferrous m.
mixtus
nervus m.
Miyoshi myopathy (MM)
Mizuho
M. aneurysm sizer-dissector
M. surgical Doppler
MKM
Mehrkoordinaten manipulator
MKM fiducial
MKM microscope
MKM stereotactic image-guided system
MKM workstation
ML
microscopic laminotomy
ML4
mucolipidosis type IV
MLC1 gene
MLD
minimal lethal dose
MLF
medial longitudinal fasciculus
MM
Miyoshi myopathy
MMA
maxillomandibular advancement
middle meningeal artery
MME
maxillomandibular expansion
M-mode electrocardiographic measurement

MMP
matrix metalloproteinase
MMPI
Minnesota Multiphasic Personality Inventory
MMS-900
MMS-900 balancing tool
MMS-900 microscope balancer
MMSE
Mini-Mental State Examination
M'Naghten test
MNC
mononuclear cell
MNCS
motor nerve conduction study
MND
motor neuron disease
mneme
mnemic, mnemenic
m. hypothesis
m. theory
mnemism
theory of m.
m. theory
mnemonics
MNGIE
mitochondrial neurogastrointestinal encephalopathy
MNTI
melanotic neuroectodermal tumor of infancy
Moban
mobile spasm
mobility
infant spine m.
Möbius
M. disease
M. syndrome
modafinil
modal dose
modality
imaging m.
therapeutic m.
mode
magnet m.
normal m.
quiet wakefulness m.
stimulated echo acquisition m. (STEAM)
syntaxic m.
transcranial Doppler B m.
model
affective schematic mental m.
affect-related schematic mental m.
affect trauma m.
Baddeley m.
biomechanical m.
biomedical m.
coherent m.
corpectomy m.
dynamic EMG-assisted biomechanical m.
finite element m.
Hitch m.
Honig working memory and brain activation m.
internal m.
jurisprudential teaching m.
kinetic m.
lumbar spine m.
Markov decision analysis m.
Mayberg limbic-cortical dysregulation m.
mental m.
multimodal treatment m.
m. 300 NCP bipolar lead
noncoherent m.
m. 100 pulse generator
m. 101 pulse generator
schematic mental m.
standard kinetic m.
subcortical dysfunction m.
m. TC2-64B pulsed-range gated Doppler instrument
treatment m.
m. U gamma knife
vitro matrigel m.
modeling
artificial disc m.
forward m.
kinetic m.
moderate dementia
mode-switching kinetics
modification
body m.
C-D screw m.
Harriluque sublaminar wiring m.
Jacobs locking hook spinal rod instrumentation m.
lifestyle m.
posttranslational m.
m. or Woodson

NOTES

M

modified
M. Autonomic Perception Questionnaire
m. Barthel Index
m. Benton Visual Retention Test
m. Bielschowsky silver stain
M. Checklist for Autism in Toddlers (M-CHAT)
m. constraint-induced therapy
m. Fischer classification
m. Gilsbach technique
m. Gomori trichrome staining
m. Harrington rod
m. McGill Pain Questionnaire
m. Rankin Scale
m. Rankin score
m. right-angled hook
m. Robert Jones dressing
m. Simpson-Angus Rating Scale
m. Stroop effect
modifier
biologic response m.
leukotriene m.
modular
m. implant system
m. instrumentation
modulation
dopaminergic m.
interneuronal calcium m.
pain m.
modulator
circadian m.
selective estrogen-receptor m. (SERM)
module
CUSA electrosurgical m.
Nd:YAG m.
Modulock posterior spinal fixation
Moduretic
Moe
M. alar hook
M. rod
M. spinal hook
M. square-ended hook
M. system
Moersch-Woltmann syndrome
mofetil
mycophenolate m.
MOG
myelin oligodendrocyte glycoprotein
mogiarthria
mogigraphia
mogilalia
mogiphonia
Moire topographic scoliosis assessment
molar behavior
molded vacuum pillow
molecular
m. approach
m. behavior
m. diagnostic technique
m. dualism
m. feedback
m. genetic aspect
m. genetics
m. layer
m. layer of cerebellar cortex
m. layer of cerebellum
m. layer of cerebral cortex
m. layer of olfactory bulb
m. layer of retina
m. layer stria
m. level
m. mimicry
m. neurosurgery
m. plexus
m. testing
molecular-based conceptual therapy
moleculare
stratum m.
molecularis
lamina m.
stria laminae m.
molecule
Abeta m.
adhesion m.
cell adhesion m. (CAM)
endothelial adhesion m.
feel-good m.
glucose transporter m.
growth-inhibiting m.
growth-promoting m.
matrix m.
nerve cell adhesion m.
neural cell adhesion m. (NCAM)
proteoglycan m.
second messenger m.
selective adhesion m. (SAM)
molecule-1
vascular cell adhesion m.-1 (VCAM-1)
molindone HCl
Mollaret meningitis
mollis
chorea m.
molluscum fibrosum
molybdenum cofactor deficiency
moment
gradient m.
macroscopic magnetization m.
magnetic m.
3-point bending m.
momentary stiffening
momentum
angular m.
Monakow
M. bundle
fasciculus aberrans of M.

M. fiber
M. nucleus
M. syndrome
M. tract
Monarch spinal system
monathetosis
monaural word repetition
monaxonic
Mondini syndrome
Mondonesi reflex
mongolian idiocy
monitor
bispectral EEG m.
Camino fiberoptic ICP m.
Camino OLM ICP m.
canopy ventilation m.
Cardiocap II pressure m.
4-channel transcranial Doppler m.
Cortexplorer cerebral blood flow m.
Datex infrared CO_2 m.
Doppler ultrasound m.
electronic m.
Hewlett-Packard pressure m.
Holter m.
ICP m.
intracranial pressure Express digital m.
Laserflow blood perfusion m.
Laserflow BPM^2 real-time cerebral perfusion m.
Medpacific LD 5000 Laser-Doppler perfusion m.
Moor MBF3D m.
Nerve Integrity M. 2
SentiLite EEG m.
SentiLite neurological m.
Sentinel-4 neurological m.
Steritek ICP mini m.
cranial nerve m.
diagnostic m.
Doppler precordial end-tidal carbon dioxide m.
ECoG m.
electronic m.
end-tidal carbon dioxide m.
end-tidal nitrogen m.
esophageal pH m.
esophageal pressure m.
fetal heart rate m.
F-wave m.
24-hour ambulatory m.
intracerebral depth electrode m.
intraoperative facial nerve m.
intraoperative neurophysiological m.
invasive electroencephalographic m.
jugular bulb oxyhemoglobin saturation m. (SjO_2)
leg movement m.
medical parameter m. (MPM)
neurophysiological m.
m. probe
real-time m.
respiratory m.
scalp EEG m.
screw position perioperative m.
seizure m.
somatosensory evoked potential m.
spinal cord function intraoperative m.
subdural grid m.
subdural ICP m.
m. technique
transcutaneous carbon dioxide m.
transcutaneous oxygen m.
video-EEG m.
video electroencephalographic m.
visual function m.
monitor-2
Xomed Nerve Integrity M.-2
monitoring
anesthetic m.
bedside multimodality m.
brain electrical activity m. (BEAM)
cardiac m.
clinical m.
closed-circuit television m.
continuous video-electroencephalogram m. (CCTV-EEG)
monoamine
m. oxidase (MAO)
m. oxidase-B inhibitor
m. oxidase inhibitor (MAOI)
m. oxidase inhibitor-serotonergic agent
monoaminergic
m. fiber
m. neuron
m. pathway
m. system
monobactam

NOTES

M

monobloc
m. advancement
butterfly-shaped m.
monobloc-type appliance
monochorea
monoclonal
m. antibody
m. antiglial fibrillary acidic protein
m. gammopathy
monocular
m. blindness
m. heads-up display imaging system
m. patching
monocystic craniopharyngioma
monocyte
monocytogenes
Listeria m.
monofilament
von Frey m.
monoganglial
monogenetic disorder
Mono-Gesic
monolayer
endothelial m.
monolithic adult block
monomelic
m. amyotrophy
m. muscular atrophy
m. paresis
monomer
acrylamide m.
monomorphic activity
monomyoplegia
mononeuralgia
mononeural lesion
mononeuric involvement
mononeuritis multiplex
mononeuropathy
entrapment m.
multifocal m.
multiple m.
m. multiplex
phrenic m.
mononuclear
m. cell (MNC)
m. leukocyte isolation
m. pleocytosis
m. pleocytosis of cerebrospinal fluid
mononucleosis
infectious m.
m. peripheral neuropathy
mononucleotide
flavin m. (FMN)
monoparesis
monoparesthesia
monophasia
monophasic
m. action potential
m. neurologic illness
m. wave
m. waveform
monophosphate
adenosine 3′,5′-cyclic m. (cAMP)
cyclic adenosine m.
guanosine m.
Monoplace hyperbaric chamber
monoplegia
crural m.
m. masticatoria
spastic m.
monoplegic cerebral palsy
monopolar
m. cathodal stimulator
m. cautery
m. electrocautery
m. needle electrode
m. stimulating electrode
m. tissue forceps
monoportal ventriculoscopy
monorail aspiration catheter
monorhythmic
m. frontal delta (MFD)
m. frontal delta activity
m. sinusoidal delta activity
monosodium
m. glutamate
m. glutamate-induced headache
m. glutamate poisoning
monosomy
chromosome (9_p) m.
monospasm
monosymptomatic hypochondriacal psychosis
monosynaptic
m. connection
m. reflex arc
m. reflex discharge
m. segmental reflex response
m. stretch reflex
monotheism
monotherapy
cabergoline m.
pramipexole m.
ropinirole m.
topiramate m.
monotonous speech
monozygotic twin
Monreal reflex hammer
Monro
M. aqueduct
M. fissure
foramen of M.
M. sulcus
montage
bipolar m.

reference m.
sleep m.
transverse bipolar m.
Monte Carlo permutation method
Montgomery and Asberg Depression Rating Scale (MADRS)
monticulus, pl. **monticuli**
m. cerebelli
clivus m.
mood
apathetic m.
m. disorder associated with sleep disorder
m. disorder with chronic insomnia
m. disturbance
m. elevation
m. regulator
m. spectrum disorder
m. stabilization
m. state
mood-stabilizing agent
Mooney face
moon facies
Moore method
Moor MBF3D monitor
mooseri
Rochalimaea m.
Morand spur
morbidity
perioperative m.
surgical m.
morbilliform rash
morcellation, morcellement
Morel-Kraepelin disease
Morgagni
M. disease
M. syndrome
M. tubercle
Morgagni-Adams-Stokes syndrome
Morgan-Russell scale
Morley peritoneocutaneous reflex
morning
m. glory syndrome
m. headache
Moro reflex
morphine
intracerebroventricular administration of m.
m. pump
morphine-Adcon-L (M-ADL)
morphine-naloxone test
morphinotherapy
intrathecal m.
morphogenesis
brainstem m.
morpholinoanthracycline
morphologic
m. change
m. feature
m. study
morphological
m. deformation
m. difference
morphology
cerebrovascular m.
injury m.
mitochondrial m.
neuronal m.
qualitative m.
quantitative m.
morphometric
m. abnormality
m. technique
morphometry
m. analysis
brain m.
pedicle m.
voxel-based m.
morphosynthesis
Morquio
M. disease
M. syndrome type A, B
Morscher
M. anterior cervical plate
M. titanium cervical plate
Morse sternal spreader
mortality
early m.
lower m.
operative m.
perioperative m.
m. rate
stroke-related m.
Morton
M. disease
M. foot
M. metatarsalgia
M. neuralgia
M. neuroma
Morvan
M. chorea
M. disease
M. syndrome

NOTES

mosaicism
germline m.
mosaic-like pattern
MOSP
myelin/oligodendrocyte-specific protein
mosquito
m. bite infection
m. clamp
m. forceps
Moss-Harms basket
Moss-Miami
M.-M. polyaxial screw
M.-M. spinal instrumentation
M.-M. spinal system
mossy
m. cell
m. fiber
m. fiber sprouting
mote-beam mechanism
moth-eaten alopecia
Mother Jones dressing
motility
m. adhesion
extraocular m.
ocular m.
motion
abnormal joint m.
active integral range of m. (AIROM)
m. artifact
brownian m.
coherent m.
m. concentration
higher order m.
m. segment
m. sense
m. sickness
spinal range of m. (SROM)
spinal segment m.
motionless stare
motivation
characteristic pattern of m.
m. factor
m. impairment
maladaptive pattern of m.
motivational
m. enhancement therapy
m. process
motivational/behavioral factor
motiveless resistance
motoceptor
motoneuron, motor neuron
alpha m.
beta m.
gamma m.
heteronymous m.
homonymous m.
peripheral m.
upper m.
motor
m. abnormality
m. activity
m. agitation
m. agraphia
m. alexia
m. amusia
m. aphasia
m. apraxia
m. ataxia
m. aura
m. cell
m. conduction
m. conduction block
m. conduction velocity (MCV)
m. control
m. control task
m. cortex
m. dapsone neuropathy
m. decussation
m. deficit
m. development examination
m. endplate
m. evoked potential (MEP)
m. fiber
m. finding
m. fluctuation
forelimb m.
m. function
m. hemideficit
m. hemiplegia
m. image
m. impairment
m. impersistence
m. intention
m. interface
m. jacksonian attack
lower m. (LM)
m. maturity
m. neglect
m. nerve conduction study (MNCS)
m. nerve terminal
m. neuron
m. neuronal pool inhibitory neuron
m. neuron disease (MND)
m. neuron disorder
m. neuron integrity
m. neuron paralysis
m. neuron senescence
m. neuron sign
m. nucleus
m. nucleus of facial nerve
m. nucleus of trigeminal nerve
m. nucleus of trigeminus
m. overflow
m. paradigm
m. pathways disease
m. phenomenon
m. point

m. point block
m. psychogenic disorder
m. recovery
m. region
m. response
m. restlessness
m. retardation
m. retardation developmental delay disorder
m. root of ciliary ganglion
m. root of mandibular nerve
m. root of spinal nerve
m. root of submandibular nerve
m. root of trigeminal nerve
m. seizure
m. slowing
m. speech area
m. speech center
m. strength
m. strip
m. subtype
m. system
m. system disease
m. system syndrome
m. thalamus
m. threshold
m. tract
m. unit (MU)
m. unit action potential (MUAP)
m. unit axon
m. unit discharge
m. unit disease
m. unit muscle
m. unit neuromuscular junction
m. unit potential (MUP)
m. unit potential amplitude potential
m. zone

motoria
decussatio m.
radix m.

motoric
m. abnormality
m. function
m. slowing

motorically impaired

motoricity

motorius
nervus m.

motor-verbal

motrice
tache m.

Motricity Index

Mount
M. laminectomy rongeur
M. syndrome

Mount-Reback syndrome

MOUSEPAD
Manchester and Oxford Universities Scale for the Psychopathological Assessment of Dementia

mouth
downturned corners of m.
m. occlusion pressure
tapir m.

movement
abnormal trunk m.
m. artifact
associated m.
bizarre asynchronous m.
choreic m.
choreiform m.
choreoathetoid m.
cocaine-induced choreoathetoid m.
conjugate contraversive eye m.
conjugated eye m.
decomposition of m.
decreased fine finger m.
discordance of m.
m. disorder
M. Disorder Society
m. duration (MD)
dysconjugate m.
dystonic m.
evasive m.
extraocular m. (EOM)
fast saccadic eye m.
fluidity of m.
habitual finger m.
head m.
horizontal eye m.
involuntary m.
lateropulsion of body m.
lateropulsion of eye m.
leg m.
Magnan trombone m.
neurobiotactic m.
nonrapid eye m. (NREM)
paradoxical abdominal m.
passive m.
peak-dose choreoathetoid dyskinetic m.
periodic leg m.
periodic limb m. (PLM)

NOTES

movement *(continued)*
psychotropic m.
purposeful m.
pursuit eye m.
quasi-purposeful m.
range of m.
rapid alternating m.
rapid eye m. (REM)
rapid fine finger m.
reaching-grasping m.
reflex m.
repetitive m.
rhythmic kicking m.
rhythmic stepping m.
saccadic pursuit eye m.
m. sense
sequential opposition finger m.
skilled finger m.
sleep-onset rapid eye m.
slow eye m. (SEM)
slow lateral eye m.
slow rolling eye m.
slow tongue m.
smooth pursuit eye m.
stereotyped m.
stereotypic m.
synchronous clonic m.
tardive m.
tongue m.
transitive limb m.
uncontrollable m.
unusual sleep m.
vergence m.
vertical eye m.
voluntary m.

movement-induced seizure

moyamoya
m. collateral enlargement
m. disease
m. syndrome

Moynihan forceps

Mozart effect

MP-35 clip material

mPFC
medial prefrontal cortex

MPM
medical parameter monitoring

MPM-1 multi-parameter monitoring system

MPPP
multidisciplinary pilot project program

MPRAGE
magnetization-prepared rapid acquisition gradient echo sequence

M-Prednisol Injection

MR
magnetic resonance
MR angiogram
gadolinium diethylenetriamine pentaacetic acid-enhanced MR
MR imaging with gadolinium enhancement
MR spectroscopy
surface coil MR
MR volumetry imaging

MRA
magnetic resonance angiography

MRC
Medical Research Council
MRC strength testing scale

MRF
melanotropin-releasing factor

MRI
magnetic resonance image
magnetic resonance imaging
brain MRI
MRI compatibility
contrast-enhanced MRI
diffusion tensor MRI
Fonar Upright MRI
FS MRI
gadolinium-enhanced MRI
MRI grade
gradient echo MRI
high-resolution MRI
high-resolution contiguous T1-weighted gradient-echo MRI
intraoperative MRI
nonproton MRI
open clam-shell MRI
perfusion-weighted MRI
MRI scan
MRI signal hyperintensity
structural MRI
thin-slice contrast MRI
3-T MRI scanner
MRI volumetry
whole-spine MRI

MRI-based brain anatomy

MRN
magnetic resonance neurography

MRS
magnetic resonance spectroscopy
multivoxel MRS

MRT
magnetic resonance tomography

MRV
magnetic resonance venography

MRZ
measles, rubella and zoster
MRZ reaction

MS
multiple sclerosis
MS etiopathogenesis
opticospinal MS
MS pathogenesis
MS pathway

pediatric MS
Rebif MS
remitting-relapsing MS
secondary progressive MS
MSA
multisystem atrophy
MSD
microsurgical discectomy
MSI
magnetic source imaging
MS-like disease state
MSLT
multiple sleep latency test
MST
multiple subpial transections
99mTc
technetium-99m
MTD
multiple-tic disorder
mtDNA
mitochondrial deoxyribonucleic acid
mtDNA depletion syndrome
MTN
medial terminal nucleus
MTS
mesial temporal sclerosis
MTS electrohydraulic piston
MU
motor unit
mu
mu opiate receptor
mu rhythm
mu wave
MUAP
motor unit action potential
MUAP on electromyogram
mucate
isometheptene m.
Much-Holzmann reaction
mucin-secreting adenocarcinoma
mucocele
clival m.
erosive sphenoid m.
m. formation
paranasal m.
sphenoid m.
mucocutaneous lymph node syndrome
mucolipidosis
mannose in m.
m. type IV (ML4)
mucopolysaccharide
mucopolysaccharidosis I–VI
mucopyocele
m. of clivus
nasal sinus m.
***Mucor* infection**
mucormycosis
Mucosil
mucosulfatidosis
mucous
m. membrane lesion
m. retention cyst
Muir
tract of Bruce and M.
mulberry-like nodule
Mulholland and Gunn criteria
Mullan
M. percutaneous trigeminal ganglion microcompression set
M. triangle
M. wire
Müller
M. fiber
M. ganglion
M. glial cell
M. law
M. muscle
M. radial cell
M. trigone
müllerian duct aplasia, renal aplasia, cervicothoracic somite dysplasia
Müller-König
M.-K. procedure
M.-K. transposition
multiarc LINAC radiosurgery
multiaxial screw
multichannel ABI
multicomponent program
multicopper ferroxidase
multicore
m. disease
m. myopathy
multicystic
m. encephalomalacia
m. encephalopathy
multidimensional
m. assessment
m. assessment of outcome
m. family therapy
m. Fourier transform
m. framework
M. Pain Inventory

NOTES

M

multidisciplinary
m. pilot project program (MPPP)
m. rehabilitation
multienzyme
pyruvate dehydrogenase m.
multifactorial
m. etiology
m. event
multifocal
m. acquired motor axonopathy
m. fibrosclerosis
m. glioma
m. leukoencephalopathy
m. mononeuropathy
m. motor neuropathy (MFMN)
m. myoclonus
m. paroxysm
m. placoid pigment epitheliopathy
m. subcortical demyelination
multiform
m. layer
m. layer of cerebral cortex
multiforme
erythema m. (E-M)
giant cell glioblastoma m.
glioblastoma m. (GBM)
stratum m.
multiforme-like
erythema m.-l.
multiformis
lamina m.
multifrequency transcranial Doppler
multiglandular hyperplasia
multiinfarct
m. dementia (MID)
m. progressive supranuclear palsy
Multi-Institutional Research in Alzheimer Genetic Epidemiology
multilead electrode
multileaf collimator
multilevel laminectomy
multilobar
m. injury
m. resection
multiloculated hydrocephalus
multimodal
m. association cortex
m. code
m. therapeutic approach
m. therapy
m. treatment model
multimodality
m. evoked potential (MEP)
m. image coregistration
multiplace chamber
multiplanar imaging
multiple
m. associations
m. buccal frenula
m. carboxylase deficiencies
m. congenital anomalies
m. cortical infarctions
m. discharges
m. endocrine neoplasia, type 1–3 (MEN 1–3)
m. focal lesions
m. genetic defects
m. impact injuries
m. intracranial aneurysms
m. line-scan imaging
m. medically unexplained symptoms
m. meningiomas
m. mononeuropathy
m. motor tics
m. mucosal neuromas syndrome
m. myeloma
m. myeloma peripheral neuropathy
m. neuritis
m. neuromas
m. operations syndrome
m. ring-enhancing lesions
m. sclerosis (MS)
m. sclerosis ataxia
m. sclerosis chronic progressive pattern
m. sclerosis dementia
m. sclerosis immunology
m. sclerosis pathophysiology
m. sclerosis plaque
m. sclerosis relapse
m. sclerosis-type organic
m. sclerosis variant
m. sensitive points
m. sleep latency test (MSLT)
m. spike population
m. subpial transections (MST)
m. synostoses
m. system atrophy
m. targeting
m. vocal tics
multiple-choice testing
multiple-dose regimen
multiple-episode patient
multiple-hook assembly
multiple-hplane imaging
multiple-loci haplotype
multiple-point sacral fixation
multiple-tic disorder (MTD)
multiple-tracer approach
multiplex
arthrogryposis congenita m.
diabetic mononeuritis m.
mononeuritis m.
mononeuropathy m.
myoclonus m.
paramyoclonus m.

multipolar
m. cell
m. neuron
multipolarity
multipore suction tip
multipotential cell
multipurpose headrest
multisegmental hyporeflexia
multispan fracture hook
multispeaker phonetic noise
Multispect 3 camera
multisynaptic pathway
multisystem
m. atrophy (MSA)
m. therapy
multisystemic
m. disorder
m. therapy
m. therapy approach
multivariate
m. analysis of variance (MANOVA)
m. technique
multivoxel
m. MRS
m. technique
multocida
Pasteurella m.
mumbling automatism
mumps
complication following vaccination for m.
m. encephalitis
m. facial nerve palsy
m. meningitis
m. meningoencephalitis
m. peripheral neuropathy
m. vaccination complication
Munchausen disease
MUP
motor unit potential
MUPS
medically unexplained physical symptoms
mural
m. nodule
m. thrombus
muramyl peptide
murine
m. double minute 2 (MDM2)
m. life span
m. typhus
m. typhus meningoencephalitis
murmur
brain m.
heart m.
Murphy
M. ball hook
M. rake retractor
MurphyScope neurologic device
Murray
M. Valley disease
M. Valley encephalitis
muscarine poisoning
muscarinic
m. acetylcholine receptor (mAChR)
m. cholinergic blockade
m. side effect
muscimol
muscle
m. absence
m. activity
agonist m.
antagonist m.
anterior scalene m.
anterior serratus m.
m. artifact
m. atonia
m. atrophy
m. biopsy
branch of glossopharyngeal nerve to stylopharyngeus m.
cervicis m.
m. contraction headache
corrugator supercilii m.
m. cramp
cranial m.
cricoarytenoid m.
cricopharyngeal m.
m. denervation
depressor anguli oris m.
digastric m.
m. dissection
distal m.
m. endplate
m. enzyme serum level
m. examination
external intercostal m.
extraocular m.
m. fascicle
m. fasciculation
m. fiber
m. fiber action potential

NOTES

M

muscle *(continued)*
m. fiber-type disproportion
m. fibrosis
m. filter
flexor carpi radialis m.
Gantzer m.
genioglossus m.
geniohyoid m.
greater rhomboid m.
homonymous m.
hyoglossus m.
hyoid m.
m. hypertrophy
iliocostal m.
iliopsoas m.
inferior rectus m.
m. inflammatory disorder
intraspinous m.
jugular foramen m.
lateral rectus m.
latissimus dorsi m.
levator palpebrae m.
limb m.
lingual m.
longus capitis m.
longus cervicis colli m.
m. mass
masseter m.
medial rectus m.
mimetic m.
motor unit m.
Müller m.
m. myotonic disorder
nuchal m.
ocular m.
omohyoid m.
orbicularis oculi m.
orbicularis oris m.
m. pain
palatoglossus m.
palatopharyngeus m.
paraspinal m.
pectoralis major m.
m. periodic paralysis
pharyngeal constrictor m.
m. phosphorylase
m. phosphorylase deficiency
platysma m.
procerus m.
m. pseudohypertrophy
psoas m.
m. psychogenic disorder
m. receptor
rectus lateralis abducens oculomotor m.
m. relaxant
m. rigidity
Rouget m.
sacrospinalis m.
scalenus anticus m.
m. sense
skeletal m.
smooth m.
somatic m.
somatic skeletal m.
m. soreness
m. spasm
m. spindle
sternocleidomastoid m.
sternohyoid m.
sternomastoid m.
sternothyroid m.
strap m.
m. strength
m. stretch reflex
striated m.
styloglossus m.
stylohyoid m.
stylopharyngeus m.
superior rectus m.
synkinetic facial m.
temporalis m.
teres major m.
m. tightness
m. tone
m. tone inhibitor system
trapezius m.
upper airway dilating m.
vascular smooth m.
m. wasting

muscle-eye-brain disease
muscle-fascia-Gelfoam combination
muscle-joint pain syndrome
muscle-paretic nystagmus
muscle-relaxing effect
muscle-splitting incision
muscular
m. anesthesia
m. branch of deep fibular nerve
m. circulation
m. dystrophy
m. fiber atrophy
m. fiber necrosis
m. hyperalgesia
m. hyperesthesia
m. hypertrophy
m. hypotonia
m. insufficiency
m. pseudohypertrophy
m. reflex
m. sense
m. trophoneurosis

muscularis
ramus m.

musculature
axial m.
bulbar m.

musculocutanei
rami musculares nervi m.
musculocutaneous
m. nerve
m. neuropathy
musculocutaneus
nervus m.
musculorum
m. deformans
dystonia m.
musculoskeletal
m. deformity
m. myopathy
m. psychogenic disorder
musculospiral
m. nerve
m. paralysis
musical
m. agraphia
m. alexia
musician's
m. cramp
m. dystonia
musicogenic
m. epilepsy
m. seizure
MuSK antibody
Mussen frame
mussitans
delirium m.
mussitation
Mustargen
mutant
m. dynactin
presenilin m.
mutase
methylmalonyl-CoA m.
phosphoglycerate m.
mutation
aprataxin gene m.
causative homozygous m.
CCM1 gene m.
deletion m.
de novo m.
m. detection
duplication m.
dynamic m.
DYT1 dystonia m.
filamin A m.
fukutin m.
genetic m.
heterozygous factor V Leiden m.
LRRK2 m.
methyltetrahydrofolate reductase m.
MGC4607 gene m.
missense m.
mitochondrial GTPase mitofusin 2 m.
nonsense m.
notch3 m.
parkin gene m.
point m.
polyglutamine m.
m. prevalence
single-point m.
sodium channel 5A m.
splicing m.
tandem double m.
transthyretin m.
truncation m.
tumor suppressor gene m.
UBE3A m.
mutilating
m. acropathy
m. leprosy
mutism
akinetic m.
apathetic akinetic m.
cerebellar m.
elective m.
hysterical m.
pure word m.
transient m.
voluntary m.
muttering delirium
MVC
maximum voluntary contraction
MVD
microvascular decompression
MVP
microvascular pressure
MwoA
migraine without aura
MWT
Maintenance of Wakefulness Test
MxA protein
myalgia cruris epidemica
myalgic asthenia
myasthenia
congenital m.
familial infantile m.
m. gravis (MG)
m. gravis evaluation
m. snarl

NOTES

myasthenic
m. crisis
m. facies
m. ptosis
m. reaction
m. syndrome
myatonia, myatony
mycetism cerebralis
mycobacteria
Mycobacterium
M. leprae
M. tuberculosis
M. tuberculosis infection
mycophenolate mofetil
Mycoplasma
M. arthritidis
M. infection
M. pneumoniae encephalitis
mycosis
mycotic
m. infection
m. intracranial aneurysm
mydriasis
alternating m.
paralytic m.
spasmodic m.
spastic m.
springing m.
mydriatic rigidity
myelalgia
myelapoplexy
myelatelia
myelauxe
myelencephalic vein
myelencephalon
myelic lesion
myelin
m. basic protein (MBP)
m. basic protein deficiency
m. body
m. breakdown
compact m.
m. decoy
m. degradation
m. figure
m. macromolecule
m. oligodendrocyte glycoprotein (MOG)
oral bovine m.
m. ovoid
peripheral nerve m.
m. sheath
m. thickening
m. thickness
m. tissue stain
myelin-associated glycoprotein (MAG)
myelinated
m. axon
m. nerve
m. nerve fiber
m. nerve fiber function
myelinating phenotype
myelination
m. of axon
central nervous system m.
peripheral nerve m.
myelin-damaging T cell
myelinic neuroma
myelinization
myelinoclasis
acute perivascular m.
postinfection perivascular m.
myelinoclastic
m. diffuse cerebral sclerosis
m. disease
myelinogenesis
myelin/oligodendrocyte glycoprotein
myelin/oligodendrocyte-specific protein (MOSP)
myelinolysis
central pontine m.
myelinopathy
myelinotoxic
myelinotoxicity
myelin-producing cell
myelitic lesion
myelitis
acute necrotizing m.
acute transverse m.
ascending m.
bulbar m.
complete transverse m.
concussion m.
demyelinated m.
dengue m.
Foix-Alajouanine m.
funicular m.
periependymal m.
postinfectious m.
postvaccinal m.
subacute necrotizing m.
syphilitic m.
systemic m.
transverse m.
m. vaccinia
viral m.
myeloarchitectonics
myelocele
myeloclast
myelocyst
myelocystic
myelocystocele
terminal m.
myelocystomeningocele
myelocyte
myelodiastasis
myelodysplasia
myelodysplastic

myeloencephalic
myeloencephalitis
eosinophilic m.
myelofibrosis
idiopathic m. (IMF)
m. osteosclerosis
myelogenesis
myelogenic sarcoma
myelogenous
myelogeny
myelogram
myelography
cervical m.
computed tomographic metrizamide m.
computer-assisted m. (CAM)
delayed computed tomographic m.
iohexol m.
lumbar m.
metrizamide m.
spinal evaluation m.
water-soluble contrast m.
myeloid elastase
myelolysis
myeloma
multiple m.
osteosclerotic m.
myeloma-associated neuropathy
myelomalacia
angiodysgenetic m.
cystic m.
myelomeningitis
myelomeningocele
lumbosacral m.
spina bifida m.
myeloneuritis
myeloneuropathy
cassava plant tropical m.
human T-cell lymphotropic virus-associated m.
tropical m.
myeloopticoneuropathy
subacute m. (SMON)
myeloparalysis
myelopathic muscular atrophy
myelopathy
acute partial m.
acute transverse m.
AIDS-associated vacuolar m.
AIDS-related m.
carcinomatous m.
cervical spondylosis without m.
cervical spondylotic m.
chronic progressive m.
compressive m.
diabetic m.
HIV m.
HTLV-I-associated m.
human T-cell lymphotropic virus-associated m.
human T-lymphotrophic virus-associated m.
m. incidence
midcervical flexion m.
necrotizing m.
paracarcinomatous m.
paraneoplastic m.
radiation m.
reducing body m.
reversible m.
spondylotic m.
subacute necrotic m.
subacute necrotizing m.
m. syndrome
systemic m.
transverse m.
traumatic m.
tropical spastic paraparesis/HTLV-I-associated m.
vacuolar m.
vascular m.
myeloperoxidase
myelopetal
myelophthisic anemia
myelophthisis
myeloplegia
myelopore
myeloproliferative disorder
myeloradiculitis
myeloradiculodysplasia
myeloradiculopathy
myeloradiculopolyneuronitis
myelorrhagia
myelorrhaphy
myeloschisis
myelosclerosis
myelosis
funicular m.
myelosyphilis
myelosyringosis
myelotome
myelotomography
myelotomy
Bischof m.

M

NOTES

myelotomy *(continued)*
commissural m.
extralemniscal m.
midline m.
T m.
myenteric plexus
Myer fiber
Myers model of perinatal asphyxia
Myerson sign
myesthesia
mylohyoideus
nervus m.
mylohyoid nerve
Myloral
myoadenylate
m. deaminase
m. deaminase deficiency
myoblast
myoblastoma
granular cell m.
Myobloc
myobradia
myocardial infarction
myocarditis
pediatric stroke from m.
myocelialgia
myoclonia
eyelid m.
fibrillary m.
myoclonic
m. absence
m. astatic petit mal epilepsy
m. astatic petit mal seizure
m. dystonia
m. encephalopathy
m. encephalopathy syndrome
m. epilepsy of adolescence
m. epilepsy of infancy
m. epilepsy with ragged red fiber myopathy
m. epilepsy with ragged red fibers (MERRF)
m. epilepsy with ragged red fiber syndrome
m. jerk
m. opsoclonus
myoclonica
dyssynergia cerebellaris m.
myoclonus
Baltic m.
benign infantile m.
benign neonatal sleep m.
cortical m.
m. epilepsy
m. epilepsy with ragged red fibers-lactic acidosis (MERRLA)
epileptic negative m.
essential m.
fragmentary m.
hereditary branchial m.
infantile jerk m.
intention m.
Mediterranean m.
multifocal m.
m. multiplex
nocturnal m.
nonepileptic m.
ocular m.
oculopalatal m.
palatal m.
palatoocular m.
paraneoplastic opsoclonus m.
postanoxic m.
postencephalitic m.
posthypoxic m.
preictal m.
propriospinal m.
m. reticular reflex
sleep m.
spinal segmental m.
stimulus-sensitive m.
tardive m.
myocutaneous flap
Myodil
myodynia
myodystony
myodystrophy, myodystrophia
myoedema
myoesthesis, myoesthesia
myofascial
m. pain
m. syndrome
myofibril
myofibrillar infantile myopathy
myofibrillary disarray
myofibroblast
myofibromatosis
infantile m.
myogenic
m. motor evoked potential
m. paralysis
m. tonus
myoglobinuria
drug-induced m.
exercise-induced m.
myogram
myography
myohypertrophia kymoparalytica
myoinositol transport mechanism
myokymia
eyelid m.
facial m.
generalized m.
hereditary m.
limb m.
superior oblique m.
myokymia-cramp syndrome
myokymic discharge

myomedulloblastoma
myonecrotic myopathy
myoneural
m. ischemia
m. junction
myoneuralgia
postural m.
myoneurasthenia
myoneurogastrointestinal encephalopathy
myoneuroma
myopalmus
myoparalysis
myoparesis
myopathic
m. atrophy
m. carnitine deficiency
m. facies
m. feature
m. gait
m. spasm
m. weakness
myopathy
acquired m.
acute steroid quadriplegic m.
adult-onset nemaline m.
alcoholic m.
bland m.
cap m.
central core m.
centronuclear m.
congenital m.
critical illness m. (CIM)
cylindrical spiral m.
cytoplasmic body m.
desmin storage m.
distal m.
endocrine m.
fingerprint body m.
HIV m.
HIV-associated nemaline m.
hyaline body m.
ICU m.
idiopathic inflammatory m. (IIM)
inclusion body m.
infantile myofibrillar m.
inflammatory m.
Kiloh-Nevin ocular m.
Kugelberg-Welander distal m.
late distal hereditary m.
late-onset rod m.
lipid storage m.
Markesbery-Griggs distal m.
metabolic m.
minicore m.
minicore-multicore m.
mitochondrial m.
Miyoshi m. (MM)
multicore m.
musculoskeletal m.
myoclonic epilepsy with ragged red fiber m.
myofibrillar infantile m.
myonecrotic m.
myotubular m.
necrotizing m.
nemaline rod m.
Nonaka distal m.
nondystrophin m.
oculoskeletal m.
polysaccharide storage m.
proximal myotonic m. (PROMM)
quadriceps m.
reducing body m.
sarcotubular m.
spheroid body m.
sporadic late-onset nemaline m.
thyrotoxic m.
trilaminar m.
tubular aggregate m.
Xp21 m.
zebra body m.
myophosphorylase deficiency
myopia
axial m.
myopsychic
myopsychopathy
myopsychosis
myorelaxant activity
myorhythmia
oculomasticatory m.
myosalgia
myoschwannoma
Myoscint
myoseism
myosin filament
myositis
cancer-associated m.
cervical tension m.
childhood m.
eosinophilic m.
inclusion body m.
influenza virus m.
necrotizing m.

NOTES

M

myositis *(continued)*
orbital m.
m. ossificans
myospasm, myospasmus
cervical m.
myotatic
m. contraction
m. contracture
m. reflex
myotome
myotomy
genioglossus advancement-hyoid m.
myotone (*var. of* myotony)
myotonia
m. acquisita
m. atrophica
Becker m.
chondrodystrophic m.
m. congenita
m. dystrophica
m. neonatorum
potassium-aggravated m. (PAM)
potassium-sensitive m.
myotonic
m. afterdischarge
m. discharge
m. dystrophy gene
m. facies
m. muscular dystrophy
m. potential
m. pupil
m. response
myotonica
dystrophia m.
myotonoid
myotonus
myotony, myotone
myotubular myopathy
myristic acid
Mysoline
Mytelase caplet
myxedema
m. ataxia
m. coma
m. depression
juvenile m.
m. madness
m. peripheral neuropathy
myxoglioma
myxoid lobule
myxoma
atrial m.
left atrial m.
myxomatous
m. cell
m. thickening
myxoneuroma
myxopapillary ependymoma
myxovirus infection

NAA
National Aphasia Association
NABTC
North American Brain Tumor Consortium
nabumetone
nAChR
nicotinic acetylcholine receptor
NADPH
nicotinamide adenine dinucleotide phosphate
NADPH-diaphorase
Naegleria
N. fowleri
N. infection
N. meningitis
Nafcil
Naffziger
N. straight midline incision
N. syndrome
N. test
Nageotte
N. bracelet
N. cell
Nager Miller syndrome
nail
intramedullary n.
Küntscher n.
n. lesion
NAIM
nasal airflow-inducing maneuver
NAIP
neuronal apoptosis inhibitory protein
naked axon
naked-eye direct vision surgery
naltrexone HCl
naltrexone-venlafaxine treatment
Namenda oral solution
naming
category-specific n.
object n.
n. objects
nandrolone decanoate
nap
diurnal n.
napsylate
naratriptan
n. HCl
n. hydrochloride
narcohypnia
narcolepsy
adolescent n.
n. characteristic
n. diagnosis
idiopathic n.
N. Network
non-REM n.
secondary n.
N. Symptoms Severity Questionnaire
narcoleptic
n. tetrad
n. triad
narcosis
CO_2 n.
nitrogen n.
narcotic
n. analgesic
n. intoxication
Nardil
NARP
neuropathy, ataxia, retinitis pigmentosa
narrative
n. data
n. speech
n. speech perception
n. speech perception impairment
narrow
n. AO dynamic compression plate
n. tripole
narrow-bite bone rongeur
narrow-blade laminar hook
narrowing
degenerative n.
disc space n.
nasal
n. airflow-inducing maneuver (NAIM)
n. bilevel ventilation
n. cannula pressure transducer
n. cavity
n. chondritis
n. congestion
n. continuous positive airway pressure
n. CPAP
n. ganglion
n. glioma
n. hemifield
n. lesion
n. mucosal sac
n. pressure measurement/monitoring
n. reconstruction
n. reflex
n. septal deviation
n. septum hematoma
n. sinus
n. sinus mucopyocele
n. surgery
NasalAire II

nasal-temporal asymmetry
nascentium
trismus n.
nascent motor unit potential
NASCET
North American Symptomatic Carotid Endarterectomy Trial
NASCIS
National Acute Spinal Cord Injury Studies
NASCIS II protocol
Nashold
N. biopsy needle
N. TC electrode
nasion
nasociliari
ramus communicans cum nervo n.
nasociliaris
nervus n.
radix n.
nasociliary
n. nerve
n. neuralgia
n. root
nasoethmoidal encephalocele
nasofrontal encephalocele
nasofrontalis
fonticulus n.
nasogastric
n. intubation
n. tube
nasomental reflex
nasoorbital encephalocele
nasopalatine
n. nerve
n. plexus
nasopalatinus
nervus n.
nasopharyngeal
n. angiofibroma
n. blastomycosis
n. cooling
n. electrode
n. electrode placement
n. malignancy
n. mucus retention cyst
nasopharyngolaryngoscopy
fiberoptic n.
nasopharyngoscopy
nasopharynx
Nasu-Hakola disease
natalizumab
Natecor
national
N. Acute Spinal Cord Injury Studies (NASCIS)
N. Adult Reading Test-Revised
N. Aphasia Association (NAA)
N. Brain Tumor Foundation
N. Comorbidity Study
N. Death Index
N. Emergency X-Radiograph Utilization Study (NEXUS)
N. Institute of Neurological and Communicative Disorders and Stroke (NINCDS)
N. Institute of Neurological Disorders and Stroke (NINDS)
N. Institute for Occupational Safety and Health (NIOSH)
N. Institutes of Health Stroke Scale (NIHSS)
N. Mental Health Association (NMHA)
N. Multiple Sclerosis Society (NMSS)
N. Rehabilitation Association
N. Society for Epilepsy (NSE)
N. Spine Network (NSN)
N. Stroke Association
N. Treatment Improvement Evaluation Study
N. Tuberous Sclerosis Association (NTSA)
natriuresis
natriuretic hormone
natural
n. chemotherapy agent
n. hearing loss
n. killer (NK)
n. killer cell
n. progesterone
naturalistic
n. design
n. followup study
nature
subcortical n.
Naturetin
navicular abdomen
navigation
intracranial n.
navigator
Operating Arm stereotactic n.
Zeiss STN surgical tool n.
Navigus
N. cranial base and cap
N. trajectory guide
Navy neurologic screening examination
NC
neurogenic claudication
NCA
nuclear cerebral angiography
NCAM
neural cell adhesion molecule
NCC
neurocysticercosis
NCCU
neurocritical care unit

NCL
neuronal ceroid lipofuscinosis
Turkish-variant NCL
NCP
NeuroCybernetic prosthesis
NCP lead
NCP programming wand
NCS
nerve conduction study
NCV
nerve conduction velocity
Nd:YAG
neodymium:yttrium-aluminum-garnet
Nd:YAG laser
Nd:YAG module
NE
neurologic examination
near
n. drowning
n. reflex spasm
n. syncope
near-infrared spectroscopy (NIRS)
nebulin
NEC
neuroendocrine carcinoma
neck
n. of aneurysm
n. circumference
fusiform aneurysm n.
ill-defined aneurysm n.
n. pain
n. righting reflex
n. sign
stiff n.
n. stiffness
n. stimulation
n. tonic reflex
transverse nerve of n.
n. weakness
wry n., wryneck
neck-tongue syndrome
necrolysis
epidermal n.
toxic epidermal n. (TEN)
necrosis
acute tubular n.
aseptic n.
avascular n.
brain radiation n.
caseous n.
cell n.
cerebral radiation n.
coagulative n.
confluent central n.
cystic medial n.
familial infantile bilateral striatal n.
full-thickness n.
gray matter n.
hemorrhagic n.
infantile bilateral striatal n.
laminar cortical n.
Marcus grading scale for avascular n.
muscular fiber n.
occlusal n.
pituitary n.
postpartum n.
pressure n.
radiation n.
segmental fibrinoid n.
selective neuronal n.
tubular n.
tumor n.
vasculitic n.
necrotic material
necrotizing
n. angiitis
n. encephalitis
n. encephalomyelitis
n. encephalomyelopathy
n. encephalopathy
n. granulomatous systemic arteritis
n. hemorrhage leukomyelitis
n. hemorrhagic leukoencephalitis
n. leukoencephalopathy
n. myelopathy
n. myopathy
n. myositis
n. retinitis
n. vasculitis
NEE
needle electrode examination
needle
Adson n.
aneurysm n.
angled n.
n. aspiration
atraumatic Sprotte n.
Backlund biopsy n.
Bier lumbar puncture n.
brain biopsy n.
butterfly n.
Colorado microdissection n.
Cone ventricular n.

N

NOTES

needle *(continued)*
Cournand arteriogram n.
Cournand-Grino arteriogram n.
Cushing ventricular n.
Dandy ventricular n.
D'Errico ventricular n.
n. dissector
n. electrode
n. electrode examination (NEE)
n. electromyography
n. EMG
epidural n.
Espocan combined spinal/epidural n.
Frazier ventricular n.
Hoen ventricular n.
n. holder
Hunstad infusion n.
insulated electrode n.
Kronecker aneurysm n.
lumbar puncture n.
Mixter ventricular n.
Nashold biopsy n.
neurography n.
Pace ventricular n.
Poppen ventricular n.
Quincke spinal n.
radioactive strontium n.
R-K n.
Scoville ventricular n.
Sedan-Nashold n.
Shaw aneurysm n.
Sheldon-Spatz vertebral arteriogram n.
Smiley-Williams arteriogram n.
spinal n.
Sprotte epidural n.
Sprotte spinal n.
stereotactic n.
straight n.
thermistor n.
titanium alloy n.
n. trephination system
Tuohy n.
n. valve
ventricular n.
ventriculostomy n.
Whitacre spinal n.
needle-in-the-eye syndrome
needle-nose rongeur
need for sleep
NEEG
normal electroencephalogram
neencephalon, neoencephalon
nefazodone
Neftel disease
negative
n. afterpotential
n. aspiration
n. change
n. dromotropism
false n.
n. feedback
n. image
n. immunosuppressive effect
n. myoclonic seizure
n. myoclonus state
n. oligoclonal band
n. picture-caption pair
n. priming effect
n. priming task
negatively
n. bathmotropic
n. correlated region
negative-pressure ventilation
negativity
early right anterior n.
mismatch n.
phonological mismatch n. (PMN)
right anterior-temporal n.
visual mismatch n. (VMMN)
neglect
emotional n.
hemispatial n.
ipsilateral n.
left visuospatial n.
n. measure
motor n.
spatial n.
thalamic n.
visuospatial n.
Negri body
Negri-Jacod syndrome
Negro
N. phenomenon
N. sign
Neisseria
N. meningitidis
N. meningitidis meningitis
Nélaton syndrome
nelfinavir
Nelson
N. rib spreader
N. syndrome
N. tumor
nemaline rod myopathy
nematode infection
Nembutal Sodium
Neo-Calglucon
neocerebellum
neocinetic
Neo-Cobefrin
Carbocaine with N.-C.
neocortex
lateral n.
n. maturation
neocortical
n. association area
n. atrophy

n. coverage
n. epilepsy
n. neurofibrillary tangle
n. region
n. temporal lobe epilepsy

NeoDerm dressing
neodymium:yttrium-aluminum-garnet (Nd:YAG)
neoencephalon (*var. of* neencephalon)
neoendorphin
neoformans
Cryptococcus n.
Neo-Iopax
neolalism
neologism
neomycin
neonatal
n. abstinence syndrome
n. adrenoleukodystrophy
n. alloimmune thrombocytopenia
n. apoplexy
n. asphyxia
n. breath-holding spell
n. cerebral hemorrhage
n. cerebral infarction
n. drug addiction
n. drug addiction seizure
n. drug addiction with cocaine
n. enterovirus infection
n. extracorporal membrane oxygenation
n. hemorrhagic disease
n. herpes simplex virus infection
n. hydrocephalus
n. hypercalcemia
n. hypertension
n. hypocalcemia
n. hypoglycemic seizure
n. hypomagnesemia
n. hypothyroidism
n. hypotonia
n. injury
n. intraventricular hemorrhage
n. kernicterus
n. language development
n. meningitis
n. myasthenia gravis
n. opiate withdrawal
n. Pelizaeus-Merzbacher disease
n. poliomyelitis
n. polycythemia
n. tetanus
n. tetany
n. tyrosinemia aminoaciduria
n. withdrawal syndrome

neonate asphyxia
neonatorum
encephalitis n.
myotonia n.
tetanus n.
trismus n.

neon occipitocervical system
neopallium
Neopap
neoplasia
adenohypophysial n.
multiple endocrine n., type 1–3 (MEN 1–3)
prostatic intraepithelial n. (PIN)

neoplasm
cranial nerve n.
de novo metachronous n.
extensive n.
frontal n.
intraaxial n.
intracranial n.
n. of lymphocytic derivation
metachronous n.
pearly n.
pineal parenchymal n.
slow-growing n.
spinal cord n.
temporal horn n.
trochlear nerve n.

neoplastic
n. aneurysm
n. angioendotheliomatosis
n. arachnoiditis
n. ataxia
n. cell
n. lesion
n. meningitis

neopterin
serum n.

Neosar Injection
neospinothalamic tract
Neosporin GU Irrigant
neostigmine test
neostriatum
Neo-Synephrine
neothalamus
neovascularization
iris n.
subretinal n.

NOTES

nephelometric assay
nephralgic crisis
nephritis
shunt n.
Nephro-Calci
nephrosis
nephrotoxicity
Néri sign
Nernst equation
nerve
abdominopelvic splanchnic n.
abducens n.
abducent n. [CN VI]
accelerator n.
accessory n. [CN XI]
accessory phrenic n.
accommodation of n.
accompanying vein of hypoglossal n.
acoustic n.
n. action potential
afferent digital n.
alveolar n.
ampullar n.
anal n.
Andersch n.
anococcygeal n.
anomalous nonrecurrent right inferior laryngeal n.
antebrachial cutaneous n.
anterior abdominal cutaneous branch of intercostal n.
anterior ampullary n.
anterior antebrachial n.
anterior auricular n.
anterior branch of axillary n.
anterior branch of thoracic n.
anterior cutaneous branch of femoral n.
anterior cutaneous branch of iliohypogastric n.
anterior cutaneous branch of intercostal n.
anterior ethmoidal n.
anterior femoral cutaneous n.
anterior interosseous n.
anterior pectoral cutaneous branch of intercostal n.
anterior pulmonary branch of vagus n.
anterior ramus of cervical n.
anterior ramus of lumbar n.
anterior ramus of sacral n.
anterior ramus of spinal n.
anterior ramus of thoracic n.
anterior root of spinal n.
anterior superior alveolar branch of infraorbital n.
aortic n.
area of facial n.
Arnold n.
articular branch of deep fibular n.
auditory n.
augmentor n.
auricular branch of vagus n.
auriculotemporal n.
autonomic n.
axillary n.
baroreceptor n.
Bell n.
n. biopsy
Bock n.
brachial cutaneous n.
buccal n.
buccinator n.
cardiac n.
caroticotympanic n.
carotid branch of glossopharyngeal n. [CN IX]
carotid sinus n.
cavernosal n.
cavernous n.
celiac n.
n. cell
n. cell adhesion molecule
n. cell body
n. center
centrifugal n.
centripetal n.
cerebral n.
cervical n.
chorda tympani n.
ciliary n.
circumflex n.
cluneal n.
coccygeal n.
cochlear part of vestibulocochlear n.
cochlear root of eighth n.
cochlear root of vestibulocochlear n.
common fibular n.
common peroneal n.
communicating branch of auriculotemporal nerve with facial n.
communicating branch of chorda tympani with lingual n.
communicating branch of facial nerve with glossopharyngeal n.
communicating branch of lacrimal nerve with zygomatic n.
communicating branch of lingual nerve with hypoglossal n.
communicating branch of median nerve with ulnar n.
communicating branch of otic ganglion to auriculotemporal n.

communicating branch of otic ganglion with medial pterygoid n.
communicating branch of radial nerve with ulnar n.
communicating branch of spinal n.
communicating branch of superficial radial nerve with ulnar n.
communicating branch of tympanic plexus with auricular branch of vagus n.
communicating branch with nasociliary n.
n. compression syndrome
n. conduction study (NCS)
n. conduction velocity (NCV)
n. conduction velocity study
Cotunnius n.
cranial n.
crural interosseus n.
cubital n.
cutaneous n.
Cyon n.
n. damage
n. deafness
n. decompression
decussation of trochlear n.
dental n.
descending tract of trigeminal n.
diaphragmatic n.
digastric n.
digital n.
n. discontinuity
dorsal root of spinal n.
dorsal scapular n.
efferent n.
eighth cranial n. [CN VIII]
eleventh cranial n. [CN XI]
encephalic n.
n. ending
n. entrapment
n. entrapment neuralgia
esodic n.
ethmoidal n.
excitor n.
excitoreflex n.
exodic n.
external popliteal n.
external sheath of optic n.
facial n. [CN VII]
n. fascicle
femoral cutaneous n.
fenestrated oculomotor n.
n. fiber
n. fiber layer hemorrhage
n. fibril
fibrous sheath of optic n.
fibular n.
n. field
fifth cranial n. [CN V]
first cranial n. [CN I]
fourth cervical n. (C4)
fourth cranial n. [CN IV]
frontal n.
furcal n.
fusimotor n.
Galen n.
gangliated n.
n. ganglion
ganglion of facial n.
ganglionic layer of optic n.
ganglionic stratum of optic n.
ganglion of intermediate n.
Gaskell n.
gastric n.
geniculum of facial n.
genitofemoral n.
genu of facial n.
glossopharyngeal cranial n. [CN IX]
gluteal n.
n. graft
greater occipital n.
greater superficial petrosal n. (GSPN)
n. growth factor (NGF)
n. growth factor antiserum
Hering sinus n.
n. hook
hypogastric n.
hypoglossal n. [CN XII]
hypoglossal cranial n.
iliohypogastric n.
ilioinguinal n.
iliopubic n.
n. implantation
n. impulse
n. impulse transmission
inferior dental n.
inferior ganglion of glossopharyngeal n.
inferior ganglion of vagus n.
inferior laryngeal n.
inferior part of vestibulocochlear n.
inferior root of vestibulocochlear n.

N

NOTES

nerve *(continued)*
infraorbital n.
infratrochlear n.
inhibitory n.
inner sheath of optic n.
N. Integrity Monitor 2
intercostal n.
intercostobrachial n.
intermediary n.
intermediate n.
internal popliteal n.
internal sheath of optic n.
interosseous branch of medial terminal branch of deep fibular n.
intervaginal space of optic n.
intracranial part of optic n.
ischiadic n.
Jacobson n.
jugular n.
labial n.
lacrimal n.
Lancisi longitudinal n.
Langley n.
laryngeal n.
Latarjet n.
lateral femoral cutaneous n.
lateral pterygoid n.
lateral root of median n.
lateral terminal branch of deep fibular n.
lesser superficial petrosal n. (LSPN)
levator ani n.
lingual n.
long thoracic n.
loop of hypoglossal n.
loop of spinal n.
Ludwig n.
lumbar n.
lumboinguinal n.
Luschka n.
mandibular n.
masseteric n.
maxillary n.
medial plantar n.
medial root of median n.
medial terminal branch of deep fibular n.
median n.
meningeal n.
mental n.
mesencephalic nucleus of trigeminal n.
mesencephalic tract of trigeminal n.
mixed n.
motor nucleus of facial n.
motor nucleus of trigeminal n.
motor root of mandibular n.
motor root of spinal n.
motor root of submandibular n.
motor root of trigeminal n.
muscular branch of deep fibular n.
musculocutaneous n.
musculospiral n.
myelinated n.
mylohyoid n.
nasociliary n.
nasopalatine n.
ninth cranial n. [CN IX]
nonmyelinated n.
nucleus of abducent n.
nucleus of accessory n.
nucleus of acoustic n.
nucleus of cranial n.
nucleus of hypoglossal n.
nucleus of oculomotor n.
nucleus of phrenic n.
nucleus of pudendal n.
nucleus of trigeminal n.
nucleus of trochlear n.
nucleus of vagus n.
obturator n.
occipital n.
oculomotor n. [CN III]
olfactory cranial n.
ophthalmic recurrent n.
optic n. [CN II]
outer sheath of optic n.
n. pain
palatine n.
n. palsy
n. papilla
parasympathetic n.
parotid n.
pathetic n.
pectineus n.
pectoral n.
perforating cutaneous n.
perineal n.
peripheral n.
perivascular n.
peroneal n.
petrosal n.
pharyngeal plexus of vagus n.
phrenic n.
phrenicoabdominal n.
pilomotor n.
piriform n.
plantar n.
n. plexus
plexus of spinal n.
pneumogastric n.
popliteal n.
posterior branch of axillary n.
posterior communicating n.
posterior interosseous n.
posterior nucleus of oculomotor n.

posterior nucleus of vagus n.
posterior pulmonary branch of vagus n.
posterior root of spinal n.
posterior tibial n.
prenatal injury to cranial n.
presacral n.
n. preservation
pressor n.
pressoreceptor n.
principal sensory nucleus of trigeminal n.
pterygoid canal n.
pterygopalatine n.
pudendal n.
quadratus femoris n.
radial n.
rectal n.
recurrent laryngeal n. (RLN)
recurrent meningeal n.
n. regrowth
n. root
n. root avulsion
n. root block
n. root compression
n. root disease
n. root edema
n. root embarrassment
root of facial n.
n. root injection
n. root injury
n. root irritation
n. root microcirculation
n. root retractor
n. root sheath effacement
root of trigeminal n.
saccular n.
sacral n.
saphenous n.
sartorius n.
scapular n.
Scarpa n.
sciatic n.
scrotal n.
second cervical n.
second cranial n. [CN II]
secretomotor n.
secretory n.
sensory ganglion of cranial n.
sensory ganglion of encephalic n.
sensory root of mandibular n.
sensory root of spinal n.
sensory root of trigeminal n.
seventh cranial n. [CN VII]
n. sheath
n. sheath tumor
n. signal conduction
sinuvertebral n.
sixth cranial n. [CN VI]
small sciatic n.
n. of smell
somatic n.
spermatic n.
sphenopalatine n.
sphincter ani n.
spinal accessory n.
spinal nucleus of accessory n.
spinal nucleus of trigeminal n.
spinal tract of trigeminal n.
splanchnic n.
stapedial n.
stapedius n.
statoacoustic n.
n. stimulator
n. stroma
n. stump
stylohyoid n.
stylopharyngeal n.
subclavian n.
subclavius n.
subcostal n.
sublingual n.
submaxillary n.
suboccipital n.
subscapular n.
n. substitution technique
sudomotor n.
sulcus of oculomotor n.
superficial petrosal n.
superior ganglion of glossopharyngeal n.
superior ganglion of vagus n.
superior laryngeal n. (SLN)
superior part of vestibulocochlear n.
superior root of vestibulocochlear n.
supraclavicular n.
supraorbital n.
suprascapular n.
supratrochlear n.
sural cutaneous n.
sural sensory n.
n. suture

NOTES

nerve *(continued)*
sympathetic n.
temporal n.
tensor tympani n.
tensor veli palatini n.
tenth cranial n. [CN X]
tentorial n.
terminal n.
third cranial n. [CN III]
thoracic splanchnic n.
thoracodorsal n.
tibial n.
Tiedemann n.
tonsillar n.
n. tract
trifacial n.
trigeminal cranial n.
trigone of auditory n.
trigone of hypoglossal n.
trigone of vagus n.
trochlear n. [CN IV]
trochlear cranial n.
tympanic n.
ulnar n.
unmyelinated n.
utricular n.
utriculoampullarly n.
vagal part of accessory n.
vaginal n.
vagus cranial n. [CN X]
Valentin n.
vascular circle of optic n.
vasoconstrictor n.
vasodilator n.
vasomotor n.
vasosensory n.
ventral branch of thoracic n.
ventral medial nucleus of
oculomotor n.
ventral ramus of thoracic n.
ventral root of spinal n.
vertebral n.
vestibular part of
vestibulocochlear n.
vestibular root of
vestibulocochlear n.
vestibulocochlear n. [CN VIII]
vidian n.
visceral nucleus of oculomotor n.
Willis n.
Wrisberg n.
n. of Wrisberg
zygomatic n.
zygomaticofacial branch of
zygomatic n.
zygomaticotemporal branch of
zygomatic n.

nerve-action current
nerveless
nerve-point massage
nervi (*pl. of* nervus)
nervimotility, neurimotility
nervimotion
nervimotor, neurimotor
nervine
nervorum
ansae n.
nervus n.

nervosa
anorexia n.
foramina n.
pars n.

nervosi
pars cranialis partis parasympathici
divisionis autonomici systematis n.
pars parasympathetica divisionis
autonomici systematis n.
pars peripherica systematis n.
pars sympathica divisionis
autonomici systematis n.

nervosum
systema n.
Willis centrum n.

nervosus
lobus n.
plexus n.
status n.

nervous
n. asthenopia
n. bladder
n. chill
n. consumption
n. discharge
n. distribution
n. fatigability
n. irritability
n. system
n. system disorder
n. system infection
n. system involvement
n. system structure
n. tissue

nervus, pl. **nervi**
n. abducens [CN VI]
n. acusticus [CN VIII]
nervi alveolares superiores
n. ampullaris anterior
n. ampullaris lateralis
n. ampullaris posterior
nervi anales inferiores
n. anococcygeus
n. articularis
nervi auriculares anteriores
n. auricularis magnus
n. auricularis posterior
n. auriculotemporalis
n. autonomicus
n. axillaris

n. buccalis
n. canalis pterygoidei
nervi cardiaci thoracici
n. cardiacus cervicalis inferior
n. cardiacus cervicalis medius
n. cardiacus cervicalis superior
nervi carotici externi
nervi caroticotympanici
n. caroticus internus
nervi cavernosi clitoridis
nervi cavernosi penis
nervi cervicales
nervi ciliares breves
nervi ciliares longi
nervi clunium inferiores
nervi clunium medii
nervi clunium superiores
n. coccygeus
n. cochlearis
nervi craniales
n. cutaneous antebrachii medialis
n. cutaneous antebrachii posterior
n. cutaneous brachii lateralis inferior
n. cutaneous brachii lateralis superior
n. cutaneous brachii medialis
n. cutaneous brachii posterior
n. cutaneous dorsalis intermedius
n. cutaneous dorsalis lateralis
n. cutaneous dorsalis medialis
n. cutaneous perforans
n. cutaneous surae lateralis
n. cutaneous surae medialis
n. cutaneus
n. cutaneus antebrachii lateralis
nervi digitales dorsales nervi radialis
nervi digitales dorsales nervi ulnaris
nervi digitales dorsales pedis
nervi digitales palmares communes nervi mediani
nervi digitales palmares communes nervi ulnaris
nervi digitales palmares proprii nervi mediani
nervi digitales palmares proprii nervi ulnaris
nervi digitales plantares communes nervi plantaris lateralis
nervi digitales plantares communes nervi plantaris medialis
nervi digitales plantares proprii nervi plantaris lateralis
nervi digitales plantares proprii nervi plantaris medialis
n. dorsalis clitoridis
n. dorsalis penis
n. dorsalis scapulae
nervi erigentes
n. ethmoidalis anterior
n. ethmoidalis posterior
n. facialis [CN VII]
n. femoralis
n. fibularis communis
n. fibularis profundus
n. fibularis superficialis
n. frontalis
n. glossopharyngeus [CN IX]
n. gluteus inferior
n. gluteus superior
n. hypogastricus
n. iliohypogastricus
n. ilioinguinalis
n. iliopubicus
n. impar
n. infraorbitalis
n. infratrochlearis
nervi intercostales
nervi intercostobrachiales
n. intermedius neuralgia
n. interosseus antebrachii anterior
n. interosseus antebrachii posterior
n. interosseus cruris
n. ischiadicus
n. jugularis
nervi labiales anteriores
nervi labiales posteriores
n. lacrimalis
n. lingualis
n. lumboinguinalis
n. mandibularis
n. massetericus
n. maxillaris
n. meatus acustici externi
n. medianus
n. meningeus medius
n. mentalis
n. mixtus
n. motorius
n. musculi obturatorii interni
n. musculi piriformis

NOTES

nervus *(continued)*
n. musculi tensoris tympani
n. musculi tensoris veli palatini
n. musculocutaneus
n. mylohyoideus
n. nasociliaris
n. nasopalatinus
n. nervorum
n. obturatorius
n. obturatorius accessorius
n. obturatorius internus
n. occipitalis major
n. occipitalis minor
n. occipitalis tertius
n. octavus [CN VIII]
n. oculomotorius [CN III]
nervi olfactorii
n. olfactorius [CN I]
n. ophthalmicus
n. opticus [CN II]
nervi palatini
nervi palatini minores
n. palatinus major
n. pectoralis lateralis
n. pectoralis medialis
nervi peroneales
n. peroneus profundus
n. peroneus profundus accessorius
n. peroneus superficialis
n. petrosus major
n. petrosus minor
n. petrosus profundus
n. pharyngeus
nervi phrenici accessorii
n. phrenicus
n. plantaris lateralis
n. plantaris medialis
n. presacralis
n. pterygoideus lateralis
n. pterygoideus medialis
nervi pterygopalatini
n. pudendus
n. quadratus femoris
n. radialis
nervi rectales inferiores
n. saccularis
nervi sacrales et nervus coccygeus
n. saphenus
n. sciaticus
nervi scrotales anteriores
nervi scrotales posteriores
n. sensorius
n. spermaticus externus
nervi spinales
n. spinosus
nervi splanchnici lumbales
nervi splanchnici lumbares
nervi splanchnici pelvici
nervi splanchnici sacrales
n. splanchnicus thoracicus imus
n. splanchnicus thoracicus major
n. splanchnicus thoracicus minor
n. stapedius
n. statoacusticus [CN VIII]
n. subclavius
n. sublingualis
n. suboccipitalis
nervi subscapulares
nervi supraclaviculares
nervi supraclaviculares intermedii
nervi supraclaviculares laterales
nervi supraclaviculares mediales
nervi supraclaviculares posteriores
n. supraorbitalis
n. suprascapularis
n. supratrochlearis
n. suralis
nervi temporales profundi
n. terminalis
n. thoracicus longus
n. thoracodorsalis
n. tibialis
n. transversus cervicalis
n. transversus colli
n. trigeminalis
n. trochlearis [CN IV]
n. tympanicus
n. ulnaris
n. utricularis
n. utriculoampullaris
nervi vaginales
nervi vasorum
n. vestibulocochlearis [CN VIII]
n. visceralis
n. zygomaticus

nesidioblastosis

nest
choristoma n.

net
n. electrochemical potential gradient
Neuro n.

netilmicin

network
matching and tuning n.
Narcolepsy N.
National Spine N. (NSN)
neural n.
neurofibrillar n.
prefrontal insular cerebellar n.
thalamocortical n.
wide area n.

Neucalm

Neuhauser syndrome

NeuraGen nerve guide

neuragmia

neural
n. activation
n. arc

n. arch
n. arch fracture
n. arch resection
n. axis
n. canal
n. capacity
n. cell adhesion molecule (NCAM)
n. cell line
n. crest
n. crest cell
n. crest precursor
n. crest syndrome
n. crest tumor localization study
n. cyst
n. cytoarchitecture
n. darwinism
n. deafness
n. discharge
n. dissector
n. ectoderm
n. fold
n. foramen
n. foramen remodeling
n. function
n. ganglion
n. groove
n. growth factor
n. hamster cell
n. imaging study
n. impulse
n. induction
n. injury
n. layer of retina
n. lobe
n. lobe of hypophysis
n. lobe of neurohypophysis
n. lobe of pituitary gland
n. maldevelopment
n. mechanism
n. migration disorder
n. network
n. noise level
n. part of hypophysis
n. pathway
n. pathway level
n. placode
n. plasticity
n. plate
n. plate formation
n. progenitor cell
n. prosthesis
n. regeneration
n. repair
n. segment
n. stalk
n. stem cell
n. structure
n. substrate
n. system
n. transplantation
n. tube
n. tube closure
n. tube defect (NTD)
n. tube development disorder
n. tube floor plate cell
n. tube formation mitosis

neuralgia

abdominal n.
atypical facial n.
atypical trigeminal n.
chronic migrainous n.
ciliary n.
cranial n.
delayed-onset postherpetic n.
epileptiform n.
facial n.
n. facialis vera
Fothergill n.
geniculate n.
glossopharyngeal n. (GPN)
hallucinatory n.
Hunt n.
hypoglossal n.
idiopathic trigeminal n. (ITN)
intercostal n.
mammary n.
migrainous cranial n.
Morton n.
nasociliary n.
nerve entrapment n.
nervus intermedius n.
occipital n.
otic n.
paratrigeminal n.
periodic migrainous n.
peripheral n.
petrosal n.
postherpetic n. (PHN)
posttraumatic n.
pterygopalatine n.
Raeder paratrigeminal n.
red n.
reminiscent n.
sciatic n.

NOTES

neuralgia *(continued)*
Sluder n.
sphenopalatine n.
stump n.
suboccipital n.
supraorbital n.
symptomatic n.
trifacial n.
trifocal n.
trigeminal n. (TN)
trigger point n.
vagoglossopharyngeal n.
Vail n.
vidian n.
neuralgic
n. amyotrophy
n. pain syndrome
neuralgiform headache
neurally mediated syncope
neuramebimeter
neuraminidase deficiency
neuranagenesis
neurapophysis
neurapraxia
peripheral nerve n.
neurarchy
neurasthenia
angioparalytic n.
angiopathic n.
gastric n.
n. gravis
n. praecox
primary n.
pulsating n.
traumatic n.
neurasthenic
n. personality
n. psychoneurosis reaction
neuraxial
neuraxis staging
neuraxon, neuraxone
neurectasis, neurectasia
neurectomy, neuroectomy
Cotte presacral n.
frontal branch n.
obturator n.
occipital n.
presacral n.
retrogasserian n.
Sonneberg n.
vestibular n.
vestibulocochlear n.
neurectopia, neurectopy
Neurelan
neurenteric cyst
neurepithelial (*var. of* neuroepithelial)
neurepithelium (*var. of* neuroepithelium)
neurergic
neurexeresis
neuriatria, neuriatry
neurilemma, neurolemma
n. sheath cell
neurilemmitis
neurilemoma
acoustic n.
Antoni type A, B n.
neurility
neurimotility (*var. of* nervimotility)
neurimotor (*var. of* nervimotor)
neurinoma
acoustic n.
dumbbell-shaped n.
trigeminal nerve n.
neurite
dystrophic n.
n. extension
n. growth
n. outgrowth
n. overgrowth
neuritic
n. cytoskeletal abnormality
n. muscular atrophy
n. plaque
neuriticum
atrophoderma n.
neuritis, pl. **neuritides**
adventitial n.
ascending n.
axial n.
brachial plexus n.
central n.
descending n.
Eichhorst n.
eighth nerve herpetic n.
endemic n.
fallopian n.
Gombault n.
heavy metal n.
herpes zoster n.
herpetic n.
inflammatory demyelinating optic n.
interdigital n.
interstitial n.
intraocular n.
ischemic n.
Leyden n.
lumbosacral plexus n.
multiple n.
occipital n.
optic n.
orbital optic n.
n. ossificans
parenchymatous n.
periaxial n.
postocular optic n.
radiation n.
radicular n.
relapsing hypertrophic n.

retrobulbar optic n.
sciatic n.
segmental n.
serum n.
shoulder-girdle n.
suboccipital n.
syphilitic n.
toxic n.
traction n.
traumatic n.
unilateral optic n.
vestibular n.

Neuro
N. net
N. N-50 lesion generator

neuroacanthocytosis
neuroactive amino acid
neuroadenolysis
neuro-AIDS
neuroallergy
neuroamebiasis
neuroanastomosis
autogenous cable graft interposition VII-VII n.

neuroanatomic
n. abnormality
n. circuit
n. connection
n. pathway

neuroanatomical
neuroanatomy of aging
neuroanesthesia
neuroanesthesiologist
neuroarthropathy
atrophic n.

neuroastrocytoma
neuroaugmentation
neuroaugmentive
NeuroAvitene applicator
neuroaxonal dystrophy
neurobehavioral
n. consequence
n. disorder
n. feature
n. manifestation
n. sequela
n. symptom
n. teratogenicity

neuro-Behçet disease
neurobiological
n. cause
n. factor
n. justification
n. mechanism
n. perspective
n. phenomenon

neurobiologist
neurobiology
n. of early childhood development
n. of sleep

neurobiotactic movement
neurobiotaxis
neuroblast
n. maturation
n. migration
n. redundancy
sympathetic n.

neuroblastoma
cerebral n.
dumbbell n.
dumbbell-type n.
intraabdominal n.
intracranial n.
occipital n.
olfactory n.
Pepper n.

Neurobloc
neuroborreliosis
late Lyme n.
Lyme n.

neurocan
neurocardiac
neurocardiogenic syncope
neurocele
NeuroCell-HD
N.-HD neural cell transplant product
N.-HD porcine fetal neural material

NeuroCell-PD
N.-PD porcine fetal neural material
N.-PD porcine neural cell transplant product

neurocentral joint of Luschka
neuroceptor
neurochemical
n. change
n. disequilibrium
n. effect
n. interaction
n. pathway
n. transmission

neurochemistry
neurochitin
neurochorioretinitis

N

NOTES

neurochoroiditis
neurocirculatory
n. asthenia
n. disorder
neurocladism
neurocognitive
n. alteration
n. dysfunction
n. impairment
n. index
n. measure
n. process
NeuroControl Freehand implant
neurocranial granulomatous arteritis
neurocristopathy
neurocritical care unit (NCCU)
neurocutaneous
n. angiomatosis
n. melanosis
n. syndrome
NeuroCybernetic
N. prosthesis (NCP)
N. Prosthesis System (NPS)
neurocysticercosis (NCC)
neurocyte
neurocytolysis
neurocytoma
central n.
neurodegeneration
glutamate receptor-mediated n.
neurodegenerative
n. dementia
n. disease
n. disorder
n. movement disorder
neurodendrite
neurodendron
neurodermal
n. sinus
n. sinus dysraphism
neurodiagnostic
n. imaging
n. investigation
n. procedure
NeuroDrape surgical drape
neurodynia
neuroectoderm
neuroectodermal
n. tumor
n. tumor desmoplastic variant
n. tumor pale island
neuroectodermatosis
neuroectomy (*var. of* neurectomy)
neuroeffector
neuroelectricity
neuroembryology
neuroencephalomyelopathy
neuroendocrine
n. carcinoma (NEC)
n. disease
n. index
n. test
n. transducer
n. transducer cell
n. tumor localization study
neuroendocrinology
neuroendoscope
Neuroview n.
neuroendoscopic third ventriculostomy
neuroendoscopy
computer-assisted n.
neuroenteric cyst
neuroepithelial, neurepithelial
n. cell
n. cell migration
n. cell proliferation
n. cyst
n. layer
n. layer of retina
n. tumor
neuroepithelioma
neuroepithelium, neurepithelium
n. of ampullary crest
n. cristae ampullaris
n. of macula
neuroferritinopathy
neurofiber
afferent n.
association n.
autonomic n.
commissural n.
efferent n.
postganglionic n.
preganglionic n.
projection n.
somatic n.
tangential n.
visceral n.
neurofibra, pl. **neurofibrae**
n. associationis
neurofibrae autonomicae
n. commissuralis
neurofibrae efferentes
neurofibrae postganglionicae
neurofibrae preganglionicae
n. projectionis
neurofibrae somaticae
neurofibrae viscerales
neurofibrarum
stratum n.
neurofibril
neurofibrillar network
neurofibrillary
n. degeneration
n. lesion
n. tangle
n. tangle score
neurofibrillatory

neurofibroma
aryepiglottic fold n.
dumbbell n.
nonplexiform cutaneous n.
orbital n.
plexiform n.
solitary n.
spinal n.
neurofibromatosis (NF)
n.-1 (NF-1)
n.-2 (NF-2)
abortive n.
central-type n.
cutaneous n.
incomplete n.
n. kyphoscoliosis
kyphoscoliosis secondary to n.
peripheral n.
segmental n.
n. type 1, 2
von Recklinghausen n.
neurofibromin
neurofibrosarcoma
neurofilament expression
Neuroform stent
neurogangliitis
neuroganglion
neurogenesis
neurogenic, neurogenetic, neurogenous
n. arthropathy
n. atrophy
n. bladder
n. cardiac toxicity
n. claudication (NC)
n. disorder
n. dysphagia
n. fiber-type group
n. fracture
n. inflammation (NI)
n. lesion
n. motor evoked potential
n. orthostatic hypotension
n. process
n. pulmonary edema (NPE)
n. thoracic outlet syndrome
n. tonus
n. torticollis
n. ulcer
neurogerontology
neuroglia
n. cell
interfascicular n.
peripheral n.
neurogliacyte
neuroglial, neurogliar
n. fiber
neurogliocytoma
neurogliomatosis
neuroglycopenia
neurogram
neurography
magnetic resonance n. (MRN)
n. needle
Neuroguard transcranial Doppler
neurohemal system
neurohistology
neurohormonal
neurohormone
neurohypophysectomy
neurohypophyseos
infundibulum n.
lobus nervosus n.
pars nervosa n.
neurohypophysial nerve terminal
neurohypophysis
neural lobe of n.
neuroid
neuroimaging
n. approach
n. assessment
3-dimensional n.
functional n.
n. manifestation
postchemotherapy n.
postradiotherapy n.
structural n.
n. study
neuroimmunology
neuroimmunomodulatory
neurointensivist
neuroinvasion
neuroinvestigational system
neurokeratin
neurokinin
neurolathyrism
neurolemma (*var. of* neurilemma)
neuroleptanalgesia
neuroleptic
n. adjunct
n. bioavailability
conventional n.
n. dosage
n. dose

NOTES

neuroleptic *(continued)*
n. dosing
n. drug
n. exposure
high-potency n.
n. malignant syndrome (NMS)
n. medication
n. sensitivity
traditional n.
typical n.
neuroleptic-free patient
neuroleptic-induced
neuroleptic-naive patient
neurolinguist
neurolinguistic programming
neurolinguistics
NeuroLink II EEG data acquisition system
Neurolite
neurologic
n. ailment
n. company
n. complication
n. complication from cardiac disease
n. deterioration
n. diagnosis
n. disorder
n. dysregulation
n. emergency
n. evaluation
n. event
n. examination (NE)
n. feature
n. function
n. history
n. illness insomnia
n. improvement
n. injury
n. manifestation
n. migraine
n. plateau
n. prognosis
n. recovery
n. rehabilitation
n. sign
n. symptom
n. syndrome
neurological
n. deficit
n. hammer
n. illness
n. sequela
neurologic-ophthalmologic history
neurologist
neurology
American Board of Psychiatry and N. (ABPN)
clinical n.
environmental n.
geriatric n.
Kyoto Multi-Institutional Study Group Pediatric N.
psychiatry and n.
restorative n.
neurology/neurosurgery intensive care unit (NNICU)
neurolymph
neurolymphomatosis
neurolysis
alcohol n.
chemical n.
internal n.
intramuscular n.
intrathecal n.
phenol n.
trigeminal n.
neurolytic block
neuroma
acoustic n.
amputation n.
n. cutis
extracanalicular acoustic n.
extrapineal pinealoma false n.
facial n.
false n.
fibrillary n.
gasserian ganglion n.
incisional n.
Joplin n.
Morton n.
multiple n.'s
myelinic n.
nevoid n.
peripheral nerve n.
plexiform n.
posttraumatic n.
stump n.
n. telangiectodes
traumatic n.
trigeminal n.
true n.
Verneuil n.
neuromagnetic response
neuromagnetometer
whole-head n.
neuromalacia
NeuroMate robotic technology
neuromatosa
elephantiasis n.
neuromatosis
neuromechanism
neuromediator
Neuromed Octrode implantable device
Neuromeet nerve approximator
neuromeningeal
neuromere
neurometabolic disorder

Neurometer CPT/C for nerve evaluation
neuromodulation
n. of sleep
n. of wakefulness
neuromodulator
neuromonitoring
intraoperative n.
neuromuscular
n. atrophy
n. attachment
n. blockade
n. blocking agent
n. condition
n. electrical stimulation
n. junction
n. junction disease
n. junction disorder
n. junction transmission
n. scoliosis
n. scoliosis orthotic treatment
n. spindle (NMS)
neuromusculoskeletal syndrome
neuromyasthenia
epidemic n.
neuromyelitis optica
neuromyopathy
carcinomatous n.
neuromyositis
neuromyotonia
neuromyotonic discharge
neuron, neurone
aberrant n.
abnormal epileptic n.
afferent n.
alpha motor n.
apoptotic nigral n.
aspiny n.
autonomic motor n.
bipolar n.
brainstem n.
burst n.
Cajal-Retzius n.
canonical n.
central respiratory n.
cerebellar granule n.
cholinergic n.
cold-sensitive n.
cortical pyramidal n.
corticobulbar motor n.
corticospinal motor n.
dopaminergic n.
dorsal horn n.
dorsal spinocerebellar tract n.
dystrophic n.
ectopic n.
epileptic n.
excitatory pyramidal n.
fetal brain transitory n.
first-order n.
GABAergic n.
gamma motor n.
ganglionic motor n.
giant n.
glutamate-containing n.
glutamatergic n.
Golgi type I, II n.
granular n.
heterotropic n.
hippocampal pyramidal n.
histaminergic n.
hNT n.
hyperexcitable n.
hypocretin n.
impaired migration of brain n.
intercalary n.
internuncial n.
ischemic n.
itch-specific central n.
layer of piriform n.
Leydig n.
lower motor n. (LMN)
magnocellular n.
mesencephalic n.
monoaminergic n.
motor neuronal pool inhibitory n.
multipolar n.
noradrenergic n.
olfactory sensory n. (OSN)
orexin-containing n.
pedunculopontine n.
peripheral sensory n.
periventricular n.
phrenic motor n.
piriform n.
polymorphic n.
postganglionic motor n.
postsynaptic n.
preganglionic motor n.
premotor n.
presynaptic n.
primary afferent n.
primary sensory n.
projection n.
pseudounipolar n.

NOTES

neuron *(continued)*
Purkinje n.
pyramidal n.
redundant n.
sacral dorsal commissural n.
secondary sensory n.
second-order n.
sensory n.
somatomotor n.
somesthetic n.
spiny n.
stellate n.
striatal n.
taste-responsive n.
thalamic reticular n.
n. theory
n. threshold
unipolar n.
upper motor n. (UMN)
visceral motor n.
vomeronasal sensory n. (VSN)
warm-sensitive n.
neuronal
n. achromasia
n. activation
n. adhesion
n. aggregate
n. apoptosis inhibitory protein (NAIP)
n. cell apoptosis
n. cell death
n. ceroid lipofuscinosis (NCL)
n. ceroid lipofuscinosis curvilinear body
n. cytoplasm
n. damage
n. degeneration
n. differentiation
n. element firing
n. excitability
n. feedback loop
n. feed-forward loop
n. function
n. heterotopia
n. hyperexcitability
n. ingrowth
n. injury
n. lipidosis
n. loss
n. lysosomal storage disorder
n. mechanism
n. membrane
n. metabolism
n. migration
n. migration abnormality
n. migration disorder
n. morphology
n. NADPH-diaphorase/NOS expression
n. nitric oxide synthase (nNOS)
n. pathology
n. plasticity
n. precursor
n. process
n. proliferation disorder
n. pruning
n. regeneration
n. reuptake
n. shrinkage
n. signal
n. size
n. somata
n. specificity
n. spike activity
n. sprouting
n. stabilizing agent
n. structure
n. subpopulation
n. tumor
n. viability
neuronavigation
frameless and armless stereotactic n.
intracranial n.
neuronavigator
3-dimensional digitizer n.
neuronavigator-guided brain surgery
neurone (*var. of* neuron)
neuronitis
vestibular n.
neuronopathy
sensory n.
X-linked recessive bulbospinal n.
neuronophage
neuronophagia, neuronophagy
neuronotropic
neuron-specific
n.-s. cytoskeletal protein
n.-s. enolase (NSE)
Neurontin
neuronyxis
neurooncology
neuroophthalmic disorder
neuroophthalmology
neurootology
neuropacemaker
neuropapillitis
neuroparalysis
neuroparalytic
n. keratitis
n. ophthalmia
neuropath
neuropathic
n. arthritis
n. arthropathy
n. atrophy
n. hyperkyphoscoliosis
n. joint

n. pain
n. phenotype
neuropathogenesis
neuropathogenicity
neuropathological lesion profile
neuropathologic examination
neuropathology
Alzheimer disease n.
postmortem n.
neuropathy
acquired demyelinative n.
acromegalic n.
acrylamide peripheral n.
acute axonal motor n.
acute ischemic brachial n.
acute motor sensory axonal sensory n.
acute sensory motor axonal n.
AIDS n.
alcoholic peripheral n.
alcohol-induced peripheral n.
alkaloid n.
amyloid n.
amyloidosis peripheral n.
anterior ischemic optic n. (AION)
anterograde fast component n.
antiretroviral toxic n.
arsenic peripheral n.
asymmetric motor n.
n., ataxia, retinitis pigmentosa (NARP)
ataxic n.
auditory n.
autonomic n.
autosympathectomy secondary to n.
avitaminosis B_{12} peripheral n.
axonal distal n.
bacterial peripheral n.
barbiturate peripheral n.
Bassen-Kornzweig peripheral n.
botulism peripheral n.
brachial plexus n.
brucellosis peripheral n.
bulbar hereditary motor n.
B vitamin deficiency n.
carcinoma peripheral n.
carcinomatous n.
chronic hepatic failure peripheral n.
chronic inflammatory demyelinating sensorimotor n.
compression n.
compressive n.
congenital hypomyelination n.
congenital sensory n.
cranial n.
Cuban epidemic n.
dapsone n.
Dejerine-Sottas peripheral n.
demyelinating n.
Denny-Brown sensory radicular n.
diabetic lumbosacral radiculoplexus n. (DLRPN)
dinitrophenol peripheral n.
diphtheria peripheral n.
diphtheritic n.
distal symmetric axonal sensorimotor n.
dying-back n.
emetine peripheral n.
entrapment n.
ethyl alcohol peripheral n.
facial n.
familial amyloid n.
femoral n.
focal n.
giant axonal n.
glossopharyngeal n.
gold peripheral n.
griseofulvin peripheral n.
Guillain-Barré postinfection peripheral n.
handcuff n.
heavy metal n.
hepatic disease-associated n.
hereditary brachial plexus n.
hereditary hypertrophic n.
hereditary motor-sensory n. (HMSN)
hereditary radicular sensory n.
hereditary sensory n. (HSN)
hereditary sensory autonomic n., type 1–4 (HSAN-1–4)
hereditary sensory motor n. (HSMN)
hereditary sensory radicular n.
heritable n.
HIV-related n.
HIV-sensory n. (HIV-SN)
huffer's n.
hyperthyroid n.
hypertrophic interstitial n.
hypoglossal n.
hypoglycemic peripheral n.
hypothyroid n.

N

NOTES

neuropathy *(continued)*
idiopathic peripheral n.
IgM paraproteinemic n.
immune-mediated n.
infantile n.
infection-related n.
infectious hepatitis peripheral n.
inflammatory demyelinating n.
inherited n.
insecticide peripheral n.
ischemic anterior optic n.
ischemic posterior optic n.
isoniazid n.
isonicotinic acid peripheral n.
Jamaican n.
lead n.
Leber hereditary optic n.
leprosy peripheral n.
leprous n.
lotus n.
lupus erythematosus peripheral n.
Lyme n.
macrocryoglobulinemia peripheral n.
macroglobulinemia peripheral n.
malabsorption syndrome peripheral n.
measles peripheral n.
mercury peripheral n.
metachromatic leukodystrophy n.
metal n.
metal-produced n.
methyl alcohol peripheral n.
mitochondrial n.
mononucleosis peripheral n.
motor dapsone n.
multifocal motor n. (MFMN)
multiple myeloma peripheral n.
mumps peripheral n.
musculocutaneous n.
myeloma-associated n.
myxedema peripheral n.
nitrofurantoin n.
nonprogressive n.
nutritional n.
occupational n.
oculomotor n.
onion bulb n.
optic n.
pantothenic acid-deficiency peripheral n.
paraneoplastic n.
paraproteinemic n.
periaxial n.
peripheral n.
peroneal entrapment n.
phrenic n.
polyarteritis nodosa peripheral n.
porphyria peripheral n.
porphyric n.
postpartum obturator n.
pressure n.
progressive hypertrophic interstitial n.
pure sensory n.
radiation n.
radicular n.
Refsum peripheral n.
relapsing n.
retrograde fast component n.
rheumatoid n.
sacral plexus n.
sarcoid n.
sarcoidosis peripheral n.
segmental n.
senile n.
sensorimotor-autonomic n.
sensorimotor peripheral n.
sensory n.
serum sickness peripheral n.
Shy-Drager n.
slow component n.
small-fiber n. (SFN)
sprue peripheral n.
steroid-sensitive n.
subacute demyelinating n.
subclinical n.
sulfonamide peripheral n.
suprascapular n.
symmetrical diffuse n.
symmetric distal n.
Tangier peripheral n.
thalidomide n.
thallium peripheral n.
therapeutic agent-related n.
tomaculous n.
toxic n.
traumatic n.
tricresyl phosphate peripheral n.
trigeminal n.
triorthocresyl phosphate n.
tropical ataxic n. (TAN)
tuberculosis peripheral n.
typhoid peripheral n.
ulnar n.
uremia peripheral n.
uremic n.
vaccination peripheral n.
vagus n.
vasculitic n.
vestibulocochlear n.
vincristine peripheral n.
vitamin B12 n.
Wegener granulomatosis-associated n.
Whipple disease peripheral n.

neuropeptide
n. change
cortistatin n.

n. gene
plasma n. Y
n. Y (NPY)
neuropharmacology
functional n.
neurophilic
neurophysin
neurophysiological
n. monitoring
n. phenotypic factor
neurophysiologic evaluation
neurophysiology
neuropil, neuropile
n. thread
neuroplasm
neuroplasmic
neuroplasticity
neuroplastic response
neuroplasty
epidural n.
neuroplegic
neuroplexus
neuropodia
neuropodium
neuropore
anterior n.
caudal n.
posterior n.
rostral n.
NeuroProbe amplifier
neuroprogenitor cell
neuroprosthesis
neuroprotection
neuroprotective
n. effect
n. therapy
neuroprotein
neuropsychiatry
Schedules for Clinical Assessment in N.
neuropsychologic
n. area
n. characteristic
n. deficit
n. disorder
n. domain
n. functioning
n. measure
n. performance
n. test
n. testing
neuropsychological
n. assessment
n. profile
n. test battery
neuropsychologically relevant task
neuropsychology
clinical n.
cognitive n.
neuroradiology
interventional n.
pediatric n.
therapeutic n.
neuroreceptor imaging
neurorecidive
neurorecurrence
neuroregeneration
neuroregulator
neurorehabilitation
neurorelapse
neuroretinal angiomatosis
neuroretinitis
neurorrhaphy
epineurial n.
neurosarcocleisis
neurosarcoidosis
meningeal n.
neurosarcoma
Neuro-Sat frameless isocentric stereotactic system
neuroschisis
neuroschwannoma
neuroscience
behavioral n.
cognitive n.
psychotherapeutic n.
neuroscientist
clinical n.
neurosecretion
neurosecretory
n. cell
n. substance
neurosegmental level
neurosensory
neuroses (*pl. of* neurosis)
neuroshunting
Neurosign 100 constant current stimulator
neurosis, pl. **neuroses**
accident n.
acute posttraumatic n.
hypochondriac n.
impulse n.

N

NOTES

neurosis *(continued)*
obsessional n.
postconcussion n.
posttraumatic n.
situation n.
situational n.
n. tarda
torsion n.
traumatic n.
neuroskeletal
neurosome
neurosonology
neurospasm
neurosplanchnic
neurospongioma
neurospongium
Neurostat-Mark
Westco N.-M. II
neurostatus
neurosteroid
neurostimulation therapy
neurostimulator
Medtronic Itrel II n.
Medtronic Xtrel n.
Synergy Versitrel n.
neurosurgeon
AANS/CNS Joint Committee of Military N.'s
The American Society of Pediatric N.'s
neurosurgery
functional n.
image n.
microscopic n.
military n.
molecular n.
stereotactic n.
neurosurgical
n. intervention
n. needle holder
n. procedure
n. stereotactic robot
neurosuture
neurosyphilis
asymptomatic n.
cerebrovascular n.
congenital n.
meningeal n.
meningitic n.
meningovascular n.
ophthalmic n.
parenchymatous n.
paretic n.
tabetic n.
neurotabes
Dejerine peripheral n.
neurotaxis
neurotendinous
n. organ
n. spindle
neurotensin
neuroterminal
neurothekeoma
neurothele
neurotherapeutics
neurotherapy
neurothlipsia, neurothlipsis
neurotic
n. anxiety state
n. depressive state
n. factor
n. manifestation
neurotica
alopecia n.
neuroticism
neurotization
neurotize
neurotmesis
neurotology
neurotome
neurotomy
radiofrequency n.
retrogasserian n.
Spiller-Frazier n.
neurotonic congestion
neurotony
neurotoxic effect
neurotoxicity
additive n.
antibiotic n.
antihistamine n.
beta-lactam antibiotic n.
boric acid n.
codeine n.
dextroamphetamine n.
diphenoxylate n.
dopamine n.
dose-dependent n.
ferrous sulfate n.
FK506 n.
glutamate n.
hydroxyquinoline n.
imipramine n.
nitric oxide-mediated n.
piperazine n.
neurotoxin
botulinus n. (BTX)
dietary n.
neurotransmission
adrenergic n.
cholinergic n.
dopamine n.
dysregulated n.
glutamatergic n.
neurotransmitter
adrenergic n.

amino acid n.
excitatory n.
false n.
inhibitory n.
n. metabolic enzyme
n. release
n. of sleep
n. transporter
n. vessel docking
n. of wakefulness

neurotransplantation

neurotrauma

Neurotrend

N. continuous multiparameter system
N. sensor

neurotripsy

neurotrophic

n. atrophy
n. factor
n. factor expression
n. keratitis
n. ulcer

neurotrophin

neurotrophy

neurotropic

n. effect
n. virus

neurotropy, neurotropism

neurotrosis

neurotubule

neurovaricosis

neurovaricosity

neurovascular

n. conflict
n. flap
n. imaging
n. relationship
n. tree

NeuroVax

neurovegetative

Neuroview

N. integrated visualization system
N. neuroendoscope

neurovirology

neurovirulence

neurovirulent

neurovisceral

neuroviscerolipidosis

familial n.

neurturin

neurulation

defined n.
primary n.
secondary n.

neururgic

neutral

n. image
n. material
n. torso posture

neutralization

anterior n.

Neutra-Phos

Neutra-Phos-K

neutropenia

neutropenic

never-medicated patient

Nevin-Jones subacute spongiform encephalopathy

nevirapine

nevoid

n. amentia
n. basal cell carcinoma syndrome
n. neuroma

nevus alveolus inferior

new

n. memory
n. variant Creutzfeldt-Jakob disease
N. York Longitudinal Study
N. York University Parkinson Disease Scale

newborn

n. drug withdrawal
hemorrhagic disease of n.
n. REM
n. screening
n. sleep

Newcastle

N. classification
N. disease virus

newer generation device

newly emergent categorical change

Newman-Keuls test

new-onset seizure

Newport collar

newtonian body

NEXUS

National Emergency X-Radiograph Utilization Study

NF

neurofibromatosis

NOTES

NF-1
neurofibromatosis-1
NF-1 gene
NF-2
neurofibromatosis-2
NF-2 gene
NGF
nerve growth factor
NHL
non-Hodgkin lymphoma
NI
neurogenic inflammation
nicardipine prolonged-release implant
Nichrome cylindrical electrode
nickel-jacketed bullet
nicking
arteriovenous n.
Nicola
N. forceps
N. pituitary rongeur
N. rasp
N. scissors
Nicolet
N. Compass EMG instrument
N. Pathfinder I
N. Pathfinder I recording device
N. Viking II electrophysiologic system
nicotinamide adenine dinucleotide phosphate (NADPH)
nicotine-induced
n.-i. insomnia
n.-i. seizure
nicotine withdrawal
nicotinic acetylcholine receptor (nAChR)
nictitans
spasmus n.
nictitate
nictitating spasm
nictitation
nidulans
Aspergillus n.
nidus
n. avis
n. definition
n. hirundinis
n. obliteration
Niemann disease
Niemann-Pick disease (type A, B, C) (NPD)
nifedipine
nifurtimox
niger
Aspergillus n.
locus n.
nucleus n.
night
n. pain
n. palsy
n. terror
nightmare
vivid n.
nighttime
n. awakening
n. pain
nigra
fetal substantia n.
substantia n. (SN)
nigrae
pars compacta substantiae n.
pars reticularis substantiae n.
rami substantiae n.
nigral TH-positve cell
nigropallidal pathway
nigrostriatal
n. denervation
n. dopaminergic system
n. dopamine system
n. pathway
n. tract
nigrostriate
n. fiber
n. tract
nigrum
tapetum n.
NIHSS
National Institutes of Health Stroke Scale
Nijmegen breakage syndrome
nimodipine
Nimotop capsule
nimustine
NINCDS
National Institute of Neurological and Communicative Disorders and Stroke
NINDS
National Institute of Neurological Disorders and Stroke
Nine-Hole Peg Test
Nintendo epilepsy
ninth cranial nerve [CN IX]
niobium-titanium
Niopam
NIOSH
National Institute for Occupational Safety and Health
Nipah
N. virus
N. virus encephalitis
Nipride
NIR Royal Advanced stent
NIRS
near-infrared spectroscopy
Nishioka system
Nishizaki-Wakabayashi suction tube
Nissl
N. body
N. degeneration

N. granule
N. substance
Nitoman
nitrate
butyl n.
gallium n.
nitrazepam
nitrazepam-induced hypotonia
nitric
n. acid
n. oxide
n. oxide-mediated neurotoxicity
n. oxide synthase (NOS)
nitrite
amyl n.
n. headache
nitrocellulose membrane
nitrofurantoin
n. neuropathy
n. polyneuropathy
nitrogen
blood urea n. (BUN)
n. metabolism
n. narcosis
n. wasting
nitroprusside
sodium n. (SNP)
nitrosoglutathione (GSNO)
nitrosourea hydrochloride
nitrous oxide
NK
natural killer
nkx gene
NMDA
N-methyl-D-aspartate
NMDA antagonist ketamine
NMDA receptor
NMDA receptor antagonist
***N*-methylspiroperidol**
NMHA
National Mental Health Association
NMR
nuclear magnetic resonance
NMS
neuroleptic malignant syndrome
neuromuscular spindle
NMSS
National Multiple Sclerosis Society
NNICU
neurology/neurosurgery intensive care unit
nNOS
neuronal nitric oxide synthase
N1, N2 receptor
Nocardia
N. asteroides
N. farcinica
N. nova
nocardial brain abscess
nocardiosis
central nervous system n.
cerebral n.
CNS n.
nociception
nociceptive
n. C fiber
n. impulse
n. pain
n. reflex
n. stimulation
nociceptor
n. activation
angry backfiring C n.
C-fiber n.
cutaneous n.
irritable n.
mechanical n.
polymodal n.
primary afferent n.
nocifensor reflex
nocturna
chorea n.
nocturnal
n. agitation
n. angina
n. awakening
n. cardiac ischemia
n. confusion
n. confusional episode
n. dyspnea
n. eating syndrome
n. event
n. frontal lobe epilepsy
n. groaning
n. hallucination
n. hypotensive episode
n. hypoxemia
n. insomnia
n. leg cramp
n. leg jerk
n. melatonin level
n. myoclonus
n. oxygen saturation

NOTES

nocturnal *(continued)*
n. pain
n. paroxysmal dystonia
n. paroxysmal wandering
n. polysomnography
n. primary enuresis
n. reflux
n. restlessness
n. seizure
n. sleep
n. sleep disturbance
n. spell
n. stridor
n. vertigo
n. vocalization
nocturnes
pavor n.
nodding spasm
node
accessory nerve lymph n.
Babès n.
flocculonodular n.
Hensen n.
hilar lymph n.
jugular chain lymph n.
local lymph n.
primitive n.
Ranvier n.
n. of Ranvier
Schmorl n.
vital n.
nodosa
periarteritis n.
polyarteritis n.
trichorrhexis n.
nodose ganglion
nodular
n. enhancement
n. headache
n. heterotopia
n. induration of temporal artery
n. mesoneuritis
n. panencephalitis
nodule
Babès n.
glial n.
iris Lisch n.
Lisch n.
mulberry-like n.
mural n.
Schmorl n.
subcutaneous n.
n. of vermis
nodulus, pl. **noduli**
n. cerebelli
vermal n.
n. vermis
noggin gene
NO-induced DNA degradation
noise
acoustic n.
n. condition
diagnostic n.
gaussian n.
multispeaker phonetic n.
phonetic n.
noise-reduction device
Nolvadex
Nomad-LE EMG
nominal
n. aphasia
n. standard dose
nonaccidental trauma
nonacoustic schwannoma
nonadapting receptor
Nonaka distal myopathy
non-Alzheimer frontal lobe-type dementia
nonamphetamine
central nervous system stimulant, n.
nonanaplastic oligodendroglioma
nonaneurysmal perimesencephalic subarachnoid hemorrhage
nonaplastic glioma
nonapneic sleep disorder
nonaxial anisotropy
nonbiological artifact
noncerebral activity
nonchromaffin paraganglioma
noncleft median face syndrome
noncoherent model
noncommunicating hydrocephalus
noncontained disc
nonconvulsive
n. seizure
n. status epilepticus
nondampened waveform
nondecalcified trabecula
nondeclarative memory
nondepolarizing
nondepressed skull fracture
nondetachable
n. endovascular balloon
n. occlusive balloon
n. silicone balloon catheter
nondominant
hand n.
n. hemisphere
n. hemisphere dysfunction
n. hemisphere function
n. hemisphere lesion
n. putaminal hemorrhage
n. temporal lobectomy
non-Duchenne smile
nondystrophin myopathy
noneloquent area
nonembolic infarction

nonencapsulated
n. nerve ending
n. nerve glomerulus
nonenteric cyst
nonentrained sleep-wake disorder
nonepileptic
n. event
n. myoclonic contraction
n. myoclonus
n. seizure
nonepileptiform activity
nonferromagnetic clip
nonferrous material
nonfluent aphasia
nonfocal elevation
non-fragilis
Bacteroides n.-f.
nonfunctional and repetitive motor behavior
nonfunctioning adenoma
nonfused spine
nongenetic chorea
nongerminoma malignant germ cell tumor
nongiant aneurysm
nonhemolytic hyperbilirubinemia
non-Hodgkin lymphoma (NHL)
nonhomonymous field defect
non-24-hour
n.-24-h. sleep phase syndrome
n.-24-h. sleep-wake disorder
noninfectious meningitis
noninvasive
n. brain imaging study
n. carotid baroceptor stimulation
n. imaging technique
n. positive pressure ventilation
nonionic contrast agent
nonketotic
n. glycine
n. hyperglycemia
n. hyperglycemic hyperosmolar coma
n. hyperglycinemia
nonlacunar syndrome
nonlanguage cognitive impairment
nonlesional cortical resection
nonlinear
n. developmental curve
n. rate-response function
nonmedullated fiber
nonmeningiomatous malignant lesion
nonmicrosurgical procedure
nonmigrainous vascular headache
nonmyelinated nerve
nonneoplastic disease
nonneural cell
nonneuropathic pain
nonolfactory cortex
nonoperative strategy
nonorganic aphonia
nonparalytic poliomyelitis
nonparetic eye valid reaction time
nonpathological dissociation
nonpenetrating trauma
nonphantom study
nonpharmacologic behavior management
nonphysiologic artifact
nonplexiform cutaneous neurofibroma
nonprogressive
n. myoclonus condition
n. neuropathy
nonproton
n. magnetic resonance imaging
n. MRI
nonpsychotic
n. Alzheimer patient
n. hallucination
n. posttraumatic brain syndrome
n. severity psychoorganic syndrome
nonpulsating headache
nonrandom rating
nonrapid
n. eye movement (NREM)
n. eye movement sleep
nonreference recording
non-REM
n.-REM narcolepsy
n.-REM sleep
nonresectable tumor
nonrheumatic atrial fibrillation
nonselective expression of transgene
nonsense mutation
nonseptic embolic brain infarction
nonshivering thermogenesis
nonsignificant protective effect
nonspastic paraparesis
nonspecific
n. encephalomyeloneuropathy
n. neck pain
n. neuronal loss
n. neurotic factor
n. response rate
n. slow potential

N

NOTES

nonspecific *(continued)*
n. stimulation
n. system
nonstereotactic PET
nonsynaptic transmission
nontoxic gene expression
nontraumatic subarachnoid hemorrhage
nonturbulence subscale
nontyphoidal salmonellosis
nonunion
n. incidence
n. rate
sacral n.
nonvasculitic autoimmune inflammatory meningoencephalitis
nonverbal
n. abstractive ability
n. communication
n. cue
n. memory
n. synthesizing ability
n. tactile attention task
nonviral infectious disease
Noonan syndrome
noradrenergic
n. effect
n. neuron
n. system function
Norcuron
Nordstadt classification
no-reflow phenomenon
norepinephrine
peripheral n.
n. toxicity
Norland digital oscilloscope
normal
n. cell
n. circuitry
n. electroencephalogram (NEEG)
n. heat defense
n. human physiology
n. mode
n. perfusion pressure breakthrough (NPPB)
n. resting potential
n. sleep
n. sleep cycle
n. thermogenesis
normal-frequency band
normalization principle
normalized whole brain volume
normal-pressure hydrocephalus (NPH)
Norman-Roberts syndrome
Norman-Wood syndrome
normative aspect
normocapnia
normokalemic periodic paralysis
normotensive hydrocephalus
normotonic
normoxic diffusion
Norpace
Norpramin
Norrie disease
North
N. American Brain Tumor Consortium (NABTC)
N. American Spine Society questionnaire
N. American Symptomatic Carotid Endarterectomy Trial (NASCET)
Northern
N. blot analysis
N. epilepsy with mental retardation
N. hybridization
N. Manhattan Stroke Study
Northwick Park Index of Independence in ADL index
nortriptyline HCl
NOS
nitric oxide synthase
NOS inhibitor
nose-bridge-lid reflex
nosecone
nose-eye reflex
nose spray test
nosocomial infection
nosotropic
notanencephalia
notch
anterior cerebellar n.
n. filter
n. gene
Kernohan n.
mamilloaccessory n.
marsupial n.
posterior cerebellar n.
preoccipital n.
semilunar n.
n. of tentorium
notch3 mutation
notched appearance of spike-wave discharge
notencephalocele
Nothnagel syndrome
notochord
notochordoma
Nottingham Health Profile
nova
Nocardia n.
Novalis shaped beam surgery
Novantrone
NovaVision VRT
novel
n. memory task
n. recall task
n. stimulus
n. task performance

novo
de n.
Novo-10a CBF measuring device
Novus
N. hydrocephalic valve
N. mini valve
noxious agent
NPD
Niemann-Pick disease (type A, B, C)
NPE
neurogenic pulmonary edema
NPH
normal-pressure hydrocephalus
NPH grading
NPH recovery rate
NPPB
normal perfusion pressure breakthrough
NPS
NeuroCybernetic Prosthesis System
NPY
neuropeptide Y
NREM
nonrapid eye movement
NSE
National Society for Epilepsy
neuron-specific enolase
NSN
National Spine Network
NT2 cell
NTD
neural tube defect
N-terminal
N-t. domain
N-t. signal
N-terminus
NTSA
National Tuberous Sclerosis Association
nuchal
n. dystonia
n. muscle
n. rigidity
nuchocephalic reflex
nuclear
n. agenesis
n. aggregate
n. aplasia
n. architecture
n. bag
n. bag fiber
n. cerebral angiography (NCA)
n. chain
n. chain fiber
n. depression
n. envelope
n. envelope protein
n. fragility
n. imaging
n. jaundice
n. layer of cerebellum
n. layer of retina
n. magnetic relaxation dispersion
n. magnetic resonance (NMR)
n. magnetization vector
n. MR scan
n. ophthalmoplegia
n. pore
n. pseudoinclusion
n. receptor
n. relaxation
n. shape
n. signal
n. spin
n. spin quantum number
n. surface
nuclei (*pl. of* nucleus)
nucleic acid metabolism
nucleocortical fiber
nucleofugal
nucleolus
nucleolysis
percutaneous laser n.
nucleon
nucleopetal
nucleoplasmic structure
nucleoplasty
nucleoside adenosine
nucleotide
guanine n.
Nucleotome
N. aspiration probe
N. Flex II flexible cutting probe
N. procedure
nucleotomy
laser n.
nucleus, pl. **nuclei**
abducens n.
n. of abducent nerve
n. accessorii nevi oculomotorii
n. accessorii tractus optici
n. accessorius columnae anterioris medullae spinalis
accessory basal amygdaloid n.
accessory cuneate n.
n. of accessory nerve

N

NOTES

nucleus *(continued)*
accessory oculomotor n.
accessory olivary n.
n. accumbens
n. accumbens septi
acoustic n.
n. of acoustic nerve
n. acusticus
aerosolized droplet n.
n. alae cinereae
almond n.
ambiguous n.
n. ambiguus
n. amygdalae
n. amygdalae basalis medialis
n. amygdalae centralis
n. amygdalae corticalis
n. amygdalae interstitialis
n. amygdalae lateralis
amygdaloid n.
n. ansae lenticularis
n. of ansa lenticularis
n. anterior corporis trapezoidei
n. anteriores thalami
anterior extremity of caudate n.
n. anterior hypothalami
anterior hypothalamic n.
anterior interpositus n.
anterior olfactory n.
anterior periventricular n.
n. anterodorsalis
n. anterodorsalis thalami
anterodorsal thalamic n.
n. anteroinferior thalami
n. anterolateralis
n. anterolateralis medullae spinalis
n. anteromedialis
n. anteromedialis nervi oculomotorii
n. anteromedialis thalami
anteromedial thalamic n.
n. anterosuperior thalami
n. anteroventralis
n. anteroventralis thalami
anteroventral thalamic n.
arcuate n.
n. arcuatus
n. arcuatus hypothalami
n. arcuatus of intermediate hypothalamic area
n. arcuatus of medulla oblongata
n. arcuatus thalami
n. areae H, H1, H2
auditory n.
autonomic oculomotor n.
autonomic visceral motor n.
basal n.
n. basales
n. basalis of Ganser
n. basalis lesion
n. basalis of Meynert
basolateral amygdaloid n.
basomedial amygdaloid n.
Bechterew n.
Blumenau n.
body of caudate n.
brain n.
branchiomotor n.
bulbar n.
Burdach n.
n. of Cajal
n. campi dorsalis
n. campi medialis
n. campi ventralis
n. camporum perizonalium
catecholaminergic n.
n. of caudal colliculus
n. caudalis centralis
n. caudalis-nucleus solitarius DREZ lesioning
caudal olivary n.
caudal pontine reticular n.
caudate n.
n. caudatus
central amygdaloid n.
central caudate n.
n. centralis lateralis
n. centralis lateralis thalami
n. centralis medialis thalami
n. centralis medullae spinalis
n. centralis superior raphes
n. centralis tegmenti superior
centromedian thalamic n.
n. centromedianus
n. centromedianus thalami
cerebellar n.
n. cerebellares
n. cerebelli
cervical n.
n. cervicalis lateralis
Clarke n.
cochlear n.
n. cochleares
n. cochlearis anterior
n. cochlearis posterior
n. coeruleus
n. colliculi caudalis
n. colliculi inferioris
n. commissurae posterioris
n. commissuralis nevi vagus
n. commissuralis rhomboidalis
n. corporis geniculati medialis
n. corporis geniculati medialis
n. corporis mamillaris
n. corporis mammillaris lateralis
n. corporis mammillaris medialis
cortical amygdaloid n.
cranial motor n.
n. of cranial nerve

cranial olivary n.
cuneate n.
n. of cuneate fasciculus
n. cuneatus
n. cuneatus accessorius
n. cuneatus pars centralis
n. cuneatus pars rostralis
n. cuneatus tubercle
cuneiform n.
n. cuneiformis
n. cuneiformis mesencephalicus
n. of Darkschewitsch
deep n.
deep cerebellar n.
Deiters n.
dentate n.
n. dentatus
n. dentatus cerebelli
depigmentation of noradrenergic brainstem n.
dorsal accessory olivary n.
dorsal cochlear n.
n. dorsales thalami
n. of dorsal field
n. dorsalis of Clarke
n. dorsalis corporis geniculati lateralis
n. dorsalis corporis geniculati medialis
n. dorsalis corporis trapezoidei
n. dorsalis hypothalami
n. dorsalis lateralis thalami
n. dorsalis nervi oculomotorii
n. dorsalis nervi vagus
n. dorsalis raphe
dorsal lateral geniculate n.
dorsal premammillary n.
dorsal raphe n.
dorsal septal n.
dorsal thoracic n.
dorsal vagal n.
dorsolateral caudate n.
n. dorsolateralis medullae spinalis
dorsomedial hypothalamic n.
n. dorsomedialis hypothalami
n. dorsomedialis hypothalamicae intermediae
n. dorsomedialis medullae spinalis
Edinger n.
Edinger-Westphal n.
electrical stimulation of centromedian thalamic n.
emboliform n.
n. emboliformis
endolemniscal n.
n. endolemniscalis
endopeduncular n.
n. endopeduncularis
external cuneate n.
extrajunctional n.
extrapyramidal n.
facial n.
facial motor n.
n. fasciculi gracilis
fastigial n.
n. fastigii
n. fibrosus lingua
filiform n.
n. filiformis
force n.
n. funiculi cuneati
n. funiculi gracilis
n. gelatinosus
gelatinous n.
geniculate n.
n. geniculati mediales
geniculatus lateralis n.
n. geniculatus lateralis
n. gigantocellularis medullae oblongatae
globose n.
n. globosus
n. of Goll
Goll column n.
gracile n.
n. gracilis tubercle
Gudden tegmental n.
gustatory n.
n. habenula
n. habenulae
habenular n.
n. habenularis lateralis
n. habenularis medialis
head of caudate n.
hilum of dentate n.
hilum of inferior olivary n.
hilum of olivary n.
hypoglossal n.
n. hypoglossalis
n. of hypoglossal nerve
hypothalamic n.
n. hypothalamicus anterior
n. hypothalamicus dorsalis
n. hypothalamicus dorsomedialis

NOTES

N

nucleus *(continued)*
n. hypothalamicus posterior
n. hypothalamicus ventrolateralis
n. hypothalamicus ventromedialis
n. of inferior colliculus
n. inferior nervi trigeminalis
inferior olivary n.
inferior salivary n.
inferior syndrome of red n.
inferior vestibular n.
n. infundibularis
intercalated n.
n. intercalatus
intercostal nerve n.
intermediolateral n.
n. intermediolateralis
intermediomedial n.
n. intermediomedialis
n. intermediomedialis medullae spinalis
interpeduncular n.
n. interpeduncularis
interposed n.
n. interpositus
n. interpositus anterior
n. interpositus posterior
interstitial amygdaloid n.
n. interstitiales fasciculi longitudinalis medialis
n. interstitiales hypothalami anterioris
intracerebellar n.
intralaminar n.
n. intralaminares thalami
ipsilateral fastigial n.
Kölliker-Fuse n.
lateral amygdaloid n.
lateral cervical n.
lateral cuneate n.
lateral dorsal tegmentum n.
lateral geniculate n. (LGN)
n. of lateral geniculate body
lateral habenular n.
n. lateralis cerebelli
n. lateralis corporis trapezoidei
n. lateralis dorsalis thalami
n. lateralis medullae oblongatae
n. lateralis posterior
n. of lateral lemniscus
lateral medullary lamina of lentiform n.
n. of lateral olfactory stria
n. of lateral olfactory tract
lateral parabrachial n.
lateral pericuneate n.
lateral posterior n.
lateral preoptic n.
lateral pulvinar n.
lateral reticular n.
lateral septal n.
lateral superior olivary n.
lateral tuberal n.
lateral vestibular n.
n. lemnisci lateralis
n. lemnisci lateralis
n. of lens
lenticular n.
lentiform n.
n. lentiformis
n. lentis
linear n.
n. linearis inferioris
n. linearis intermedius
n. linearis superior
n. of Luys
magnocellular reticular n.
magnus raphe n.
main cuneate n.
n. mamillaris medialis
n. of mamillary body
n. masticatorius
masticatory n.
medial accessory olivary n.
medial amygdaloid n.
n. mediales thalami
n. of medial field
medial geniculate n. (MGN)
n. of medial geniculate body
medial habenular n.
n. medialis centralis thalami
n. medialis cerebelli
n. medialis corporis trapezoidei
n. medialis magnocellularis
n. medialis magnocellularis corporis geniculati
medial magnocellular n.
medial medullary lamina of lentiform n.
medial parabrachial n.
medial pericuneate n.
medial preoptic n.
medial septal n.
medial superior olivary n.
medial terminal n. (MTN)
medial ventral n.
medial vestibular n.
median preoptic n.
median raphe n.
mediodorsal n.
n. mediodorsalis
n. medioventralis
medullary raphe n.
mesencephalic n.
n. mesencephalicus nervi trigemini
n. mesencephalicus trigeminalis
Monakow n.
motor n.
n. motorius nervi trigemini

n. motorius trigeminalis
N. 24 multichannel auditory brainstem implant
n. nervi abducentis
n. nervi cochlearis
n. nervi cranialis
n. nervi facialis
n. nervi glossopharyngei
n. nervi hypoglossi
n. nervi phrenici
n. nervi pudendi
n. nervi trigeminalis
n. nervi trigemini
n. nervi trochlearis
n. nervi vagus
n. nervi vestibulocochlearis
n. nervorum cranialium
n. niger
oculomotor n.
n. oculomotorii accessorii
n. oculomotorii autonomici
n. oculomotorius
n. of oculomotor nerve
n. olfactorius anterior
n. olivares inferiores
n. olivaris
n. olivaris accessorius dorsalis
n. olivaris accessorius medialis
n. olivaris accessorius posterior
n. olivaris cranialis
n. olivaris inferior
n. olivaris principalis
n. olivaris rostralis
n. olivaris superior
n. olivaris superior lateralis
n. olivaris superior medialis
olivary n.
Onuf n.
Onufrowicz n.
oral pontine reticular n.
n. of origin
n. originis
oval hyperchromatic n.
pallidal raphe n.
n. pallidus raphes
parabigeminal n.
n. parabigeminalis
parabrachial n.
n. parabrachiales
n. parabrachialis lateralis
n. parabrachialis medialis
n. paracentralis thalami
parafascicular n.
n. parafascicularis thalami
n. paragigantocellular lateralis
paralemniscal n.
n. paralemniscalis
paramedial reticular n.
paramedian n.
n. paramedianus dorsalis
n. paramedianus posterior
paranigral n.
n. paranigralis
parapeduncular n.
n. parapeduncularis
n. parasympathici sacrales
paraventricular n.
n. paraventriculares thalami
n. paraventricularis hypothalami
pars magnocellularis n.
pedunculopontine tegmental n.
n. pericuneatus lateralis
n. pericuneatus medialis
perifornical n.
n. perifornicalis
perihypoglossal n.
n. periolivares
periolivary n.
peripeduncular n.
n. peripeduncularis
peritrigeminal n.
n. peritrigeminalis
n. periventricularis posterior
n. periventricularis ventralis
periventricular preoptic n.
n. of perizonal field
Perlia n.
phrenic motor n.
n. of phrenic nerve
n. phrenicus columnae anterioris medullae spinalis
pontine raphe n.
pontine reticular n.
n. pontis raphes
pontobulbar n.
n. pontobulbaris
postbulbar motor n.
posterior accessory olivary n.
n. of posterior commissure
n. posteriores thalami
n. posterior hypothalami
posterior hypothalamic n.
posterior interpositus n.
n. posterior nervi vagus

N

NOTES

nucleus *(continued)*
posterior periventricular n.
posterior raphe n.
n. posterior raphes
posterior thoracic n.
posterolateral n.
n. posterolateralis medullae spinalis
posteromedial n.
n. posteromedialis medullae spinales
precommissural septal n.
pregeniculate n.
n. premammillaris dorsalis
n. premammillaris ventralis
preoptic n.
n. preopticus lateralis
n. preopticus medialis
n. preopticus medianus
n. preopticus periventricularis
n. prepositus hypoglossi
prerubral n.
n. of prerubral field
pretectal n.
n. pretectales
n. principalis nervi trigemini
principal olivary n.
n. proprius
prosthetic disc n. (PDN)
n. of pudendal nerve
n. pulposus
n. pulposus disci intervertebralis
pulvinar n.
n. pulvinares
n. pulvinares thalami
pyknotic n.
n. pyramidalis
raphe n.
n. raphe obscurus
n. raphes magnus
n. raphes medianus
n. raphes pallidus
n. raphes pontis
n. raphes posterior
red n.
reticular n.
n. reticulares medullae oblongatae
n. reticulares mesencephali
n. reticulares pontis
n. reticulares raphes
n. reticularis intermedius gigantocellularis
n. reticularis intermedius medullae oblongatae
n. reticularis intermedius pontis inferioris
n. reticularis intermedius pontis superioris
n. reticularis lateralis medullae oblongatae
n. reticularis magnocellularis
n. reticularis paragigantocellularis
n. reticularis paramedianus
n. reticularis parvocellularis
n. reticularis pontis caudalis
n. reticularis pontis oralis
n. reticularis pontis rostralis
n. reticularis tegmenti pontis
n. reticularis thalami
n. reticularis trigeminalis pedunculopontinus
n. reticulatus thalami
reticulotegmental n.
n. retroambiguus
retrodorsal n.
retrofacial n.
retroposterior lateral n.
retroposterolateralis n.
n. retroposterolateralis medulla spinalis
n. reuniens
rhombencephalic gustatory n.
rhomboid n.
n. robustus archistriatalis
Roller n.
roof n.
rostral interstitial n.
rostral olivary n.
n. ruber
sacral dorsal commissural n. (SDCN)
sacral parasympathetic n.
n. saguli
sagulum n.
n. salivarius inferior
n. salivarius superior
salivary n.
n. salivatorius inferior
n. salivatorius superior
Schwalbe n.
Schwann n.
secondary sensory n.
n. semilunaris
n. sensorius inferior nervi trigeminalis
n. sensorius principalis nervi trigemini
n. sensorius superior nervi trigemini
sensory n.
septal n.
n. septalis lateralis
n. septalis medialis
n. septalis precommissuralis
septofimbrial n.
Siemerling n.
sole n.
n. solitarii
n. solitarius
n. of solitary tract

somatomotor n.
somesthetic relay n.
special visceral efferent n.
special visceral motor n.
spherical n.
n. spinalis nervi accessorii
n. spinalis nervi trigemini
spinal trigeminal n.
Spitzka n.
Staderini n.
Stilling n.
n. striae terminalis
striate n.
subcaeruleus n.
n. subcoeruleus
subcortical limbic n.
subcuneiform n.
n. subcuneiformis
subhypoglossal n.
n. subhypoglossalis
sublingual n.
subparabrachial n.
n. subparabrachialis
subthalamic n. (STN)
n. subthalamicus
superior central raphe n.
superior central tegmental n.
superior olivary n.
superior salivary n.
superior salivatory n.
superior vestibular n.
suprachiasmatic n.
n. suprachiasmaticus
supralemniscal n.
n. supralemniscalis
n. supramammillaris
supramammillary n.
supraoptic n.
n. supraopticus
n. supraopticus hypothalami
tail of caudate n.
tectal n.
n. tecti
n. tegmentales anteriores
n. tegmentalis pedunculopontinus
n. tegmentalis posterolateralis
tegmental pedunculopontine reticular n.
n. tegmenti
n. tegmenti pontis caudalis
n. tegmenti pontis oralis
terminal n.
n. terminales
n. terminationis
n. terminationis
thalamic gustatory n.
thoracic n.
n. thoracicus
n. thoracicus dorsalis
n. thoracicus posterior
n. tractus mesencephalici nervi trigeminalis
n. tractus mesencephali nervi trigemini
n. tractus olfactorii lateralis
n. tractus spinalis nervi trigemini
n. of trapezoid body
triangular n.
n. triangularis
n. triangularis septi
triangular septal n.
trigeminal mesencephalic n.
trigeminal motor n.
n. of trigeminal nerve
trochlear n.
n. of trochlear nerve
tuberal n.
n. tuberales
n. tuberales laterales
tubercle of cuneate n.
n. tuberomammillaris
tuberomammillary n.
n. vagalis dorsalis
n. of vagus nerve
vein of caudate n.
ventral anterior n.
n. ventrales laterales thalami
n. ventrales mediales thalami
n. ventrales thalami
n. of ventral field
ventral intermediate n. (VIM)
ventral intermediate thalamic n.
n. ventralis anterior
n. ventralis anterior thalami
n. ventralis corporis geniculi lateralis
n. ventralis corporis trapezoidei
n. ventralis intermedius
n. ventralis intermedius thalami
n. ventralis lateralis
n. ventralis posterior intermedius thalami
n. ventralis posterior thalami
n. ventralis posterolateralis

NOTES

nucleus *(continued)*
n. ventralis posterolateralis thalami
n. ventralis posteromedialis
n. ventralis posteromedialis thalami
ventral lateral geniculate n.
ventral posterior n.
ventral posteroinferior n.
ventral posterolateral n.
ventral posteromedial n.
ventral premammillary n.
ventral principal n.
ventral tier thalamic n.
ventrobasal n.
n. ventrobasales
ventrocaudal n.
n. ventrolateralis hypothalami
n. ventrolateralis medullae spinalis
ventromedial hypothalamic n.
n. ventromedialis hypothalami
n. ventromedialis medullae spinalis
vestibular n.
n. vestibulares
n. vestibularis caudalis
n. vestibularis inferior
n. vestibularis lateralis
n. vestibularis medialis
n. vestibularis rostralis
n. vestibularis superior
vestibulocochlear n.
n. viscerales nervi oculomotorii
Voit n.
VPI n.
VPL n.
Westphal n.
null
n. cell adenoma
n. condition detection threshold
n. gene
nulling
gradient moment n.
null-position nystagmus
numb
n. cheek syndrome
n. chin syndrome
n. gene
number
dissociation of n.'s
n. of excitation
nuclear spin quantum n.
quantum n.
Reynolds n.
wave n.
number-recency measure
numbing symptom
numbness
emotional n.
facial n.
periodic hemilingual n.
sudden n.
waking n.
Nurick score
Nurolon suture
Nurrl protein
nursing home placement
nut alignment guide
nutans
chorea n.
epilepsia n.
head nodding in spasmus n.
spasmus n.
nutation
nutraceutical
n. data
n. product
nutrient vessel
nutrition
parenteral n.
n. risk
total parenteral n. (TPN)
nutritional
n. change
n. neuropathy
n. polyneuropathy
n. status
nutritional-type cerebellar atrophy
nyctalgia
Nymox urinary test
Nyquist
N. frequency
N. sampling criteria
Nyssen-van Bogaert syndrome
nystagmoid jerk
nystagmus
abduction n.
acquired n.
alternating n.
apogeotropic n.
asymmetric optokinetic n.
bow-tie n.
Bruns n.
caloric n.
central n.
cerebellar n.
circular n.
coarse n.
congenital n.
conjugate n.
contralateral monocular n.
convergence-evoked n.
convergence-retraction n.
diagonal n.
dissociated n.
downbeat n.
down-moving optokinetic n.
drug-induced n.
dysjunctive n.
elliptical n.

end-gaze physiologic n.
end-point n.
n. examination
fine rapid n.
first-degree n.
fixation n.
gaze-evoked n.
gaze-paretic n.
horizontal pendular n.
irregular n.
jelly n.
jerky seesaw n.
lateral gaze n.
left-bearing n.
lid n.
miner's n.
muscle-paretic n.
null-position n.
oblique n.
ocular bobbing n.
ocular dysmetria n.
ocular flutter n.
oculomasticatory myorhythmia n.
opsoclonus n.
optokinetic n. (OKN)
palatal n.
paretic n.
paroxysmal positional n.
party n.
pendular n.
periodic alternating n. (PAN)
peripheral n.
phasic n.
positional n.
postrotational n.
railway n.
rapid n.
rebound n.
refractory convergence n.
resilient n.
retraction n.
retraction-convergence n.
n. retractorius
reversed optokinetic n.
right-bearing n.
rotary n.
rotatory n.
second-degree n.
seesaw n. (SSN)
sensory-deprivation n.
spasmus mutans n.
spontaneous n.
third-degree continuous spontaneous n.
torsional n.
toxic n.
transient n.
true n.
unidirectional n.
upbeating n.
vertical n.
vestibular end-organ n.
voluntary n.

nystagmus-myoclonus

NOTES

N

OBAS
Oregon Brain Aging Study
OBD
organic brain disease
obdormition
Obersteiner-Redlich
O.-R. line
O.-R. zone
Oberto mouth prop
obesity
hyperplastic-hypertrophic o.
hypertrophic o.
hypothalamic o.
o. hypoventilation syndrome
Obex plugging
object
o. agnosia
o. blindness
dissociation of o.'s
functional o.
linkage o.
metal o.
minute o.
o. naming
naming o.'s
pointed o.
primary o.
retained foreign o.
objective
o. assessment
o. measure
o. motor score
o. pulsatile tinnitus
o. sensation
o. severity
o. severity of illness
o. trauma characteristic
o. vertigo
objectivism
oblique
o. bundle of pons
o. flow misregistration
o. gastric fiber
o. nystagmus
o. pontine fasciculus
o. sagittal gradient-echo MR imaging
o. screw insertion
o. transcorporeal approach
obliquus reflex
obliterans
thromboangiitis o.
obliterated
o. arteriovenous malformation
o. basal cistern
obliteration
aneurysm o.
cortical o.
nidus o.
transcatheter o.
obliterative
o. arachnoiditis
o. arteritis
oblongata
anterior column of medulla o.
anterior median fissure of medulla o.
dorsal median fissure of medulla o.
gigantocellular nucleus of medulla o.
gracile fasciculus of medulla o.
lateral nucleus of medulla o.
median raphe of medulla o.
medulla o.
nucleus arcuatus of medulla o.
posterior median fissure of medulla o.
posterior median sulcus of medulla o.
pyramid of medulla o.
raphe mediana medullae o.
reticular nucleus of medulla o.
sensory decussation of medulla o.
vein of medulla o.
ventral median fissure of medulla o.
oblongatae
fasciculus gracilis medullae o.
fissura mediana anterior medullae o.
fissura mediana ventralis medullae o.
foramen caecum medullae o.
formatio reticularis medullae o.
funiculus lateralis medullae o.
funiculus posterior medullae o.
nucleus gigantocellularis medullae o.
nucleus lateralis medullae o.
nucleus reticulares medullae o.
nucleus reticularis intermedius medullae o.
nucleus reticularis lateralis medullae o.
pyramis medullae o.
raphe medullae o.
sulcus anterolateralis medullae o.
sulcus dorsolateralis medullae o.

oblongatae *(continued)*
sulcus medianus dorsalis medullae o.
sulcus medianus posterior medullae o.
sulcus posterolateralis medullae o.
sulcus ventrolateralis medullae o.
tractus solitarius medullae o.
venae medullae o.
oblongatal
OBS
organic brain syndrome
obscurus
nucleus raphe o.
obsessional
o. compulsive inventory alpha
o. neurosis
o. Q factor
o. reaction
o. thinking
obstacle sense
obstetric
o. hand
o. palsy
o. paralysis
obstetrical
o. hand
o. paralysis
obstructing hydrocephalus
obstruction
airway o.
cranial venous o.
incomplete upper airway o.
retinal venous o.
retrolingual o.
upper airway o.
venous outflow o.
venular o.
obstructive
o. arrhythmia
o. dementia
o. hydrocephalus
o. sleep apnea (OSA)
o. sleep apnea-hypopnea (OSAH)
o. sleep apnea-hypopnea syndrome (OSAHS)
o. sleep apnea syndrome (OSAS)
OBT
Olivier-Bertrand-Tipal
OBT stereotactic frame
obtained finding
obtundation
obturans
keratosis o.
obturator
blunt o.
o. nerve
o. nerve lesion
o. neurectomy
obturatorii
rami musculares rami anterioris nervi o.
rami musculares rami posterioris nervi o.
ramus anterior nervi o.
ramus cutaneus lateralis pectoralis nervi o.
ramus posterior nervi o.
obturatorius
nervus o.
occasional headache
occipital
o. alpha
o. artery
o. association
o. association cortical area
o. bitranstentorial/falcine approach
o. bone
o. bone-jugular incisure
o. bone malformation
o. bossing
o. cortex
o. cortex damage
o. cortex tissue
o. cortical dysplasia of Taylor
o. corticectomy
o. dominant intermittent rhythmic delta activity
o. encephalocele
o. eye field
o. forceps
o. glioblastoma
o. gray matter
o. groove
o. gyrus
o. headache
o. hematoma
o. horn
o. interhemispheric approach
o. intermittent rhythmic delta activity (OIRDA)
o. lesion
o. line
o. lobe
o. lobe of cerebrum
o. lobectomy
o. lobe epilepsy
o. lobe infarction
o. lobe seizure
o. lobe tumor
o. nerve
o. neuralgia
o. neurectomy
o. neuritis
o. neuroblastoma
o. operculum
o. pain
o. part of corpus callosum

o. plexus
o. pole
o. pole of cerebrum
o. resection
o. sinus
o. stripe
o. transtentorial approach
o. white matter
occipital-atlas-axis ligament
occipitalis
arteria o.
forceps o.
incisura jugularis ossis o.
lobus o.
polus o.
processus intrajugularis ossis o.
processus jugularis ossis o.
sinus o.
stria o.
occipitoatlantoaxial
o. complex
o. fusion
o. instability
occipitocervical
o. arthrodesis
o. dissociation (OCD)
o. fixation
o. fusion
o. instability
o. stabilization
occipitocervicothoracic (OCT)
occipitocollicular tract
occipitofrontal fasciculus
occipitofrontalis
fasciculus o.
occipitomastoid suture
occipitonuchal region
occipitoparietal artery occlusion
occipitopontile tract
occipitopontinae
fibrae o.
occipitopontine
o. fiber
o. tract
occipitopontinus
tractus o.
occipitotectal
o. fiber
o. tract
occipitotectales
fibrae o.
occipitotemporal
o. convolution
o. cortex
o. sulcus
occipitotemporalis
ramus o.
sulcus o.
occipitothalamic radiation
occiput
flat o.
o. flattening
occluded superior sagittal sinus
occluder
Heifetz carotid o.
occlusal necrosis
occlusion
aneurysm o.
aqueductal o.
o. balloon catheter with silicone balloon
balloon test o.
carotid o.
carotid artery o. (CAO)
chronic o.
o. coil
distal o.
dural sinus o.
endosaccular o.
endovascular balloon o.
internal carotid artery balloon test o.
intracranial o.
intraoperative balloon o.
intravascular balloon o.
luminal o.
middle cerebral artery o.
occipitoparietal artery o.
posterotemporal artery o.
prerolandic artery o.
proximal balloon o.
retinal arterial o.
retinal artery o.
sinovenous o.
sinus o.
superior sagittal sinus o.
thrombotic o.
transtorcular o.
transverse sinus o.
vascular o.
ventral spinal artery o.
ventricular catheter o.
vertebral artery o.

NOTES

occlusion/stenosis
occlusive
o. cerebrovascular disease
o. hyperemia
o. meningitis
occulomotor pathway
occult
o. abnormality
o. cerebrovascular malformation (OCVM)
o. frontal focus
o. hydrocephalus
o. presenile dementia
o. spinal dysraphism
o. vascular malformation (OVM)
occulta
spina bifida o.
occultum
cranium bifidum o.
occupancy
D2 o.
preferential o.
receptor o.
occupation
ligand o.
occupational
o. exposure
o. lifting task
o. neuropathy
o. neurotic disorder
o. risk factor
o. spasm
o. therapy
OCD
occipitocervical dissociation
ochronosis
OCT
occipitocervicothoracic
1-octanol
octapeptide
cholecystokinin o. (CCK-8)
octapolar lead
octavi
pars cochlearis nevi o.
pars vestibularis nervi o.
octavus
nervus o. [CN VIII]
Octopus visual field analyzer
OctreoScan scanner
octreotide
intrathecal o.
ocular
o. abnormality
o. alignment
o. bobbing
o. bobbing nystagmus
o. contrapulsion
o. cup
o. deviation
o. dipping
o. dyskinesia
o. dysmetria
o. dysmetria nystagmus
o. flutter
o. flutter nystagmus
o. hypotonia
o. ipsipulsion
o. ischemic syndrome
o. lateropulsion
o. lesion
o. malalignment
o. metastasis
o. motility
o. motility examination
o. muscle
o. muscle dysfunction
o. myasthenia gravis
o. myoclonus
o. pain
o. palsy
o. paralysis
o. perfusion pressure
o. photoreceptor
o. pneumoplethysmography
o. pseudomyasthenia
o. pulse
o. tilt reaction
o. torsion
o. torticollis
o. toxoplasmosis
o. vertigo
o. vesicle
oculi
pars orbitalis musculi orbicularis o.
tapetum o.
Oculinum
oculoauricular reflex
oculocephalic
o. reflex
o. test
oculocephalogyric
o. crisis
o. reflex
oculocerebrorenal syndrome
oculocraniosomatic disease
oculocutaneous albinism
oculoencephalic angiomatosis
oculogastrointestinal muscular dystrophy
oculographic artifact
oculography
infrared reflection o.
oculogyric crisis
oculomasticatory
o. myorhythmia
o. myorhythmia nystagmus
oculomotor
o. abnormality
o. apraxia

o. ataxia
o. delayed-response task
o. disturbance
o. nerve [CN III]
o. nerve examination
o. nerve paralysis
o. nerve paresis
o. neuropathy
o. nuclear complex
o. nucleus
o. nucleus raphes
o. ptosis
o. reflex
o. response
o. root of ciliary ganglion
o. sulcus
o. sulcus of mesencephalon
o. system
o. trigone

oculomotorii
nuclei accessorii nevi o.
nuclei viscerales nervi o.
nucleus anteromedialis nervi o.
nucleus dorsalis nervi o.
ramus inferior nervi o.
ramus superior nervi o.
sulcus nervi o.

oculomotorius
nervus o. [CN III]
nucleus o.
sulcus o.

oculomotor syndrome
oculopalatal myoclonus
oculopharyngeal
o. muscular dystrophy (OPMD)
o. syndrome

oculoplethysmography
oculorespiratory reflex
oculoskeletal myopathy
oculospinal reflex
oculosympathetic
o. dysfunction
o. ptosis

oculovestibular reflex
OCVM
occult cerebrovascular malformation

odaxesmus
Oden syndrome
ODI
oxygen desaturation index

ODN
oligodeoxynucleotide

odogenesis
Odom score
odonterism
odontoblast
odontogenic infection
odontoid
o. dysplasia
o. fracture
o. fracture internal fixation
o. fracture stabilization
o. process
o. process osteosynthesis
o. process resection
o. screw placement

odontoideum
os o.

odontoneuralgia
odor
o. detection
o. discrimination

odorant receptor (OR)
OEC-Diasonics mobile C-arm image intensifier
OEF
oxygen extraction fraction

off-period dystonia
offset frequency
Ogura operation
6-OHDA
6-hydroxydopamine

ohm
Ohtahara syndrome
OI
osteogenesis imperfecta

oil
brominated o.
ethiodized o.
evening primrose o. (EPO)
iodized o.
Lorenzo o.

OIRDA
occipital intermittent rhythmic delta activity
OIRDA on electroencephalogram

Ojemann cortical stimulator
okadaic acid
OKAN
optokinetic afternystagmus

Oklahoma tick fever virus
OKN
optokinetic nystagmus

NOTES

OKS
optokinetic stimulation
OKT3
OKT3 monoclonal antibody
OKT3 uremic
olanzapine
olanzapine-associated DKA
OLC
oligodendrocyte-like cell
old
o. memory
o. nerve injury
Oldberg
O. brain retractor
O. dissector
O. intervertebral disc rongeur
O. pituitary forceps
O. pituitary rongeur
old-sergeant syndrome
olecranon reflex
olfaction
olfactology
olfactometer
olfactometry
olfactoria
fila o.
hyperesthesia o.
idiosyncrasia o.
olfactoriae
striae o.
olfactorii
nervi o.
vena gyri o.
olfactorium
organum o.
trigonum o.
tuberculum o.
olfactorius
bulbus o.
nervus o. [CN I]
sulcus o.
tractus o.
olfactory
o. amnesia
o. anesthesia
o. area
o. aura
o. axonal growth
o. brain
o. bulb
o. bundle
o. coefficient
o. cortex
o. cranial nerve
o. deficit
o. dysfunction
o. ensheathing cell
o. epithelium
o. esthesioneuroblastoma
o. filum
o. function
o. glomerulus
o. groove
o. groove meningioma
o. groove tumor
o. gyrus
o. hair
o. hallucination
o. hyperesthesia
o. hypesthesia
o. knob
o. lobe
o. nerve examination
o. nerve layer
o. neuroblastoma
o. organ
o. pathway
o. peduncle
o. perception
o. pyramid
o. receptor
o. receptor cell
o. rod
o. root
o. sensation
o. sensory neuron (OSN)
o. sheathing cell
o. stria
o. sulcus
o. system
o. tract
o. trigone
o. tubercle
o. vestibule
olfactus
organum o.
oligemia
hippocampal o.
oligemic
oligoastrocytoma
mixed o.
oligoblast
oligoclonal band
oligodendria
oligodendroblast
oligodendroblastoma
oligodendrocyte
o. lineage cell
o. progenitor (OP)
o. progenitor recruitment
oligodendrocyte-like cell (OLC)
oligodendroglia cell
oligodendroglial lineage cell
oligodendroglioma
anaplastic o.
nonanaplastic o.

pleomorphic o.
supratentorial o.
oligodeoxynucleotide (ODN)
oligomer
beta-amyloid o.
oligonucleotide
antisense o.
oligopeptidase
brain prolyl o.
prolyl o.
oligosaccharide chain
oligosynaptic
O-linked glycan
Oliphant
oliva, pl. **olivae**
o. inferior
siliqua olivae
o. superior
olivare
amiculum o.
corpus o.
olivaris
hilum nuclei o.
nucleus o.
olivarum
commissura o.
olivary
o. body
o. degeneration
o. eminence
o. nucleus
olive
accessory o.
amiculum of inferior o.
inferior o.
superior o.
Olivecrona
O. aneurysm clamp
O. brain spatula
O. clip
O. clip applier
O. dura dissector
O. dura scissors
O. rasp
O. rongeur
O. trigeminal knife
O. trigeminal scissors
O. wire saw
Olivecrona-Gigli saw
Olivecrona-Toennis clip-applying forceps
Olivier-Bertrand-Tipal (OBT)
O.-B.-T. frame
olivifugal
olivipetal
olivocerebellar
o. fiber
o. tract
olivocerebellaris
tractus o.
olivocochlear
o. bundle
o. bundle of Rasmussen
o. tract
olivocochlearis
tractus o.
olivopontocerebellar
o. ataxia
o. atrophy
o. degeneration
olivospinal
o. fiber
o. tract
olivospinales
fibrae o.
Ollier disease
Olmsted County Study
O-mannosyl glycan synthesis
Omersch-Woltman syndrome
Ommaya
O. reservoir
O. ventriculoperitoneal shunt
Omni
O. clip gun
O. 2 microscope
Omnipaque
omnipresent dysphoria
Omniscan
Omni-Vent
omohyoid muscle
omphalocele-exstrophy-imperforate anus-spinal defects complex
OMS
opsoclonus-myoclonus syndrome
oncocytoma
oncogene
ras o.
oncolytic virus
oncoprotein
c-erbB-2-encoded o.
OncoScint
OncoTrac
Oncovin
ondansetron
Ondine curse

NOTES

O

one-and-a-half syndrome
oneiric, oniric
o. hyperesthesia
oneiroid
ongoing
o. cognitive process
o. neuroleptic treatment
onion
o. bulb change
o. bulb formation
o. bulb neuropathy
onion-skin distribution
oniric (*var. of* oneiric)
ONL
outer nuclear layer
onlay
o. collagen matrix
o. dural graft
on-off
o.-o. flushing reservoir
o.-o. motor fluctuation
o.-o. phenomenon
on-period dystonia
ONSD
optic nerve sheath decompression
onset
age of o.
locus of o.
wake after sleep o. (WASO)
ontogenesis
central nervous system o.
ontogenic process
ontogeny
Onuf nucleus
Onufrowicz nucleus
ONYX-015 virus
Onyx liquid embolic agent
Oort
bundle of O.
OP
oligodendrocyte progenitor
opacification
contrast o.
Opalski cell
open
o. angiography
o. C-D hook
o. clam-shell MRI
o. cordotomy
o. exit foramen
o. head injury
o. loop reflex
o. magnet
o. skull fracture
o. stereotactic craniotomy
open-door laminoplasty
opening
apraxia of eyelid o.
o. of aqueduct of midbrain
o. of cerebral aqueduct
o. pressure
open-label trial
open-mouthed anteroposterior tomogram
operant
tact o.
operating
O. Arm stereotactic navigator
o. microscope VM 900
operation
aneurysmal clipping o.
Ball o.
Brooks-Gallie cervical o.
Brooks-Jenkins cervical o.
cingulate o.
Cloward o.
concrete o.
Cotte o.
Dana o.
Dandy o.
decompression o.
floating-forehead o.
Frazier-Spiller o.
Gardner o.
Hartley-Krause o.
Horsley o.
Hunter o.
Keen o.
Killian o.
Koerte-Ballance o.
Krause o.
Leriche o.
Matas o.
Mikulicz o.
Ogura o.
partial debulking o.
Schloffer o.
Smith-Robinson o.
stereotactic o.
Stoffel o.
Stookey-Scarff o.
synchrocyclotron o.
tongue-in-groove o.
Torkildsen o.
operative
o. microscope
o. mortality
o. stabilization
o. trajectory
o. wedge frame
opercula (*pl. of* operculum)
opercular
o. cortex
o. epilepsy
o. part
opercularis
pars o.
operculum, pl. **opercula**
frontal o.

o. frontale
frontoparietal o.
o. frontoparietale
insula o.
medial o.
occipital o.
parietal o.
o. parietale
rolandic o.
sylvian o.
temporal o.
o. temporale

O-PET
optical positron emission tomography
O-PET technique

OPG
osteoprotegerin

ophryosis

ophthalmencephalon

ophthalmia
neuroparalytic o.

ophthalmic
o. artery
o. artery aneurysm
o. disorder
o. migraine
o. neurosyphilis
o. plexus
o. recurrent nerve
o. segment
o. segment aneurysm
o. system
o. vein
o. vesicle
o. zoster
o. zoster infection

ophthalmica
vesicula o.
zona o.

ophthalmici
ramus meningeus recurrens nervi o.
ramus tentorii nervi o.

ophthalmicus
caliculus o.
herpes zoster o.
nervus o.

ophthalmodynamometer
Bailliart o.
compression o.

ophthalmodynamometry
suction o.

ophthalmologic examination

ophthalmoneuritis

ophthalmoneuromyelitis

ophthalmoparesis
progressive external o.

ophthalmopathy
Graves o.

ophthalmoplegia
chronic progressive external o. (CPEO)
o. externa
fascicular o.
infectious o.
o. interna
internal o.
internuclear o. (INO)
o. internuclearis
intranuclear o.
latent o.
nuclear o.
orbital o.
o. and paralysis
Parinaud o.
o. partialis
o. plus
o. progressiva
progressive external o. (PEO)
pseudointernuclear o.
supranuclear o.
o. totalis

ophthalmoplegic migraine

ophthalmoplethysmography

ophthalmoscopy

opiate receptor

opioid
o. intoxication
o. peptide
o. peptide in seizure
o. poisoning
o. precursor protein
o. withdrawal

opiophagorum
tremor o.

opisthion

opisthotonic

opisthotonoid

opisthotonos, opisthotonus
o. position

OPLL
ossification of posterior longitudinal ligament

OPMD
oculopharyngeal muscular dystrophy

NOTES

OPMI
O. microscopic drape
O. surgical microscope
O. Vario/NC 33 system
Oppenheim
O. disease
O. reflex
O. sign
O. syndrome
opportunistic CNS infection
opprobrium
OPSI
orthogonal polarized spectral imaging
opsialgia
OpSite dressing
opsoclonus, opsoclonia
myoclonic o.
o. nystagmus
opsoclonus-myoclonus syndrome (OMS)
optic
o. agnosia
o. aphasia
o. ataxia
o. canal
o. chiasm
o. chiasmal syndrome
o. chiasm compression
o. chiasm tumor
o. cup
o. decussation
o. disc
o. disc edema
o. disc edema with macular star
o. disc pallor
o. disc swelling
o. fissure
o. glioma
o. layer
o. lobe
o. nerve astrocytoma
o. nerve atrophy
o. nerve [CN II]
o. nerve examination
o. nerve glioma
o. nerve hypoplasia
o. nerve infarction
o. nerve injury
o. nerve lesion
o. nerve sheath decompression (ONSD)
o. nerve sheath decompression surgery
o. nerve sheath hematoma
o. nerve sheath meningioma
o. neuritis
o. neuropathy
o. part of retina
o. pathway glioma
o. pathway tumor
o. radiation
o. recess
o. tectum
o. thalamus
o. tract
o. tract compression
o. tract syndrome
o. vesicle
optica
hyperesthesia o.
neuromyelitis o.
radiatio o.
optical
o. alexia
o. densitometry
o. device
o. digitizer
o. image-guided surgery system with dynamic referencing
o. positron emission tomography (O-PET)
o. righting reflex
o. shingle
o. system
optici
circulus vasculosus nervi o.
nuclei accessorii tractus o.
pars canalis nervi o.
pars intracranialis nervi o.
pars intraocularis nervi o.
pars orbitalis nervi o.
radix lateralis tractus o.
radix medialis tractus o.
rami tractus o.
stratum ganglionare nervi o.
vaginae nervi o.
vagina externa nervi o.
vagina interna nervi o.
opticocarotid triangle
opticocerebral syndrome
opticochiasmatic cistern
opticociliary shunt vessel
opticofacial reflex
opticokinetic (*var. of* optokinetic)
opticopyramidal syndrome
opticospinal MS
opticostriate region
opticum
brachium o.
chiasma o.
stratum o.
opticus
nervus o. [CN II]
recessus o.
tractus o.
optimal
o. group size
o. treatment strategy
Optiray

optochiasmic arachnoiditis
optokinetic, opticokinetic
o. afternystagmus (OKAN)
o. disorder
o. nystagmus (OKN)
o. reflex dysfunction
o. stimulation (OKS)
Optotrak motion and position measurement system
OR
odorant receptor
Oracle Delivery System
Oragrafin
oral
o. administered drug
o. administration
o. alimentary automatism
o. antiviral agent
o. appliance
o. appliance guideline
o. appliance prognosis
o. appliance safety
o. appliance selection
o. appliance side effect
o. appliance therapy
o. apraxia
o. atresia
o. biting period
o. bovine myelin
Calciferol O.
o. cavity
o. contraceptive-induced chorea
o. corticosteroid
Cytoxan O.
Dormarex O.
o. dose
Drisdol O.
o. dyskinesia
o. hemangioma
o. herpes lesion
o. intubation
Mephyton O.
o. pontine reticular nucleus
o. progesterone
o. retraction
o. supplementation
o. ulceration
VitaCarn O.
oral-buccal-lingual dyskinesia
oral-facial-digital syndrome
oralis
nucleus reticularis pontis o.
nucleus tegmenti pontis o.
Oramorph
Orap
Orascoptic
O. fiberoptic headlight
O. loupe extension
Orbeli effect
orbicularis
o. oculi muscle
o. oculi reflex
o. oris muscle
o. pupillary reflex
sign of o.
o. sign
Orbis-Sigma
O.-S. cerebrospinal fluid shunt valve
O.-S. valve (OSV)
O.-S. valve II
orbital
o. apex syndrome
o. blood flow
o. cephalocele
o. chemosis
o. decompression
o. disease
o. dystopia
o. ecchymosis
o. encephalocele
o. floor fracture
o. floor syndrome
o. granulocytic sarcoma
o. hypertelorism
o. myositis
o. neurofibroma
o. ophthalmoplegia
o. optic neuritis
o. osteotomy
o. part
o. part of inferior frontal gyrus
o. plate
o. prefrontal cortex
o. pseudotumor
o. region
o. schwannoma
o. solitary fibrous tumor
o. sulcus
o. varix
o. vein

NOTES

orbital *(continued)*
o. venous approach
o. zygomatic craniotomy
orbitales
gyri o.
sulci o.
orbitalis
pars o.
orbitofrontal
o. activity
o. approach
o. area
o. cortex
o. epilepsy
o. syndrome
orbitomedial/cingulate lesion
orbitopathy
thyroid o.
orbitotomy
orbitozygomatic
o. mandibular osteotomy
o. temporopolar approach
orderly nerve cell transmission
Oregon Brain Aging Study (OBAS)
orexin A
orexin-containing neuron
organ
anulospiral o.
auditory o.
Bidder o.
circumventricular o.
Corti o.
effector o.
encapsulated end o.
end o.
Golgi tendon o. (GTO)
gustatory o.
intromittent o.
o. jargon
lateral line o.
neurotendinous o.
olfactory o.
parapineal o.
parietal o.
reinnervation of target o.
Ruffini o.
sense o.
sensory o.
o. of smell
o. of special sense
spiral o.
statoacoustic o.
subcommissural o.
subfornical o.
tactile o.
o. of taste
terminal o.
o. of touch
o. transplantation
vestibular o.
vestibulocochlear o.
o. of vision
visual o.
vomeronasal o.
o. of Zuckerkandl
organa (*pl. of* organum)
organelle
cellular o.
cytoplasmic o.
membrane-bound o.
organic
o. acidemia
o. aciduria
o. affective syndrome
o. amnesia
o. amnestic syndrome
o. anxiety disorder
o. brain disease (OBD)
o. brain disorder
o. brain syndrome (OBS)
o. contracture
o. delusional disorder
o. delusional syndrome
o. dysfunction
o. etiology
o. hallucinosis syndrome
o. headache
o. mental disorder
o. mental syndrome
o. mood disorder
o. mood syndrome
multiple sclerosis-type o.
o. pain
o. personality disorder
o. psychiatric disorder
o. solvent
o. toxic disorder
o. toxin
o. vertigo
organism
causative o.
cryptococcal o.
o. embolus
organism-specific antibody index
organization
cortical o.
memory o.
postmigratory cortical o.
spatial o.
World Health O. (WHO)
organizer
o. gene
Spemann o.
organochlorine
organoleptic
organophosphate
o. exposure
o. pesticide poisoning

organophosphorus insecticide poisoning
organotypic brain slice
organum, pl. **organa**
o. auditus
o. gustatorium
o. gustus
o. olfactorium
o. olfactus
organa sensoria
organa sensuum
o. spirale
o. subcommissurale
o. tactus
o. vasculosum
o. vasculosum laminae terminalis
o. vestibulocochleare
o. visus
Orgaran
orgasmic headache
Orgogozo Stroke Scale
oriens
o. layer
o. layer of hippocampus
stratum o.
orientation
body spatial o.
coronal o.
ideological o.
religious o.
reverse o.
sagittal o.
spatial o.
theoretical o.
transverse o.
whole focus o.
oriented
alert and o. (AAO)
o. and alert
o. in all spheres
awake, alert, and o.
orienting
o. reflex
o. response
origin
anomalous o.
apparent o.
deep o.
ectal o.
intrapsychic o.
nuclei of o.
psychodynamic o.
psychogenic o.
real o.
Schwann cell o.
superficial o.
unifocal o.
originis
nucleus o.
Orinase
Orion anterior cervical plate
ornithine
o. decarboxylase
o. transcarbamoylase
o. transcarbamoylase deficiency (OTCD)
ornithine-ketoacid
o.-k. aminotransferase
o.-k. aminotransferase deficiency
ornithinemia
ornithosis lymphocytic meningitis
orofacial-digital syndrome
orofacial movement without vocalization
orolingual-buccal dyskinesia
oromandibular dystonia
oromotor dyspraxia
oropharyngeal
o. airway space
o. dystonia
o. reconstruction
o. reflex
orotic acid urine level
Orozco cervical plate
orphan
enteric cytopathic human o. (ECHO)
o. train
orphenadrine
Orpington Prognosis Scale
Orthawear antiembolism stockings
orthochorea
orthodox sleep
orthodromic
orthodromically
Orthofix Cervical-Stim stimulator
orthogenics
orthognathic surgery
orthogonal
o. angiography
o. combination
o. depression factor
o. film
o. laser
o. polarized spectral imaging (OPSI)

O

NOTES

orthogonal *(continued)*
o. square Helmholtz coil
o. x-ray
orthograde degeneration
orthographic
o. lexicon
o. process
o. regularity
orthomyxovirus infection
Orthopedic Systems, Inc. (OSI)
orthosis, pl. **orthoses**
cervicothoracic o.
CranioCap custom-made cranial o.
EZBrace o.
Flex Foam o.
halo o.
Malibu o.
postoperative lumbosacral o.
thoracolumbar standing o.
thoracolumbosacral o.
orthostatic
o. edema
o. epileptoid
o. fluctuation
o. hypertension
o. hypotension
o. stability
o. syncope
o. tremor
orthosympathetic branch
orthotonos, orthotonus
o. position
orthotopic liver transplantation
Orthotrac pneumatic vest
OSA
obstructive sleep apnea
OSAH
obstructive sleep apnea-hypopnea
OSAHS
obstructive sleep apnea-hypopnea syndrome
Osaka telesensor
OSAS
obstructive sleep apnea syndrome
Osborn band
Os-Cal 500
oscillating microsaw
oscillation
high-frequency o.
oscillator
sleep-wake o.
oscillatory brain activity
oscillopsia
oscilloscope
Norland digital o.
Tektronix 2214 o.
OSI
Orthopedic Systems, Inc.
OSI modular table system
Osler-Rendu-Weber syndrome
Osler-Weber-Rendu arteriovenous malformation
osmatic
osmesis
osmesthesia
osmicate
osmics
osmoceptor, osmoreceptor
osmole
idiogenic o.
osmology
osmophobia
osmophore group
osmoreceptor (*var. of* osmoceptor)
osmosis
osmotherapy
osmotic
o. dehydrating agent
o. demyelination
o. demyelination syndrome
o. mechanism
OSN
olfactory sensory neuron
os odontoideum
osphresiology
osphretic
OssaTron device
ossea
crura o.
leontiasis o.
Osserman criteria
ossicle
Tutoplast auditory o.
ossificans
fibrodysplasia o.
meningitis o.
myositis o.
neuritis o.
ossification
heterotopic o.
o. of posterior longitudinal ligament (OPLL)
ossifying
o. arachnoiditis
o. fibroma
osteitis deformans
osteoblastoma
Osteocalcin Injection
osteochondral spinal column
osteochondroma
osteochondrosis
intervertebral o.
osteoclastic
osteodiastasis
osteogenesis imperfecta (OI)
osteogenic sarcoma
osteoid osteoma
osteointegration

osteolysis
osteoma
choroidal o.
osteoid o.
osteomalacia
Osteomed
osteomyelitis
cranial o.
pyogenic o.
spinal o.
osteonecrosis
syphilitic o.
osteopathic
o. scoliosis
o. spinal manipulation
osteopetrosis
cranial o.
osteophyte formation
osteoplastic
o. bone flap
o. craniotomy
o. laminectomy
osteoporosis
o. circumscripta
o. circumscripta cranii
disuse o.
glucocorticoid-induced o.
posttraumatic o.
steroid-induced o.
osteoporotic spine
osteoprotegerin (OPG)
osteoradionecrosis
osteosarcoma
osteosclerosis
myelofibrosis o.
osteosclerotic myeloma
OsteoSet
OsteoStim
O. cervical allograft spacer
O. DBM putty
O. resorbable bone graft substitute
O. Skelite
osteosynthesis
anterior column o.
cranial o.
facial o.
lumbar spine vertebral o.
odontoid process o.
plate-screw o.
posterior column o.
thoracic spine vertebral o.
thoracolumbar spine vertebral o.
vertebral o.
wire o.
osteotome
Cherry o.
Cloward spinal fusion o.
osteotomy
craniofacial o.
ethmoidal o.
frontonasomaxillary o.
frontoorbital o.
glabellar exposure o.
LeFort o.
mandibular o.
maxillary o.
orbital o.
orbitozygomatic mandibular o.
Tessier o.
ostium tympanicum tubae auditivae
OSV
Orbis-Sigma valve
OSV II Smart Valve system
Oswestry
O. Disability score
O. Low Back Pain Disability Questionnaire
otalgia
geniculate o.
tabetic o.
OTCD
ornithine transcarbamoylase deficiency
otic
o. abscess
o. capsule
o. ganglion
o. hydrocephalus
o. meningitis
o. neuralgia
otici
radix parasympathica ganglii o.
radix sensoria ganglii o.
oticum
ganglion o.
rami ganglionares nervi maxillaris ad ganglion o.
oticus
herpes zoster o.
otitis
malignant external o.
o. media
o. with headache
otocerebritis
otoconial plug

O

NOTES

otocyst
otoencephalitis
otoganglion
otolithic crisis of Tumarkin
otologic implant
otoneuralgia
otoneurology
otorhinorrhea
otorrhea
  cerebrospinal fluid o.
  CSF o.
otosclerosis
Ototome irrigation kit
ototoxic
  o. antibiotic
  o. drug
ototoxicity
otx gene
Ouchterlony double-diffusion technique
outcome
  o. assessment
  caregiver o.
  global o.
  o. of illness
  long-term o.
  o. measure
  multidimensional assessment of o.
  overall management o.
  premature infant neurodevelopmental o.
  primary efficacy o.
  psychosocial symptom o.
  secondary o.
  seizure-free o.
  o. strata
  o. study
  therapeutic o.
  treatment o.
outer
  o. band of Baillarger
  o. cone fiber
  o. limiting layer
  o. line of Baillarger
  o. mesaxon of myelin sheath
  o. nuclear layer (ONL)
  o. plexiform layer
  o. sheath of optic nerve
  o. sphenoid ridge meningioma
outfolding
outgrowth
  chemoattractant axonal o.
  neurite o.
outlet
  o. syndrome
  thoracic o.
out-of-phase
  o.-o.-p. deflection
  o.-o.-p. image
  o.-o.-p. waveform
output
  cortical motor o.
  sympathetic o.
outside-in signaling
outward focus
oval
  o. area of Flechsig
  o. corpuscle
  o. curette
  o. fasciculus
  o. hyperchromatic nucleus
ovale
  centrum o.
  foramen o.
  patent foramen o.
  white matter of centrum o.
ovalis
  fossa o.
ovarian
  o. androgen secretion
  o. function
overall
  o. cognitive functioning
  o. cognitive measure
  o. disability
  o. management outcome
  o. risk index
  o. survival
overconcern with sleep
overdrainage syndrome
overflow
  motor o.
  receiver o.
overgrowth
  brain o.
  early brain o.
  neurite o.
overhang
  bony o.
overlap
  o. syndrome
  o. syndrome in polymyositis
overlapping agitation
overlay
  emotional o.
  psychosocial o.
overload
  receiver o.
  sensory o.
over-right hypertropia
oversecretion
  hydrocephalus o.
overshooting
  saccadic o.
overt
  o. agitation
  o. hallucination
  o. weeping
Overtime tablet

overuse phenomenon
OVM
occult vascular malformation
postirradiation OVM
ovoid
myelin o.
Owen gauze dressing
Owsley acid
oxacillin
oxalate
escitalopram o.
oxalic acid urine level
oxaloacetate
oxazepam
oxcarbazepine
Oxfordshire Community Stroke Project classification
oxidant
endogenous o.
oxidase
cytochrome *c* o.
monoamine o. (MAO)
xanthine o.
oxidation
alpha-ketoglutarate o.
fatty acid o.
pyruvate o.
o. state
oxidative
o. cellular injury
o. damage
o. degeneration
o. phosphorylation
o. stress
o. stress signaling
oxide
exogenous nitric o.
magnesium o.
nitric o.
nitrous o.
superparamagnetic iron o.
oxidized
o. cotton
o. regenerated cellulose
oxidronate
technetium-99m o.
oxime
hexamethylpropyleneamine oxime (HMPAO)
^{99m}Tc-hexamethylpropyleneamine o.
oximeter
INVOS transcranial cerebral o.
pulse o.
Somanetics INVOS 3100 cerebral o.
oximetry
continuous venous o.
pulse o.
oxolinic acid
oxoprolinuria
oxyacoia
oxyaphia
oxybarbiturate
oxybate
sodium o.
oxybutynin chloride
Oxycel
oxycellulose
oxycephalic, oxycephalous
oxycephaly, oxycephalia
oxychlorosene
OxyContin
oxyecoia
oxyesthesia
oxygen
arterial o.
brain tissue o.
cerebral metabolic rate of o. ($CMRO_2$)
o. desaturation index (ODI)
o. extraction fraction (OEF)
o. free radical
hyperbaric o. (HBO)
o. inhalation
partial venous gas tension of o.
o. radical attack
o. radical-induced cellular injury
regional cerebral metabolic rate of o.
saturation of o. (SaO2)
supplemental o.
o. tension
o. therapy
oxygenation
brain o.
cerebral hemodynamics and o.
extracorporeal membrane o.
neonatal extracorporal membrane o.
sleep-related o.
oxygeusia
oxylate
sodium o.
oxymetazoline nasal spray
oxyosmia

NOTES

O

oxyosphresia
oxyphenbutazone
oxyphencyclimine hydrochloride
oxytocin

1p
chromosome 1p
6p
chromosome 6p
p170 glycoprotein
P3 probe
p53 gene
PA
plasminogen activator
tissue-type PA
urokinase-type PA
Pabenol
pacchionian
p. body
p. corpuscle
p. foramen
p. gland
p. granulation
Pacchioni foramen
Paced Auditory Serial Addition test
pacemaker
circadian p.
Pace ventricular needle
Pachon test
pachydermatocele
pachygyria
pachygyria-type cortical neuronal migration disorder
pachyleptomeningitis
pachymeninges (*pl. of* pachymeninx)
pachymeningitis
p. cranialis hypertrophica
p. externa
hemorrhagic p.
hypertrophic cervical p.
hypertrophic chromic p. (HCP)
hypertrophic cranial p.
idiopathic hypertrophic cranial p.
idiopathic intracranial p.
p. interna
intracranial p.
p. intralamellaris
meningeal p.
purulent p.
pyogenic p.
spinal p.
syphilitic cerebral hypertrophic p.
pachymeningopathy
pachymeninx, pl. **pachymeninges**
pacificus
Ixodes p.
pacinian
p. corpuscle
p. mechanoreceptor
Pacini corpuscle
packer
Woodson dura p.
packing
Avitene p.
endosaccular p.
Vaseline gauze p.
pack-year exposure
paclitaxel
PAD
primary afferent depolarization
pad
cotton p.
Gelfoam p.
parapharyngeal fat p.
pharyngeal fat p.
Padgett baseline pinch gauge
PAE
pediatric and adolescent epilepsy
PAF
platelet-activating factor
Paget disease
pain
p. apprehension
p. asymbolia
atypical facial p.
back p.
bone p.
brain central p.
causalgic p.
central post-stroke p.
chronic intractable p.
congenital insensitivity to p.
core p.
deafferentation p.
deliberate infliction of p.
dermatome p.
diabetic neuropathy neuralgia p.
p. disorder
effected p.
electrically evoked p.
end-zone p.
extraterritorial spontaneous p.
eye p.
facial p.
faciocephalic p.
p. fiber
functional p.
gate control theory of p.
p. generator
girdle p.
Goody's Body P.
hemicranial p.
heterotopic p.
homotopic p.
ice pick p.

P

pain *(continued)*
ice pick-like p.
inescapable p.
p. intensity threshold
intractable chronic p.
intractable somatic p.
intractable unilateral p.
lancinating p.
law of referred p.
leg p.
level of psychological p.
low back p. (LBP)
lumbar puncture p.
masking p.
migratory p.
p. modulation
muscle p.
myofascial p.
neck p.
nerve p.
neuropathic p.
night p.
nighttime p.
nociceptive p.
nocturnal p.
nonneuropathic p.
nonspecific neck p.
occipital p.
ocular p.
organic p.
paroxysmal evoked p.
P. Patient Profile
P. Perception Profile
peripheral deafferentation p.
phantom limb p.
phantom tooth p.
physical p.
pinprick p.
posttraumatic p.
psychogenic chest p.
psychogenic pelvic p.
psychogenic precordial p.
radicular distribution of p.
p. reaction
recurrent p.
referred p.
rest p.
retroorbital p.
root p.
sciatic p.
p. sense
short-lasting unilateral neuralgiform p.
skin graft harvesting p.
somatic p.
somatoform p.
spinal cord p.
p. spot
subclinical neck p.
tabetic p.
tactile p.
p. and temperature pathway
terebrating p.
thalamic p.
p. threshold reduction
p. tolerance
p. tract
p. transduction
transient p.
unilateral p.
p. unpleasantness
venipuncture p.
visceral p.
viscerogenic referred p.

PainBuster infusion pump management kit

Paine retinaculatome

painful
p. anesthesia
p. erection
p. legs and moving fingers syndrome
p. legs and moving toes syndrome
p. paraplegia

painless
p. aura
p. vision loss

pain-sensitive vessel

pain-transmitting
p.-t. nerve fiber
p.-t. tract

pair
coherent negative picture-caption p.
coherent positive picture-caption p.
control picture-caption p.
Maxwell p.
negative picture-caption p.
picture-caption p.
positive picture-caption p.
reference picture-caption p.

paired
p. electrode recording
p. gene
p. helical filament

paired-pulse
p.-p. inhibition
p.-p. transcranial magnetic stimulation

pairwise intensity

palatal
p. lift prosthesis
p. mucosal eruption
p. mucosal incision
p. myoclonus
p. nystagmus
p. paresis
p. reflex
p. split

p. surgery
p. syndrome
palatine nerve
palatini
levator p.
nervi p.
nervus musculi tensoris veli p.
tensor veli p.
palatinum
velum p.
palatoglossus muscle
palatooccipital line
palatoocular myoclonus
palatopharyngeal
p. flap
p. paralysis of Avellis
palatopharyngeus muscle
palatopharyngoplasty
palatoplasty
laser-assisted p.
radiofrequency p.
palatoplegia
paleencephalon
paleocerebellum
paleocortex
paleokinetic
paleostriatal syndrome
paleostriatum
paleothalamus
paligraphia
palikinesia, palicinesia
palilogia
palindrome
palindromic encephalopathy
palingnosticum
delirium p.
palinopsia
palinoptic hallucination
palinphrasia, paliphrasia
Palladone
pallanesthesia
pallesthesia
pallesthetic sensibility
pallidal
p. atrophy
p. degeneration
p. lesion
p. raphe nucleus
p. syndrome
pallidectomy
pallidi
rami globi p.
pallidoamygdalotomy
pallidoansection
pallidoansotomy
pallidofugal
pallidostriatal feedback loop
pallidotomy
Leksell posteroventral p.
posteroventral p.
stereotactic p.
ventroposterolateral p.
ventroposteromedial p.
VPL p.
pallidum
dorsal p.
p. dorsale
p. I, II
posteroventral sensorimotor p.
Treponema p.
ventral p.
p. ventrale
pallidus
globus p.
nucleus raphes p.
ventral globus p.
pallii
impressio petrosa p.
Pallister-Hall syndrome
Pallister-Killian syndrome
pallium
petrosal impression of p.
pallor
optic disc p.
palmar
p. crease
p. grasp reflex
p. hyperhidrosis
Palmaz-Schatz stent
Palmaz stent
palm-chin reflex
palmic
palmitate
palmitic acid
palmitoylation
palmitoyltransferase
carnitine p.
serine p.
palmodic
palmomental
p. reflex
p. test
palmus
palpatometry

NOTES

P

palsy
abducens nerve p.
American Academy of Cerebral P.
ataxic cerebral p.
athetoid cerebral p.
atonic cerebral p.
backpack p.
Bell p.
bilateral gaze p.
birth p.
brachial birth p.
bridegroom's p.
bulbar p.
cerebellar cerebral p.
cerebral p.
choreoathetoid cerebral p.
congenital cerebral p.
craft p.
cranial nerve p.
creeping p.
crutch p.
Dejerine-Klumpke p.
diabetic oculomotor p.
diabetic third nerve p.
double elevator p.
dystonic cerebral p.
Erb p.
Erb-Duchenne p.
extraocular muscle p.
extrapyramidal cerebral p.
facial p.
feeding difficulties in cerebral p.
Féréol-Graux p.
fourth nerve p.
gaze p.
hereditary neuropathy with liability to pressure p. (HNPP)
hereditary neuropathy with susceptibility to pressure p.
horizontal gaze p.
hypertonic cerebral p.
hypoglossal nerve p.
hypotonic cerebral p.
idiopathic facial nerve p.
ipsilateral facial p.
ipsilateral gaze p.
isolated radial nerve p.
Klumpke p.
labioglossolaryngeal p.
lateral gaze p.
lateral rectus p.
lead p.
long thoracic p.
mixed form cerebral p.
monoplegic cerebral p.
multiinfarct progressive supranuclear p.
mumps facial nerve p.
nerve p.
night p.
obstetric p.
ocular p.
peripheral nerve pressure p.
peripheral occulomotor p.
peroneal nerve p.
persistent facial p.
pharyngeal-brachial p.
postganglionic oculosympathetic p.
posticus p.
postinfectious abducens p.
pressure p.
progressive infantile bulbar p.
progressive supranuclear p. (PSP)
pseudoabducens p.
pseudobulbar p.
pure athetoid p.
pure spastic p.
pyramidal cerebral p.
right sixth nerve p.
saccadic p.
Saturday night p.
scrivener's p.
seventh nerve p.
shaking p.
sixth cranial nerve p.
spastic bulbar p.
spastic cerebral p.
spinal accessory p.
stimulation program in cerebral p.
supranuclear gaze p.
Tapia vagohypoglossal p.
tardy median p.
tardy ulnar nerve p.
third nerve p.
trembling p.
trochlear nerve p.
vertical gaze p.
wasting p.

PAM
potassium-aggravated myotonia

pamabrom

pamidronate

pamoate
hydroxyzine p.

PAN
periodic alternating nystagmus

panacea

Panama cut

panasthenia

panautonomic

Panayiotopoulos syndrome

pancerebellar ataxia

panchreston

Pancoast
P. syndrome
P. tumor

pancreatic
p. beta cell

p. carcinoma
p. encephalopathy
pancreaticus
plexus p.
pancreatitis
pancuronium bromide
pancytopenia
PANDAS
pediatric autoimmune neuropsychiatric disorder associated with streptococcus
pandemic
p. epidemiology
influenza A p.
pandiculation
Pandy maturation
pandysautonomia
acquired p.
acute p.
panel
12-hour fasting lipid p.
panencephalitis
measles p.
nodular p.
Pette-Döring p.
progressive rubella p.
rubella p.
sclerosing p.
subacute sclerosing p. (SSPE)
panesthesia
panesthetic
Panevril
pang
brow p.
Pang-type agenesis
panhypopituitarism
panicogenic effect
Panlor
panneuritis endemica
panodic
panplegia
panpotency
Pansch fissure
PANSS
Positive and Negative Syndrome Scale
PANSS-EC
Positive and Negative Syndrome Scale–Excitement Component
pansynostosis
pantalgia
pantanencephaly, pantanencephalia
panthodic
panting center
Pantopaque
Pantopon
pantothenic acid-deficiency peripheral neuropathy
PAP
positive airway pressure
papaverine hydrochloride
papaverine-soaked Gelfoam
paper stop artifact
Papez
P. circle
P. circuit
papilla, pl. **papillae**
acoustic p.
clavate papillae
fungiform papillae
nerve p.
papillary
p. meningioma
p. mucosal hyperplasia
p. response
papilledema
axoplasmic flow and p.
intracranial hypertension without p. (IHWOP)
papilliferous cystoma
papillitis
papilloma
choroid plexus p.
papillomatosis
juvenile p.
papillomatous
papillophlebitis
papovavirus
papulosis
malignant atrophic p.
paraballism
parabigeminalis
nucleus p.
parabigeminal nucleus
parabrachiales
nuclei p.
parabrachial nucleus
paracarcinomatous
p. encephalomyelopathy
p. myelopathy
paracenesthesia
paracentesis
paracentral
p. fissure
p. gyrus
p. hemianopia

NOTES

P

paracentral *(continued)*
p. lobule
p. nucleus of thalamus
p. scotoma
p. sulcus
paracentralis
gyrus p.
lobulus p.
sulcus p.
paracerebellar
paracetamol
parachiasmal epidermoid tumor
parachlorophenylalanine
parachute
p. reaction
p. reflex
p. response
paracinesia (*var. of* parakinesia)
paracinesis (*var. of* parakinesis)
paraclinoid internal carotid artery aneurysm
Paracoccidioides brasiliensis
paracrine mechanism
paracusis, paracousis, paracusia
paradigm
awake language p.
complex p.
event-related innocuous somatosensory stimulation p.
gap p.
memory p.
motor p.
positive-going p.
risk p.
stimuli p.
3-stimulus p.
task p.
paradox
calcium p.
pH p.
paradoxica
kinesia p.
paradoxical
p. abdominal movement
p. air embolism
p. cerebral embolism
p. cold response
p. combination
p. contraction
p. depression
p. diaphragm phenomenon
p. effect
p. extensor reflex
p. flexor reflex
p. ipsilateral hemiparesis
p. patellar reflex
p. phenomenon of dystonia
p. pupil
p. pupillary phenomenon
p. pupillary reflex
p. sleep
p. stimulation
p. triceps reflex
paraepilepsy
paraequilibrium
paraesthesia (*var. of* paresthesia)
parafalcine region
parafalx
parafascicular nucleus
paraffin embedding
paraflocculus
ventral p.
p. ventralis
parafollicular cell
paraganglioma
intrasellar p.
intravagal p.
nonchromaffin p.
parageusia
parageusic
paragigantocellularis
nucleus reticularis p.
paragloboside
sulfated glucuronyl p. (SGPG)
sulfate-3-glucuronyl p.
sulfoglucuronyl lactosaminyl p.
paragonimiasis
p. lymphocytic meningitis
p. trematode
Paragonimus westermani
paragrammatism
paragraphia
parahaemolyticus
Vibrio p.
parahippocampal
p. activation
p. gyrus
p. white matter
parahippocampalis
gyrus p.
uncus gyri p.
parahippocampus
parahypophysis
parainfluenzae
Haemophilus p.
parainfluenza virus infection
paraisopropyliminodiacetic acid (PIPIDA)
parakinesia, paracinesia
parakinesis, paracinesis
parakinetic
paralalia
paraldehyde
paralemniscalis
nucleus p.
paralemniscal nucleus
paraleprosis
paralexia
paralexic

paralgesia
paralgesic
paralgia
paralimbic
p. cortex
p. region
paralinguistic feature
parallel
p. fiber
p. pathways of metabolism
p. subsystem
paralogism
paralogistic
paralysis, pl. **paralyses**
abducens nerve p.
acute ascending p.
acute atrophic p.
p. agitans
ascending p.
Avellis p.
backpack p.
Benedikt ipsilateral oculomotor p.
botulism with p.
Brown-Séquard p.
bulbar p.
central p.
chronic basal meningitis with cranial nerve p.
complete flaccid extremity p.
compression p.
conjugate p.
contralateral facial p.
crossed p.
crutch p.
Cruveilhier p.
decubitus p.
deglutition p.
Dejerine-Klumpke p.
diaphragm p.
diphtheritic p.
Duchenne p.
Duchenne-Erb p.
Erb-Duchenne p.
Erb spinal p.
extraocular p.
facial nerve p.
familial dyskalemic periodic p.
familial hypokalemic periodic p.
faucial p.
flaccid p.
gaze p.
generalized p.
ginger p.
global p.
glossolabiolaryngeal p.
glossolabiopharyngeal p.
glossopalatolabial p.
glossopharyngeal nerve p.
glossopharyngeolabial p.
Gubler p.
hyperkalemic periodic p.
hypokalemic periodic p.
hysterical p.
immunological p.
infranuclear p.
ipsilateral facial p.
Jackson vagoaccessory hypoglossal p.
jake p.
Klumpke p.
Klumpke-Dejerine p.
Kussmaul p.
Kussmaul-Landry p.
labial p.
labioglossolaryngeal p.
labioglossopharyngeal p.
Landry p.
lead p.
lingual p.
Lissauer p.
lower motor neuron p.
mimetic p.
mixed p.
motor neuron p.
muscle periodic p.
musculospiral p.
myogenic p.
normokalemic periodic p.
obstetric p.
obstetrical p.
ocular p.
oculomotor nerve p.
ophthalmoplegia and p.
partial flaccid extremity p.
periodic p.
peripheral facial p.
peroneal p.
phonetic p.
phrenic nerve p.
physiologic sleep p.
postdiphtheritic p.
postepileptic p.
posthemiplegic p.
posticus p.

NOTES

P

paralysis *(continued)*
Pott p.
predominantly predormital sleep p.
pressure p.
progressive bulbar p.
pseudobulbar p.
pseudohypertrophic muscular p.
radial p.
Ramsay Hunt p.
rectus p.
reflex p.
Remak p.
residual p.
rotating p.
rucksack p.
saccade p.
sensory p.
Simmer p.
sleep p.
sodium-responsive periodic p.
spastic spinal p.
spinal p.
spinomuscular p.
supranuclear p.
tegmental mesencephalic p.
thyrotoxic periodic p. (TPP)
tick p.
Todd postepileptic p.
transient flaccid p.
trigeminal p.
trochlear nerve p.
upper motor neuron p.
vasomotor p.
vocal cord p.
vocal fold p.
waking p.
wasting p.
West Nile virus-induced p.
Zenker p.
paralytic
p. chorea
p. dementia
p. ileus
p. miosis
p. mydriasis
p. poliomyelitis
p. pontine exotropia
p. psychosomatic disorder
p. ptosis
p. scoliosis
p. stroke
paralytica
aphonia p.
chorea p.
dementia p.
keratitis p.
paralyticus
ictus p.
paralytogenic
paralyzed limb
paralyzing
p. depression
p. vertigo
paramagnetic
p. contrast
p. contrast enhancement
p. contrast injection
p. relaxation
paramedial reticular nucleus
paramedian
p. durotomy
p. infarction
p. lobule
p. mesencephalic syndrome
p. nucleus
p. pontine reticular formation (PPRF)
p. region
p. thalamopeduncular artery
p. thalamus
p. triangle
paramedianus
lobulus p.
nucleus reticularis p.
parameningeal mass
parameter
aberrant laboratory p.
dichotomous p.
pharmacokinetic p.
psychiatric p.
stimulation p.
suprasegmental p.
treatment intensity p.
paramethadione
paramethoxyamphetamine
parametric mapping
parametrismus
paramimia
paramusia
paramyoclonus multiplex
paramyotonia
ataxic p.
p. congenita
congenital p.
symptomatic p.
paramyxovirus infection
paranalgesia
paranasal
p. mucocele
p. sinus
p. sinus tumor
paraneoplastic
p. cerebellar degeneration
p. cerebral degeneration
p. encephalomyelitis
p. encephalomyelopathy
p. myelopathy
p. neurological disease

p. neurologic disease
p. neurologic disorder
p. neurologic syndrome
p. neuropathy
p. opsoclonus myoclonus
p. pain syndrome
p. polyneuropathy
p. syndrome

paranesthesia

paraneurone

paranigralis
nucleus p.

paranigral nucleus

paranodal region

paranoia
hypochondriac p.
Kraepelina p.

paranoid
p. involutional reaction
p. state
p. thinking
p. type

paranoid-type
p.-t. arteriosclerotic
p.-t. arteriosclerotic dementia
p.-t. presenile dementia
p.-t. psychoorganic syndrome
p.-t. senile dementia

paranormal capacity

paranuclear

paraolfactorii
sulci p.

paraolfactory cortical area

paraorbital lesion

paraparesis
acute-onset p.
chronic p.
flaccid p.
hereditary spastic p. (HSP)
HTLV-associated myelopathy/tropical spastic p.
human T-cell lymphotropic virus type 1-associated myelopathy/tropical spastic p. (HAM/TSP)
nonspastic p.
spastic p.
tropical spastic p.
X-linked spastic p.

paraparetic gait

parapeduncularis
nucleus p.

parapeduncular nucleus

parapharyngeal
p. fat pad
p. wall

paraphasia, paraphrasia
central p.
literal p.
phonemic p.
semantic p.
thematic p.

paraphasic error

paraphia

paraphilia

paraphrasia (*var. of* paraphasia)

paraphrenic

paraphysial, paraphyseal
p. body
p. cyst

paraphysis, pl. **paraphyses**

parapineal organ

paraplectic

paraplegia
American Spinal Injury Association/International Medical Society of P. (ASIA/IMSOP)
ataxic p.
congenital spastic p.
p. dolorosa
Erb syphilitic spastic p.
p. in extension
familial spastic p.
p. in flexion
hereditary spastic p.
infantile spastic p.
painful p.
peripheral p.
postoperative p.
Pott p.
senile p.
spastic p.
superior p.
syphilitic p.
tetanoid p.
toxic p.
tropical spastic p.

paraplegic
p. idiocy
p. spasm
p. spastic gait

paraplegiform

paraplegin

parapraxis, parapraxia

NOTES

paraprotein
IgM-lambda p.
light chain p.
paraproteinemia
paraproteinemic neuropathy
parareflexia
parasagittal
p. cerebral injury
p. falx
p. groove
p. intracranial mass
p. lesion
p. meningioma
p. section
p. tumor
parasellar
p. cistern
p. dysgerminoma
p. lesion
p. mass
p. region
p. tentorial meningioma
p. tumor
parasinoidal
p. sinus
p. space
parasitic
p. brain abscess
p. infection
p. meningitis
parasomnia
parasomniac
paraspecific stimulation
paraspinal
p. infection
p. muscle
p. muscle block
p. rod application
Parastep I System
parastriate
p. area
p. cortex
parasubiculum
parasympathetic
p. nerve
p. nerve injury
p. nervous system
p. part
p. root of ciliary ganglion
p. root of otic ganglion
p. root of pterygopalatine ganglion
p. root of sublingual ganglion
p. root of submandibular ganglion
parasympathica
pars p.
parasympathotonia
parataxic
paraterminal
p. body
p. gyrus
paraterminale
corpus p.
paraterminalis
gyrus p.
parathyreopriva
tetania p.
parathyroid
p. gland
p. hormone (PTH)
p. hormonelike protein (PLP)
p. insufficiency
p. tetany
parathyroprival tetany
paratonia progressiva
paratonic rigidity
Paratrend 7 sensor
paratrigeminal
p. neuralgia
p. syndrome
paraventricular
p. cyst
p. fiber
p. nucleus
p. nucleus of hypothalamus
paraventriculohypophysialis
tractus p.
paraventriculohypophysial tract
paravertebral
p. ganglion
p. venous plexus
paraxial mesenchyme
parchment crackling
Parcopa
parectropia
parencephalia
parencephalitis
parencephalocele
parencephalous
parenchyma
brain p.
spinal cord p.
parenchymal
p. bacillary peliosis
p. cerebral hemorrhage
p. granuloma
p. matrix
parenchymatous
p. atrophy
p. cell of corpus pineale
p. cerebellar degeneration
p. hematoma
p. hemorrhage
p. neuritis
p. neurosyphilis
p. syphilis

parent
p. artery
p. vessel
parental consanguinity
parenteral
p. alimentation
p. formula
p. nutrition
paresis
abducens nerve p.
accessory nerve p.
ascending p.
asymmetrical palatal p.
bibrachial p.
canal p.
central facial p.
cerebral gaze p.
congenital suprabulbar p.
crural p.
distal motor p.
downgaze p.
downward gaze p.
elevation p.
extraocular muscle p.
flaccid p.
gaze p.
general p.
horizontal gaze p.
hypoglossal nerve p.
ipsilateral facial p.
limb-girdle-trunk p.
monomelic p.
oculomotor nerve p.
palatal p.
postictal p.
progressive extraocular p.
pseudoabducens nerve p.
saccadic p.
spastic p.
Todd p.
trochlear nerve p.
upward gaze p.
vertical gaze p.
watershed area p.
zoster p.
paresthesia, paraesthesia
Berger p.
Bernhardt p.
transient facial p.
paresthetica
brachialgia statica p.
cheiralgia p.
gonyalgia p.
meralgia p.
paresthetic pseudopolycythemia
paretic
p. agraphia
p. analgesia
p. dementia
p. eye
p. jerk
p. neurosyphilis
p. nystagmus
pargyline hydrochloride
paries, pl. **parietes**
p. vestibularis ductus cochlearis
parietal
p. body
p. cell vagotomy
p. cortex
p. cortex damage
p. cortex lesion
p. corticectomy
p. craniotomy
p. encephalocele
p. eye field
p. foramen
p. gyrus
p. hypoperfusion
p. lobe
p. lobe of cerebrum
p. lobe epilepsy
p. lobe lesion
p. lobe syndrome
p. lobe tumor
p. lobule
p. meningioma
p. neocortical association area
p. operculum
p. organ
p. pathology
p. plane
p. tissue
p. vein
parietale
operculum p.
parietales
venae p.
parietalis
lobus p.
parietes (*pl. of* paries)
parietooccipital
p. craniotomy
p. fissure

NOTES

P

parietooccipital *(continued)*
p. hypoperfusion
p. infarction
p. lesion
p. sulcus
parietooccipitalis
arcus p.
arteriae p.
fissura p.
ramus p.
sulcus p.
parietooccipitotemporal hypometabolism
parietopontinae
fibrae p.
parietopontine
p. fiber
p. tract
parietopontinus
tractus p.
parietosquamous suture
parietotemporal area
Parinaud
P. ophthalmoplegia
P. sign
P. syndrome
park bench position
Parkes Weber syndrome
parkin
p. carrier
p. disease
p. gene
p. gene mutation
p. protein
parkin-related disease
Parkinson
P. disease
P. disease and lateral sclerosis-dementia complex
P. Disease Quality of Life Scale (PDQUALIF)
P. Disease Questionnaire-39 (PDQ-39)
P. facies
P. mask
P. Research The Organized Genetic Initiative (PROGENI)
P. Research The Organized Genetic Initiative study
P. sign
P. Study Group (PSG)
P. triangle
parkinsonian
p. crisis
p. dysarthria
p. gait
p. postmenopausal women
p. symptom
p. syndrome
parkinsonism
amyotrophy p.
atypical p.
autosomal recessive juvenile p. (ARJP)
deprenyl and tocopherol antioxidative therapy of p. (DATATOP)
drug-induced p.
hypersomnia p.
juvenile p.
postencephalitic p.
p. tremor
vascular p.
parkinsonism-dementia
Parkinson-plus syndrome
Parlodel
Parnate
parolfactory, parolfactoria
p. area
p. sulcus
parolivary body
parosmia
parotid
p. dissection
p. duct
p. nerve
p. plexus
p. tumor
parotideus
plexus p.
parotitis
paroxetine
paroxysm
childhood epilepsy with occipital p.
multifocal p.
paroxysmal
p. alpha activity
p. atrial fibrillation
p. bursting
p. cerebral dysrhythmia
p. convulsion
p. dystonic choreoathetosis of Mount and Reback
p. epileptiform discharge
p. evoked pain
p. exertional dyskinesia
p. hemicrania
p. hypertension
p. kinesigenic choreoathetosis
p. kinesigenic dyskinesia
p. migraine
p. migraine headache
p. nocturnal dystonia
p. nocturnal hemoglobinuria
p. nonkinesigenic dyskinesia (PNKD)
p. positional nystagmus
p. positional vertigo

p. sleep
p. sleep disorder
p. torticollis

Parrot
P. disease
P. mask
P. sign

Parry-Romberg
P.-R. disease
P.-R. syndrome

pars
p. abdominalis autonomica
p. abdominalis systematis
p. anterior
p. anterior commissurae anterioris
p. anterior commissurae rostralis
p. anterior faciei diaphragmatis hepatis
p. anterior facies diaphragmatis
p. anterior fornicis vaginae
p. anterior fornix vaginae
p. anterior lobuli quadrangularis anterioris
p. anterior pedunculi cerebri
p. anterior pontis
p. autonomica systematis nervosi peripherici
p. basilaris pontis
p. basolateralis corporis amygdaloidei
p. canalis nervi optici
p. caudalis
p. caudalis nervi vestibularis
p. centralis ventriculi lateralis
p. cervicalis arteriae carotidis internae
p. cervicalis ductus thoracici
p. cervicalis esophagi
p. cervicalis medullae spinalis
p. coccygea medullae spinalis
p. cochlearis
p. cochlearis nervi vestibulocochlearis
p. cochlearis nevi octavi
p. compacta
p. compacta substantiae nigrae
p. corticalis
p. corticomedialis corporis amygdaloidei
p. cranialis partis parasympathici divisionis autonomici systematis nervosi
p. cupularis
p. cupularis recessus epitympanici
p. distalis
p. distalis adenohypophyseos
p. dorsalis corporis geniculati lateralis
p. dorsalis corporis geniculati medialis
p. dorsalis lobuli quadrangularis anterioris
p. dorsalis pedunculi cerebri
p. dorsalis pontis
p. duralis fili terminalis
p. flaccida
p. frontalis corporis callosi
p. inferior alae lobuli centralis
p. inferior nervi vestibularis
p. inferoposterior lobuli quadrangularis
p. infraclavicularis plexus brachialis
p. infundibularis
p. insularis
p. interarticularis
p. intermedia
p. intermedia adenohypophyseos
p. intermedia commissura bulborum
p. intermedia lobi anterioris hypophyseos
p. intracranialis nervi optici
p. intralaminaris nervi optici intraocularis
p. intraocularis nervi optici
p. lateralis nuclei accumbentis
p. lumbalis diaphragmatis
p. lumbalis medullae spinalis
p. magnocellularis nucleus
p. medialis nuclei accumbentis
p. nervosa
p. nervosa hypophyseos
p. nervosa neurohypophyseos
p. occipitalis corporis callosi
p. olfactoria corporis amygdaloidei
p. opercularis
p. opercularis gyri frontalis inferioris
p. optica retinae
p. orbitalis
p. orbitalis glandulae lacrimalis
p. orbitalis gyri frontalis inferioris
p. orbitalis musculi orbicularis oculi
p. orbitalis nervi optici

NOTES

P

pars *(continued)*
p. orbitalis ossis frontalis
p. parasympathetica divisionis autonomici systematis nervosi
p. parasympathica
p. parasympathica divisionis automaticae systematis nervosi peripherici
p. parvocellularis nuclei rubri
p. pelvica autonomica
p. pelvica systematis autonomici
p. peripherica
p. peripherica systematis nervosi
p. pharyngea hypophyseos
p. pialis fili terminalis
p. plana
p. plicata
p. posterior commissurae anterioris
p. posterior commissurae rostralis
p. posterior facies diaphragmatis hepatis
p. posterior fornix vaginae
p. posterior lobuli quadrangularis anterioris
p. postlaminalis nervi optici vaginae
p. precommunicalis arteriae cerebri anterioris
p. prelaminaris nervi optici intraocularis
p. reticularis substantiae nigrae
p. reticulata
p. retrolentiformis capsulae internae
p. retrolentiformis cruris posterior
p. rostralis nervi vestibularis
p. sacralis medullae spinalis
p. sellaris
p. sphenoidalis arteriae cerebralis mediae
p. spinalis nervi accessorii
p. sublentiformis capsulae internae
p. sublentiformis cruris posterioris
p. superior ali lobuli centralis
p. superior nervi vestibularis
p. supraclavicularis plexus brachialis
p. sympathica
p. sympathica divisionis autonomici systematis nervosi
p. tensa
p. thalamolenticularis capsulae internae
p. thoracica aortae
p. thoracica autonomica
p. thoracica ductus thoracici
p. thoracica esophagi
p. thoracica medullae spinalis
p. thoracica systematis autonomici
p. triangularis
p. triangularis gyri frontalis inferioris
p. tuberalis
p. vagalis
p. vagalis nervi accessorii
p. vascularis
p. vasculosa
p. ventralis corporis geniculati lateralis
p. ventralis corporis geniculati medialis
p. ventralis lobuli quadrangularis anterioris
p. ventralis pedunculi cerebri
p. ventralis pontis
p. vertebralis
p. vestibularis nervi octavi
p. vestibularis nervi vestibulocochlearis

Parsidol

Parsitan

Parsonage-Aldren-Turner syndrome

Parsonage-Turner
P.-T. disease
P.-T. syndrome

part
autonomic p.
cupular p.
cupulate p.
infundibular p.
intermediate p.
opercular p.
orbital p.
parasympathetic p.
sympathetic p.
triangular p.
vertebral p.

partial
p. agenesis
p. arousal event
p. arterial gas tension of carbon dioxide
p. central hypophysectomy
p. complex epilepsy
p. complex seizure
p. debulking operation
p. disability
p. embolization
p. facetectomy
p. flaccid extremity paralysis
p. flip-angle imaging
p. Fourier imaging
p. hemianopia
p. hemilaminectomy
p. homonymous field defect
p. labyrinthectomy petrous apicectomy approach
p. lipodystrophy phenotype
p. nominal aphasia

p. oxygen pressure of brain tissue ($PbrO_2$)
p. pressure
p. saturation
p. temporal lobe epilepsy
p. thromboplastin time (PTT)
p. venous gas tension of oxygen
p. visual loss

partialis
ophthalmoplegia p.
rachischisis p.

partially clipped aneurysm

partial-onset seizure

partial-thickness craniectomy

particle
p. beam
p. beam radiosurgery
p. domain
electron transport p. (ETP)
Ivalon p.
polyvinyl alcohol p.
proteinaceous infectious p.
signal recognition p. (SRP)
viral p.

particulate embolization

partition
brain-blood p.
low blood gas p.

party nystagmus

parvalbumin (PV)

parvocellularia
strata p.

parvocellularis
nucleus reticularis p.

PAS
periodic acid-Schiff

Pascal Law

PAS-positive circular body

PASS
portal access surgical system
Postural Assessment Scale for Stroke

passage
adiabatic fast p.
wire p.

passer
Malis ligature p.

passive
p. extension
p. flexion
p. movement
p. tremor

paste
calcium phosphatase bone p.
M-ADL p.

Pasteurella
P. meninigitis
P. multocida
P. ureae meningitis

past head injury

Patau syndrome

patch
acetylsalicylic acid p.
blood p.
Dura-Guard dural repair p.
lidocaine transdermal p.
p. pattern
retinal achromic p.
selegiline p.
shagreen p.
striosome p.
Tissue-Guard bovine pericardial p.
transdermal p.
Tutoplast Dura p.

patch-clamp
whole-cell p.-c.

patched gene

patching
lysolecithin p.
monocular p.

patchy retrograde amnesia

patellar
p. clonus
p. plexus
p. tendon reflex

patelloadductor reflex

patellometer

patency
valve p.

patent foramen ovale

pathema

pathematic aphasia

pathergy phenomenon

pathetic nerve

PathFinder
P. pedicle screw system
P. polyaxial screw

pathfinder
Nicolet P. I

pathogen
meningeal p.

pathogenesis
biologic p.

NOTES

pathogenesis *(continued)*
MS p.
poliomyelitis p.
pathogenetic theory
pathogenic
p. dystonia
p. factor
pathognomonic sign
pathologic
p. hyperreflexia
p. intoxication
p. spondylolisthesis
p. spontaneous activity
pathological
p. aggression
p. change
p. communication
p. dissociation
p. drowsiness
p. feature
p. finding
p. grief reaction
p. intoxication
p. level
p. mendicancy
p. mood state
p. personality
p. response
p. sleepiness
p. study
pathology
alpha-synuclein p.
Alzheimer-like p.
anatomic p.
beta-amyloid p.
borderline p.
cerebrovascular p.
cognitive p.
cortical p.
deep white matter p.
dental p.
Down syndrome p.
dual p.
incidental dual p.
ischemic p.
neuronal p.
parietal p.
personality p.
phenotype p.
pontine p.
secondary dual p.
subcortical p.
true dual p.
white matter p.
pathomechanics
kyphotic deformity p.
spinal fusion p.
pathophysiologic
p. factor
p. process
pathophysiological
p. basis
p. cascade
p. role
pathophysiology
p. of delirium
p. of headache
ischemic stroke p.
multiple sclerosis p.
tremor p.
pathway
abducens p.
accessory conduction p. (ACP)
afferent p.
amygdalofugal p.
auditory p.
basal forebrain cholinergic p.
basic brain p.
biochemical p.
brain dopaminergic p.
catabolic p.
catalase p.
catecholaminergic p.
central auditory p.
cerebellar p.
cerebrospinal fluid p.
corticobulbar p.
corticofugal p.
corticospinal motor p.
CSF outflow p.
descending motor p.
dopamine p.
dopaminergic tuberoinfundibular p.
dorsal column sensory p.
efferent p.
extrapyramidal p.
extrathymic p.
final common p.
frontopontocerebellar p.
frontostriatal p.
geniculocortical p.
geniculostriate p.
glutamatergic p.
graviceptive p.
gustatory p.
heat-loss p.
indirect striatopallidal p.
internuncial p.
intracellular metabolic p.
intracortical facilitatory p.
lemniscal p.
limbic system p.
lipoxygenase p.
magnocellular p.
mesocortical dopamine p.
mesolimbic dopamine p.

metabolic p.
migratory p.
monoaminergic p.
MS p.
multisynaptic p.
neural p.
neuroanatomic p.
neurochemical p.
nigropallidal p.
nigrostriatal p.
occulomotor p.
olfactory p.
pain and temperature p.
pentose phosphate p. (PPP)
peptidergic p.
perforant p.
perforating p.
pilomotor p.
pontine cholinergic p.
pyramidal p.
ras signaling p.
reticulocortical p.
retinal p.
retrochiasmal visual p.
sensory p.
serotonergic p.
signal transduction p.
startle p.
stretch reflex p.
sympathoexcitatory brainstem p.
synaptic p.
thalamocortical p.
thymidine salvage p.
trigeminovascular p.
tuberoinfundibular p.
ubiquitin p.
vasoconstrictor p.
ventral amygdalofugal p.
visceromotor p.
visual p.

patient

adult scoliosis p.
akinetic p.
amnesic p.
p. autonomy
bipolar p.
borderline p.
catatonic p.
delirious p.
demented p.
dementia p.
disruptive psychotic p.
dissociative p.
drug-naïve p.
dysphoric p.
first-episode p.
full-dose-treated p.
high-functioning p.
infliximab-treated p.
manic p.
multiple-episode p.
neuroleptic-free p.
neuroleptic-naive p.
never-medicated p.
nonpsychotic Alzheimer p.
peregrinating p.
placebo-treated p.
p. placement criterion
p. positioning
psychotic Alzheimer p.
rapid metabolizer p.
skeletally immature p.
sleepy p.
slow metabolizer p.
suicidal depressed p.
symptomatic p.
treatment-intolerant p.
unipolar p.
variable screw placement system-plated p.

patient-centered approach

patient-controlled analgesia (PCA)

patient-matched

hard tissue replacement-p.-m.
p.-m. implant

Patil

P. stereotactic head frame
P. stereotactic headholder
P. stereotactic system II

Patrick

P. sign
P. test

pattern

aberrant gamma burst p.
alpha p.
anomalous parental vocal p.
Antoni type A, B p.
atypical curve p.
atypical sleep p.
beaten copper p.
breathing p.
p. of care
catamenial seizure p.
change in sleep p.

NOTES

P

pattern *(continued)*
chicken-wire vascular p.
chronic p.
complex fracture p.
connectivity p.
convergence-divergence p.
dermatoglyphic p.
desynchronized discharge p.
discharge p.
double major curve p.
Down syndrome dermatoglyphic p.
EEG alpha p.
electroencephalogram burst suppression p.
electroencephalographic p.
electromyographic incomplete interference p.
p. of expression
field p.
fixed-action p.
p. generator
glycosylation p.
gullwing p.
hair whorl p.
hippocampal p.
hypsarrhythmic electroencephalographic p.
ictal cerebral perfusion p.
ictal EEG p.
ictal epileptiform p.
ineffective communication p.
interictal p.
iris stellate p.
irregular sleep-wake p.
laser speckle p.
left thoracolumbar major curve p.
Lennox-Gastaut p.
localized electroencephalographic seizure p.
maladaptive p.
mendelian p.
mosaic-like p.
multiple sclerosis chronic progressive p.
patch p.
polygenic threshold p.
radiofrequency homogeneity p.
recruitment p.
repeating p.
p. of repetitive behavior
right thoracic left lumbar curve p.
right thoracic minor curve p.
seizure p.
sleep-wake p.
speech p.
spike-and-wave p.
storiform p.
syndromic p.
temporal p.
type II curve p.
unstable injury p.
whorling p.

patterned
p. alopecia
p. stimulus

pattern-induced epilepsy

patterning
gene conservation in p.
gene families in p.
homeoboxes in p.
retinoic acid in p.
p. synaptic connection
transcription factor in p.

pattern-reversal stimulus

pattern-sensitive
p.-s. epilepsy
p.-s. seizure

patting automatism

patty
polyclot p.

pauciimmune necrotizing vasculitis

paucisynaptic

Pauli exclusion principle

Paulus trocar

pause
apneic p.
respiratory p.

paving stone degeneration

Pavlov method

pavor nocturnes

Pavulon

pax gene

Paxil

Paykel classification

Payne syndrome

PBD
peroxisome biogenesis disorder

PBI
protein-bound iodine

PBMC
peripheral blood mononuclear cell

$PbrO_2$
partial oxygen pressure of brain tissue
$PbrO_2$ monitoring probe

PBS
phosphate-buffered saline

PC12 cell

PC-2048B positron emission tomograph

PCA
patient-controlled analgesia
DAT for PCA

PCD
programmed cell death

PCMRA
phase-contrast magnetic resonance angiography

PCNSL
primary central nervous system lymphoma
PComA
posterior communicating artery
PCP
posterior clinoid process
PCR
polymerase chain reaction
false-negative PCR
frataxin gene PCR
X25 PCR
PCV
procarbazine, lomustine (CCNU), vincristine
PCV chemotherapy
PD
phenyldichloroarsine
cyclothymic PD
PDA
polymorphic delta activity
PDA on electroencephalogram
PDD
pervasive development disorder
PDGF
platelet-derived growth factor
PDH
pyruvate dehydrogenase
PDH complex
PDN
prosthetic disc nucleus
PDN device
PDN prosthetic disc
PDQ-39
Parkinson Disease Questionnaire-39
PDQUALIF
Parkinson Disease Quality of Life Scale
PDSS
pediatric daytime sleepiness scale
PE
plasma exchange
PEA
percentage of error in amplitude
peak
p. absorption spike
p. behavioral effect
p. bone mass
Bragg ionization p.
p. expiratory flow rate
P. polyaxial anterior cervical fixation system
p. score
p. systolic velocity
peak-dose
p.-d. choreoathetoid dyskinetic movement
p.-d. dyskinesia
peak-to-peak amplitude
Péan
P. clamp
P. forceps
peapod intervertebral disc forceps
pear bur
pearl
p. chain appearance
p. tumor
pearl-and-string sign
pearly
p. neoplasm
p. tumor
pear-shaped nerve hook
Pearson syndrome
pectineus nerve
pectoral
p. nerve
p. reflex
pectoralgia
pectoralgic
p. migraine
p. migraine headache
pectoralis major muscle
pectoris
Prinzmetal vasospastic angina p.
pediatric
p. and adolescent epilepsy (PAE)
p. autoimmune neuropsychiatric disorder associated with streptococcus (PANDAS)
p. brainstem glioma
p. brain tumor
p. C-D hook
p. Cotrel-Dubousset rod
p. cranium
p. daytime sleepiness scale (PDSS)
p. headrest
p. moyamoya disease
p. MS
p. neurological surgery
p. neuroradiology
p. polypharmacy
p. polysomnography
p. respiratory definition
P. Sleep Questionnaire (PSQ)

NOTES

P

pediatric *(continued)*
p. sleep survey
p. spinal anatomy
p. spinal column injury
p. spinal cord injury
p. stroke from leukemia
p. stroke from Libman-Sacks endocarditis
p. stroke from myocarditis
p. stroke from rheumatic heart disease
p. stroke from septal defect
p. stroke from systemic lupus erythematosus
p. stroke from Takayasu arteritis
p. stroke from thrombocytopenia
p. supratentorial hemispheric tumor
p. TSRH hook
p. Wada testing
pedication
pedicle
p. anatomy
p. awl
p. axis angle
p. C-D hook
p. cortex disruption
p. diameter
p. dimension
p. entrance point
p. evaluation
p. landmark
p. localization
p. location
lower thoracic p.
p. marker
p. morphometry
p. perforation
rigid p.
p. screw
p. screw breakage
p. screw chord length
p. screw construct
p. screw construct peg
p. screw hardware prominence
p. screw insertion
p. screw linkage design
p. screw malformation
p. screw path length
p. screw plating
p. screw pullout strength
p. screw-rod fixation
p. sounding probe
thoracic p.
pedicled pericranial flap
pedicular fixation
pedi-gravity assisted valve
pedionalgia, pedioneuralgia
pedis
nervi digitales dorsales p.
peduncle
caudal cerebellar p. (CCP)
cerebellar p.
cerebral p.
p. of corpus callosum
cranial cerebellar p.
decussation of superior cerebellar p.
p. of flocculus
inferior cerebellar p.
inferior thalamic p.
lateral thalamic p.
p. of mamillary body
middle cerebellar p.
olfactory p.
pineal p.
pontine cerebellar p.
rostral cerebellar p.
superior cerebellar p.
thalamic p.
ventral thalamic p.
peduncular
p. ansa
p. loop
p. vein
pedunculares
rami p.
venae p.
peduncularis
ansa p.
pedunculi (*pl. of* pedunculus)
pedunculomamillaris
fasciculus p.
pedunculomammillary fasciculus
pedunculopontine
p. cholinergic group
p. neuron
p. tegmental nucleus
p. tegmentum
pedunculopontinus
nucleus reticularis trigeminalis p.
nucleus tegmentalis p.
pedunculotomy
pedunculus, pl. **pedunculi**
basis p.
p. cerebellaris caudalis
p. cerebellaris inferior
p. cerebellaris medius
p. cerebellaris superior
pedunculi cerebelli
p. cerebralis
p. cerebri
p. corporis callosi
p. corporis mamillaris
p. corpus pinealis
p. flocculus
pes p.
p. of pineal body
p. thalami inferior

p. thalami lateralis
p. thalami ventralis
PEEP
positive end-expiratory pressure
Peet splanchnic resection
peg
p. electrode
fibular p.
pedicle screw construct p.
Peganone
Peiper-Beyer laminectomy rongeur
peliosis
parenchymal bacillary p.
Pelizaeus-Merzbacher
P.-M. disease
P.-M. leukodystrophy
P.-M. sclerosis
pellagra
Casal necklace appearance in p.
p. dementia
pellet
air gun p.
shotgun p.
pellucidi
cavitas septi p.
cavum septi p.
lamina septi p.
vena anterior septi p.
vena posterior septi p.
pellucidum
anterior vein of septum p.
cavity of septum p.
cavum septum p.
lamina of septum p.
posterior vein of septum p.
septum p.
vein of septum p.
Pelorus
P. stereotactic frame
P. surgical system
pelvic
p. fixation
p. ganglion
p. plexus
pelvica
ganglia p.
pelvici
nervi splanchnici p.
pelvicorum
radix parasympathica gangliorum p.
pelvicus
plexus p.
pelvina
ganglia p.
plexus p.
pelvis
crossed reflex of p.
kyphotic p.
pelvofemoral muscular dystrophy
PEMF
pulsed electromagnetic field
pemoline
Pena-Shokeir syndrome
pencil-grip instrument
Pende sign
pendetide
satumomab p.
Pendred syndrome
pendular nystagmus
pendulum of diagnosis
penetrating
p. brain injury
p. neck wound
p. spinal injury
p. trauma
penetration
anterior cortex p.
antibiotic p.
dural p.
facioorbital p.
spinal canal p.
vertebral body anterior cortex p.
Penfield hypothesis
penicillamine
penicillamine-induced myasthenia gravis
penile
p. reflex
p. tumescence
penis
nervi cavernosi p.
nervus dorsalis p.
p. reflex
Penn cube function formula
pentaacetate
pentastarch
pentobarbital
p. coma
p. in status epilepticus
pentose phosphate pathway (PPP)
pentoxifylline
pentylenetetrazol
penumbra
ischemic p.
penumbral region

NOTES

PEO
progressive external ophthalmoplegia
Pepper
P. neuroblastoma
P. syndrome
P. tumor
peptide
Abeta p.
alpha beta p.
amyloid beta p.
atrial natriuretic p. (ANP)
brain natriuretic p. (BNP)
calcitonin gene-related p. (CGRP)
p. cotransmitter
C-type natriuretic p.
p. inhibitor
muramyl p.
opioid p.
vasoactive intestinal p.
peptidergic
p. fiber
p. pathway
percentage of error in amplitude (PEA)
perception
altered spatial p.
altered time p.
p. analysis
auditory p.
complex visual p.
p. of disability
figure-ground p.
heightened sensory p.
narrative speech p.
olfactory p.
spatial p.
speech p.
taste quality p.
time p.
perceptorium
perceptual
p. aspect
p. disturbance
p. emotive stimulus
p. error
p. filtering
p. identification test
p. level
p. motor skill
p. process
perceptual/cognitive mechanism
perceptual-motor ability impairment
perchlorate extract
Perclose closure device
percussion
distal tingling on p. (DTP)
p. hammer
percutaneous
p. approach
p. assisted technique
p. balloon commissurotomy
p. cabling
p. cordotomy
p. discoscope
p. electrode array
p. endoscopic recanalization
p. epidural electrode
p. intraarterial embolization
p. laser nucleolysis
p. radiofrequency gangliolysis
p. radiofrequency retrogasserian rhizotomy (PRFR)
p. radiofrequency rhizolysis
p. radiofrequency sympathectomy
p. retrogasserian glycerol chemoneurolysis
p. retrogasserian glycerol rhizolysis (PRGR)
p. retrogasserian glycerol rhizotomy
p. spinal endoscope
p. stimulation
p. thecoperitoneal shunt
p. thermocoagulation
p. transvenous coil embolization
p. trigeminal nerve compression
peregrinating patient
perencephaly
Perez reflex
perfection
manie de p.
perfluorocarbon
perfluorooctyl bromide
perforans
nervus cutaneous p.
perforant pathway
perforatae
habenulae p.
perforated space
perforating
p. bur
p. cutaneous nerve
p. pathway
perforation
esophageal p.
pedicle p.
vascular p.
perforator
Acra-Cut cranial p.
Aesculap skull p.
cranial p.
Cushing cranial p.
Heifetz cranial p.
Heifetz skull p.
Hudson p.
powered automatic skull p.
Raney p.
perforatum
hypericum p.

performance
cognitive p.
error-free p.
p. level
memory p.
memory-continuous p.
neuropsychologic p.
novel task p.
P. Oriented Balance and Mobility Assessment
recall p.
P. Scale Score
task p.
Taylor complex figure task p.
vocational p.
work p.
Perf-Plate cranial plate
perfusate
p. drip
luminal p.
perfusion
cerebral p.
critical p.
p. deficit
frontal brain p.
luxury p.
microcirculatory p.
misery p.
transcardiac p.
perfusion-weighted
p.-w. imaging
p.-w. MRI
pergolide mesylate
perhexiline maleate
periamygdaloid
p. area
p. cortex
perianal reflex
perianeurysmal hemorrhage
periapical abscess
periaqueductal
p. central gray
p. glioma
p. gray matter
p. gray substance
p. hemorrhage
p. pneumatization
periarterial
p. plexus of choroid artery
p. sympathectomy
periarterialis
plexus p.
periarteritis nodosa
periaxial
p. neuritis
p. neuropathy
periaxialis
encephalitis p.
periaxonal
pericallosa
cisterna p.
pericallosal
p. azygos artery
p. cistern
pericapillary encephalorrhagia
pericardial reflex
pericentromeric region of chromosome 16q
pericephalic edema
periclaustral lamina
pericorpuscular synapse
pericranial temporalis flap
pericranii
sinus p.
pericranitis
pericranium
pericyte edema generation
pericytosis
peridendritic
peridural
peridurale
spatium p.
periencephalitis
periependymal myelitis
perifascicular
p. atrophy
p. migration
perifocal edema
periforaminal
perifornical
p. area
p. nucleus
perifornicalis
nucleus p.
perigangliitis
periganglionic
perigemmal cell
periglomerular cell
perihematomal
perihypoglossal
p. nuclear complex
p. nucleus
perikaryon, pl. **perikarya**
perilesional inhibitory cortex

NOTES

P

perilimbal flush
perilymph
p. bathing
p. fistula (PLF)
perilymphatic
p. duct
p. fistula
perilymphaticus
ductus p.
perilymph fistula (PLF)
perimedullary venous system
perimeningitis
perimesencephalic
p. cistern
p. nonaneurysmal subarachnoid hemorrhage
perimetry
Goldman p.
kinetic p.
perimyelitis
perimysium
perinatal
p. anoxia
p. asphyxia
p. clavicle fracture
p. craniocerebral trauma
p. development
p. event in history
p. humerus fracture
p. obturator nerve injury
p. trauma infarction
p. unilateral cerebral ischemic insult
perineal
p. nerve
p. post
perineural
p. anesthesia
p. fibroblastoma
p. infiltration
perineuria (*pl. of* perineurium)
perineurial cyst
perineuritis
perineurium, pl. **perineuria**
perineuronal
p. end foot
p. space
perinuclear
period
absolute refractory p.
amblyogenic p.
apneustic p.
cluster p.
ictal p.
interictal p.
latent p.
p. line
major risk p.
oral biting p.
readout p.
relative refractory p.
sensorimotor p.
silent p.
sleep onset p. (SOP)
sleep-onset rapid eye movement p. (SOREMP)
treatment p.
periodic
p. acid-Schiff (PAS)
p. acid-Schiff-hematoxylin stain
p. alternating gaze
p. alternating nystagmus (PAN)
p. breathing
p. edema
p. hemilingual numbness
p. lateralizing epileptiform discharge (PLED)
p. leg movement
p. limb movement (PLM)
p. limb movement disorder (PLMD)
p. limb movement during sleep (PLMS)
p. migrainous neuralgia
p. paralysis
p. sharp-wave complex
p. vestibular ataxia (PVA)
periolivares
nuclei p.
periolivary nucleus
perioperative
p. anoxia
p. cisternography
p. complication
p. morbidity
p. mortality
p. reduction
perioptic
p. meningioma
p. subarachnoid space
perioral eruption
periorbital ecchymosis
periosteal
p. elevator
p. reflex
periostitis interna cranii
peripachymeningitis
peripapillary nerve fiber layer
peripapullar astrocyte
peripartum stroke
peripatetic
peripeduncularis
nucleus p.
peripeduncular nucleus
peripheral
p. antimuscarinic side effect
p. aromatization
p. avulsion

p. benzodiazepine receptor
p. blood lymphocyte
p. blood mononuclear cell (PBMC)
p. catecholamine
p. catecholamine receptor
p. chemoreceptor
p. cholinergic activity
p. deafferentation pain
p. dysarthria
p. electromyographic activity
p. facial paralysis
p. glioma
p. motoneuron
p. myelin protein 22
p. nerve
p. nerve axotomy
p. nerve cell
p. nerve disease
p. nerve entrapment syndrome
p. nerve fascicle
p. nerve injury
p. nerve lesion
p. nerve level motor impairment
p. nerve myelin
p. nerve myelination
p. nerve neurapraxia
p. nerve neuroma
p. nerve pressure palsy
p. nerve regeneration
p. nerve regeneration conduit
p. nerve sheath tumor
p. nerve trauma
p. nervous system (PNS)
p. nervous system disorder
p. neuralgia
p. neuroectodermal tumor
p. neurofibromatosis
p. neuroglia
p. neuropathic pain syndrome
p. neuropathy
p. nociceptor activation
p. nociceptor sensitization
p. norepinephrine
p. nystagmus
p. occulomotor palsy
p. oculomotor lesion
p. paraplegia
p. part of nervous system
p. sensory loss
p. sensory neuron
p. steroid hormone
p. tabes
p. tissue
p. trigeminal nerve branch
p. vascular disease
p. vasomotor disturbance
p. vertigo
p. vestibular system

peripherally
p. acting anticholinergic medication
p. inserted central catheter (PICC)

peripheraphose

peripherica
pars p.

peripherici
divisio autonomica systematis nervosi p.
pars autonomica systematis nervosi p.
pars parasympathica divisionis automaticae systematis nervosi p.

periphericum
systema nervosum p.

periphery dose

periphlebitis retinae

perirolandic parietal cortex

perisinusoidal lacuna

perispondylitis

perissodactylous

peristriate
p. area
p. cortex

perisylvian
p. cortex
p. microgyria
p. polymicrogyria
p. region
p. ulegyria

perithelial small cell sarcoma

peritoneal catheter

peritoneum

peritorcular meningioma

peritraumatic predictor

peritrigeminalis
nucleus p.

peritrigeminal nucleus

Peritrode

peritumoral
p. band
p. brain edema

periungual fibroma

perivascular
p. change
p. cuff

NOTES

perivascular *(continued)*
p. cuffing
p. end foot
p. gliosis
p. macrophage
p. mononuclear cell
p. nerve
p. nerve-ending stimulation
p. sheath
p. space
periventricular
p. disease
p. fiber
p. gray (PVG)
p. gray matter
p. gray matter area
p. gray region
p. gray substance
p. hyperintense lesion
p. hyperintensity
p. leukemia
p. leukomalacia (PVL)
p. neuron
p. nodular heterotopia
p. preoptic nucleus
p. radiolucency
p. white matter
p. white matter lesion
p. zone
periventriculares
fibrae p.
periventricular-intraventricular hemorrhage (PIH)
periventricularis
nucleus preopticus p.
zona p.
perivenular inflammation
perizonalium
nuclei camporum p.
Perlia
convergence nucleus of P.
P. nucleus
Perls stain
permanent
p. cranial nerve deficit
p. injury
p. magnet
p. section
p. sympathectomy
p. vegetative state
p. visual loss
Permax
permissive substrate
Perneczky-designed microscope-assisting endoscope
pernicious anemia
peroneal
p. entrapment neuropathy
p. muscular atrophy
p. nerve
p. nerve lesion
p. nerve palsy
p. paralysis
p. phenomenon
p. sign
p. somatosensory evoked potential
peroneales
nervi p.
peroxidase
glutathione p.
peroxidation
lipid p.
peroxisomal
p. disease
p. metabolic disorder
peroxisome biogenesis disorder (PBD)
peroxynitrite anion
perpendicular fasciculus
perphenazine and amitriptyline hydrochloride
Perroncito
P. apparatus
P. spiral
perseverative agraphia
persistence
cerebral artery fetal p.
persistent
p. clonus
p. daily headache
p. developmental stuttering
p. facial palsy
p. hyperplastic primary vitreous (PHPV)
p. primary insomnia
p. primitive carotid-basilar artery anastomosis
p. rumination
p. tremor
p. trigeminal artery anastomosis
p. vegetative state (PVS)
personality
abnormal p.
p. abnormality
amoral p.
brooding p.
p. change
p. dimension
p. disorder instrument
interictal epileptic p.
mixed-type psychopathic p.
neurasthenic p.
pathological p.
p. pathology
p. theory
perspective
behavioral p.
biologic p.
developmental p.

functional anatomical p.
linear p.
neurobiological p.
psychoanalytic p.
psychosocial p.
religious p.
symptomatic p.
perspective-taking skill
perspiration artifact
persuades
glutathione p. (GSHPx)
Perthes-Bankart lesion
Pertofrane
Pertscan 99m
perturbation
p. magnitude
postural p.
torque-pulse p.
pertussis-toxin-catalyzed ADP-ribosylation
pertussis vaccination encephalopathy
pervasive
p. developmental disorder
p. development disorder (PDD)
p. inhibition
pes
p. anserinus
p. cavus deformity
p. cavus in Friedreich ataxia
p. hippocampus
p. pedunculus
pesticide exposure
pestis
Yersinia p.
PET
positron emission tomography
PET image
nonstereotactic PET
PET scan
PET technique
***Petasites hybridus* root**
petechia, pl. **petechiae**
petechial hemorrhage
PET-FDG
positron emission tomography-fluorodeoxyglucose
PET-guided stereotactic biopsy
pethidine
petit
p. mal
p. mal epilepsy
p. mal seizure
p. mal status
p. mal variant
P. syndrome
petroclinoclival meningioma
petroclinoid fold
petroclival
p. cholesterol granuloma
p. lesion
p. meningioma
p. tumor
petroclivotentorial meningioma
petrooccipitalis
fissura p.
petrosa
vena p.
petrosal
p. approach
p. draining group
p. ganglion
p. impression of pallium
p. nerve
p. neuralgia
p. sinus
p. sinus sampling
petrosectomy
petrositis
petrosphenoidal ligament
petrosphenoid syndrome
petrosquamosal sinus
petrosquamous
p. sinus
p. suture
petrous
p. apex
p. apex mass
p. bone
p. bone tumor
p. carotid artery
p. carotid-to-intradural carotid saphenous vein graft
p. ganglion
p. ridge chemodectoma
Pette-Döring
P.-D. disease
P.-D. panencephalitis
petty durotomy
Peyronie disease
Peyton brain spatula
Pfeiffer syndrome
Pfuhl sign
PGD
phosphogluconate dehydrogenase
P-glycoprotein

NOTES

PGR
psychogalvanic response
phacoma, phakoma
phacomatosis, phakomatosis
phagocytosis
phakoma (*var. of* phacoma)
phalangeal cell
Phalen
P. maneuver
P. sign
P. test
phantom
p. absence seizure
p. arm
p. base
Compass stereotactic p.
3-dimensional SPECT p.
gelatin p.
p. hand
hot-spot p.
p. image
p. limb
p. limb pain
p. limb phenomenon
Plexiglas p.
radiological p.
sensory p.
p. shock syndrome
p. tooth pain
phantosmia
PHA-P
phytohemagglutinin A-P
pharmaceutical
unconventional p.
pharmacodynamic interaction
pharmacogenomics
pharmacokinetic
p. interaction
p. parameter
protein-binding p.
pharmacologic
p. agent
p. factor
p. impact
p. intervention
p. sensitivity
pharmacological
p. agent
p. antagonism
p. approach
p. armamentarium
p. blockade
p. difference
p. intervention
p. mechanism
p. predictor
p. property
p. stimulus
pharmacology of sleep
pharmacoresistent epilepsy
pharmacotherapy
conventional p.
p. regimen
pharyngeal
p. airway
p. anesthesia
p. cleft
p. constrictor muscle
p. fat pad
p. hypophysis
p. plexus of vagus nerve
p. pouch
p. reflex
p. tissue
p. tubercle
p. wall
p. weakness
pharyngeal-brachial palsy
pharyngeus
nervus p.
pharyngismus
pharyngoplegia
pharyngospasm
pharyngotympanic cephalalgia
phase
absolute construction of p.
p. angle
ascension p.
p. cancellation
p. coherence
p. cycling
delayed sleep p.
p. encoding
extradural p.
p. instability
intradural p.
p. mapping
p. position
postambivalent p.
recovery p.
reference p.
relaxation p.
p. reversal
p. reversal potential
rising p.
p. shift
tonic p.
transverse magnetization p.
treatment p.
vector p.
walking swing p.
phase-contrast
p.-c. magnetic resonance angiography (PCMRA)
p.-c. map
p.-c. method
p.-c. technique

phased-array
p.-a. coil
p.-a. color-flow ultrasound system
phase-dependent
phase-encoding
p.-e. direction
p.-e. gradient
phase-sensitive
p.-s. detector
p.-s. gradient-echo MR imaging
phase-shift effect
phasic
p. alertness
p. nystagmus
p. reflex
p. twitching
phenacemide
phenacetin
phencyclidine
p. and amphetamine/methamphetamine
p. delirium
p. hydrochloride
p. intoxication
methylenedioxymethamphetamine and p.
p. thiophene
phenobarbital
ephedrine, theophylline, p.
very high dose p.
phenol
p. motor point block
p. neurolysis
phenolphthalein
phenolsulfonphthalein (PSP)
phenomena (*pl. of* phenomenon)
phenomenalistic causality
phenomenological
p. characteristic
p. measure
phenomenology
clinical p.
delirium p.
phenomenon, pl. **phenomena**
alien limb p.
arm p.
Babinski p.
baked brain p.
Bell p.
bilateral motor phenomena
breakthrough p.
centralization p.
cervicolumbar p.
cheek p.
clasp-knife p.
clinical p.
cogwheel p.
crankshaft p.
crossed phrenic p.
Cushing p.
Dandy-Walker p.
Dejerine hand p.
Dejerine-Lichtheim p.
doll's eye p.
doll's head p.
Duckworth p.
embolic p.
Erben p.
escape p.
facialis p.
finger p.
freezing p.
Galassi pupillary p.
Gibbs p.
Gowers p.
Grasset p.
Grasset-Gaussel p.
Gunn p.
halo p.
hemifield slide p.
hidden observer p.
hip p.
hip-flexion p.
Hochsinger p.
Hoffmann p.
Holmes p.
Holmes-Stewart p.
Hunt paradoxic p.
interictal p.
intracranial steal p.
ischemic p.
jaw-winking p.
Kernohan notch p.
Kienböck p.
knee p.
Kohnstamm p.
Kühne p.
leg p.
Leichtenstern p.
Lhermitte p.
Lust p.
Marcus Gunn p.
Mayer-Gross closing-in p.
mental p.

NOTES

P

phenomenon *(continued)*
misdirection p.
motor p.
Negro p.
neurobiological p.
no-reflow p.
on-off p.
overuse p.
paradoxical diaphragm p.
paradoxical pupillary p.
pathergy p.
peroneal p.
phantom limb p.
Philippe-Gombault p.
polyspike-spike wave p.
Pool p.
psychomotor p.
psychotic-like p.
Pulfrich p.
Queckenstedt p.
radial p.
Raynaud p.
rebound p.
release p.
Riddoch p.
Ritter-Rollet p.
Rust p.
Schiff-Sherrington p.
Schlesinger p.
Schramm p.
Schüller p.
seizurelike p.
Sherrington p.
soft psychotic-like p.
Souques p.
springlike p.
staircase p.
steal p.
Strümpell p.
suction p.
tibial p.
toe p.
tongue p.
transient visual p.
Trousseau p.
twilight p.
Uhthoff p.
vacuum p.
visual p.
warmup p.
wearing-off p.
Wedensky p.
Wernicke hemianopic pupillary p.
Westphal p.
Westphal-Piltz p.
Wever-Bray p.

phenomenon/syndrome
Fregoli p./s.
jet lag p./s.

phenothiazine toxic effect

phenotype
alcohol-related p.
Charcot-Marie-Tooth p.
clinical p.
DMD p.
headache p.
malignant p.
membrane p.
myelinating p.
neuropathic p.
partial lipodystrophy p.
p. pathology

phenotypic
p. expression
p. factor
p. heterogenicity
p. marker
p. study

phenoxybenzamine

phenylalanine
p. hydroxylase deficiency
p. hydroxylase therapy in phenylketonuria
p. serum level

phenylalaninemia

phenylalanine-restricted diet

phenylbutazone

phenylbutyrate

phenyldichloroarsine (PD)

phenylethylmalonamide

phenylketonuria (PKU)
p. genetic factor
phenylalanine hydroxylase therapy in p.
p. treatment

phenylpiperazine

phenylpiperidine

phenylpropanolamine

phenylpropylamine

phenyl-*t*-butyl-nitrone

Phenytek

phenytoin-induced
p.-i. chorea
p.-i. choreoathetosis

phenytoin interaction with other drugs

pheochromocytoma and neuroblastoma localization study

pheromonal

pheromone

Philadelphia
P. collar
P. halo

Philippe-Gombault phenomenon

Philippe triangle

Philips
P. Gyroscan S5, S15
P. linear accelerator
1.5T P. Intera-NT system

P. Tomoscan
P. 400 transmission electron microscope
Philly bolt
Phineas Gage syndrome
phi rhythm
phlebitis
sinus p.
phlebography
PHN
postherpetic neuralgia
phobia
blood/injection p.
isolated p.
p. reaction
universal p.
phobia-induced migraine headache
phobic
p. postural vertigo
p. reaction
Phoenix
P. ancillary valve
P. Anti-Blok ventricular catheter
P. cranial drill
P. cruciform valve
P. fifth ventricle system
pholcodine
phonatory spasm
phonemic paraphasia
phonetic
p. input
p. noise
p. paralysis
p. stimulus
phonic spasm
phonoangiography
quantitative spectral p.
phonologic
p. assembly impairment
p. syntactic syndrome
phonological
p. agraphia
p. mismatch negativity (PMN)
p. process
phonomyoclonus
phonomyography
phonophobia
phonoreceptor
phoria
phosphatase
alkaline p.
pyruvate dehydrogenase p.
tyrosine p.
phosphate
p. buffer
dibasic calcium p.
disopyramide p.
p. disorder
Hexadrol P.
Hydrocortone P.
p. metabolism
nicotinamide adenine dinucleotide p. (NADPH)
potassium phosphate and sodium p.
sodium p.
triorthocresyl p. (TOCP)
phosphate-buffered saline (PBS)
phosphate-regulating gene
phosphate-wasting syndrome
phosphatidylinositol
phosphatidylserine (PO)
phosphene
3′-phosphoadenosine 5′-phosphosulfate
phosphofructokinase transferase deficiency
phosphogluconate dehydrogenase (PGD)
phosphoglycerate
p. kinase
p. kinase deficiency
p. mutase
p. mutase deficiency
phosphoinositol metabolite
phosphokinase
creatine p.
phospholipid
p. hydroperoxide
membrane p.
phospholipid-related signal transduction
phosphoribosyl pyrophosphate synthetase superactivity
phosphoribosyltransferase
hypoxanthine guanine p.
phosphorus
p. nuclear magnetic resonance spectroscopy
serum p.
phosphorylase
p. deficiency
p. kinase
liver p.
muscle p.
phosphorylate tau protein

NOTES

P

phosphorylation
oxidative p.
posttranslation p.
protein tyrosine p.
tau p.
5′-phosphosulfate
adenosine 5′-p. (APS)
3′-phosphoadenosine 5′-p.
phosphotungstic acid hematoxylin (PTAH)
photalgia
photesthesia
photic
p. afterdischarge
p. driving
p. stimulation
p. stimulation activating technique
p. stimulus
photic-induced epileptiform activity
photic-sneeze reflex
photism
photoaffinity labeling
photochemically induced graded spinal cord infarction
photocoagulation
laser p. (LPC)
in situ p.
photoconvulsive
photodynamic therapy
photodynia
photodysphoria
photoesthetic
photofrin porfimer sodium
photogenic epilepsy
photographic memory
photometrazol
photomicrograph
photomicroscope
Zeiss IIIRS p.
photomyoclonic jerk
photomyoclonus
hereditary p.
photon
p. beam radiosurgery
p. knife
p. radiosurgery system
p. ray
photonic radiosurgical system
photoparoxysmal response (PPR)
photophobia
photophobic
photopsia
photoptarmosis
photoradiation therapy
photoreceptor
ocular p.
photosensitive seizure
photosensitivity
photosensitizer
photothrombosis
arterial p.
photothrombotic infarction
phototransduction
humoral p.
pH paradox
PHPV
persistent hyperplastic primary vitreous
phrenalgia
phrenectomy (*var. of* phrenicectomy)
phrenemphraxis
phrenic
p. ganglion
p. mononeuropathy
p. motor neuron
p. motor nucleus
p. nerve
p. nerve conduction time
p. nerve injury
p. nerve lesion
p. nerve paralysis
p. neuropathy
p. nucleus of anterior column of spinal cord
p. plexus
phrenica
ganglia p.
phrenicectomy, phrenectomy, phrenicoexeresis
phrenici
nucleus nervi p.
rami phrenicoabdominales nervi p.
ramus pericardiacus nervi p.
phreniclasia
phrenicoabdominal nerve
phrenicoexeresis (*var. of* phrenicectomy)
phreniconeurectomy
phrenicotomy
phrenicotripsy
phrenicus
nervus p.
phrenoglottic
phrenologist
phrenology
phrenoplegia
phrenospasm
phrenotropic agent
phthisica
spes p.
phthisis bulbus
***Phycomycetes rhizopus* infection**
phylogenetic predecessor
phylogeny of sleep
Phynox cobalt alloy clip material
physaliphore
physaliphorous cell
physical
p. activity
p. attack

p. comorbid disorder
p. danger
p. disturbance
p. exercise
p. functioning
p. injury
p. integrity
p. pain
p. skill
p. therapy
physicochemical
p. interaction
p. principle
physiognomic
physiologic
p. epilepsy
p. sleep paralysis
p. slowing
p. tetanus
p. tremor
p. vertigo
p. zero
physiological
p. antagonism
p. arousal
p. artifact
p. component
p. drive
p. hyperarousal
p. reflex
physiology
age-related sleep p.
normal human p.
respiratory p.
p. of women
physiopsychic
physiotherapy treatment
physocephaly
phytanic acid level
phytohemagglutinin A-P (PHA-P)
phytol metabolism
phytonadione
pi
pi procedure
pi rhythm
pia
p. mater
p. mater cranialis
p. mater encephali
p. mater spinalis
pia-arachnoid cell
pial
p. arteriovenous malformation
p. artery
p. cortical vessel
p. funnel
p. part of filum terminale
p. terminal filament
p. tissue
p. vascular plexus
pial-glial membrane
pianist's cramp
piarachnitis
piarachnoid
PICA
posterior inferior cerebellar artery
posterior inferior communicating artery
PICA aneurysm
PICA index
PICC
peripherally inserted central catheter
Pick
P. atrophy
P. body
P. bundle
P. cell
P. disease
P. inclusion
P. syndrome
Picker scanner
Picornaviridae
picornavirus
pictorial aphasia
picture
Allen p.
compromised neurologic p.
picture-caption pair
picture-in-picture technique
piesesthesia
piesimeter, piezometer
piezoelectric
p. band
p. potential
piezoresistive transducer
PIF
prolactin-inhibiting factor
pigment
acute posterior multifocal placoid p.
p. epithelial lesion
p. gene
melanin p.
pigmentary retinopathy

NOTES

pigmentation
pigmentation-related gene
pigmented
p. layer of retina
p. villonodular synovitis (PVS)
pigmenti
incontinentia p.
pigmentosa
neuropathy, ataxia, retinitis p. (NARP)
retinitis p.
pigmentosum
xeroderma p.
PIH
periventricular-intraventricular hemorrhage
pili torti
pillar
p. cell
p. cell of Corti
Corti p.
p. of fornix
pillar-and-post microsurgical retractor
pillow
Mediflow p.
molded vacuum p.
pill-rolling tremor
pilocytic juvenile astrocytoma
piloid
p. astrocytoma
p. gliosis
pilomatrixoma
pilomotor
p. fiber
p. nerve
p. pathway
p. reflex
pilomyxoid astrocytoma
pilonidal sinus
pilot program
Piltz sign
pimethixene
pimozide
PIN
prostatic intraepithelial neoplasia
PIN entrapment
pin
AO guide p.
p. fixation headrest
halo p.
p. headholder
Kirschner p.
p. loosening
Mayfield disposable skull p.
Mayfield skull cap p.
p. sensation
Steinmann p.
Synthes guide p.
torlone fixation p.
pincer grip
pinch
digital p.
pindolol
pineal
p. body
p. cell
p. cell tumor
p. cyst
p. germinoma
p. gland
p. habenula
p. lesion
p. meningioma
p. parenchymal neoplasm
p. parenchymal tumor
p. peduncle
p. recess
p. region
p. regional choriocarcinoma
p. region mass
p. region teratoma
p. region tumor
p. stalk
p. ventricle
pineale
chief cell of corpus p.
corpus p.
parenchymatous cell of corpus p.
pinealectomy
pinealis
glandula p.
pedunculus corpus p.
recessus p.
pinealoblastoma
pinealocyte
pinealocytoma
pinealoma
ectopic p.
extrapineal p.
pinealopathy
pineoblastoma
pineocytoma
ping-pong
p.-p. appearance
p.-p. fracture
p.-p. gaze
pinion
p. headholder
Mayfield p.
pinocytosis
pinocytotic vesicle
pinprick
p. pain
p. response
skin surface p.
pins-and-needles sensation
pinwheel
Safe-T-Wheel p.

Piotrowski sign
pipecolic acid level
piperazine neurotoxicity
piperidine
piperidyl
pipe stemming of ankle-brachial index
PIPIDA
paraisopropyliminodiacetic acid
technetium-99m PIPIDA
pipradrol
PI-R
plasma immunoreactive
piracetam
piribedil
piriform, pyriform
p. area
p. cortex
p. lobe
p. nerve
p. neuron
p. neuron layer
p. softening
piriformis
nervus musculi p.
p. syndrome
piriformium
stratum neuronorum p.
pirlindole
Pisces electrode
Pisces-Quad electrode
pistol-grip instrument
piston
MTS electrohydraulic p.
Pitanguy
P. oval skin resection
P. plastic surgery
pitch contour
Pitt-Rogers-Dank syndrome
Pittsburgh
P. gamma knife group
P. Sleep Quality Index
pituicyte
pituicytoma
pituitaria
glandula p.
pituitary
p. abscess
p. adamantinoma
p. adenoma
p. adiposity
p. ameloblastoma
p. apoplexy
p. autoimmunity
p. basophilia
p. cachexia
p. curette
p. dwarfism
p. dysfunction
p. dystopia
p. forceps
p. gland
hyaline body of p.
p. hypoplasia
p. infarction
p. macroadenoma
p. microadenoma
p. necrosis
p. portal system
p. prolactin release
p. replacement therapy
p. spoon
p. stalk
p. stalk lesion
p. stalk section
p. tumor
PIVKA
protein induced by vitamin K absence
pivotal role
pizotifen
PKC
protein kinase C
PKU
phenylketonuria
placebo-controlled
p.-c. drug study
p.-c. trial
placebo response rate
placebo-treated patient
4-place laminectomy
placement
bone graft p.
carotid artery angioplasty and stent p.
clip p.
computer-assisted p.
endosaccular coil p.
International 10–20 system of electrode p.
Kirschner wire p.
K-wire p.
nasopharyngeal electrode p.
nursing home p.
odontoid screw p.
plate p.

NOTES

P

placement *(continued)*
posterolateral bone graft p.
rod p.
sacral screw p.
screw p.
shunt p.
subdural electrode p.
therapeutic school p.
therapeutic vocational p.
variable screw p.
placing reaction
placode
neural p.
placoid pigment epitheliopathy
PLACS
protease-linked activation cloning system
plagiocephaly
lambdoid p.
plain
Citanest P.
p. forceps
p. radiography
p. tomography
p. x-ray
plana
pars p.
planar
p. reconstruction
p. spin imaging
p. stereotaxic atlas of human brain
plane
Aeby p.
arachnoid p.
coronal insonation p.
frontal p.
frontoparallel p.
parietal p.
sagittal p.
sensitive p.
subplatysmal p.
superior temporal p.
vertical p.
planning
comprehensive treatment p.
conceptual p.
image-integrated surgery treatment p.
inverse treatment p.
preoperative p.
spatial p.
plant
p. toxic disorder
p. toxin
plantalgia
plantar
p. grasp reflex
p. muscle reflex
p. nerve
planum
fetal p.
p. polare
p. sphenoidale
p. temporale
p. temporale asymmetry
plaque
Abeta-centered neuritic p.
amylase p.
amyloid p.
argyrophil p.
atherosclerotic p.
beta-amyloid p.
chronic p.
cortical neuritic p.
cotton-wool p.
fibromyelinic p.
fibrous p.
p. heterogeneity
Hollenhorst p.
Lichtheim p.
multiple sclerosis p.
neuritic p.
Redlich-Fisher miliary p.
p. reduction assay
p. rupture
sclerotic p.
senile p.
shadow p.
tuberculoma en p.
plasma
p. amyloid beta 40
delta-function arterial p.
p. dopamine beta hydroxylase
p. elastase
p. exchange (PE)
p. factor
p. fatty acid
p. fibrinolytic enzyme system
p. glutamate concentration
p. homocysteine level
p. immunoreactive (PI-R)
p. leptin level
p. membrane dopamine transporter
p. neuropeptide Y
p. protein
p. thromboplastin
plasmacytoma
intracranial p.
primary intracranial p.
plasmapheresis
Plasmatein
plasmin-antiplasmin complex
plasminogen
p. activator (PA)
p. activator inhibitor
Plasmodium falciparum
Plastazote cervical collar

plastic
p. collar
p. compensatory mechanism
p. reorganization
p. scalp clip
plastic-covered hydrogel disc
plasticity
axonal p.
brain p.
cortical p.
dendritic p.
experience-induced cortical p.
lesion-induced cortical p.
neural p.
neuronal p.
somatosensory p.
synapse p.
synaptic p.
plate
alar p.
American Optical Hardy-Rand-Rittler color p.
AO dynamic compression p.
AO reconstruction p.
ASIF broad dynamic compression bone p.
ASIF T p.
basal p.
bone p.
broad AO dynamic compression p.
butterfly-shaped monobloc vertebral p.
cartilage p.
Caspar anterior cervical p.
Caspar trapezoidal p.
cervical p.
commissural p.
contoured anterior spinal p.
cortical p.
cranial bone fixation p.
craniocervical p.
cranioplasty p.
cribriform p.
3D titanium mini bone p.
end p.
E-Z Flap cranial bone p.
p. fixation
floor p.
Hardy-Rand-Rittler p.
Harm posterior cervical p.
Howmedica microfixation cranial p.
Ishihara p.
Kühne terminal p.
Leibinger 3D p.
Leibinger Micro Plus p.
Leibinger Micro System cranial fixation p.
Lorenz cranial p.
Lorenz titanium screws and p.
Luhr microfixation cranial p.
Luhr pan p.
medullary p.
metal p.
Mini Orbita p.
Morscher anterior cervical p.
Morscher titanium cervical p.
narrow AO dynamic compression p.
neural p.
orbital p.
Orion anterior cervical p.
Orozco cervical p.
Perf-Plate cranial p.
p. placement
prochordal p.
Profile anterior spinal p.
Profil-O-Plastic p.
quadrigeminal p.
roof p.
round hole p.
Roy-Camille p.
skull p.
sole p.
spinous process p.
stainless steel preformed skull p.
Steffee p.
Storz Microsystems cranial fixation p.
symmetrical sacral p.
symmetrical thoracic vertebral p.
Synthes cervical p.
Synthes Microsystem cranial fixation p.
tantalum preformed skull p.
tectal p.
terminal p.
thoracolumbosacral p.
titanium p.
TSRH p.
vascular foot p.
vertebral p.
Vitallium p.
wing p.

NOTES

plateau
neurologic p.
platelet
p. count
p. glycoprotein Ia/IIa deficiency
p. glycoprotein IIb/IIIa
p. thromboxane release
platelet-activating factor (PAF)
platelet-derived growth factor (PDGF)
platelet-fibrin embolus
platelet-shaped knife
plate-screw
p.-s. fixation
p.-s. osteosynthesis
plate-spacer washer
platform
positioning p.
StealthStation treatment guidance p.
plating
anterior spinal p.
Caspar p.
pedicle screw p.
posterior spinal p.
Steffee p.
variable spinal p. (VSP)
Platinol
platinum
p. coil
p. coil embolization
p. Dacron microcoil
p. microwire electrode
P. Plus guidewire
p. ring
platinum-based drug
platybasia
platysmal reflex
platysma muscle
Plavix
PLED
periodic lateralizing epileptiform discharge
synchronous bilateral PLED
pledget
cotton p.
cottonoid p.
Gelfoam p.
latex-covered p.
pleiotrophin
pleocytosis
cerebrospinal fluid p.
p. of cerebrospinal fluid
lymphocytic p.
mononuclear p.
pleomorphic
p. adenoma
p. oligodendroglioma
p. xanthoastrocytoma (PXA)
Pletal
plethysmograph
plethysmography
air p.
respiratory inductance p.
venous occlusion p. (VOP)
pleura, pl. **pleurae**
pleurodynia
pleurothotonos, pleurothotonus
plexectomy
plexiform
p. layer
p. layer of cerebral cortex
p. layer of retina
p. neurofibroma
p. neuroma
plexiformis
stria laminae p.
Plexiglas phantom
plexitis
brachial p.
plexopathy
brachial p.
lumbar p.
median sternotomy brachial p.
radiation p.
radiation-induced p.
sacral p.
plexus, pl. **plexus, plexuses**
abdominal aortic p.
anterior cerebral artery p.
anular p.
p. aorticus abdominalis
p. aorticus thoracalis
p. aorticus thoracicus
ascending pharyngeal p.
Auerbach p.
autonomic p.
p. autonomici
p. autonomicus
Batson p.
brachial p.
p. brachialis
cardiac p.
p. cardiacus
p. caroticus communis
p. caroticus externus
p. caroticus internus
carotid p.
cavernous p.
celiac p.
cervical p.
p. cervicalis
choroid p.
p. of choroid artery
p. choroideus
p. choroideus ventriculi lateralis
p. choroideus ventriculi quarti
p. choroideus ventriculi tertii
ciliary ganglionic p.
coccygeal p.

p. coccygeus
p. coeliacus
common carotid nervous p.
communicating branch of facial nerve with tympanic p.
communicating branch of intermediate nerve with tympanic p.
crural p.
Cruveilhier p.
p. deferentialis
p. dentalis inferior
p. dentalis superior
diaphragmatic p.
p. of ductus deferens
p. entericus
epidural venous p.
epigastric p.
Erb-Duchenne-Klumpke injury to brachial p.
esophageal p.
Exner p.
external maxillary p.
external vertebral venous p.
facial p.
p. femoralis
ganglion of autonomic p.
gastric coronary p.
p. gastrici
gastroepiploic p.
p. hypogastricus
p. hypogastricus inferior
p. hypogastricus superior
ileocolic p.
p. iliacus
incisive p.
inferior choroid p.
inferior thyroid p.
infraorbital p.
p. intermesentericus
internal vertebral venous p.
interradial p.
intramural p.
p. intraparotideus
ischiadic p.
Jacobson p.
lienal p.
p. lienalis
lingual p.
p. lumbalis
lumbar p.
p. lumbaris
lumboaortic intermesenteric p.
p. lumbosacralis
maxillary p.
p. of medial cerebral artery
Meissner p.
meningeal p.
p. meningeus
p. mesentericus inferior
p. mesentericus superior
middle hemorrhoidal p.
molecular p.
myenteric p.
nasopalatine p.
nerve p.
p. nervorum spinalium
p. nervosus
p. nervosus celiacus
occipital p.
ophthalmic p.
p. pancreaticus
paravertebral venous p.
parotid p.
p. parotideus
patellar p.
pelvic p.
p. pelvicus
p. pelvina
p. periarterialis
p. pharyngeus nervi vagus
phrenic p.
pial vascular p.
popliteal p.
posterior auricular p.
prevertebral p.
prostatic p.
p. prostaticus
pterygoid p.
p. pulmonalis
rachial p.
p. rectalis inferior
p. rectalis medius
p. rectalis superior
sacral p.
p. sacralis
sagittal p.
Santorini p.
sciatic p.
solar p.
spermatic p.
p. of spinal nerve
spinal nerve p.
p. splenicus

NOTES

plexus *(continued)*
p. subclavius
subdermal p.
submucous intestinal p.
subsartorial p.
p. subserosus
subtrapezius p.
superficial temporal p.
superior hemorrhoidal p.
superior thyroid p.
supraradial p.
p. suprarenalis
sympathetic p.
tentorial p.
thoracic aortic p.
tonsillar p.
p. tympanicus
p. uretericus
p. uterovaginalis
vaginal p.
vascular p.
p. vascularis
venous p.
vertebral p.
p. vertebralis
vesical p.
p. vesicalis
vidian p.
visceral p.
p. visceralis
PLF
perilymph fistula
plica choroidea
plicata
pars p.
pliers
Howmedica microfixation system p.
Leibinger Micro System p.
Luhr microfixation system p.
PLIF
posterior lumbar interbody fusion
PLM
periodic limb movement
PLMD
periodic limb movement disorder
PLMS
periodic limb movement during sleep
PLMS index
PLOSL
polycystic lipomembranous osteodysplasia with sclerosing leukoencephalopathy
plot
funnel p.
PLP
parathyroid hormonelike protein
plug
methylmethacrylate cranioplastic p.
otoconial p.
soaked fat p.
soaked muscle p.
plugging
Obex p.
plumbism
plumbline
coronal p.
sagittal p.
plus
APAP P.
generalized epilepsy with febrile seizures p. (GEFS+)
Medtronic Pisces Quad P.
ophthalmoplegia p.
REMstar P.
Siemens Somatom P.
PME
progressive myoclonus epilepsy
PML
polymorphonuclear leukocyte
progressive multifocal leukoencephalopathy
PMN
phonological mismatch negativity
PMP-22 gene
PMR
polymyalgia rheumatica
PNET
primitive neuroectodermal tumor
pneumatic
p. chair lift
p. cylinder
p. microscope
p. splint mechanism
pneumatization
periaqueductal p.
pneumatocele
p. cranii
extracranial p.
intracranial p.
pneumatorrhachis (*var. of* pneumorrhachis)
pneumatosis
epidural p.
pneumobulbar
pneumocele
extracranial p.
intracranial p.
pneumocephalus
epidural p.
tension p.
pneumococcal
p. infection
p. meningitis
p. pneumonia
pneumocranium
Pneumocystis carinii
pneumoencephalocele
pneumoencephalogram

pneumoencephalography
pneumogastric nerve
pneumogram
pneumograph
pneumonia
hospital-acquired p.
pneumococcal p.
pneumoniae
drug-resistant *Streptococcus p.* (DRSP)
Streptococcus p.
pneumonitis
pneumoorbitography
pneumoplethysmography
ocular p.
pneumorrhachis, pneumatorrhachis
pneumosinus dilatans
pneumotachogram
pneumotachograph
pneumotachometer
pneumotaxic
p. center
p. center of Lumsden
p. localization
pneumotonometry
pneumoventricle
PNF
proprioceptive neuromuscular facilitation
PNF exercise
PNKD
paroxysmal nonkinesigenic dyskinesia
PNS
peripheral nervous system
PO
phosphatidylserine
podospasm, podismus, podospasmus
POEMS
polyneuropathy, organomegaly, endocrinopathy, monoclonal gammopathy, skin changes
POEMS syndrome
point
acupuncture p.
anchoring p.
anterior commissure-posterior commissure reference p.
apophysary p.
apophysial p.
ashi p.
Baker p.
Barker p.
Crutchfield drill p.
entry p.
Erb p.
hysteroepileptogenous p.
p. imaging
Keen p.
Kocher p.
motor p.
multiple sensitive p.'s
p. mutation
pedicle entrance p.
powered automatic-stopping drill p.
pressure p.
pressure-arresting p.
pressure-exciting p.
retromandibular tender p.
sacral brim target p.
p. scanning
self-stopping drill p.
sensitive p.
supraclavicular p.
supraorbital p.
surface p.
sylvian p.
tender p.
time p.
trigger p.
Trousseau p.
Valleix p.
Vogt p.
Vogt-Hueter p.
Ziemssen motor p.
3-point
3-p. bending moment
3-p. fixation frame
3-p. headholder
3-p. headrest
3-p. skull clamp
pointed
p. awl
p. object
pointes
torsades de p.
pointing test
point-resolved spectroscopy (PRESS)
7-point scale
Poiseuille
P. equation
P. law
poisoning
acute alcohol p.
alcoholic p.
arsenic p.

NOTES

P

poisoning *(continued)*
barbiturate p.
carbon monoxide p.
carbon tetrachloride p.
cholinesterase inhibitory p.
curare p.
cyanide p.
ethylene glycol p.
iron p.
Jamaica ginger p.
lead p.
mercury vapor p.
methanol p.
methotrexate p.
methyl alcohol p.
monosodium glutamate p.
muscarine p.
opioid p.
organophosphate pesticide p.
organophosphorus insecticide p.
pyrimethamine p.
strychnine p.
thallium p.
valproic acid p.
poison risk
poker spine
Poland syndrome
polar
p. artery
p. coordinate system
p. spongioblastoma
p. sulcus
polare
planum p.
spongioblastoma p.
Polaris
P. adjustable spinal cage implant
P. camera system
P. position tracker
polarity
dynamic p.
reverse p.
Polar-Mate coagulator
pole
frontal p.
occipital p.
temporal p.
PoleStar
P. magnet
P. N-10 iMRI
poliencephalitis
poliencephalomyelitis
polio
French p.
polioclastic
poliodystrophia
p. cerebri
p. cerebri progressiva infantilis
poliodystrophy
cerebral p.
progressive cerebral p.
progressive infantile p.
polioencephalitis
p. infectiva
inferior p.
superior hemorrhagic p.
polioencephalomeningomyelitis
polioencephalomyelitis
polioencephalopathy
polioencephalotropic
poliomyelencephalitis
poliomyelitis
abortive p.
acute anterior p.
acute bulbar p.
acute lateral p.
acute paralytic p.
anterior p.
ascending p.
bulbar p.
cerebral p.
chronic anterior p.
endemic p.
epidemic p.
p. infection
neonatal p.
nonparalytic p.
paralytic p.
p. pathogenesis
postinoculation p.
postvaccinal p.
spinal paralytic p.
p. treatment
poliomyelitis-induced respiratory failure
poliomyeloencephalitis
poliomyelopathy
poliovirus infection
pollakiuria episode
polus
p. frontalis
p. frontalis hemispherii cerebri
p. occipitalis
p. occipitalis hemispherii cerebri
p. temporalis
p. temporalis cerebri
p. temporalis hemispherii
polyamine biosynthesis inhibitor
polyangiitis
microscopic p.
polyanhydride biodegradable polymer wafer
polyanhydroglucuronic acid
polyarteritis
p. nodosa
p. nodosa group
p. nodosa peripheral neuropathy
polyaxial screw

polyaxonic
polychondritis
relapsing p.
Polycillin-N
Polycitra-K
polyclonal antibody
polyclonia
polyclot patty
polycystic
p. lipomembranous osteodysplasia with sclerosing leukoencephalopathy (PLOSL)
p. ovary syndrome
polycythemia
neonatal p.
p. vera
polydipsia
hysterical p.
polyene thread
polyesthesia
polyethylene
p. intravenous catheter
p. sleeve
ultra-high molecular weight p. (UHMWPE)
polyganglionic mass
polygenic threshold pattern
polyglot
polyglucosan storage disease
polyglutamine
p. disease
p. mutation
p. stretching
p. string
polygram
ictal p.
polygraphic recording
polygyria
polyhydramnios
polyhydroxyethylmethacrylate
polylactic
p. acid
p. acid mesh
polyleptic
polymer
cellulose acetate p.
p. drug delivery
p. encapsulation
HTR p.
Hydrolene p.
implanted p.
polymerase
p. chain reaction (PCR)
p. chain reaction technique
polymerization
polymethylmethacrylate
polymicrogyria
congenital bilateral perisylvian p.
perisylvian p.
polymicrogyric cortex
polyminimyoclonus
polymodal nociceptor
polymorphic
p. delta activity (PDA)
p. epilepsy of childhood
p. neuron
polymorphism
insertion/deletion p.
MAO-A gene p.
restriction fragment length p. (RFLP)
sequence p.
polymorphonuclear leukocyte (PML)
polymorphous layer
polymyalgia
p. arteritica
p. rheumatica (PMR)
polymyoclonus
dentatorubral cerebellar atrophy with p.
polymyositis
interstitial p.
overlap syndrome in p.
polymyositis/dermatomyositis
polymyxin
polyneural
polyneuralgia
polyneuritiformis
heredopathia atactica p.
polyneuritis
acute febrile p.
acute idiopathic p.
acute infective p.
acute postinfective p.
anemic p.
chronic familial p.
cranial p.
erythredema p.
Guillain-Barré p.
infectious p.
Jamaica ginger p.
leprous p.
postinfectious p.

NOTES

P

polyneuromyositis
polyneuronitis
polyneuropathy
acute inflammatory p.
acute inflammatory demyelinating p. (AIDP)
acute painful p.
acute postinfectious p.
alcoholic p.
amyloid p.
anemic p.
arsenic p.
arsenical p.
autoimmune demyelinating p. (AIDP)
axonal p.
axon loss p.
buckthorn p.
carcinomatous p.
chronic inflammatory demyelinating p. (CIDP)
chronic relapsing p.
cranial p.
critical illness p.
demyelinating p.
diabetic sensorimotor p.
diphtheric p.
disimmune p.
distal sensory p. (DSP)
distal symmetric p.
dying-back p.
familial amyloidotic p.
Finnish-type familial amyloid p.
gait disorder, autoantibody, late-age onset p.
generalized p.
gestational p.
idiopathic p.
Indiana-type familial amyloid p.
inflammatory demyelinating p. (IDP)
isoniazid p.
Japanese-type familial amyloid p.
Maryland-type familial amyloid p.
Meretoja-type familial amyloid p.
mitochondrial encephalomyopathy with sensorimotor p.
nitrofurantoin p.
nutritional p.
p., ophthalmoplegia, leukoencephalopathy, and intestinal
p., organomegaly, endocrinopathy, monoclonal gammopathy, skin changes (POEMS)
paraneoplastic p.
porphyric p.
Portuguese-type familial amyloid p.
recurrent p.
Rukavina-type familial amyloid p.
sarcoid p.
segmental demyelinating p.
sensorimotor axonal p.
subacute p.
symmetric p.
symmetrical sensory p.
thallium p.
uremic p.
Van Allen-type familial amyloid p.

polyomavirus
polyopia, polyopsia
polyp
antrochoanal p.

polypectomy
polypeptide
calcitonin gene-related p.
p. hormone gene
vasoactive intestinal p. (VIP)

polypeptidorrhachia
polypharmacy
pediatric p.
rational p.

polyphasic motor unit
polyplegia
polypneic center
polypropylene suture
polyQ
p. ataxia
p. gene

polyradiculitis
polyradiculomyelitis
CMV p.
cytomegalovirus p. (CMV-PRAM)

polyradiculomyopathy
polyradiculoneuritis
acute idiopathic demyelinating p. (AIDP)

polyradiculoneuropathy
acute inflammatory demyelinating p.
chronic inflammatory demyelinating p. (CIDP)
chronic relapsing p.
demyelinating p.
inflammatory demyelinating p.

polyradiculopathy
acute inflammatory demyelinating p.
chronic inflammatory demyelinating p.
diabetic p.

polyrhythmic activity
polysaccharide storage myopathy
polysensitivity
polysensory
polyserositis
polysomnogram
polysomnograph (PSG)
polysomnographic
p. abnormality
p. study

polysomnography
Atlas of p.
digital p.
full-night p.
nocturnal p.
pediatric p.
polysomy
chromosomal p.
polyspike-and-wave
p.-a.-w. activity
p.-a.-w. discharge
polyspike-spike wave phenomenon
polyspike-wave complex
polysynaptic discharge
polytetrafluoroethylene
expanded p. (ePTFE)
polytherapy
rational p.
p. regimen
polytomography
polytrauma
polyvinyl
p. acetate emulsion
p. alcohol
p. alcohol foam
p. alcohol particle
polyvitamin
Pompe disease, type 1, 2
pond fracture
ponesiatrics
ponograph
pons, pl. **pontes**
p. abnormality
anterior part of p.
basilar part of p.
p. cerebelli
dorsal part of p.
p. et cerebellum
pontes grisei caudolenticulares
p. hypertrophy
lower p.
median raphe of p.
oblique bundle of p.
raphe of p.
p. reticular formation
reticular nucleus of p.
tegmentum of p.
transverse fiber of p.
upper p.
p. varolii
vein of p.
ventral part of p.
pontem
rami ad p.
ponticulus promontorii
pontine
p. angioma
p. angle
p. angle tumor
p. apoplexy
p. artery
p. cerebellar peduncle
p. cholinergic pathway
p. cistern
p. corticonuclear fiber
p. flexure
p. glioma
p. gray matter
p. hemianesthesia
p. hemorrhage
p. hydatid cyst
p. hypertrophy
p. infarction
p. lateral gaze center
p. lesion
p. paramedian reticular formation
p. parareticular formation
p. pathology
p. raphe nucleus
p. reticular nucleus
p. sign
p. syndrome
p. tegmentum
p. tractotomy
p. vein
pontis
basis p.
brachium p.
cisterna p.
fasciculi longitudinales p.
fasciculus obliquus p.
fibrae corticonucleares p.
formatio reticularis tegmenti p.
nuclei reticulares p.
nucleus raphes p.
nucleus reticularis tegmenti p.
pars anterior p.
pars basilaris p.
pars dorsalis p.
pars ventralis p.
raphe p.
sulcus basilaris p.
taenia p.

NOTES

pontis *(continued)*
tegmentum p.
venae p.
pontobulbar
p. body
p. nucleus
p. sulcus
pontobulbare
corpus p.
pontobulbaris
nucleus p.
pontocerebellar
p. fiber
p. recess
p. trigone
pontocerebellare
trigonum p.
pontocerebellares
fibrae p.
pontocerebellaris
angulus p.
cisterna p.
pontocerebellum
pontomedullary
p. epidermoid cyst
p. groove
p. junction
p. separation
p. sulcus
pontomesencephalic
p. cavernous hemangioma
p. junction
p. vein
pontomesencephalica
vena p.
pontopeduncular sulculus
pontoreticulospinalis
tractus p.
pontoreticulospinal tract
pontosubicular degeneration
pool
blood p. (BP)
P. phenomenon
Pool-Schlesinger sign
poor
p. balance
p. coordination
p. pronunciation
popliteal
p. artery
p. nerve
p. plexus
Poppen
P. intervertebral disc laminectomy rongeur
P. ventricular needle
Poppen-Blalock carotid clamp
Poppen-Gelpi laminectomy retractor

population
high-risk p.
multiple spike p.
p. stratification
target p.
population-controlled study
Porch Index of Communicative Ability
porcine
p. cell transplantation
p. dopaminergic cell
pore
gustatory p.
nuclear p.
taste p.
porencephalia (*var. of* porencephaly)
porencephalic, porencephalous
p. cyst
porencephalitis
porencephaly, porencephalia
congenital p.
encephaloclastic p.
schizencephalic p.
porocarcinoma
poroelasticity
poroma
malignant eccrine p.
porosis, pl. **poroses**
cerebral p.
porphobilinogen
p. deaminase
urinary p.
porphyria
acute intermittent p.
delta-aminolevulinate dehydratase p.
hepatic p.
intermittent acute p. (IAP)
p. peripheral neuropathy
p. synthesizing enzyme
variegate p.
porphyric
p. neuropathy
p. polyneuropathy
porphyrin
p. compound
p. metabolism
port
lumbar p.
p. wine stain
porta, pl. **portae**
portal
p. access surgical system (PASS)
integrated sideport access p.
p. systemic encephalopathy
3-portal video-assisted thoracoscopic sympathectomy
Portnoy
P. DPV device
P. ventricular cannula
P. ventricular catheter

portosystemic
p. shunt
p. shunting
Portuguese-Azorean disease
Portuguese-type familial amyloid polyneuropathy
porus
p. acusticus
p. gustatorius
Poser criteria
position
p. agnosia
angular p.
p. of attack
body p.
brow-down p.
decubitus p.
emprosthotonos p.
equinus p.
fetal p.
Hollingshead Index of Social P.
joint p.
knee-chest p.
k-space reordered by inversion time at each slice p.
lateral recumbent p.
p. loss
lounging p.
opisthotonos p.
orthotonos p.
park bench p.
phase p.
prone p.
reverse Trendelenburg p.
semi-Fowler p.
p. sensation
p. sense
sitting p.
supine p.
translational p.
Trendelenburg p.
tuck p.
positional
p. nystagmus
p. obstructive sleep apnea
p. therapy
p. vertigo
p. vertigo of Bárány
positioning
patient p.
p. platform
proper neck p.
position-specific tremor
positive
p. ability
p. afterpotential
p. airway pressure (PAP)
p. dromotropism
p. effect
p. end-expiratory pressure (PEEP)
false p.
p. feedback
p. image
p. ion
P. and Negative Stroke Scale
P. and Negative Syndrome Scale (PANSS)
P. and Negative Syndrome Scale–Excitement Component (PANSS-EC)
p. occipital sharp transient
p. occipital sharp transients of sleep (POSTS)
p. picture-caption pair
p. result
p. score
p. sharp wave
p. symptom
p. symptom dimension
positive-going paradigm
positively
p. bathmotropic
p. correlated region
positron
p. emission tomography (PET)
p. emission tomography-fluorodeoxyglucose (PET-FDG)
p. emission tomography technique
post
p. baseline visit
Caspar retraction p.
p. hoc analysis
p. hoc stimulation
p. hoc stratification
p. hoc test
p. hoc testing
iliac p.
Isola spinal implant system iliac p.
Luque-Galveston p.
perineal p.
p. pertussis vaccination encephalopathy
p. rabies vaccination encephalopathy
p. recovery

NOTES

postactivation
p. depression
p. exhaustion
p. facilitation
postadrenalectomy syndrome
postambivalence
postambivalent
p. phase
p. phase stage
postanoxic
p. coma
p. dystonia
p. encephalopathy
p. myoclonus
postapoplectic epilepsy
postbasic stare
postbulbar motor nucleus
postcardiotomy
postcentral
p. area
p. fissure
p. gyrus
p. resection
p. sulcus
postcentralis
gyrus p.
sulcus p.
postchemotherapy neuroimaging
postclival
p. fissure
p. sulcus
postcommissurales
fibrae p.
postcommissural fiber
postconcussion
p. amnesia
p. headache
p. neurosis
p. syndrome
postconcussive amnesia
postcontusional brain syndrome
postcontusion syndrome encephalopathy
postdiphtheritic paralysis
post-ECT
postelectroconvulsive therapy
postembolization
p. angiogram
p. bleeding rate
postencephalitic
p. behavior syndrome
p. myoclonus
p. parkinsonism
postepileptic paralysis
4-poster frame
posterior
p. accessory olivary nucleus
p. acoustic stria
p. alexia
p. aphasia
area hypothalamica p.
arteria cerebelli inferior p.
arteria cerebri p.
arteria choroidea p.
arteria spinalis p.
arteria temporalis p.
p. atlantoaxial arthrodesis
p. auricular plexus
p. beaten copper appearance
p. bone graft
p. branch of axillary nerve
p. callosal vein
p. callosotomy
p. canal line
p. central convolution
p. central gyrus
p. cerebellar artery
p. cerebellar notch
cerebellomedullaris p.
p. cerebellomedullary cistern
p. cerebral artery
p. cerebral commissure
p. cerebral territory infarction
p. cervical fixation
p. cervical spinal instrumentation
p. choroidal artery
p. cingulate
p. cingulate gyrus
p. cingulate region
p. circle of Willis
p. circulation
p. circulation aneurysm
p. circulation ischemia
cisterna cerebellomedullaris p.
p. clinoid process (PCP)
columna p.
p. column cordotomy
p. column dysfunction gait
p. column lesion
p. column osteosynthesis
p. column of spinal cord
p. column syndrome
commissura alba p.
commissura grisea p.
p. communicating aneurysm
p. communicating artery (PComA)
p. communicating nerve
p. compartment lesion
p. construct
p. cranial fossa
p. craniocervical junction
p. decompression
decussatio tegmentalis p.
p. distraction instrumentation
p. dominant activity
ductus semicircularis p.
p. ecchymosis
p. external arcuate fiber
fasciculus longitudinalis p.

p. fasciculus proprius
p. fixation system biomechanics
forceps p.
p. fossa aneurysm
p. fossa approach
p. fossa-atrial shunt
p. fossa craniotomy
p. fossa dural arteriovenous fistula
p. fossa extradural hematoma
p. fossa mass
p. fossa mass lesion
p. fossa meningioma
p. fossa syndrome
p. fossa tumor
p. funiculus
p. fusiform gyrus
p. gray commissure
gyrus paracentralis p.
gyrus temporalis transversalis p.
p. hippocampal activation
p. hook-rod spinal instrumentation
p. horn
p. hypothalamic area
p. hypothalamic nucleus
p. hypothalamic region
incisura cerebelli p.
p. inferior cerebellar artery (PICA)
p. inferior cerebellar artery syndrome
p. inferior communicating artery (PICA)
p. inferior communicating artery aneurysm
p. intercavernous sinus
p. intermediate groove
p. intermediate sulcus
p. interosseous nerve
p. interpositus nucleus
p. interspinous wiring
p. joint syndrome
p. lacerate foramen
p. language area lesion
p. language cortex
p. leukoencephalopathy syndrome
p. ligamentous complex
p. limb of internal capsule
p. lobe of cerebellum
p. lobe of hypophysis
p. lobe of pituitary gland
p. longitudinal bundle
p. longitudinal ligament
p. lower cervical spine stabilization
p. lower cervical spine surgery
p. lumbar interbody fusion (PLIF)
p. lumbar interbody fusion surgery
p. lumbar spine and sacrum surgery
p. lunate lobule
p. marginal vein
p. medial nucleus of thalamus
p. median fissure
p. median fissure of medulla oblongata
p. median fissure of spinal cord
p. median sulcus of medulla oblongata
p. median sulcus of spinal cord
p. medullary velum
nervus ampullaris p.
nervus auricularis p.
nervus cutaneous antebrachii p.
nervus cutaneous brachii p.
nervus ethmoidalis p.
nervus interosseus antebrachii p.
p. neuropore
p. notch of cerebellum
p. nuclear complex of thalamus
nucleus cochlearis p.
nucleus hypothalamicus p.
p. nucleus of hypothalamus
nucleus interpositus p.
nucleus lateralis p.
p. nucleus of oculomotor nerve
nucleus olivaris accessorius p.
nucleus paramedianus p.
nucleus periventricularis p.
nucleus raphes p.
nucleus thoracicus p.
p. nucleus of vagus nerve
p. occipitocervical approach
p. odontoid surface
p. paracentral gyrus
p. parietal cortex (PPC)
p. parolfactory sulcus
pars retrolentiformis cruris p.
p. peduncle of thalamus
p. perforated substance
p. pericallosal vein
p. periventricular nucleus
p. pillar of fornix
p. pituitary fossa
p. pituitary gland ectopia
posterioris apex cornus p.
p. primary ramus

NOTES

P

posterior *(continued)*
p. pulmonary branch of vagus nerve
p. pyramid of medulla
p. quadrantic dysplasia
p. quadrigeminal body
p. rachischisis
radiatio thalamica p.
radix p.
p. raphe nucleus
p. recess
p. recess of interpeduncular fossa
recessus p.
regio hypothalamica p.
p. rhizotomy
p. rhythm
p. rod system
p. root
p. root of ansa cervicalis
p. root ganglion
p. root of spinal nerve
p. segmental fixation
p. semicircular canal (PSC)
sinus intercavernosus p.
spina bifida p.
p. spinal artery
p. spinal cord syndrome
p. spinal fusion
p. spinal plating
p. spinal sclerosis
p. spinocerebellar tract
stria cochlearis p.
p. subscapular approach
substantia perforata p.
sulcus intermedius p.
sulcus lateralis p.
sulcus parolfactorius p.
p. superior fissure
p. surgical exposure of sacrum and coccyx
p. tegmental decussation
p. thalamic radiation
p. thalamic tubercle
p. thoracic nucleus
p. tibial nerve
p. tibial nerve evoked potential
tractus spinocerebellaris p.
tractus trigeminothalamicus p.
p. transcallosal approach
p. transverse temporal gyrus
p. trigeminothalamic tract
p. truncal vagotomy
truncus vagalis p.
p. upper cervical spine surgery
p. vagal trunk
p. vein of corpus callosum
p. vein of septum pellucidum
vena septi pellucidi p.
ventralis oralis p.
p. vermis syndrome
p. vomer

posteriores
fibrae arcuatae externae p.
nervi labiales p.
nervi scrotales p.
nervi supraclaviculares p.
rami temporales p.

posterioris
apex cornus p.
p. apex cornus posterior
bulbus cornus p.
cervix columnae p.
nucleus commissurae p.
pars sublentiformis cruris p.
rami gastrici posteriores trunci vagalis p.
rami perineales nervi cutanei femoris p.
ramus occipitalis nervi auricularis p.
vena cornus p.

posterius
cornu p.
corpus quadrigeminum p.
foramen caecum p.

posteroinferior

posterolateral
p. approach
p. bone graft
p. bone grafting
p. bone graft placement
p. costotransversectomy
p. costotransversectomy incision
p. costotransversectomy technique
p. fissure
p. groove
p. lumbar spinal fusion
p. lumbosacral fusion
p. nucleus
p. sclerosis
p. spinal artery
p. spinal fusion
p. sulcus
p. tract
ventral p. (VPL)

posterolateralis
fissura p.
nucleus tegmentalis p.
nucleus ventralis p.
sulcus p.
tractus p.

posteromedial
ventral p. (VPM)

posteromedialis
nucleus ventralis p.
ramus frontalis p.
ventralis p.

posteromedial nucleus

posteromedian column of spinal cord
posteroparietal
posterotemporal artery occlusion
posteroventral
p. pallidotomy
p. sensorimotor pallidum
postexertional malaise
postextubation croup
postfundibular eminence
postganglionic
p. efferent activity
p. motor neuron
p. nerve fiber
p. neurofiber
p. oculosympathetic palsy
postganglionicae
neurofibrae p.
posthemiplegic
p. athetosis
p. chorea
p. paralysis
posthemorrhagic hydrocephalus
postherpetic
p. neuralgia (PHN)
p. neuralgia prophylaxis
posthippocampal fissure
posthypnotic amnesia
posthypophysectomy traction syndrome
posthypoxic myoclonus
postictal
p. blood flow switch
p. cognitive dysfunction
p. confusion
p. impairment
p. migrainous headache
p. paresis
p. slowing
p. state
p. suppression
p. symptom
posticus
locus perforatus p.
p. palsy
p. paralysis
tetanus p.
postinduction occipital cortex
postinfection
p. encephalomyelopathy
p. perivascular myelinoclasis
postinfectious
p. abducens palsy
p. brainstem encephalitis
p. cerebellitis
p. disseminated encephalomyelitis
p. hydrocephalus
p. leukoencephalitis
p. myelitis
p. polyneuritis
postinfective encephalitis
postinoculation poliomyelitis
postirradiation OVM
postischemic seizure
postjunctional
postlaminectomy
p.-l. kyphosis
p.-l. 2-level spondylolisthesis
p.-l. syndrome
postleucotomy syndrome
postlingual fissure
postlumbar
p. puncture headache
p. puncture syndrome
postlunate fissure
postmalaria neurologic syndrome
postmeningitic hydrocephalus
postmenopausal seizure
postmigratory cortical organization
postmortem
p. brain tissue
p. data
p. finding
p. neuropathology
p. spinal cord
p. study
p. technique
postmovement beta desynchronization
postnatal injury
postneuritic atrophy
postnodular sulcus
postocular optic neuritis
postoperative
p. angiogram
p. angiography
p. arachnoiditis
p. aseptic meningitis
p. bracing
p. care
p. confusion
p. corticosteroid
p. extubation
p. hydrocephalus
p. immobilization
p. infection
p. intellectual development

NOTES

P

postoperative *(continued)*
p. lumbosacral orthosis
p. paraplegia
p. regimen
p. skull defect
p. tetany
postparainfectious encephalomyelitis
postparalytic
postpartum
p. necrosis
p. obturator neuropathy
p. pituitary necrosis syndrome
postpolio
p. sequela
p. syndrome
postpoliomyelitis syndrome
postprandial
postpsychotic
postpuberty
postpubescence
postpump seizure
postpyramidal
p. fissure
p. sulcus
postradiation fibrosis
postradiotherapy neuroimaging
postrema
area p.
postrhinal fissure
postrolandic area
postrotational nystagmus
POSTS
positive occipital sharp transients of sleep
POSTS on electroencephalogram
postspike facilitation
poststress ankle/arm Doppler index
poststroke
p. dementia
p. depression
p. epilepsy
postsurgical infection rate
postsylvian
postsynaptic
p. compensatory mechanism
p. cortical neuronal potential
p. disorder
p. enhancement
p. excitation
p. fold
p. 5-HT2 receptor
p. 5-HT3 receptor
p. neuromuscular junction
p. neuron
p. neuronal membrane
p. stimulation
posttest level
posttetanic
p. exhaustion
p. facilitation
p. potentiation (PTP)
post-TIA depression
posttranslational modification
posttranslation phosphorylation
posttraumatic
p. amnesia
p. amnestic syndrome
p. apoplexy
p. apoplexy of Bollinger
p. brain histology
p. brain syndrome
p. delirium
p. dementia
p. epilepsy
p. epileptiform activity
p. frontal lesion
p. headache
p. hydrocephalus
p. insomnia
p. intradiploic pseudomeningocele
p. kyphosis
p. leptomeningeal cyst
p. mental disturbance
p. neck syndrome
p. neuralgia
p. neuroma
p. neurosis
p. osteoporosis
p. pain
p. pain syndrome
p. spinal deformity
p. stress symptom
p. symptom formation
p. vertigo
postural
P. Assessment Scale for Stroke (PASS)
p. element
p. hypertension
p. inflexibility
p. instability
p. myoneuralgia
p. orthostatic tachycardia syndrome
p. perturbation
p. reaction
p. reflex
p. stability
p. syncope
p. tremor
p. unsteadiness
p. vertigo
posture
p. agnosia
cervical resting p.
erect torso p.
p. examination
excessively erect p.
flexed p.

habitual p.
p. interaction
neutral torso p.
p. reflex abnormality
p. sense
stooped p.
torso flexion p.
trunk p.
universal flexion p.
unstable p.
wide-based p.

posturing
axial p.
bizarre p.
decerebrate p.
decorticate p.
unilateral dystonic p.

posturography

postvaccinal
p. encephalitis
p. encephalomyelitis
p. encephalomyelopathy
p. encephalopathy
p. leukoencephalitis
p. myelitis
p. poliomyelitis

potassium (K)
p. acetate
p. acetate, potassium bicarbonate, and potassium citrate
p. bicarbonate
p. bicarbonate and potassium chloride, effervescent
p. bicarbonate, potassium chloride, and potassium citrate
p. bicarbonate and potassium citrate, effervescent
p. bromide
p. channel
p. channel gene
p. chloride
p. chloride and potassium gluconate
p. citrate and citric acid
p. citrate and potassium gluconate
p. disorder
p. imbalance
low p.
p. phosphate and sodium phosphate
p. salicylate
serum p.

potassium-aggravated myotonia (PAM)

potassium-sensitive myotonia

potatorum
tremor p.

potency
antidopaminergic p.

potential
abuse p.
acoustic evoked p.
action p.
auditory compound action p.
auditory evoked p.
biphasic action p.
bizarre high-frequency p.
brain p.
brainstem auditory evoked p. (BAEP)
brainstem evoked p.
cerebral p.
click-evoked vestibular myogenic p.
cochlear microphonic p.
cognitive p.
compound motor action p. (CMAP)
compound muscle action p. (CMAP)
compound nerve action p. (CNAP)
p. correlation
cortical somatosensory evoked p.
p. cumulative trauma disorder
demarcation p.
dermatosensory evoked p.
direct auditory compound actional p.
direct cortical stimulation and somatosensory evoked p. (SSEP)
electrical evoked p.
electromyographic p.
endplate p. (EPP)
equal p.
event-related p.
evoked p. (EP)
excitatory postsynaptic p. (EPSP)
extracellular action p.
extrapyramidal symptom p.
extreme somatosensory evoked p.
fasciculation p.
fibrillation p.
generator p.
giant motor unit action p.
glossokinetic p.
heartbeat p.
inhibitory postsynaptic p. (IPSP)
injury p.

NOTES

P

potential *(continued)*
latency-evoked p.
localized evoked p.
median mixed nerve action p.
membrane p.
miniature endplate p. (MEPP)
monophasic action p.
motor evoked p. (MEP)
motor unit p. (MUP)
motor unit action p. (MUAP)
motor unit potential amplitude p.
multimodality evoked p. (MEP)
muscle fiber action p.
myogenic motor evoked p.
myotonic p.
nascent motor unit p.
nerve action p.
neurogenic motor evoked p.
nonspecific slow p.
normal resting p.
peroneal somatosensory evoked p.
phase reversal p.
piezoelectric p.
posterior tibial nerve evoked p.
postsynaptic cortical neuronal p.
p. predisposing factor
pretreatment binding p.
prothrombotic p.
pudendal somatosensory evoked p.
receptor p.
resting membrane p.
rhythmic repetitive muscle p.
satellite p.
scalp electrical p.
sensory compound action p.
sensory evoked p. (SEP)
sensory nerve action p. (SNAP)
serrated action p.
small motor unit p.
somatosensory evoked p. (SSEP)
spike p.
spinal sensory evoked p.
steady-state visual evoked p.
summating p.
sural sensory p.
transcranial motor evoked p.
transmembrane p. (TMP)
trigeminal evoked p. (TEP)
visual evoked p. (VEP)
visual evoked cortical p.
weight gain p.

potentially curable lesion

potentiation
late-phase long-term p. (L-LTP)
posttetanic p. (PTP)
short-term p. (STP)

potentiometer
angle position p.

Pott
P. abscess
P. disease
P. paralysis
P. paraplegia
P. puffy tumor

Potter syndrome

Potzl syndrome

pouch
Blake p.
pharyngeal p.
Rathke p.
spinal extradural arachnoid p.

Pourfour du Petit syndrome

pouting reflex

poverty
Liddle psychomotor p.
p. of speech

povidone-iodine
aqueous p.-i.

Powassan
P. encephalitis
P. virus

powder
antibiotic p.
Avitene p.

power
p. amplifier
combined predictive p.
p. drill
p. dynamic
global field p. (GFP)
mind p.
predictive p.
processing p.
p. router
p. spectral analysis

powered
p. automatic skull perforator
p. automatic-stopping drill
p. automatic-stopping drill point

7p13-p15
chromosome 7p13-p15

PPA
primary progressive aphasia

PPC
posterior parietal cortex

PPP
pentose phosphate pathway

PPPMA
progressive postpolio muscle atrophy

PPR
photoparoxysmal response

PPRF
paramedian pontine reticular formation

practiced task

Prader-Willi syndrome

praecox
dementia p.
neurasthenia p.
pragmatagnosia
pragmatamnesia
pramipexole
p. dihydrochloride
p. monotherapy
p. study
praxis
visual constructional p.
praxis-induced seizure
preacher's hand
prealbumin protein
preamplifier
epoxy-mounted p.
preataxic
precalibrated pointing device
precapillary end foot
precaution
spine p.
Precedex
precentral
p. area
p. cerebellar vein
p. fissure
p. gyrus
p. sulcus
precentralis
fissura p.
gyrus p.
sulcus p.
precession
fast imaging with steady p. (FISP)
Larmor p.
steady-state free p.
precessional frequency
prechiasmatic sulcus
prechiasmaticus
sulcus p.
precipitating
p. factor
p. stimulus
precipitation
p. by hyperventilation
p. by photic stimulation
preclinical stage
preclival
p. fissure
p. sulcus
Preclude
P. dura substitute prosthesis
P. spinal membrane
precollagenous filamentous material
precoma
precommissural
p. bundle
p. septal area
p. septal nucleus
p. septum
precommissurales
fibrae p.
precommissuralis
nucleus septalis p.
preconditioning
ischemic p.
preconsciousness
precontoured unit rod
preconvulsive
precoronal bur hole
preculminalis
fissura p.
preculminate fissure
precuneal fissure
precunealis
arteria p.
precuneate
precuneus
precursor
neural crest p.
neuronal p.
p. sign to rupture of aneurysm
precursory symptom
predecessor
phylogenetic p.
predementia
predictive
p. characteristic
p. factor
p. power
p. property
p. relationship
p. saccade
predictor
back pain p.
clinical p.
peritraumatic p.
pharmacological p.
symptom-related p.
predisposition
fundamental p.
genetic p.

NOTES

P

predominantly predormital sleep paralysis
predorsal bundle
preexcision spike
preexisting
p. cognitive impairment
p. dementia
p. representation
preference
gaze p.
preferential
p. anosmia
p. occupancy
prefixed chiasm
prefrontal
p. cortex
p. cortex activation
p. cortex of brain
p. cortical area
p. cortical volume
p. flow
p. hypometabolism
p. insular cerebellar network
p. leukotomy
p. lobe
p. lobotomy
p. metabolism
p. region
p. vein
prefrontales
venae p.
pregabalin
preganglionic
p. autonomic fiber
p. efferent activity
p. motor neuron
p. nerve fiber
p. neurofiber
preganglionicae
neurofibrae p.
pregeniculate nucleus
prehemiplegic chorea
preictal
p. headache
p. myoclonus
preinduction
p. occipital cortex
p. thickness
preinsular gyrus
preischemic blood glucose
prelemniscal radiation
preliminary analysis
prematura
alopecia p.
premature
p. closure
p. confrontation
p. discharge
p. infant bowing reflex
p. infant head circumference measurement
p. infant hydrocephalus
p. infant hypocalcemia
p. infant hypothyroidism
p. infant kernicterus
p. infant meningitis
p. infant neurodevelopmental outcome
p. infant periventricular leukomalacia
p. infant pontosubicular degeneration
p. infant seizure
p. infant spastic hemiparesis
p. infant subarachnoid hemorrhage
p. infant tyrosinemia
premedullary
p. arteriovenous fistular
p. cistern
premenstrual dysphoria
PremiCron nonabsorbable suture
Premier anterior cervical plate system
premonitory
p. headache
p. stage
p. symptom
premorbid
p. ability
p. cognition
p. dementia
p. functioning
p. personality trait
p. trauma
premotor
p. area
p. cortex
p. neuron
p. syndrome
prenatal injury to cranial nerve
prenodular fissure
preoccipital
p. incisure
p. notch
preoccipitalis
incisura p.
preoperative
p. angiogram
p. angiography
p. evaluation
p. planning
p. preparation
p. sedation
p. tomography
preoptic
p. area
p. hypothalamus
p. nucleus

p. recess
p. region
preoptica
area p.
preorgasmic headache
preparalytic
preparation
facet joint p.
preoperative p.
rod contour p.
wire contour p.
prepiriform
p. cortex
p. gyrus
prepontine
p. cistern
p. lesion
p. region
prepyramidal
p. fissure
p. sulcus
p. tract
prepyramidalis
fissura p.
prerolandic
p. artery occlusion
p. sulcus
prerubral
p. field
p. nucleus
prerupture of aneurysm
presacral
p. nerve
p. neurectomy
p. sympathectomy
presacralis
nervus p.
presaturation pulse
presbyacusis, presbycusis
prescription drug therapy
presenile dementia
presenilin (PS)
p. 1 (PS1)
p. 2 (PS2)
p. mutant
preservation
carotid p.
lordosis p.
lumbar lordosis p.
nerve p.
p. technique
zone of partial p.
preservative-free normal saline
preserved conduction velocity
presigmoid approach
PRESS
point-resolved spectroscopy
press
environmental p.
pressor
p. fiber
p. nerve
pressoreceptive
pressoreceptor
p. nerve
p. reflex
p. system
pressosensitive
pressure
p. algesiometer
p. anesthesia
autoadjusting positive airway p. (APAP)
p. autoregulation
p. autoregulatory status
autotitrating continuous positive airway p.
bilevel positive airway p. (BiPAP)
carbon dioxide arterial p.
central venous p.
cerebral perfusion p.
cerebrospinal fluid p.
closure p.
colloid oncotic p.
p. cone
continuous positive airway p. (CPAP)
cranial perfusion p.
diastolic blood p.
p. distension technique
exhalation positive airway p. (EPAP)
feeding mean arterial p. (FMAP)
p. gauge
increased intracranial p.
inspiratory positive airway p. (IPAP)
intracranial p. (ICP)
intracranial epidural p.
intraocular p.
intraspinal epidural p.
intravascular p.
mean arterial blood p.
microvascular p. (MVP)

NOTES

P

pressure *(continued)*
mouth occlusion p.
nasal continuous positive airway p.
p. necrosis
p. neuropathy
ocular perfusion p.
opening p.
p. palsy
p. paralysis
partial p.
p. point
positive airway p. (PAP)
positive end-expiratory p. (PEEP)
pulmonary capillary wedge p.
raised intracranial p.
p. rating
p. receptor
regional cerebral perfusion p. (rCPP)
p. sense
p. of speech
supraglottic p.
tentorial p.
touch p.
transdiaphragmatic p.
transducer-measured intracranial venous p.
valve opening p.
variable positive airway p. (VPAP)
pressure-arresting point
pressure-exciting point
pressure-gradient change
pressure-volume index
Preston ligamentum flavum forceps
prestriate area
prestroke dementia
presubiculum
presumptive basis
presurgical
p. assessment
p. investigation
presylvian fissure
presynaptic
p. congenital myasthenic syndrome
p. disorder
p. membrane
p. membrane protein
p. nerve ending
p. neuron
p. stimulation
p. terminal
presyncope
pretectal
p. area
p. lesion
p. nucleus
p. region
p. syndrome
pretectales
nuclei p.
pretectalis
area p.
pretectoolivares
fibrae p.
pretectoolivary fiber
pretectum
prethymectomy
pretraumatic
p. amnesia
p. risk factor
p. vulnerability
pretreatment
p. binding potential
p. measure
prevalence
epilepsy p.
mutation p.
prevention
infection p.
rod rotation p.
preventive therapy
preverbal attentional processing
prevertebral
p. ganglion
p. plexus
Prévost sign
PRF
prolactin-releasing factor
PRFR
percutaneous radiofrequency retrogasserian rhizotomy
PRGR
percutaneous retrogasserian glycerol rhizolysis
PRH
prolactin-releasing hormone
primary
p. active compound
p. afferent depolarization (PAD)
p. afferent loss
p. afferent neuron
p. afferent nociceptor
p. alveolar hypoventilation
p. amebic meningoencephalitis
p. amenorrhea
p. aminoaciduria
p. angiitis
p. antiphospholipid antibody syndrome
p. auditory cortex
p. axotomy
p. brain lymphoma
p. brain tumor
p. brain vesicle
p. central nervous system lymphoma (PCNSL)
p. clip

p. CNS lymphoma
p. cough headache
p. drive
p. dystonia
p. effect
p. efficacy outcome
p. encephalitis
p. ending
p. end-to-end anastomosis
p. enduring negative symptom
p. enuresis
p. epidural cyst
p. epileptogenic zone
p. fibromyalgia syndrome
p. fissure of cerebellum
p. generalized epilepsy
p. generalized seizure
p. group
p. headache associated with sexual activity
p. hydrocephalus
p. hyperoxaluria
p. idiopathic seizure
p. insomnia
p. intracranial plasmacytoma
p. intramedullary lymphoma
p. lateral sclerosis
p. leptomeningeal lymphoma
p. mechanism
p. motor area
p. motor cortex
p. neurasthenia
p. neuroectodermal tumor
p. neuronal cell
p. neuronal degeneration
p. neurulation
p. nonenduring negative symptom
p. object
p. optic atrophy
p. orthostatic tremor
p. pharmacological approach
p. pontine hemorrhage
p. process
p. progressive amyotrophy
p. progressive aphasia (PPA)
p. progressive cerebellar degeneration
p. progressive multiple sclerosis
p. receiving area
p. receptive area
p. rhinencephalic psychomotor epilepsy
p. risk factor
p. senile dementia
p. sensation
p. sensorimotor cortex
p. sensory cortex
p. sensory neuron
p. shock
p. Sjögren syndrome
p. snoring
p. somatic problem
p. somatomotor area
p. somatosensory area
p. somatosensory cortex
p. stabbing headache
p. subarachnoid supratentorial hemorrhage
p. synaptic cleft
p. thought disorder
p. thunderclap headache
p. trunk syndrome
p. vertigo
p. victim
p. visual area
p. visual cortex
p. vitreous

primary/secondary distinction

primer instrument

primidone

priming dose

primitiva

meninx p.

primitive

p. contagion
p. emotional level
p. lamina terminalis
p. maxillary vein
p. meninx
p. neural cell
p. neuroectodermal tumor (PNET)
p. neuroepithelial tumor
p. node
p. otic artery
p. reflex
p. streak
p. trigeminal artery
p. trigeminal artery variant

primordial inferior hypophysial artery

principal

p. olivary nucleus
p. sensory nucleus of trigeminal nerve
p. sensory nucleus of trigeminus

NOTES

P

principal-components analysis
principalis
nucleus olivaris p.
principle
p. of debridement
image formation p.
normalization p.
Pauli exclusion p.
physicochemical p.
Tarasoff p.
wellness p.
Pringle disease
prinomastat
Prinzmetal vasospastic angina pectoris
prion
p. analog
p. disease
p. protein (PrP)
p. protein gene
prism
Fresnel paste-on p.
PRL
prolactin
proaccelerin
proapoptotic
proband
p. condition
p. status
probe
bipolar cautery p.
Bipolar Circumactive P. (BICAP)
Bunnell dissecting p.
Bunnell forwarding p.
Dandy p.
Doppler p.
electromagnetic flow p.
electromagnetic focusing field p.
extended sector ultrasonic p.
fluoroptic thermometry p.
gearshift p.
hemispherical contact p.
indirect p.
intraoperative ultrasonic p.
Jacobson p.
Jannetta p.
Laserflo Doppler p.
LED p.
monitoring p.
Nucleotome aspiration p.
Nucleotome Flex II flexible cutting p.
P3 p.
$PbrO_2$ monitoring p.
pedicle sounding p.
right-angle blunt p.
SpineStat p.
TCD p.
Transonics flow p.
ultrasonic p.
Vasamedics laser Doppler flow p.
virtual p.
problem
conceptual p.
core p.
Daily Record of Severity of P.'s
fundamental conceptual p.
graft-related p.
integrative p.
primary somatic p.
sleep p.
p. sleepiness
somatic p.
subtle memory p.
problem-solving skill
Probst bundle
Procanbid
procarbazine
p. hydrochloride
p., lomustine (CCNU), vincristine (PCV)
procedural memory
procedure
ablative central neurosurgical p.
ablative spinal cord p.
aborted p.
activation p.
Albee shelf p.
analysis p.
anterior stabilization p.
assessment p.
Bonferroni-Dunn p.
Buschke Free and Cued Selective Reminding P.
Caldwell-Luc p.
carotid ablative p.
carotid Amytal p.
cervical spine stabilization p.
clinical p.
Cloward p.
cloze p.
coiling p.
Colonna shelf p.
debulking p.
demyelinating p.
Dewar posterior cervical fixation p.
DREZ p.
EDAS p.
EEG activating p.
egg-shelling p.
electrophysiological p.
Epley p.
extracranial-to-intracranial bypass p.
fetal shunt p.
genioglossus advancement p.
Gill p.
Hacker p.
Heifetz p.
Hoffmann and Mohr p.

hydrocephalus shunt p.
IDET p.
immunoperoxidase p.
instillation p.
intradiscal electrothermal p.
intrauterine shunt p.
Jaeger-Hamby p.
Jannetta microvascular decompression p.
Kestenbaum p.
Koerte p.
LDD p.
lower cervical spine p.
microoperative p.
microsurgical p.
Mitofsky-Aaksberg random digit dialing p.
Müller-König p.
neurodiagnostic p.
neurosurgical p.
nonmicrosurgical p.
Nucleotome p.
pi p.
prototype matching p.
psychophysical p.
Q-sort p.
radiosurgical lesioning p.
rating p.
retrogasserian p.
Scaramella p.
shunt p.
single bur hole p.
single-stage p.
Smith-Robinson p.
2-stage p.
standard rating p.
2-step p.
surgical p.
transnasal septal displacement p.
upper cervical spine p.
Wada p.

Proceed hemostatic agent

procerus

p. muscle
p. sign

process

absent spinous p.
active pathophysiologic p.
affective p.
age-related deterioration p.
age-related developmental p.
anterior clinoid p.
apical p.
autoimmune p.
axonal p.
BioCleanse tissue sterilization p.
brain p.
central timing p.
clinoid p.
clinoidal p.
common central p.
continuous inflammatory p.
declarative memory p.
deficient spinous p.
Deiters p.
dendritic p.
deterioration p.
developmental p.
diagnostic p.
emotional memory p.
environmental p.
executive p.
falciform p.
fundamental cognitive p.
GFAP-stained p.
identification p.
implicit p.
intact spinous p.
intracellular metabolic p.
kindling p.
lexical p.
mastoid p.
memory p.
metabolic p.
motivational p.
neurocognitive p.
neurogenic p.
neuronal p.
odontoid p.
ongoing cognitive p.
ontogenic p.
orthographic p.
pathophysiologic p.
perceptual p.
phonological p.
posterior clinoid p. (PCP)
primary p.
secondary p.
semantic p.
sensory p.
spinous p.
stress illness p.
sucker p.
uncinate p.

NOTES

process *(continued)*
viscerosensory p.
withdrawal p.
processing
affective p.
affect-related p.
altered tau p.
p. area
beta-amyloid p.
cell p.
declarative emotional memory p.
emotional information p.
emotional memory p.
information p.
memory p.
p. power
preverbal attentional p.
receptive language p.
signal p.
speech p.
speed of p.
tau p.
temporal p.
p. time
visual motor p.
word p.
processus
p. intrajugularis ossis occipitalis
p. intrajugularis ossis temporalis
p. jugularis ossis occipitalis
prochlorperazine maleate
prochordal plate
procoagulant
endothelial cell-derived p.
proconvulsant effect
proctalgia fugax
proctoparalysis
proctoplegia
proctospasm
procursiva
aura p.
procursive
p. chorea
p. epilepsy
procyclidine
prodromal psychotic symptom
prodrome
dementia p.
epileptic p.
product
gene p.
NeuroCell-HD neural cell transplant p.
NeuroCell-PD porcine neural cell transplant p.
nutraceutical p.
Valleylab neurosurgical p.
production
adrenal androgen p.
eicosanoid p.
emotion p.
endolymph p.
lexical word p.
word p.
prodynorphin
proencephalon (*var. of* prosencephalon)
proenkephalin
Proetz test
Pro-Fast
P.-F. HS capsule
P.-F. SR capsule
profile
P. anterior plate system
P. anterior spinal plate
Aphasia Diagnostic P.
cognitive p.
Communication Skills P.
conversion V p.
demyelinative spinal fluid p.
Derogatis Stress P.
diagnostic p.
Emory Functional Ambulation P.
eye-motor-verbal p.
Functional Limitation P. (FLP)
Life Skills P.
P. Lite
microsomal isoenzyme metabolism p.
P. of Mood States, Vigor
neuropathological lesion p.
neuropsychological p.
Nottingham Health P.
Pain Patient P.
Pain Perception P.
Q-score p.
risk-benefit p.
Sickness Impact P. (SIP)
symptom p.
therapeutic p.
velocity p.
P. VS
profiling
facial p.
Profil-O-Plastic plate
profound hypercapnia
profunda
cisterna intercruralis p.
vena cerebri media p.
profundae
fibrae pontis p.
venae cerebri p.
profundi
nervi temporales p.
rami musculares nervi fibularis p.
rami musculares nervi peronei p.
profundum
stratum album p.

stratum griseum p.
stratum medullare p.
profundus
nervus fibularis p.
nervus peroneus p.
nervus petrosus p.
PROGENI
Parkinson Research The Organized Genetic Initiative
PROGENI study
progenitor
p. cell
oligodendrocyte p. (OP)
temperature-sensitive neural p.
progestational activity
progesterone
p. effect
p. level
luteal phase p.
natural p.
oral p.
p. receptor
p. secretion
synthetic p.
progestin
prognosis
Kleine-Levin syndrome p.
neurologic p.
oral appliance p.
prognostic
p. factor
p. scale
p. status
p. variable
Prograf
program
cerebral palsy infant stimulation p.
clinical intervention p.
coercion p.
Leksell GammaPlan computerized p.
Leksell SurgiPlan computerized p.
multicomponent p.
multidisciplinary pilot project p. (MPPP)
pilot p.
research p.
standard bone algorithm p.
treatment p.
programmable
p. pulse generator
p. valve
p. valve pressure setting
programmed cell death (PCD)
programming
genetic p.
neurolinguistic p.
P. Wand
progressing stroke
progression
backward p.
clinical p.
cross-legged p.
curve p.
dementia p.
symptom p.
progression-free survival
progressiva
dementia paratonia p.
dysbasia lordotica p.
dyssynergia cerebellaris p.
dystonia deformans p.
dystrophia musculorum p.
p. infantilis
leukodystrophia cerebri p.
ophthalmoplegia p.
paratonia p.
progressive
P. Alzheimer Disease Assessment Scale-cognitive subscale
p. ataxia
p. brain disease
p. bulbar palsy of childhood
p. bulbar paralysis
p. bulbar paralysis of childhood
p. cerebellar tremor
p. cerebral
p. cerebral poliodystrophy
p. circumscribed cerebral atrophy
p. cognitive decline
p. deformity
p. degenerative subcortical encephalopathy
P. Deterioration Scale
p. dialysis encephalopathy
p. dysarthria
p. epilepsy with mental retardation
p. epileptogenesis
p. external ophthalmoparesis
p. external ophthalmoplegia (PEO)
p. extraocular paresis
p. facial atrophy
p. familial myoclonic epilepsy

NOTES

progressive *(continued)*
p. flaccid quadriparesis
p. headache
p. hereditary nerve deafness
p. hydrocephalus
p. hypertrophic interstitial neuropathy
p. infantile bulbar palsy
p. infantile poliodystrophy
p. infantile spinal muscular atrophy
p. kyphosis
p. leptomeningeal fibrosis
p. lingual hemiatrophy
p. multifocal leukoencephalopathy (PML)
p. muscle relaxation
p. muscular dystrophy
p. myoclonus epilepsy (PME)
p. necrotizing leukoencephaly
p. neurological disease
p. neurologic compromise
p. neurologic deterioration
p. neuromuscular atrophy
p. neuromuscular disease
p. neuropathic muscle atrophy
p. nonfluent aphasia
p. nuclear amyotrophy
p. posthemorrhagic ventriculomegaly
p. postpolio muscle atrophy (PPPMA)
p. rubella panencephalitis
p. spinal amyotrophy
p. spongiform encephalopathy
p. subcortical encephalopathy
p. subcortical gliosis
p. supranuclear palsy (PSP)
p. systemic sclerosis
p. torsion spasm
p. traumatic encephalopathy
p. ventricular dilation
p. visual loss

ProHance

project
Harvard Atherosclerosis Reversibility P. (HARP)

projection
anteroposterior p.
p. area
axial p.
Caldwell p.
cerebrocerebellar p.
dopamine p.
dopaminergic p.
feedback p.
feedforward p.
p. fiber
filtered-back p.
ipsilateral p.
lateral p.
maximum intensity p.
minimum intensity p.
p. neurofiber
p. neuron
retrospective p.
sagittal p.
p. system
thalamocortical p.

projectionis
neurofibra p.

projective test

prokinetic drug therapy

prolactin (PRL)
p. elevation
p. release
p. response
serum p.

prolactin-inhibiting
p.-i. factor (PIF)
p.-i. hormone

prolactinoma

prolactin-producing adenoma

prolactin-releasing
p.-r. factor (PRF)
p.-r. hormone (PRH)

prolactin-secreting
p.-s. pituitary adenoma
p.-s. pituitary tumor

prolapse
disc p.
mitral valve p.

proliferation
cell p.
dendrite p.
fibroblastic p.
granule cell p.
neuroepithelial cell p.
smooth muscle p.

proliferative malignant glial cell

proline urine level

Prolixin

Prolo function-economic rating scale

prolongation
pulse repetition time p.

prolonged
p. exposure
p. febrile seizure
p. nocturnal sleep
p. sedation

prolotherapy
p. injection
p. protocol

prolyl oligopeptidase

promethazine
p. hydrochloride
meperidine and p.

prominence
pedicle screw hardware p.
tongue base p.

prominent
p. dementia
p. phobic anxiety component
PROMM
proximal myotonic myopathy
promontorii
ponticulus p.
subiculum p.
promoter
endogenous chromosomal p.
pronation sign
pronator
p. reflex
p. teres syndrome
prone
p. position
p. to relapse
p. straight leg raising test
pronucleus, pl. **pronuclei**
pronunciation
p. disorder
poor p.
proopiomelanocortin
prop
Oberto mouth p.
propagation
p. of activity
ictal p.
propallylonal
propanolamine
propantheline
proparacaine hydrochloride
Propavan
propentofylline
proper
p. fasciculus
p. neck positioning
properdin
property
affective p.
androgenic p.
anxiolytic p.
mirrorlike p.
pharmacological p.
predictive p.
receptor-binding p.
reinforcing p.
sedative p.
shape p.
thermoregulatory p.
thermosensory p.
prophylactic
p. anticonvulsant therapy
p. craniospinal irradiation
p. hypertensive hypervolemic hemodilution
p. medication
prophylaxis
anaphylactic shock p.
anticonvulsant p.
antimicrobial p.
postherpetic neuralgia p.
stroke p.
propionic
p. acidemia
p. aciduria
propionyl-CoA carboxylase
proplexus
propofol infusion
proportional sensitivity
propranolol
p. hydrochloride
p. and hydrochlorothiazide
propria
dura p.
proprii
fasciculi p.
proprioceptive
p. nervous system
p. neuromuscular facilitation (PNF)
p. reflex
p. sense
p. sensibility
p. sensory deficit
p. vertigo
proprioceptor
propriospinal
p. myoclonus
p. system
proprius
anterior fasciculus p.
fasciculus anterior p.
fasciculus lateralis p.
lateral fasciculus p.
nucleus p.
posterior fasciculus p.
proptosis
propulsive gait
propylene glycol toxicity
propyliodone
prosencephalon, proencephalon
prosocele
prosocoele

NOTES

prosopagnosia
prosopalgia
prosopodiplegia
prosoponeuralgia
prosopoplegia
prosopospasm
prospective
p. experimental study design
p. memory
prostacyclin
prostaglandin
Prostaphlin
prostate-specific antigen (PSA)
prostatic
p. intraepithelial neoplasia (PIN)
p. plexus
prostaticus
plexus p.
prosthesis, pl. **prostheses**
acrylic p.
articulating disc p.
auditory p.
ball-type disc p.
Bristol disc p.
Bryan cervical disc p.
Charité disc p.
composite disc p.
Cummins disc p.
elastic-type disc p.
hydraulic-type disc p.
Lee disc p.
Link SB Charité disc p.
mechanical-type disc p.
neural p.
NeuroCybernetic p. (NCP)
palatal lift p.
Preclude dura substitute p.
sacral segmental nerve stimulation implantable neural p.
spinal disc p.
prosthetic
p. disc nucleus (PDN)
p. disc nucleus device
p. heart valve
Prostigmin test
protease
cysteine p.
p. inhibitor
membrane-anchored aspartyl p.
serine p.
protease-linked activation cloning system (PLACS)
protection
airway p.
cerebral p.
protective
p. effect
p. laryngeal reflex
protector
Adson dural p.
protein
p. 2
Abeta p.
acetylcholine-binding p.
alpha-synuclein p.
Alzheimer precursor p. (APP)
amyloid beta p.
amyloid precursor p. (APP)
antiapoptotic p.
antiglial fibrillary acidic p.
argyrophil organizer region p.
astrotactin p.
ataxin-1 p.
B amyloid p.
basement membrane p.
Bence Jones p.
beta amyloid p.
betaB-Trace p. (beta-B-TP)
bifunctional p.
p. binding
p. binding interaction
bone morphogenetic p. (BMP)
bone morphogenic p. (BMP)
brain-enriched hyaluronan binding p.
cAMP receptor p.
cAMP response element binding p.
capsid p.
caveolin-3 p.
cellular prion p. (PrP^c)
cerebrospinal fluid p.
p. concentration
connexin 32 p.
C-reactive p. (CRP)
CREB binding p.
p. C, S deficiency
cyclin-dependent kinase inhibitory p.
cytoskeletal p.
dynein p.
p. electrophoresis
encephalitogenic p.
estrogen-related p.
extracellular matrix p.
extracellular signal-regulated p.
FAK p.
filament p.
FOS p.
fukutin p.
G p.
gamma carboxylated p.
glial fibrillary acidic p. (GFAP)
growth-associated p.
heat shock p.
hemostasis-related p.
high animal p.
HIV-1-envelope p.

homeodomain p.
human prion p.
huntingtin p.
p. induced by vitamin K absence (PIVKA)
inhibitory p.
intracellular p.
56 kD p.
p. kinase
p. kinase B
p. kinase C (PKC)
p. kinase C inhibitor
lamina-associated p.
late endosomal p.
lipoprotein receptor-related p.
matrix p.
membrane-associated p.
methyl-CpG-binding p.
microtubule-associated p.
mitogen-activated p. (MAP)
monoclonal antiglial fibrillary acidic p.
MxA p.
myelin basic p. (MBP)
myelin/oligodendrocyte-specific p. (MOSP)
neuronal apoptosis inhibitory p. (NAIP)
neuron-specific cytoskeletal p.
nuclear envelope p.
Nurrl p.
opioid precursor p.
parathyroid hormonelike p. (PLP)
parkin p.
peripheral myelin p. 22
phosphorylate tau p.
plasma p.
prealbumin p.
presynaptic membrane p.
prion p. (PrP)
proteinlike p.
proteoglycan p.
proteolipid p.
ras p.
reelin p.
p. S-100b
S-100 beta p.
Schwann cell p.
serum p.
small heat shock p.
synaptosome-associated p.
p. synthesis
tau p.
transporter p.
transthyretin p.
triad p.
tubbylike p.
p. tyrosine phosphorylation
voltage-sensitive p.
wild-type p.
p. zero

protein-2
bone morphogenetic p.-2

proteinaceous infectious particle

proteinase
aspartic p.
cysteine p.
serine p.

protein-binding pharmacokinetic

protein-bound iodine (PBI)

protein-energy malnutrition

proteinlike protein

proteinosis
lipoid p.

proteoglycan
aggrecan p.
biglycan p.
brevican p.
chondroitin sulfate p.
disc matrix p.
extracellular matrix p.
p. molecule
p. protein
versican p.

proteolipid protein

proteolysis

proteolytic fragment

proteomic

proteosome
extracellular p.

Proteus
P. meningitis
P. syndrome

prothrombin time (PT)

prothrombotic
p. disorder
p. potential

protirelin

protocol
brain death p.
CANVAS p.
Computer-Aided Neurovascular Analysis and Simulation p.
Dana-Farber Cancer Institute p.

NOTES

P

protocol *(continued)*
Dysphagia Evaluation P.
exercise p.
formal dose-escalation p.
fractionation p.
Gliadel wafer treatment p.
imaging p.
NASCIS II p.
prolotherapy p.
steroid p.
surveillance p.
treatment p.
Wada p.
web-based neuropsychological test p.
protocol-driven treatment
proton
p. beam
p. beam radiation
p. density
p. density weighting
p. imaging
p. magnetic resonance spectroscopy
p. nuclear magnetic resonance spectroscopy
p. relaxation time
p. spectrum
proton-electron dipole-dipole interaction
proton-weighted image
Protopam
protopathic sensibility
protoplasmaticum
astrocytoma p.
protoplasmic
p. astrocyte
p. astrocytoma
protoporphyria
erythrocyte p.
protoporphyrin IX
protospasm
prototaxic
prototype
p. matching
p. matching procedure
protozoan infection
protracta
catatonia p.
protriptyline
protruded disc
protrusio defect
protrusion
anular p.
coil p.
disc p.
mass p.
medullary p.
pseudopodial p.
protuberans
dermatofibrosarcoma p.
protuberantia occipitalis interna
Providence scoliosis system
Provigil
provocative testing
prowazekii
Rochalimaea p.
Prowler
P. double-tipped microcatheter
P. Plus catheter
Prowler-14 microcatheter
proximal
p. axonopathy
p. balloon occlusion
p. carotid ring
p. clipping
p. myotonic myopathy (PROMM)
p. segment retraction
PrP
prion protein
P. gene
PrP^c^
cellular prion protein
Pruitt-Inahara shunt
pruning
neuronal p.
pruritus
localized p.
p. vulvae
PS
presenilin
PS Medical Flow Control valve
PS1
presenilin 1
PS2
presenilin 2
PSA
prostate-specific antigen
psalterii
cavum p.
psalterium, pl. **psalteria**
psammocarcinoma
psammoma
p. body
Virchow p.
psammomatoid ossifying fibroma
psammomatous meningioma
PSC
posterior semicircular canal
P segment
pselaphesia, pselaphesis
pseudagraphia, pseudoagraphia
Pseudallescheria boydii
pseudaphia
pseudarthrosis
documented p.
failed back syndrome with documented p.
p. rate
p. repair

pseudesthesia, pseudoesthesia
pseudoabducens
p. nerve paresis
p. palsy
pseudoagrammatism
pseudoagraphia (*var. of* pseudagraphia)
pseudoaneurysm
pseudoapoplexy
pseudoapraxia
pseudo-Argyll Robertson pupil
pseudoarthritis
pseudoataxia
pseudoathetosis
pseudoauthenticity
pseudo-battered child syndrome
pseudobulbar
p. palsy
p. paralysis
p. speech
pseudocele
pseudocephalocele
pseudocholinesterase
pseudochorea
pseudochromesthesia
pseudoclonus
pseudocoma
pseudocyesis
pseudocyst
secreting glial p.
pseudocystic
p. degeneration
p. hypodense lesion
pseudodementia
p. of depression
depressive p.
hysterical p.
pseudoephedrine
pseudoepileptic seizure
pseudoesthesia (*var. of* pseudesthesia)
pseudofracture
pseudoganglion
Bochdalek p.
Cloquet p.
Valentin p.
pseudogene
pseudogeusesthesia
pseudogeusia
pseudo-Graefe sign
pseudo-Hurler
p.-H. disease
p.-H. syndrome
pseudohydrocephaly
pseudohypersomnia
pseudohypertrophic
p. muscular atrophy
p. muscular dystrophy
p. muscular paralysis
pseudohypertrophy
muscle p.
muscular p.
pseudohypoparathyroidism
pseudoinclusion
nuclear p.
pseudointernuclear ophthalmoplegia
pseudologia
pseudolumen
pseudomalignancy
pseudomedial longitudinal fasciculus lesion
pseudomeningitis
pseudomeningocele
posttraumatic intradiploic p.
traumatic p.
Pseudomonas
P. aeruginosa
P. aeruginosa meningitis
P. exotoxin
pseudomotivation
pseudomotor cerebri
pseudomuscular hypertrophy
pseudomyasthenia
ocular p.
pseudomyotonia
Debré-Sémélaigne p.
p. disease
pseudoneoplasm
pseudoneurological symptom grouping
pseudoneuroma
pseudoneuronophagia
pseudonymity
pseudonymous
pseudoobstruction
pseudopalisading astrocytoma
pseudopapilledema
pseudoparalysis
arthritic general p.
congenital atonic p.
pseudoparaplegia
Basedow p.
pseudoparesis
pseudoperiodic discharge
pseudophotesthesia
pseudoplegia
pseudopodial protrusion

NOTES

P

pseudopolycythemia
paresthetic p.
pseudopsammoma body
pseudopseudohypoparathyroidism
pseudoptosis
pseudopuberty
pseudorandom
pseudoreminiscence
pseudorosette
pseudosauthenticity
pseudosclerosis
Westphal p.
Westphal-Strümpell p.
pseudoseizure
pseudosplenium
pseudo status epilepticus
pseudosubluxation
pseudotabes
diabetic p.
pupillotonic p.
pseudotetanus
pseudotrismus
pseudotrisomy 13 syndrome
pseudotumor
p. cerebri
idiopathic orbital p.
orbital p.
pseudotumoral lymphocytic hypophysitis
pseudounipolar
p. ganglion cell
p. neuron
pseudoventricle
pseudovertigo
pseudovomiting
pseudo-Wernicke syndrome
pseudoxanthoma elasticum
pseudo-Zellweger syndrome
PSG
Parkinson Study Group
polysomnograph
Albert Grass Heritage PSG
psittacosis encephalitis
psoas
p. abscess
p. muscle
psoriasis spondylitica
psoriatic arthritis
PSP
phenolsulfonphthalein
progressive supranuclear palsy
PSQ
Pediatric Sleep Questionnaire
psychedelic drug
psychiatric
p. effect
p. medication
p. parameter
p. syndrome
psychiatry
American Association for Geriatric P. (AAGP)
Association of Directors of Medical Student Education in P.
p. and neurology
psychic
p. blindness
p. seizure
p. slowness
p. tic
p. wound
psychical
p. aura
p. manner
psychoactive
p. chemical
p. substance-induced organic mental disorder
psychoanalytic perspective
psychocardiac reflex
psychodynamic
p. effect
p. origin
psychogalvanic
p. reaction
p. reflex
p. reflex/response
p. response (PGR)
psychogenic
p. amnesia
p. chest pain
p. duodenal ulcer
p. dystonia
p. effort syndrome
p. epilepsy
p. event
p. fatigability
p. gastric ulcer
p. headache
p. hearing impairment
p. learning disorder
p. limb disorder
p. motor disorder
p. muscle disorder
p. musculoskeletal disorder
p. neurocirculatory disorder
p. nonepileptic seizure
p. obsessional disorder
p. origin
p. pain disorder
p. pelvic pain
p. peptic ulcer
p. precordial pain
p. respiratory disorder
p. rheumatic disorder
p. skin disorder
p. sleep disorder
p. stomach disorder

p. torticollis
p. tremor
p. vertigo

psychological
p. consequence
p. construct
p. effect
p. response
p. state
p. strength
p. symptom
p. trauma
p. weakness

psychological/physiological arousal

psychologic test

psychometric
p. advantage
p. testing of sleeplessness

psychomotor
p. abnormality
p. attack
p. behavioral disturbance
p. delay
p. development
p. dysadaptation syndrome
p. epilepsy
p. impairment
p. phenomenon
p. retardation
p. seizure
p. slowing
p. speed
p. status
p. stress reaction
p. stupor
p. swelling

psychoneurotic depressive reaction

psychoorganic syndrome

psychopathic trait

psychopathologic accompaniment

psychopathology rating scale

psychopathy
autistic p.

psychopharmacologic agent

psychophysical procedure

psychophysiologic
p. insomnia
p. manifestation
p. vertigo

psychophysiological insomnia

psychosensory aphasia

psychosine accumulation

psychosis
monosymptomatic hypochondriacal p.

psychosocial
p. function
p. overlay
p. perspective
p. stressor
p. symptom outcome

psychosomatic symptom score

psychotherapeutic
p. approach
p. neuroscience
p. therapy

psychotic
p. Alzheimer patient
p. brain syndrome
p. choreoathetosis
p. depressive reaction
p. relapse

psychotic-like phenomenon

psychotomimetic agent

psychotropic
p. agent
p. effect
p. medication
p. metabolism
p. movement

psychroalgia

psychroesthesia

psychrophobia

PT
prothrombin time

PTAH
phosphotungstic acid hematoxylin

ptc gene

6-PT deficiency

pterion

pterional
p. approach
p. craniotomy

pterygoid
p. canal nerve
p. fossa
p. plexus

pterygoidei
nervus canalis p.

pterygomaxillary suture

pterygopalatine
p. fossa
p. ganglion

NOTES

pterygopalatine *(continued)*
p. nerve
p. neuralgia
pterygopalatini
nervi p.
radix intermedia ganglii p.
radix parasympathica ganglii p.
radix sensoria ganglii p.
radix sympathica ganglii p.
rami orbitales ganglii p.
ramus pharyngeus ganglii p.
pterygopalatinum
ganglion p.
rami ganglionares nervi maxillaris ad ganglion p.
PTH
parathyroid hormone
ptosis, pl. **ptoses**
cerebral p.
eyelid p.
Horner p.
myasthenic p.
oculomotor p.
oculosympathetic p.
paralytic p.
p. sympathetica
ptotic
PTP
posttetanic potentiation
PTS-Ultrason
PTT
partial thromboplastin time
pudendal
p. nerve
p. SEP
p. somatosensory evoked potential
pudendi
nucleus nervi p.
pudendus
nervus p.
Pudenz
P. shunt
P. valve
P. ventricular catheter
Pudenz-Heyer-Schulte valve
Pudenz-Heyer shunt system
puerperal eclampsia
puffer fish
pugilistica
dementia p.
Pulfrich phenomenon
pullout
screw p.
p. strength
pull test
pull-test technique
pulmonale
glomus p.
pulmonalis
plexus p.
rami pulmonales plexus p.
pulmonary
p. arteriovenous fistula
p. arteriovenous shunt
p. capillary wedge pressure
p. edema
p. embolism
p. encephalopathy
p. glomus
p. medication
p. tuberculosis
pulmonocoronary reflex
pulp
vertebral p.
pulposus
herniated nucleus p.
nucleus p.
Pulsar infusion pump
pulsatile
p. mass
p. tinnitus
pulsatility
Gosling p.
p. index
pulsating
p. electromagnetic field
p. headache
p. neurasthenia
p. visual halo
pulsation
p. artifact
carotid p.
pulse
entoptic p.
p. flip angle
p. generator
p. length
ocular p.
p. oximeter
p. oximetry
presaturation p.
radiofrequency p.
p. rate
p. repetition time
p. repetition time prolongation
RF p.
p. sequence
p. synchronous sound
p. timing diagram
p. transit time
p. wave artifact
p. wave Doppler
p. width
pulsed
p. Doppler
p. Doppler imaging
p. electromagnetic field (PEMF)

p. fluorography
p. gradient
pulsed-field gel electrophoresis
pulsed-range gated Doppler instrument
pulse-gated cine phase contrast sequence
pulseless disease
pulselessness
pulsion theory
pulvinar
p. nucleus
p. nucleus of thalamus
p. thalami
pulvinares
nuclei p.
pulvinotomy
pump
Cordis Secor implantable p.
drug infusion p.
implanted infusion p.
InDura intrathecal catheter and p.
Infusaid M400 constant-flow p.
infusion p.
intraaortic balloon p.
Medrad infusion p.
Medtronic SynchroMed implantable p.
miniosmotic infusion p.
morphine p.
Pulsar infusion p.
Shiley-Infusaid p.
SynchroMed model 8611H prototype implantable p.
volumetric infusion p.
punch
bone p.
Cone skull p.
disc p.
dural p.
Fehling TOP ejector p.
Ferris Smith-Kerrison p.
Hajek-Koffler p.
Hajek laminectomy p.
Hardy sellar p.
intervertebral p.
Kerrison bone p.
Raney laminectomy p.
p. rongeur
sellar p.
skull p.
punch-drunk syndrome
puncta (*pl. of* punctum)
punctata
rhizomelic chondrodysplasia p.
punctate
p. cavernous malformation
p. white matter hyperintensity
punctual stimulation
punctum, pl. **puncta**
p. dolorosum
p. luteum
p. vasculosum
puncture
Bernard p.
brain p.
cisternal p.
cranial p.
failed lumbar p.
intracisternal p.
lumbar p. (LP)
Quincke p.
spinal p.
stereotactic p.
sternal p.
thecal p.
ventricle p.
ventricular p.
Puno-Winter-Byrd (PWB)
P.-W.-B. system
pupil
absent p.
Adie-Holmes p.
Adie tonic p.
Argyll Robertson p.
blown p.
Bumke p.
consensual response p.
corn-picker's p.
dilated poorly reactive p.
enlarged p.
fixed p.
Holmes-Adie p.
Hutchinson p.
inverse Argyll Robertson p.
isocoric p.
p. light-near dissociation
Marcus Gunn p.
myotonic p.
paradoxical p.
pseudo-Argyll Robertson p.
p. reactivity
p. response
rigid p.
Robertson p.

NOTES

P

pupil *(continued)*
p. size
p. size disparity
tonic p.
tonically dilated p.
pupillary
p. abnormality
p. light reflex
p. light response
p. reactivity
pupillary-skin reflex
pupillatonia
pupillometry
pupillomotor
pupilloplegia
pupillotonic pseudotabes
purchase
bony p.
pure
p. absence
p. agraphia
p. alexia
p. aphasia
p. athetoid palsy
p. autonomic failure
p. depression
p. germinoma
p. hemisensory stroke
p. limb apraxia
p. motor hemiparesis
p. motor hemiplegia
p. sensory neuropathy
p. sensory stroke
p. spastic palsy
p. word deafness
p. word mutism
pure-tone
p.-t. audiogram
p.-t. audiometry
p.-t. average
p.-t. discrimination
p.-t. hearing loss
p.-t. hearing threshold
purine
p. metabolic disorder
p. metabolism
p. nucleotide phosphorylase deficiency
Purkinje
P. cell
P. cell degeneration
P. cell layer
P. corpuscle
P. neuron
Purmann method
Puros Accugraft allograft
purposeful movement
purpura
brain p.
Henoch-Schönlein p.
idiopathic thrombocytopenic p. (ITP)
immune thrombocytopenic p. (ITP)
malignant p.
thrombocytopenic p.
thrombotic thrombocytopenic p.
purpurea
Claviceps p.
pursuit
p. defect
p. eye movement
saccadic vertical smooth p.
smooth p.
p. system
purulent
p. encephalitis
p. meningitis
p. pachymeningitis
pusher
Jacobson suture p.
putamen
ventral p.
putaminal
p. hemorrhage
p. infarction
putative
p. effect
p. endogenous ligand
p. insult
p. mechanism
putatively poor-prognosis deficit syndrome
Putnam-Dana syndrome
putty
Bishop p.
OsteoStim DBM p.
Puusepp reflex
PV
parvalbumin
PV foam
PVA
periodic vestibular ataxia
PVG
periventricular gray
PVL
periventricular leukomalacia
PV-positive cell
PVS
persistent vegetative state
pigmented villonodular synovitis
PWB
Puno-Winter-Byrd
PXA
pleomorphic xanthoastrocytoma
pyelography
pyencephalus
pyknoepilepsy, pyknolepsy
pyknoleptic petit mal

pyknomorphous, pyknomorphic
pyknotic nucleus
pyla
pylar
pyocephalus
circumscribed p.
external p.
internal p.
pyogenes
Streptococcus p.
pyogenic
p. brain abscess
p. discitis
p. meningitis
p. osteomyelitis
p. pachymeningitis
pyogenica
encephalitis p.
Pyramesh case
pyramid
anterior p.
cerebellar p.
decussation of p.
Malacarne p.
p. of medulla
p. of medulla oblongata
olfactory p.
P. Scale
p. sign
syndrome of p.
p. of tympanum
p. of vermis
pyramidal
p. cell
p. cell layer
p. cerebral palsy
p. decussation
p. eminence
p. fiber
p. neuron
p. pathway
p. radiation
p. system
p. tract
p. tract disease
p. tract dysfunction
p. tract lesion
p. tractotomy
p. tract sign
p. trocar
p. weakness
pyramidale
stratum p.
pyramidales
fibrae p.
pyramidalis
eminentia p.
nucleus p.
radiatio p.
tractus p.
pyramidis, pl. **pyramides**
fasciculus circumolivaris p.
pyramidotomy
medullary p.
spinal p.
pyramidum
decussatio p.
pyramis
p. bulbus
p. of cerebellum
p. medullae oblongatae
p. tympani
p. vermis
pyranocarboxylic acid class
pyrazinamide
pyrazolopyrimidine
pyrexial headache
pyridostigmine bromide
pyridoxine deficiency
pyridoxine-deficiency seizure
pyridoxine-dependent epilepsy
pyriform (*var. of* piriform)
pyrimethamine
p. poisoning
p. sulfadoxine
pyrimidine metabolic disorder
pyrogen
endogenous p. (EP)
pyroglutamic aciduria
pyromaniac
pyrophosphate
technetium-99m p.
technetium stannous p.
pyruvate
p. carboxylase
p. carboxylase deficiency
p. dehydrogenase (PDH)
p. dehydrogenase complex
p. dehydrogenase multienzyme
p. dehydrogenase phosphatase
glycogen-derived p.
p. kinase deficiency
p. oxidation

NOTES

pyruvate-mediated anaplerosis

Q

Q

Q factor
Q fever
Q fever infection
Q score
Q test

2q
chromosome 2q

2q21-33
chromosome 2q21-33

2q24
chromosome 2q24

5q33-55
chromosome 5q33-55

6q
chromosome 6q

6q24
chromosome 6q24

7q21.2
chromosome 7q21.2

8q
chromosome 8q

8q13-21
chromosome 8q13-21

8q24
chromosome 8q24

10q22-24
chromosome 10q22-24

16q
chromosome 16q
pericentromeric region of chromosome 16q

16q24.1
chromosome 16q24.1

19q11-13
chromosome 19q11-13

19q13.3
chromosome 19q13.3

20q
chromosome 20q

20q13.2
chromosome 20q13.2

20q13.3
chromosome 20q13.3

21q22.1
chromosome 21q22.1

21q22.3
chromosome 21q22.3

QALE
quality-adjusted life expectancy

QEEG
quantitative electroencephalogram

QNP
quinpirole

3q25.2-q27
chromosome 3q25.2-q27

Q-SART
Quantitative Sudomotor Axon Reflex Test

Q-score profile

Q-sort
Q-s. method
Q-s. procedure
Q-s. technique

QST
quantitative sensory test

Q-Sweat

QTL
quantitative trait locus

Quad electrode

Quadramet

quadrangularis
lobulus q.
pars inferoposterior lobuli q.

quadrangular lobule

quadrantanopia, quadrantanopsia
upper homonymous q.

quadrantic hemianopia

quadrate
q. gyrus
q. lobe
q. lobe of cerebral hemisphere
q. lobule

quadrature
q. detector
q. head coil

quadratus
q. femoris nerve
lobulus q.

quadriceps
q. gait
q. jerk
q. muscle biopsy
q. myopathy
q. reflex

quadrigemina
corpora q.
lamina q.

quadrigeminal
q. arachnoid cyst
q. body
q. cistern
q. cistern lipoma
q. lamina
q. plate

quadrigeminalis
cisterna q.

quadrigeminum

Quadrilite 6000 fiberoptic headlight

quadriparesis
progressive flaccid q.
spastic q.
quadriplegia
spastic q.
static spastic q.
quadriplegic injury
quadrupedal extensor reflex
quadruple sectoranopia
qualitative morphology
quality
compulsive q.
Q. of Crisis Support Scale
q. factor
hypomanic q.
image q.
Q. of Life in Epilepsy-89 Inventory
q. of life measure
Q. of Life Scale
sleep q.
quality-adjusted
q.-a. life expectancy (QALE)
q.-a. life-year (QUALY)
quality-of-life measurement
QUALY
quality-adjusted life-year
quantal release deficiency
quantification
color velocity imaging q.
q. ultrasound
quantitative
q. computerized tomography
q. data
q. EEG analysis
q. electroencephalogram (QEEG)
q. functional test
q. imaging
q. measure
q. morphology
q. morphometric technique
q. morphometric tool
q. motor unit potential analysis
q. receptor autoradiography
Q. Scoring System
q. sensory test (QST)
q. spectral phonoangiography
Q. Sudomotor Axon Reflex Test (Q-SART)
q. sweat measurement system
q. trait locus (QTL)
quantum
q. mechanics
q. number
quarta
crista q.
macula cribrosa q.
quarti
apertura lateralis ventriculi q.
apertura mediana ventriculi q.
foramen lateralis ventriculi q.
plexus choroideus ventriculi q.
ramus choroideus ventriculi q.
recessus lateralis ventriculi q.
striae medullares ventriculi q.
sulcus limitans ventriculi q.
sulcus medianus ventriculi q.
tegmen ventriculi q.
tela choroidea ventriculi q.
tenia ventriculi q.
ventriculi q.
quartus
ventriculus q.
Quartzo device
quasi-purposeful movement
quavering voice
quazepam
Queckenstedt
Q. phenomenon
Q. sign
Q. test
Queckenstedt-Stookey test
quench
magnet q.
question mark-shaped incision
questionnaire
Abbreviated Life Event Q.
Ages and Stages Q.'s
Autism Screening Q.
Berlin Sleep Q.
children's sleep habits q.
Cognitive Failures Q.
Communications Profile Q.
Cree Q.
Dysexecutive Q.
Edinburgh Q.
Frankfurt Complaint Q.
Functional Outcomes of Sleep Q. (FOSQ)
Horne-Ostberg q.
Kenney Self-Care Q.
Leeds Sleep Evaluation Q. (LSEQ)
McGill Pain Q.
Modified Autonomic Perception Q.
modified McGill Pain Q.
Narcolepsy Symptoms Severity Q.
North American Spine Society q.
Oswestry Low Back Pain Disability Q.
Parkinson Disease Q.-39 (PDQ-39)
Pediatric Sleep Q. (PSQ)
Roland-Morris disability q.
Short-Form McGill Pain Q. (SF-MPQ)
Short Portable Mental Status Q.
sleep q.
Sleep Timing Q. (STQ)
Stanford Acute Stress Reaction Q.

St. George Anxiety Q.
St. Mary's Hospital Sleep Q. (SMHSQ)
quetiapine fumarate
Quick
Q. Connect twist drill
Q. neurological screening test
QuickAnchor
Resolve Q.
QuickStart
Beckman Coulter Q.
quiet
q. sleep
q. sleep characteristic
q. wakefulness mode
quinacrine fluorescent banding
Quincke
Q. disease
Q. edema
Q. puncture
Q. spinal needle
quinidine
quinine ascorbate
quinolinate
quinolinic acid
quinolone
quinpirole (QNP)
quintana
Rochalimaea q.
quintus
ventriculus q.
quinuclidinyl benzilate
quisqualic acid
quotient
Ayala q.
brain-age q.
intelligence q. (IQ)

NOTES

RA
RAATE
Recovery Attitude and Treatment Evaluator
RAATE score
RAB
remote afterloading brachytherapy
rabbit syndrome
rabic tubercle
rabies virus
Rabiner neurological hammer
Rabot disease
raccoon eye
racemase deficiency
Racetrack Microtron MM50 accelerator
rachial plexus
rachicentesis
rachidial
rachidian
rachigraph
rachilysis
rachiocentesis
rachiochysis
rachiometer
rachiomyelitis
rachiopathy
rachioplegia
rachioscoliosis
rachiotome, rachitome
rachiotomy, rachitomy
lateral r.
rachischisis
r. partialis
posterior r.
r. totalis
rachitome (*var. of* rachiotome)
Racz Tun-L-Kath catheter
radial
r. artery
r. artery graft
r. artery harvesting (RAH)
r. glia
r. glial cell
r. nerve
r. nerve trauma
r. paralysis
r. phenomenon
r. reflex
radialis
flexor carpi r. (FCR)
nervi digitales dorsales nervi r.
nervus r.
rami musculares nervi r.
ramus communicans ulnaris nervi r.
ramus profundus nervi r.
ramus superficialis nervi r.
r. sign
radiant layer
radiata
corona r.
radiate
r. crown
r. layer of hippocampus
radiatio, pl. **radiationes**
r. acustica
r. corporis callosi
r. inferior thalami
r. optica
r. pyramidalis
r. thalami anterior
r. thalamica posterior
radiation
acoustic r.
r. angiopathy
anterior thalamic r.
auditory r.
r. beam
beta-emitting r.
Bragg peak r.
central thalamic r.
r. of corpus callosum
r. dose
r. effect
electromagnetic r.
r. exposure
external r.
fibrosis r.
r. field
focal r.
geniculocalcarine r.
Gratiolet r.
inferior thalamic r.
r. injury
r. injury headache
leukoencephalopathy r.
low-energy gamma r.
r. myelopathy
r. necrosis
r. neuritis
r. neuropathy
occipitothalamic r.
optic r.
r. plexopathy
posterior thalamic r.
prelemniscal r.
proton beam r.
pyramidal r.
r. retinopathy
single-fraction r.
stereotactic gamma r.

radiation *(continued)*
tegmental r.
temporal lobe r.
thalamic r.
thalamostriate r.
thalamotemporal r.
r. therapy
r. vasculitis
r. vasculopathy
Wernicke r.
radiation-induced
r.-i. glioma
r.-i. morphologic change
r.-i. plexopathy
r.-i. vasculopathy
radiatum
stratum r.
radical
r. debridement
r. decompressive craniotomy
diflavin free r.
r. disc excision
free r.
r. fringe
hydroxyl r.
r. induced brain injury
oxygen free r.
r. prefrontal lobotomy
superoxide anion r.
radices (*pl. of* radix)
radicotomy
radiculalgia
radicular
r. cyst
r. distribution of pain
r. fiber
r. filum
r. hyporeflexia
r. motor deficit
r. neuritis
r. neuropathy
r. syndrome
r. vein
radicularia
fila r.
radicularis magna
radiculectomy
radiculitis
acute brachial r.
radiculoganglionitis
radiculomedullary
r. fistula
r. syndrome
radiculomeningeal spinal vascular malformation
radiculomeningomyelitis
radiculomyelopathy
radiculoneuritis
radiculoneuropathy
radiculopathy
cervical r.
diabetic thoracic r.
hereditary sensory r.
lumbosacral r.
spondylotic caudal r.
radiculospinal artery
Radifocus
R. guidewire
R. introducer B kit
radioactive
r. count
r. iodide
r. strontium needle
r. tracer
r. yttrium (^{90}Y)
r. yttrium seed
radiobicipital reflex
radiobinding assay
radiocapitellar joint ganglion
radioencephalogram
radioencephalography
radiofluoroscopy
televised r.
radiofrequency (RF)
r. eddy current
r. electromagnetic field
r. generator
r. head coil
r. heating
r. homogeneity pattern
r. lesion
r. lesioning
r. needle electrode system
r. neurotomy
r. palatoplasty
r. pulse
r. rhizotomy
r. spoiling
r. thermocoagulation
r. thoracic sympathectomy
r. transmitter
R. Triage System (RAFTS)
radiofrequency-induced echo
radiograph
cephalometric r.
Waters view r.
radiography
digital r. (DR)
lateral cephalometric r.
plain r.
radiohumeral joint
radioimmunoassay
radioimmunoprecipitation (RIP)
radioimmunotherapy
radioisotope
r. cisternogram
r. cisternography

r. scan
r. uptake
radiolabeled neurotrophic factor
radiolabeling
radiologic abnormality
radiological
r. phantom
r. pressure-volume index
radiology
interventional r. (IR)
radiolucency
hydrocephalic periventricular r.
periventricular r.
radiolucent
r. cranial pin headholder
r. operating room table extension
radionecrosis
radioneuritis
Radionics
R. bipolar coagulation unit
R. bipolar instrument
R. CRW stereotactic head frame
R. RF lesion generator
radionucleotide (RN)
r. scanning
radionuclide
r. bone scan
r. cisternography
r. imaging
r. study
radiopaque fiducial
radioperiosteal reflex
radiopharmaceutical
radioreceptor
radiosensitizer
radiosignal line
radiosurgery
advanced design LINAC r.
arteriovenous malformation r.
Bragg peak r.
charged particle r.
cranial r.
extracranial r.
gamma knife r. (GKRS)
hypofractionated r.
image-guided robotic r.
LINAC r.
linear accelerator r.
multiarc LINAC r.
particle beam r.
photon beam r.
repeat r.
single-dose r.
stereotactic r. (SRS)
trunnion-guided r.
radiosurgical
r. corpus callosotomy
r. dosage
r. lesioning procedure
r. management
r. technique
radiotherapy
r. brain mapping
conformal r.
external beam r. (EBRT)
fractionated r.
heavy particle r.
hyperfractionated r.
interstitial r.
mathematical optimization and logical dimensioning for r.
stereotactic linear accelerator r.
whole-brain r.
radiotracer
radius of angulation
radix, pl. **radices**
r. anterior
r. anterior ansae cervicalis
r. anterior nervi spinalis
r. brevis ganglii ciliaris
r. cochlearis
r. cochlearis nervi vestibulocochlearis
radices craniales
r. cranialis nervi accessorii
r. dorsalis
r. dorsalis nervi spinalis
r. inferior ansae cervicalis
r. inferior nervi vestibulocochlearis
r. intermedia ganglii pterygopalatini
r. lateralis nervi mediani
r. lateralis tractus optici
r. longa ganglii ciliaris
r. medialis nervi mediani
r. medialis tractus optici
r. motoria
r. motoria nervi spinalis
r. nasociliaris
r. nasociliaris ganglii ciliaris
r. nervi facialis
radices nervi trigemini
r. oculomotoria ganglii ciliaris
r. parasympathica ganglii ciliaris
r. parasympathica ganglii otici

NOTES

radix *(continued)*
r. parasympathica ganglii pterygopalatini
r. parasympathica ganglii sublingualis
r. parasympathica ganglii submandibularis
r. parasympathica gangliorum pelvicorum
radices plexus brachialis
r. posterior
r. posterior ansae cervicalis
r. posterior nervi spinalis
r. sensoria ganglii otici
r. sensoria ganglii pterygopalatini
r. sensoria ganglii submandibularis
r. sensoria nervi spinalis
r. sensoria nervi trigemini
radices spinales
r. spinalis nervi accessorii
r. superior ansae cervicalis
r. superior nervi vestibulocochlearis
r. sympathica ganglii ciliaris
r. sympathica ganglii pterygopalatini
r. ventralis
r. ventralis nervi spinalis
r. vestibularis
r. vestibularis nervi vestibulocochlearis
Radovici sign
Raeder
R. paratrigeminal neuralgia
R. paratrigeminal syndrome
RAFTS
Radiofrequency Triage System
ragged red fiber (RRF)
RAH
radial artery harvesting
RAI
respiratory arousal index
railway nystagmus
Raimondi
R. infant scalp hemostatic forceps
R. low-pressure shunt
R. peritoneal catheter
R. spring catheter
R. ventricular catheter
Rainin clip-bending spatula
raised intracranial pressure
raloxifene
Rambaud syndrome
ramelteon
rami (*pl. of* ramus)
ramicotomy
ramisection
ramitis
ramp stimulation
Ramsay
R. Hunt paralysis
R. Hunt syndrome, type I, II
R. Hunt type of inherited dentatorubral degeneration
ramus, pl. **rami**
rami ad pontem
rami albus nevi spinalis
rami alveolares superiores anteriores nervi maxillaris
rami alveolares superiores posteriores nervi maxillaris
rami alveolaris superiores medius nervi maxillaris
anterior ascending r.
rami anteriores nervorum cervicalium
rami anteriores nervorum lumbalium
rami anteriores nervorum sacralium
rami anteriores nervorum thoracicorum
anterior horizontal r.
r. anterior nervi auricularis
r. anterior nervi coccygei
r. anterior nervi cutanei antebrachii medialis
r. anterior nervi obturatorii
r. anterior nervi spinalis
r. anterior sulci lateralis cerebri
r. articularis
r. articularis nervi vagus
r. ascendens sulci lateralis cerebri
r. autonomicus
rami bronchiales anteriores nervi vagus
rami bronchiales posteriores nervi vagus
rami buccales nervi facialis
rami calcanei laterales nervi suralis
rami calcanei mediales nervi tibialis
rami cardiaci cervicales inferiores nervi vagus
rami cardiaci cervicales superiores nervi vagus
rami cardiaci thoracici
rami cardiaci thoracici nervi vagus
rami caudae nuclei caudati
rami celiaci nervi vagus
rami centrales anteromediales
rami cervicalis nervi facialis
r. chiasmaticus
rami choroidei
r. choroidei posteriores laterales
r. choroidei posteriores mediales
r. choroidei ventriculi lateralis
r. choroidei ventriculi tertii
r. choroideus ventriculi quarti
r. cingularis
rami clivales

rami clunium inferiores
rami clunium mediales
rami clunium superiores
r. colli nervi facialis
r. communicans
r. communicans albus nervi spinalis
r. communicans cochlearis nervi vestibularis
r. communicans cum nervo glossopharyngeo
r. communicans cum nervo nasociliari
r. communicans fibularis nervi fibularis communis
r. communicans griseus nervi spinalis
r. communicans nervi facialis cum nervo glossopharyngeo
r. communicans nervi glossopharyngei cum chorda tympani
r. communicans nervi glossopharyngei cum nervo auriculotemporali
r. communicans nervi glossopharyngei ramo auriculari nervi vagus
r. communicans nervi glossopharyngei ramo meningeo nervi vagus
r. communicans nervi intermedii cum nervo vagus
r. communicans nervi intermedii cum plexu tympanico
r. communicans nervi lacrimalis cum nervo zygomatico
r. communicans nervi laryngei inferioris cum ramo laryngeo interno
r. communicans nervi laryngei superioris cum nervo laryngeo inferiore
r. communicans nervi lingualis cum chorda tympani
r. communicans nervi mediani com nervo ulnari
r. communicans nervi nasociliaris cum ganglio ciliari
r. communicans nervi vagi cum nervo glossopharyngeo
r. communicans peroneus nervi peronei communis
r. communicans ulnaris nervi radialis
r. communicantes
rami communicantes nervi auriculotemporalis cum nervi faciali
rami communicantes nervi lingualis cum nervo hypoglosso
rami communicantes nervorum spinalium
rami corporis amygdaloidei
r. corporis callosi dorsalis
rami corporis geniculati lateralis
rami cruris posterioris capsulae internae
rami cutanei anteriores nervi femoralis
rami cutanei cruris medialis nervi sapheni
r. cutaneus
r. cutaneus anterior abdominalis nervi intercostalis
r. cutaneus anterior nervi iliohypogastrici
r. cutaneus anterior pectoralis nervi intercostalis
r. cutaneus lateralis abdominalis nervi intercostalis
r. cutaneus lateralis nervi iliohypogastrici
r. cutaneus lateralis pectoralis nervi intercostalis
r. cutaneus lateralis pectoralis nervi obturatorii
rami dentales inferiores plexus dentalis inferioris
rami dentales superiores plexus dentalis superiores
r. digastricus nervi facialis
dorsal r.
rami dorsales nervorum cervicalium
rami dorsales nervorum lumbalium
rami dorsales nervorum sacralium
rami dorsales nervorum thoracicorum
r. dorsalis nervi coccygei
r. dorsalis nervi spinalis
r. dorsalis nervi ulnaris
rami esophagei nervi laryngei recurrentis
r. externus nervi accessorii
r. externus nervi laryngei superioris

NOTES

ramus *(continued)*
rami fauciales nervi lingualis
r. femoralis nervi genitofemoralis
r. frontalis anteromedialis
r. frontalis intermediomedialis
r. frontalis posteromedialis
rami ganglionares nervi lingualis ad ganglion submandibulare
rami ganglionares nervi maxillaris ad ganglion oticum
rami ganglionares nervi maxillaris ad ganglion pterygopalatinum
rami gastrici anteriores trunci vagalis anterioris
rami gastrici nervi vagus
rami gastrici posteriores trunci vagalis posterioris
r. genitalis nervi genitofemoralis
rami genus capsulae internae
rami gingivales inferiores plexus dentalis inferioris
rami gingivales nervi mentalis
rami gingivales superiores plexus dentalis superioris
rami glandulares ganglii submandibularis
rami globi pallidi
rami gluteales inferiores
rami gluteales mediales
r. gluteales superiores
gray r.
rami hepatici trunci vagalis anterioris
r. hypothalamicus
rami inferiores nervi transversi colli
r. inferior nervi oculomotorii
r. infrapatellaris nervi sapheni
rami interganglionares trunci sympathici
r. internus nervi accessorii
r. internus nervi laryngei superioris
rami isthmi faucium nervi lingualis
rami labiales nervi mentalis
rami labiales superiores nervi infraorbitalis
rami laryngopharyngei ganglii cervicalis superioris
r. lateralis nervi supraorbitalis
r. lateralis rami posterioris nervi cervicalis
r. lateralis rami posterioris nervi lumbalis
r. lateralis rami posterioris nervi sacralis
r. lateralis rami posterioris nervi thoracici
rami linguales nervi glossopharyngei
rami linguales nervi hypoglossi
rami linguales nervi lingualis
r. lingualis nervi facialis
rami mammarii laterales rami cutanei lateralis pectoralis nervi intercostalis
rami mammarii mediales rami cutanei anterioris pectoralis nervi intercostalis
r. marginalis
r. marginalis mandibularis nervi facialis
r. medialis nervi supraorbitalis
r. medialis rami posterioris nervi cervicalis
r. medialis rami posterioris nervi lumbalis
r. medialis rami posterioris nervi sacralis
r. medialis rami posterioris nervi thoracici
rami medullares laterales
rami medullares mediales
r. membranae tympani nervi auriculotemporalis
r. meningeus nervi mandibularis
r. meningeus nervi maxillaris
r. meningeus nervi spinalis
r. meningeus nervi vagus
r. meningeus recurrens nervi ophthalmici
rami mentales nervi mentalis
rami musculares nervi femoralis
rami musculares nervi fibularis profundi
rami musculares nervi ischiadici
rami musculares nervi mediani
rami musculares nervi musculocutanei
rami musculares nervi nervorum intercostalium
rami musculares nervi peronei profundi
rami musculares nervi peronei superficialis
rami musculares nervi radialis
rami musculares nervi tibialis
rami musculares nervi ulnaris
rami musculares plexus lumbalis
rami musculares rami anterioris nervi obturatorii
rami musculares rami externi nervi accessorii
rami musculares rami posterioris nervi obturatorii
r. muscularis
r. musculi stylopharyngei nervi glossopharyngei

rami nasales externi nervi infraorbitalis
rami nasales interni laterales nervi ethmoidalis anterioris
ram nasales interni mediales nervi ethmoidalis anterioris
rami nasales interni nervi infraorbitalis
rami nasales nervi ethmoidalis anterioris
rami nasales posteriores inferiores nervi palatini majoris
rami nasales posteriores superiores laterales nervi maxillaris
rami nasales posteriores superiores mediales nervi maxillaris
r. nasalis externus nervi ethmoidalis anterioris
r. nervi oculomotorii ganglii ad ciliare
rami nucleorum hypothalamicorum
r. occipitalis nervi auricularis posterioris
r. occipitotemporalis
rami orbitales ganglii pterygopalatini
rami orbitales nervi maxillaris
r. palmaris nervi mediani
r. palmaris nervi ulnaris
rami palpebrales inferiores nervi infraorbitalis
rami palpebrales nervi infratrochlearis
r. parietooccipitalis
rami parotidei nervi auriculotemporalis
rami partis retrolentiformis capsulae internae
rami pedunculares
r. pericardiacus nervi phrenici
rami perineales nervi cutanei femoris posterioris
ram pharyngeal nervi glossopharyngei
rami pharyngei nervi laryngei recurrentis
r. pharyngeus ganglii pterygopalatini
r. pharyngeus nervi vagus
rami phrenicoabdominales nervi phrenici
rami posteriores nervorum cervicalium
rami posteriores nervorum lumbalium
rami posteriores nervorum sacralium
rami posteriores nervorum thoracicorum
r. posterior nervi auricularis magni
r. posterior nervi coccygei
r. posterior nervi cutanei antebrachii medialis
r. posterior nervi obturatorii
r. posterior nervi spinalis
posterior primary r.
r. posterior sulci lateralis cerebri
r. profundus nervi plantaris lateralis
r. profundus nervi radialis
r. profundus nervi ulnaris
rami pulmonales plexus pulmonalis
rami pulmonales thoracici gangliorum thoracicorum
r. recurrens nervi spinalis
rami renales nervi vagus
rami renales plexus coeliaci
r. renalis nervi splanchnici minoris
r. sinus carotici
r. sinus carotici nervi glossopharyngei
r. stylohyoideus nervi facialis
rami substantiae nigrae
r. superficialis nervi plantaris lateralis
r. superficialis nervi radialis
r. superficialis nervi ulnaris
rami superiores nervi transversi colli
r. superior nervi oculomotorii
r. sympathicus ad ganglion submandibulare
r. sympathicus ganglii ciliaris
rami temporales anteriores
rami temporales intermedii
rami temporales posteriores
rami temporales superficiales nervi auriculotemporalis
r. tentorii nervi ophthalmici
rami thalamici
r. thalamicus
r. thyrohyoideus ansae cervicalis
r. tonsillae cerebellae
rami tonsillares nervi glossopharyngei
rami tonsillares nervorum palatinorum minorum

NOTES

ramus *(continued)*
rami tracheales nervi laryngei recurrentis
rami tractus optici
r. tubarius plexus tympanici
rami tuberis cinerei
ventral r.
rami ventrales nervorum cervicalium
rami ventrales nervorum lumbalium
rami ventrales nervorum sacralium
rami ventrales nervorum thoracicorum
r. ventralis nervi coccygei
r. ventralis nervi spinalis
r. visceralis
white r.
rami zygomatici nervi facialis
r. zygomaticofacialis nervi zygomatici
r. zygomaticotemporalis nervi zygomatici

Rand
R. Functional Limitations Battery
R. Physical Capacities Battery

random
r. digital dialing
r. urine testing
r. wave

randomized
r. clinical trial
r. controlled trial
R. Trial of Tirilazad Mesylate in Patients With Acute Stroke (RANTTAS)

Raney
R. coagulating forceps
R. laminectomy punch
R. laminectomy rongeur
R. perforator
R. rongeur forceps
R. scalp clip
R. scalp clip applier
R. scalp clip-applying forceps
R. stirrup-loop curette

range
alpha frequency r.
dose r.
extreme r.
frequency r.
r. of movement
significant r.
subclinical r.
therapeutic r.

ranine

ranitidine

Rankin
R. Disability Index
R. score

Ransford loop

RANTES
regulated on activation, normal T-cell expressed and secreted

RANTTAS
Randomized Trial of Tirilazad Mesylate in Patients With Acute Stroke
RANTTAS study

Ranvier
R. cross
node of R.
R. node
R. segment
R. tactile disc

rapamycin

RAPD
relative afferent pupillary defect

raphe
r. corporis callosi
dorsal r.
r. mediana medullae oblongata
r. medullae oblongatae
medullary r.
r. nuclei region
r. nucleus
nucleus dorsalis r.
r. of pons
r. pontis
serotonergic dorsal r.
Stilling r.

raphes
nuclei reticulares r.
nucleus centralis superior r.
nucleus pallidus r.
nucleus pontis r.
nucleus posterior r.
oculomotor nucleus r.

raphespinal fiber

rapid
r. acquisition radiofrequency-echo steady-state imaging
r. alternating movement
r. eye movement (REM)
r. eye movement deprivation
r. eye movement-onset blinking
r. eye movement sleep
r. eye movement-sleep behavior
r. eye movement sleep-locked headache
r. fine finger movement
r. fluctuating course
r. metabolizer patient
r. nystagmus
r. plasma reagin (RPR)
r. spin echo (RSE)
r. time-zone change syndrome
R. Transit catheter
R. Transit microcatheter

rapsyn gene

raptus
status r.
rarefaction
r. stimulation
r. stimulus
RAS
reticular activating system
ras
r. oncogene
r. protein
r. signaling pathway
rasagiline mesylate
rash
bull's-eye r.
butterfly r.
heliotrope r.
maculopapular r.
morbilliform r.
scarlatiniform r.
target r.
Rasmussen
bundle of R.
R. chronic focal encephalitis
R. nerve fiber
olivocochlear bundle of R.
R. olivocochlear bundle
R. syndrome
rasp
Jansen r.
Nicola r.
Olivecrona r.
Yasargil r.
raspatory
rate
alternate motion r. (AMR)
bleeding r.
cerebral metabolic r.
clearance r.
compliance r.
decline r.
erythrocyte sedimentation r. (ESR)
exacerbation r.
false-positive r.
fusion nonunion r.
implant survival r.
intrathecal IgG synthetic r.
limbic neuronal firing r.
metabolic r.
mortality r.
nonspecific response r.
nonunion r.
NPH recovery r.
peak expiratory flow r.
placebo response r.
postembolization bleeding r.
postsurgical infection r.
pseudarthrosis r.
pulse r.
r. of recovery
r. of recovery at discharge
relapse r.
respiratory r.
seizure-free r.
specific absorption r.
r. of speech
spinal load r.
transverse relaxation r.
treatment completion r.
treatment response r.
T2 relaxation r.
vertebral osteosynthesis fusion r.
rate-limiting enzyme
Rathke
R. cleft cyst
R. pouch
R. pouch cyst
R. pouch tumor
rating
baseline r.
Clinical Dementia R. (CDR)
clinician r.
dimensional r.
hyperintensity r.
r. instrument
intent r.
maximum intent r.
maximum lethality r.
r. method
nonrandom r.
pressure r.
r. procedure
ratio
absolute terminal innervation r.
bicaudate r.
CD4/CD8 r.
choline/*N*-acetyl-aspartate r.
Cho/NAA r.
contrast-to-noise r. (CNR)
Cre + Cho r.
CSF to serum glucose r.
cup-to-disc r.
distribution volume r. (DVR)
embolus-to-blood r.
estrogen-to-progesterone r.

NOTES

ratio *(continued)*
Evans r.
functional terminal innervation r.
guanine/cytosine r.
gyromagnetic r.
international normalized r. (INR)
Lindegaard hemispheric r.
magnetic transfer r.
magnetization transfer r.
risk r.
risk-benefit r.
signal-to-noise r. (SNR)
T r.
^{99m}Tc HMPAO T/C r.
Torg r.
tumor/cerebellum r.
tumor/healthy tissue r.
rational
r. polypharmacy
r. polytherapy
r. problem solving
Ratliff avascular necrosis classification
raw
r. Q score
r. speckled image
r. volume
ray
R. brain spatula
R. brain spatula spoon
gamma r.
photon r.
R. pituitary curette
R. RRE-TM thermistor electrode
R. TFC
R. threaded fusion cage
Raymond
R. apoplexy
R. syndrome
Raymond-Cestan syndrome
Raynaud
R. disease
R. phenomenon
R. syndrome
Rayport
R. dura and knife dissector
R. dural dissector and knife
Ray-Tec sponge
ray-tracing reconstruction
Rayvist
RBE
relative biologic effectiveness
RBS
right brain stroke
RC
real contour
rCBF
regional cerebral blood flow
rCBV
relative cerebral blood volume
rCPP
regional cerebral perfusion pressure
RDD
Rosai-Dorfman disease
RDI
respiratory disturbance index
reaching-grasping movement
reaction
abnormal r.
acute dystonic r. (ADR)
acute organic r.
affective r.
agitated r.
allergic r.
amplification r.
anaphylactoid r.
arousal r.
Arthus r.
aseptic meningeal r.
Asian alcohol flush r.
astrocytic r.
autoimmune r.
axon r.
axonal r.
Bechterew r.
catastrophic r.
chronic paranoid r.
compulsive r.
consciousness stress r.
contrast dye r.
conversion r.
r. of degeneration
delayed hypersensitivity r.
depressive psychoneurotic r.
depressive psychotic r.
depressive situational r.
dissociative psychoneurotic r.
doll's eye r.
drug r.
dystonic r.
echo r.
exogenous r.
Fenton r.
galvanic skin r.
gemistocytic r.
glial r.
heel-tap r.
hyperkinetic r.
hypochondriacal r.
hypochondriac psychoneurotic r.
idiosyncratic r.
initial stress r.
intracutaneous r.
involutional paranoid r.
involutional psychotic r.
Jarisch-Herxheimer fever r.
Jolly r.
lengthening r.
R. Level Scale

magnet r.
Marchi r.
MRZ r.
Much-Holzmann r.
myasthenic r.
neurasthenic psychoneurosis r.
obsessional r.
ocular tilt r.
pain r.
parachute r.
paranoid involutional r.
pathological grief r.
phobia r.
phobic r.
placing r.
polymerase chain r. (PCR)
postural r.
psychogalvanic r.
psychomotor stress r.
psychoneurotic depressive r.
psychotic depressive r.
retrograde axon r.
reverse transcriptase-polymerase chain r. (RT-PCR)
situational stress r.
sleeplessness associated with acute emotional conflicts or r.
sleeplessness associated with intermittent emotional conflicts or r.
r. speed
startle r.
stress r.
tendon r.
r. time
Wernicke r.

reaction/response
startle r./r.

reactivation
varicella-zoster virus r.
VZV r.

reactive
r. astrocyte
r. cell
r. gliosis
r. oxygen species (ROS)
r. seizure

reactivity
emotional r.
pupil r.
pupillary r.

reader
kinetic microplate r.

reading seizure

readout
r. delay
r. gradient
r. period

reagin
rapid plasma r. (RPR)

real
r. contour (RC)
r. origin

reality
r. distortion
r. therapy

real-life stimulus

real-time
r.-t. color Doppler imaging
r.-t. guidance
r.-t. monitoring

reaming awl

reanimation
facial r.

reasoning
visuospatial r.

Reback
paroxysmal dystonic choreoathetosis of Mount and R.

Rebif MS

rebleed
aneurysmal r.

rebleeding of aneurysm

rebound
r. effect
r. hyperthermia
r. insomnia
r. nystagmus
r. phenomenon
REM r.
r. suppression

reboxetine mesylate

recalcitrant

recall
event r.
r. failure
r. memory
r. performance
recognition versus r.
remote r.
r. of similarities
word r.
r. of word list

NOTES

recall-accuracy
code substitution-immediate r.-a.
recalled-delay
recanalization
angiographic r.
percutaneous endoscopic r.
TCD r.
receiver
r. bandwidth
r. coil
r. limitation
r. operating characteristic (ROC)
r. overflow
r. overload
r. saturation
recency effect
recent memory
receptive
r. aphasia
r. area
r. dysphagia
r. dysprosody
r. language processing
receptoma
receptor
A1 adenosine r.
acetylcholine r. (AChR)
ACH r.
activated estrogen r.
adenosine r.
adrenergic r.
r. affinity
AI adenosine r.
airway mucosal r.
alpha-adrenergic r.
alpha-2 adrenergic r.
AMPA r.
androgen r.
benzodiazepine postsynaptic r.
calcitonin receptor-like r. (CRLR)
catecholamine r.
central benzodiazepine r.
cerebral acetylcholine nicotinic r.
chemosensory r.
cold r.
contact r.
cutaneous r.
D2 r.
D3 r.
r. density
r. dimerization
dopamine D_2 r.
epidermal growth factor r. (EGFR)
epsilon opiate r.
estrogen r.
excitatory amino acid r.
extrasynaptic r.
fibroblast growth factor r. (FGFR)
fibroblast growth factor r. 2 (FGFR2)
GABA r.
$GABA_A$ r. (GABAR)
$GABA_B$ r.
glutamate r. 1 (GluR1)
G-protein-coupled r. (GPCR)
gustatory r.
H1 r.
hair follicle r.
heterodimeric r.
hormonal r.
5-HT1 r.
5-HT2 r.
5-HT3 r.
5-HT2C r.
5HTIA r.
human poliovirus r. (hPVR)
Iggo r.
intranuclear r.
intraperitoneal r.
J r.
joint r.
juxtapulmonary r.
kainate r.
kappa opiate r.
r. ligand
limbic dopamine r.
low-density lipoprotein r.
mechanical r.
metabotropic glutamate r.
N-methyl-D-aspartate r.
mu opiate r.
muscarinic acetylcholine r. (mAChR)
muscle r.
nicotinic acetylcholine r. (nAChR)
NMDA r.
N1, N2 r.
nonadapting r.
nuclear r.
r. occupancy
odorant r. (OR)
olfactory r.
opiate r.
peripheral benzodiazepine r.
peripheral catecholamine r.
postsynaptic 5-HT2 r.
postsynaptic 5-HT3 r.
r. potential
pressure r.
progesterone r.
r. protein tyrosine phosphatase zeta/beta
retroviral CB r.
ryanodine r.
sensory neuron-specific G protein-coupled r. (SNSRs)
serotonin 5-HT2 r.

signal transducing r.
stretch r.
striatal r.
subsensitization of presynaptic r.'s
r. subunit
tactile r.
thermal r.
touch r.
Trk r.
tumor necrosis factor r. (TNFR)
tyrosine-kinase r.
tyrosine kinase A r.
r. up-regulation
urokinase plasminogen activator r.
vanilloid VR1 r.
VCAM-1 r.
very low density lipoprotein r.
viral r.
warmth r.

receptor-binding property

receptor-mediated current

recess
anterior r.
cerebellopontine r.
chiasmatic r.
cochlear r.
cupular part of epitympanic r.
frontoethmoidal r.
infundibular r.
optic r.
pineal r.
pontocerebellar r.
posterior r.
preoptic r.
Reichert cochlear r.
sphenoethmoidal r.
spherical r.
supraoptic r.
suprapineal r.
Tarin r.
triangular r.

recessive
autosomal r.
r. dystonia musculorum deformans

recessus
r. anterior
r. cochlearis
r. infundibularis
r. infundibuli
r. lateralis ventriculi quarti
r. opticus
r. pinealis
r. posterior
r. supraopticus
r. suprapinealis
r. triangularis

Rechtschaffen

recipiomotor

reciprocal
r. circuitry
r. connection
r. innervation
r. translocation

recognition
covert face r.
environmental sound r.
face r.
facial r.
impaired face r.
impaired object r.
r. memory
R. Memory Test (RMT)
taste quality r.
r. test
r. time
r. versus recall
word r.

recombinant
r. DNA technique
r. human tumor necrosis factor-alpha
r. tau isoform
r. tissue plasminogen activator (RTPA)

reconstruction
craniofacial r.
3-dimensional r.
maximum intensity pixel r.
nasal r.
oropharyngeal r.
planar r.
ray-tracing r.
split bone graft r.
surface r.

record
Candidate Profile R.
r. electrode

recorder
SnoreSat sleep r.

recording
ambulatory EEG r.
concurrent video-EEG r.
continuous electromyographic r.
continuous online r.

NOTES

recording *(continued)*
deep brain microelectrode r.
depth r.
r. electrode
intracranial r.
jerk-locked back-averaged r.
magnetic search coil r.
microelectrode r.
nonreference r.
paired electrode r.
polygraphic r.
videocassette r.
video-EEG r.
whole-cell r.
recovered memory
recovery
R. Attitude and Treatment Evaluator (RAATE)
fluid-attenuated inversion r. (FLAIR)
functional language r.
inversion r.
motor r.
neurologic r.
r. phase
post r.
rate of r.
saturation r.
short tau inversion r.
short TI inversion r. (STIR)
short time inversion r.
r. sleep
r. of vision
recruiting response
recruitment
r. line
oligodendrocyte progenitor r.
r. pattern
sibling r.
recta
vasa r.
rectal nerve
rectangle
Hartshill r.
Luque r.
rectangular
r. awl
r. brain spatula
rectocardiac reflex
rectolaryngeal reflex
rectus
gyrus r.
r. lateralis abducens oculomotor muscle
r. paralysis
sinus r.
r. spike artifact
recurrence
headache r.
seizure r.
recurrens
arteria r.
recurrent
r. artery of Heubner
r. concussion
r. course
r. encephalopathy
r. enteric cyst
r. headache
r. insomnia
r. laryngeal nerve (RLN)
r. meningeal nerve
r. mood disorder
r. pain
r. panic attack
r. perforating artery
r. polyneuropathy
r. subluxation
r. tumor
recurrentis
rami esophagei nervi laryngei r.
rami pharyngei nervi laryngei r.
rami tracheales nervi r.
rami tracheales nervi laryngei r.
recurring
r. headache
r. symptom
recutita
Matricaria r.
recycling
lipid r.
red
r. cell folic acid level
r. eye
r. man syndrome
r. neck syndrome
r. neuralgia
r. nucleus
r. softening
red/blue pulsatile mass
redifferentiation
Redlich-Fisher miliary plaque
redox factor-1
reduced tremor
reducer
Cloward cervical dislocation r.
reducing
r. body myelopathy
r. body myopathy
reductase
aldose r.
dihydropteridine r.
r. inhibitor
reduction
r. of amplitude
CBF r.

contrast sensitivity r.
cumulative medication r.
dose r.
r. fixation
fracture r.
fracture-dislocation r.
r. glossectomy
medication r.
meditation-based stress r.
r. method
pain threshold r.
perioperative r.
ritual r.
smoking-related r.
spondylolisthesis r.
r. stabilization
striatal binding r.
swan-neck deformity r.
symptom r.
r. technique

reductionism
biologic r.

redundancy
neuroblast r.
synapse r.

redundant neuron

reelin
r. gene
r. immunoreactive band
r. protein

reference
r. electrode
r. measurement
r. montage
r. phase
r. picture-caption pair

referencing
dynamic r.
optical image-guided surgery system with dynamic r.

referral
sleep center r.

referred
r. pain
r. sensation

ReFix
R. noninvasive fixation
R. stereotactic head fixator
R. stereotactic headholder

refixation saccade

reflectance spectrophotometry

reflectometry

reflex
abdominal r.
abdominocardiac r.
abnormal nocturnal respiratory r.
Abrams heart r.
Achilles r.
acoustic r.
acousticopalpebral r. (APR)
acoustic startle r.
acquired r.
acromial r.
r. action
adductor foot r.
adductor thigh r.
affective startle r.
allied r.
anal r.
ankle r.
r. anosmia
r. anoxic seizure
antagonistic r.
anticus r.
antigravity r.
aponeurotic r.
r. arc
asymmetric tonic neck r.
attenuation r.
attitudinal r.
auditory oculogyric r.
auriculopalpebral r.
auropalpebral r.
axon r.
Babinski r.
back of foot r.
Barkman r.
basal joint r.
Bechterew deep r.
Bechterew-Mendel r.
behavior r.
Benedek r.
Bezold-Jarisch r.
biceps femoris r.
Bing r.
bladder r.
blink r.
body righting r.
bone r.
bowing r.
brachioradial r.
brachioradialis r.
brain r.
brainstem r.

NOTES

reflex *(continued)*
bregmocardiac r.
Brissaud r.
Brudzinski r.
bulbocavernosus r.
bulbomimic r.
bulbospongiosus r.
carotid sinus r.
cephalopalpebral r.
cervicocollic r.
C-fiber r.
Chaddock r.
chain r.
r. change
chin r.
Chodzko r.
ciliospinal r.
r. circuit
clasp-knife r.
closed loop r.
cochleopalpebral r.
cochleopupillary r.
cochleostapedial r.
concealed r.
conditioned r. (CR)
contralateral r.
r. control
convulsive r.
coordinated r.
corneal r.
corneomandibular r.
corneomental r.
corneopterygoid r.
costal arch r.
costopectoral r.
cough r.
cranial r.
craniocardiac r.
cremasteric r.
crossed adductor r.
crossed extension r.
crossed knee r.
crossed spinoadductor r.
cry r.
cuboidodigital r.
Cushing r.
cutaneous pupil r.
dartos r.
darwinian r.
deep abdominal r.
deep tendon r. (DTR)
defense r.
deglutition r.
Dejerine r.
delayed r.
depressed corneal r.
depressed gag r.
depressor r.
detrusor r.
diffused r.
digital r.
r. disorder
diving r.
doll's eye r.
dorsal r.
dorsum pedis r.
elbow r.
enterogastric r.
epigastric r.
r. epilepsy
Erben r.
erector-spinal r.
Escherich r.
esophagosalivary r.
external auditory meatus r.
external oblique r.
eye-closure r.
facial r.
faucial r.
femoral r.
femoroabdominal r.
finger-thumb r.
flexor r.
foot r.
forced grasping r.
front-tap r.
gag r.
Galant r.
galvanic skin r. (GSR)
gastrocolic r.
gastroileac r.
Geigel r.
Gifford r.
glabellar r.
gluteal r.
Golda r.
Golgi r.
Gordon r.
grasp r.
grasping r.
great toe r.
Guillain-Barré r.
gustatory-sudorific r.
gustolacrimal r.
H r.
hand grasp r.
r. headache
heart r.
Hering-Breuer r.
Hirschberg r.
Hoffmann r.
Hughes r.
hyperactive tendon r.
hypochondrial r.
hypogastric r.
inborn r.
indirect r.
infraspinatus r.

inguinal r.
innate r.
interscapular r.
intersegmental r.
intrasegmental r.
intrinsic r.
inverted radial r.
investigatory r.
ipsilateral r.
r. iridoplegia
Jacobson r.
jaw-jerk r.
jaw-winking r.
jaw-working r.
Joffroy r.
Juster r.
Kehrer r.
Kisch r.
knee r.
knee-jerk r.
Kocher r.
labyrinthine righting r.
lacrimal r.
lacrimogustatory r.
Landau r.
laryngospastic r.
latent r.
laughter r.
Liddell-Sherrington r.
lip r.
local r.
Lovén r.
lower abdominal periosteal r.
lumbar r.
Lust r.
magnet r.
Magnus and de Kleijn neck r.
mandibular r.
Marinesco-Radovici r.
mass r.
masseter r.
Mayer r.
McCarthy r.
McCormac r.
mediopubic r.
Mendel-Bechterew r.
Mendel dorsal foot r.
Mendel instep r.
metacarpohypothenar r.
metacarpothenar r.
metatarsal r.
micturition r.
milk-ejection r.
Mondonesi r.
monosynaptic stretch r.
Morley peritoneocutaneous r.
Moro r.
r. movement
muscle stretch r.
muscular r.
myoclonus reticular r.
myotatic r.
nasal r.
nasomental r.
neck righting r.
neck tonic r.
r. neurogenic bladder
r. neurologic activity
nociceptive r.
nocifensor r.
nose-bridge-lid r.
nose-eye r.
nuchocephalic r.
obliquus r.
oculoauricular r.
oculocephalic r.
oculocephalogyric r.
oculomotor r.
oculorespiratory r.
oculospinal r.
oculovestibular r.
olecranon r.
open loop r.
Oppenheim r.
optical righting r.
opticofacial r.
orbicularis oculi r.
orbicularis pupillary r.
orienting r.
oropharyngeal r.
palatal r.
palmar grasp r.
palm-chin r.
palmomental r.
parachute r.
paradoxical extensor r.
paradoxical flexor r.
paradoxical patellar r.
paradoxical pupillary r.
paradoxical triceps r.
r. paralysis
patellar tendon r.
patelloadductor r.
pectoral r.

NOTES

reflex *(continued)*
penile r.
penis r.
Perez r.
perianal r.
pericardial r.
periosteal r.
pharyngeal r.
phasic r.
photic-sneeze r.
physiological r.
pilomotor r.
plantar grasp r.
plantar muscle r.
platysmal r.
postural r.
pouting r.
premature infant bowing r.
pressoreceptor r.
primitive r.
pronator r.
proprioceptive r.
protective laryngeal r.
psychocardiac r.
psychogalvanic r.
pulmonocoronary r.
pupillary light r.
pupillary-skin r.
Puusepp r.
quadriceps r.
quadrupedal extensor r.
radial r.
radiobicipital r.
radioperiosteal r.
rectocardiac r.
rectolaryngeal r.
regional r.
Remak r.
respiratory r.
Riddoch mass r.
righting r.
Roger r.
rooting r.
Rossolimo r.
Ruggeri r.
Saenger r.
scapular r.
scapulohumeral r.
scapuloperiosteal r.
Schäffer r.
scratch r.
segmental medullary r.
r. seizure
semimembranosus r.
semitendinosus r.
r. sensation
simple r.
sinus r.
skin r.
skin-muscle r.
skin-pupillary r.
snapping r.
Snellen r.
snout r.
sole tap r.
somatointestinal r.
r. spasm
spinal monosynaptic r.
spinoadductor r.
stapes r.
Starling r.
startle r.
static r.
statokinetic r.
statotonic r.
sternobrachial r.
sternutatory r.
Stookey r.
stretch r.
Strümpell r.
styloradial r.
suck r.
superficial r.
supination r.
supinator longus r.
supraorbital r.
suprapatellar r.
suprapubic r.
supraumbilical r.
swallowing r.
r. sympathetic dystrophy (RSD)
r. sympathetic dystrophy syndrome (RSDS)
synchronous r.
r. syncope
tarsophalangeal r.
tendo Achillis r.
tendon r.
testicular compression r.
r. testing
r. therapy
Throckmorton r.
thumb r.
tibioadductor r.
toe r.
tonic r.
trace conditioned r.
trained r.
triceps surae r.
trigeminofacial r.
trochanter r.
Trömner r.
ulnar r.
unconditioned r.
upper abdominal periosteal r.
upper airway r.
urinary r.
utricular r.

vagus r.
vasopressor r.
venorespiratory r.
vesical r.
vestibular r.
vestibuloocular r. (VOR)
vestibulospinal r.
virile r.
visceral r.
viscerogenic r.
visceromotor r.
viscerosensory r.
visual grasp r.
visual orbicularis r.
vomiting r.
Weingrow r.
Westphal pupillary r.
wink r.
withdrawal r.
wrist clonus r.
zygomatic r.

reflexive
r. saccade inhibition
r. saccade triggering

reflexogenic, reflexogenous
r. syncope
r. zone

reflexograph

reflexology

reflexometer

reflexophil, reflexophile

reflexotherapy

reflex/response
psychogalvanic r./r.

reflux
nocturnal r.
sleep-related gastroesophageal r.
vesicoureteral r.

reformatted image

reformulation
sequential diagrammatic r.

refractoriness
medication r.

refractory
r. convergence nystagmus
r. erectile dysfunction
r. localization-related seizure
r. migraine
r. partial epilepsy
r. state
r. status epilepticus

Refsum
R. disease
R. peripheral neuropathy
R. syndrome

regenerate nerve sprouting

regeneration
aberrant r.
axon r.
axonal r.
cranial nerve r.
neural r.
neuronal r.
peripheral nerve r.

regimen
drug r.
holistic r.
medication r.
multiple-dose r.
pharmacotherapy r.
polytherapy r.
postoperative r.
steady-state r.
treatment r.

regio
r. hypothalamica anterior
r. hypothalamica dorsalis
r. hypothalamica intermedia
r. hypothalamica lateralis
r. hypothalamica posterior

region
anterior head r.
anterior hypothalamic r.
anterior insula r.
auditory r.
basal forebrain r.
bridge r.
Broca r.
carboxyl-terminal r.
central gray matter r.
cerebellar r.
cerebral r.
circumscribed r.
cortical gray r.
craniocervical r.
deep white matter r.
dopamine-innervated limbic r.
dorsal anterior cingulate r.
dorsal hypothalamic r.
dorsal limbic r.
dorsal neocortical r.
dorsolateral r.
extrapolar r.

NOTES

region *(continued)*
frontal brain r.
germ cell tumor with synchronous lesions in pineal and suprasellar r.'s
gray matter r.
iliosacral r.
inferior parietal r.
infragranular r.
infratentorial r.
infundibulotubular r.
interconnected cerebral r.
r. of interest (ROI)
intermediate hypothalamic r.
interolivary r.
lateral cerebellar r.
lateral hypothalamic r.
limbic brain r.
limbic-related r.
locus coeruleus r.
mamillary r.
medullary inhibitory r.
motor r.
negatively correlated r.
neocortical r.
occipitonuchal r.
opticostriate r.
orbital r.
parafalcine r.
paralimbic r.
paramedian r.
paranodal r.
parasellar r.
penumbral r.
perisylvian r.
periventricular gray r.
pineal r.
positively correlated r.
posterior cingulate r.
posterior hypothalamic r.
prefrontal r.
preoptic r.
prepontine r.
pretectal r.
15q11-13 r.
raphe nuclei r.
rolandic r.
sacrococcygeal r.
sellar r.
sensory r.
septal r.
silver-staining nucleolar organizer r.
speech perception r.
subcortical gray r.
subgenual cingulate r.
subicular r.
supraoptic r.
suprasellar r.
temporal speech r.
temporomesial r.
terminal r.
thalamic r.
transentorhinal r.
ventral paralimbic r.
visual r.
watershed r.
Wernicke r.
white matter r.

regional
r. brain lactate
r. brain parenchymal volume
r. cerebral blood flow (rCBF)
r. cerebral blood flow scintigraphy
r. cerebral metabolic rate of oxygen
r. cerebral perfusion pressure (rCPP)
r. distribution
r. glucose metabolism
r. glucose metabolism at rest
r. hypothermia
r. oxygen extraction fraction
r. oxygen saturation (rSO_2)
r. reflex

registration
r. error
image r.
imperfect image r.
segmental r.
surface vessel r.

registry
Acoustic Neuroma R.
Alzheimer Disease Patient R. (ADPR)
Brain Tumor R.
Familial Amyloid Polyneuropathy World Transplant R.
Mayo Alzheimer Disease Center/Alzheimer Disease Patient R.
Rush Alzheimer R.

Regitine

Regonol Injection

regression
r. analysis
autism with r.

regressive electric shock therapy (REST)

regrowth
axon r.
nerve r.

regular
r. eating schedule
r. sleeping schedule
r. waking schedule

regularity
orthographic r.

regulated on activation, normal T-cell expressed and secreted (RANTES)
regulation
cerebrovascular r.
emotional r.
top-down r.
volume r.
weight r.
regulator
r. gene
mood r.
suction Regugauge r.
regulatory
r. center
r. input
r. role
Regulus frameless stereotactic system
regurgitant lesion
rehabilitation
aquatic r.
functional r.
geriatric r.
learning-based r.
multidisciplinary r.
neurologic r.
r. strategy
Rehbein rib spreader
Reichert
R. cochlear recess
R. stereotaxy system
R. substance
substantia innominata of R.
Reichert-Mundinger
R.-M. apparatus
R.-M. stereotactic head frame
R.-M. syndrome
R.-M. technique
Reichert-Mundinger-Fischer stereotactic head frame
Reid baseline
Reil
R. ansa
R. band
circular sulcus of R.
insula of R.
island of R.
limiting sulcus of R.
R. ribbon
substantia innominata of R.
R. sulcus
taeniola corporis callosi of R.
threshold of island of R.
R. triangle
R. trigone
Reilly body
reinforcement
drug r.
homogenous r.
Teflon mesh r.
reinforcing
r. agent
r. drug response
r. effect
r. property
r. stimulus
reinnervated
r. fiber
r. motor unit
reinnervation of target organ
Reintegration
R. to Normal Living (RNL)
R. to Normal Living Index
Reissner fiber
Reiter syndrome
relapse
acute r.
r. mechanism
multiple sclerosis r.
prone to r.
psychotic r.
r. rate
r. therapy
relapse-prevention
relapsing
r. fever
r. hypertrophic neuritis
r. neuropathy
r. polychondritis
relapsing-remitting (RR)
r.-r. multiple sclerosis (RRMS)
relation
afferent r.
dose-response r.
efferent r.
stress-strain r.
relational
r. alliance
r. efficacy
r. threshold
relationship
attachment r.
brain-behavior r.
cause-effect r.
complainant-listener r.

NOTES

relationship *(continued)*
complex r.
counterintuitive r.
dose-response r.
forced r.
genetic r.
human r.
intrinsic r.
neurovascular r.
predictive r.
r. tool
relative
r. afferent pupillary defect (RAPD)
r. band amplitude
r. biological effectiveness
r. biologic effectiveness (RBE)
r. cerebral blood volume (rCBV)
first-degree r.
r. hyperemia
r. hypoxia
r. optical density (ROD)
r. refractory period
relaxant
muscle r.
relaxation
applied r.
r. constant
dipole-dipole r.
intramolecular r.
longitudinal r.
nuclear r.
paramagnetic r.
r. phase
progressive muscle r.
r. rate enhancement
r. response
spin-lattice r.
spin-spin r.
state of mindful r.
stress r.
T1 r.
T2 r.
r. theory
r. time
transverse r.
relaxation/tension
relaxometry
relay
spinothalamic r.
thalamic r.
thalamocortical r.
release
dopamine r.
extended r. (ER)
r. of information
neurotransmitter r.
r. phenomenon
pituitary prolactin r.
platelet thromboxane r.
prolactin r.
sustained r. (SR)
voltage-dependent neurotransmitter r.
Relefact TRH injection
relevance
clinical r.
reliability
split-half r.
relief
headache r.
religious
r. difference
r. dynamic
r. orientation
r. perspective
reln gene
Relpax
Relton-Hall frame
REM
rapid eye movement
REM deprivation
REM latency
newborn REM
REM rebound
REM sleep behavior disorder
REM sleep-locked headache
REM sleep-related disorder
remacemide
remaining aneurysm
Remak
R. fiber
R. ganglion
R. paralysis
R. reflex
R. sign
R. symptom
Remeron SolTab
remifentanil hydrochloride
reminiscent
r. aura
r. neuralgia
Reminyl
remission
full r.
remitting-relapsing MS
remodeled forehead
remodeling
bone r.
craniofacial r.
neural foramen r.
REM-onset blinking
remote
r. afterloading brachytherapy (RAB)
r. cerebellar hemorrhage
r. memory
r. recall
r. symptomatic seizure
removal
Arana-Iniquez intracranial cyst r.

implant r.
metastatic tumor r.
rib r.
transsphenoidal r.

remoxipride

REM-sleep behavior

REMstar
R. Auto
R. Auto with heated humidification
R. Plus
R. Plus with C-Flex
R. Plus with C-Flex and heated humidification
R. Pro with C-Flex
R. Pro with C-Flex and heated humidification

remyelinate

remyelination

renal
r. amino acid transport disorder
r. dysfunction
r. function
r. ganglion
r. insufficiency

renalia
ganglia r.

Renaut body

Rendu-Osler angiomatosis

Rendu-Osler-Weber disease

renin
long-term vasomotor tone r.

renin-angiotensin

renitent

Renografin

Renografin-60, -76

Reno-M

Reno-M-30, -60

Reno-M-Dip

Renovue

Renshaw cell

ReoPro

reorganization
cortical r.
plastic r.
somatotopographic r.

repair
cranial nerve r.
dural r.
Gardner meningocele r.
neural r.
pseudarthrosis r.
rod fracture r.

reparative response

repeat
r. concussion
microtubule-binding r.
r. radiosurgery
trinucleotide r.

repeated
r. FID
r. measure (rm)

repeating pattern

3-repeat isoform

4-repeat isoform

repellent apraxia

repetition
monaural word r.
r. time

repetitive
r. discharge
r. lifting task
r. motion injury (RMI)
r. motion syndrome (RMS)
r. movement
r. nerve stimulation
r. rumination
r. seizures
r. stimulus
r. temporalis muscle temperature
r. transcranial magnetic stimulation (rTMS)
r. watching

rephasing
even-echo r.
r. gradient

replacement
Bristol disc r.
disc r.
elastic-type disc r.
facet r.
hard tissue r. (HTR)
hormone r.
hydraulic-type disc r.
hydrogel disc r.
joint r.
low-dose estrogen r.
spinal disc r.
tile plate facet r.
valve r.
vertebral body r. (VBR)

repolarization

repositioner
mandibular r.

NOTES

representation
Cartesian coordinate r.
internal r.
preexisting r.
spherical coordinate r.
representational
abstract versus r.
reprocessing
eye movement desensitization and r. (EMDR)
reproducible target imaging
repulsive axon guidance signal
Requip
requirement
energy r.
rerupture of aneurysm
Rescriptor
rescue
autologous bone marrow r.
bone marrow r.
r. medication
r. screw
research
Australian Council for Education R.
biologic r.
construct r.
cross-sectional r.
empirical r.
epidemiological r.
European Society for Sleep R.
r. interview
Japanese Society of Sleep R.
r. program
taxonomic r.
twin r.
resectable tumor
resection
anterior craniofacial r.
anterior mesial temporal r. (AMTR)
anteromedial temporal lobe r.
asleep-awake-asleep surgical r.
Badgley iliac wing r.
caudal lamina r.
condyle r.
cortical r.
craniofacial r.
dorsolateral r.
electroencephalography-guided cortical r.
en bloc r.
extratemporal r.
focal r.
gross total r.
hippocampal r.
iliac crest r.
image-complete r.
intracranial meningioma r.
lateral temporal r.
lobar r.
meningioma r.
microsurgical r.
multilobar r.
neural arch r.
nonlesional cortical r.
occipital r.
odontoid process r.
Peet splanchnic r.
Pitanguy oval skin r.
r. of pituitary tumor, transfacial approach
postcentral r.
seizure focus r.
surgical r.
temporal r.
transcranial r.
transoral odontoid r.
transthoracic vertebral body r.
tumor r.
vertebral r.
volumetric r.
resective epilepsy surgery
reserpine
reserve
cognitive r.
cross-flow r.
reservoir
Accu-Flo CSF r.
Braden flushing r.
McKenzie r.
Ommaya r.
on-off flushing r.
retromastoid Ommaya r.
Rickham r.
Salmon Rickham ventriculostomy r.
side-port flat-bottomed Ommaya r.
r. sign
suboccipital Ommaya r.
ventricular catheter r.
ventricular Ommaya r.
residual
r. aneurysm
r. aura
r. autoparalytic syndrome
r. dense nasal defect
r. hemiparesis
r. language function
r. latency
r. negative symptom
r. paralysis
r. positive symptom
r. tumor
r. vertigo
r. weakness
resilient nystagmus
resin
Spurr epoxy r.

resistance
cerebrovascular r.
estimated cerebrovascular r.
galvanic skin r. (GSR)
manifestation of r.
motiveless r.
upper airway r.
r. vessel
resistant
r. epilepsy
treatment r.
resistive magnet
resolution threshold
Resolve QuickAnchor
resolving ischemic neurologic deficit (RIND)
resonance
fast-scan magnetic r.
localized magnetic r.
magnetic r. (MR)
nuclear magnetic r. (NMR)
stochastic r.
resonant frequency
resonator
birdcage r.
respiration
ataxic r.
Biot r.
Cheyne-Stokes r.
corneal r.
diffusion r.
electrophrenic r.
internal r.
tissue r.
respirator
r. brain
Drinker tank r.
respiratory
r. acidosis
r. alkalosis
r. anosmia
r. arousal index (RAI)
r. arousal response
r. ataxia
r. center
r. chain
r. chain complex I deficiency
r. complex
r. disturbance index (RDI)
r. effort amplitude
r. effort-related arousal
r. embarrassment
r. event arousal
r. inductance plethysmography
r. insufficiency
r. monitoring
r. pause
r. physiology
r. rate
r. reflex
r. system
r. variability
respiratory-related arousal
respite care
respondent condition
response
abnormal muscle r.
achromatic r.
acute genomic r.
acute nociceptive r.
adverse autonomic r.
A-fiber evoked r.
agitation r.
alpha r.
altered immune r.
AMPA receptor-mediated r.
amperometric r.
amygdala r.
angiogenic r.
antidromic r.
antigen-specific T-cell r.
antiparkinsonian r.
auditory brainstem r. (ABR)
auditory brainstem evoked r.
auditory evoked r.
auditory visual-evoked r.
automated brainstem auditory evoked r. (ABAER)
automatic auditory brainstem r.
average evoked r.
axon r.
Babinski r.
biphasic locomotor r.
blink r.
Bobath r.
brain metabolic r.
brainstem auditory evoked r. (BAER)
brainstem evoked r.
bulldog r.
buttress r.
caffeine r.
cellular immune r.
C-fiber evoked r.

NOTES

response *(continued)*
chronic r.
cingulate r.
clasp-knife r.
clinical r.
conditioned drug r.
consistent r.
coping r.
Cushing r.
decremental r.
discrete emotional r.
dissociative r.
dorsal horn neuronal r.
dysregulated stress r.
electromyographic r.
evoked cortical r.
exaggerated r.
extensor plantar r.
extensor toe r.
eye-blink r.
fastigial pressor r.
fatigue failure r.
fetal r.
finger r.
galvanic skin r. (GSR)
genital r.
glutamatergic r.
H r.
heat defense r.
host immune r.
humoral immune r.
hyperactive sympathetic r.
hyperadrenergic r.
hypercapnic ventilatory r. (HCVR)
hyperemic r.
hypocapnic ventilatory r.
hypoxic ventilatory r.
immune r.
inconsistent r.
incremental r.
inflammatory r.
inhibited r.
Janz r.
light touch r.
loss of r.
low-key r.
M r.
meningitis inflammatory r.
metabolic r.
monosynaptic segmental reflex r.
motor r.
myotonic r.
neuromagnetic r.
neuroplastic r.
oculomotor r.
orienting r.
papillary r.
parachute r.
paradoxical cold r.
pathological r.
photoparoxysmal r. (PPR)
pinprick r.
r. processing time
prolactin r.
psychogalvanic r. (PGR)
psychological r.
pupil r.
pupillary light r.
recruiting r.
reinforcing drug r.
relaxation r.
reparative r.
respiratory arousal r.
reward-irrelevant r.
segmentary r.
skin conductance r.
somatosensory evoked r. (SER)
sonomotor r.
spatial r.
spinally elicited peripheral nerve r. (SEPNR)
steady-state r. (SSR)
stepping r.
suboptimal r.
supramaximal r.
sympathetic skin r.
syntagmatic r.
thalamic r.
therapeutic r.
thermoeffector r.
thermoregulatory r.
theta r.
tissue-type metabolic r.
tonic neck r.
unconditioned r.
visual evoked r. (VER)

response-produced cue

responsiveness
absence of emotional r.
hypercapnic r.

REST
regressive electric shock therapy
REST condition

rest
aneurysmal r.
metabolism at r.
r. pain
regional glucose metabolism at r.
r. tremor

Restcue bed

restiform
r. body
r. eminence

restiforme
corpus r.

restiformis
eminentia r.

resting
r. ankle/arm Doppler index
r. anterior cingulate flow
r. membrane potential
r. motor threshold
r. PET study
r. state
r. T cell
r. tone
r. tremor
restless
r. legs
r. leg syndrome (RLS)
restlessness
motor r.
nocturnal r.
Reston
R. dressing
R. foam-padded headrest
restorative neurology
Restore neurostimulation system
Restoril
restraint law
restricted
r. focus
r. interest
restriction
r. endonuclease
r. fragment length polymorphism (RFLP)
gown r.
r. of inward gaze
salt r.
sleep r.
restrictive
r. criterion
r. lung disease
result
anomalous r.
biometric r.
concordant r.
long-term r.
positive r.
Resume electrode
resuscitation
hemodynamic r.
retained
r. bullet fragment
r. foreign object
retainer
tongue r.
retardata
ejaculatio r.
retardation
fetal growth r.
mental r.
mild mental r.
motor r.
Northern epilepsy with mental r.
progressive epilepsy with mental r.
psychomotor r.
Spastic Paraplegia, Ataxia, Mental R. (SPAR)
rete
carotid r.
r. mirabile
r. mirabile caroticum
retention
brain r.
fluid r.
sodium-water r.
reticula (*pl. of* reticulum)
reticular
r. activating system (RAS)
r. formation
r. nucleus
r. nucleus of brainstem
r. nucleus of medulla oblongata
r. nucleus of mesencephalon
r. nucleus of pons
r. nucleus of thalamus
r. substance
reticularis
formatio r.
livedo r.
substantia r.
reticulata
pars r.
substantia nigra pars r. (sNr)
reticulocerebellar tract
reticulocortical pathway
reticulocytosis
cerebroside r.
reticulopituicyte
reticulospinalis
tractus r.
reticulospinal tract
reticulotegmental nucleus
reticulotomy
reticulum, pl. **reticula**
r. cell sarcoma
endoplasmic r.
Kölliker r.

NOTES

reticulum *(continued)*
sarcoplasmic r.
smooth endoplasmic r.
r. stain
retigabine
retina
blood and thunder r.
cerebral layer of r.
cone cell of r.
external nuclear layer of r.
ganglion cell of r.
ganglionic cell layer of r.
granular layer of r.
horizontal cell of r.
molecular layer of r.
neural layer of r.
neuroepithelial layer of r.
nuclear layer of r.
optic part of r.
pigmented layer of r.
plexiform layer of r.
rod cell of r.
sustentacular fiber of r.
retinaculatome
Paine r.
retinae
fovea centralis r.
macula r.
pars optica r.
periphlebitis r.
strata nuclearia externa et interna r.
stratum cerebrale r.
stratum ganglionare r.
stratum moleculare r.
stratum neuroepitheliale r.
stratum nucleare externum et internum r.
stratum pigmenti r.
stratum plexiforme externum et internum r.
retinal
r. achromic patch
r. angioma
r. arterial occlusion
r. artery occlusion
r. cone
r. cyst
r. degeneration
r. detachment
r. embolism
r. ganglion cell (RGC)
r. hemorrhage
r. infarction
r. migraine
r. migraine headache
r. pathway
r. pigment epitheliopathy
r. pigment epithelium
r. stroke
r. vasculitis
r. venous obstruction
retinitis
necrotizing r.
r. pigmentosa
retinoblastoma
ectopic intracranial r.
r. gene
retinocerebral angiomatosis
retinocochleocerebral arteriolopathy
retinofugal target
retinohypothalamic tract (RHT)
retinoic
r. acid
r. acid in patterning
retinoneuropathy
toxic r.
retinopathy
arterial occlusive r.
hypotensive r.
infectious r.
melanoma-associated r. (MAR)
pigmentary r.
radiation r.
stasis r.
venous stasis r.
retinotopic map
retracting suture
retraction
brain r.
cerebellar r.
eyelid r.
r. injury
mandibular r.
r. nystagmus
oral r.
proximal segment r.
sigmoid sinus r.
soft palate r.
temporal lobe r.
retraction-convergence nystagmus
retraction-induced cerebral damage
retractor
Adson-Anderson cerebellar r.
Adson hemilaminectomy r.
Anderson-Adson scalp r.
angled nerve root r.
Apfelbaum r.
Army-Navy r.
Badgley laminectomy r.
Ballantine hemilaminectomy r.
Beckman r.
Beckman-Eaton laminectomy r.
Beckman-Weitlaner laminectomy r.
r. blade
Bookwalter r.
brain r.
Budde halo ring r.

Burford r.
Campbell nerve root r.
Caspar cervical r.
cerebellar r.
Cherry brain r.
Cherry laminectomy r.
Cloward blade r.
Cloward brain r.
Cloward-Cushing vein r.
Cloward dural r.
Cloward-Hoen laminectomy r.
Cloward lumbar lamina r.
Cloward nerve root r.
Cloward skin r.
Cloward small cervical r.
Cloward tissue r.
collapsible tissue r.
Cone laminectomy r.
Cone scalp r.
Cottle-Neivert r.
Crile r.
Crockard r.
Cushing bivalve r.
Cushing decompressive r.
Cushing nerve r.
Cushing subtemporal r.
Cushing vein r.
Davis brain r.
Davis scalp r.
Deaver r.
deep r.
D'Errico-Adson r.
D'Errico nerve root r.
double fishhook r.
Downing r.
dural r.
fan r.
Farley r.
Finochietto r.
flexible arm r.
Frazier laminectomy r.
Frazier lighted brain r.
French brain r.
Fukushima r.
Gelpi r.
Glaser automatic laminectomy r.
Greenberg r.
Greenberg-Sugita r.
r. handle Cloward dural hook
Hardy lip r.
Holscher nerve root r.
House-Fisch dural r.
Inge laminectomy r.
intradural r.
Jannetta posterior fossa r.
Jansen mastoid r.
Jansen scalp r.
Jansen-Wagner r.
Kennerdell-Maroon orbital r.
Kobayashi r.
Leyla brain r.
LightWare micro r.
Love nerve root r.
Malis brain r.
Markham-Meyerding
 hemilaminectomy r.
Martin nerve root r.
mastoid r.
METRx X-Tube r.
Meyerding laminectomy r.
Miskimon cerebellar r.
Murphy rake r.
nerve root r.
Oldberg brain r.
pillar-and-post microsurgical r.
Poppen-Gelpi laminectomy r.
Roos brachial plexus root r.
Schwartz laminectomy r.
Scoville cervical disc r.
Scoville-Haverfield
 hemilaminectomy r.
Scoville hemilaminectomy r.
Scoville nerve root r.
Scoville-Richter laminectomy r.
self-retaining brain r.
Senn r.
Sheldon hemilaminectomy r.
single-hook r.
Smith nerve root suction r.
Spurling nerve root r.
stereotactic r.
Stuck laminectomy r.
Sugita r.
Taylor r.
Teflon-coated brain r.
Temple-Fay laminectomy r.
Tew cranial spinal r.
titanium wound r.
Tuffier laminectomy r.
Tuffier-Raney r.
Weary nerve root r.
Weitlaner r.
Weitlaner-Beckman r.
Wiltse-Gelpi r.

NOTES

retractor *(continued)*
Yasargil r.
Yasargil-Leyla brain r.
retractorius
nystagmus r.
retraining
breathing r.
vestibuloocular r.
retrieval
word r.
retroactive amnesia
retroambiguus
nucleus r.
retroauricular edema
retrobulbar
r. hemorrhage
r. injection
r. lesion
r. optic neuritis
r. orbital metastasis
retrochiasmal
r. lesion
r. visual pathway
retrochiasmatic
r. area
r. lesion
retrochiasmatica
area r.
retrocochlear
r. deafness
r. hearing loss
r. lesion
retrocursive absence
retrodorsal nucleus
retrofacial nucleus
retroflex
r. bundle of Meynert
r. fasciculus
retroflexus
fasciculus r.
retrogasserian
r. anhydrous glycerol injection therapy
r. injection
r. neurectomy
r. neurotomy
r. procedure
r. rhizotomy
retrognathism, retrognathia
retrograde
r. axon reaction
r. blood flow
r. chromatolysis
r. degeneration
r. fast component neuropathy
r. memory
r. transport
retrography
retrogressive differentiation
retrolabyrinthine-presigmoid approach
retrolabyrinthine-transsigmoid approach
retrolental fibroplasia
retrolenticular
r. limb of internal capsule
r. part of internal capsule
retrolentiform limb of internal capsule
retrolingual obstruction
retrolisthesis
retromandibular tender point
retromastoid
r. approach
r. craniotomy
r. Ommaya reservoir
r. suboccipital craniectomy
retromembranous hematoma
retroocular
retroolivaris
retroolivary groove
retroorbital pain
retroparotid space syndrome
retroperitoneal
r. approach
r. fibrosis
retropharyngeal
r. abscess
r. approach
r. hemangioma
r. hematoma
r. space
retroposterior lateral nucleus
retroposterolateralis nucleus
retropulsed bone excision
retropulsion
retrosigmoid
r. approach
r. craniectomy
r. craniotomy
retrospection
retrospective
r. experimental study design
r. projection
retrotarsal fold
retrotonsillar fissure
retrovesical center
retroviral CB receptor
retrovirus infection
retrusion
midface r.
Rett syndrome
Retzius
R. fiber
R. foramen
foramen of Key and R.
R. gyrus
sheath of Key and R.
reuniens
canaliculus r.
canalis r.

ductus r.
nucleus r.
reuptake
r. blockade
neuronal r.
revascularization
brain r.
cerebral r.
reverberating circuit
reversal
deficit r.
homuncular organization phase r.
phase r.
reverse
r. analgesia
r. causality
r. genetics
r. learning function
r. ocular bobbing
r. orientation
r. polarity
r. transcriptase-polymerase chain reaction (RT-PCR)
r. Trendelenburg position
reverse-angled curette
reversed optokinetic nystagmus
reversible
r. C-arm
r. cognitive impairment of depression
r. decortication
r. dementia
r. encephalopathy
r. intoxication
r. ischemia
r. ischemic neurologic deficit (RIND)
r. ischemic neurologic disability (RIND)
r. motor neuron disease
r. myelopathy
r. posterior leukoencephalopathy syndrome (RPLS)
r. shock
r. uvulopalatal flap
Reversol Injection
ReVia
Revilliod sign
revised
Bracken Basic Concept Scale, R.
Clymer-Barrett Readiness Test, R.
Comprehensive Identification Process, R.
Continuous Visual Memory Test, R.
Derogatis Affects Balance Scale, R.
Herrmann Brain Dominance Instrument, R.
R. Physical Anhedonia Scale
R. Trauma Score
revision
Fast Health Knowledge Test, 1986 R.
UltraPower r.
revolving door syndrome
reward
r. circuitry
r. system
reward-irrelevant response
rewinder gradient
Rexed
lamina of R.
R. lamina
Rey Auditory Verbal Learning test
Reye-like syndrome
Reye syndrome
Reynolds
R. number
R. skull traction tongs
Rey-Osterrieth complex
RF
radiofrequency
RF coil
RF electrocoagulation
RF needle electrode system
RF pulse
RFG-3C radiofrequency lesion generator system
RFLP
restriction fragment length polymorphism
RGC
retinal ganglion cell
rhabdoid
r. meningioma
r. tumor
rhabdomyolysis
rhabdomyoma
cardiac r.
rhabdomyosarcoma
intrasellar r.
rhabdovirus infection
rhenium-186

NOTES

rheoencephalogram
rheoencephalography
rheologic therapy
rheology
cerebral blood flow r.
rheolytic catheter
rheumatic
r. carditis
r. chorea
r. fever
r. fever cerebral embolism
r. tetany
r. torticollis
rheumatica
polymyalgia r. (PMR)
tetania r.
rheumatism
lumbar r.
rheumatoid
r. arteritis
r. arthritis
r. factor
r. neuropathy
r. spondylitis
Rheumatrex
rhinal
r. fissure
r. sulcus
rhinalis
sulcus r.
rhinencephalic mamillary body
rhinencephalon
rhinitis
vasomotor r.
viral r.
rhinocele
rhinocerebral zygomycosis
rhinolalia aperta
rhinoplasty
external r.
rhinorrhea
cerebrospinal fluid r.
CSF r.
rhinoseptal approach
rhinosinusitis
rhinotomy
lateral r.
rhizolysis
percutaneous radiofrequency r.
percutaneous retrogasserian glycerol r. (PRGR)
rhizomelic chondrodysplasia punctata
rhizomeningomyelitis
rhizopathy
***Rhizopus* infection**
rhizotomy
anterior r.
bilateral ventral r.'s
chemical r.
Dana posterior r.
dorsal r.
facet r.
Frazier-Spiller r.
glycerol r.
intracranial r.
percutaneous radiofrequency retrogasserian r. (PRFR)
percutaneous retrogasserian glycerol r.
posterior r.
radiofrequency r.
retrogasserian r.
selective dorsal r. (SDR)
thermal r.
trigeminal r.
rho
Spearman r.
r. wave
rho-aminosalicylic acid
Rhodesian trypanosomiasis
Rhodococcus rodochrous
rhombencephali
isthmus r.
tegmentum r.
rhombencephalic
r. gustatory nucleus
r. isthmus
r. tegmentum
rhombencephalitis
rhombencephalon
tegmentum of r.
ventricle of r.
rhombencephalosynapsis
rhombic lip
rhombocele
rhomboid
r. fossa
medial eminence of r.
r. nucleus
rhomboidalis
nucleus commissuralis r.
sinus r.
rhomboidal sinus
rhomboidea
fossa r.
rhomboideae
eminentia medialis fossae r.
striae medullares fossae r.
sulcus limitans fossae r.
Rhoton
R. ball dissector
R. blunt-ring curette
R. dissecting forceps
R. loop curette
R. microcurette
R. microdissector
R. microhook
R. spatula

R. spoon curette
R. suction tip
Rhoton-Cushing forceps
Rhoton-Merz suction tube
Rhoton-Tew bipolar forceps
RHT
retinohypothalamic tract
rhythm
alpha r.
background r.
Berger r.
beta r.
breach r.
cardiac r.
circadian r.
circannual r.
delta r.
EEG alpha r.
electroencephalogram r.
endogenous circadian r.
fast field-potential r.
focal slowing of background r.
gamma r.
heart r.
idiojunctional r.
infradian r.
r. of lags and spurts in development
light effect on circadian r.
low-amplitude circadian r.
mu r.
phi r.
pi r.
posterior r.
rolandic mu r.
sleep-wake r.
Society for Light Therapy and Biological R.'s
theta r.
time-locked occipital r.
ultradian r.
wake r.
well-formed electroencephalogram r.
wicket r.
rhythmic
r. artifact
r. chorea
r. delta activity
r. discharge
r. kicking movement
r. midtemporal burst of drowsiness
r. midtemporal theta of drowsiness (RMTD)
r. movement disorder
r. repetitive muscle potential
r. spindle-shaped activity
r. stepping movement
r. teeth grinding
rhythmical midtemporal discharge
rhythmicity
circadian r.
sleep-wake r.
vegetative circadian r.
rib
r. cranioplasty
r. fracture
r. graft
r. removal
vertical expandable prosthetic titanium r. (VEPTR)
ribavirin
ribbed hook
ribbon
r. blade
Reil r.
Ribes ganglion
riboflavin deficiency
ribonucleic acid (RNA)
ribosuria
Ribot
R. gradient
R. law
R. law of memory
Richards
R. curette
R. tamp
Richardson-Steele-Olszewski syndrome
Richards-Rundle syndrome
Riche-Cannieu anastomosis
Richmond
R. bolt
R. subarachnoid screw instrument
Richter laminectomy punch forceps
rickets
tumor-associated r.
rickettsial infection
rickettsii
Rochalimaea r.
Rickham reservoir
Riddoch
R. mass reflex
R. phenomenon
Ridenol

NOTES

ridge
apical ectodermal r.
mamilloaccessory r.
supraorbital r.
transverse r.
triangular r.
ridging
spondylitic r.
Ridley
R. circle
R. sinus
ridleyi
circulus venosus r.
Riedel thyroiditis
Rieger syndrome
Rienhoff-Finochietto rib spreader
Rienhoff rib spreader
rifampin
Rift Valley fever
right
r. anterior-temporal negativity
r. basilar mesial temporoparietal cortex
r. brain stroke (RBS)
r. ear advantage
r. frontal craniotomy for gross total resection of tumor
r. frontal lobe
r. frontoparietal infarction
r. hemiplegia
r. hemisphere dominance
r. hemisphere mechanism
r. hepatic vein
r. parietal lobe syndrome
r. parietal occipital vertex craniotomy
r. sixth nerve palsy
r. temporoparietal craniotomy
r. thalamus
r. thoracic curve
r. thoracic curve scoliosis
r. thoracic curve with hypokyphosis
r. thoracic curve with junctional kyphosis
r. thoracic left lumbar curve pattern
r. thoracic left lumbar scoliosis
r. thoracic left thoracolumbar scoliosis
r. thoracic minor curve pattern
r. ventricle
r. ventricular activation (RVA)
r. and wrong test
right-angle
r.-a. bipolar cautery
r.-a. blunt probe
r.-a. booster clip
r.-a. bur
r.-a. drill
r.-a. screwdriver
right-bearing nystagmus
righting reflex
right-left confusion
right-sided
r.-s. submandibular transverse incision
r.-s. thoracotomy
right-to-left shunt (RLS)
rightward saccade
rigid
r. body transformation matrix
r. cantilever beam construct
r. curve
r. curve scoliosis
r. dysarthria
r. frame
r. internal fixation
r. internal fixation technique
r. pedicle
r. pedicle screw
r. pupil
r. rod-lens endoscope
r. spine disease
r. spine muscular dystrophy
r. spine syndrome
r. ventriculoscope
rigidity
catatonic r.
C-D instrumentation r.
cerebellar r.
clasp-knife r.
cogwheel r.
Cotrel pedicle screw r.
decerebrate r.
decorticate r.
extrapyramidal r.
gamma r.
hemiplegic r.
lead-pipe r.
muscle r.
mydriatic r.
nuchal r.
paratonic r.
spastic r.
spinal fixation r.
Riley-Day syndrome
Riley-Smith syndrome
riluzole
rim
r. degeneration
supraorbital r.
rimula
RIND
resolving ischemic neurologic deficit
reversible ischemic neurologic deficit
reversible ischemic neurologic disability

ring
apophysial r.
atrial r.
r. block anesthesia
Brown-Roberts-Wells base r.
Budde halo r.
carotid r.
r. chromosome
Cosman-Roberts-Wells stereotactic r.
cricoid r.
r. curette
dural r.
enhancing r.
r. fracture
Gibbs r.
halo r.
head r.
hemosiderin r.
Kayser-Fleischer corneal r.
Luque r.
platinum r.
proximal carotid r.
tentorial r.
vascular r.
V1 halo r.
ringed formed forceps
Ringer lactate
ring-wall lesion
Rinne test
Rio Bravo virus
RIP
radioimmunoprecipitation
rippling muscle disease
risedronate
rise time
rising phase
risk
bleeding r.
disc at r.
driving r.
fall r.
home safety r.
nutrition r.
r. paradigm
poison r.
r. ratio
r. score
seizure r.
stroke r.
trivial r.
wander r.
risk-benefit
r.-b. assessment
r.-b. profile
r.-b. ratio
Risperdal Consta
Risser-Cotrel body cast
Risser localizer
risus
r. caninus
r. sardonicus
Ritadex
Ritalin LA extended-release capsule
Ritchie index
ritonavir
Ritter
R. law
R. opening tetanus
Ritter-Rollet phenomenon
ritual reduction
rituximab
rivastigmine tartrate
Rivermead
R. ADL index
R. Mobility Index
R. Motor Assessment
R. Perceptual Assessment Battery
rizatriptan benzoate
R-K needle
RLN
recurrent laryngeal nerve
RLS
restless leg syndrome
right-to-left shunt
rm
repeated measure
RMI
repetitive motion injury
RMS
repetitive motion syndrome
RMT
Recognition Memory Test
RMTD
rhythmic midtemporal theta of drowsiness
RMTD on electroencephalogram
RN
radionucleotide
RN scanning
RNA
ribonucleic acid
RNA expression
RNA virus

NOTES

RNL
Reintegration to Normal Living
RNL index
Robaxin
robertsonian chromosome translocation
Robertson pupil
Robert syndrome
Robinow syndrome
Robin sequence micrognathia
Robinson
R. anterior cervical discectomy
R. anterior cervical fusion
robot
Evolution 1 precision r.
Grenoble stereotactic r.
Lausanne stereotactic r.
Long Beach stereotactic r.
Mayo Clinic stereotactic r.
neurosurgical stereotactic r.
stereotactic r.
robotic
r. microscope
r. system
ROC
receiver operating characteristic
Rocaltrol
Rochalimaea
R. henselae
R. mooseri
R. prowazekii
R. quintana
R. rickettsii
R. tsutsugamushi
Rochester lamina dissector
Rocky
R. Mountain spotted fever
R. Mountain spotted fever meningoencephalitis
ROD
relative optical density
rod
aluminum master r.
r. bending
r. cell of retina
cerebellomesoencephalic fissure Perspex r.
compression r.
compressive r.
r. contour preparation
Corti r.
Cotrel-Dubousset r.
Delrin r.
distraction r.
double-L spinal r.
Edwards-Levine r.
Edwards modular system universal r.
r. fiber
r. fixation
r. fracture repair
Harrington r.
Hartshill rectangle r.
Isola spinal implant system eye r.
Jacobs locking hook spinal r.
Knodt r.
Kostuik r.
r. linkage
Luque r.
r. migration
modified Harrington r.
Moe r.
olfactory r.
pediatric Cotrel-Dubousset r.
r. placement
precontoured unit r.
r. rotation prevention
screw alignment r.
spinal r.
unit spinal r.
Wiltse system aluminum master r.
Wiltse system spinal r.
rodenticide
rod-hook construct
rodochrous
Rhodococcus r.
rod-sleeve
Edwards modular system spinal r.-s.
r.-s. instrumentation
Roeder manipulative aptitude test device
roentgen knife stereotactic radiosurgical device
roentgenogram
biplane r.
lateral r.
roentgenographic opaque marker
rofecoxib
Roger
R. reflex
R. symptom
Rogozinski spinal rod system
Rohon-Beard cell body
ROI
region of interest
Rolandi
substantia gelatinosa R.
rolandic
r. area
r. benign epilepsy of childhood with centrotemporal spike
r. cortex
r. epilepsy
r. epileptiform discharge
r. line
r. mu rhythm
r. operculum
r. paroxysmal focus

r. region
r. seizure
r. vein syndrome
rolandica
zona r.
Roland-Morris disability questionnaire
Rolando
R. angle
R. area
R. cell
R. column
fissure of R.
R. gelatinous substance
R. tubercle
rolandoparietal glioma
role
adultomorphic behavior r.
central r.
etiologic r.
integral r.
intrinsic transverse connector r.
pathophysiological r.
pivotal r.
regulatory r.
r. strain
roll
Fluftex gauze r.
laminectomy r.
r. plane sign
Roller nucleus
rolling
eye r.
roll-off filter
Romano-Ward syndrome
Romberg
R. disease
facial hemiatrophy of R.
R. sign
R. spasm
R. symptom
R. syndrome
R. test
R. trophoneurosis
Romberg-Howship symptom
rombergism
rongeur
Adson cranial r.
Bacon cranial r.
Beyer laminectomy r.
bone-biting r.
Bucy laminectomy r.
Cherry-Kerrison laminectomy r.
Cloward disc r.
Cloward-English laminectomy r.
Codman-Harper laminectomy r.
Codman-Kerrison laminectomy r.
Codman-Leksell laminectomy r.
Codman-Schlesinger cervical laminectomy r.
cranial r.
Cushing cranial r.
Cushing intervertebral disc r.
Dahlgren cranial r.
DeVilbiss cranial r.
disc r.
double-action r.
Echlin laminectomy r.
Echlin-Luer r.
Elekta Leksell r.
Ferris Smith-Kerrison laminectomy r.
Fulton laminectomy r.
gooseneck r.
Grünwald neurosurgical r.
Hajek-Koffler laminectomy r.
Hoen intervertebral disc r.
Hoen pituitary r.
Horsley r.
Hudson cranial r.
Husk bone r.
Jansen r.
Jansen-Middleton r.
Jarit-Kerrison laminectomy r.
Jarit-Liston bone r.
Jarit-Ruskin bone r.
Kerrison r.
Leksell r.
Love-Gruenwald cranial r.
Love-Gruenwald disc r.
Love-Gruenwald pituitary r.
Love-Kerrison laminectomy r.
Love pituitary r.
Mayfield r.
micropituitary r.
Mount laminectomy r.
narrow-bite bone r.
needle-nose r.
Nicola pituitary r.
Oldberg intervertebral disc r.
Oldberg pituitary r.
Olivecrona r.
Peiper-Beyer laminectomy r.
Poppen intervertebral disc laminectomy r.

NOTES

rongeur *(continued)*
punch r.
Raney laminectomy r.
Schlesinger laminectomy r.
Selverstone intervertebral disc r.
Smith-Petersen laminectomy r.
Spence intervertebral disc r.
Spurling-Kerrison laminectomy r.
Stille-Luer r.
Stookey cranial r.
upbiting/downbiting pituitary r.
Weil-Blakesley intervertebral disc r.
Yasargil pituitary r.
roof
r. of fourth ventricle
r. nucleus
r. plate
roof-patch graft
Roos brachial plexus root retractor
Roosen clamp
root
r. of ansa cervicalis
anterior r.
r. avulsion
conjoined nerve r.'s
cranial r.
developmental r.
dorsal spinal r.
entering r.
r. entry zone
r. entry zone lesion
facial r.
r. of facial nerve
r. filament
ganglion cell of dorsal spinal r.
r. level motor impairment
r. mean square error
nasociliary r.
nerve r.
olfactory r.
r. of olfactory tract, lateral and medial
r. of otic ganglion
r. pain
Petasites hybridus r.
posterior r.
selective nerve r. (SNR)
r. sleeve fibrosis
spinal nerve r.
symptomatic r.
r. syndrome
trigeminal r.
r. of trigeminal nerve
ventral spinal r.
vestibular r.
rooting reflex
rootlet
glossopharyngeal nerve r.
ropinirole
r. hydrochloride
r. monotherapy
r. study
ROS
reactive oxygen species
Rosai-Dorfman disease (RDD)
rose bengal test
Rosenbach
R. law
R. sign
Rosenberg-Chutorian syndrome
Rosen bur
Rosenmüller
fossa of R.
Rosenthal
basal vein of R. (BVR)
R. degeneration
R. fiber
R. fiber formation
R. vein
Rosenthal-Rosenthal syndrome
roseola
r. infantum
r. infection
rosette
Homer Wright r.
Rosser crypt hook
Rossolimo
R. contraction
R. reflex
R. sign
rostra (*pl. of* rostrum)
rostrad
rostral
r. basilar artery syndrome
r. brainstem
r. brainstem ischemia
caudal to r.
r. cerebellar peduncle
r. cingulotomy
r. colliculus
r. colliculus commissure
r. interstitial nucleus
r. lamina
r. layer
r. lobe of cerebellum
r. medial prefrontal cortex
r. medullary vellum frenulum
r. midbrain
r. neuropore
r. olivary nucleus
r. posterior fossa
r. spinal axon
r. subcortical target
r. supplementary motor area
r. tegmentum
r. transtentorial herniation
r. ventrolateral medulla

rostral-central tegmentum
rostralis
area hypothalamica r.
brachium colliculi r.
colliculus r.
commissura colliculi r.
frenulum veli medullaris r.
lamina r.
lobulus semilunaris r.
nucleus cuneatus pars r.
nucleus olivaris r.
nucleus reticularis pontis r.
nucleus vestibularis r.
pars anterior commissurae r.
pars posterior commissurae r.
substantia perforata r.
rostrocaudal
r. contact array
r. epidural array
rostrum, pl. **rostra**
r. corporis callosi
r. of corpus callosum
sphenoid r.
Rotablator rotating bur
Rotafix lumbar cage
rotary
r. atlantoaxial luxation
r. nystagmus
r. vertigo
rotating
r. hemostatic valve
r. mechanism
r. paralysis
rotation
axial r.
gantry r.
lateral r.
varimax r.
rotational
r. correction
r. injury
r. vertebral artery syndrome (RVAS)
rotationally
r. induced shear-strain injury
r. induced shear-strain lesion
rotator
Jarit r.
rotatoria
chorea r.
rotatory
r. acceleration
r. dislocation
r. epilepsy
r. luxation
r. nystagmus
r. spasm
r. tic
rotavirus encephalitis
Roth
R. disease
R. spot
R. syndrome
Roth-Bernhardt syndrome
rotigotine
rotoscoliosis
rotundum
foramen r.
rotundus
fasciculus r.
Rouget muscle
rouleaux formation
round
r. bur
r. eminence
r. fasciculus
r. hole plate
round-handled forceps
round-tipped periosteal elevator
Roussy-Dejerine syndrome
Roussy-Lévy
R.-L. disease
R.-L. hereditary areflexic dystasia
R.-L. syndrome
router
power r.
routine
complex finger r.
complex hand r.
rovelizumab
Rowland
criteria of R.
Roy-Camille
R.-C. plate
R.-C. posterior screw plate fixation
R.-C. posterior screw plate fixation biomechanics
R.-C. technique
Rozerem
RPLS
reversible posterior leukoencephalopathy syndrome

NOTES

RPR
rapid plasma reagin
RPR test
RPTP zeta/beta
RR
relapsing-remitting
RRF
ragged red fiber
RRMS
relapsing-remitting multiple sclerosis
R1, R2 wave
RSD
reflex sympathetic dystrophy
RSDS
reflex sympathetic dystrophy syndrome
RSE
rapid spin echo
rSO_2
regional oxygen saturation
rTMS
repetitive transcranial magnetic stimulation
RTPA
recombinant tissue plasminogen activator
RT-PCR
reverse transcriptase-polymerase chain reaction
rubber button
rubella
congenital r.
r. infection
r. panencephalitis
r. vaccination complication
r. virus
rubeosis iridis
ruber
nucleus r.
Rubinstein-Taybi syndrome
Rubin vase
rubral tremor
rubri
pars parvocellularis nuclei r.
rubrobulbaris
tractus r.
rubrobulbar tract
rubroolivares
fibrae r.
rubroolivary fiber
rubropontine tract
rubropontinus
tractus r.
rubroreticular
r. fasciculus
r. tract
rubroreticulares
fasciculi r.
rubrospinal
r. decussation
r. syndrome
r. tract
rubrospinalis
tractus r.
rubrothalamic fiber
rucksack paralysis
rudimentary
r. brainstem
r. sympathetic innervation
rudimentum, pl. **rudimenta**
r. hippocampus
Ruffini
R. corpuscle
R. cylinder
R. ending
flower-spray organ of R.
R. mechanoreceptor
R. organ
rufinamide
Ruggeri
R. reflex
R. sign
Ruggles Surgical Instrument
Rukavina syndrome
Rukavina-type familial amyloid polyneuropathy
rule
advanced sleep staging r.
Allen r.
anatomic r.
Bergman r.
Jackson r.
3-minute r.
r. of 2
r. of Spence
ruling in tic
rumination
manie de r.
persistent r.
repetitive r.
ruminative depression
runner
intrinsic-negative r.
intrinsic-positive r.
running
r. commentary hallucination
r. seizure
runs of activity
rupture
aneurysmal r.
anular radial r.
disc r.
intervertebral disc r.
intraoperative r.
longitudinal ligament r.
lumbar disc r.
membranous labyrinth r.
plaque r.

surgical r.
vein patch r.
ruptured
r. disc
r. saccular aneurysm
Rush Alzheimer Registry
Russell
hooked bundle of R.
R. syndrome
uncinate bundle of R.
uncinate fasciculus of R.
R. viper venom time
Russell-Rubinstein cerebrovascular malformation classification
Russian
R. autumnal encephalitis
R. autumn encephalitis
R. endemic encephalitis
R. forest spring encephalitis
R. spring-summer encephalitis
R. tick-borne encephalitis
R. vernal encephalitis
Rust
R. disease
R. phenomenon
Ruvalcaba-Myhre syndrome
RVA
right ventricular activation
RVAS
rotational vertebral artery syndrome
ryanodine receptor

NOTES

S
S incision
S phase cell
S sleep
S-100
S-100 beta protein
S-100 tumor marker
SAB
subarachnoid block
SAB anesthesia
sabeluzole
Saber CBF-ICP trauma sensor
Sabin-Feldman dye test
Sabril
sac
aneurysm s.
dural s.
endolymphatic s.
nasal mucosal s.
thecal s.
saccade
s. amplitude
anticipatory s.
contrapulsion of s.
hypometric s.
s. impairment
s. inhibition
intentional visually guided s.
leftward s.
memory-guided s.
s. paralysis
predictive s.
refixation s.
rightward s.
successive s.'s
s. velocity
vertical conjugate s.
visually guided s.
saccadic
s. abnormality
s. contraversive head turning
s. dysmetria
s. overshooting
s. palsy
s. paresis
s. pursuit eye movement
s. slowing
s. velocity
s. vertical smooth pursuit
saccharopinuria
saccular
s. aneurysm
s. nerve
s. spot
saccularis
nervus s.
sacculi
macula s.
sacculus communis
Sachs
S. brain suction tip
S. brain suction tube
S. dural hook
S. dural separator
S. nerve separator-spatula
S. nerve spatula
sacral
s. agenesis
s. agenesis dysraphism
s. alar screw
s. brim target point
s. dimple
s. docking sheath
s. dorsal commissural neuron
s. dorsal commissural nucleus (SDCN)
s. foraminal approach
s. ganglion
s. hemangioma
s. insufficiency fracture
s. meningocele
s. nerve
s. nerve root cyst
s. nerve stimulation
s. nerve stimulation therapy
s. nonunion
s. parasympathetic nucleus
s. pedicle screw
s. pedicle screw fixation
s. plexopathy
s. plexus
s. plexus avulsion
s. plexus neuropathy
s. screw placement
s. segmental nerve stimulation implantable neural prosthesis
s. slope
s. sparing
s. spine
s. spine decompression
s. spine fixation
s. spine fusion
s. spine modular instrumentation
s. spine stabilization
s. spine Universal instrumentation
s. stress fracture
s. vertebra

sacrales
nervi splanchnici s.
nuclei parasympathici s.
sacralia
ganglia s.
sacralis
ansa s.
plexus s.
ramus lateralis rami posterioris nervi s.
ramus medialis rami posterioris nervi s.
segmentum medullae spinalis s.
sacralium
rami anteriores nervorum s.
rami dorsales nervorum s.
rami posteriores nervorum s.
rami ventrales nervorum s.
sacrifice
carotid artery s.
endovascular carotid s.
sacrococcygeal
s. agenesis
s. myxopapillary ependymoma
s. region
s. spine
s. teratoma
sacroiliac joint
sacroiliitis
sacrolisthesis
sacrolumbar
sacroposterior (SP)
sacrospinalis muscle
sacrum fusion screw fixation
SAD
seasonal affective disorder
saddle
Cloward surgical s.
s. coil
s. nose deformity
tubercle of s.
saddle-area sensory loss
saddleback fever
saddle-shaped anesthesia
Saenger
S. reflex
S. sign
Saethre-Chotzen syndrome
Safe-T-Wheel pinwheel
safety
oral appliance s.
sagittal
s. anatomic alignment
s. craniosynostosis
s. deformity
s. flexion angle
s. groove
s. orientation
s. pedicle angle
s. pedicle diameter
s. plane
s. plane instability
s. plexus
s. plumbline
s. projection
s. sinus
s. sinus thrombosis
s. slice fracture
s. spin-echo image
s. synostosis
s. T1-weighted SE image
s. T1-weighted spin echo image
saguli
nucleus s.
sagulum nucleus
SAH
subarachnoid hemorrhage
angiogram-negative SAH
Saint
S. Anthony dance
S. Guy dance
S. Vitus dance
Sakoda complex
salaam
s. attack
s. convulsion
s. seizure
s. spasm
Sala cell
salazosulfapyridine
salbutamol
Salibi carotid artery clamp
salicylate
magnesium s.
potassium s.
serum s.
sodium s.
s. toxic effect
triethanolamine s.
salient loading
saline
s. injection
phosphate-buffered s. (PBS)
preservative-free normal s.
s. torch
saline-soaked sponge
salivary
s. gland
s. gland dysfunction
s. nucleus
saliva screen for alcohol
salivation
copious s.
excessive s.
Salla disease
Salmonella
S. meningitis
S. typhi

salmonellosis
nontyphoidal s.
Salmonine Injection
Salmon Rickham ventriculostomy reservoir
Salpix
salt
Earle s.'s
s. restriction
s. wasting
saltation
saltatorial conduction
saltatoric spasm
saltatory
s. chorea
s. conduction
s. spasm
salvage chemotherapy
SAM
S-adenosylmethionine
selective adhesion molecule
synthetic aperture magnetometry
SAM inhibitor
samarium-EDTMP
SAMe
S-adenosylmethionine
sampling
chorionic villus s. (CVS)
petrosal sinus s.
Samuels-Weck hemoclip
sanatorium disease
sand
s. body
brain s.
s. tumor
Sandhoff disease
Sandifer syndrome
Sandostatin
sandwich
fascia-muscle-fascia s.
Sanfilippo
S. disease
S. syndrome
Sanger Brown ataxia
sanguinis
ictus s.
Sano clip applier
Santavuori disease
Santavuori-Haltia disease
Santavuori-Haltia-Hagberg disease
Santorini plexus
SaO2
saturation of oxygen
sapheni
falciformis hiatus s.
rami cutanei cruris medialis nervi s.
ramus infrapatellaris nervi s.
saphenous
s. nerve
s. vein
s. vein bypass graft
s. vein patch graft
saphenus
cornu inferius hiatus s.
nervus s.
sapophore group
Sapporo shunt tube
saquinavir
SARA
SQUID array for reproductive assessment
sarcoglycan deficiency
sarcoid
s. neuropathy
s. polyneuropathy
sarcoidosis
intracranial s.
s. neuromuscular involvement
s. peripheral neuropathy
sarcolemma membrane
sarcoma
angiolithic s.
Ewing s.
fibrous s.
granulocytic s.
juxtacortical s.
Kaposi s.
myelogenic s.
orbital granulocytic s.
osteogenic s.
perithelial small cell s.
reticulum cell s.
sarcomatous
s. leptomeningitis
s. tumor
sarcomere
sarcoplasmic reticulum
sarcosinemia
sarcotubular myopathy
Sardinian multiple sclerosis
sardonic

S

NOTES

sardonicus
risus s.
trismus s.
sartorius nerve
SAS
sleep apnea syndrome
Sassouni analysis
satellite
s. cell
s. potential
satellitosis
satiety
s. center
early s.
Sativex
satumomab pendetide
saturation
arterial oxygen s.
jugular bulb venous oxygen s.
nocturnal oxygen s.
s. of oxygen (SaO2)
partial s.
receiver s.
s. recovery
regional oxygen s. (rSO_2)
s. transfer
venous oxygen s.
Saturday night palsy
saturnine
s. encephalopathy
s. tremor
Saunders cervical HomeTrac
saver
Cell S.
intraoperative cell s.
saw
Adson wire s.
Bier s.
Cushing s.
DeMartel wire s.
Gigli s.
Midas Rex craniotomy s.
Olivecrona-Gigli s.
Olivecrona wire s.
spinal s.
threadwire s.
triton reciprocating s.
undercutting s.
sawtooth wave
Sayre head sling (SHS)
S-100b
protein S-100b
SCA
spinocerebellar ataxia
SCA gene
SCA1–7
spinocerebellar ataxia gene encoding types 1–7
SC-AcuFix Anterior Cervical Plate System
scala, pl. **scalae**
s. media
s. vestibuli
scale
Abnormal Involuntary Movement S.
absolute s.
Alzheimer Disease Assessment S. (ADAS)
Alzheimer Disease Rating S. (ADRS)
American Musculoskeletal Tumor Society rating s.
American Spinal Injury Association/International Medical Society of Paraplegia Impairment S.
Aminoff S.
AO S.
Aphasia Language Performance S.
Ashworth s.
Barthel Activities of Daily Living S.
Basic Living Skills S.
Behavior Pathology in Alzheimer Disease Rating S.
Berg Balance S. (BBS)
Black grading s.
Blessed Dementia S.
Blessed-Roth Dementia S.
Bricklin Perceptual S.
Brief Cognitive Rating S.
British Ability S.
Brown-Goodwin s.
Burke-Fahn-Marsden Dystonia Rating S.
Bush-Francis Catatonia Rating S.
Canadian Neurological S. (CNS)
CDR S.
Chapman s.
Cincinnati Stroke S.
Clinical Adaptive Test/Clinical Linguistic and Auditory Milestone S. (CAT/CLAMS)
Clinical Dementia Rating S.
Clinical Global Improvement S.
Clinical Linguistic Auditory Milestone S.
Clinician Global Rating S.
clinician-rated s.
Cognitive Abilities Screening S.
coma s.
Community-Oriented Programs Environment S.
Comprehensive Level of Consciousness S.
Conversational Skills Rating S.
Daily Rating S.

DBD S.
Delirium Rating S. (DRS)
Dementia Mood Assessment S.
Derogatis Affects Balance S.
Differential Ability S.
digital vernier s.
Drooling Rating S.
Drooling Severity and Frequency S.
Dystonia Movement S.
Edinburgh 2 Coma S.
efficacy s.
Engel Seizure Outcome S.
Epworth Sleepiness S. (ESS)
European Stroke S. (ESS)
EuroQol visual analog s.
Expanded Disability Status S. (EDSS)
Fahn-Tolosa-Marin tremor rating s.
Fränkel s.
Functional Ergonomic Prolo S.
Gait Abnormality Rating S.
Geriatric Depression S.
Gesell Developmental S.
Glasgow Outcome S.
global clinician-rated s.
global dementia rating s.
Global Deterioration S. (GDS)
Guy Neurological Disability S.
Hachinski ischemic s.
Hague Seizure Severity S.
Hasegawa Dementia S.
Hoehn and Yahr Disability S.
Hollingshead-Redlich s.
House-Brackmann Facial Nerve Function Grading S.
Hunt and Hess Stroke S.
Hunt-Hess subarachnoid hemorrhage s.
injury severity s.
Internal State S.
International Cooperative Ataxia Rating S.
Iowa Conners s.
3-Item Delirium S.
Johns Hopkins Severity S.
Karnofsky performance s.
Karnofsky rating s.
Karolinska Sleepiness S.
Kurtzke Expanded Disability Status S.
Kurtzke multiple sclerosis disability s.
Leeds Anxiety S.
Level of Functioning S.
linear s.
manual vernier s.
Maryland coma s.
Mathew Stroke S.
Mattis Dementia Rating S.
Memorial Delirium Assessment S. (MDAS)
Memorial Symptom Assessment S.
Modified Rankin S.
modified Simpson-Angus Rating S.
Montgomery and Asberg Depression Rating S. (MADRS)
Morgan-Russell s.
MRC strength testing s.
National Institutes of Health Stroke S. (NIHSS)
New York University Parkinson Disease S.
Orgogozo Stroke S.
Orpington Prognosis S.
Parkinson Disease Quality of Life S. (PDQUALIF)
pediatric daytime sleepiness s. (PDSS)
7-point s.
Positive and Negative Stroke S.
Positive and Negative Syndrome S. (PANSS)
prognostic s.
Progressive Deterioration S.
Prolo function-economic rating s.
psychopathology rating s.
Pyramid S.
Quality of Crisis Support S.
Quality of Life S.
Reaction Level S.
Revised Physical Anhedonia S.
Shipley-Hartford S.
Smith Extrapyramidal S.
Social and Occupational Functioning S.
Spetzler-Martin grading s.
Stanford Sleepiness S.
state-dependent psychopathology rating s.
St. Paul-Ramsey S.
Strauss-Carpenter s.
Stroke Impact S. (SIS)

NOTES

scale *(continued)*
Teasdale and Jennett s.
Thurston s.
total s.
Tourette Syndrome Association Unified Tic Rating S.
Tremor Clinical Rating S.
tremor self-rating s.
Unified Huntington Disease Rating S. (UHDRS)
Unified Parkinson Disease Rating S. (UPDRS)
UPDRS s.
verbal analog pain s.
Vineland Adaptive Behavior S.
Vineland percentile s.
visual analog s. (VAS)
WFNS s.
Women's Health Initiative Insomnia Rating S.
World Federation of Neurological Surgeons s.
Yale Global Tic Severity S. (YGTSS)
Yale Tic Severity S.
Zung Anxiety S.
Zung Self-Rating Depression S.

Scale–Cognition
Alzheimer Disease Assessment S.-C. (ADAS-Cog)

scaled
s. score
s. stereotactic atlas section

scalenectomy

scalenotomy

scalenus
s. anterior syndrome
s. anticus
s. anticus muscle

Scale-Revised
Hasegawa Dementia S.-R.

scalp
s. clip
s. clip applicator
s. clip forceps
s. closure
s. contusion
s. EEG monitoring
s. electrical potential
s. electrode
s. flap
s. flap forceps
s. hematoma
s. ictal electroencephalography
s. incision
s. infection
s. laceration
s. sensation

scalp-derived EEG activity

scalp-sphenoidal electroencephalography

scan
attenuation coefficient on MRI s.
attenuation value on MRI s.
baseline s.
bone density s.
bone window CT s.
brain SPECT s.
CAT s.
computerized tomography s.
contrast-enhanced CT s.
CT s.
echo planar diffusion- and perfusion-weighted imaging s.
fast spin-echo s.
fluorodopa positron emission tomographic s.
gallium s.
genome-wide admixture s.
instant s.
intrathecal contrast-enhanced CAT s.
Iso-C s.
longitudinal s.
MRI s.
nuclear MR s.
PET s.
radioisotope s.
radionuclide bone s.
sequential computed tomographic s.
single-photon emission CT s.
SPECT s.
standardized A s.
s. time
triple-phase bone s.
T1-weighted inversion recovery s.
T2-weighted magnetic resonance s.

scanner
General Electric CT 9800 s.
General Electric Hi-Speed Advantage helical s.
General Electric Hi-Speed Spiral CT S.
General Electric Signa 1.5-Tesla magnetic resonance s.
Magnetom Open s.
Magnetom Vision s.
OctreoScan s.
Picker s.
Siemens Magnetom Harmony s.
Siemens Symphony 1.5-T s.
Siemens Vision s.
SilkTouch CO_2 laser s.
3-T MRI s.

scanner-assisted target localization

scanning
CAT s.
computerized axial tomography s.
confocal laser s.

diffusion-weighted s.
duplex s.
s. electron microscopy
functional activation PET s.
GE Signa s.
GE Vector s.
line s.
point s.
radionucleotide s.
RN s.
s. speech
visual s.
XeCT s.
xenon CT s.
xenon-enhanced CT s.
scaphocephaly
scaphohydrocephalus
scaphohydrocephaly
scapulae
levator s.
nervus dorsalis s.
scapular
s. nerve
s. reflex
scapularis
Ixodes s.
scapulohumeral
s. atrophy
s. muscular dystrophy
s. reflex
scapuloperiosteal reflex
scapuloperoneal
s. muscular atrophy
s. muscular dystrophy
s. syndrome
scar
glia s.
hemosiderin s.
Scaramella procedure
scarf sign
scarlatiniform rash
Scarpa
S. ganglion
S. method
S. nerve
scarred dura
scarring
glial s.
scattered
s. dysrhythmic slow activity
s. dysrhythmic slow activity on EEG
scattergram
scattering
Compton s.
scavenger
free radical s.
SCD
spinocerebellar degeneration
Scedosporium apiospermum
scelalgia
Sceratti arc
SCG
superior cervical ganglion
Schacher ganglion
Schaffer
S. collateral axon
S. collateral cell
Schäffer reflex
Schaltenbrand-Wahren stereotactic atlas
Scharff microbipolar and suction forceps
Schaumberg disease
schedule
altered sleep s.
Autism Diagnostic Observation S.
S.'s for Clinical Assessment in Neuropsychiatry
Glasgow Assessment S.
s. II substance
medical taper s.
medication taper s.
regular eating s.
regular sleeping s.
regular waking s.
sleep-wake s.
Scheie
S. disease
S. syndrome
schema, pl. **schemata**
body s.
Kraepelin s.
schematic mental model
scheme
Guiot s.
schenckii
Sporothrix s.
Scheuermann
S. disease
S. kyphosis
Schiff-Sherrington phenomenon
Schilder
S. disease
S. encephalitis

NOTES

Schilling test
Schindler disease
Schinzel-Giedion syndrome
Schirmer
S. syndrome
S. test
schistorrhachis
Schistosoma mansoni
schistosomiasis trematode
schizaxon
schizencephalic
s. microcephaly
s. porencephaly
schizencephaly
schizogyria
schizophrenia
Bleulerian s.
childhood s.
schizophrenia-related sleep disturbance
Schlesinger
S. laminectomy rongeur
S. phenomenon
S. sign
Schlichter test
Schloffer operation
Schlösser treatment
Schmidt-Fischer angle
Schmidt-Lanterman
S.-L. cleft
S.-L. incisure
S.-L. segment
Schmidt vagoaccessory syndrome
Schmitt disease
Schmorl
S. node
S. nodule
Schneider first-rank symptom
Schnidt clamp
Schober measurement
Scholz disease
Schramm phenomenon
Schreiber maneuver
Schrötter chorea
Schüller phenomenon
Schultze
S. cell
comma bundle of S.
comma tract of S.
S. comma tract
S. scissors
S. sign
Schultze-Chvostek sign
Schumacher criteria
Schütz
S. bundle
S. fasciculus
tract of S.
S. tract
Schwabach test
Schwalbe
S. corpuscle
S. fissure
S. foramen
S. nucleus
S. space
Schwann
S. cell
S. cell body
S. cell differentiation
S. cell implant
S. cell marker
S. cell origin
S. cell protein
S. cell tumor
S. cell unit
S. membrane
S. nucleus
sheath of S.
S. white substance
schwannoglioma
schwannoma
acoustic s.
cerebellopontine angle s.
intracranial s.
intralabyrinthine s.
intraosseous s.
jugular foramen s.
nonacoustic s.
orbital s.
spinal intradural s.
synchronous facial s.
trigeminal s.
vestibular s.
schwannomatosis
familial s.
schwannosis
Schwartz
S. aneurysm clip
S. laminectomy retractor
S. temporary intracranial artery clamp
S. tractotomy
Schwartz-Jampel syndrome
SCI
spinal cord injury
sciatic
s. nerve
s. nerve lesion
s. nerve trauma
s. neuralgia
s. neuritis
s. notch syndrome
s. pain
s. plexus
s. scoliosis
sciatica
sciaticus
nervus s.

scientific empiricism
scieropia
scintiangiography
scintigram
  ^{99m}Tc-HMPAO leukocyte s.
scintigraphy
  Ga s.
  indium-111 octreotide s.
  leukocyte s.
  regional cerebral blood flow s.
  ^{99m}Tc-HMPAO leukocyte s.
  ^{201}Tl s.
scintillating visual scotoma
scintillation camera
scintiphotography
scissoring walk
scissors
  Adson ganglion s.
  Aslan endoscopic s.
  bipolar cautery s.
  Codman s.
  Dandy neurological s.
  Dandy neurosurgical s.
  Dandy trigeminal nerve s.
  DeBakey endarterectomy s.
  Decker alligator s.
  Decker microsurgical s.
  dural s.
  Frazier dural s.
  s. gait
  Harrington s.
  Jacobson microneurosurgical s.
  Jannetta-Kurze dissecting s.
  Jansen-Middleton s.
  Kurze dissection s.
  Malis bipolar cautery s.
  Malis neurological s.
  Mayo s.
  Metzenbaum s.
  Nicola s.
  Olivecrona dura s.
  Olivecrona trigeminal s.
  Schultze s.
  Smellie s.
  Strully neurological s.
  Sweet pituitary s.
  Taylor brain s.
  Taylor dural s.
  Toennis dissecting s.
  Yasargil bayonet s.
SCIWORA
  spinal cord injury without radiographic abnormality
sCJD
  sporadic Creutzfeldt-Jakob disease
sclerencephaly, sclerencephalia
scleritis
sclerodactyly, sclerodactylia
scleroderma
sclerodermatomyositis
sclerosing
  s. leukoencephalitis
  s. panencephalitis
sclerosis, pl. **scleroses**
  acute lateral s. (ALS)
  Alzheimer s.
  Ammon horn s.
  amyotrophic lateral s. (ALS)
  ash-leaf spot in tuberous s.
  Baló concentric s.
  Bourneville tuberous s.
  Canavan s.
  cerebral s.
  combined s.
  concentric s.
  congenital hippocampal s.
  diffuse cerebral s.
  diffuse infantile familial s.
  discogenic s.
  disseminated s.
  epidemic multiple s.
  Erb s.
  familial amyotrophic lateral s. (FALS)
  familial centrolobar s.
  familial form of amyotrophic lateral s.
  focal s.
  hippocampal s.
  human herpesvirus 6/multiple s. (HHV6-MS)
  insular s.
  ipsilateral mesial temporal s.
  Krabbe diffuse s.
  laminar cortical s.
  lateral spinal s.
  lobar s.
  mantle s.
  mesial temporal s. (MTS)
  multiple s. (MS)
  myelinoclastic diffuse cerebral s.
  Pelizaeus-Merzbacher s.

S

NOTES

sclerosis *(continued)*
posterior spinal s.
posterolateral s.
primary lateral s.
primary progressive multiple s.
progressive systemic s.
relapsing-remitting multiple s. (RRMS)
Sardinian multiple s.
secondary progressive multiple s. (SPMS)
subchondral s.
sudanophilic cerebral s.
systemic s.
tuberous s.
ventrolateral s.
s. of white matter
sclerotherapy
transvenous retrograde nidus s.
sclerotic
s. area
s. plaque
sclerotome area
SCM
sternocleidomastoid
SCN1B gene
scoliosis
adult s.
atypical idiopathic s.
compensatory s.
congenital s.
degenerative lumbar s.
double major curve s.
double thoracic curve s.
early-onset s.
fracture with s.
idiopathic thoracic s.
King type I–V s.
Lenke classification of adolescent idiopathic s.
lumbar s.
neuromuscular s.
osteopathic s.
paralytic s.
right thoracic curve s.
right thoracic left lumbar s.
right thoracic left thoracolumbar s.
rigid curve s.
sciatic s.
thoracic curve s.
thoracolumbar idiopathic s.
thoracolumbar spine s.
scoliotic
s. curve fixation
s. paralytic deformity
scoop
Cushing pituitary s.
Scoville intervertebral disc s.
Yasargil s.
scopolamine
score
Abbreviated Injury S.
Abnormal Involuntary Movement S.
Acute Physiology S.
Aminoff disability s.
Apgar s.
Barnes global s.
brain relaxation s.
Champion Trauma S.
Children's Coma S.
Clinician Awareness S.
cognitive s.
conservative cutoff s.
cutoff s.
elevated s.
emotional memory s.
end-point CGI s.
event recall s.
factor s.
FOUR coma s.
Galante disc degeneration s.
general knowledge s.
Glasgow Coma S. (GCS)
Glasgow Outcome S. (GOS)
global AIMS s.
global clinical impression s.
Global Tic Rating S.
Hachinski ischemic s.
House-Brackmann S.
impairment rating s.
Informant Awareness S.
injury severity s.
kappa s.
Karnofsky performance s. (KPS)
Kurtzke s.
Lahey s.
leukoaraiosis s.
logarithm of odds s.
logical memory subtest s.
mean total weighted sum s.
mean weighted s.
modified Rankin s.
neurofibrillary tangle s.
Nurick s.
objective motor s.
Odom s.
Oswestry Disability s.
peak s.
Performance Scale S.
positive s.
psychosomatic symptom s.
Q s.
RAATE s.
Rankin s.
raw Q s.
Revised Trauma S.
risk s.
scaled s.

Simpson-Angus total s.
standard s.
stroke s.
subtest scale s.
T s.
Tegner s.
Thoracolumbar Injury Classification and Severity S. (TLICS)
total AIMS s.
total emotional memory s.
total symptom s.
total weighted sum s.
verbal recall s.
verbal weighted sum s.
Wada memory s.
weighted sum s.

scoring coefficient

scotodinia

scotoma, pl. **scotomata**
scotomata of action
bilateral centrocecal s.
cecocentral s.
flittering s.
hemianopic s.
homonymous scintillating s.
paracentral s.
scintillating visual s.

Scott
S. cannula
S. silicone ventricular catheter

scotty dog sign

Scoville
S. blade
S. brain clip-applying forceps
S. brain spatula
S. brain spatula forceps
S. cervical disc retractor
S. clip
S. dissector
S. hemilaminectomy retractor
S. intervertebral disc scoop
S. nerve root hook
S. nerve root retractor
S. ruptured disc curette
S. skull trephine
S. ventricular needle

Scoville-Haverfield hemilaminectomy retractor

Scoville-Richter laminectomy retractor

scrapie form

scratching automatism

scratch reflex

screen
Los Angeles Prehospital Stroke S. (LAPSS)

screener
closed head injury s.

screening
anencephaly s.
autism s.
blood s.
bone density s.
developmental disorder s.
Down syndrome s.
genetic s.
metabolic disorder s.
newborn s.
Tay-Sachs disease s.
urine s.
Wyatt s.

screw
alar s.
s. alignment bar
s. alignment rod
s. angulation
s. backout
bone s.
s. breakage
Camino subdural s.
cancellous s.
cannulated s.
Caspar cervical s.
cervical pedicle s.
cortical s.
Cotrel pedicle s.
Edwards sacral s.
s. fixation
fixed-head s.
iliac s.
iliosacral s.
s. implantation
s. insertion
s. insertion technique
Isola spinal implant system iliac s.
KLS-Martin center drive s.
Kostuik s.
lateral mass s.
Leibinger Micro Plus s.
Lorenz cranial s.
lumbar pedicle s.
s. malposition
Micro Plus s.
Mille Pattes s.
Mini Würzburg s.

S

NOTES

screw *(continued)*
Moss-Miami polyaxial s.
multiaxial s.
PathFinder polyaxial s.
pedicle s.
s. placement
s. plate approach
polyaxial s.
s. position perioperative monitoring
s. pullout
s. pullout strength
rescue s.
rigid pedicle s.
sacral alar s.
sacral pedicle s.
self-tapping s.
set s.
s. stabilization
stainless steel s.
Steinhauser cranial s.
s. stripout
subarachnoid s.
subdural pressure s.
superior thoracic pedicle s.
Synthes s.
Texas Scottish Rite Hospital pedicle s.
thoracolumbar pedicle s.
TiMesh s.
transarticular s.
transpedicular cannulated s.
triangulated pedicle s.
tulip pedicle s.
Vari-Angle s.
screwdriver
right-angle s.
Stab-and-Grab s.
screw-related complication
screw-to-screw compression construct
scrivener's palsy
scrotal nerve
SD
semantic dementia
sleep deprivation
stimulus drive
SDAT
senile dementia of Alzheimer type
SDAVF
spinal dural arteriovenous fistula
SDCN
sacral dorsal commissural nucleus
SDEEG
stereotactic depth electroencephalogram
stereotactic depth electroencephalography
SDR
selective dorsal rhizotomy
SDS
Shy-Drager syndrome
sodium dodecyl sulfate
SE
status epilepticus
sealant
cyanoacrylate polymer s.
fibrin adhesive s.
FloSeal Matrix hemostatic s.
FocalSeal-S surgical s.
tissue fibrin s.
seamstress's cramp
search
face s.
Seashore test
seasonal
s. affective disorder (SAD)
s. migraine
s. migraine headache
seat
Wayne laminectomy s.
seatbelt fracture
Seattle Longitudinal Study
sebaceous, sebaceus
s. adenoma
sebaceum
adenoma s.
seborrheic keratosis
Sechrist monoplace hyperbaric chamber
Seconal
second
s. cervical nerve
s. cranial nerve [CN II]
s. harmonic imaging (SHI)
s. impact syndrome
s. messenger molecule
s. somatosensory area
s. temporal convolution
s. visual area
secondarily generalized tonic-clonic seizure
secondary
s. axotomy
s. bilateral synchrony
s. brain injury
s. bruxism
s. cognitive task
s. degeneration
s. delirium
s. disorder
s. drive
s. dual pathology
s. dystonia
s. effect
s. encephalitis
s. ending
s. epileptogenesis
s. epileptogenic focus
s. fissure of cerebellum
s. generalized epilepsy
s. headache
s. hydrocephalus

s. insomnia
s. narcolepsy
s. neurulation
s. outcome
s. periodic leg movement of sleep
s. posttraumatic syringomyelia
s. process
s. progressive MS
s. progressive multiple sclerosis (SPMS)
s. restless leg syndrome
s. seizure
s. sensory cortex
s. sensory neuron
s. sensory nucleus
s. somatosensory area
s. somatosensory cortex
s. symptom
s. synaptic cleft
s. tumor
s. verbal memory
s. visual area
s. visual cortex

second-degree nystagmus

second-line
s.-l. agent
s.-l. therapy

second-order neuron

Secor system

secretase
alpha s.
beta s.
gamma s.

secreted
s. protein acidic and rich in cysteine
regulated on activation, normal T-cell expressed and s. (RANTES)

secretin

secreting glial pseudocyst

secretion
androgen s.
endocrine s.
gastrointestinal s.
leptin s.
ovarian androgen s.
progesterone s.

secretomotor nerve

secretomotory

secretory
s. function
s. meningioma
s. nerve

section
attached cranial s.
axial s.
callosal s.
coronal s.
detached cranial s.
histologic s.
midsagittal s.
parasagittal s.
permanent s.
pituitary stalk s.
scaled stereotactic atlas s.
trigeminal root s.
vestibular nerve s.

sectioning
cryomicrotome s.

sectoranopia
quadruple s.

Secure Balance

SecureStrand
S. cable
S. cervical fusion system

Sedan cannula

Sedan-Nashold needle

sedation
preoperative s.
prolonged s.

sedation/apathy

sedative
s. activity
s. antihistamine
hypnotic s.
s. intoxication
s. property
s. withdrawal

seed
^{125}I s.
radioactive yttrium s.

seeding
meningeal s.
subarachnoid s.
surgical s.

SEEG
stereoelectroencephalography

Seeligmüller sign

seesaw nystagmus (SSN)

SEF
spectral edge frequency
supplementary eye field

NOTES

segment
adjacent s.
adrenal s.
clinoidal s.
exiting s.
globus pallidus external s.
globus pallidus internal s.
initial s.
interannular s.
internodal s.
intracanalicular s.
intracranial prechiasmatic s.
intradural s.
Lanterman s.
M s.
M2 artery s.
medullary s.
motion s.
neural s.
ophthalmic s.
P s.
Ranvier s.
Schmidt-Lanterman s.
s. of spinal cord
sympathetic s.
traversing s.
segmenta (*pl. of* segmentum)
segmental
s. anesthesia
s. arterial disorganization
s. compression construct
s. conduction abnormality
s. demyelinating polyneuropathy
s. demyelination
s. dystonia
s. ectasia
s. fibrinoid necrosis
s. fixation
s. medullary reflex
s. neuritis
s. neurofibromatosis
s. neuropathy
s. registration
s. sensory deficit
s. sensory disassociation with brachial muscular atrophy
s. spinal instrumentation (SSI)
s. vulnerability
segmentary
s. response
s. syndrome
segmentation
volume s.
segmentum, pl. **segmenta**
s. cervicalia 1–8
s. cervicalia medullae spinalis
s. coccygea 1–3
s. coccygea medullae spinalis
s. internodale
s. lumbalia 1–5
s. lumbalia medullae spinalis
s. lumbaria
s. medullae spinalis
s. medullae spinalis cervicalia
s. medullae spinalis coccygea
s. medullae spinalis lumbalis
s. medullae spinalis sacralis
s. medullae spinalis thoracica
s. sacralia 1–5
s. sacralia medullae spinalis
s. thoracica 1–12
s. thoracica medullae spinalis
segregation
mitotic s.
Séguin
S. sign
S. signal symptom
SEH
spinal epidural hematoma
seipin gene
Seitelberger disease
seizure
absence s.
s. activity
afebrile s.
affective symptom of s.
alcohol-related s.
alcohol withdrawal s.
alimentary s.
amygdala s.
anosognosic s.
astatic s.
asymmetric tonic s.
atonic s.
atypical absence s.
atypical petit mal s.
audiogenic s.
auditory s.
automotor s.
autonomic s.
catamenial s.
cerebellar fit s.
chemically induced s.
childhood absence epilepsy with generalized tonic-clonic s.
s. classification
clinical s.
clonic s.
clonicotonic s.
complex febrile s.
complex motor s.
complex partial nocturnal s.
convulsive s.
dileptic s.
drop s.
drug-resistant localization-related s.
drug withdrawal s.
early s.

eating s.
eclamptic s.
electroconvulsive s.
electrographic s.
encephalotrigeminal angiomatosis s.
epileptic s.
s. evaluation
evoked s.
s. exacerbation
exercise-induced s.
extratemporal s.
febrile s.
fictitious s.
first-trimester maternal s.
focal motor s.
s. focus resection
s. free
s. frequency
frontal lobe s.
gelastic s.
generalized atypical absence s.
generalized epilepsy plus febrile s.
generalized tonic-clonic s. (GTCS)
grand mal s.
habitual s.
hippocampal slice model of s.
HIV-related s.
hypermotor s.
hyperventilation s.
hypoglycemic s.
hypomotor s.
hysterical s.
ictal confusional s.
idiopathic s.
s. induced by flickering light
s. induced by thinking
International Classification of S.'s
intractable partial s.
jackknife s.
jacksonian s.
Janz juvenile myoclonic s.
juvenile absence s.
kindled s.
language-induced s.
late s.
laughing s.
localization-related s.
major motor s.
s. management
maternal s.
maximal electroshock s. (MES)
maximal electroshock-induced s.
medically refractory partial s.
medication-induced s.
midtemporal s.
minor motor s.
s. monitoring
motor s.
movement-induced s.
musicogenic s.
myoclonic astatic petit mal s.
negative myoclonic s.
neonatal drug addiction s.
neonatal hypoglycemic s.
new-onset s.
nicotine-induced s.
nocturnal s.
nonconvulsive s.
nonepileptic s.
occipital lobe s.
opioid peptide in s.
partial complex s.
partial-onset s.
s. pattern
pattern-sensitive s.
petit mal s.
phantom absence s.
photosensitive s.
postischemic s.
postmenopausal s.
postpump s.
praxis-induced s.
premature infant s.
primary generalized s.
primary idiopathic s.
prolonged febrile s.
pseudoepileptic s.
psychic s.
psychogenic nonepileptic s.
psychomotor s.
pyridoxine-deficiency s.
reactive s.
reading s.
s. recurrence
reflex s.
reflex anoxic s.
refractory localization-related s.
remote symptomatic s.
repetitive s.'s
s. risk
rolandic s.
running s.
salaam s.

NOTES

seizure *(continued)*
secondarily generalized tonic-clonic s.
secondary s.
s. semiology
serial motor s.'s
simple febrile s.
simple partial s.
single s.
s. in sleep
sound-sensitive s.
spontaneous s.
stimulant-related s.
subclinical s.
subtle s.
supplementary motor s.
suspected s.
sylvian s.
symptomatic s.
temporal lobe s.
tonic s.
tonic-clonic s.
s. trigger
s. triggered by somatosensory sensation
typical absence s.
unclassified epileptic s.
unilateral s.
unprovoked s.
versive s.
vestibulogenic s.
video monitoring of s.

seizure-alerting dog

seizure-free
s.-f. outcome
s.-f. rate
s.-f. state

seizurelike
s. activity
s. phenomenon

seizure-related behavior

Seldinger
S. angiogram
S. method
S. retrograde wire/intubation technique

selection
bone plate s.
Edwards modular system construct s.
internal s.
ligand s.
oral appliance s.
slice s.

selective
s. adhesion molecule (SAM)
s. amnesia
s. auditory agnosia
s. dorsal rhizotomy (SDR)
s. embolization
s. estrogen-receptor modulator (SERM)
s. excitation
s. focusing on environmental stimulus
s. imaging and graphics for stereotactic surgery (SIGSS)
s. irradiation
s. memory
s. microadenomectomy
s. nerve root (SNR)
s. neuronal necrosis
s. norepinephrine reuptake inhibitor
s. phosphodiesterase inhibitor
s. reading disability
s. relaxation enhancement
S. Reminding test
s. serotonin reuptake inhibitor (SSRI)
s. speech perception alteration
s. thoracic spine fusion
s. T2 shortening
s. vagotomy

selectivity
mesolimbic s.

selector
Leksell s.
S. ultrasonic aspirator

selegiline
s. HCl
s. patch

self-adhering electrode

self-attaching electrode

self-care task

self-induced
s.-i. artifactual skin disease
s.-i. dermatitis artefacta
s.-i. epilepsy

self-inflicted damage

self-injurious motor tic

self-object transference

Self-Ordered Pointing Test

self-perceived cognitive disorder

self-perpetuated disease

self-retaining brain retractor

self-stopping drill point

self-sustaining hyperexcitability

self-tapping screw

sella
ballooning of s.
diaphragm of s.
empty s.
s. punch forceps
tuberculum s.
s. turcica
s. turcica diaphragm

sellae
diaphragma s.

sellar
s. aneurysm
s. anomaly
s. cyst
s. entrance
s. gangliocytoma
s. punch
s. region
s. tumor
sellaris
pars s.
Selter disease
Selverstone
S. clamp
S. cordotomy hook
S. intervertebral disc rongeur
S. Semmes curette sensor
SEM
slow eye movement
standard error of mean
semantic
s. aphasia
s. cue
s. cueing
s. decision task
s. dementia (SD)
s. memory
s. memory function
s. memory impairment
s. paraphasia
s. process
semialdehyde
succinic s.
semicircular
s. canal
s. duct
semicirculares
ductus s.
semicircularis
crus membranaceum simplex ductus s.
ductus s.
tenia s.
semicircularium
canalium s.
crura ossea canalium s.
crus membranaceum commune ductuum s.
semicoma
semicomatose
semiconscious
semi-Fowler position
semiinvasive electrode
semilobar holoprosencephaly
semilunar
s. fasciculus
s. ganglion
s. lobe
s. lobule
s. notch
s. nucleus of Flechsig
s. tract
semilunare
velum s.
semilunares
lobuli s.
semilunaris
fasciculus s.
hiatus s.
nucleus s.
semimembranosus reflex
seminoma
intracranial s.
semiology
ictal s.
seizure s.
semioval center
semiovale
centrum s.
Vicq d'Azyr centrum s.
semiplegia
semipurposeful
s. activity
s. behavior
semirigid pedicle screw-plate fixation
semispinalis capitis
semisynthetic sphingolipid
semitendinosus reflex
Semliki Forest encephalitis
Semmes curette
Semmes-Weinstein esthesiometer
Semon-Hering theory
Semon law
semustine
senescence
motor neuron s.
senescent
s. fibroblast
s. forgetfulness
senile
s. chorea
s. delirium
s. dementia

NOTES

senile *(continued)*
s. dementia of Alzheimer type (SDAT)
s. gait disorder
s. leukoencephalopathic lesion
s. memory
s. neuropathy
s. paranoid state
s. paraplegia
s. plaque
s. tremor
Senn retractor
sensate focus approach
sensation
abnormal tactile s.
altered s.
cincture s.
cutaneous s.
delayed s.
epicritic s.
fine touch s.
general s.
girdle s.
objective s.
olfactory s.
pin s.
pins-and-needles s.
position s.
primary s.
referred s.
reflex s.
scalp s.
seizure triggered by somatosensory s.
shocking s.
special s.
subjective s.
s. of swelling
tingling s.
transferred s.
vascular s.
sense
s. of alienation
body s.
contact s.
s. of control
distance s.
s. epithelium
s. of equilibrium
s. of fatigue
internal s.
joint s.
kinesthetic s.
motion s.
movement s.
muscle s.
muscular s.
obstacle s.
s. organ
organ of special s.
pain s.
position s.
posture s.
pressure s.
proprioceptive s.
seventh s.
sixth s.
somatic s.
space s.
special s.
static s.
tactile s.
taste s.
temperature s.
thermal s.
thermic s.
thoroughness, reliability, efficiency, analytic s.
time s.
vestibular s.
vibration s.
visceral s.
weight s.
s. of wellness
s. of wholeness
sensibility
articular s.
bone s.
common s.
cortical s.
deep s.
dissociation s.
electromuscular s.
epicritic s.
mesoblastic s.
pallesthetic s.
proprioceptive s.
protopathic s.
splanchnesthetic s.
vibratory s.
sensible hemideficit
sensiferous
sensigenous
sensimeter
sensitiva
trichosis s.
sensitive
s. measure
s. plane
s. point
steroid s.
s. volume
sensitivity
age-associated s.
cold s.
enhanced s.
feedback s.
gluten s.

high s.
loss of s.
neuroleptic s.
pharmacologic s.
proportional s.
somatosensory s.
s. threshold
warm s.

sensitization
central s.
peripheral nociceptor s.

sensomobile

sensomobility

sensomotor (*var. of* sensorimotor)

sensor
CardioSearch s.
DC SQUID s.
DermaTemp infrared thermographic s.
disposable Doppler-constant thermocouple s.
measuring s.
MEG s.
Neurotrend s.
Paratrend 7 s.
s. position indicator
Saber CBF-ICP trauma s.
Selverstone Semmes curette s.
telemetric intracranial pressure s.
Watson angular rate s.
zero drift of s.

sensoria
decussatio s.
ganglia craniospinalia s.
organa s.

sensorial area

sensoriglandular

sensorimotor, sensomotor
s. area
s. axonal polyneuropathy
s. behavior
s. grating
s. period
s. peripheral neuropathy
s. strip
s. stroke

sensorimotor-autonomic neuropathy

sensorimuscular

sensorineural
s. acuity level masking technique
s. deafness

sensorium commune

sensorius
nervus s.

sensorivascular

sensorivasomotor

sensory
s. alexia
s. amusia
s. aphasia
s. apraxia
s. association area
s. ataxia
s. aura
s. axon
s. cell
s. compound action potential
s. compound action potential amplitude
s. cortex
s. crossway
s. cueing
s. decussation of medulla oblongata
s. deficit
s. deprivation
s. dimension
s. distribution
s. dysprosody
s. dystaxia
s. epithelium
s. evoked potential (SEP)
s. function
s. ganglion of cranial nerve
s. ganglion of encephalic nerve
s. gating
s. hair
s. image
s. impairment
s. inattention
s. information
s. integration dysfunction
s. interface
s. jacksonian attack
s. latency
s. load
s. loss
s. myelinated fiber
s. nerve action potential (SNAP)
s. nerve action potential amplitude
s. neurogenic arthropathy
s. neuron
s. neuronopathy
s. neuron-specific G protein-coupled receptor (SNSRs)

NOTES

sensory *(continued)*
s. neuropathy
s. nucleus
s. organ
s. overload
s. paralysis
s. pathway
s. perceptual examination
s. phantom
s. process
s. processing area
s. region
s. root of ciliary ganglion
s. root of mandibular nerve
s. root of otic ganglion
s. root of spinal nerve
s. root of submandibular ganglion
s. root of trigeminal nerve
s. speech center
s. tract
s. transduction
sensory-deprivation nystagmus
sensory-precipitated epilepsy
sensual dysarthria
sensuosity
sensuum
organa s.
senticosus
Eleutherococcus s.
SentiLite
S. EEG monitor
S. neurological monitor
sentinel
s. leak
s. spinous process fracture
S. system
Sentinel-4 neurological monitor
Seoul virus
SEP
sensory evoked potential
pudendal SEP
separans
funiculus s.
separation
articular mass s.
atlantoaxial s.
atlantooccipital s.
growth plate s.
pontomedullary s.
separator
Davis dural s.
Davis nerve s.
Dorsey dural s.
dural s.
Frazier dural s.
Hoen dural s.
Horsley dural s.
Hunter dural s.
Sachs dural s.
synovial s.
Woodson dural s.
separator-spatula
Davis nerve s.-s.
Sachs nerve s.-s.
Woodson dural s.-s.
sepiapterin reductase deficiency
SEPNR
spinally elicited peripheral nerve response
Sepracor
sepsis
septa (*pl. of* septum)
septal
s. area
s. nucleus
s. region
septation
intraventricular s.
septi
nuclei triangularis s.
nucleus accumbens s.
septic
s. embolus
s. encephalitis
s. encephalopathy
s. meningitis
s. shock
s. thrombosis
s. venous vasculitis
septicemia
septofimbrial nucleus
septomarginal
s. fasciculus
s. tract
septomarginalis
fasciculus s.
septooptic dysplasia
septooptic-pituitary dysplasia
septum, pl. **septa**
s. cervicale intermedium
dural s.
intermediate cervical s.
s. lingua
lingual s.
s. lucidum
s. medianum dorsale medullae spinalis
s. medianum posterius medullae spinalis
s. pellucidum
s. pellucidum cave
precommissural s.
subarachnoidal s.
s. of tongue
transparent s.
transverse s.

triangular nucleus of s.
s. verum
sequela, pl. **sequelae**
caffeine s.
caffeine-related s.
clinical s.
clinically adverse s.
neurobehavioral s.
neurological s.
postpolio s.
sequence
Carr-Purcell s.
Carr-Purcell-Meiboom-Gill s.
3-dimensional spoiled GRASS s.
s. of events
fast low-angle shot s.
fast spin-echo inversion recovery s.
gradient-refocused s.
hemisphere s.
magnetization-prepared rapid acquisition gradient echo s. (MPRAGE)
s. polymorphism
pulse s.
pulse-gated cine phase contrast s.
short-tau inversion recovery MRI s.
SPGR s.
spin-density s.
spin-warp pulse s.
spoiled gradient echo s.
STEAM s.
stimulated spin-echo s.
STIR s.
s. time
T2-weighted spin echo s.
sequencing
s. deletion breakpoint
s. task
sequential
s. compression device
s. computed tomographic scan
s. diagrammatic reformulation
s. dose
s. gradient-recalled acquisition in the steady state
s. GRASS
s. opposition finger movement
s. plane imaging
s. point imaging
s. ultrasonography
sequestrate
sequestrated disc
sequestrectomy
Williams s.
SER
somatosensory evoked response
sera (*pl. of* serum)
Serax
serial
s. CT
s. imaging
s. motor seizures
s. percutaneous needle drainage
s. position effects
s. reaction time (SRT)
series
Leksell gamma knife target s.
serine
s. palmitoyltransferase
s. protease
s. proteinase
SERM
selective estrogen-receptor modulator
seroepidemiological study
seronegative
s. myasthenia gravis
s. spondyloarthropathy
Seroquel
serosa
s. meningitis
meninx s.
serositis
serotonergic
s. activity
s. agent
s. dorsal raphe
s. dysfunction
s. pathway
s. side effect
s. system
serotonin
s. antagonist
s. excess disorder
s. 5-HT1
s. 5-HT2 receptor
s. 5-HT receptor agonist
s. norepinephrine reuptake inhibitor
s. receptor assay
s. stimulation
s. syndrome
s. system
serotonin/dopamine antagonist

NOTES

serotoninergic
s. cell body
s. syndrome
serous
s. apoplexy
s. meningitis
serpentine aneurysm
serpiginous mass
Serralnyl suture
Serralsilk suture
serrated action potential
serration
dentated s.
sertindole
Sertoli cell
sertraline hydrochloride
serum, pl. **sera**
s. albumin
s. ammonia level
s. androgen level
s. bicarbonate
s. bromide
s. caffeine level
s. calcium
s. ceruloplasmin
s. chloride
s. copper
s. cotinine
s. creatinine kinase
s. enzyme determination
s. ferritin
s. folate
s. folic acid
s. folic acid level
s. glutamic oxaloacetic transaminase
s. glutamic-pyruvic transaminase
s. glutamyl transaminase
s. heavy metal intoxication
s. lead level evaluation
s. lipid
s. lipid concentration
s. lipoprotein disorder
s. marker
s. neopterin
s. neuritis
s. phosphorus
s. potassium
s. prolactin
s. protein
s. protein binding
s. salicylate
s. sickness peripheral neuropathy
s. sodium
s. vitamin B12
s. von Willebrand factor
service
sleep disorder s.
servohydraulic test frame
servomechanism
Serzone
sestamibi
technetium-99m s.
set
aluminum contouring template s.
Bremer halo crown traction s.
empty s.
Greenberg retractor s.
Hudson cranial drill s.
Lyon data s.
Mira Mark III cranial drill s.
Mira Mark V craniotome s.
Mullan percutaneous trigeminal ganglion microcompression s.
s. screw
Weber human genome screening s.
setting
limit s.
programmable valve pressure s.
setting-sun sign
settling
cranial s.
seventh
s. cranial nerve [CN VII]
s. cranial nerve transposition
s. nerve injury
s. nerve palsy
s. sense
severe
s. childhood autosomal recessive muscular dystrophy
s. dementia
s. headache
s. head injury
s. head trauma
s. impairment
s. kyphoscoliosis
s. postanoxic encephalopathy
s. rigid right thoracic curve
severity
APACHE II measure of disease s.
baseline s.
concussion s.
dementia s.
depression s.
s. grading for hemorrhage
hyperintensity s.
objective s.
tremor s.
sevoflurane anesthesia
sewing spasm
sex
s. chromosome abnormality
s. headache
s. hormone
s. hormone-binding globulin (SHBG)
sexual dysfunction

SF
Kaochlor SF
SFEMG
single-fiber electroencephalography
single-fiber EMG
SF-MPQ
Short-Form McGill Pain Questionnaire
SFN
small-fiber neuropathy
SFr-TMS
slow-frequency repetitive transcranial magnetic stimulation
SGPG
sulfated glucuronyl paragloboside
shadowing
acoustical s.
shadow plaque
shaft
dendritic s.
shagreen
s. patch
s. spot
shaken baby syndrome
shaken-impact syndrome
shaking palsy
sham block
sham-movement vertigo
shampoo
chlorhexidine s.
shank clipping
Shannon bur
shape
s. analysis
dendritic s.
nuclear s.
s. property
Shapiro-Wilk test
sharing
Edwards modular system load s.
Sharplan
S. laser
S. Ultra ultrasonic aspirator
sharp wave
sharp-wave complex
shaving cramp
Shaw
S. aneurysm needle
S. catheter
SHBG
sex hormone-binding globulin
Shealy theory
shear
s. fracture
s. stress
shearing
s. force
s. injury
shear-strain deformation
sheath
arachnoid s.
Avanti s.
axillary s.
carotid s.
dural s.
femoral introducer s.
ganglionic cyst in synovial tendon s.
Henle s.
s. of Key and Retzius
lamellar s.
Mauthner s.
medullary s.
myelin s.
nerve s.
outer mesaxon of myelin s.
perivascular s.
sacral docking s.
s. of Schwann
threaded s.
s. tumor
Sheehan syndrome
sheet
beta-B-structure s.
beta-pleated s.
MacroPore s.
Sheffield
S. collimator helmet
S. gamma unit
Sheldon hemilaminectomy retractor
Sheldon-Spatz vertebral arteriogram needle
Sherrington
S. law
S. phenomenon
shh gene
SHI
second harmonic imaging
shield
design for vision side s.
Faraday s.
shielding
magnet s.

NOTES

shift
brain s.
chemical s.
fat/water chemical s.
field s.
frequency s.
gaze refixational s.
midline s.
s. of midline structure
phase s.
transmembrane ionic s.
s. work-related sleep disorder
s. work sleep disorder
shiga toxin
***Shigella dysenteriae* infection**
Shiley
S. catheter
S. catheter distention system
S. distention kit
Shiley-Infusaid pump
shim coil
shimmering light with aura
shingle
optical s.
shingles-related stroke
Shipley-Hartford Scale
Shirley drain
shivering thermogenesis
shock
anaphylactic s.
break s.
cardiogenic s.
deferred s.
delayed s.
delirious s.
hemorrhagic s.
hypovolemic s.
primary s.
reversible s.
septic s.
spinal s.
vasogenic s.
shocking sensation
short
s. association fiber
s. gyrus of insula
s. insular gyrus
s. inversion recovery imaging
S. Portable Mental Status Questionnaire
s. pulse repetition time/echo time image
s. pulse repetition time/short echo time
s. root of ciliary ganglion
s. segment spinal fusion
s. sleep (SS)
s. sleeper
s. tau inversion recovery
s. TI inversion recovery (STIR)
s. time inversion recovery
short-acting
s.-a. benzodiazepine
s.-a. block
s.-a. hypnotic agent
s.-a. local anesthetic
shortening
selective T2 s.
spine s.
T2 s.
Short-Form McGill Pain Questionnaire (SF-MPQ)
short-interval intracortical inhibition (SICI)
short-lasting
s.-l. unilateral neuralgiform headache with conjunctival injection and tearing
s.-l. unilateral neuralgiform pain
s.-l. unilateral neuralgiform pain with conjunctival injecting and tearing (SUNCT)
short-latency SSEP
short-tau inversion recovery MRI sequence
short-term
s.-t. bleeding
s.-t. declarative memory
s.-t. hypoxia
s.-t. insomnia
s.-t. memory task
s.-t. potentiation (STP)
s.-t. therapy
s.-t. treatment
s.-t. vasomotor tone
s.-t. visual memory
shot
fast low-angle s. (FLASH)
shotgun pellet
shoulder
s. jerking
s. shrugging
shoulder-girdle
s.-g. neuritis
s.-g. syndrome
shoulder-hand syndrome
shrapnel wound
shrinkage
neuronal s.
tumor s.
shrinking retrograde amnesia
shrugging
shoulder s.
SHS
Sayre head sling
sleep hypopnea syndrome
shuffling gait

shunt
Accura s.
artery-to-vein s.
s. assessment
AV s.
s. blockage
cerebrospinal fluid s.
cisternal-peritoneal s.
cisternal-pleural s.
CSF s.
cystoatrial s.
Delta valve in ventriculoperitoneal s.
Denver hydrocephalus s.
s. dependent
Diamond valve flow-regulating s.
differential pressure s.
Edwards/Barbaro syringo-peritoneal s.
extracranial s.
s. filter
Hakim-Cordis ventriculoperitoneal s.
Heyer-Schulte neurosurgical s.
intratumoral arteriovenous s.
Javid s.
left-to-right s.
lumbar arachnoid peritoneal s.
lumboatrial s.
lumboperitoneal s.
s. malfunction
s. nephritis
Ommaya ventriculoperitoneal s.
percutaneous thecoperitoneal s.
s. placement
portosystemic s.
posterior fossa-atrial s.
s. procedure
Pruitt-Inahara s.
Pudenz s.
pulmonary arteriovenous s.
Raimondi low-pressure s.
right-to-left s. (RLS)
Spetzler lumboperitoneal s.
spinal cord arteriovenous s.
subdural-pleural s.
subduroperitoneal s.
Sundt carotid s.
Sundt loop s.
syringoperitoneal s.
syringosubarachnoid s.
syrinx s.
s. tap
thecoperitoneal Pudenz-Schulte s.
Torkildsen s.
T-shaped Edwards-Barbaro syringeal s.
T-tube s.
valve-regulated s.
ventriculoatrial s.
ventriculocisternal s.
ventriculoperitoneal s.
ventriculopleural s.
ventriculovenous s.
VJ s.
VP s.
zero ICP ventricle s.

shunted hydrocephalus

shunting
lumbar-peritoneal s.
portosystemic s.
syringosubarachnoid s.
ventriculoamniotic s.
ventriculoperitoneal s.

shunt-related complication

Shy-Drager
S.-D. disease
S.-D. neuropathy
S.-D. syndrome (SDS)

SIADH
syndrome of inappropriate secretion of antidiuretic hormone

sialic
s. acid
s. acid storage disease

sialidase gene

sialidosis type I, II

sialocele

sialodochitis

sialorrhea

sialosis

sibling
discordant s.
s. recruitment

siboroxime
technetium-99m s.

Sicard syndrome

sicca
hypophysis s.
keratoconjunctivitis s.

SICI
short-interval intracortical inhibition

sick
s. building syndrome

NOTES

sick *(continued)*
s. headache
s. sinus syndrome
sickle
s. cell disease
s. cell trait
s. flap
s. hemoglobinopathy
sickness
acute African sleeping s.
acute mountain s. (AMS)
African sleeping s.
chronic African sleeping s.
decompression s.
decompressive s.
East African sleeping s.
S. Impact Profile (SIP)
Jamaican vomiting s.
laughing s.
motion s.
sleeping s.
West African sleeping s.
sidebent
extended, rotated, s. (ERS)
extended, rotated, s. left (ERSL)
extended, rotated, s. right (ERSR)
side-cutting cannula
1-sided chorea
side-glance
side-opening laminar hook
side-port flat-bottomed Ommaya reservoir
sideroblastic anemia
siderosis
superficial s.
side-to-end hypoglossal-facial nerve attachment
sidewise flexion
Siegert sign
Siemens
S. couch
S. Magnetom Harmony scanner
S. Neurostar digital subtraction angiographic system
S. Somatom Plus
S. Somatom Plus DCT system
S. Symphony 1.5-T scanner
S. Vision scanner
S. Vision system
Siemerling-Creutzfeldt disease
Siemerling nucleus
sighing dyspnea
sight blindness
sigma
sigma activity
sigmoid
s. sinus (SS)
s. sinus retraction
sigmoideus
sinus s.
sign
Abadie s.
alien hand s.
alien limb s.
anterior tibialis s.
anticus s.
Babinski s.
Baillarger s.
Bamberger s.
Bamberger-Pins-Ewart s.
Barré pyramidal s.
Bastian-Bruns s.
Battle s.
Bechterew s.
Beevor s.
Bell s.
Berger s.
Biernacki s.
Biot breathing s.
s. blindness
Bonhoeffer s.
Bonnet s.
Bouchet-Gsell s.
Bragard s.
brim s.
Brown-Séquard s.
Brudzinski s.
Bruns s.
buckling s.
Cantelli s.
cap s.
cardinal s.
Castellani-Low s.
Chaddock s.
Charcot s.
Chvostek s.
Chvostek-Weiss s.
clinical s.
cogwheel s.
Collier s.
contralateral s.
cotton-wool s.
coughing s.
cracked pot s.
cranial cracked pot s.
Crichton-Browne s.
crossed adductor s.
Crowe s.
Cupid's bow s.
Czarnecki s.
Dejerine s.
Demianoff s.
doll's eye s.
double fragment s.
Duchenne s.
Duckworth s.
early warning s.

empty delta s.
empty sella s.
empty triangle s.
Erb s.
Erben s.
Erb-Westphal s.
Escherich s.
external malleolar s.
extrapyramidal s. (EPS)
eyelash s.
facial s.
Fajersztajn crossed sciatic s.
false localizing s.
Falx s.
fan s.
flat tire s.
focal neurologic s.
focal neurological s.
focal sensorimotor s.
forearm s.
formication s.
Fränkel s.
Froment paper s.
Froment prehensile thumb s.
Goldstein toe s.
Goldthwait s.
Gordon s.
Gorlin s.
Gottron s.
Gowers s.
Graefe s.
Grasset s.
Grasset-Bychowski s.
Grasset-Gaussel-Hoover s.
Griesinger s.
Guilland s.
Gunn s.
Hahn s.
head impulse s.
Heilbronner s.
Hennebert s.
Hirschberg s.
Hitselberger s.
Hochsinger s.
Hoffmann s.
Holmes s.
Homans s.
Hoover s.
Horsley s.
Hoyt-Spencer s.
Huntington s.
Hutchinson s.
hyperkinesis s.
ipsilateral cerebellar s.
ipsilateral corticospinal tract s.
Jackson s.
Joffroy s.
jugular s.
Kernig s.
Kernohan s.
Kerr s.
Kleist s.
Klippel-Weil s.
Lasègue s.
leg s.
Legendre s.
Leichtenstern s.
Leri s.
Leser-Trélat s.
Lhermitte s.
Lichtheim s.
Linder s.
Livierato s.
local s.
Lust s.
Macewen s.
Magendie-Hertwig s.
Magnan s.
Mannkopf s.
Marcus Gunn s.
Marie-Foix s.
Marie quadrilateral s.
Marinesco s.
Masini s.
matchbox s.
Mayerson s.
medullary s.
Mendel-Bechterew s.
meningeal s.
mesencephalic s.
Minor s.
motor neuron s.
Myerson s.
neck s.
Negro s.
Néri s.
neurologic s.
Oppenheim s.
s. of orbicularis
orbicularis s.
Parinaud s.
Parkinson s.
Parrot s.
pathognomonic s.

NOTES

sign *(continued)*
Patrick s.
pearl-and-string s.
Pende s.
peroneal s.
Pfuhl s.
Phalen s.
Piltz s.
Piotrowski s.
pontine s.
Pool-Schlesinger s.
Prévost s.
procerus s.
pronation s.
pseudo-Graefe s.
pyramid s.
pyramidal tract s.
Queckenstedt s.
radialis s.
Radovici s.
Remak s.
reservoir s.
Revilliod s.
roll plane s.
Romberg s.
Rosenbach s.
Rossolimo s.
Ruggeri s.
Saenger s.
scarf s.
Schlesinger s.
Schultze s.
Schultze-Chvostek s.
scotty dog s.
Seeligmüller s.
Séguin s.
setting-sun s.
Siegert s.
Signorelli s.
Simon s.
soft s.
Souques s.
spine s.
Spurling s.
stairs s.
Stellwag s.
Stewart-Holmes s.
Straus s.
string s.
Strümpell s.
Summerskill s.
sunset s.
swinging flashlight s.
telltale s.
Theimich lip s.
Thomas s.
Throckmorton s.
tibialis s.
Tinel s.
toe s.
tram track s.
Trendelenburg s.
Trousseau s.
Turyn s.
Uhthoff s.
upper extremity pronator s.
upper extremity scarf s.
Vanzetti s.
von Graefe s.
Waddell s.
Wartenberg s.
Weber s.
Weiss s.
Wernicke s.
Westphal s.
Westphal-Erb s.
yaw plane s.

signal
s. analysis
anchorage-dependent s.
astrocytic s.
contralateral routing of s.
costimulatory s.
s. detection
electrical s.
feedback s. (FBS)
s. filtering
free induction s.
high-density transient s.
high-intensity s.
s. hyperintensity
increased s.
s. intensity curve
intracellular s.
leptin s.
s. loss
magnetic resonance s.
microembolic s.
neuronal s.
N-terminal s.
nuclear s.
s. processing
s. recognition particle (SRP)
repulsive axon guidance s.
s. strength
s. symptom
s. transducing receptor
s. transducing receptor component
s. transduction
s. transduction inhibitor
s. transduction pathway
vestibulospinal s.
s. void
s. voltage waveform

signaling
chemical s.
downstream s.
inside-out s.

outside-in s.
oxidative stress s.
signal-noise characteristic
signal-to-noise
s.-t.-n. ratio (SNR)
s.-t.-n. threshold
significant
s. displacement
s. range
s. subjective distortion
Signorelli sign
SIGSS
selective imaging and graphics for stereotactic surgery
Silapap
Children's S.
Silastic
S. catheter
S. device
S. sponge
S. stent
S. tube
S. wick
sildenafil
silence
electrical s.
electrocerebral s. (ECS)
silent
s. area
s. infarction
s. intracerebral hemorrhage
s. microembolism
s. period
s. stroke
silicone
s. balloon
Codman ventricular s.
s. implant
s. sponge
siliconosis
siliqua olivae
SilkTouch CO_2 laser scanner
SilverHawk
S. catheter
S. device
S. plaque excision system
Silverman placement of electrode
silver-silver chloride electrode
silver-staining nucleolar organizer region
simethicone
aluminum hydroxide with magnesium hydroxide and s.
simiae
Herpesvirus s.
simian
s. crease
s. fissure
s. hand
s. line
s. virus 40 (SV40)
similarities subtest
similarity
recall of s.'s
Simmerlin dystrophy
Simmer paralysis
Simmons
S. catheter
S. cervical spine fusion
S. method
S. plating system
Simon
S. sign
S. task
simple
s. absence
s. chorea
s. decompression
s. febrile seizure
s. hallucination
s. lobule
s. membranous limb of semicircular duct
s. partial seizure
s. partial status
s. primitive aura
s. reflex
s. skull fracture
simplex
crus membranaceum s.
herpes s.
lobulus s.
toxoplasmosis, other infections, rubella, cytomegalovirus, and herpes s. (TORCH)
Simpson
S. catheter
S. grade
S. grading
Simpson-Angus total score
simulation
conscious s.
simulator
BTE work s.
Tepper proprioceptor s.

NOTES

S

simultanagnosia, simultagnosia
simultaneous volume imaging
Simvastatin Survival Study
sincalide
sinciput, pl. **sincipita**
Sinemet CR
Sinequan
singe
main en s.
single
s. bur hole procedure
s. enhancing CT lesion
s. seizure
s. synostosis
single-agent oral strategy
single-dose radiosurgery
single-fiber
s.-f. electroencephalography (SFEMG)
s.-f. electromyography
s.-f. EMG (SFEMG)
single-fraction radiation
single-hook retractor
single-level
s.-l. decompressive laminectomy
s.-l. ligamentous instability
s.-l. spinal fusion
single-photon
s.-p. emission computed tomography (SPECT)
s.-p. emission CT scan
single-point mutation
single-rod construct
single-stage procedure
single-voxel
s.-v. magnetic resonance spectroscopy (SV-MRS)
s.-v. technique
sinica
Ephedra s.
sinistral
sinistrality
sinistrocerebral
sinistromanual
sinistropedal
sinking brain syndrome
sinodural angle
sinogenic meningitis
Sinografin
sinography
sinonasal
s. cavity
s. psammomatoid ossifying fibroma
sinovenous
s. occlusion
s. stroke
s. thrombosis
sinus
anterior intercavernous s.
s. arrest
s. bradycardia
Breschet s.
s. cavernosus
cavernous s.
cerebral s.
circular s.
s. circularis
confluence of s.
cranial dermal s.
dermal s.
dilated intercavernous s.
dural venous s.
s. of dura mater
endodermal s.
ethmoid s.
s. headache
Henle rhomboid s.
s. histiocytosis
inferior longitudinal s.
inferior petrosal s.
inferior sagittal s.
s. intercavernosus anterior
s. intercavernosus posterior
intercavernous s.
intracranial venous s.
lateral s.
marginal s.
s. marginalis
maxillary s.
nasal s.
s. nerve of Hering
neurodermal s.
occipital s.
s. occipitalis
occluded superior sagittal s.
s. occlusion
paranasal s.
parasinoidal s.
s. pericranii
petrosal s.
petrosquamosal s.
petrosquamous s.
s. petrosus inferior
s. petrosus superior
s. phlebitis
pilonidal s.
posterior intercavernous s.
s. rectus
s. reflex
rhomboidal s.
s. rhomboidalis
Ridley s.
sagittal s.
s. sagittalis inferior
s. sagittalis superior
sigmoid s. (SS)
s. sigmoideus
space of cavernous s.

sphenoid s.
sphenoidal s.
sphenoparietal s.
s. sphenoparietalis
sphenotemporal s.
spinal dermal s.
s. squeeze
straight s.
subarachnoidal s.
superior longitudinal s.
superior petrosal s. (SPS)
superior sagittal s.
tentorial s.
thrombosis of venous s.
transverse s. (TS)
s. transversus durae matris
s. vein thrombosis
s. venosi duralis
venous dural s.

sinusitis with headache
sinusoidal
sinuum
confluens s.

sinuvertebral nerve
SIP
Sickness Impact Profile

siphon effect
SIS
Stroke Impact Scale

site
binding s.
bone graft harvest s.
dopamine uptake s.
entry s.
enzymatic binding s.
exit s.
graft s.
HealosMP52-treated fusion s.
high-affinity binding s.
hook s.
uptake s.

sitting
s. balance
s. position

situ
carcinoma in s.

situation
s. neurosis
social s.

situational
s. neurosis
s. stress reaction
s. tic variation
s. variable

situation-related epilepsy
sixth
s. cranial nerve [CN VI]
s. cranial nerve palsy
s. sense
s. ventricle

size
aneurysm s.
effect s.
fiber s.
internal architecture neuronal s.
neuronal s.
optimal group s.
pupil s.

sizer-dissector
Mizuho aneurysm s.-d.

sizing clamp
SjO_2
jugular bulb oxyhemoglobin saturation monitoring

Sjogren-Larsson syndrome
Sjögren syndrome
Sjöqvist tractotomy
skein
choroid s.

Skelaxin
skeletal
s. amyloidosis
s. deformity
s. maturation
s. muscle
s. muscle injury

skeletally immature patient
Skelite
OsteoStim S.

skill
abstraction s.
ambulation s.
basic s.
Canadian Test of Cognitive S.'s
Clinical Observations of Motor and Postural S.'s
communication s.
graphomotor s.
improved communication s.
intact reading s.
perceptual motor s.
perspective-taking s.
physical s.
problem-solving s.

NOTES

skill *(continued)*
spatial conceptualization s.
visuoconstructive s.
visuomotor problem-solving s.
visuoperceptual s.
visuospatial s.
vocabulary s.
skilled finger movement
skin
s. breakdown
s. conductance response
s. depth
s. flap
glabrous s.
glossy s.
s. graft harvesting pain
s. incision
s. reflex
s. surface pinprick
skin-muscle reflex
skin-pupillary reflex
skip lesion
SK-N-SH cell
Skoog release of Dupuytren contracture
skull
s. base
s. base foramina
s. base malignancy
s. base surgery
s. bone graft
cloverleaf s.
s. fracture
lacunar s.
maplike s.
s. plate
s. punch
steeple s.
tower s.
s. transillumination
skullcap
Skytron bed
slant
antimongoloid s.
slap
foot s.
SLE
systemic lupus erythematosus
sleep
active s.
s. activity
American Association for the Psychophysiological Study of S.
anteroposterior hypothalamic s.
anticonvulsant effect on s.
s. apnea
s. apnea subtype
s. apnea syndrome (SAS)
s. architecture
s. attack
autonomic change in s.
benign epileptiform transients of s. (BETS)
brain areas generating s.
brain region for s.
s. breathing
s. bruxism
s. bruxism episode
cardiovascular effect of s.
s. center referral
s. characteristic
s. chewer
components of s.
continuous spike and wave during s.
core s.
crescendo s.
curtailed s.
s. cycle
daily living activities affecting s.
decreased need for s.
s. deficit
delta s.
s. deprivation (SD)
desynchronized s.
s. diary
s. disorder associated with mental disorder
s. disorder facility
disorder of initiation and maintenance of s.
s. disorder service
s. disruption
s. dissociation
s. disturbance
s. disturbance associated with mania
s. disturbance in major depression
disturbed s.
s. and dream alteration
dreaming s.
s. drive
s. drunkenness
Dysfunctional Beliefs and Attitudes about S. (DBAS)
s. efficiency
electrical status epilepticus of s.
electrical status epilepticus during slow s.
electrotherapeutic s.
s. epilepsy
erratic s.
s. feature
s. fragmentation
fragmentation of nocturnal s.
function of s.
s. hallucination
S. Heart Health Study
s. history

s. hygiene
s. hygiene abnormality
s. hyperhidrosis
s. hypopnea syndrome (SHS)
s. hypoventilation syndrome
s. inertia
infant REM s.
s. initiation insomnia
insufficient s.
s. latency
light s.
s. log
long s. (LS)
maintaining s.
s. maintenance insomnia
medication effect on s.
s. montage
s. myoclonus
need for s.
neurobiology of s.
neuromodulation of s.
neurotransmitter of s.
newborn s.
nocturnal s.
nonrapid eye movement s.
non-REM s.
normal s.
s. onset period (SOP)
orthodox s.
overconcern with s.
paradoxical s.
s. paralysis
paroxysmal s.
periodic limb movement during s. (PLMS)
s. period time
pharmacology of s.
s. phase delay syndrome
phylogeny of s.
s. position indicator (SPI)
positive occipital sharp transients of s. (POSTS)
s. problem
prolonged nocturnal s.
s. psychogenic disorder
s. quality
s. questionnaire
quiet s.
rapid eye movement s.
recovery s.
S. Research Society
s. restriction
s. restriction therapy
S s.
secondary periodic leg movement of s.
seizure in s.
short s. (SS)
slow sharp spike of s. (SSSS)
slow-wave s. (SWS)
s. spindle
stage s.
stage 1–4 s.
s. stage 1–4
s. staging
s. starts
s. state
s. state misperception
supine s.
synchronized s.
s. talking
s. technique
s. terror disorder
S. Timing Questionnaire (STQ)
waveform of s.

sleep-awake
s.-a. activity inventory
s.-a. cycle

sleep-deprived EEG

sleep-disordered breathing

sleeper
long s.
short s.

sleep-generating center

sleep-induced apnea

sleepiness
s. consequence
s. countermeasure
daytime s.
determining s.
diurnal s.
excessive daytime s. (EDS)
measuring s.
medication-related s.
pathological s.
problem s.

sleeping sickness

sleeplessness
s. analysis
s. associated with acute emotional conflicts or reaction
s. associated with conditional arousal

NOTES

sleeplessness *(continued)*
s. associated with intermittent emotional conflicts or reaction
daytime consequences of s.
evaluating s.
s. log
psychometric testing of s.
sleep-onset
s.-o. association disorder
s.-o. rapid eye movement
s.-o. rapid eye movement period (SOREMP)
sleep-related
s.-r. abnormal swallowing
s.-r. asthma
s.-r. breathing disorder (SRBD)
s.-r. condition
s.-r. epilepsy
s.-r. gastroesophageal reflux
s.-r. headache
s.-r. oxygenation
s.-r. painful erection
s.-r. respiratory disturbance
s.-r. respiratory dysregulation
s.-r. ventilation
sleep-starts disorder
sleep-state misconception
sleeptalking disorder
sleep-wake
S.-W. Activity Inventory (SWAI)
s.-w. cycle
s.-w. cyclicity
s.-w. oscillator
s.-w. pattern
s.-w. rhythm
s.-w. rhythmicity
s.-w. schedule
s.-w. schedule disturbance
s.-w. transition disorder
sleepwalker
sleepwalking
anticholinergic for s.
sleepy patient
sleeve
s. adapter
arachnoid s.
arachnoidal root s.
s. graft
polyethylene s.
slender
s. fasciculus
s. lobule
SLEV
St. Louis encephalitis virus
slice
corticostriatal s.
digital subtraction venous angiography s.
3-dimensional s.
s. fracture
hippocampal s.
organotypic brain s.
s. selection
s. thickness
slice-select encoding gradient
slide
Superfrost microscope s.
Slimline clip
Slim-LOC anterior cervical plate system
sling
clip-reinforced cotton s.
fascia lata s.
Sayre head s. (SHS)
static s.
slipped disc
slipping clutch syndrome
slit
s. hemorrhage
s. valve
s. ventricle
s. ventricle syndrome
slit-lamp examination
SLN
superior laryngeal nerve
slope
gradient s.
sacral s.
Slosson
slot fracture
slotted
s. hammer
s. suction tip
slow
s. axonal transport
s. channel syndrome
s. component neuropathy
s. double taper
s. eye movement (SEM)
s. lateral eye movement
s. metabolizer patient
s. rolling eye movement
s. sharp spike of sleep (SSSS)
s. tongue movement
s. virus infection
slowed mentation
slow-frequency
s.-f. repetitive transcranial magnetic stimulation (SFr-TMS)
s.-f. wave
slow-growing
s.-g. neoplasm
s.-g. tumor
slowing
age-dependent s.
cognitive s.
diffuse bilateral s.
focal s.
frontotemporal s.

generalized s.
intermittent focal s.
motor s.
motoric s.
physiologic s.
postictal s.
psychomotor s.
saccadic s.
temporal s.

slowness
psychic s.

slow-wave
s.-w. abnormality
s.-w. activity (SWA)
s.-w. complex
s.-w. generation
s.-w. sleep (SWS)
s.-w. stupor

Sluder
S. neuralgia
S. syndrome

slug gene

Sluijter-Mehta
S.-M. SMK-C10 cannula
S.-M. thermocouple electrode

slurred speech

Sly
S. disease
S. syndrome

SMA
spinal muscular atrophy type 1–4
supplementary motor area

small
s. bowel carcinoid tumor
s. cell carcinoma
s. centrum ovale infarction
s. deep recent infarction
s. heat shock protein
s. intensely fluorescent cell
s. lacunar infarction
s. motor unit potential
s. penetrator infarction (SPI)
s. sciatic nerve
s. sharp spike
s. vessel disease
s. vessel infarction

small-angle double-incidence angiogram

small-fiber
s.-f. dysfunction
s.-f. neuropathy (SFN)

smallpox vaccination complication

small-step gait

small-volume correction (SVC)

smear
acid-fast bacilli s.
fungal s.
Tzanck s.

smell
s. blindness
s. brain
s. disorder
s. identification
s. identification test
nerve of s.
organ of s.

smell-brain

Smellie scissors

SMHSQ
St. Mary's Hospital Sleep Questionnaire

smile
Duchenne s.
non-Duchenne s.
spontaneous s.

Smiley-Williams arteriogram needle

Smith
S. air craniotome
S. Extrapyramidal Scale
S. nerve root suction retractor

Smith-Lemli-Opitz syndrome

Smith-Magenis syndrome

Smith-Petersen laminectomy rongeur

Smith-Robinson
S.-R. approach
S.-R. operation
S.-R. procedure
S.-R. technique

Smithwick
S. button hook
S. dissector
S. ganglion hook
S. sympathectomy
S. sympathectomy hook

SMN
SMN gene
SMN system

smoker
former s.

smoker's stroke

smoking
cigarette s.
s. habit

smoking-related reduction

NOTES

SMON
subacute myeloopticoneuropathy
smooth
s. endoplasmic reticulum
s. muscle
s. muscle proliferation
s. muscle tumor
s. pursuit
s. pursuit defect
s. pursuit eye movement
smooth-bordered cystic mass
SN
substantia nigra
SNAP
sensory nerve action potential
SNAP amplitude
SNAP on electromyogram
snap finger
snapping reflex
snapshot
cross-sectional s.
snarl
myasthenia s.
SNc
substantia nigra pars compacta
SNE
subacute necrotizing encephalomyelopathy
Sneddon syndrome
Snellen reflex
sniffing strength
sniff test
snore
s. guard
S. Guard mandibular repositioning device
SnoreSat sleep recorder
snoring
primary s.
snout reflex
snowshoe hare virus
SNP
sodium nitroprusside
SNR
selective nerve root
signal-to-noise ratio
sNr
substantia nigra pars reticulata
SNSRs
sensory neuron-specific G protein-coupled receptor
snuffbox
anatomical s.
soaked
s. fat plug
s. muscle plug
Soaker catheter
soapsuds cyst
SOC
social
s. activity
s. cognition
s. disinterest
s. impairment
s. intelligence
s. interaction
S. and Occupational Functioning Scale
s. situation
s. therapy
s. toxicity
s. viscosity
socially stigmatizing utterance
societal force
Society
American Epilepsy S.
American Pain S.
American Thoracic S.
Behavior Therapy and Research S.
European Sleep Research S.
International Headache S. (IHS)
Latin American Sleep S.
S. for Light Therapy and Biological Rhythms
Movement Disorder S.
National Multiple Sclerosis S. (NMSS)
S. for Quantitative Analyses of Behavior
Sleep Research S.
World Federation of Neurosurgical S.'s (WFNS)
Socon spinal system
SOD
superoxide dismutase
sodium
s. acetate
s. aminobenzoate
s. amytal
s. ascorbate
s. bicarbonate
s. bromide
s. channel 5A mutation
s. channel beta subunit
s. channel disorder
s. chloride
danaparoid s.
dantrolene s.
divalproex s.
s. dodecyl sulfate (SDS)
s. dodecyl sulfate-polyacrylamide gel electrophoresis
extended phenytoin s.
high s.
s. imbalance
indigotin disulfonate s.
ioxaglate s.
s. lactate

liothyronine s.
lipophilic s.
methotrexate s.
Nembutal S.
s. nitroprusside (SNP)
s. oxybate
s. oxylate
s. phosphate
photofrin porfimer s.
s. salicylate
serum s.
technetium-99m pertechnetate s.
thiopental s.
s. thiosalicylate
s. thiosulfate

sodium-potassium ATPase
sodium-responsive periodic paralysis
sodium-water retention
Soemmerring
S. ganglion
S. spot
SOF
superior orbital fissure
Sofamor-Danek stealth system
Sofamor spinal instrument device
Sof-Rol dressing
soft
s. disc herniation
s. line
s. palate retraction
s. psychotic-like phenomenon
s. sign
s. sign in neurologic examination
s. tissue abnormality
s. tissue contrast
s. tissue dissection
s. tissue injury
s. tissue stretching
softening
s. of brain
hemorrhagic s.
piriform s.
red s.
white s.
yellow s.
soft/spongy endplate
software
BrainVoyager s.
3-dimensional postprocessing s.
Sof-Wick dressing
Sofwire spinal fixation
soiling
fecal s.
Sokoda complex
solar
s. ganglion
s. plexus
sole
s. nucleus
s. plate
s. tap reflex
solenoid coil
sole-plate ending
solid
s. fusion
s. gray velocity trace
solid-phase extraction (SPE)
solid-state
s.-s. coagulator
s.-s. instrument
solitarii
nuclei s.
nuclei tractus s.
solitariospinalis
tractus s.
solitariospinal tract
solitarius
fasciculus s.
funiculus s.
nucleus s.
tractus s.
solitary
s. aggressive-type conduct disorder
s. bundle
s. extranodal lymphoma
s. fasciculus
s. fibrous tumor
s. hydatid cyst
s. neurofibroma
s. tract
solium
Taenia s.
Solomon-Bloembergen equation
Solstice balloon
SolTab
Remeron S.
soluble specific substance (SSS)
solute transport
solution
ferumoxide injectable s.
Formula EM oral s.
Hanks buffered saline s.

NOTES

S

solution *(continued)*
hydroxyethyl methacrylate polymerizing s.
image-guided s.
major s.
Namenda oral s.
volumetric s. (VS)
Zenker s.
solution-focused therapy
solvent
organic s.
solving
frontal lobe abstraction/problem s.
rational problem s.
Somanetics
S. INVOS 3100 cerebral oximeter
S. INVOS cerebral oximeter device
SomaSensor device
somata
neuronal s.
somatagnosia agnosia
somatalgia
somatesthesia, somesthesia
somatesthetic area
somatic
s. afferent fiber
s. block
s. category
s. depression
s. efferent fiber
s. muscle
s. nerve
s. nerve fiber
s. nervous system
s. neurofiber
s. neurologic manifestation
s. pain
s. problem
s. sense
s. skeletal muscle
somaticae
neurofibrae s.
Somatics monitoring electrode
somatization disorder
somatizing
somatochrome
somatodendritic excitability
somatoform
s. disorder
s. pain
s. vertigo
somatognosis
somatointestinal reflex
somatomotor
s. component
s. neuron
s. nucleus
somatosensory
s. area
s. aura
s. component
s. cortex
s. cued task
s. dysfunction
s. evoked magnetic
s. evoked potential (SSEP)
s. evoked potential monitoring
s. evoked response (SER)
s. homunculus
s. map
s. mapping
s. plasticity
s. sensitivity
somatostatin
somatotopic
somatotopographic reorganization
somatotopy
somatotroph
s. cell
s. hyperplasia
somatotropin
somatotypology
somesthesia (*var. of* somatesthesia)
somesthetic
s. area
s. cortex
s. dysarthria
s. neuron
s. relay nucleus
s. system
SOMI
sternooccipital-mandibular immobilization
SOMI Jr. brace
somite
embryonic cervical s.
sommeil
tic de s.
Sommer
hypoxia-susceptible sector of S.
somnambulance (*var. of* somnambulism)
somnambulant
somnambulate
somnambulic epilepsy
somnambulism, somnambulance
somnambulist
somniloquy
somnocinematograph
somnofluoroscopy
somnolence
daytime s.
disorders of excessive s. (DOES)
excessive daytime s.
s. syndrome
treatment-emergent s.
somnolency
somnolent
somnolentia

somnoplasty
Sonata
Songer
S. cable
S. cable system
sonic stereometry
Sonneberg neurectomy
Sonocut ultrasonic aspirator
sonography
color-flow Doppler s.
Doppler s.
TCD s.
transcranial color-coded duplex s.
transcranial color-coded real-time s.
sonomotor response
Sonopuls 190
SonoWand
S. intraoperative imaging system
S. ultrasound-based neuronavigation system
SOP
sleep onset period
Sophy
S. adjustable pressure valve
S. mini programmable pressure valve
sopor
soporific
soporose, soporous
SOREMP
sleep-onset rapid eye movement period
soreness
muscle s.
sotalol
Sotos syndrome
sound
coconut s.
contralateral routing of s.
s. memory
pulse synchronous s.
sound-sensitive seizure
Souques
S. phenomenon
S. sign
source
Arclite light s.
calorigenic s.
embolic s.
external s.
s. image
interstitial radiation s.
Maxenon 300-watt xenon light s.
Maxillume 250-watt quartz halogen light s.
Minimax 200-watt light s.
spike s.
Zeiss Super Lux 40 light s.
201-source
201-s. cobalt-60 gamma knife
201-s. cobalt-60 gamma unit
South African tick-bite fever
Southern blot
Southwestern immunohistochemistry
SP
sacroposterior
space
anterior cavernous sinus s.
arachnoid s.
brain s.
s. of cavernous sinus
s. context
craniospinal s.
dead s.
detail response to small white s.
disc s.
dorsal subcutaneous s.
enclosed s.
epicerebral s.
epidural s.
epispinal s.
extracellular s.
extradural s.
frontal interhemispheric s.
His perivascular s.
incisural s.
intercrural s.
intermeningeal s.
interpeduncular s.
Magendie s.
Malacarne s.
Marie quadrilateral s.
Meckel s.
oropharyngeal airway s.
parasinoidal s.
perforated s.
perineuronal s.
perioptic subarachnoid s.
perivascular s.
retropharyngeal s.
Schwalbe s.
s. sense
subarachnoid s.
subdural s.
subepicranial s.

NOTES

space *(continued)*
subgaleal s.
synaptic s.
Talairach s.
Tarin s.
Virchow-Robin s.
***k*-space**
space-form blindness
space-occupying brain lesion
spacer
Allograft s.
ceramic vertebral s.
methylmethacrylate s.
OsteoStim cervical allograft s.
telescopic plate s.
SPAMM
spatial modulation of magnetization
span
auditory s.
life s.
liver s.
murine life s.
spanning
transmembrane s.
SPAR
Spastic Paraplegia, Ataxia, Mental Retardation
sparing
macular s.
sacral s.
spark-gap instrument
spasm
affect s.
athetoid s.
Bell s.
canine s.
carpopedal s.
cervical muscle s.
clonic s.
convergence s.
cryptogenic hemifacial s.
cynic s.
dancing s.
dystonic s.
epileptic s.
facial habit s.
fixed s.
functional s.
habit s.
head s.
hemifacial s. (HFS)
infantile s.
intention s.
jackknife s.
lightning attacks in infantile s.
lock s.
malleatory s.
massive s.
masticatory s.
mimic s.
mixed s.
mobile s.
muscle s.
myopathic s.
near reflex s.
nictitating s.
nodding s.
occupational s.
paraplegic s.
phonatory s.
phonic s.
progressive torsion s.
reflex s.
Romberg s.
rotatory s.
salaam s.
saltatoric s.
saltatory s.
sewing s.
spasmogenic s.
spasmophile s.
synclonic s.
tailor's s.
tetanic s.
s.'s and tics
tonic s.
tonicoclonic s.
torsion s.
toxic s.
vascular s.
vasomotor s.
winking s.
spasmodic
s. apoplexy
s. diathesis
s. mydriasis
s. tic
s. torticollis
spasmodica
dysarthria syllabaris s.
tabes s.
spasmogen
spasmogenic spasm
spasmology
spasmolygmus
spasmolysis
spasmolytic
spasmophile spasm
spasmophilia
spasmophilic diathesis
spasmus
s. agitans
s. caninus
s. coordinatus
s. mutans nystagmus
s. nictitans
s. nutans

spastic
s. abasia
s. aphonia
s. ataxia
s. bulbar palsy
s. cerebral palsy
s. diplegia
s. dysarthria
s. dystonia
s. equinus foot
s. gait
s. hemiparesis
s. hemiplegia
s. hyperreflexia
s. miosis
s. monoplegia
s. mydriasis
s. paraparesis
s. paraplegia
S. Paraplegia, Ataxia, Mental Retardation (SPAR)
s. paresis
s. quadriparesis
s. quadriplegia
s. rigidity
s. spinal paralysis
s. triplegia
spastica
dysphonia s.
torticollis s.
spasticity
Ashworth score of muscle s.
clasp-knife s.
sphincter s.
s. vertical suspension test
spatia (*pl. of* spatium)
spatial
s. agraphia
s. bias
s. conceptualization
s. conceptualization skill
s. frequency
s. frequency grating
s. homogeneity
s. localization
s. memory
s. modulation of magnetization (SPAMM)
s. neglect
s. organization
s. orientation
s. perception
s. planning
s. response
s. span backward (SSB)
s. span forward (SSF)
s. span test
spatial-temporal context
spatiotemporal
s. brain mapping
s. source analysis
spatium, pl. **spatia**
s. epidurale
s. extradurale
s. leptomeningeum
s. peridurale
s. subarachnoideum
s. subdurale
spatula
brain s.
Children's Hospital brain s.
curved-tipped s.
Cushing brain s.
Davis brain s.
Davis nerve s.
D'Errico brain s.
s. dissector
double-vector brain s.
duck-billed anodized s.
House-Fisch dural s.
Jacobson endarterectomy s.
Mayfield brain s.
Olivecrona brain s.
Peyton brain s.
Rainin clip-bending s.
Ray brain s.
rectangular brain s.
Rhoton s.
Sachs nerve s.
Scoville brain s.
S-shaped brain s.
tapered brain s.
SPE
solid-phase extraction
speaking
sudden difficulty s.
Spearman
S. correlation coefficient
S. 2-factor theory
S. rank correlation coefficient test
S. rho
spear tackler's spine
special
s. sensation

NOTES

special *(continued)*
s. sense
s. somatic afferent (SSA)
s. somatic afferent column
s. visceral efferent column
s. visceral efferent nucleus
s. visceral motor nucleus
species
allopatric s.
reactive oxygen s. (ROS)
specific
s. absorption rate
s. curve
s. effect
s. irritability
s. sensory cue
s. symptom
s. system
specificity
criterion of s.
neuronal s.
specimen
flash-frozen tumor s.
s. staining
tumor s.
speckle
laser s.
SPECT
single-photon emission computed tomography
SPECT analysis
dual-isotope SPECT
high-resolution brain SPECT
SPECT image
SPECT scan
^{99m}Tc HMPAO SPECT
^{201}Tl SPECT
spectra (*pl. of* spectrum)
spectral
s. analysis
s. density
s. density function
s. edge frequency (SEF)
s. peak frequency of activity
s. velocity
spectrometer
mass s.
spectrometry
gas chromatography mass s.
spectrophotometer
Hitachi s.
spectrophotometric assay
spectrophotometry
reflectance s.
spectropolarimeter
Jasco S.
spectroscopy
Fourier s.
laser Doppler s.
magnetic resonance s. (MRS)
MR s.
near-infrared s. (NIRS)
phosphorus nuclear magnetic resonance s.
point-resolved s. (PRESS)
proton magnetic resonance s.
proton nuclear magnetic resonance s.
single-voxel magnetic resonance s. (SV-MRS)
in vivo 1H magnetic resonance s.
in vivo optical s. (INVOS)
s. voxel
spectrum, pl. **spectra**
autism s.
s. disorder
Doppler frequency s.
fortification s.
impulsive s.
proton s.
in vitro spectra
speculum
bivalved s.
Cushing-Landolt s.
Halle nasal s.
Hardy bivalve s.
Killian septum s.
Landolt pituitary s.
transsphenoidal s.
speech
absent s.
s. apraxia
aprosody of s.
s. aprosody
s. arrest
s. center
cerebellar s.
cluttering in s.
comprehensible s.
s. developmental disorder
digressed s.
s. discrimination test
disorganized s.
s. disturbance
s. dyspraxia
echo s.
ejaculatory s.
emotional s.
excessive s.
explosive s.
external s.
fluent s.
s. hallucination
ictal s.
increased s.
s. and language cluttering
monotonous s.
s. and motor mapping

narrative s.
s. pattern
s. perception
s. perception region
s. perception system
poverty of s.
pressure of s.
s. processing
s. processing alteration
s. processing impairment
pseudobulbar s.
rate of s.
s. reception threshold
s. recognition threshold
scanning s.
slurred s.
staccato s.
s. structure
s. stuttering
subvocal s.
syllabic s.
telegraphic s.
s. tracking
s. tracking alteration
s. tracking task
unintelligible s.
unstoppable flow of s.

Speech-Sounds Perception Test

speed
s. of conduction
gait s.
mental s.
s. of processing
psychomotor s.
reaction s.

speed-dependent treadmill training (STT)

SpeedReducer instrument

spelencephaly

spell
akinetic drop s.
apnea-like s.
breath-holding s.
intractable paroxysmal s.
neonatal breath-holding s.
nocturnal s.
staring s.

Spemann organizer

Spence
S. intervertebral disc rongeur
rule of S.

Spencer
S. biopsy forceps
S. probe depth electrode

Spens syndrome

spermatic
s. nerve
s. plexus

spes phthisica

Spetzler
S. lumboperitoneal shunt
S. system
S. titanium aneurysm clip

Spetzler-Martin
S.-M. classification
S.-M. classification of arteriovenous malformation
S.-M. grade
S.-M. grade III medium-size lesion with deep venous drainage
S.-M. grade II small lesion with deep venous drainage
S.-M. grading scale
S.-M. grading system

SpF-PLUS spinal fusion stimulator

SpF spinal fusion stimulator

SpF-XL stimulator

SPGR sequence

S-phase fraction

sphenocavernous syndrome

sphenoethmoidal
s. encephalocele
s. meningoencephalocele
s. recess

sphenoethmoidectomy

sphenoid
s. encephalocele
s. mucocele
s. ridge meningioma
s. rostrum
s. sinus
s. wing
s. wing dysplasia
s. wing meningioma

sphenoidal
s. electrode
s. electrode insertion
s. encephalocele
s. fossa
s. herniation
s. sinus

sphenoidale
planum s.

NOTES

sphenoidectomy
sphenoiditis
sphenoidostomy
sphenoidotomy
sphenomaxillary
s. encephalocele
s. ganglion
sphenooccipitalis
fissura s.
sphenoorbital
s. encephalocele
s. meningioma
s. meningoencephalocele
sphenopalatine
s. ganglion
s. ganglionectomy
s. nerve
s. neuralgia
s. test
sphenoparietalis
sinus s.
sphenoparietal sinus
sphenopharyngeal meningoencephalocele
sphenotemporal sinus
sphere
infrared light-reflecting s.
oriented in all s.'s
spheresthesia
spherical
s. bur
s. coordinate representation
s. nucleus
s. recess
spheroid
axonal s.
s. body myopathy
spherule
sphincter
anal s.
s. ani nerve
s. control
s. disturbance
s. dysfunction
s. electromyography
s. spasticity
s. tone
urinary s.
sphincteric disturbance
sphingolipid
s. metabolism disorder
semisynthetic s.
sphingolipidosis
cerebral s.
sphingomyelinase
sphingomyelin lipidosis
sphingosine
Sphrintzen syndrome
SPI
sleep position indicator
small penetrator infarction
spicule
spider cell
Spiegelberg
S. epidural balloon
S. intracranial pressure monitoring system
Spiegel-Wycis human apparatus
Spielmeyer acute swelling
Spielmeyer-Sjögren disease
Spielmeyer-Vogt disease
Spielmeyer-Vogt-Sjögren disease
Spigelius lobe
spike
anterior temporal focal s.
benign childhood epilepsy with centrotemporal s.
benign partial epilepsy with centrotemporal s. (BPECTS)
chasing s.
s. detection
s. discharge
s. frequency
6-hertz s.
high-voltage centrotemporal s.
injury s.
interictal epileptiform s.
middle temporal focal s.
peak absorption s.
s. potential
preexcision s.
rolandic benign epilepsy of childhood with centrotemporal s.
small sharp s.
s. source
train of s.'s
wicket s.
spike-and-wave
s.-a.-w. activity
s.-a.-w. complex
s.-a.-w. electroencephalographic discharge
s.-a.-w. pattern
s.-a.-w. trait
spike-initiation zone
spikelike artifact
spike-wave
s.-w. complex
s.-w. discharge
spiking activity
Spiller-Frazier
S.-F. neurotomy
S.-F. technique
spin
s. density
s. echo
Iso-C s.

s. magnetization
nuclear s.
s. velocity

spina, pl. **spinae**
s. bifida
s. bifida anterior
s. bifida aperta
s. bifida cystica
s. bifida dysraphism
s. bifida manifesta
s. bifida myelomeningocele
s. bifida occulta
s. bifida posterior
s. dorsalis

spinal
s. accessory nerve
s. accessory nerve-facial nerve anastomosis
s. accessory palsy
s. anesthesia
s. angiography
s. apoplexy
s. arachnoid
s. arachnoid mater
s. arteriography
s. ataxia
s. automatism
s. axis
s. blastomycosis
s. canal
s. canal compromise
s. canal encroachment
s. canal hydatid cyst
s. canal penetration
s. catheter
s. column
s. column stability
s. cord
s. cord abscess
s. cord angioma
s. cord arachnoid cyst
s. cord arachnoiditis
s. cord arteriovenous malformation
s. cord arteriovenous shunt
s. cord arteritis
s. cord artery
s. cord blood flow
s. cord blood supply
s. cord cavitation
s. cord compression
s. cord concussion
s. cord contusion
s. cord disease
s. cord disorder
s. cord function
s. cord function intraoperative monitoring
s. cord glioma
s. cord gray matter
s. cord hemisection
s. cord hemorrhage
s. cord infarction
s. cord infection
s. cord inflammation
s. cord injury (SCI)
s. cord injury trauma
s. cord injury without radiographic abnormality (SCIWORA)
s. cord lateral horn
s. cord lesion
S. Cord Motor Index and Sensory Indices
s. cord neoplasm
s. cord pain
s. cord parenchyma
s. cord reticular formation
s. cord segmentation in embryonic development
s. cord stimulation
s. cord terminal cone
s. cord terminal ventricle
s. cord tissue
s. cord tumor
s. cord tumor with lymphoma
s. cord ventral horn
s. cord ventricular funiculus
s. cord white matter blood flow
s. coronal plane deformity
s. decompression
s. deformity/instability
s. deformity treatment
s. dermal sinus
s. dermal sinus tract
s. disc degeneration
s. disc prosthesis
s. disc replacement
s. distraction instrument
s. drainage
s. dural arteriovenous fistula (SDAVF)
s. dysraphism
s. embolism
s. endodermal cyst
s. ependymoma

NOTES

S

spinal *(continued)*
s. epidural abscess
s. epidural angiolipoma
s. epidural empyema
s. epidural hematoma (SEH)
s. epidural hemorrhage
s. evaluation myelography
s. extradural arachnoid pouch
s. fixation
s. fixation rigidity
s. fluid
s. fluid analysis
s. fusion
s. fusion gouge
s. fusion pathomechanics
s. fusion technique
s. growth
s. hemangioblastoma
s. hemangioma
s. hemianesthesia
s. hemiplegia
s. herniation
s. immobilization
s. implant design
s. implant load to failure
s. injury operative stabilization
s. instability
s. instrumentation
s. intradural schwannoma
s. lamina II
s. lemniscus
s. level
s. lipoma
s. loading
s. load rate
s. mass lesion
s. maturation
s. mechanics
s. meningitis
s. meningocele
s. metastasis
s. metastatic disease
s. monosynaptic reflex
s. muscular atrophy type 1–4 (SMA)
s. needle
s. nerve level motor impairment
s. nerve plexus
s. nerve root
s. nerve root filament
s. neurenteric cyst
s. neurofibroma
s. nucleus of accessory nerve
s. nucleus of trigeminal nerve
s. nucleus of trigeminus
s. osteomyelitis
s. osteotomy stabilization
s. pachymeningitis
s. paralysis
s. paralytic poliomyelitis
s. perforating forceps
s. pia mater
s. puncture
s. puncture headache
s. pyramidotomy
s. range of motion (SROM)
s. reflex arc
s. rod
s. rod cross-bracing
s. saw
s. screw and rod system
s. segmental myoclonus
s. segment motion
s. sensory evoked potential
s. shock
s. stenosis
s. stroke
s. subarachnoid block
s. subarachnoid hemorrhage
s. subdural hemorrhage
s. synovial cyst
s. syphilis
s. tap
s. teratoma
s. tractotomy
s. tract of trigeminal nerve
s. trigeminal nucleus
s. tuberculosis
s. wind-up

SpinaLase neodymium:yytrium-aluminum-garnet surgical laser system

spinale
filum s.
tache s.

spinales
nervi s.
nucleus posteromedialis medullae s.
radices s.

spinalis
apex cornus dorsalis medullae s.
apex cornus posterioris medullae s.
arachnoidea mater s.
basis cornus dorsalis medullae s.
basis cornus posterioris medullae s.
cervix cornus dorsalis medullae s.
cervix cornus posterioris medullae s.
chorda s.
columna anterior medullae s.
columna dorsalis medullae s.
columnae griseae medullae s.
columna intermedia medullae s.
columna intermediolateralis medullae s.
columna posterior medullae s.
columna ventralis medullae s.
commissura alba anterior medullae s.

commissura alba posterior medullae s.
commissura grisea anterior medullae s.
commissura grisea anterior/posterior medullae s.
commissura grisea posterior medullae s.
commotio s.
cornu anterius medullae s.
cornu dorsalis medullae s.
cornu laterale medullae s.
cornu posterius medullae s.
cornu ventrale medullae s.
dura mater s.
fasciculus gracilis medullae s.
fasciculus proprius anterior medullae s.
fasciculus proprius dorsalis medullae s.
fasciculus proprius lateralis medullae s.
fasciculus proprius posterior medullae s.
fila radicularia nervi s.
filum durae matris s.
fissura mediana anterior medullae s.
fissura mediana ventralis medullae s.
formatio reticularis medullae s.
funiculi medullae s.
funiculus ventralis medullae s.
ganglion sensorium nervi s.
hydrocele s.
lamina s. II
lemniscus s.
medulla s.
meningitis serous s.
nucleus accessorius columnae anterioris medullae s.
nucleus anterolateralis medullae s.
nucleus centralis medullae s.
nucleus dorsolateralis medullae s.
nucleus dorsomedialis medullae s.
nucleus intermediomedialis medullae s.
nucleus phrenicus columnae anterioris medullae s.
nucleus posterolateralis medullae s.
nucleus retroposterolateralis medulla s.
nucleus ventrolateralis medullae s.
nucleus ventromedialis medullae s.
pars cervicalis medullae s.
pars coccygea medullae s.
pars lumbalis medullae s.
pars sacralis medullae s.
pars thoracica medullae s.
pia mater s.
radix anterior nervi s.
radix dorsalis nervi s.
radix motoria nervi s.
radix posterior nervi s.
radix sensoria nervi s.
radix ventralis nervi s.
ramus albus nevi s.
ramus anterior nervi s.
ramus communicans albus nervi s.
ramus communicans griseus nervi s.
ramus dorsalis nervi s.
ramus meningeus nervi s.
ramus posterior nervi s.
ramus recurrens nervi s.
ramus ventralis nervi s.
segmentum cervicalia medullae s.
segmentum coccygea medullae s.
segmentum lumbalia medullae s.
segmentum medullae s.
segmentum sacralia medullae s.
segmentum thoracica medullae s.
septum medianum dorsale medullae s.
septum medianum posterius medullae s.
substantia alba medullae s.
substantia gelatinosa centralis medullae s.
substantia gelatinosa cornu posterioris medullae s.
substantia grisea medullae s.
substantia intermedia centralis medullae s.
sulcus dorsolateralis medullae s.
sulcus intermedius dorsalis medullae s.
sulcus intermedius posterior medullae s.
sulcus medianus dorsalis medullae s.
sulcus medianus posterior medullae s.
sulcus posterolateralis medullae s.

NOTES

spinalis *(continued)*
sulcus ventrolateralis medullae s.
tabes s.
theca medullare s.
truncus nervi s.
ventriculus terminalis medullae s.
spinalium
ansae nervorum s.
plexus nervorum s.
rami communicantes nervorum s.
spinally elicited peripheral nerve response (SEPNR)
SpinaLogic bone growth stimulator
Spinal-Stim Lite
spin-density sequence
spindle
alpha s.
s. cell
s. cell tumor
s. coma
EEG alpha s.
Kühne s.
muscle s.
neuromuscular s. (NMS)
neurotendinous s.
sleep s.
tendon s.
spindle-shaped cyst
spine
bamboo s.
s. biomechanics
caroticojugular s.
cervical s.
CID Picture S.
cleft s.
dendritic s.
developing s.
dorsal s.
fused s.
Henle s.
human cadaveric s.
internal fixation of s.
kinetic cervical s.
laminectomized s.
s. load
lower cervical s.
lower lumbar s.
lower thoracic s.
nonfused s.
osteoporotic s.
poker s.
s. precaution
sacral s.
sacrococcygeal s.
s. shortening
s. sign
spear tackler's s.
suprameatal s.
thoracic s.
thoracolumbar s.
s. tuberculosis
tumor metastatic to s.
upper thoracic s.
variable screw placement system-instrumented lumbar s.
young s.
SpineCATH
spin-echo
s.-e. imaging
long pulse repetition time/long echo time s.-e.
s.-e. T1-weighted plan image
SpineLink-II independent intrasegmental spine fixation system
SpineLink system
SpineScope
Clarus S.
SpineStat probe
spinifugal
spinipetal
spin-lattice
s.-l. relaxation
s.-l. relaxation time
spinoadductor reflex
spinobulbar
spinocerebellar
s. ataxia (SCA)
s. ataxia 1–7
s. ataxia gene encoding types 1–7 (*SCA1–7*)
s. degeneration (SCD)
s. tract
spinocerebellum
spinocervicalis
tractus s.
spinocervical tract
spinocervicothalamic tract
spinocollicular
spinocortical
spinocranial meningioma
spinocuneatae
fibrae s.
spinocuneate fiber
spinogalvanization
spinogracile fiber
spinograciles
fibrae s.
spinography
digitized s.
spinohypothalamicae
fibrae s.
spinohypothalamic fiber
spinolamellar line
spinomesencephalicae
fibrae s.
spinomesencephalic fiber
spinomuscular paralysis

spinoolivares
fibrae s.
spinoolivaris
tractus s.
spinoolivary
s. fiber
s. tract
spinopelvic
s. transiliac fixation (STIF)
s. transiliac fixation technique
spinoperiaqueductales
fibrae s.
spinoperiaqueductal fiber
spinopetal
spinopontine degeneration
spinoreticular
s. fiber
s. tract
spinoreticulares
fibrae s.
spinospinalis tract
spinosum
foramen s. (FS)
spinosus
nervus s.
spinotectal
s. fiber
s. tract
spinotectales
fibrae s.
spinotectalis
tractus s.
spinothalamic
s. cordotomy
s. fiber
s. relay
s. tract
s. tractotomy
spinothalamicus
tractus s.
spinous
s. interlaminar line
s. process
s. process fracture
s. process plate
s. process-splitting laminoplasty
s. process wire
s. process wiring
spinovestibularis
tractus s.
spinovestibular tract
spin-spin
s.-s. coupling
s.-s. relaxation
s.-s. relaxation time
spin-warp
s.-w. imaging
s.-w. pulse sequence
spiny neuron
spiral
Archimedes s.
s. cochlear ganglion
S. Flute cranioblade
s. foraminous tract
s. ganglion of cochlea
s. membrane
s. organ
Perroncito s.
spirale
organum s.
spiramycin
spirochetal
s. aneurysm
s. infection
spirochete
spirohydantoin
spirometry
spiromustine
spironolactone
hydrochlorothiazide and s.
Spitz-Holter shunt system
Spitzka
S. marginal tract
S. marginal zone
S. nucleus
Spitzka-Lissauer
S.-L. column
S.-L. tract
SPL
superior parietal lobule
splanchnesthesia
splanchnesthetic sensibility
splanchnic
s. anesthesia
s. circulation
s. ganglion
s. motor component
s. nerve
s. sensory component
splanchnicectomy
splanchnici
ganglion nevi s.
splanchnicotomy

NOTES

splanchnicum
ganglion thoracicum s.
splaying
facet joint s.
splenial
s. artery
s. gyrus
splenicus
plexus s.
splenium
callosal s.
s. corporis callosi
s. of corpus callosum
s. tissue
splenius
s. capitis
s. cervicis
splenomegaly
splicing
exon s.
s. mutation
splinter hemorrhage
split
s. bone graft reconstruction
s. brain
s. calvarial graft
s. notochord syndrome
palatal s.
vermian s.
split-brain syndrome
split-cord malformation
split-half reliability
split-thickness calvarial graft
SPM
statistical parametric map
SPMS
secondary progressive multiple sclerosis
spoiled
s. gradient echo
s. gradient echo sequence
spoiling
radiofrequency s.
spoken
s. language disorder
s. language impairment
spondylalgia
spondylarthritis
spondylectomy
en bloc s.
spondylitica
psoriasis s.
spondylitic ridging
spondylitis
ankylosing s.
cryptococcal s.
s. deformans
Kümmell s.
rheumatoid s.
tuberculous s.
spondyloarthropathy
seronegative s.
s. syndrome
spondylodesis
ventral derotation s. (VDS)
spondylodiscitis
spondylolisthesis
degenerative s.
dysplastic s.
grade I–IV s.
high-grade s.
isthmic s.
pathologic s.
postlaminectomy 2-level s.
s. reduction
s. reduction fixation
symptomatic s.
traumatic s.
spondylolisthetic crisis
spondylolysis
spondylomalacia
spondylopathy
spondyloptosis
spondylopyosis
spondyloschisis
spondylosis
cervical s.
s. deformans
degenerative s.
degenerative lumbar s.
hyperostotic s.
lumbar s.
thoracolumbar s.
spondylosyndesis
spondylotic
s. caudal radiculopathy
s. headache
s. myelopathy
spondylotomy
sponge
absorbable gelatin s.
gelatin s.
Ivalon embolic s.
Ray-Tec s.
saline-soaked s.
Silastic s.
silicone s.
thrombin-soaked gelatin s.
sponge-holding forceps
spongiform
s. leukodystrophy
s. virus encephalopathy
spongioblast
spongioblastoma
polar s.
s. polare
unipolar s.
s. unipolare
spongiocyte

spongiosa
substantia s.
spongiosus
status s.
spongy
s. bone
s. degeneration
s. degeneration of cerebral white matter
s. degeneration of infancy
s. degeneration leukodystrophy
s. substance
spontaneous
s. activity
s. echo contrast
s. exacerbation
s. flexion
s. improvement
s. intracranial hypotension
s. nystagmus
s. occlusion of circle of Willis
s. panic attack
s. seizure
s. smile
s. spinal epidural hematoma (SSEH)
spoon
brain s.
Cushing brain spatula s.
Cushing pituitary s.
Hardy pituitary s.
pituitary s.
Ray brain spatula s.
sporadic
s. ALS
s. ataxia
s. chorea
s. Creutzfeldt-Jakob disease (sCJD)
s. depression
s. fatal insomnia prion protein gene
s. late-onset nemaline myopathy
s. nerve root involvement
Sporothrix schenckii
sports-related
s.-r. concussion
s.-r. spinal injury
spot
acoustic s.
ash-leaf s.
blind s.
Brushfield s.
café au lait s.
central direct-current bright s.
cherry-red s.
cotton-wool s.
Graefe s.
hot s.
hypnogenic s.
pain s.
Roth s.
saccular s.
shagreen s.
Soemmerring s.
temperature s.
Trousseau s.
utricular s.
warm s.
yellow s.
spotted fever
spray
air plasma s.
butorphanol tartrate nasal s.
dihydroergotamine mesylate nasal s.
Miacalcin Nasal S.
oxymetazoline nasal s.
sumatriptan nasal s.
Zomig nasal s.
spread
centripetal s.
spreader
Bailey rib s.
Blount laminar s.
Bobechko s.
Burford-Finochietto rib s.
Caspar disc space s.
Cloward cervical vertebra s.
Cloward lamina s.
Davis rib s.
DeBakey rib s.
Doyen rib s.
Favaloro-Morse sternal s.
Finochietto rib s.
Gerbode-Burford rib s.
Haight-Finochietto rib s.
Haight rib s.
Harken rib s.
Harrington s.
Inge cervical lamina s.
Inge laminectomy s.
lamina s.
Landolt s.
Lemmon sternal s.
Lilienthal rib s.

NOTES

spreader *(continued)*
Miltex rib s.
Morse sternal s.
Nelson rib s.
Rehbein rib s.
Rienhoff-Finochietto rib s.
Rienhoff rib s.
Texas Scottish Rite Hospital eyebolt s.
Tuffier rib s.
vertebra s.
Weinberg rib s.
Wilson rib s.
Wiltberger spinous process s.
spreading
s. cortical depression theory
s. depression
spring
coiled s.
compression s.
s. finger
Gruca-Weiss s.
internal fixation s.
s. mechanism
springing mydriasis
springlike phenomenon
spring-loaded electrode
Sprotte
S. epidural needle
S. spinal needle
sprouting
collateral nerve s.
hippocampal s.
mossy fiber s.
neuronal s.
regenerate nerve s.
sympathetic s.
synaptic s.
sprue peripheral neuropathy
SPS
superior petrosal sinus
spur
calcarine s.
Morand s.
traction s.
spurious
s. finding
s. meningocele
s. torticollis
Spurling
S. maneuver
S. nerve root retractor
S. sign
S. test
Spurling-Kerrison laminectomy rongeur
Spurr epoxy resin
squamous cell carcinoma
square-ended hook
square wave
square-wave jerk
squeeze
sinus s.
s. technique
SQUID
superconducting quantum interference device
SQUID array for reproductive assessment (SARA)
SR
sustained release
SRBD
sleep-related breathing disorder
Src inhibitor
SREDA
subclinical rhythmic EEG discharge of adults
SRF
sustained high-frequency repetitive firing
SROM
spinal range of motion
SRP
signal recognition particle
SRS
stereotactic radiosurgery
SRT
serial reaction time
substrate reduction therapy
SS
short sleep
sigmoid sinus
SSA
special somatic afferent
SSB
spatial span backward
SSC
superior semicircular canal
SSEH
spontaneous spinal epidural hematoma
SSEP
direct cortical stimulation and somatosensory evoked potential
somatosensory evoked potential
short-latency S.
SSF
spatial span forward
SSH
suppression subtractive hybridization
S-shaped brain spatula
SSI
segmental spinal instrumentation
anterior-posterior fusion with SSI
SSN
seesaw nystagmus
SSPE
subacute sclerosing panencephalitis
SSPT
steady-state probe topography

SS-QOL
Stroke Specific Quality of Life Measure
SSR
steady-state response
SSRI
selective serotonin reuptake inhibitor
SSRI-induced bruxism
SSS
soluble specific substance
SSSS
slow sharp spike of sleep
SST
stereotactic subcaudate tractotomy
St.
St. George Anxiety Questionnaire
St. John's Wort
St. Louis encephalitis
St. Louis encephalitis virus (SLEV)
St. Martin disease
St. Mary's Hospital Sleep Questionnaire (SMHSQ)
St. Paul-Ramsey Scale
STA
superficial temporal artery
Stab-and-Grab screwdriver
stability
axial compression s.
biomechanical s.
clinical s.
extension s.
flexion s.
lateral bending s.
long-term s.
lumbar spine rotational s.
mechanical s.
orthostatic s.
postural s.
spinal column s.
temporal s.
torsion s.
stabilization
anterior internal s.
anterior short-segment s.
s. approach
atlantoaxial s.
atlantooccipital s.
cervical spine s.
cervicothoracic junction s.
flexion-compression spine injury s.
fracture s.
iliac crest bone graft s.
lower cervical spine posterior s.
lumbar spine s.
mood s.
occipitocervical s.
odontoid fracture s.
operative s.
posterior lower cervical spine s.
reduction s.
sacral spine s.
screw s.
spinal injury operative s.
spinal osteotomy s.
subluxation s.
thoracolumbar spine s.
TSRH crosslink s.
wire s.
stable
s. alignment
s. cervical spine injury
s. fracture
s. vision
s. xenon CT
stab wound
staccato speech
stackable cage corpectomy
Staderini nucleus
stage
apoptotic s.
attritional s.
Braak s.
concrete operational s.
confrontation s.
delta activity s.
ideoplastic s.
initial s.
manipulation s.
postambivalent phase s.
preclinical s.
premonitory s.
s. sleep
s. 1–4 sleep
sleep s. 1–4
staged
s. bilateral stereotactic thalamotomy
s. embolization
s. surgical approach
2-stage procedure
staggering gait
staging
Braak & Braak s.
Braak neurofibrillary s.
Hoehn and Yahr Parkinson s.
infant sleep s.

S

NOTES

staging *(continued)*
neuraxis s.
sleep s.
stagnant hypoxia
Stagnara wake-up test
stain
acid-fast s.
CSF Gram s.
Elastica-Masson s.
Elastica-van Gieson s.
Elastica-Verhoeff s.
eosin s.
Fite s.
Gomori trichrome s.
Gordon and Sweet silver reticulin s.
Gram s.
Grocott s.
hematoxylin-eosin s.
Hortega neuroglia s.
Klüver-Barrera Luxol fast blue s.
Masson-Fontana s.
Masson trichrome s.
modified Bielschowsky silver s.
myelin tissue s.
periodic acid-Schiff-hematoxylin s.
Perls s.
port wine s.
reticulum s.
trichrome s.
Verhoeff-Van Gieson s.
staining
CD34 s.
Golgi s.
immunoperoxidase s.
modified Gomori trichrome s.
specimen s.
Sudan black s.
terminal deoxynucleotidyl transferase-mediated dUTP nick end-labeling s.
Weigert s.
stainless
s. steel equipment
s. steel implant
s. steel preformed skull plate
s. steel screw
staircase phenomenon
stairs sign
Stalevo
stalk
cerebral s.
s. effect
hypophysial s.
infundibular s.
neural s.
pineal s.
pituitary s.
s. of thalamus
STA-MCA
superficial temporal artery-middle cerebral artery
STA-MCA anastomosis
STA-MCA bypass
stammering of bladder
stamp test
stance
adultomorphic s.
walking s.
stand
Brown-Roberts-Wells floor s.
Contraves s.
Mayo s.
Yasargil OptiMat floor s.
standard
s. antipsychotic therapy
s. bone algorithm program
s. care
s. of care
s. dose
s. dose administration
s. error of mean (SEM)
s. kinetic model
s. laboratory test
s. rating procedure
s. retroperitoneal flank approach
s. retroperitoneal flank incision
s. score
s. thoracotomy
s. valve
s. Würzburg titanium mini-plating system
standardized
s. A scan
s. assessment
S. Assessment of Concussion
standing balance
Stanford
S. Acute Stress Reaction Questionnaire
S. Sleepiness Scale
stanozolol
STA-PCA
superficial temporal artery-posterior cerebral artery
STA-PCA bypass
stapedial
s. artery
s. nerve
stapedius
s. muscle fatigue
s. nerve
nervus s.
stapes
footplate of s.
s. reflex

staphylococcal
s. infection
s. meningitis
Staphylococcus
S. aureus
S. epidermidis
staphylococcus, pl. **staphylococci**
coagulase-negative s.
methicillin-resistant s.
staphyloma
staphyloplegia
star
s. array
optic disc edema with macular s.
stare
manic s.
motionless s.
postbasic s.
staring
s. spell
vacant s.
Starling
S. reflex
S. resistor model of upper airway
startle
s. disease
s. disorder
s. epilepsy
s. pathway
s. reaction
s. reaction/response
s. reflex
s. syndrome
starts
sleep s.
STA-SCA
superficial temporal artery-superior cerebellar artery
STA-SCA bypass
stasis
s. retinopathy
venous s.
state
absent s.
active s.
acute confusional s.
affective s.
s. of alertness
alpha s.
amnesic s.
anelectrotonic s.
apallic s.
appetitive s.
calm wakefulness s.
catelectrotonic s.
central excitatory s.
cognitive s.
confabulatory amnestic s.
confusional s.
convulsive s.
crepuscular s.
deafferented s.
decerebrate s.
decorticate s.
depressive mixed s.
dreamlike s.
dreamy s.
drug-induced hallucinatory s.
drug-induced paranoid s.
drug-induced semihypnotic s.
drug-like desire s.
dysphoric manic s.
elusive illness s.
entatic s.
epileptic clouded s.
epileptic twilight s.
explosive psychotic s.
s. factor
general mood s.
gradient-recalled acquisition in steady s. (GRASS)
homozygous s.
hyperadrenergic s.
hypercoagulable s.
hyperdopaminergic s.
hypnagogic s.
hypnoidal s.
hysterical fugue s.
hysteric coma-like s.
lacunar s.
local excitatory s.
Markov transition s.
migraine-free s.
s. of mindful relaxation
minimally conscious s.
mixed bipolar s.
mood s.
MS-like disease s.
negative myoclonus s.
neurotic anxiety s.
neurotic depressive s.
oxidation s.
paranoid s.
pathological mood s.

NOTES

state *(continued)*
permanent vegetative s.
persistent vegetative s. (PVS)
postictal s.
psychological s.
refractory s.
resting s.
seizure-free s.
senile paranoid s.
sequential gradient-recalled acquisition in the steady s.
sleep s.
subacute delirious s.
subacute irritable depressive s.
subcortical dysexecutive s.
trancelike s.
twilight s.
vegetative s.
visceral emotional s.
state-dependent
s.-d. measure
s.-d. psychopathology rating scale
state-of-the-art
s.-o.-t.-a. analysis
s.-o.-t.-a. analysis technique
state-trait interaction
static
s. acoustic impedance
s. allodynia
s. ataxia
s. convulsion
s. and dynamic sitting balance
s. and dynamic standing balance
s. hyperplasia
s. intervention
s. magnetic field
s. reflex
s. sense
s. sling
s. spastic quadriplegia
s. suspension
s. tremor
stationary visual stimulus
station test
statistical
s. artifact
s. parametric map (SPM)
statoacoustic
s. nerve
s. organ
statoacusticus
nervus s. [CN VIII]
statokinetic reflex
statotonic reflex
status
acute change in mental s.
altered mental s.
s. aura
s. choreicus
cognitive s.
complex partial s.
s. convulsivus
s. cribrosus
s. criticus
s. dysmyelinisatus
s. dysraphicus
s. epilepticus (SE)
functional s.
general cognitive s.
s. hemicranicus
s. hypnoticus
s. lacunaris
s. lacunosus
s. marmoratus
s. migraine
s. migrainosus
s. nervosus
nutritional s.
petit mal s.
pressure autoregulatory s.
proband s.
prognostic s.
psychomotor s.
s. raptus
simple partial s.
s. spongiosus
triad of altered mental s.
s. typhosus
s. vertiginosus
visuomotor s.
stauroplegia
staurosporine
stavudine
steady-state
s.-s. dose
s.-s. free precession
s.-s. method
s.-s. probe topography (SSPT)
s.-s. regimen
s.-s. response (SSR)
s.-s. visual evoked potential
steal
cerebral ischemia s.
s. effect
s. index
intracerebral s.
s. phenomenon
subclavian s.
vascular s.
Stealth Image Guided System
StealthStation
S. image-interactive system
S. system real-time guidance
S. treatment guidance platform
STEAM
stimulated echo acquisition mode
STEAM sequence
steam-shaping mandrel

steatosis
microvesicular s.
Stecher arachnoid knife
steel-containing bullet
Steele-Richardson-Olszewski
S.-R.-O. disease
S.-R.-O. syndrome
steep-dose gradient
steeple skull
Steffee
S. instrumentation
S. pedicle screw-plate system
S. plate
S. plating
Steinert
S. disease
S. myotonic dystrophy
Steinhauser cranial screw
Stein-Leventhal syndrome
Steinmann pin
stellate
s. astrocyte
s. cell of cerebral cortex
s. endplate fracture
s. ganglion
s. ganglion block
s. neuron
s. skull fracture
stellatum
ganglion s.
stellectomy
Stellwag sign
stem
s. cell-based remyelinating therapy
s. cell transplantation
infundibular s.
s. serotonergic cell
stem-completion test
stenogyria
stenosis, pl. **stenoses**
acquired spinal s.
aqueductal s.
asymptomatic carotid artery s.
canal s.
carotid artery s.
cervical spinal s.
foraminal s.
high-grade s.
lateral recess s.
lumbar spinal s.
spinal s.
stomal s.
thoracolumbar spinal canal s.
Stensen duct
stent
Acculink s.
Gianturco-Roubin II s.
Jostent graft s.
Memotherm s.
Neuroform s.
NIR Royal Advanced s.
Palmaz s.
Palmaz-Schatz s.
Silastic s.
Symbiot covered s.
Wallstent s.
stent-assisted carotid angioplasty
stenting
carotid artery s.
intracranial s.
vertebral origin angioplasty and s.
stent-supported coil embolization
stepdown connector
step fracture
Stephenson-Gibbs reference electrode
Stephen syndrome
steppage gait
stepping response
2-step procedure
stercoralis
Strongyloides s.
stereoadapter
Laitinen s.
stereoagnosis
stereoanesthesia
stereocognosy
stereoelectroencephalography (SEEG)
stereoencephalometry
stereoencephalotomy
stereognosis
stereoguide collimator
stereo-isomer
stereomagnification angiography
stereometry
sonic s.
stereoselective glomerulus
stereotactic, stereotaxic
s. anatomic target localization
s. angiography
s. anteroposterior and lateral metrizamide ventriculography
s. arc
s. atlas

NOTES

stereotactic *(continued)*
s. biopsy
s. biopsy exploration
s. brachytherapy
s. catheter drainage
s. cingulotomy
s. coordinate system
s. cordotomy
s. depth electroencephalogram (SDEEG)
s. depth electroencephalography (SDEEG)
s. frame
s. gamma radiation
s. gamma unit
s. guidance
s. guide
s. implantation
s. instrument
s. instrumentation
s. intracystic injection
s. intratumoral photodynamic therapy
s. irradiation
s. lesionectomy
s. linear accelerator
s. linear accelerator radiotherapy
s. microsurgical approach
s. microsurgical craniotomy
s. needle
s. needle aspiration
s. neurosurgery
s. operation
s. pallidotomy
s. PET image
s. puncture
s. radiation therapy treatment
s. radiosurgery (SRS)
s. retractor
s. robot
s. subcaudate tractotomy (SST)
s. surgery
s. surgical ablation
s. surgical guidance system
s. technique
s. thermocoagulation
s. tractotomy
s. VL thalamotomy
stereotactic-assisted
s.-a. radiation therapy
s.-a. radiation therapy kit
stereotactic-focused radiation therapy
stereotactic-guided craniotomy
stereotaxic (*var. of* stereotactic)
stereotaxis
image-guided s.
stereotaxy
frame s.
frameless s.
functional s.
volumetric s.
stereotyped
s. movement
s. movement disorder
stereotypic
s. movement
s. movement disorder
Steri-Dent dry heat sterilizer
sterile
s. abscess
s. meningitis
s. meningoencephalitis
sterilizer
Steri-Dent dry heat s.
Steripaque
Steripaque-BR
Steripaque-V
Steritek ICP mini monitor
sternal puncture
sternobrachial reflex
sternocleidomastoid (SCM)
branch to s.
s. muscle
s. muscle testing in spinal accessory nerve examination
s. muscle weakness
sternohyoid muscle
sternomastoid muscle
sternooccipital-mandibular immobilization (SOMI)
sternothyroid muscle
sternotomy
sternum-splitting approach
sternutatory
s. absence
s. reflex
steroid
s. dosage
s. hormone
insomnia with s.'s
lumbar epidural s.
s. protocol
s. sensitive
s. therapy
steroid-induced osteoporosis
steroid-sensitive neuropathy
stethoparalysis
stethospasm
Stevens-Johnson syndrome
Stewart-Holmes sign
Stewart-Morel syndrome
STGC
syncytiotrophoblastic giant cell
Stickler syndrome
sticky platelet syndrome
STIF
spinopelvic transiliac fixation
STIF technique

stiff-baby syndrome
stiffening
bilateral tonic s.
momentary s.
stiff-man syndrome
stiff neck
stiffness
axial s.
fusion s.
hemiparkinsonian s.
jaw s.
neck s.
torsional s.
stiff-person syndrome
stigma, pl. **stigmata**
medication s.
Stille bur
Stille-Luer rongeur
Stilling
S. column
S. fiber
S. fleece
S. gelatinous substance
S. nucleus
S. raphe
Stim neuromuscular stimulation system
Stimson dressing
stimulant
chimeric s.
dopaminergic s.
s. therapy
s. treatment
stimulant-dependent sleep disorder
stimulant-related seizure
stimulated
s. echo acquisition mode (STEAM)
s. spin-echo sequence
stimulating electrode
stimulation
abnormal response to sensory s.
antidromic s.
areal s.
audiovisual s.
audiovisual-tactile s.
brain s.
carotid baroceptor s.
click s.
Computer-Aided Neurovascular Analysis and S. (CANVAS)
condensation s.
s. condition
conditioned s.
cortical s.
cutaneous electrical s.
deep brain s. (DBS)
direct brain s.
discrete locus s.
dopamine s.
dorsal column s.
dorsal cord s.
electrical cortical s.
electromyogram-triggered neuromuscular s.
electrophysiological s.
EMG-triggered neuromuscular s.
emotional s.
epileptogenic s.
extraspinal nerve s.
fast-frequency repetitive transcranial magnetic s.
s. fatigability
fixed-dose s.
functional electrical s.
functional neuromuscular s.
galvanic vestibular s.
high-intensity click s.
intermittent photic s.
intraoperative electrical cortical s. (IOECS)
macro s.
macroelectrical s.
magnetoelectric s.
s. mapping
mesh glove s.
minimizing s.
neck s.
neuromuscular electrical s.
nociceptive s.
noninvasive carotid baroceptor s.
nonspecific s.
optokinetic s. (OKS)
paired-pulse transcranial magnetic s.
paradoxical s.
s. parameter
paraspecific s.
percutaneous s.
perivascular nerve-ending s.
s. PET study
photic s.
post hoc s.
postsynaptic s.
precipitation by photic s.
presynaptic s.
s. program in cerebral palsy

NOTES

stimulation *(continued)*
punctual s.
ramp s.
rarefaction s.
repetitive nerve s.
repetitive transcranial magnetic s. (rTMS)
sacral nerve s.
serotonin s.
slow-frequency repetitive transcranial magnetic s. (SFr-TMS)
spinal cord s.
STN s.
subthalamic nucleus deep brain s. (STN-DBS)
supramaximal rapid s.
supranormal s.
sympathetic s.
tactile s.
tetanic s.
thalamic s.
therapeutic electric s.
therapeutic electrical s.
thorax s.
threshold electrical s. (TES)
thyrotropin-releasing hormone s.
s. time
transcranial high-frequency repetitive electrical s.
transcranial magnet s. (TMS)
transcranial magnetic s.
transcutaneous electrical nerve s.
transfer direct current s.
trigeminal s.
vagal nerve s. (VNS)
vagus nerve s. (VNS)

stimulation-related adverse effect

stimulator
Axostim nerve s.
Caldwell high-speed magnetic s.
8-channel muscle s.
constant current s.
dorsal column s.
electronic s.
EMG s.
Grass s. S44
Hilger facial nerve s.
Intrel II spinal cord s.
magnetic s.
Magstim 200 s.
Magstim Rapid magnetic s.
Micro-Z neuromuscular s.
monopolar cathodal s.
nerve s.
Neurosign 100 constant current s.
Ojemann cortical s.
Orthofix Cervical-Stim s.
SpF-PLUS spinal fusion s.
SpF spinal fusion s.
SpF-XL s.
SpinaLogic bone growth s.
Toennis ES standalone constant-current electrical s.
vagus nerve s.

stimulatory effect

2-stimuli task

stimulus, pl. **stimuli**
adequate s.
ambiguous external s.
anxiogenic s.
anxiolytic s.
s. artifact
auditory s.
binocular flash s.
chemosensory s.
conditioned s. (CS)
costimulatory s.
deviant s.
discriminant s.
s. drive (SD)
s. duration
emotional s.
emotive s.
excitatory s.
external speech s.
heterologous s.
homologous s.
inadequate s.
ionic s.
irrelevant s.
liminal s.
maximal s.
Michotte visual s.
novel s.
patterned s.
pattern-reversal s.
perceptual emotive s.
pharmacological s.
phonetic s.
photic s.
precipitating s.
rarefaction s.
real-life s.
reinforcing s.
repetitive s.
selective focusing on environmental s.
stationary visual s.
subliminal s.
subthreshold s.
summation of s.
supraliminal s.
supramaximal s.
suprathreshold s.
tactile s.
taste s.
test s.
s. threshold

train-of-4 s.
unconditioned s.
s. word
stimulus-control therapy
3-stimulus paradigm
stimulus-response time
stimulus-sensitive myoclonus
stinger injury
STIR
short TI inversion recovery
STIR sequence
stiripentol
STM
supratentorial meningioma
STN
subthalamic nucleus
STN stimulation
STN-DBS
subthalamic nucleus deep brain stimulation
stochastic resonance
stock
bone s.
stocking
s. anesthesia
Orthawear antiembolism s.'s
Vairox high-compression vascular s.'s
stocking-glove
s.-g. anesthesia
s.-g. distribution
s.-g. sensory loss
Stoffel operation
stoichiometric change
stoker's cramp
Stokes-Adams
S.-A. attack
S.-A. disease
S.-A. syndrome
Stokes law
stoma blast
stomachal vertigo
stomal stenosis
stomodeum
Stookey
S. cranial rongeur
S. reflex
Stookey-Scarff operation
stooped posture
stop
unexpected gait s.
stopcock
Luer-Lok s.
stop-start technique
storage disease
store
cellular s.
high-energy cellular s.
storiform
s. pattern
s. whorl
Storz
S. Microsystem microplate
S. Microsystems cranial fixation plate
S. Microsystems drill bit
STP
short-term potentiation
STQ
Sleep Timing Questionnaire
strabismus
convergent s.
kinetic s.
Strachan syndrome
straight
s. aneurysm clip
s. cannula with locking dilator
s. connector
s. filament
s. gyrus
s. incision
s. knot-tying forceps
s. leg raising test
s. microscissors
s. needle
s. needle electrode
s. nerve hook
s. ring curette
s. sinus
straightening cannula
straight-in ventriculostomy
straight-line bayonet forceps
strain
alpha wave s.
s. birefringence
s. gauge
Lister s.
role s.
strand break
strangalesthesia
strap muscle
strategy
acceptance s.

NOTES

strategy *(continued)*
adjunctive s.
age-appropriate s.
antisense s.
candidate gene s.
coactive s.
combination s.
coping s.
dose reduction s.
genetic s.
loading s.
low-dose s.
memory retrieval s.
minimalist surgical s.
nonoperative s.
optimal treatment s.
rehabilitation s.
single-agent oral s.
therapeutic s.
treatment s.
visual representation s.
stratification
Davidoff age s.
population s.
post hoc s.
stratum, pl. **strata**
Strata adjustable Delta valve
s. album profundum
s. cerebrale retinae
s. cinereum colliculi superioris
s. ganglionare nervi optici
s. ganglionare retinae
s. ganglionicum
s. gangliosum cerebelli
s. granulare
s. granulosum corticis cerebelli
s. griseum intermedium
s. griseum intermedium colliculus superioris
s. griseum medium
s. griseum profundum
s. griseum profundum colliculi superioris
s. griseum superficiale
s. griseum superficiale colliculi superioris
strata gyri dentati
strata hippocampi
s. interolivare lemniscus
s. limitans externum
s. limitans internum
s. lucidum hippocampus
strata magnocellularia
s. medullare intermedium
s. medullare intermedium colliculi superioris
s. medullare profundum
s. medullare profundum colliculi superioris
s. moleculare
s. moleculare corticis cerebelli
s. moleculare et substratum lacunosum
s. moleculare hippocampus
s. moleculare retinae
s. multiforme
s. neuroepitheliale retinae
s. neurofibrarum
s. neuronorum piriformium
s. nucleare externum
s. nucleare externum et internum retinae
s. nucleare internum
strata nuclearia externa et interna retinae
s. opticum
s. opticum colliculi superioris
s. oriens
s. oriens hippocampus
outcome strata
strata parvocellularia
s. pigmenti bulbus
s. pigmenti retinae
s. plexiforme cerebelli
s. plexiforme externum
s. plexiforme externum et internum retinae
s. plexiforme internum
s. purkinjense corticis cerebelli
s. pyramidale
s. pyramidale hippocampus
s. radiatum
s. radiatum hippocampus
s. segmentorum externorum et internorum
s. zonale
s. zonale colliculi superioris
s. zonale thalami
Strauss-Carpenter scale
Straus sign
streak
angioid s.
fatty s.
meningitic s.
primitive s.
stream
dorsal s.
ventral s.
streaming
s. birefringence
intravascular s.
strength
axial gripping s.
bending s.
bone-screw interface s.
C-D instrumentation fixation s.
Cotrel pedicle screw fixation s.
field s.

human s.
masseter s.
motor s.
muscle s.
pedicle screw pullout s.
psychological s.
pullout s.
screw pullout s.
signal s.
sniffing s.
torsional gripping s.
s. training

strength-duration curve

streptococcal
s. infection
s. meningitis

Streptococcus
S. agalactiae
S. agalactiae meningitis
S. aureus meningitis
S. pneumoniae
S. pneumoniae meningitis
S. pyogenes
S. viridans

streptococcus
group A beta-hemolytic s.
group B s.
microaerophilic s.
pediatric autoimmune neuropsychiatric disorder associated with s. (PANDAS)
viridans s.

streptokinase

streptomycin

stress
acute foot shock s.
caregiver s.
heat s.
s. illness process
ischemic s.
major life s.
measured s.
oxidative s.
s. reaction
s. relaxation
shear s.
tensile s.
thermal s.
transient emotional s.
s. ulcer

stressed-induced iNOS

stressor
biological s.
cumulative s.
psychosocial s.

stress-strain relation

stretch
s. receptor
s. reflex
s. reflex pathway

stretching
polyglutamine s.
soft tissue s.
s. syncope

stria, pl. **striae**
acoustic s.
anterior acoustic s.
auditory s.
s. cochlearis anterior
s. cochlearis intermedia
s. cochlearis posterior
s. diagonalis
diagonalis s.
striae distensae
s. fornicis
Gennari s.
intermediate acoustic s.
s. of internal granular layer
s. of internal pyramidal layer
Kaes s.
Kaes-Bechterew s.
s. laminae granularis externae
s. laminae granularis internae
s. laminae molecularis
s. laminae plexiformis
s. laminae pyramidalis internae
striae lancisi
lateral longitudinal s.
lateral olfactory s.
s. longitudinalis lateralis
s. longitudinalis lateralis corporis callosi
s. longitudinalis medialis
s. longitudinalis medialis corporis callosi
medial longitudinal s.
medial olfactory s.
striae medullares
striae medullares acusticae
striae medullares fossae rhomboideae
striae medullares ventriculi quarti
s. medullaris

S

NOTES

stria *(continued)*
s. medullaris thalami
molecular layer s.
s. of molecular layer
nucleus of lateral olfactory s.
s. occipitalis
striae olfactoriae
s. olfactoria lateralis
s. olfactoria medialis
olfactory s.
posterior acoustic s.
tectal s.
s. tectum
terminal s.
s. terminalis
s. terminalis fiber
ventral acoustic s.
s. ventriculi tertii
striatae
venae s.
striatal
s. binding reduction
s. dopamine
s. dopaminergic abnormality
s. dopamine transporter density
s. hand
s. lesion
s. metabolism
s. neuron
s. receptor
s. target
s. toe
striate
s. area
s. body
s. cortex
s. hemorrhage
s. nucleus
s. vein
striated muscle
striati
cauda s.
lamina medullaris lateralis corporis s.
lamina medullaris medialis corporis s.
striation
striational autoantibody
striatocapsular infarction
striatofrontal
s. circuitry
s. dysfunction
striatonigral
s. degeneration
s. degeneration type
s. fiber
striatum
corpus s.
dorsal s.
s. dorsale
lateral medullary lamina of corpus s.
medial medullary lamina of corpus s.
vein of corpus s.
ventral s.
s. ventrale
striatus-orbitofrontal metabolism
stricture
clip-induced s.
stridor
nocturnal s.
3 strikes law
string
polyglutamine s.
s. sign
striocerebellar tremor
striomotor column
strionigral tract
striosome patch
strip
Ad-Tech electrode s.
motor s.
sensorimotor s.
stripe
s. area
s. of Gennari
occipital s.
Vicq d'Azyr s.
stripout
screw s.
stroboscope
stroboscopic light activating technique
stroke
acute s.
S. and the Alzheimer Disease and Related Disorders Association
anterior circulation s.
cardioembolic s.
caudal s.
completed s.
cryptogenic s.
S. Data Bank Neurologic Rush Alzheimer Registry Examination
developing s.
early-onset ischemic s.
embolic s.
s. in evolution
hemisphere s.
hemispheric s.
hemorrhagic s.
S. Impact Scale (SIS)
ipsilateral s.
ischemic s.
lacunar s.
late-onset ischemic s.
migraine-associated s.
migraine-induced s.

National Institute of Neurological and Communicative Disorders and S. (NINCDS)
National Institute of Neurological Disorders and S. (NINDS)
paralytic s.
peripartum s.
Postural Assessment Scale for S. (PASS)
progressing s.
s. prophylaxis
pure hemisensory s.
pure sensory s.
Randomized Trial of Tirilazad Mesylate in Patients With Acute S. (RANTTAS)
retinal s.
right brain s. (RBS)
s. risk
s. score
sensorimotor s.
shingles-related s.
silent s.
sinovenous s.
smoker's s.
S. Specific Quality of Life Measure (SS-QOL)
spinal s.
subinsular s.
s. subtype
s. syndrome
thalamic s.
The S. Council of The American Heart Association
thromboembolic s.
thrombotic s.

strokelike episode
stroke-related mortality
stroma, pl. **stromata**
s. ganglii
s. ganglionicum
nerve s.
tumor s.

Stromeyer cephalhematocele
Strong Vocational Interest Blank (SVIB)
Strongyloides stercoralis
strongyloidiasis
strontium-89
Stroop
S. Color-Word Interference Task
S. Color-Word Test

structural
s. abnormality
s. autosomal anomaly
s. brain lesion
s. change
s. family therapy
s. gene
s. intracranial disease
s. magnetic resonance imaging
s. malformation
s. MRI
s. neuroimaging

structure
alteration of memory s.
brain s.
brainstem s.
cerebral s.
cortical s.
craniofacial s.
cytoskeletal s.
dorsal stream s.
dysphoric character s.
hypoactive limbic s.
intraarachnoid neurovascular s.
ipsilateral mesial temporal s.
limbic system s.
medial temporal s.
mesencephalic premotor s.
mesial cerebral s.
nervous system s.
neural s.
neuronal s.
nucleoplasmic s.
shift of midline s.
speech s.
subcortical s.
uniform pore s.
vascular s.
white matter s.

Strully neurological scissors
Strümpell
S. disease
S. phenomenon
S. reflex
S. sign

Strümpell-Leichtenstern
S.-L. disease
S.-L. encephalitis

Strümpell-Lorrain disease
Strümpell-Marie disease
Strümpell-Westphal disease

NOTES

strut
allograft s.
corticocancellous s.
s. fusion technique
s. graft
s. grafting
miniplate s.
Struthers ligament
strychnine
lysergic acid diethylamide and s.
s. poisoning
Stryker
S. bed
S. drill
S. frame
STS
superior temporal sulcus
STT
speed-dependent treadmill training
Stuart-Power factor
Stuck laminectomy retractor
Student-Newman-Keuls test
study
AANS/CNS Joint Section Lumbar Disc Herniation S.
air contrast s.
antiphospholipid antibody in stroke s.
asymptomatic carotid atherosclerosis s.
audiologic s.
audiometric s.
autopsy-based neurochemical s.
autoradiographic s.
baseline s.
biochemical s.
biophysical s.
Brain Matters Stroke Initiative Edinburgh Artery S.
brain perfusion s.
brain potential s.
brain structure s.
Bronx Aging S.
cabergoline s.
Carotid Artery Stenosis with Asymptomatic Narrowing: Operation Versus Aspirin S.
CASANOVA S.
case s.
CBF s.
cerebral blood flow s.
chromosome s.
clinical comparison s.
clinicopathologic s.
cost-of-illness s.
crossover s.
cross-sectional s.
cytogenetic s.
double-blind drug s.
early treatment diabetic retinopathy s.
ECA s.
efficacy s.
electrodiagnostic s.
electroencephalogram s.
electrophysiologic s.
empirical s.
epidemiological s.
Epidemiological Catchment Area S.
event-related brain potential s.
experimental s.
first seizure s. (FIR.S.T.)
fluorodeoxyglucose PET s.
Framingham Eye S.
Framingham Heart S.
functional brain imaging s.
functional MRI s.
GenePD s.
Global Burden of Disease S.
histochemical s.
ICA-occluded stable Xe/CT CBF s.
imaging s.
immunohistochemical s.
indium-diethylene triamine pentaacetic acid s.
Isle of Wight S.
laboratory s.
Life Span S.
light microscopy s.
long-term naturalistic s.
Marcé s.
Mayo Asymptomatic Carotid Endarterectomy S.
metrizamide contrast s.
morphologic s.
motor nerve conduction s. (MNCS)
National Acute Spinal Cord Injury S.'s (NASCIS)
National Comorbidity S.
National Emergency X-Radiograph Utilization S. (NEXUS)
National Treatment Improvement Evaluation S.
naturalistic followup s.
nerve conduction s. (NCS)
nerve conduction velocity s.
neural crest tumor localization s.
neural imaging s.
neuroendocrine tumor localization s.
neuroimaging s.
New York Longitudinal S.
noninvasive brain imaging s.
nonphantom s.
Northern Manhattan Stroke S.
Olmsted County S.
Oregon Brain Aging S. (OBAS)
outcome s.

Parkinson Research The Organized Genetic Initiative s.
pathological s.
phenotypic s.
pheochromocytoma and neuroblastoma localization s.
placebo-controlled drug s.
polysomnographic s.
population-controlled s.
postmortem s.
pramipexole s.
PROGENI s.
radionuclide s.
RANTTAS s.
resting PET s.
ropinirole s.
Seattle Longitudinal S.
seroepidemiological s.
Simvastatin Survival S.
Sleep Heart Health S.
stimulation PET s.
time-motion s.
Tirilazad Efficacy Stroke S. (TESS)
transcatheter s.
ultrastructural s.
in vitro molecular s.
Wisconsin Sleep Cohort S.
XeCT CBF s.

stump
distal sympathetic s.
s. embolization syndrome
s. hallucination
nerve s.
s. neuralgia
s. neuroma

stupor
benign s.
catatonic s.
daytime s.
depressive s.
frank catatonic s.
idiopathic recurring s.
malignant s.
psychomotor s.
slow-wave s.

Sturge
S. disease
S. syndrome

Sturge-Kalischer-Weber syndrome

Sturge-Weber
S.-W. disease
S.-W. syndrome (SWS)

Sturge-Weber-Dimitri syndrome

stuttering
persistent developmental s.
speech s.

stylet, stylette
Frazier s.

styloglossus muscle

stylohyoid
s. muscle
s. nerve

stylomastoid foramen

stylopharyngeal nerve

stylopharyngeus muscle

styloradial reflex

stylus-type sensor wand

subacute
s. angle-closure glaucoma
s. cerebellar degeneration
s. cerebral infarction
s. combined degeneration
s. combined degeneration of spinal cord
s. delirious state
s. demyelinating neuropathy
s. hemorrhage
s. inclusion body encephalitis
s. irritable depressive state
s. measles encephalitis
s. meningitis
s. meningitis syndrome
s. myeloopticoneuropathy (SMON)
s. necrotic myelopathy
s. necrotizing encephalomyelitis
s. necrotizing encephalomyelopathy (SNE)
s. necrotizing myelitis
s. necrotizing myelopathy
s. periventricular necrotizing encephalopathy
s. polyneuropathy
s. psychoorganic syndrome
s. sclerosing leukoencephalitis
s. sclerosing leukoencephalopathy
s. sclerosing panencephalitis (SSPE)
s. spongiform encephalopathy

subarachnoid
s. block (SAB)
s. blood layer
s. bolt

NOTES

subarachnoid *(continued)*
s. cavity
s. cistern
s. cysticerci
s. drain
s. drainage
s. ependymal cyst
s. hemorrhage (SAH)
s. lipoma
s. screw
s. seeding
s. space
s. space metastasis
subarachnoidal
s. cistern
s. septum
s. sinus
subarachnoidea
cavitas s.
subarachnoideae
cisternae s.
subarachnoideales
cisternae s.
subarachnoideum
cavum s.
spatium s.
subcaeruleus nucleus
subcalcarine
subcallosa area s.
subcallosa
area s.
s. area subcalcarine
subcallosal
s. area
s. fasciculus
s. gyrus
s. layer
subcallosus
fasciculus s.
gyrus s.
subcapsular epithelium
subcaudate tractotomy
subcellular localization
subchondral sclerosis
subchoroidal approach
subclavia
ansa s.
subclavian
s. artery
s. loop
s. nerve
s. steal
s. steal syndrome
subclavius
s. nerve
nervus s.
plexus s.
subclinical
s. absence
s. depressive symptom
s. neck pain
s. neuropathy
s. range
s. rhythmic EEG discharge
s. rhythmic EEG discharge of adults (SREDA)
s. rhythmic epileptiform discharge of adult
s. seizure
s. status epilepticus induced by sleep in children
s. syndrome
subcoeruleus
nucleus s.
subcollateral gyrus
subcommissurale
organum s.
subcommissural organ
subconjunctival hemorrhage
subcoracoid-pectoralis minor tendon syndrome
subcortex
subcortical
s. arteriosclerotic encephalopathy
s. atrophy
s. band heterotopia
s. band heterotopia/double cortex
s. cerebrovascular disease
s. condition
s. deficit
s. disequilibrium
s. dysexecutive state
s. dysfunction model
s. ectopic cortex
s. encephalomalacia
s. gray matter
s. gray matter area
s. gray matter hyperintensity
s. gray region
s. hemorrhage
s. infarction
s. ischemic vascular dementia
s. laminar heterotopia
s. lesion
s. leukoencephalopathy
s. limbic nucleus
s. motor aphasia
s. nature
s. pathology
s. protoplasmic astrocytoma
s. sensory aphasia
s. small vessel disease
s. structure
s. syndrome
s. U fiber
s. vascular encephalopathy
subcortical/frontal lobe abnormality
subcorticalis chronica encephalitis

subcostal nerve
subcranial
subcuneiformis
nucleus s.
subcuneiform nucleus
subcutaneous
s. lipoma
s. nodule
s. pentylenetetrazol seizure test
s. sacrococcygeal myxopapillary ependymoma
subdelirium
subdental synchondrosis
subdermal plexus
subdivision
hippocampal formation s.
subdural
s. abscess
s. button
s. cavity
s. effusion
s. effusion with hydrocephalus
s. electrode array
s. electrode placement
s. electroencephalography
s. empyema
s. grid
s. grid electrode
s. grid implantation
s. grid monitoring
s. hematoma
s. hematorrhachis
s. hemorrhage
s. hygroma
s. ICP monitoring
s. meningioma
s. pressure screw
s. space
s. strip electrode
s. tap
s. tumor
subdurale
cavum s.
spatium s.
subdural-pleural shunt
subduroperitoneal shunt
subendocardial myocardial infarction
subendymal
subependymal
s. diffuse heterotopia
s. extension
s. giant cell astrocytoma
s. glomerate astrocytoma
s. hamartoma
s. hemorrhage
s. mixed glioma
s. tuber
s. tumor
subependymoma
subepicranial space
subepicranium
subfalcial herniation
subfalcine herniation
subfolium
subfornical organ
subfrontal
s. craniotomy
s. fissure
s. meningioma
s. transbasal approach
subgaleal
s. abscess
s. cerebrospinal fluid
s. drain
s. emphysema
s. hematoma
s. hemorrhage
s. space
subgenual cingulate region
subgrundation
subhyaloid hemorrhage
subhypoglossalis
nucleus s.
subhypoglossal nucleus
subicular region
subiculum, pl. **subicula**
s. cornu ammonis
s. hippocampus
s. promontorii
subinsular stroke
subintimal hemorrhage
subitum
exanthem s.
subjective
s. depression
s. distortion
s. effect
s. insomnia
s. memory decline
s. mood change
s. sensation
s. vertigo
s. vision
s. well-being

NOTES

sublabial
s. midline rhinoseptal approach
s. transseptal transsphenoidal approach
sublaminar
s. fixation
s. wire
s. wiring
sublenticular
s. limb of internal capsule
s. part of internal capsule
sublentiform limb of internal capsule
subligamentous disc herniation
subliminal stimulus
sublingual
s. ganglion
s. nerve
s. nucleus
sublinguale
ganglion s.
sublingualis
nervus s.
radix parasympathica ganglii s.
subluxation
atlantoaxial rotatory s.
cervical s.
degenerative s.
irreducible s.
recurrent s.
s. stabilization
unilateral interfacetal dislocation or s.
vertebral s.
submandibulare
ganglion s.
rami ganglionares nervi lingualis ad ganglion s.
ramus sympathicus ad ganglion s.
submandibular ganglion
submandibularis
radix parasympathica ganglii s.
radix sensoria ganglii s.
rami glandulares ganglii s.
submaxillary
s. ganglion
s. nerve
submucous intestinal plexus
subneural
s. apparatus
s. cleft
subnucleus
amygdala s.
s. caudalis
suboccipital
s. craniectomy
s. craniotomy
s. decompression
s. encephalocele
s. headache
s. nerve
s. neuralgia
s. neuritis
s. Ommaya reservoir
s. posterior fossa approach
s. transmeatal approach
suboccipitale
malum vertebrale s.
suboccipitalis
nervus s.
suboptimal
s. imaging
s. response
s. treatment
subparabrachialis
nucleus s.
subparabrachial nucleus
subparalytic
subparietalis
sulcus s.
subparietal sulcus
subperiosteal
s. corticotomy
s. cyst
s. dissection
s. hematoma
subpial transection
subplate zone
subplatysmal plane
subpopulation
neuronal s.
subretinal neovascularization
subsartorial plexus
subscale
ADAS noncognitive s.
Alzheimer Disease Assessment Scale-Cognition s.
Alzheimer disease noncognitive s.
nonturbulence s.
Progressive Alzheimer Disease Assessment Scale-cognitive s.
subscapulares
nervi s.
subscapular nerve
subsensitization of presynaptic receptors
subserosus
plexus s.
substance
s. abuse
anterior perforated s.
basophil s.
basophilic s.
black s.
central gray s.
central and lateral intermediate s.
chromophil s.
s. dependence
exophthalmos-producing s. (EPS)
gelatinous s.

gray s.
I s.
innominate s.
s. intoxication
lateral intermediate s.
medullary s.
neurosecretory s.
Nissl s.
s. P
periaqueductal gray s.
periventricular gray s.
posterior perforated s.
Reichert s.
reticular s.
Rolando gelatinous s.
schedule II s.
Schwann white s.
soluble specific s. (SSS)
spongy s.
Stilling gelatinous s.
tigroid s.
transmitter s.
vasoactive s.
white s.

substance-induced
s.-i. delirium
s.-i. organic mental disorder

substance-related syndrome

substantia, pl. **substantiae**
s. alba
s. alba medullae spinalis
basal s.
s. basalis
s. basophilia
s. cinerea
s. ferruginea
s. gelatinosa
s. gelatinosa centralis
s. gelatinosa centralis medullae spinalis
s. gelatinosa cornu posterioris medullae spinalis
s. gelatinosa Rolandi
s. grisea centralis
s. grisea medullae spinalis
s. innominata
s. innominata of Reichert
s. innominata of Reil
s. intermedia centralis
s. intermedia centralis et lateralis
s. intermedia centralis medullae spinalis
s. medullaris
s. nigra (SN)
s. nigra disorder
s. nigra pars compacta (SNc)
s. nigra pars reticulata (sNr)
s. perforata anterior
s. perforata interpeduncularis
s. perforata posterior
s. perforata rostralis
s. reticularis
s. spongiosa
s. trabecularis

substitute
Allomatrix bone s.
disc s.
human dural s.
OsteoStim resorbable bone graft s.

substituted benzamide

substitutive agent therapy

substrate
artificial blood s.
biologic s.
brain s.
extramuscular s.
neural s.
permissive s.
s. reduction therapy (SRT)
s. transport

subsultus
s. clonus
s. tendinum

subsynaptic web

subsyndromal
s. depression
s. mood symptom

subsystem
cognitive s.
parallel s.
visual s.

subtalar arthralgia

subtelomeric anomaly

subtemporal
s. basal approach
s. decompression
s. dissection
s. fissure
s. infratemporal approach
s. keyhole approach

subtentorial lesion

subtest
s. scale score
similarities s.

NOTES

subtetanic
subthalamic
s. fasciculus
s. nucleus (STN)
s. nucleus deep brain stimulation (STN-DBS)
s. tegmentum
subthalamicum
corpus s.
subthalamicus
fasciculus s.
nucleus s.
subthalamus
subtherapeutic dose
subthreshold stimulus
subtle
s. memory problem
s. seizure
s. structural abnormality
s. symptom
subtraction
s. imaging
s. technique
subtrapezius plexus
subtype
clinical s.
glutamate receptor s.
insomnia categories of s.'s
motor s.
sleep apnea s.
stroke s.
subungual fibroma
subunit
glutamide receptor s.
receptor s.
sodium channel beta s.
subventricular zone
subvocal speech
subwakefulness syndrome
succedaneum
caput s.
successive saccades
succimer
technetium-99m s.
succinate
chloramphenicol sodium s.
cortisol and sodium s.
frovatriptan s.
methylprednisolone and sodium s.
succinic
s. semialdehyde
s. semialdehyde dehydrogenase deficiency
succinylcholine
succulente
main s.
sucker
s. apparatus
s. foot
s. process
suck reflex
suction
s. cautery
s. dissection
Ferguson s.
Frazier s.
s. injury
s. ophthalmodynamometry
s. phenomenon
s. Regugauge regulator
s. tube
Sudan black staining
sudanophilic
s. cerebral sclerosis
s. leukodystrophy
sudden
s. confusion
s. difficulty speaking
s. difficulty walking
s. dizziness
s. infant death syndrome
s. loss of balance
s. loss of coordination
s. numbness
s. severe headache
s. unexplained death in epilepsy (SUDEP)
s. unexplained nocturnal death syndrome (SUNDS)
s. vision difficulty
s. weakness
sudden-onset headache
Sudeck
S. atrophy
S. syndrome
SUDEP
sudden unexplained death in epilepsy
sudomotor
s. component
s. fiber
s. nerve
sudorific center
Suetens-Gybels-Vandermeulen angiographic localizer
sufentanil citrate
suffocation hysterica
Sugita
S. aneurysm clip
S. cross-legged clip
S. fork
S. head clamp
S. headholder
S. multipurpose head frame
S. retractor
S. side-curved bayonet clip
S. temporary straight clip
S. Titanium

Sugita-Ikakogyo clip
suicidal depressed patient
sulbactam
sulcal
s. atrophy
s. enlargement
s. prefrontal cortex
sulci (*pl. of* sulcus)
sulcocommissural artery
sulcomarginalis
fasciculus s.
sulcomarginal tract
sulculus, pl. **sulculi**
pontopeduncular s.
sulcus, pl. **sulci**
anterior intermediate s.
anterior parolfactory s.
anterolateral s.
s. anterolateralis
s. anterolateralis medullae oblongatae
artery of central s.
artery of postcentral s.
artery of precentral s.
s. basilaris
s. basilaris pontis
basilar pontine s.
bulbopontine s.
s. bulbopontis
calcarine s.
s. calcarinus
callosal s.
callosomarginal s.
s. callosomarginalis
central cerebral s.
s. centralis
s. centralis cerebri
s. centralis insula
cerebellar s.
cerebral s.
sulci cerebrales
chiasmatic s.
s. chiasmaticus
s. chiasmatis
cingulate s.
s. cinguli
s. of cingulum
s. circularis insula
collateral s.
s. collateralis
s. corporis callosi
s. of corpus callosum
cortical s.
dorsal intermediate s.
dorsal median s.
dorsolateral s.
s. dorsolateralis medullae oblongatae
s. dorsolateralis medullae spinalis
s. effacement
fimbriodentate s.
s. fimbriodentatus
s. frontalis inferior
s. frontalis medius
s. frontalis superior
s. frontomarginalis
s. habenula
habenular s.
s. habenularis
hippocampal s.
s. hippocampalis
s. hippocampus
hypothalamic s.
s. hypothalamicus
inferior frontal s.
inferior temporal s.
sulci interlobares cerebri
s. intermedius anterior
s. intermedius dorsalis medullae spinalis
s. intermedius posterior
s. intermedius posterior medullae spinalis
interparietal s.
intragracile s.
s. intragracilis
intraparietal s.
s. intraparietalis
lateral cerebral s.
s. lateralis anterior
s. lateralis mesencephali
s. lateralis pedunculi cerebri
s. lateralis posterior
lateral occipital s.
s. limitans
s. limitans fossae rhomboideae
s. limitans of insula
s. limitans ventriculi quarti
limiting s.
lunate s.
s. lunatus
s. lunatus cerebri
marginal branch of cingulate s.
s. marginalis

S

NOTES

sulcus *(continued)*
s. medialis cruris cerebri
median frontal s.
s. medianus dorsalis medullae oblongatae
s. medianus dorsalis medullae spinalis
s. medianus posterior medullae oblongatae
s. medianus posterior medullae spinalis
s. medianus ventriculi quarti
medullopontine s.
middle frontal s.
middle temporal s.
Monro s.
s. nervi oculomotorii
s. nervi petrosi majoris
s. nervi petrosi minoris
s. occipitalis lateralis
s. occipitalis superior
s. occipitalis transversus
occipitotemporal s.
s. occipitotemporalis
oculomotor s.
s. oculomotorius
s. of oculomotor nerve
s. olfactorius
s. olfactorius lobi frontalis
olfactory s.
orbital s.
sulci orbitales
sulci orbitales lobi frontalis
paracentral s.
s. paracentralis
sulci paraolfactorii
parietooccipital s.
s. parietooccipitalis
s. parolfactorius anterior
s. parolfactorius posterior
parolfactory s.
polar s.
pontobulbar s.
pontomedullary s.
postcentral s.
s. postcentralis
postclival s.
posterior intermediate s.
posterior parolfactory s.
posterolateral s.
s. posterolateralis
s. posterolateralis medullae oblongatae
s. posterolateralis medullae spinalis
postnodular s.
postpyramidal s.
precentral s.
s. precentralis
prechiasmatic s.
s. prechiasmaticus
preclival s.
prepyramidal s.
prerolandic s.
Reil s.
rhinal s.
s. rhinalis
subparietal s.
s. subparietalis
superior frontal s.
superior occipital s.
superior temporal s. (STS)
suprasplenial s.
s. sylvii
sulci temporales transversi
s. temporalis inferior
s. temporalis medius
s. temporalis superior
s. temporalis transversus
transverse occipital s.
transverse temporal s.
Turner s.
s. valleculae
s. ventralis
ventrolateral s.
s. ventrolateralis medullae oblongatae
s. ventrolateralis medullae spinalis
vermicular s.
s. verticalis

sulfadoxine
pyrimethamine s.

sulfamethoxazole

sulfatase
s. A
N-acetylgalactosamine-4-sulfate s.
N-acetylglucosamine-6-sulfate s.
s. A deficiency
cerebroside s.
galactose-6-sulfate s.
iduronate s.

sulfate
amphetamine s.
barium s.
bleomycin s.
dehydroepiandrosterone s. (DHEA-S)
dermatan s.
dimethylamine s. (DMAS)
ephedrine s.
guanethidine s.
heparin s.
iron ferrous s.
keratan s.
magnesium s.
sodium dodecyl s. (SDS)
tranylcypromine s.
vinblastine s.
vincristine s.

sulfate-3-glucuronyl paragloboside
sulfated glucuronyl paragloboside (SGPG)
sulfatide
s. accumulation
s. lipidosis
sulfatidosis
sulfinpyrazone
sulfite oxidase deficiency aminoaciduria
sulfoglucuronyl lactosaminyl paragloboside
sulfonamide peripheral neuropathy
sulfosuccinate
dioctyl sodium s.
sulfoxide
dimethyl s. (DMSO)
sulfur metabolism defect
Sullivan VPAP III
sulodexide
sumatriptan
intranasal s.
s. nasal spray
s. succinate injection
summating potential
summation of stimulus
summer encephalitis
Summerskill sign
Summit occipito-cervico-thoracic spinal fixation system
sunburst mechanism
SUNCT
short-lasting unilateral neuralgiform pain with conjunctival injecting and tearing
Sunderland classification
sundowner effect
sundowning
s. behavior
s. syndrome
SUNDS
sudden unexplained nocturnal death syndrome
Sundt
S. AVM microclip system
S. booster clip
S. carotid shunt
S. carotid ulceration classification
S. cross-legged clip
S. loop shunt
S. straddling clip
Sundt-Kees
S.-K. encircling patch clip
S.-K. graft clip
S.-K. Slimline clip
sunset sign
Sun workstation
superactivity
phosphoribosyl pyrophosphate synthetase s.
superantigen
superconducting
s. magnet
s. quantum interference device (SQUID)
0.5-T s. magnet
1.5 T s. system
superconductor
type 2 s.
superficial
s. gray layer of superior colliculus
s. middle cerebral vein
s. origin
s. petrosal nerve
s. reflex
s. siderosis
s. siderosis of the central nervous system
s. temporal artery (STA)
s. temporal artery-middle cerebral artery (STA-MCA)
s. temporal artery to middle cerebral artery bypass
s. temporal artery-posterior cerebral artery (STA-PCA)
s. temporal artery to posterior cerebral artery bypass
s. temporal artery-superior cerebellar artery (STA-SCA)
s. temporal artery to superior cerebral artery bypass
s. temporal plexus
s. temporal vein
superficiale
stratum griseum s.
superficiales
venae cerebri s.
superficialis
fibrae pontis s.
nervus fibularis s.
nervus peroneus s.
rami musculares nervi peronei s.
vena cerebri media s.
superfine fiberscope
superfrontal fissure

NOTES

Superfrost microscope slide
superior
s. alternating hemiplegia
s. anastomotic vein
s. aperture of axillary fossa
area vestibularis s.
arteria cerebelli s.
s. basal vein
s. central raphe nucleus
s. central tegmental nucleus
s. cerebellar artery
s. cerebellar artery syndrome
s. cerebellar peduncle
s. cerebral vein
s. cervical ganglion (SCG)
s. cervical ganglionectomy
s. choroid vein
s. cistern
s. colliculus
s. colliculus layer
fasciculus longitudinalis s.
fasciculus occipitofrontalis s.
fissura posterior s.
s. fovea
s. frontal convolution
s. frontal gyrus
s. frontal sulcus
s. ganglion of glossopharyngeal nerve
s. ganglion of vagus nerve
gyrus frontalis s.
gyrus temporalis s.
s. hemorrhagic polioencephalitis
s. hemorrhoidal plexus
s. hypophysial artery
s. intradural approach
s. laryngeal artery
s. laryngeal nerve (SLN)
s. laryngeal nerve external branch
s. limb of ansa cervicalis
lobulus parietalis s.
lobulus semilunaris s.
s. longitudinal fasciculus
s. longitudinal sinus
s. long-term memory
macula cribrosa s.
s. medullary velum
s. mesenteric artery syndrome
s. mesenteric ganglion
nervus cardiacus cervicalis s.
nervus cutaneous brachii lateralis s.
nervus gluteus s.
nucleus centralis tegmenti s.
nucleus linearis s.
nucleus olivaris s.
nucleus salivarius s.
nucleus salivatorius s.
nucleus vestibularis s.
s. oblique myokymia
s. oblique tendon sheath syndrome
s. occipital gyrus
s. occipital sulcus
s. occipitofrontal fasciculus
oliva s.
s. olivary complex
s. olivary nucleus
s. olive
s. ophthalmic vein
s. ophthalmic vein approach
s. orbital fissure (SOF)
s. orbital fissure tumor
s. paraplegia
s. parietal gyrus
s. parietal lobule (SPL)
s. part of vestibulocochlear nerve
s. peduncle of thalamus
pedunculus cerebellaris s.
s. periventricular white matter
s. petrosal sinus (SPS)
plexus dentalis s.
plexus hypogastricus s.
plexus mesentericus s.
plexus rectalis s.
s. pontine syndrome
s. pulmonary sulcus tumor
s. quadrigeminal brachium
s. rectus muscle
s. root of ansa cervicalis
s. root of cervical loop
s. root of vestibulocochlear nerve
s. sagittal sinus
s. sagittal sinus occlusion
s. salivary nucleus
s. salivatory nucleus
s. semicircular canal (SSC)
s. semilunar lobule
sinus petrosus s.
sinus sagittalis s.
sulcus frontalis s.
sulcus occipitalis s.
sulcus temporalis s.
s. surface of cerebellar hemisphere
tela choroidea s.
s. temporal artery-middle cerebral artery anastomosis
s. temporal auditory cortical area
s. temporal convolution
s. temporal fissure
s. temporal lobe gyrus
s. temporal plane
s. temporal sulcus (STS)
s. thalamostriate vein
s. thoracic pedicle screw
s. thyroid artery
s. thyroid plexus
s. thyroid vein
s. vein of cerebellar hemisphere
s. vein of vermis

vena anastomotica s.
s. vena cava syndrome
vena choroidea s.
vena thalamostriata s.
vena vermis s.
s. vestibular area
s. vestibular nucleus

superiores
nervi alveolares s.
nervi clunium s.
rami clunium s.
rami dentales superiores plexus dentalis s.
rami gluteales s.
venae cerebri s.
venae hemispherii cerebelli s.

superior-inferior submucous tunnel

superioris
brachium colliculi s.
cisterna s.
commissura colliculi s.
frenulum veli medullaris s.
nucleus reticularis intermedius pontis s.
rami gingivales superiores plexus dentalis s.
rami laryngopharyngei ganglii cervicalis s.
ramus externus nervi laryngei s.
ramus internus nervi laryngei s.
stratum cinereum colliculi s.
stratum griseum intermedium colliculus s.
stratum griseum profundum colliculi s.
stratum griseum superficiale colliculi s.
stratum medullare intermedium colliculi s.
stratum medullare profundum colliculi s.
stratum opticum colliculi s.
stratum zonale colliculi s.

superiorum
decussatio pedunculorum cerebellarium s.

superius
brachium quadrigeminum s.
frenulum veli medullaris s.
ganglion cervicale s.
ganglion mesentericum s.
velum medullare s.

supermotility

supernatant

superolateral
s. cerebral surface
s. face of cerebral hemisphere
s. surface of cerebrum

superomedialis
margo s.

superoxide
s. anion
s. anion radical
s. dismutase (SOD)

superparamagnetic iron oxide

superparamagnetism

superselective
s. angiography
s. catheterization
s. embolization

supersensitivity
disuse s.

supination reflex

supinator
s. jerk
s. longus reflex

supine
s. position
s. sleep

supplemental
s. oxygen
s. steroid hormone

supplementary
s. eye field (SEF)
s. motor area (SMA)
s. motor area epilepsy
s. motor cortex
s. motor seizure

supplementation
glycine s.
oral s.

supply
cochlear vascular s.
collateral blood s.
spinal cord blood s.

supporter
Malis vessel s.

suppressant
vestibular s.

suppression
apoptosis s.
bone marrow s.
burst s.
electroencephalographic burst s.

NOTES

suppression *(continued)*
medication-induced REM sleep s.
postictal s.
rebound s.
s. subtractive hybridization (SSH)
vestibuloocular reflex s.
suppressor
s. area
s. gene
suppurative
s. cerebritis
s. encephalitis
suprabrow
s. approach
s. transorbital roof craniotomy
supracallosal gyrus
supracerebellar
s. approach
infratentorial s.
supracerebral
suprachiasmatic nucleus
suprachiasmaticus
nucleus s.
supraclavicular
s. approach
s. nerve
s. point
supraclaviculares
nervi s.
supraclinoid
s. aneurysm
s. internal carotid artery
supraglottic pressure
supraglottis
supralemniscalis
nucleus s.
supralemniscal nucleus
supraliminal stimulus
supramammillaris
nucleus s.
supramammillary nucleus
supramarginal
s. convolution
s. gyrus
supramarginalis
gyrus s.
supramastoid crest
supramaximal
s. rapid stimulation
s. response
s. stimulus
suprameatal spine
supraneuroporica
lamina s.
supranormal stimulation
supranuclear
s. gaze palsy
s. lesion
s. ophthalmoplegia
s. paralysis
s. vertical gaze impairment
supraoptic
s. commissure
s. fiber
s. nucleus
s. nucleus of hypothalamus
s. recess
s. region
supraopticae
commissurae s.
fibrae s.
supraopticohypophysiales
fibrae s.
supraopticohypophysialis
tractus s.
supraopticohypophysial tract
supraopticus
nucleus s.
recessus s.
supraorbital
s. nerve
s. neuralgia
s. pericranial flap
s. point
s. pterional approach
s. reflex
s. ridge
s. rim
supraorbitalis
nervus s.
ramus lateralis nervi s.
ramus medialis nervi s.
suprapatellar reflex
suprapinealis
recessus s.
suprapineal recess
suprapubic reflex
supraradial plexus
suprarenal ganglion
suprarenalis
plexus s.
suprascapular
s. nerve
s. nerve entrapment
s. neuropathy
suprascapularis
nervus s.
suprasegmental parameter
suprasellar
s. adenoma
s. aneurysm
s. area
s. capsule
s. cistern
s. cyst
s. extension
s. lesion
s. mass

s. meningioma
s. region
suprasplenial sulcus
suprastriate layer
suprasylvian
supratentorial
s. approach
s. arteriovenous malformation
s. astrocytoma
s. brain
s. cavernous angioma
s. craniotomy
s. dura
s. glioma
s. lobar ependymoma
s. mass
s. meningioma (STM)
s. oligodendroglioma
s. primary malignant brain tumor
s. primitive neuroectodermal tumor
s. structural lesion
s. subdural hemorrhage
s. symptom
s. system
suprathreshold
s. stimulus
s. taste intensity estimation
suprathreshold stimulus
supratrochlearis
nervus s.
supratrochlear nerve
supraumbilical reflex
supreme intercostal artery
sural
s. cutaneous nerve
s. nerve biopsy
s. nerve bridge graft
s. nerve cable graft
s. sensory nerve
s. sensory potential
suralis
nervus s.
rami calcanei laterales nervi s.
Suramin
surface
s. affability
s. coil
s. coil array
s. coil MR
s. coil spectroscopic imaging
curved vertebral s.
s. dyslexia
s. electrode
s. epitope
s. fiducial marker
inferior cerebral s.
s. landmark
s. matching
medial cerebral s.
mesial s.
nuclear s.
s. point
posterior odontoid s.
s. reconstruction
s. scalp electroencephalogram
superolateral cerebral s.
tentorial s.
s. thalamic vein
s. vessel registration
Surgairtome II drill halo
surgeon
American Association of Neurological Surgeons/Congress of Neurological S.'s (AANS/CNS)
Congress of Neurological S.'s
surgery
acoustic neuroma s.
adult scoliosis s.
aneurysm s.
anterior cervicothoracic junction s.
anterior cranial fossa s.
anterior lower cervical spine s.
anterior radical s.
awake brain s.
cerebellopontine angle s.
cervical decompression s.
cervicothoracic junction s.
computer-assisted s. (CAS)
computer-assisted stereotactic s. (CASS)
craniofacial s.
cytoreductive s.
decompressive s.
direct vision s.
DREZ s.
ECA-PCA bypass s.
endoscopic endonasal transsphenoidal s.
endoscopic sinus s.
endoscopic skull-base s.
epilepsy s.
s. evaluation
extracranial-intracranial bypass s.

NOTES

surgery *(continued)*
Foundation for International Education in Neurological S. (FIENS)
gastric bypass s.
hypotensive s.
International Cooperative Study on the Timing of Aneurysm S.
intradural tumor s.
intraorbital s.
keyhole s.
laser s.
lower posterior lumbar spine and sacrum s.
microscopic endoscopy s.
minimum incision s.
naked-eye direct vision s.
nasal s.
neuronavigator-guided brain s.
Novalis shaped beam s.
optic nerve sheath decompression s.
orthognathic s.
palatal s.
pediatric neurological s.
Pitanguy plastic s.
posterior lower cervical spine s.
posterior lumbar interbody fusion s.
posterior lumbar spine and sacrum s.
posterior upper cervical spine s.
resective epilepsy s.
selective imaging and graphics for stereotactic s. (SIGSS)
skull base s.
stereotactic s.
telepresence s.
thoracic and thoracolumbar spine s.
tongue reduction s.
transsphenoidal s.
untethering s.
vascular s.
video-assisted thorascopic s.
weight-loss s.

surgical
s. anatomy
s. arthrodesis
s. clipping
s. correction
s. decompression
s. dressing
s. epilepsy
s. exploration
s. exposure
s. hearing loss
S. Interbody Research Group
s. microscope
s. microscope navigator system
s. morbidity
s. procedure
s. resection
s. rupture
s. seeding
s. technique

Surgicel
S. fibrillar absorbable hemostat
S. Nu-Knit dressing

Surgiflo hemostatic matrix

SurgiScope
S. image-guided system
S. robotic microscope
S. stereotactic system

Surgi-Spec telescope

Surgivac drain

Surmontil

Surrogate Outcome Measure

surveillance
developmental s.
s. imaging
s. protocol

survey
Medical Outcomes Study Short Form Health S.
pediatric sleep s.

survival
cell s.
s. curve
s. motor neuron gene
overall s.
progression-free s.
s. time

survivor
Alzheimer s.
trauma s.

Susac syndrome

susceptibility
s. agent
s. artifact
s. effect
environmental s.
s. factor
genetic s.
magnetic s.

suspected seizure

suspended embryonic astrocyte

suspension
hyoid s.
magnesium hydroxide s.
static s.

sustained
s. ankle clonus
s. compliance
s. fatigability
s. high-frequency repetitive firing (SRF)
s. release (SR)

sustentacular fiber of retina

sustention/intention tremor

Sustiva
suture
American silk s.
Bondek s.
s. clamp
coronal s.
cranial s.
Czerny s.
s. diastasis
dural tack-up s.
lambdoidal s.
Mersilk black silk s.
metopic s.
Micrins microsurgical s.
Millipore s.
nerve s.
Nurolon s.
occipitomastoid s.
parietosquamous s.
petrosquamous s.
polypropylene s.
PremiCron nonabsorbable s.
pterygomaxillary s.
retracting s.
Serralnyl s.
Serralsilk s.
tacking s.
tension s.
tentalum wire tension s.
tympanosquamous s.
Vicryl Rapide s.
sutureless onlay graft
Suzuki classification
SV40
simian virus 40
SVC
small-volume correction
SVIB
Strong Vocational Interest Blank
SV-MRS
single-voxel magnetic resonance spectroscopy
SWA
slow-wave activity
SWAI
Sleep-Wake Activity Inventory
swallow
s. artifact
s. syncope
swallowing
s. automatism
s. center
s. disorder
s. dysfunction
s. reflex
sleep-related abnormal s.
s. threshold
Swan-Ganz catheter
swan-neck
s.-n. deformity
s.-n. deformity reduction
Swanson scaphoid awl
Swash-Schwartz disease
sway
body s.
s. velocity
swaying
broad-based gait with s.
sweat
s. artifact
s. center
sweating
abnormal s.
s. test
Swedish gamma knife group
Sweet
S. disease
S. pituitary scissors
S. 2-point discrimination
swelling
axonal s.
blennorrhagic s.
brain s.
ischemic hemispheric s.
optic disc s.
psychomotor s.
sensation of s.
Spielmeyer acute s.
tympanic s.
swim goggle headache
swimmer's view
swineherd disease
swinging
s. flashlight sign
s. flashlight test
Swischuk line
switch
postictal blood flow s.
wake s.
swollen axon
SWS
slow-wave sleep
Sturge-Weber syndrome

NOTES

Sydenham
S. chorea
S. disease
syllabic
s. blindness
s. speech
sylvian
s. angle
s. approach
s. aqueduct
s. aqueduct syndrome
s. cistern
s. dissection
s. fissure
s. fossa
s. hematoma
s. line
s. operculum
s. point
s. seizure
s. ventricle
sylvian/rolandic junction
sylvii
aqueductus s.
cistern s.
cisterna fossae s.
sulcus s.
vallecula s.
Sylvius
S. angle
aqueduct of S.
cerebral aqueduct of S.
fissure of S.
fossa of S.
iter of S.
ventricle of S.
S. ventricle
Symadine
Symax-SR caplet
Symbiot covered stent
Symmetrel
symmetric
s. cleavage
s. distal neuropathy
s. polyneuropathy
symmetrical
s. diffuse neuropathy
s. sacral plate
s. sensory polyneuropathy
s. thoracic vertebral plate
symmetry
S. angioplasty balloon
facial s.
Hermetian s.
Symonds headache
sympathectomy, sympathetectomy, sympathicectomy
cervical perivascular s.
chemical s.
s. effect
Leriche s.
lumbar s.
percutaneous radiofrequency s.
periarterial s.
permanent s.
3-portal video-assisted thoracoscopic s.
presacral s.
radiofrequency thoracic s.
Smithwick s.
thoracic endoscopic s.
video-assisted endoscopic s.
visceral s.
sympathetic
s. block
s. blockade
s. chain
s. discharge
s. dystrophy syndrome
s. ganglion
s. hypertonia
s. imbalance
s. iridoplegia
s. meningitis
s. nerve
s. nerve burst
s. nerve ending
s. nervous system
s. nervous system-medicated vasoconstriction
s. neuroblast
s. output
s. part
s. plexus
s. reflex dystrophy
s. segment
s. skin response
s. sprouting
s. stimulation
s. trunk
sympathetica
ptosis s.
sympathetically
s. independent pain syndrome
s. mediated pain syndrome
sympatheticum
ganglion s.
sympatheticus
truncus s.
sympathetoblastoma
sympathica
meningitis s.
pars s.
sympathicectomy (*var. of* sympathectomy)
sympathici
ganglia trunci s.
rami interganglionares trunci s.

sympathicoblast
sympathicoblastoma
sympathicogonioma
sympathicolysis
sympathicolytic
sympathicomimetic
sympathiconeuritis
sympathicopathy
sympathicotripsy
sympathicotrope
sympathicotropic
sympathicum
ganglion s.
sympathicus
truncus s.
sympathoblastoma
sympathoexcitatory brainstem pathway
sympathogonioma
sympatholytic
sympathomimetic
s. agent
s. drug
s. toxicity
sympathomimetic-induced thermogenesis
sympathotonic orthostatic hypotension
Symphony platelet concentrate system
symptom
affective s.
s. amplification
Anton s.
arousal s.
array of s.
s. assessment
autism-related s.
behavioral s.
bizarre s.
bodily s.
body-related obsessive-like s.
Bonhoeffer s.
Brauch-Romberg s.
s. categorization
S. Checklist-90
s. checklist
S. Checklist 90-Revised Global Severity Index
clinical s.
clinician-rated cognitive s.
cluster of s.
cluster C, D s.
cognitive s.
s. complex
cranial autonomic s.
s. crystallization
debilitating dysphoric s.
s. dimension
disaster-related avoidant s.
disaster-related intrusive s.
discrete s.
disorganization s.
dissociation s.
drug-induced negative s.
eclamptic s.
Epstein s.
s. exacerbation
extrapyramidal s. (EPS)
extrapyramidal syndrome s.
first-rank s.
Frenkel s.
generic negative s.
Gordon s.
Haenel s.
hyperarousal s.
ill-defined s.
induced factitious s.
intrusive s.
inventory of s.'s
Kerandel s.
s. level
longstanding s.
Macewen s.
manifest s.
s. measure
medically unexplained physical s.'s (MUPS)
migrainous s.
mild subsyndromal s.
multiple medically unexplained s.'s
neurobehavioral s.
neurologic s.
numbing s.
parkinsonian s.
positive s.
postictal s.
posttraumatic stress s.
precursory s.
premonitory s.
primary enduring negative s.
primary nonenduring negative s.
prodromal psychotic s.
s. profile
s. progression
psychological s.
recurring s.
s. reduction

NOTES

symptom *(continued)*
Remak s.
residual negative s.
residual positive s.
Roger s.
Romberg s.
Romberg-Howship s.
Schneider first-rank s.
secondary s.
Séguin signal s.
signal s.
specific s.
subclinical depressive s.
subsyndromal mood s.
subtle s.
supratentorial s.
tic s.
total s.
Trendelenburg s.
Ulthoff s.
vegetative s.
visual s.
Wartenberg s.
worrying s.
s. worsening
symptomatic
s. depression
s. dystonia
s. extrapulmonary disease
s. headache
s. hydrocephalus
s. neuralgia
s. palatal tremor
s. paramyotonia
s. partial epilepsy
s. patient
s. perspective
s. root
s. seizure
s. spondylolisthesis
s. tetany
s. torticollis
s. vasospasm
symptom-related predictor
symptoms
synalgia
synalgic
synangiosis
synaphoceptor
synapse
axoaxonic s.
axodendritic s.
axodendrosomatic s.
axosomatic s.
dendrodendritic s.
electrotonic s.
Gray type I, II s.
hebbian potentiation of s.
inhibitory s.
loop s.
s. loss
pericorpuscular s.
s. plasticity
s. redundancy
viable s.
synapsis
synaptic
s. activity
s. bouton
s. cleft
s. conduction
s. connection
s. degeneration
s. density
s. ending
s. glomerulus
s. knob
s. loss
s. mechanism
s. membrane
s. pathway
s. plasticity
s. protein level
s. space
s. sprouting
s. terminal
s. trough
s. vesicle
synaptogenesis
dendrite s.
synaptology
synaptophysin
synaptosome
brain s.
synaptosome-associated protein
syncheiria, synchiria
synchondrosis
basilar subdental s.
subdental s.
synchrocyclotron operation
SynchroMed
S. drug administration device
S. model 8611H prototype implantable pump
synchronization
thalamocortical s.
synchronized
s. neuronal discharge
s. sleep
synchronous
s. bilateral PLED
s. clonic movement
s. corticofugal epileptic discharge
s. epileptiform activity
s. facial schwannoma
s. lesion
s. reflex
s. spike-and-wave discharge

synchrony
- bilateral s.
- interhemispheric s.
- secondary bilateral s.

synclonic spasm
synclonus
syncopal
- s. migraine
- s. migraine headache

syncope
- Adams-Stokes s.
- cardiac s.
- carotid sinus hypersensitivity-induced s.
- convulsive s.
- cough s.
- digital s.
- hysterical s.
- idiopathic s.
- laryngeal s.
- local s.
- micturition s.
- near s.
- neurally mediated s.
- neurocardiogenic s.
- orthostatic s.
- postural s.
- reflex s.
- reflexogenic s.
- stretching s.
- swallow s.
- tussive s.
- vasodepressor s.
- vasomotor s.
- vasovagal s.

syncopic
syncytial
- s. island
- s. meningioma

syncytiotrophoblastic giant cell (STGC)
syncytium
syndactyly
syndesmosis
syndrome
- Aarskog-Scott s. (ASS)
- ABC s.
- abdominal compartment s.
- abolic s.
- achalasia, adrenocortical insufficiency, alacrimia s. (AAAS)
- acquired epileptiform opercular s.
- acquired hepatocerebral s.
- acquired immunodeficiency s. (AIDS)
- acrocallosal s.
- acromegaloid-hypertelorism-pectus carinatum s.
- acroparesthesia s.
- acute disconnection s.
- acute organic brain s.
- acute psychoorganic s.
- Adams-Stokes s.
- Adie tonic pupil s.
- adiposogenital s.
- adult respiratory distress s.
- adult Reye s. (ARS)
- advanced sleep-phase s. (ASPS)
- age-dependent epilepsy s.
- agitated delirium s.
- Aicardi s.
- Aicardi-Goutières s.
- akinetic-rigid s.
- Alagille s.
- Alajouanine s.
- Albright s.
- Aldrich s.
- Alice in Wonderland s.
- alien hand s.
- Allgrove s.
- Alport s.
- ALS-like s.
- Alstrom-Hallgren s.
- alveolar hypoventilation s.
- amnesic s.
- anatomicoclinical s.
- Andermann s.
- Andersen s.
- Andrade s.
- aneusomy s.
- Angelman s. (AS)
- Angelucci s.
- angular gyrus s.
- anterior bulb s.
- anterior cervical cord s.
- anterior cingulate prefrontal s.
- anterior cornual s.
- anterior interosseus s.
- anterior spinal artery s.
- anterior spinal cord s.
- anterior vermis s.
- antiepileptic drug hypersensitivity s.
- antiphospholipid s.
- Antley-Bixler s.
- Anton s.

S

NOTES

syndrome *(continued)*
Anton-Babinski s.
aortic arch s.
apallic s.
Apert s.
Arnold-Chiari s.
Arnold nerve reflex cough s.
arterial thoracic outlet s.
Asperger s.
ataxia-telangiectasia s.
audiovestibular s.
auriculotemporal nerve s.
Avellis s.
axonopathic neurogenic thoracic outlet s.
Babinski s.
Babinski-Nageotte s.
Balint s.
Baller-Gerold s.
Baltic s.
Bannayan s.
Bannwarth s.
barber chair s.
Bardet-Biedl s.
Barlow s.
Barré-Lieou s.
Barth s.
Bartter s.
basal cell nevus s.
basal ganglia s.
basilar artery thrombosis s.
Bassen-Kornzweig s.
Basser s.
Beckwith-Wiedemann s.
Behçet s.
Benedikt s.
benzodiazepine discontinuation s.
Berardinelli s.
Bernard s.
Bernard-Horner s.
Bernhardt-Roth s.
Bessman-Baldwin s.
Beuren s.
Biedl-Moon-Laurence s.
Biemond s.
bilateral acoustic neuromas s.
Bing-Horton s.
Bing-Neel s.
biopercular s.
Björeson s.
Bloch-Sulzberger s.
Bloom s.
blue diaper s.
bobble-head doll s.
body of Luys s.
Bonhoeffer s.
Bonnet-Dechaume-Blanc s.
Bonnevie-Ullrich s.
Bonnier s.
Börjeson-Forssman-Lehmann s.
brachial-basilar insufficiency s.
brachialgia and cord s.
Brachmann-de Lange s.
Bradbury-Eggleston s.
brainstem s.
Brauch-Romberg s.
bright thalamus s.
Briquet s.
Brissaud s.
Brissaud-Marie s.
Brissaud-Sicard s.
Broca s.
Brown s.
Brown-Séquard s.
Brown-Vialetto-van Laere s.
Brueghel s.
Brugada s.
Bruns s.
Brushfield-Wyatt s.
bulbar s.
burner s.
burning feet s.
burning hands s.
C2 s.
calf compartment s.
Call-Fleming s.
Camurati-Engelmann s.
carbohydrate-deficient glycoprotein s.
cardiofacial s.
carotid sinus s.
carpal tunnel s. (CTS)
Carpenter s.
cataract-oligophrenia s.
catch-22 s.
cauda equina s.
caudal regression s.
cavernous sinus s.
Cayler s.
central alveolar hypoventilation s.
central anticholinergic s.
central cord injury s.
central hypoventilation s.
central sleep apnea s.
cerebellar cognitive affective s.
cerebellar hemisphere s.
cerebellar hemorrhage s.
cerebellomedullary malformation s.
cerebellopontine angle s.
cerebral salt wasting s.
cerebral steal s.
cerebrofaciothoracic dysplasia s.
cerebrohepatorenal s.
cerebrovascular s.
cervical compression s.
cervical disc s.
cervical fusion s.
cervical rib and band s.

cervical tension s.
cervicobrachial s.
Cestan s.
Cestan-Chenais s.
Cestan-Raymond s.
Charcot-Marie s.
Charcot-Weiss-Baker s.
CHARGE s.
Charles Bonnet s.
Charlevoix-Saguenay s.
Charlin s.
Chediak-Higashi s.
cherry-red spot myoclonus s.
Chiari II s.
chiasma s.
chiasmal s.
chiasmatic s.
childhood-onset Tourette s.
Chinese paralytic s.
choreic s.
chronic fatigue and immune dysfunction s.
chronic hyperventilation s.
chronic paroxysmal hemicrania-tic s.
Churg-Strauss s.
classic cervical rib s.
Claude s.
Claude-Bernard s.
Clerambault s.
clinical s.
clinically isolated s.
closed head s.
cloverleaf skull s.
clumsy child s.
clumsy hand s.
cluster-tic s.
Cobb s.
cochleovestibular compression s.
Cockayne s.
Coffin-Lowry s. (CLS)
Coffin-Siris s.
Cogan s.
Cohen s.
Collet s.
Collet-Sicard s.
comorbid s.
compartment s.
complex regional pain s.
compression s.
congenital bilateral perisylvian s.
congenital central hypoventilation s.
congenital Horner s.
congenital myasthenic s. (CMS)
Conradi s.
Conradi-Hünermann s.
contiguous gene s.
continuous muscle fiber activity s.
conus medullaris s.
cord s.
Cornelia de Lange s.
corpus striatum s.
cortical disconnection s.
Costen s.
costoclavicular s.
coxsackievirus infection paralytic s.
CPH-tic s.
craniocerebellocardiac s.
creatinine deficiency s.
CREST s.
cri du chat s.
Crigler-Najjar s.
crocodile tears s.
Crouzon s.
Crow-Fukase s.
crying-cat s.
CSF pressure s.
cubital tunnel s.
Curschmann-Steinert s.
Cushing s.
cyclic vomiting s.
DaCosta s.
DAF s.
Dandy-Walker s.
Davidenkow s.
Davidoff-Dyke-Masson s.
deafferentation pain s.
Debre-Sémélaigne s.
deficit s.
Dejerine anterior bulb s.
Dejerine-Klumpke s.
Dejerine-Roussy s.
Dejerine-Sottas s.
Dejerine-Thomas s.
de Lange s.
delayed sleep-phase s.
delusional and hallucinatory s.
delusional misidentification s.
dementia s.
de Morsier s.
denervation pain s.
Denis Browne s.
Denny-Brown s.
depressive s.

NOTES

syndrome *(continued)*
De Sanctis-Cacchione s.
De Toni-Fanconi s.
developmental quotient in Down s.
dialysis disequilibrium s.
dialysis encephalopathy s.
DiGeorge s.
disc s.
disconnection s.
Divry-van Bogaert s.
DNA repletion s.
Doose s.
dorsal column s.
dorsal mesencephalic s.
dorsal midbrain s.
dorsolateral prefrontal s.
dorsomedial mesencephalic s.
Down s.
Dravet s.
droopy shoulder s.
drug-induced organic personality s.
dry eye s.
Duane retraction s.
Duchenne s.
Duchenne-Davidoff-Masson s.
Duchenne-Erb s.
Duncan s.
Dyke-Davidoff s.
Dyke-Davidoff-Mason s.
dysarthria-clumsy hand s.
dysexecutive s.
dysgenetic s.
dysmnesic s.
dysmorphic s.
Eagle s.
Eaton-Lambert s.
ectopic ACTH s.
Edwards s.
effort s.
Ehlers-Danlos s. (EDS)
eight-and-a-half s.
Eisenlohr s.
Ekbom s.
elfin facies s.
E-M s.
empty sella s.
encephalotrigeminal vascular s.
eosinophilia-myalgia s.
epidermal nevus s.
epilepsy s.
episodic dyscontrol s.
Erb-Duchenne s.
Escobar s.
Evans s.
exploding head s.
extrapyramidal s.
facet joint s.
Fahr s.
failed back surgery s.
familial dysautonomia s.
familial restless leg s.
Fanconi s.
fast channel s.
fatty degeneration in Reye s.
FAV s.
Fazio-Londe s.
Felty s.
fetal alcohol s. (FAS)
fetal valproic acid s.
Figueira s.
filum terminale s.
Fischer s.
Fisher s.
flashing pain s.
flat back s.
floppy head s.
floppy infant s.
flu-like s.
Flynn-Aird s.
focal brain s.
Foix s.
Foix-Alajouanine s.
Foix-Cavany-Marie s.
Förster s.
Foster Kennedy s.
Foville s.
fragile X s.
fragmented s.
Freeman-Sheldon s.
Frey s.
Friderichsen-Waterhouse s.
Friedmann vasomotor s.
Froin s.
frontal lobe s.
Fryns s.
Fukuhara s.
Fukuyama s.
full s.
full-blown s.
fulminant neuroleptic malignant s.
functional psychiatric s.
Garcin s.
Gardner s.
Gass s.
Gélineau s.
Gerstmann s.
Gerstmann-Sträussler s.
Gerstmann-Sträussler-Scheinker s.
Geschwind s.
Gilles de la Tourette s.
glioma-polyposis s.
Godtfredsen s.
Goebel s.
Goldberg-Shprintzen s.
Goldenhar s.
Goldenhar-Gorlin s.
Goliath s.
Gorlin s.

Gowers s.
Gradenigo s.
graviceptive brainstem s.
gray baby s.
Greig cephalopolysyndactyly s.
Gubler s.
Guillain-Barré s.
Guillain-Barré-Strohl s.
Guillain-Garcin s.
Gulf War s.
Gunn s.
gustatory sweating s.
Haddad s.
Hajdu-Cheney s.
Hakim s.
half base s.
Hallermann-Streiff s.
Hallervorden s.
Hallervorden-Spatz s.
hallucinatory transient organic s.
hand-shoulder s.
Harris s.
headache s.
head-bobbing doll s.
Heidenhain s.
hemibasal s.
hemichorea-hemiballism s.
hemiconvulsion-hemiplegia-epilepsy s. (HHES)
hemineglect s.
hemisensory s.
hemispheric disconnection s.
hemolytic uremia s.
hemolytic-uremic s.
hereditary ataxic s.
hereditary spinocerebellar ataxia s.
herniation s.
Herrmann s.
HHE s.
Hick s.
HID s.
Hoffmann-Werdnig s.
Holmes-Adie s.
Hopkins s.
Horner s.
Horner-Bernard s.
Horton s.
Hunt s.
Hunter s.
Hunter-McAlpine s.
Hurler s.
Hurler-Scheie s.
Hutchinson-Gilford progeria s.
Hutchison s.
hyperabduction s.
hypereosinophilic s.
hyperkinetic s.
hypernychthemeral s.
hyperosmolar hyperglycemic nonketotic s.
hyperperfusion s.
hypertrophied frenuluum s.
hyperviscosity s.
hypokinetic s.
hypoperfusion s.
hypophysial s.
hypophysiosphenoidal s.
hypothalamic savage s.
idiopathic ataxic s.
idiopathic generalized epilepsy s.
idiopathic Parsonage-Turner s.
iliac crest s.
s. of inappropriate secretion of antidiuretic hormone (SIADH)
indifference to pain s.
indomethacin-responsive headache s.
infantile tremor s.
infectious polyneuritis s.
inferior pontine s.
infratentorial neoplastic s.
infratentorial structural s.
insufficient sleep s.
interictal behavior s.
intermediolateral mesencephalic s.
internal capsule s.
International Classification of Epilepsies and Epileptic S.'s
intracranial steal s.
inverse Anton s.
inversed jaw-winking s.
irritable s.
Isaac s.
Isaacs-Mertens s.
jabs-and-jolts s.
Jackson-Weiss s.
Jacod s.
Jahnke s.
s. of Janz
Janz s.
Jarcho-Levin s.
jaw-winking s.
Jefferson s.
jerking stiff-person s.
Jervell-Lange-Nielsen s.

NOTES

syndrome *(continued)*
Johanson-Blizzard s.
Joubert s.
jugular foramen s.
Kabuki s.
Kahn s.
Kallmann s.
Kartagener s.
Kasabach-Merritt s.
Kearns-Sayre s.
Kennedy s.
Kernohan notch s.
Kiloh-Nevin s.
Kinsbourne s.
Kjellin s.
Kleine-Levin s.
Klinefelter s.
Klippel-Feil s.
Klippel-Trenaunay s.
Klippel-Trenaunay-Weber s.
Klumpke-Dejerine s.
Klüver-Bucy s.
Kocher-Debré-Semelaigne s.
Koerber-Salus-Elschnig s.
Kohlmeier-Degos s.
Korsakoff s.
Krabbe s.
Kugelberg-Welander s.
Labbé neurocirculatory s.
labyrinthine concussion s.
lacunar s.
Lambert s.
Lambert-Eaton s. (LES)
Lambert-Eaton myasthenic s. (LEMS)
Lance-Adams s.
Landau s.
Landau-Kleffner s.
Landry s.
Landry-Guillain-Barré s.
Landry-Guillain-Barré-Strohl s.
Langer-Giedion s.
Lasègue s. I, II
lateral inferior pontine s.
lateral medullary s.
lateral midpontine s.
lateral superior pontine s.
late whiplash s.
Laurence-Biedl s.
Laurence-Moon s.
Laurence-Moon-Bardet-Biedl s.
Laurence-Moon-Biedl s.
Lawford s.
Leach-Nyhan s.
Leigh s.
Lemieux-Neemeh s.
Lennox s.
Lennox-Gastaut s.
Leopard s.
Leriche s.
Lesch-Nyhan s.
Levine-Critchley s.
Lev-Lenègre s.
Lévy-Roussy s.
Leyden-Möbius s.
Lichtheim s.
Li-Fraumeni s.
lissencephalic s.
lissencephaly s.
locked-in s.
loculation s.
Louis-Bar s.
low back s.
Lowe s.
lower motor neuron s.
lower radicular s.
Lowry-MacLean s.
lumbar flat back s.
luxury perfusion s.
Lyell s.
Mackenzie s.
Mad Hatter s.
Maffucci s.
Magendie-Hertwig s.
magnesium deficiency infantile tremor s.
major psychiatric s.
malignant neuroleptic s.
malnutrition infantile tremor s.
manic s.
man-in-a-barrel s.
mapped epilepsy s.
Marchiafava-Bignami s.
Marcus Gunn s.
Marfan s.
marfanoid craniosynostosis s.
Marin Amat s.
Marinesco-Garland s.
Marinesco-Sjögren s.
marker X s.
Maroteaux-Lamy s.
Martin-Bell s.
maternal deprivation s.
May-White s.
McLeod s.
Meckel-Gruber s.
medial frontal lobe s.
medial inferior pontine s.
medial medullary s.
median cleft face s.
median face s.
medication-induced depressive s.
medullary s.
Meige s.
MELAS s.
Melkersson s.
Melkersson-Rosenthal s.
Melnick-Fraser s.

Ménière s.
Menkes kinky hair s.
Meretoja s.
MERRF s.
MERRLA s.
metameric s.
microdeletion s.
microvascular compression s.
middle radicular s.
midface hypoplasia s.
midline s.
midpontine s.
Millard-Gubler s.
Miller-Dieker s.
Miller-Fisher s. (MFS)
Miller-Fisher variant of Guillain-Barré s.
Milles s.
mitochondrial depletion s.
mixed headache s.
Möbius s.
Moersch-Woltmann s.
Monakow s.
Mondini s.
Morgagni s.
Morgagni-Adams-Stokes s.
morning glory s.
Morquio s. type A, B
Morvan s.
motor system s.
Mount s.
Mount-Reback s.
moyamoya s.
mtDNA depletion s.
mucocutaneous lymph node s.
multiple mucosal neuromas s.
multiple operations s.
muscle-joint pain s.
myasthenic s.
myelopathy s.
myoclonic encephalopathy s.
myoclonic epilepsy with ragged red fiber s.
myofascial s.
myokymia-cramp s.
Naffziger s.
Nager Miller s.
neck-tongue s.
needle-in-the-eye s.
Negri-Jacod s.
Nélaton s.
Nelson s.
neonatal abstinence s.
neonatal withdrawal s.
nerve compression s.
Neuhauser s.
neural crest s.
neuralgic pain s.
neurocutaneous s.
neurogenic thoracic outlet s.
neuroleptic malignant s. (NMS)
neurologic s.
neuromusculoskeletal s.
nevoid basal cell carcinoma s.
Nijmegen breakage s.
nocturnal eating s.
noncleft median face s.
non-24-hour sleep phase s.
nonlacunar s.
nonpsychotic posttraumatic brain s.
nonpsychotic severity psychoorganic s.
Noonan s.
Norman-Roberts s.
Norman-Wood s.
Nothnagel s.
numb cheek s.
numb chin s.
Nyssen-van Bogaert s.
obesity hypoventilation s.
obstructive sleep apnea s. (OSAS)
obstructive sleep apnea-hypopnea s. (OSAHS)
ocular ischemic s.
oculocerebrorenal s.
oculomotor s.
oculopharyngeal s.
Oden s.
Ohtahara s.
old-sergeant s.
Omersch-Woltman s.
one-and-a-half s.
Oppenheim s.
opsoclonus-myoclonus s. (OMS)
optic chiasmal s.
opticocerebral s.
opticopyramidal s.
optic tract s.
oral-facial-digital s.
orbital apex s.
orbital floor s.
orbitofrontal s.
organic affective s.
organic amnestic s.

NOTES

syndrome *(continued)*
organic brain s. (OBS)
organic delusional s.
organic hallucinosis s.
organic mental s.
organic mood s.
orofacial-digital s.
Osler-Rendu-Weber s.
osmotic demyelination s.
outlet s.
overdrainage s.
overlap s.
painful legs and moving fingers s.
painful legs and moving toes s.
palatal s.
paleostriatal s.
pallidal s.
Pallister-Hall s.
Pallister-Killian s.
Panayiotopoulos s.
Pancoast s.
paramedian mesencephalic s.
paraneoplastic neurologic s.
paraneoplastic pain s.
paranoid-type psychoorganic s.
paratrigeminal s.
parietal lobe s.
Parinaud s.
Parkes Weber s.
parkinsonian s.
Parkinson-plus s.
Parry-Romberg s.
Parsonage-Aldren-Turner s.
Parsonage-Turner s.
Patau s.
Payne s.
Pearson s.
Pena-Shokeir s.
Pendred s.
Pepper s.
peripheral nerve entrapment s.
peripheral neuropathic pain s.
Petit s.
petrosphenoid s.
Pfeiffer s.
phantom shock s.
Phineas Gage s.
phonologic syntactic s.
phosphate-wasting s.
Pick s.
piriformis s.
Pitt-Rogers-Dank s.
POEMS s.
Poland s.
polycystic ovary s.
pontine s.
postadrenalectomy s.
postconcussion s.
postcontusional brain s.
postencephalitic behavior s.
posterior column s.
posterior fossa s.
posterior inferior cerebellar artery s.
posterior joint s.
posterior leukoencephalopathy s.
posterior spinal cord s.
posterior vermis s.
posthypophysectomy traction s.
postlaminectomy s.
postleucotomy s.
postlumbar puncture s.
postmalaria neurologic s.
postpartum pituitary necrosis s.
postpolio s.
postpoliomyelitis s.
posttraumatic amnestic s.
posttraumatic brain s.
posttraumatic neck s.
posttraumatic pain s.
postural orthostatic tachycardia s.
Potter s.
Potzl s.
Pourfour du Petit s.
Prader-Willi s.
premotor s.
presynaptic congenital myasthenic s.
pretectal s.
primary antiphospholipid antibody s.
primary fibromyalgia s.
primary Sjögren s.
primary trunk s.
pronator teres s.
Proteus s.
pseudo-battered child s.
pseudo-Hurler s.
pseudotrisomy 13 s.
pseudo-Wernicke s.
pseudo-Zellweger s.
psychiatric s.
psychogenic effort s.
psychomotor dysadaptation s.
psychoorganic s.
psychotic brain s.
punch-drunk s.
putatively poor-prognosis deficit s.
Putnam-Dana s.
s. of pyramid
rabbit s.
radicular s.
radiculomedullary s.
Raeder paratrigeminal s.
Rambaud s.
Ramsay Hunt s., type I, II
rapid time-zone change s.
Rasmussen s.
Raymond s.
Raymond-Cestan s.

Raynaud s.
red man s.
red neck s.
reflex sympathetic dystrophy s. (RSDS)
Refsum s.
Reichert-Mundinger s.
Reiter s.
repetitive motion s. (RMS)
residual autoparalytic s.
restless leg s. (RLS)
retroparotid space s.
Rett s.
reversible posterior leukoencephalopathy s. (RPLS)
revolving door s.
Reye s.
Reye-like s.
Richardson-Steele-Olszewski s.
Richards-Rundle s.
Rieger s.
right parietal lobe s.
rigid spine s.
Riley-Day s.
Riley-Smith s.
Robert s.
Robinow s.
rolandic vein s.
Romano-Ward s.
Romberg s.
root s.
Rosenberg-Chutorian s.
Rosenthal-Rosenthal s.
rostral basilar artery s.
rotational vertebral artery s. (RVAS)
Roth s.
Roth-Bernhardt s.
Roussy-Dejerine s.
Roussy-Lévy s.
Rubinstein-Taybi s.
rubrospinal s.
Rukavina s.
Russell s.
Ruvalcaba-Myhre s.
Saethre-Chotzen s.
Sandifer s.
Sanfilippo s.
scalenus anterior s.
scapuloperoneal s.
Scheie s.
Schinzel-Giedion s.
Schirmer s.
Schmidt vagoaccessory s.
Schwartz-Jampel s.
sciatic notch s.
secondary restless leg s.
second impact s.
segmentary s.
serotonin s.
serotoninergic s.
shaken baby s.
shaken-impact s.
Sheehan s.
shoulder-girdle s.
shoulder-hand s.
Shy-Drager s. (SDS)
Sicard s.
sick building s.
sick sinus s.
sinking brain s.
Sjögren s.
Sjogren-Larsson s.
sleep apnea s. (SAS)
sleep hypopnea s. (SHS)
sleep hypoventilation s.
sleep phase delay s.
slipping clutch s.
slit ventricle s.
slow channel s.
Sluder s.
Sly s.
Smith-Lemli-Opitz s.
Smith-Magenis s.
Sneddon s.
somnolence s.
Sotos s.
Spens s.
sphenocavernous s.
Sphrintzen s.
split-brain s.
split notochord s.
spondyloarthropathy s.
startle s.
Steele-Richardson-Olszewski s.
Stein-Leventhal s.
Stephen s.
Stevens-Johnson s.
Stewart-Morel s.
Stickler s.
sticky platelet s.
stiff-baby s.
stiff-man s.
stiff-person s.

S

NOTES

syndrome *(continued)*
Stokes-Adams s.
Strachan s.
stroke s.
stump embolization s.
Sturge s.
Sturge-Kalischer-Weber s.
Sturge-Weber s. (SWS)
Sturge-Weber-Dimitri s.
subacute meningitis s.
subacute psychoorganic s.
subclavian steal s.
subclinical s.
subcoracoid-pectoralis minor tendon s.
subcortical s.
substance-related s.
subwakefulness s.
sudden infant death s.
sudden unexplained nocturnal death s. (SUNDS)
Sudeck s.
sundowning s.
superior cerebellar artery s.
superior mesenteric artery s.
superior oblique tendon sheath s.
superior pontine s.
superior vena cava s.
Susac s.
sylvian aqueduct s.
sympathetically independent pain s.
sympathetically mediated pain s.
sympathetic dystrophy s.
syringomyelic cord s.
Tapia s.
tarsal tunnel s.
tegmental s.
Terson s.
tethered spinal cord s.
thalamic pain s.
Thévenard s.
thoracic outlet s. (TOS)
thyrohypophysial s.
tight filum terminale s.
tin ear s.
Tolosa-Hunt s.
top of basilar s.
TORCH s.
Torré s.
Torsten Sjögren s.
Tourette s.
toxic shock s.
trapped ventricle s.
traumatic central cord s.
Treacher Collins s.
triad of Dejerine s.
triangular s.
triple A s. (AAAS)
trisomy 8, 13, 20, 21 s.
trisomy C, D s.
trisomy 9 mosaic s.
Trousseau s.
Troyer s.
true neurogenic thoracic outlet s.
tuberous sclerosis s.
Turcot s.
Turner s.
Ulrich-Turner s.
unilateral facial pain s.
Unverricht-Lundborg s.
upper airway resistance s. (UARS)
upper radicular s.
Usher s.
uveomeningeal s.
uveomeningoencephalic s.
vaccine-associated Guillain-Barré s.
vagoaccessory s.
vagoaccessory-hypoglossal s.
Vail s.
Van Allen s.
van der Knaap s.
vasovagal s.
velocardiofacial s.
ventral medial mesencephalic s.
Vernet s.
vertebrobasilar s.
vertebrogenic pain s.
very low density s.
VHL s.
vibration s.
Villaret s.
Villaret-Mackenzie s.
visual paraneoplastic s.
Vogt s.
Vogt-Koyanagi-Harada s.
von Hippel-Lindau s.
Waardenburg s.
Walker s.
Walker-Warburg s.
Wallenberg s.
Warburg s.
warfarin s.
Waring blender s.
wasting s.
Waterhouse-Friderichsen s.
Watson s.
Weber s.
Weber-Leyden s.
Welander s.
Wermer s.
Wernicke s.
Wernicke-Korsakoff s.
West s. (WS)
whiplash shaken infant s.
white-out s.
Wildervanck s.
Williams s.
Wilson s.

withdrawal emergent s.
Wohlfart-Kugelberg-Welander s.
Wolf-Hirschhorn s.
Wolfram s.
Wright s.
Wyburn-Mason s.
X-linked lymphoproliferative s.
XXX s.
yo-yo s.
Zellweger s.
Zinsser-Cole-Engman s.
Zollinger-Ellison s.

syndrome-related epilepsy
syndromic
s. depression
s. pattern
synencephalocele
synergia
synergic control
synergistic divergence
synergy
cervical flexor s.
gene s.
S. neurostimulation system
S. Versitrel neurostimulator
synesthesia
s. algica
auditory s.
synesthesialgia
synkinesia
synkinesis
synkinetic facial muscle
synostosis, pl. **synostoses**
coronal s.
cranial s.
lambdoid s.
metopic s.
multiple synostoses
sagittal s.
single s.
tribasilar s.
unicoronal s.
synovial
s. cyst
s. separator
synovitis
pigmented villonodular s. (PVS)
synreflexia
syntactical aphasia
syntactic manipulation
syntagmatic response
syntaxic mode
synthase
endothelial nitric oxide s.
immunologic nitric oxide s.
isoform of NO s. (iNOS)
neuronal nitric oxide s. (nNOS)
nitric oxide s. (NOS)
Synthes
S. cervical plate
S. guide pin
S. Microsystem cranial fixation plate
S. Microsystem drill bit
S. Microsystem microplate
S. screw
S. universal spinal system
synthesis, pl. **syntheses**
adenosine triphosphate s.
de novo s.
dopamine s.
fibronectin s.
Fourier s.
heme s.
illegal drug s.
intrathecal immunoglobulin s.
O-mannosyl glycan s.
protein s.
synthetase
alanyl-tRNA s.
glutathione s.
holocarboxylase s.
synthetic
s. aperture magnetometry (SAM)
s. corticotropin-releasing factor
s. intervertebral disc
s. progesterone
syphilis
cerebrospinal s.
Hutchison triad in s.
s. infection
meningeal s.
meningovascular s.
parenchymatous s.
spinal s.
syphilitic
s. amyotrophy
s. cerebral hypertrophic pachymeningitis
s. meningoencephalitis
s. meningomyelitis
s. meningovasculitis
s. myelitis
s. neuritis

S

NOTES

syphilitic *(continued)*
- s. osteonecrosis
- s. paraplegia

Syracuse
- S. anterior I-plate
- S. anterior I-plate insertion

syringeal
syringe grip
syringes (*pl. of* syrinx)
syringobulbia
syringocele
syringocephalus
syringocisternostomy
syringocystadenoma
syringoencephalia
syringoencephalomyelia
syringohydromyelia
syringoid
syringomeningocele
syringomyelia
- ape hand of s.
- cervical s.
- s. dysraphism
- secondary posttraumatic s.
- traumatic s.

syringomyelia-Chiari complex
syringomyelic
- s. cavity
- s. cord syndrome
- s. dissociation
- s. hemorrhage

syringomyelobulbia
syringomyelocele
syringomyelomeningocele
syringomyelus
syringoperitoneal shunt
syringopontia
syringosubarachnoid
- s. shunt
- s. shunting

syrinx, pl. **syringes**
- s. cavity
- s. drainage
- s. formation
- s. shunt

syrup
- Mestinon S.

system
- ABC anterior cervical plating s.
- ABC cervical plating s.
- Accusway balance measurement s.
- Acragun system
- Activa tremor control s.
- adaptive control of thought s.
- adrenergic s.
- Allen and Ferguson classification s.
- angiographic reference s.
- AngioJet rapid thrombectomy s.
- Anspach 65K instrument s.
- Anspach 65K neuro s.
- anterior Kostuik-Harrington distraction s.
- anterolateral s.
- antioxidant s.
- arc-centered guidance s.
- arc guidance s.
- arc-quadrant stereotactic s.
- arc radius s.
- Ariel computerized exercise s.
- ascending neurotransmitter s.
- ascending reticular activating s. (ARAS)
- ascending reticular arousal s.
- ASIA grading s.
- Aspen ultrasound s.
- association s.
- Atavi atraumatic spine fusion s.
- Atlantis anterior cervical plate s.
- auditory s.
- automatic positioning s.
- autonomic division of nervous s.
- autonomic nervous s. (ANS)
- autonomic part of peripheral nervous s.
- axial spinal s.
- Bactiseal antimicrobial-impregnated catheter s.
- BAK/cervical interbody fusion s.
- BAK/C interbody fusion s.
- Balance Error Scoring S.
- Balance Master-training and assessment s.
- behavior s.
- Betaseron needle-free delivery s.
- bilateral variable screw placement s.
- Biojector 2000 needle-free injection management s.
- Boston brace s.
- Boston Classification S.
- brain cooling s.
- brain dopaminergic s.
- BrainLAB VectorVision neuronavigational s.
- brain neurochemical s.
- BrainSCAN computer planning s.
- BrainSCAN LINAC radiosurgery s.
- Bremer halo crown s.
- Brown-Roberts-Wells arc s.
- Brown-Roberts-Wells stereotactic s.
- Bruker Biospec s.
- Bruker S 200 MR s.
- Bryan cervical disc s.
- Budde halo retractor s.
- Budde surgical s.
- bulbosacral s.
- 6-camera Vicon motion capture s.

Camino intracranial pressure monitoring s.
Case IV S.
CASS whole-brain mapping s.
CD Horizon Eclipse spinal s.
CD Horizon Sextant percutaneous screw-rod s.
cellular s.
central cholinergic s.
central nervous s. (CNS)
central vestibular s.
centrencephalic integrating s.
cerebrospinal s.
Cervive anterior cervical plating s.
cholinergic s.
circadian s.
classification s.
clinically relevant classification s.
CMA 600 neuromonitoring s.
CMS AccuProbe 450 s.
Coblation-based spinal surgery s.
Codman anterior cervical plate s.
Codman Bactiseal antimicrobial impregnated catheter s.
Codman neurological headrest s.
Compass arc-quadrant stereotactic s.
Compass frame-based stereotactic s.
computer-assisted image-guided s.
computer-controlled neurological stimulation s.
computer navigation s.
conceptual s.
Cordis-Hakim shunt s.
Cosman-Roberts-Wells stereotactic s.
Cotrel-Dubousset distraction s.
Cotrel-Dubousset screw-rod s.
cranial osteosynthesis s.
cranial plating s.
craniomaxillofacial plating s.
craniosacral nervous s.
Crock-Yamagishi s.
CRW arc s.
CRW stereotactic s.
C-TEK anterior cervical plate s.
C-Tek anterior cervical plate s.
CUSA CEM s.
CyberKnife planning s.
CyberKnife robotic radiosurgery s.
CyberKnife stereotactic radiosurgery/radiotherapy s.
Cygnus PFS Image-Guided s.
Das-Naglieri Cognitive Assessment S.
data acquisition s.
Daumas-Duport astrocytoma grading s.
Daumas-Duport tumor grading s.
Delis-Kaplan Executive Function S.
Developmental Observation Checklist S.
Dingman oral retraction s.
Doc ventral cervical stabilization s.
Dogbone anterior cervical plate fixation s.
dopamine s.
dopamine-modulating transmitter s.
dopaminergic s.
double-detector Vertex s.
double-donut s.
double-pore vent s.
drug risk analysis message s.
Dual Quattrode spinal cord stimulation s.
dysfunctional dopamine s.
Eagle rigid anterior cervical plate s.
EasyGuide Neuro image-guided surgery s.
EBI Array spinal s.
EBI Omega21 spinal fixation s.
Edwards modular s.
Elan-E electronic motor s.
Electri-Cool cold therapy s.
Endeavor Instructional Rating S.
endocrine s.
entorhinal-hippocampal s.
Envision anterior cervical plate s.
E9000 Power S.
Epstein staging s.
Equinox EEG neuromonitoring s.
esthesiodic s.
external support s.
exteroceptive nervous s.
exterofective s.
extracorticospinal s.
extralemniscal s.
extrapyramidal motor s.
E-Z flap cranial flap fixation s.
feedback s.
fetal cerebrovascular s.
Fielding and Hawkins classification s.
Fischer stereotaxy s.

S

NOTES

system *(continued)*
flavin-containing mono-oxygenase metabolic s.
FluoroNav virtual fluoroscopic s.
FluoroNav virtual fluoroscopy s.
fluoroptic thermometry s.
frame-based radiosurgical s.
frameless stereotaxy s.
Fränkel grading s.
Freehand neuroprosthetic s.
Galassi classification s.
gamma efferent s.
gamma motor s.
Gardner and Robertson classification s.
GE 9800 CT s.
GliaSite radiation therapy s.
glucose-6-phosphate transport s.
Golgi s.
GoodKnight 420G Nasal CPAP S.
Gordon Diagnostic S.
Greenberg retracting s.
Guglielmi detachable coil s.
Haid universal bone plate s.
Hakim programmable valve s.
Halifax interlaminar clamp s.
halo retractor s.
Hannover s.
Harrington rod and hook s.
heads-up imaging s.
Hematome s.
hemodynamic s.
hemoglobin glutamer-250[bovine] oxygen-based therapeutic s.
Hemopure oxygen-based therapeutic s.
Hermetic external ventricular drainage s.
Hermetic II drainage management s.
Hermetic lumbar drainage s.
high-force Sundt clip s.
high-resolution brain SPECT s.
s. high-speed microdrill
Hoehn and Yahr staging s.
humoral immune s.
Hunt-Hess aneurysm grading s.
hypocretin s.
hypophyseoportal s.
hypophysial portal s.
hypothalamic-pituitary s.
hypothalamic-pituitary-adrenocortical s.
hypothalamohypophysial portal s.
immune s.
incentive s.
Indiana tome carpal tunnel release s.
InFix interbody fusion s.
Innovative Magnetic Resonance Imaging S.
InstaTrak guidance s.
integrated ECT s.
interactive voice response s.
internal fixation plate-screw s.
interoceptive nervous s.
interofective s.
intraoperative neuroinvestigational s.
intraspinal drug infusion s.
Intrel II spinal cord stimulation s.
involuntary nervous s.
INVOS 3100 cerebral oximeter monitoring s.
Ionic spine spacer s.
irrigation bipolar s.
ISG Wand navigation s.
Isola spinal implant s.
isolated angiitis of central nervous s.
Itrel 3 Spinal Cord Stimulation S.
Java arthrodesis s.
juvenile justice s.
Kaneda anterior spinal s.
Kaneda anterior spinal/scoliosis s.
Kaneda SR spinal s.
K-Centrum anterior spinal fixation s.
Kelly-Goerss Compass stereotactic s.
Kelly stereotactic s.
Kernohan s.
Komet K-wire/Steinman pin and delivery tray s.
Komet Medical/Brasseler USA XK-95 high-speed drill s.
Kostuik-Harrington distraction s.
Ladd fiberoptic s.
Laitinen stereotactic s.
large-scale neural s.
lateralized brain language s.
LDD delivery s.
Legend high-speed pneumatic s.
Leibinger titanium mini-Würzburg implant s.
Leksell Micro-Stereotactic s.
lemniscal s.
Lenke scoring s.
limbic s.
LINAC-based radiosurgical s.
LINAC radiosurgery s.
linear accelerator s.
Liquid Embolic S.
Lorenz Neuro/skull base titanium osteosynthesis s.
3M Agee carpal tunnel release s.
Magellan electromagnetic navigation s.
Magerl hook-plate s.

Magerl plate-screw s.
Magnes MEG s.
Magnetom SP 4000 1.5-Tesla s.
magnocellular visual s.
malevolent thought s.
Malis CMC-III electrosurgical s.
mammalian olfactory s.
mammalian vomeronasal s.
M-2 anterior plate s.
maxillofacial plating s.
Mayfield headrest s.
Mayfield surgical s.
McGuire screw s.
medial temporal memory s.
medical value s.
Medisorb drug delivery s.
MedNext bone dissecting s.
Medtronic Midas Rex Legend s.
MEG head-based coordinate s.
memory s.
mesocortical dopaminergic s.
mesolimbic dopamine s.
metameric nervous s.
METRx s.
microcatheter s.
MicroChoice electric-powered surgical s.
microelectromechanical s. (MEMS)
microendoscopic discectomy s.
MicroGuide microelectrode recording s.
Micro-Plus titanium plating s.
Midas Rex instrumentation s.
Midas Rex Legend S.
Midas Rex power s.
mini-Würzburg implant s.
mirror s.
MKM stereotactic image-guided s.
modular implant s.
Moe s.
Monarch spinal s.
monoaminergic s.
monocular heads-up display imaging s.
Moss-Miami spinal s.
motor s.
MPM-1 multi-parameter monitoring s.
muscle tone inhibitor s.
needle trephination s.
neon occipitocervical s.
nervous s.
neural s.
NeuroCybernetic Prosthesis S. (NPS)
neurohemal s.
neuroinvestigational s.
NeuroLink II EEG data acquisition s.
Neuro-Sat frameless isocentric stereotactic s.
Neurotrend continuous multiparameter s.
Neuroview integrated visualization s.
Nicolet Viking II electrophysiologic s.
nigrostriatal dopamine s.
nigrostriatal dopaminergic s.
Nishioka s.
nonspecific s.
oculomotor s.
olfactory s.
ophthalmic s.
OPMI Vario/NC 33 s.
optical s.
Optotrak motion and position measurement s.
Oracle Delivery S.
OSI modular table s.
OSV II Smart Valve s.
Parastep I S.
parasympathetic nervous s.
PathFinder pedicle screw s.
Patil stereotactic s. II
Peak polyaxial anterior cervical fixation s.
Pelorus surgical s.
perimedullary venous s.
peripheral nervous s. (PNS)
peripheral part of nervous s.
peripheral vestibular s.
phased-array color-flow ultrasound s.
Phoenix fifth ventricle s.
photonic radiosurgical s.
photon radiosurgery s.
pituitary portal s.
plasma fibrinolytic enzyme s.
polar coordinate s.
Polaris camera s.
portal access surgical s. (PASS)
posterior rod s.
Premier anterior cervical plate s.

NOTES

system *(continued)*
pressoreceptor s.
Profile anterior plate s.
projection s.
proprioceptive nervous s.
propriospinal s.
protease-linked activation cloning s. (PLACS)
Providence scoliosis s.
Pudenz-Heyer shunt s.
Puno-Winter-Byrd s.
pursuit s.
pyramidal s.
Quantitative Scoring S.
quantitative sweat measurement s.
radiofrequency needle electrode s.
Radiofrequency Triage S. (RAFTS)
Regulus frameless stereotactic s.
Reichert stereotaxy s.
respiratory s.
Restore neurostimulation s.
reticular activating s. (RAS)
reward s.
RFG-3C radiofrequency lesion generator s.
RF needle electrode s.
robotic s.
Rogozinski spinal rod s.
SC-AcuFix Anterior Cervical Plate S.
Secor s.
SecureStrand cervical fusion s.
Sentinel s.
serotonergic s.
serotonin s.
Shiley catheter distention s.
Siemens Neurostar digital subtraction angiographic s.
Siemens Somatom Plus DCT s.
Siemens Vision s.
SilverHawk plaque excision s.
Simmons plating s.
Slim-LOC anterior cervical plate s.
SMN s.
Socon spinal s.
Sofamor-Danek stealth s.
somatic nervous s.
somesthetic s.
Songer cable s.
SonoWand intraoperative imaging s.
SonoWand ultrasound-based neuronavigation s.
specific s.
speech perception s.
Spetzler s.
Spetzler-Martin grading s.
Spiegelberg intracranial pressure monitoring s.
SpinaLase neodymium:yytrium-aluminum-garnet surgical laser s.
spinal screw and rod s.
SpineLink s.
SpineLink-II independent intrasegmental spine fixation s.
Spitz-Holter shunt s.
standard Würzburg titanium mini-plating s.
Stealth Image Guided S.
StealthStation image-interactive s.
Steffee pedicle screw-plate s.
stereotactic coordinate s.
stereotactic surgical guidance s.
Stim neuromuscular stimulation s.
Summit occipito-cervico-thoracic spinal fixation s.
Sundt AVM microclip s.
superficial siderosis of the central nervous s.
supratentorial s.
surgical microscope navigator s.
SurgiScope image-guided s.
SurgiScope stereotactic s.
sympathetic nervous s.
Symphony platelet concentrate s.
Synergy neurostimulation s.
Synthes universal spinal s.
table-fixed retractor s.
Talairach bicommissural reference s.
Talairach stereotactic s.
Talairach-Tournoux s.
Taylor and Abrams diagnostic s.
Telefactor beehive s.
Telescopic Plate Spacer spinal s.
temporolimbic s.
tesla MRI s.
Texas Scottish Rite Hospital crosslink s.
Texas Scottish Rite Hospital screw-rod s.
thermoregulatory s.
Thompson-Farley spinal retractor s.
thoracolumbar s.
thoracolumbosacroiliac implant s.
Thoracoport trocar s.
TiMesh LP cranial miniplate and screw s.
TiMesh titanium bone plating s.
TiMX low back s.
titanium alloy screw and rod s.
titanium hollow screw plate s.
titanium micro s.
1.5T Philips Intera-NT s.
transdermal methylphenidate s.
transmitter s.
Trinity polyaxial pedicle screw s.
TS s.

TSRH universal spinal instrumentation s.
1.5 T superconducting s.
ubiquitin-proteosome s. (UPS)
UltraPower basic drill s.
UltraPower bur guard drill s.
UltraPower revision drill s.
UltraPower surgical drill s.
unilateral variable screw placement s.
Universal bone screw insertion/extraction s.
Universal cannulated screw s.
Valleylab CUSA CEM s.
value s.
valve s.
variable screw placement s.
VariGrip spine fixation s.
VectorVision image-guided surgery s.
vegetative nervous s.
VenaFlow compression s.
venous s.
Ventrix fiberoptic ventricular drainage s.
Ventrix fiberoptic ventricular monitoring s.
Ventrix tunnelable ventricular ICP monitoring and drainage s.
Ventrix tunnelable ventricular intracranial pressure monitoring s.
vergence s.
VertAlign spinal support s.
vertebrobasilar s.
Vertex reconstruction s.
vestibular s.
Viewing Wand image guided s.
viral vector s.
visceral nervous s.
visual s.
V-tunnel drill s.
VueLock anterior cervical spine s.
VuePASS portal access surgical s.
welfare s.
wet bipolar s.
whole-cortex MEG/EEG s.
Wiltse s.
Winquist tibial/femoral extraction s.
Würzburg implant s.
Würzburg titanium plating s.
Xia hook s.
Xia spinal s.
XK-PRO100 high-speed drill s.
X-Trel spinal cord stimulation s.
ZD stereotactic s.
Zeiss Image Guided S.
Zeiss stereotactic tool navigator s.
Zephir anterior cervical plate s.
Zeppelin micro-motor s.
Z-plate fixation s.

systema, pl. **systemata**
s. nervosum
s. nervosum autonomicum
s. nervosum centrale
s. nervosum periphericum

systematic
s. drug administration
s. family therapy
s. followup
s. vertigo

systematis
pars abdominalis s.

systemic
s. chemotherapy
s. giant cell disorder
s. impact
s. inflammatory disease
s. lupus erythematosus (SLE)
s. mastocytosis
s. multifocal fibrosclerosis
s. myelitis
s. myelopathy
s. neoplastic disease
s. sclerosis
s. vasculature
s. vasculitis

System-Loc back brace

NOTES

T
T cell
T fiber
T myelotomy
T ratio
T regulatory cell
T score
T1
T1 hypointense lesion
T1 relaxation
T1 relaxation constant
T1 weighting
T2
T2 hyperintense lesion
T2 relaxation
T2 relaxation constant
T2 relaxation rate
T2 shortening
T2 weighting
T_4
thyroxine
tabes
t. diabetica
t. dorsalis
t. ergotica
Friedreich t.
peripheral t.
t. spasmodica
t. spinalis
tabetic
t. arthropathy
t. crisis
t. cuirass
t. dissociation
t. gait
t. mask
t. neurosyphilis
t. otalgia
t. pain
tabetiform
table
activator t.
American Sterilizer operating t.
Jackson spine t.
T-shaped Edwards-Barbaro syringeal shunt t.
table-fixed retractor system
tablet
20-20 t.
357 HR Magnum t.
Koala Pad graphics t.
Overtime t.
taboparalysis
taboparesis
tabula interna
tabulation
allophone t.
Tac
T. gel for EMS unit
T. gel for TENS unit
tache
t. cerebrale
t. motrice
t. spinale
tachistoscopic constant reading test
tachistoscopy viewing
tachykinin
tachyphemia
tachyphylaxis
tacking suture
tacrine HCl
tacrolimus
Tacticon peripheral neuropathy screening device
tactile
t. agnosia
t. alexia
t. amnesia
t. anesthesia
t. anomia
t. aphasia
t. bisection task
t. cell
t. corpuscle
t. disc
t. hallucination
t. hyperesthesia
t. image
t. meniscus
t. naming test
t. organ
t. pain
t. perception test
t. performance test
t. receptor
t. sense
t. stimulation
t. stimulus
t. transfer deficit
tactile-kinesthetic training
tactometer
tact operant
tactus
corpuscula t.
corpusculum t.
meniscus t.
organum t.
taenia
t. choroidea
t. pontis

taenia *(continued)*
T. solium
t. tela
t. thalami
taeniae acusticae
taeniola
t. corporis callosi
t. corporis callosi of Reil
taftian therapy
Tag complex
tail
acetylcholinesterase collagen t.
t. of caudate nucleus
t. of dentate gyrus
dural t.
embryonic t.
tailor's
t. cramp
t. spasm
Takayasu
T. arteritis
T. arteritis vasculitis
T. disease
Talairach
T. bicommissural reference system
T. space
T. stereotactic frame
T. stereotactic system
T. whole-brain mapping
Talairach-Tournoux system
talampanel
talipes
talipexole
talking
sleep t.
Talma disease
talocalcaneal
anteroposterior t.
tamoxifen therapy
tamp
KyphX Xpander inflatable bone t.
Richards t.
tampon
Merocel t.
TAN
tropical ataxic neuropathy
tandem
t. clipping technique
t. connector
t. double mutation
tangential
t. incision
t. nerve fiber
t. neurofiber
tangentiales
tangent screen examination
Tangier
T. disease
T. peripheral neuropathy
tangle
t. fragment
intraneural neurofibrillary t.
intraneuronal fibrillary t.
neocortical neurofibrillary t.
neurofibrillary t.
tannate
vasopressin t.
tantalum
t. ball
t. cranioplasty
t. mesh
t. powder contrast agent
t. preformed skull plate
tanycyte
tap
bloody t.
front t.
glabellar t.
heel t.
shunt t.
spinal t.
subdural t.
traumatic t.
tape
Mersiline t.
taper
double t.
slow double t.
tapered
t. blade
t. brain spatula
tapering
drug t.
medication t.
tapetum
t. corporis callosi
t. nigrum
t. oculi
Tapia
T. syndrome
T. vagohypoglossal palsy
tapir
bouche de t.
t. mouth
tapping
foot t.
t. memory
TaqMan assay
Tarasoff principle
tarbagan
Tarbell-Loeffler-Cosman frame
Tarceva
tarda
epilepsia t.
neurosis t.
tardive
t. dystonia
t. movement

t. myoclonus
t. oral dyskinesia
t. orobuccal dyskinesia
t. tic
t. tremor

tardy
t. epilepsy
t. median palsy
t. ulnar nerve palsy

target
t. acquisition
brain t.
bullying t.
t. localization
t. localization error
t. population
t. rash
t. registration error (TRE)
retinofugal t.
rostral subcortical t.
striatal t.
therapeutic t.
t. velocity
t. weight

targeted
t. approach
t. brain biopsy
t. intervention

targeting
angiographic t.
multiple t.

targetry
angiographic t.

Tarin
T. fascia
T. recess
T. space
T. tenia
T. valve

tarini
valvula semilunaris t.
velum t.

Tarinus valve

Tarlov cyst

tarsal
t. tunnel
t. tunnel syndrome

tarsophalangeal reflex

tarsorrhaphy
bilateral temporary t.'s
lateral t.

tartrate
butorphanol t.
ergotamine t.
levallorphan t.
metoprolol t.
rivastigmine t.
thorium t.
zolpidem t.

Tarui disease

task
antisaccade t.
auditory continuous performance t.
auditory responsive naming t.
auditory word/nonword discrimination t.
chronometric and force generation t.
cognitive t.
complex t.
developmental t.
dot-probe t.
finger-tapping t.
handgrip t.
t.'s of independent living
light-prompted button t.
memory t.
motor control t.
negative priming t.
neuropsychologically relevant t.
nonverbal tactile attention t.
novel memory t.
novel recall t.
occupational lifting t.
oculomotor delayed-response t.
t. paradigm
t. performance
practiced t.
repetitive lifting t.
secondary cognitive t.
self-care t.
semantic decision t.
sequencing t.
short-term memory t.
Simon t.
somatosensory cued t.
speech tracking t.
2-stimuli t.
Stroop Color-Word Interference T.
tactile bisection t.
theory of mind t.
time reproduction t.
transitive inference t.

NOTES

task *(continued)*
verbal memory encoding t.
visually guided pointing t. (VGPT)
visual object-naming t.
work-related t.
task-accuracy
continuous performance t.-a.
task-efficiency
continuous performance t.-e.
tasking
dual t.
task-specific tremor
taste
t. blindness
t. bud
t. cell
t. change
color t.
t. corpuscle
t. disorder
t. distinction
franklinic t.
t. hair
organ of t.
t. pore
t. quality perception
t. quality recognition
t. receiving area
t. sense
t. stimulus
taste-responsive neuron
TAT
thematic apperception test
tau
fetal t.
t. gene
hyperphosphorylated t.
t. phosphorylation
t. processing
t. protein
tau-negative nerve cell
taurine detection
tautological
tautology
tautomeral cell
tautomeric fiber
taxonomic research
Taylor
T. and Abrams diagnostic system
T. brain scissors
T. complex figure task performance
T. dural scissors
T. halter device
occipital cortical dysplasia of T.
T. percussion hammer
T. retractor
T. series linearization method
Tay-Sachs
T.-S. disease
T.-S. disease screening
TBI
traumatic brain injury
^{99m}Tc
technetium-99m
^{99m}Tc HMPAO SPECT
^{99m}Tc HMPAO T/C ratio
Tc-99m HMPAO cerebral perfusion SPECT imaging
TCA
tricarboxylic acid
TCB
transcallosal band
TCC
traditional circulatory criteria
TCD
transcranial Doppler
TCD probe
TCD pulsatility index
TCD recanalization
TCD sonography
TCD ultrasound
TCDB
trauma coma databank
T-cell
T-c. alpha chemoattractant (ITAC)
T-c. function
^{99m}Tc-hexamethylpropyleneamine oxime
TcHIDA
^{99m}Tc-HMPAO
^{99m}Tc-HMPAO leukocyte scintigram
^{99m}Tc-HMPAO leukocyte scintigraphy
^{99m}Tc HMPAO SPECT imaging
TCI
transient cognitive impairment
TCOF1 gene
TCT
transcallosal conduction time
TE
echo time
toxoplasmic encephalitis
Te
effective half time
tellurium
tear
anular t.
dural t.
intraoperative dural t.
teardrop
t. dissector
t. fracture
tearing
short-lasting unilateral neuralgiform headache with conjunctival injection and t.

short-lasting unilateral neuralgiform pain with conjunctival injecting and t. (SUNCT)
Teasdale and Jennett scale
teboroxime
technetium-99m t.
Teca Sapphire EMG machine
Techneplex
technetium
t. albumin colloid
t. etidronate
t. stannous pyrophosphate
^{99m}technetium
technetium-99m (99mTc, ^{99m}Tc)
t.-99m albumin aggregated
t.-99m bicisate
t.-99m disofenin
t.-99m ferpentetate
t.-99m furifosmin
t.-99m gluceptate
t.-99m HIDA
t.-99m iron-ascorbate-DTPA
t.-99m lidofenin
t.-99m macroaggregated albumin
t.-99m medronate
t.-99m mertiatide
t.-99m oxidronate
t.-99m pertechnetate sodium
t.-99m PIPIDA
t.-99m pyrophosphate
t.-99m sestamibi
t.-99m siboroxime
t.-99m succimer
t.-99m sulfur colloid
t.-99m teboroxime
t.-99m tetrofosmin
technique
Abbott fluorescence polarization immunoassay t.
active t.
advanced imaging t.
Agee t.
angiographic road-mapping t.
Arana-Iniquez intracranial cyst removal t.
Asher physical build assessment t.
avidin-biotin stain t.
Barbour t.
Bayesian t.
biportal t.
blood oxygenation level-dependent contrast t.
Bohlman cervical fusion t.
boost irradiation t.
Brooks t.
Brown-Roberts-Wells t.
carotid preservation t.
cervical screw insertion t.
cervical spondylotic myelopathy fusion t.
chaining t.
chromosomal banding t.
clinical monitoring t.
Cloward t.
Cobb t.
cognitive t.
composite addition t.
Cone-Grant t.
continuous-wave t.
contoured anterior spinal plate t.
cooling t.
Cushing t.
CyberKnife t.
decortication t.
destructive interference t.
direct screw fixation t.
Dolenc t.
double-rod t.
Drake tandem clipping t.
drilling t.
Drummond spinous wiring t.
effective t.
electroencephalogram BEAM t.
electroencephalogram brain electrical activity method t.
endovascular t.
entubulation t.
ex vivo t.
facet excision t.
fast gradient recalled spectroscopic imaging t.
fat-suppression t.
fiber dissection t.
finger fracture t.
fixation t.
flow detection t.
Fourier transform t.
frameless stereotactic t.
functional imaging t.
fusion t.
Gallie-Rodgers t.
Gallie wiring t.
gradient-recalled echo t.
Håkanson t.

NOTES

technique *(continued)*
Halstead modified t.
Harms t.
Harriluque t.
Hartel t.
Hirsch endonasal t.
homogenate t.
Hood masking t.
Hunt-Early t.
hyperventilation activating t.
immunoelectrotransfer blot t.
immunohistochemical t.
implantation t.
interspinous segmental spinal instrumentation t.
intravenous oxygen-15 water bolus t.
ipsilateral transcallosal t.
Jacobs locking hook spinal rod t.
Kennerdell-Maroon t.
Lamaze t.
Leksell t.
loss-of-resistance t.
Luque instrumentation concave t.
Luque instrumentation convex t.
Luque sublaminar wiring t.
macroelectrode t.
mandibular swing t.
Meyer sublaminar wiring t.
microsurgical t.
midface degloving t.
Mille Pattes t.
mini-open t.
t. of Miyazaki and Kato
modified Gilsbach t.
molecular diagnostic t.
monitoring t.
morphometric t.
multivariate t.
multivoxel t.
nerve substitution t.
noninvasive imaging t.
O-PET t.
Ouchterlony double-diffusion t.
percutaneous assisted t.
PET t.
phase-contrast t.
photic stimulation activating t.
picture-in-picture t.
polymerase chain reaction t.
positron emission tomography t.
posterolateral costotransversectomy t.
postmortem t.
preservation t.
pressure distension t.
pull-test t.
Q-sort t.
quantitative morphometric t.
radiosurgical t.
recombinant DNA t.
reduction t.
Reichert-Mundinger t.
rigid internal fixation t.
Roy-Camille t.
screw insertion t.
Seldinger retrograde wire/intubation t.
sensorineural acuity level masking t.
single-voxel t.
sleep t.
Smith-Robinson t.
Spiller-Frazier t.
spinal fusion t.
spinopelvic transiliac fixation t.
squeeze t.
state-of-the-art analysis t.
stereotactic t.
STIF t.
stop-start t.
stroboscopic light activating t.
strut fusion t.
subtraction t.
surgical t.
tandem clipping t.
terminal deoxynucleotide transferase-mediated nick end-labeling t.
thin-slab acquisition t.
thoracolumbar spondylosis surgical t.
tilted optimized nonsaturating excitation t.
time-of-flight t.
Todd-Wells t.
transcortical t.
transfemoral artery t.
triple-wire t.
vagus nerve stimulation t.
in vivo t.
Whitesides-Kell cervical t.
whole-cell patch clamp t.
wire removal t.
^{133}Xe intravenous injection t.

technology
Cogent microillumination t.
EBI V-Force thread t.
information t.
minimal access spinal t. (MAST)
NeuroMate robotic t.
wafer t.
work evaluation systems t.
Zydis drug delivery t.

tecta (*pl. of* tectum)

tectal
t. germinoma
t. glioma
t. lesion
t. lipoma

t. nucleus
t. plate
t. plate tumor
t. stria
tecti
lamina t.
nucleus t.
tectobulbaris
tractus t.
tectobulbar tract
tectocerebellar
t. dysraphism
t. tract
tectoolivares
fibrae t.
tectoolivary fiber
tectopontinae
fibrae t.
tectopontine
t. fiber
t. tract
tectopontinus
tractus t.
tectoreticulares
fibrae t.
tectoreticular fiber
tectospinal
t. decussation
t. tract
tectospinalis
tractus t.
tectum, pl. **tecta**
beaked t.
lamina of mesencephalic t.
t. mesencephali
t. of midbrain
optic t.
stria t.
tenia t.
teddy bear gait
teeth grinding
teeth-grinding event
Teflon
T. mesh
T. mesh reinforcement
T. tube graft
Teflon-coated brain retractor
tegmen
t. cruris
t. ventriculi quarti
tegmenta (*pl. of* tegmentum)
tegmental
t. decussation
t. field of Forel
t. glioma
t. mesencephalic paralysis
t. pedunculopontine reticular nucleus
t. radiation
t. reticular formation
t. syndrome
t. tract
tegmenti
nuclei t.
tractus centralis t.
tegmentospinal tract
tegmentotomy
tegmentum, pl. **tegmenta**
lateral dorsal t.
t. mesencephali
mesencephalic t.
midbrain t.
t. of midbrain
pedunculopontine t.
t. of pons
pontine t.
t. pontis
t. rhombencephali
rhombencephalic t.
t. of rhombencephalon
rostral t.
rostral-central t.
subthalamic t.
ventral t.
Tegner score
Tegopen
Tegretol
teichopsia
Tektronix 2214 oscilloscope
tela, pl. **telae**
t. choroidea
t. choroidea of fourth ventricle
t. choroidea inferior
t. choroidea of lateral ventricle
t. choroidea superior
t. choroidea of third ventricle
t. choroidea ventriculi lateralis
t. choroidea ventriculi quarti
t. choroidea ventriculi tertii
tenia telae
t. vasculosa
telalgia

NOTES

telangiectasia
calcinosis, Raynaud phenomenon, esophageal motility disorders, sclerodactyly, and t. (CREST)
capillary t.
cephalooculocutaneous t.
hereditary hemorrhagic t.
telangiectasis, pl. **telangiectases**
telangiectatic
t. angiomatosis
t. change
t. discectomy vessel
t. glioma
telangiectodes
glioma t.
neuroma t.
Telebrix
teleceptive
teledendrite
teledendron
Telefactor beehive system
telegraphic speech
telemetric intracranial pressure sensor
telemetry
closed-circuit television electroencephalographic t.
telencephali
fasciculus medialis t.
fibrae commissurales t.
telencephalic
t. flexure
t. vein
t. ventriculofugal artery
t. vesicle
telencephalization
telencephalon
teleneurite
teleneuron
teleopsia
Telepaque
telepresence surgery
teleradiotherapy unit
telereceptor
telergy
telescope
High-Vision surgical t.
Luxtec illuminated surgical t.
Surgi-Spec t.
telescopic
t. plate spacer
T. Plate Spacer spinal system
telesensor
in-line t.
Osaka t.
Telestill photo adapter
televised
t. radiofluoroscopic control
t. radiofluoroscopy
television-induced epilepsy
telltale sign
tellurium (Te)
telodendria
telodendron
teloglia
teloreceptor
telovelotonsillar
temazepam
temerity
Temodar
temozolomide
temperature
core t.
elevated core t.
t. fluctuation
intracranial pressure-t. (ICP-T)
t. irritation
repetitive temporalis muscle t.
t. sense
t. spot
temporalis muscle t.
temperature-sensitive neural progenitor
Tempium
template
Damasio and Damasio t.
diagnostic t.
Marchac forehead t.
Temple-Fay laminectomy retractor
temporal
t. arachnoid cyst
t. arteritis
t. artery
t. artery biopsy
t. bone
t. bone-jugular incisure
t. characteristic
t. cortex
t. cortex damage
t. course
t. craniotomy
t. dispersion
t. dynamic
t. fossa
t. fossa floor
t. gyrus
t. headache
t. horn
t. horn atrophy
t. horn neoplasm
left planum t.
t. lobe
t. lobe abscess
t. lobe atrophy
t. lobectomy
t. lobe dysfunction
t. lobe epilepsy
t. lobe herniation
t. lobe impairment
t. lobe infarction

t. lobe metabolism
t. lobe radiation
t. lobe retraction
t. lobe seizure
t. lobe tumor
medial superior t.
t. neocortical association area
t. nerve
t. operculum
t. pattern
t. pole
t. pole of cerebrum
t. processing
t. processing acuity (TPA)
t. resection
t. slowing
t. speech region
t. stability
t. tissue

temporal-cerebral arterial anastomosis

temporale
operculum t.
planum t.

temporalis
impressio trigeminalis ossis t.
incisura jugularis ossis t.
lobus t.
t. muscle
t. muscle temperature
polus t.
processus intrajugularis ossis t.
Tutoplast fascia t.

temporary
t. clip
t. edema
t. percutaneous SCS electrode
t. personality disorder

temporofrontal tract

temporolimbic
t. area
t. epilepsy
t. system

temporomandibular
t. joint (TMJ)
t. joint arthralgia
t. joint dislocation

temporomesial region

temporooccipital craniotomy

temporoparietal
t. aphasia
t. association area
t. defect
t. hypoperfusion
t. junction (TPJ)

temporopolar artery (TPA)

temporopontinae
fibrae t.

temporopontine
t. fiber
t. tract

temporopontinus
tractus t.

temporospatial orientation disturbance

temporosuboccipital bone graft

TEN
toxic epidermal necrolysis

tendency
autism t.
cognitive t.
dissociative t.

tender
t. line
t. point
t. zone

tenderness
midline cervical t.

tendineus

tendinum
subsultus t.
tremor t.

tendo Achillis reflex

tendon
t. jerk
t. reaction
t. reflex
t. spindle
Tutoplast anterior tibialis t.

tendril fiber

tenebric vertigo

tenia, pl. **teniae**
t. choroidea
t. fimbriae
t. fornicis
t. of fourth ventricle
t. hippocampi
medullary teniae
t. semicircularis
Tarin t.
t. tectum
t. telae
t. terminalis
t. thalami
thalamic t.

NOTES

T

tenia *(continued)*
 t. ventriculi quarti
 t. ventriculi tertii
Ten-K
tenoreceptor
Tenoretic
tenosynovectomy
tenoxicam
tensa
 pars t.
tensile stress
Tensilon
 T. Injection
 T. test
tensiometer
tension
 carbon dioxide t.
 conjugal t.
 t. hydrocephalus
 oxygen t.
 t. pneumocephalus
 t. suture
 t. vascular headache
tension-type headache
tensor
 t. tympani
 t. tympani nerve
 t. veli palatini
 t. veli palatini nerve
tentalum wire tension suture
tenth cranial nerve [CN X]
tentorial
 t. angle
 t. apex meningioma
 t. draining group
 t. herniation
 t. hiatus
 t. incisura
 t. incisure
 t. leaf meningioma
 t. nerve
 t. plexus
 t. pressure
 t. ring
 t. sinus
 t. surface
 t. traversal
tentorii
 incisura t.
tentorium
 cerebellar t.
 t. cerebelli
 t. of hypophysis
 notch of t.
Tenuate Dospan
tenuis
 meninx t.
TEP
 trigeminal evoked potential
Tepanil
tephromalacia
tephrylometer
Tepper proprioceptor simulator
teratogenicity
 neurobehavioral t.
teratoid-rhabdoid tumor
teratoid tumor
teratoma
 atypical t.
 hCG-secreting suprasellar immature t.
 immature t.
 malignant t.
 mature t.
 pineal region t.
 sacrococcygeal t.
 spinal t.
terbutaline
terebrating pain
teres
 eminentia t.
 funiculus t.
 t. major muscle
terete eminence
terfenadine
terminal
 t. anoxia
 axon t.
 t. bouton
 cerebrocortical nerve t.
 t. cognitive decline
 t. cylinder
 t. deoxynucleotide transferase-mediated nick end-labeling
 t. deoxynucleotide transferase-mediated nick end-labeling technique
 t. deoxynucleotidyl transferase-mediated dUTP nick end-labeling staining
 t. filament
 t. filum
 t. ganglion
 t. hydrolase
 hypolemmal nerve t.
 t. insomnia
 t. latency
 motor nerve t.
 t. myelocystocele
 t. nerve
 t. nerve corpuscle
 neurohypophysial nerve t.
 t. nucleus
 t. organ
 t. plate
 presynaptic t.
 t. region
 t. stria

synaptic t.
t. thread
t. vein
t. ventricle
t. ventriculostomy

terminale
corpusculum nervosum t.
dural part of filum t.
filum t.
ganglion t.
pial part of filum t.
velum t.

terminales
nuclei t.

terminalia
corpuscula nervosa t.

terminalis
bed nucleus of stria t.
cisterna laminae t.
cistern of lamina t.
conus t.
fibrae striae t.
lamina t. (LT)
nervus t.
nucleus striae t.
organum vasculosum laminae t.
pars duralis fili t.
pars pialis fili t.
primitive lamina t.
stria t.
tenia t.
vascular organ of lamina t.
vena t.
ventriculus t.

termination
diet t.

terminationes nervorum liberae

terminationis
nuclei t.
nucleus t.

terra firma

terreus
Aspergillus t.

terror
anticholinergic for night t.
night t.

Terson syndrome

tertiary neuron lesion

tertii
plexus choroideus ventriculi t.
ramus choroidei ventriculi t.
stria ventriculi t.
tela choroidea ventriculi t.
tenia ventriculi t.

tertius
nervus occipitalis t.
ventriculus t.

TES
threshold electrical stimulation

tesla MRI system

TESS
Tirilazad Efficacy Stroke Study

Tessier osteotomy

test
ability t.
Action Research Arm t.
AD7C cerebrospinal fluid t.
ADL t.
adrenaline-Mecholyl t.
Adson t.
air conduction t.
Alcock t.
Allen t.
alpha t.
alternate binaural loudness balance t.
amobarbital t.
ancillary t.
Animal Naming t.
Annett t.
Anstie t.
anti-GM_1 antibody t.
antimicrobial susceptibility t.
antinuclear antibody t.
axial manual traction t.
axon reflex t.
Ayer t.
Ayer-Tobey t.
Babinski t.
balloon occlusion t.
Bankson Language T. 2
Bárány pointing t.
baseline t.
Bechterew t.
Bender Gestalt Visual Motor t.
Benton Naming t.
Benton Visual Retention T. (BVRT)
Bero t.
Bielschowsky head tilt t.
binaural distorted speech t.
blind t.
Bloomer Learning t.
Boston Naming t.

NOTES

test *(continued)*
Box and Block timed manipulation t.
Bragard sign t.
bromocriptine t.
Buschke Free and Cued Selective Reminding T.
Buschke-Fuld Selective Memory t.
caloric t.
Canadian Cognitive Abilities T., Form 7
cardiac function t.
Carrow Auditory-Visual Abilities t.
category fluency t.
7C Gold t.
clock drawing t.
Cognitive Abilities T., Form 5
complement fixation antibody t.
Contextual Memory t.
Continuous Performance t. (CPT)
contralateral straight leg raising t.
Controlled Oral Word Association t.
Coombs t.
corroborative t.
countercurrent immunoelectrophoresis t.
cover t.
CO_2-withdrawal seizure t.
craniocervical flexion t.
C-reactive protein t.
creative reasoning t.
Crithidia IFA t.
Cross-Cultural Smell Identification t.
Crossing-Off t.
cryptococcal polysaccharide antigen t.
Culture Fair Intelligence t.
deductive reasoning t.
Delayed List Recall t.
Denver-II Developmental screening t.
dexamethasone suppression t.
Deyerle sciatic tension t.
Discourse Comprehension t.
Dix-Hallpike t.
Dunnett t.
Ebbinghaus t.
edrophonium chloride t.
electrophysiologic t.
electrophysiology t.
ELISA t.
Elsberg t.
excitability t.
eye blink conditioning t.
femoral nerve stretch t.
ferritin t.
finger-nose t.
finger tapping t.
finger-to-finger t.
finger-to-nose t.
Fisher exact t.
fluorescent treponemal antibody absorption t.
forced choice of recognition t.
Frenchay Aphasia Screening t.
F-wave t.
Gaenslen t.
gag reflex t.
Galveston Orientation and Awareness t.
glycerol t.
Goldscheider t.
grip-strength t.
Guthrie t.
Hallpike t.
Halstead-Wepman Aphasia Screening t.
Hammill Multiability Achievement t.
Hand Dynamometer t.
Hand T., Revised 1983
Harding W87 t.
Hausa Speaking t.
head-dropping t.
head impulse t.
head-thrust t.
heel-knee t.
heel-knee-shin t.
heel-tap t.
heel-to-knee-to-toe t.
heel-to-shin t.
Hendler t.
Hess screen t.
Hirschberg t.
Hollander t.
Holter monitor t.
homovanillic acid t.
Hopkins Verbal Learning t.
H-wave t.
hyperventilation t.
incomplete-sentence t.
insulin hypoglycemia t.
internal carotid balloon t.
intrathecal infusion t.
ischemic forearm exercise t. (IFET)
isoproterenol tilt table t.
Janet t.
Jolly t.
Katzman t.
Kennedy disease t.
Kernig t.
Krimsky t.
Kruskal-Wallis t.
Kruskal-Wallis H t.
Kveim t.
labyrinthine fistula t.

Lasègue t.
latex particle agglutination t.
L-dopa stimulation t.
leg-raising t.
letter fluency t.
Liddle dexamethasone suppression t.
lidocaine t.
Linder t.
liver function t.
Lombard voice-reflex t.
Maintenance of Wakefulness T. (MWT)
Mann-Whitney t.
Mann-Whitney U t.
Mantoux interdermal tuberculin skin t.
Matas t.
Matching to Simple t.
Maze t.
melatonin t.
mental alternation t.
MES t.
metyrapone t.
MFD t.
microhemagglutination-*Treponema pallidum* t.
Miller-Fisher t.
M'Naghten t.
modified Benton Visual Retention t.
morphine-naloxone t.
multiple sleep latency t. (MSLT)
Naffziger t.
neostigmine t.
neuroendocrine t.
neuropsychologic t.
Newman-Keuls t.
Nine-Hole Peg t.
nose spray t.
Nymox urinary t.
oculocephalic t.
Paced Auditory Serial Addition t.
Pachon t.
palmomental t.
Patrick t.
perceptual identification t.
Phalen t.
pointing t.
post hoc t.
Proetz t.
projective t.
prone straight leg raising t.
Prostigmin t.
psychologic t.
pull t.
Q t.
quantitative functional t.
quantitative sensory t. (QST)
Quantitative Sudomotor Axon Reflex T. (Q-SART)
Queckenstedt t.
Queckenstedt-Stookey t.
Quick neurological screening t.
recognition t.
Recognition Memory T. (RMT)
Rey Auditory Verbal Learning t.
right and wrong t.
Rinne t.
Romberg t.
rose bengal t.
RPR t.
Sabin-Feldman dye t.
Schilling t.
Schirmer t.
Schlichter t.
Schwabach t.
Seashore t.
Selective Reminding t.
Self-Ordered Pointing T.
Shapiro-Wilk t.
smell identification t.
sniff t.
spasticity vertical suspension t.
spatial span t.
Spearman rank correlation coefficient t.
speech discrimination t.
Speech-Sounds Perception T.
sphenopalatine t.
Spurling t.
Stagnara wake-up t.
stamp t.
standard laboratory t.
station t.
stem-completion t.
t. stimulus
straight leg raising t.
Stroop Color-Word t.
Student-Newman-Keuls t.
subcutaneous pentylenetetrazol seizure t.
sweating t.
swinging flashlight t.
tachistoscopic constant reading t.

T

NOTES

test *(continued)*
tactile naming t.
tactile perception t.
tactile performance t.
Tensilon t.
thematic apperception t. (TAT)
thenar weakness t.
thermoregulatory sweat t.
thyroid function t.
tilt-table t.
Timed Tandem Walk t.
Timed Up and Go t.
Tobey-Ayer t.
transmission disequilibrium t.
Treponema pallidum immobilization t.
Tukey t.
tuning fork t.
tyramine challenge t.
University of Pennsylvania Smell t.
VDRL t.
Venereal Disease Research Laboratory t.
vertical suspension t.
very short Minnesota differential aphasia t.
von Frey t.
Wada memory t.
Waddell t.
Warrington Recognition Memory t.
Watson-Schwartz t.
Weber t.
Weinstein Enhanced Sensory t.
Western blot t.
Wilcoxon rank sum t.
3-word recall t.
X-O t.
Benton Visual Form Discrimination T.

tester
Komet medical battery t.
West hand and foot nerve t.

testicular
t. atrophy
t. compression reflex
t. insufficiency

testing
adult Wada t.
Amsler grid t.
autoantibody assay t.
bedside t.
biomechanical t.
caloric t.
cerebellar aggregation culture for teratogenicity t.
cognitive t.
conduction t.
confrontation t.
continuous cognitive t.
coordination t.
corneal reflex t.
Diamox challenge t.
electrodiagnostic t.
electrophysiologic t.
eye movement t.
flexion reflex t.
genetic t.
head-up tilt t.
hypoglossal nerve t.
intraarterial Amytal t.
intracarotid amobarbital t.
intracarotid sodium Amytal memory t.
isokinetic dynamometric t.
Medical Research Council scale for strength t.
metabolic t.
molecular t.
multiple-choice t.
neuropsychologic t.
pediatric Wada t.
post hoc t.
provocative t.
random urine t.
reflex t.
urine t.
visual field t.
Wada language lateralization t.
Wada language and memory t.

testobulbar tract
testosterone enanthate
testosterone-estradiol-binding globulin
test-revised
National Adult Reading T.-r.

Tesuloid
tetani
Clostridium t.

tetania
t. epidemica
t. gastrica
t. gravidarum
t. parathyreopriva
t. rheumatica

tetanic
t. contraction
t. convulsion
t. spasm
t. stimulation

tetaniform
tetanigenous
tetanism
tetanization
tetanize
tetanoid
t. chorea
t. paraplegia

tetanometer
tetanomotor

tetanospasmin
tetanus
t. anticus
t. antitoxin
apyretic t.
benign t.
cephalic t.
cerebral t.
complete t.
t. completus
t. dorsalis
drug t.
extensor t.
flexor t.
generalized t.
head t.
hydrophobic t.
imitative t.
intermittent t.
local t.
neonatal t.
t. neonatorum
physiologic t.
t. posticus
Ritter opening t.
toxic t.
t. toxoid
traumatic t.
tetany
t. of alkalosis
duration t.
epidemic t.
gastric t.
hyperventilation t.
hypoparathyroid t.
infantile t.
latent t.
manifest t.
neonatal t.
parathyroid t.
parathyroprival t.
postoperative t.
rheumatic t.
symptomatic t.
tethered
t. conus medullaris
t. spinal cord
t. spinal cord syndrome
tetrabenazine
tetrabromophenolphthalein
tetrad
classic narcolepsy t.
narcoleptic t.
tetrahydroaminoacridine
tetrahydrobiopterin metabolism
tetrahydrocannabinol
tetrahydronaphthalene
tetrahydropyridine
tetraiodophenolphthalein
tetraparalysis
tetraparesis
tetrapeptide
cholecystokinin t. (CCK-4)
tetraplegia
tetraplegic
tetrathiomolybdate
ammonium t.
tetrodotoxin (TTX)
tetrofosmin
technetium-99m t.
Tew cranial spinal retractor
Texas
T. Scottish Rite Hospital (TSRH)
T. Scottish Rite Hospital buttressed laminar hook
T. Scottish Rite Hospital circular laminar hook
T. Scottish Rite Hospital corkscrew device
T. Scottish Rite Hospital crosslink
T. Scottish Rite Hospital crosslink system
T. Scottish Rite Hospital double-rod construct
T. Scottish Rite Hospital eyebolt spreader
T. Scottish Rite Hospital hook holder
T. Scottish Rite Hospital hook inserter
T. Scottish Rite Hospital I-bolt
T. Scottish Rite Hospital instrumentation
T. Scottish Rite Hospital mini-corkscrew device
T. Scottish Rite Hospital pedicle hook
T. Scottish Rite Hospital pedicle screw
T. Scottish Rite Hospital rod fixation

T

NOTES

Texas *(continued)*
T. Scottish Rite Hospital screw-rod system
T. Scottish Rite Hospital trial hook
T. Scottish Rite Hospital wrench
text blindness
TFC
threaded fusion cage
Ray TFC
TFNE
transient focal neurologic event
6TG
6-thioguanine
TGA
transient global amnesia
TGF
transforming growth factor
T-group
TH1
TH1 cell
TH1 cytokine
TH2
TH2 cell
TH2 cytokine
thalamectomy
thalamencephalic
thalamencephalon
thalami
laminae medullares t.
nuclei anteriores t.
nuclei dorsales t.
nuclei intralaminares t.
nuclei mediales t.
nuclei paraventriculares t.
nuclei posteriores t.
nuclei pulvinares t.
nuclei ventrales t.
nuclei ventrales laterales t.
nuclei ventrales mediales t.
nucleus anterodorsalis t.
nucleus anteroinferior t.
nucleus anteromedialis t.
nucleus anterosuperior t.
nucleus anteroventralis t.
nucleus arcuatus t.
nucleus centralis lateralis t.
nucleus centralis medialis t.
nucleus centromedianus t.
nucleus dorsalis lateralis t.
nucleus lateralis dorsalis t.
nucleus medialis centralis t.
nucleus paracentralis t.
nucleus parafascicularis t.
nucleus reticularis t.
nucleus reticulatus t.
nucleus ventralis anterior t.
nucleus ventralis intermedius t.
nucleus ventralis posterior t.
nucleus ventralis posterior intermedius t.
nucleus ventralis posterolateralis t.
nucleus ventralis posteromedialis t.
pulvinar t.
radiatio inferior t.
stratum zonale t.
stria medullaris t.
tenia t.
tuberculum anterius t.
thalamic
t. aphasia
t. astrocytoma
t. circulation
t. fasciculitis
t. fasciculus
t. glioma
t. gustatory nucleus
t. hemorrhage
t. hyperesthetic anesthesia
t. infarction
t. lesion
t. neglect
t. pain
t. pain syndrome
t. peduncle
t. radiation
t. region
t. relay
t. response
t. reticular neuron
t. stimulation
t. stroke
t. tenia
t. tumor
thalamici
rami t.
thalamic-subthalamic hemorrhage
thalamicus
fasciculus t.
ramus t.
thalamocaudate
t. arteriovenous malformation
t. artery
thalamocortical
t. axon
t. connection
t. excitability
t. fiber
t. network
t. pathway
t. projection
t. relay
t. synchronization
thalamogeniculate artery
thalamolenticular
thalamomamillaris
fasciculus t.
thalamomamillary bundle

thalamomammillaris
fasciculus t.
thalamoolivary tract
thalamoparietales
thalamopeduncular infarction
thalamoperforating artery
thalamoperforator
thalamostriate
t. radiation
t. vein
thalamotegmental
thalamotemporal radiation
thalamotomy
anterior t.
dorsomedial t.
gamma t.
staged bilateral stereotactic t.
stereotactic VL t.
ventrolateralis t.
Vim t.
VL t.
thalamus
anterior nucleus of t.
anterior peduncle of t.
anterior tubercle of t.
anterodorsal nucleus of t.
anteromedial nucleus of t.
arcuate nucleus of t.
caudal peduncle of t.
central lateral nucleus of t.
central peduncle of t.
dorsal t.
t. dorsalis
dorsal nucleus of t.
lateral nucleus of t.
medial central nucleus of t.
medial dorsal nucleus of t.
medullary lamina of t.
medullary layer of t.
medullary stria of t.
medullary tenia of t.
motor t.
optic t.
paracentral nucleus of t.
paramedian t.
posterior medial nucleus of t.
posterior nuclear complex of t.
posterior peduncle of t.
pulvinar nucleus of t.
reticular nucleus of t.
right t.
stalk of t.
superior peduncle of t.
t. tissue
ventral anterior nucleus of t.
ventral anterior nucleus of t.
ventral intermediate nucleus of t.
t. ventralis
ventral lateral complex of t.
ventral lateral nucleus of t.
ventral medial complex of t.
ventral posterior intermediate nucleus of t.
ventral posterior lateral nucleus of t.
ventral posterolateral nucleus of t.
ventral posteromedial nucleus of t.
ventrobasal complex of the t.
Vim t.
zonal layer of t.
thalassemia
thalidomide neuropathy
thallium
t. intoxication
t. peripheral neuropathy
t. poisoning
t. polyneuropathy
t. toxic disorder
t. toxicity
thallium-201 (^{201}Tl)
thalposis
thalpotic
THAM
tromethamine
THAM Injection
THAM-E Injection
thanatobiologic
thanatognomonic
thanatophoric dysplasia
thanatopsis
thanatotic
T-handle
T-h. bone awl
T-h. Jacob chuck
T-h. nut wrench
T-h. screw wrench
Thane method
theca, pl. **thecae**
t. medullare spinalis
t. vertebralis
thecal
t. abscess
t. puncture

NOTES

thecal *(continued)*
t. sac
t. sac compression
thecoperitoneal Pudenz-Schulte shunt
Theiler murine encephalomyelitis
Theimich lip sign
thematic
t. apperception test (TAT)
t. paraphasia
thenar
t. eminence
t. weakness test
theophylamine
theophylline
theoretical orientation
theory
advanced wakefulness t.
affective arousal t.
avalanche t.
birth trauma t.
Burn and Rand t.
Cannon t.
Cannon-Bard t.
causal-attributional t.
clinical t.
convergence projection t.
crowding t.
deontologic t.
emotive t.
ERG t.
etiology t.
existential-humanistic t.
flow t.
gate control t.
Golgi t.
hydrodynamic t.
local circuit t.
mass action t.
McLone and Knepper etiological t.
Melzack and Wall gate t.
memory reinforcement t.
t. of mind task
mnemic t.
t. of mnemism
mnemism t.
neuron t.
pathogenetic t.
personality t.
pulsion t.
relaxation t.
Semon-Hering t.
Shealy t.
Spearman 2-factor t.
spreading cortical depression t.
thermostat t.
traction t.
trigeminovascular t.
vasogenic t.
Wolff vasogenic t.
Wollaston t.
Young-Helmholtz trichromacy t.
Thera
T. Cane
T. Pulse bed
therapeutic
t. advantage
t. agent
t. agent-related neuropathy
t. approach
t. connection
t. contribution
t. efficacy
t. electrical stimulation
t. electric stimulation
t. embolism
t. embolization
t. exploration
t. intervention
t. malaria
t. measure
t. modality
t. neuroradiology
t. outcome
t. profile
t. range
t. response
t. school placement
t. strategy
t. target
t. vocational placement
therapy
abortive t.
Activa tremor control t.
adjunctive t.
adjuvant whole-brain radiation t.
albendazole t.
alternative t.
analytic t.
analytical t.
anticoagulation t.
anticonvulsant t.
antifibrinolytic t.
antimicrobial t.
antimigraine t.
antioxidant t.
antiplatelet t.
antireflux t.
antiretroviral t.
antiviral t.
aspirin t.
attractor field t. (AFT)
behavior modification t.
biofeedback t.
boron neutron capture t. (BNCT)
Bragg peak proton beam t.
brain gene t.
bright light t.
cellular t.

cerebral protective t.
chelation t.
cholesterol-lowering t.
cholinergic t.
cholinomimetic t.
chronic corticosteroid t.
cloaca t.
clozapine t.
cognitive analytic t.
cognitive behavioral group t.
cognitive enhancement t.
computer-aided t.
computer-guided t.
constraint-induced t.
convulsive t.
cooling t.
corticosteroid t.
cytosine arabinoside t.
diet t.
disease-modifying agent t.
DMA t.
dopaminergic t.
electric differential t.
electroconvulsive t.
electrotherapeutic sleep t.
emotional control t.
emotional release t.
empirical t.
endovascular t.
enzyme replacement t.
estrogen replacement t. (ERT)
experimental t.
first-line t.
fluorouracil t.
focused radiation t.
fractionated radiation t.
functional occupational t. (FOT)
gene t.
Gerson t.
global gene replacement t.
HBO t.
highly active antiretroviral t. (HAART)
hormonal t.
hormone replacement t. (HRT)
hyperbaric oxygen t.
hypertensive, hypervolemic, hemodilutional t.
image-guided minimally invasive t. (IGMIT)
immunosuppressive t.
implosion t.
inadequate t.
intensity-modulated radiation t.
interstitial radiation t.
intradiscal electrothermal t. (IDET)
intrathecal drug t.
intravenous immune globulin humoral t.
iron replacement t.
isoniazid t.
IT-MS infusion t.
language t.
lifelong t.
localization-related t.
localized restorative central nervous system gene t.
magnetic seizure t.
massage t.
melatonin-replacement t.
modified constraint-induced t.
molecular-based conceptual t.
motivational enhancement t.
multidimensional family t.
multimodal t.
multisystem t.
multisystemic t.
neuroprotective t.
neurostimulation t.
occupational t.
oral appliance t.
oxygen t.
photodynamic t.
photoradiation t.
physical t.
pituitary replacement t.
positional t.
postelectroconvulsive t.
prescription drug t.
preventive t.
prokinetic drug t.
prophylactic anticonvulsant t.
psychotherapeutic t.
radiation t.
reality t.
reflex t.
regressive electric shock t. (REST)
relapse t.
retrogasserian anhydrous glycerol injection t.
rheologic t.
sacral nerve stimulation t.
second-line t.
short-term t.

NOTES

therapy *(continued)*
sleep restriction t.
social t.
solution-focused t.
standard antipsychotic t.
stem cell-based remyelinating t.
stereotactic-assisted radiation t.
stereotactic-focused radiation t.
stereotactic intratumoral photodynamic t.
steroid t.
stimulant t.
stimulus-control t.
structural family t.
substitutive agent t.
substrate reduction t. (SRT)
systematic family t.
taftian t.
tamoxifen t.
third-line t.
thrombolytic t.
transvenous t.
Triple-H t.
ultrasonic t.
VAC T.
video t.
viral vector-mediated t.
virtual reality t.
vision restoration t. (VRT)
VNS t.
whole-brain radiation t. (WBRT)
x-ray t. (XRT)
thermal
t. ablation
t. anesthesia
t. drive
t. lesioning
t. receptor
t. rhizotomy
t. sense
t. stress
thermalgesia
thermalgia
thermesthesia
thermesthesiometer
thermhyperesthesia
thermhypesthesia
thermic
t. anesthesia
t. sense
thermistor
t. electrode
t. needle
thermistry
thermoalgesia
thermoanalgesia, thermoanesthesia
thermocoagulation
percutaneous t.
radiofrequency t.
stereotactic t.
thermocouple
Copper-Constantan t.
thermoeffector
t. activity
antagonistic t.
t. function
t. response
thermoesthesia
thermoesthesiometer
thermoexcitory
thermogenesis
catecholamine-induced t.
nonshivering t.
normal t.
shivering t.
sympathomimetic-induced t.
thermogenic
t. component
t. effect
t. mechanism
t. tissue mass
thermography
infrared t. (IRT)
thermohyperalgesia
thermohyperesthesia
thermohypesthesia, thermohypoesthesia
thermoluminescent dosimeter
thermometry
cerebral t.
thermoreceptor
thermoregulatory
t. center
t. function
t. property
t. response
t. sweat test
t. system
thermorhizotomy
thermosensory
t. information
t. property
thermostat
hypothalamic t.
t. theory
theta
t. activity
t. peak frequency
t. response
t. rhythm
t. wave
Thévenard syndrome
thiabendazole
thiamine
t. deficiency
t. deficiency encephalopathy
thiamylal
thiazide-induced hypokalemia

thickening
hyaline t.
myelin t.
myxomatous t.
thickness
anulus t.
lumbosacral junction cortical t.
myelin t.
preinduction t.
slice t.
thick-skinned
thick-witted
thienobenzodiazepine
thigh
driver's t.
Heilbronner t.
thigh-high alternating compression air boot
thigmesthesia
thinking
abnormal t.
clinical t.
disorganized t.
magic t.
obsessional t.
paranoid t.
seizure induced by t.
thin-layer agarose gel electrophoresis
thinning
blood t.
thin-section image
thin-slab acquisition technique
thin-slice contrast MRI
thin-wall introducer catheter
thiobarbituric acid
thioflavin-positive fibril
6-thioguanine (6TG)
thiopental sodium
thiophene
analog of phencyclidine t.
phencyclidine t.
thioridazine
thiosalicylate
sodium t.
thiosulfate
sodium t.
thiotepa
thiothixene
thioxanthene
third
t. cranial nerve [CN III]
law of t.'s
t. nerve avulsion
t. nerve palsy
t. temporal convolution
t. ventricle
t. ventricle floor
t. ventricle width
t. ventricular hemangioblastoma
t. ventriculostomy
t. visual area
third-degree continuous spontaneous nystagmus
third-generation cephalosporin
third-line therapy
third-person auditory hallucination
thirst center
Thomas sign
Thompson carotid clamp
Thompson-Farley spinal retractor system
Thomsen
T. disease
T. dystrophy
thoracalis
plexus aorticus t.
thoracic
t. aortic plexus
t. column
t. cord lesion
t. curve scoliosis
t. dermatome
t. discectomy
t. disc herniation
t. duct injury
t. endoscopic sympathectomy
t. hypokyphosis
t. inlet
t. interspace
t. kyphosis
t. meningioma
t. nucleus
t. outlet
t. outlet syndrome (TOS)
t. outlet syndrome dissection
t. part of aorta
t. part of esophagus
t. part of spinal cord
t. part of thoracic duct
t. pedicle
t. pedicle marker
t. spinal fusion
t. spine
t. spine biopsy

NOTES

thoracic *(continued)*
t. spine decompression
t. spine fracture
t. spine injury
t. spine lordosis
t. spine pedicle diameter
t. spine scoliotic deformity
t. spine vertebral osteosynthesis
t. splanchnic ganglion
t. splanchnic nerve
t. and thoracolumbar spine surgery
t. tumor
t. vertebra
thoracica
columna t.
ganglia t.
segmentum t. 1–12
segmentum medullae spinalis t.
thoracici
nervi cardiaci t.
pars cervicalis ductus t.
pars thoracica ductus t.
rami cardiaci t.
ramus lateralis rami posterioris nervi t.
ramus medialis rami posterioris nervi t.
thoracicorum
rami anteriores nervorum t.
rami dorsales nervorum t.
rami posteriores nervorum t.
rami pulmonales thoracici gangliorum t.
rami ventrales nervorum t.
thoracicus
nucleus t.
plexus aorticus t.
thoracoabdominal approach
thoracodorsalis
nervus t.
thoracodorsal nerve
thoracolumbar
t. burst fracture
t. curve
t. degenerative disease
t. gibbus deformity
t. idiopathic scoliosis
T. Injury Classification and Severity Score (TLICS)
t. junction
t. junction surgical exposure
t. kyphoscoliosis
t. kyphosis
t. pedicle screw
t. retroperitoneal approach
t. spinal canal stenosis
t. spine
t. spine anterior exposure
t. spine decompression
t. spine flexion-distraction injury
t. spine fracture-dislocation
t. spine scoliosis
t. spine stabilization
t. spine vertebral osteosynthesis
t. spondylosis
t. spondylosis surgical technique
t. standing orthosis
t. system
t. trauma
t. vertebra
thoracolumbosacral
t. orthosis
t. plate
thoracolumbosacroiliac
t. implant system
t. implant system thread
Thoracoport trocar system
thoracoscopic anterior discectomy
thoracostomy
thoracotomy
left-sided t.
right-sided t.
standard t.
thorax stimulation
Thorazine
thorium
t. dioxide
t. tartrate
thorn
dendritic t.
Thornton-Griggs-Moxley disease
Thorotrast
thoroughness, reliability, efficiency, analytic sense
Thor-Prom
thread
neuropil t.
polyene t.
terminal t.
thoracolumbosacroiliac implant system t.
threaded
t. fusion cage (TFC)
t. fusion cage (TFC)
t. mandrel
t. sheath
threadwire saw
threshold
absolute t.
afterdischarge t.
apneic t.
arousal t.
auditory t.
cold detection t.
t. of consciousness
convulsant t.
current perception t. (CPT)
differential t.

double-point t.
t. effect
t. electrical stimulation (TES)
electroshock seizure t.
heat pain t.
high arousal t.
insular t.
t. of island of Reil
low anger t.
mechanical sensory t.
motor t.
neuron t.
null condition detection t.
pain intensity t.
pure-tone hearing t.
relational t.
resolution t.
resting motor t.
sensitivity t.
signal-to-noise t.
speech reception t.
speech recognition t.
stimulus t.
swallowing t.
touch perception t. (TPT)
vibration detection t.
warmth sensory t.

Throckmorton
T. reflex
T. sign

thrombi (*pl. of* thrombus)

thrombin
topical t.

Thrombinar

thrombin-soaked
t.-s. gelatin sponge
t.-s. Gelfoam

thromboangiitis obliterans

thrombocythemia

thrombocytopenia
neonatal alloimmune t.
pediatric stroke from t.
t. venous-sinus

thrombocytopenic purpura

thrombocytosis
essential t.

thromboelastography

thromboembolectomy

thromboembolic stroke

thromboembolism

Thrombogen

thrombogenic
t. coil
t. ferrous mixture

thrombolysis
intracisternal t.
intraluminal t.

thrombolytic therapy

thrombomodulin-protein

thrombophlebitis
cavernous sinus t.

thromboplastin
plasma t.

thrombosed
t. giant aneurysm
t. thick-walled vein

thrombosinusitis

thrombosis, pl. **thromboses**
acute t.
arterial t.
catheter-induced subclavian vein t.
cavernous sinus t.
cerebral artery t.
cerebral vein t.
cerebral venous t.
cerebrovascular arterial t.
cerebrovascular venous t.
cortical venous t.
deep vein t.
deep venous t.
dural venous sinus t.
fistula-induced sinus t.
iliofemoral t.
intracranial sinus t.
lateral sinus t.
marasmic t.
middle cerebral artery t. (MCAT)
sagittal sinus t.
septic t.
sinovenous t.
sinus vein t.
venous sinus t.
t. of venous sinus
wire t.

thrombospondin

Thrombostat

thrombotic
t. apoplexy
t. hydrocephalus
t. occlusion
t. stroke
t. thrombocytopenic purpura

NOTES

thromboxane synthase inhibitor
thrombus, pl. **thrombi**
chronic t.
fibrin t.
longitudinal sinus t.
marasmic t.
mural t.
through-and-through gunshot wound
thrusting
tongue t.
thumbprinting appearance
thumb reflex
Thumb-Saver introducer clamp
thunderclap headache
Thurston scale
Thymapad stimulus electrode
thymectomy
thymergasia
thymic
t. involution
t. myoid cell
thymidine
t. kinase gene (TK2)
t. salvage pathway
thymine
thymocyte apoptosis
thymogenic drinking
thymoleptic
thymoma
thymopathy
Thypinone
thyrocervical trunk of subclavian artery
thyroglobulin
thyroglossal duct cyst
thyrohypophysial syndrome
thyroid
t. cartilage
t. deficiency
t. disease
t. function test
t. gland
t. orbitopathy
thyroideae
cartilaginis t.
cornu inferius cartilaginis t.
thyroiditis
autoimmune t.
Riedel t.
thyroid-stimulating
t.-s. hormone (TSH)
t.-s. hormone level
thyrotoxic
t. coma
t. encephalopathy
t. myopathy
t. periodic paralysis (TPP)
thyrotoxicosis
apathetic t.
endogenous t.
thyrotoxicosis-induced
t.-i. chorea
t.-i. choreoathetosis
thyrotroph cell
thyrotrophic axis
thyrotropin
thyrotropin-producing adenoma
thyrotropin-releasing
t.-r. hormone (TRH)
t.-r. hormone stimulation
thyroxine (T_4)
Thytropar
TIA
transient ischemic attack
tiagabine
t. HCl
t. hydrochloride
tiapride
Tibex
tibial
t. nerve
t. phenomenon
tibialis
nervus t.
rami calcanei mediales nervi t.
rami musculares nervi t.
t. sign
tibioadductor reflex
tic
chronic t.
compulsive spasms and t.'s
convulsive t.
t. de sommeil
diaphragmatic t.
t. disorder
t. douloureux
facial t.
glossopharyngeal t.
habit t.
local t.
maladie des t.
mimic t.
multiple motor t.'s
multiple vocal t.'s
psychic t.
rotatory t.
ruling in t.
self-injurious motor t.
spasmodic t.
spasms and t.'s
t. symptom
tardive t.
TICA
traumatic intracranial aneurysm
tick
deer t.
t. paralysis

tick-borne
t.-b. encephalitis (Central European subtype)
t.-b. encephalitis (Eastern subtype)
t.-b. meningopolyneuritis
t.-b. relapsing fever
tic-like
tic-related obsessive-compulsive disorder
tidal volume (VT)
tidembersat
Tiedemann nerve
tier
Adson knot t.
Tigan
tight
t. brain
t. filum terminale syndrome
tightener
Love-Adson wire t.
tightness
muscle t.
tigroid
t. body
t. mass
t. substance
tigrolysis
TIL
tumor-infiltrating leukocyte
tumor-infiltrating lymphocyte
Tilcotil
tile plate facet replacement
tilt
head t.
head-down t. (HDT)
T. and Turn Paragon bed
tilted optimized nonsaturating excitation technique
tilting of visual image
tilt-table test
tiludronate
1.5-T imager
time
Achilles tendon reflex t.
acquisition t.
association t.
t. axis
biologic t.
bleeding t.
central somatosensory conduction t.
cochlear response t.
conduction t.
t. constant
t. context
correlation t.
dilute Russell viper venom t. (DRVVT)
echo t. (TE)
effective half t. (Te)
image acquisition t.
inertia t.
interhemispheric propagation t.
interpulse t.
t. interval
inversion t.
kaolin clotting t.
long pulse repetition time/long echo t.
mass doubling t.
nonparetic eye valid reaction t.
partial thromboplastin t. (PTT)
t. perception
phrenic nerve conduction t.
t. point
processing t.
prothrombin t. (PT)
proton relaxation t.
pulse repetition t.
pulse transit t.
reaction t.
recognition t.
relaxation t.
repetition t.
t. reproduction task
response processing t.
rise t.
Russell viper venom t.
scan t.
t. sense
sequence t.
serial reaction t. (SRT)
short pulse repetition time/short echo t.
sleep period t.
spin-lattice relaxation t.
spin-spin relaxation t.
stimulation t.
stimulus-response t.
survival t.
transcallosal conduction t. (TCT)
vigilance reaction t.
timed
T. Tandem Walk Test
T. Up and Go test
time-density curve

NOTES

T

time-dependent behavior
time-locked occipital rhythm
time-motion study
time-of-flight
t.-o.-f. angiography
t.-o.-f. effect
t.-o.-f. positron emission tomographic camera
t.-o.-f. technique
time-on-task effect
time-out
involuntary t.-o.
voluntary t.-o.
TiMesh
T. hardware
T. LP cranial miniplate and screw system
T. screw
T. titanium bone plating system
time-variance imaging (TVI)
timing
circadian t.
t. of decompression
Timofeew corpuscle
Timo headrest
timolol maleate
TIMP
tissue inhibitor of metalloproteinase
TiMX low back system
tin ear syndrome
Tinel sign
tingling
t. sensation
t. with aura
tinnitus
objective pulsatile t.
pulsatile t.
tip
Adson brain suction t.
bipolar diathermy forceps t.
CUSA t.
Ferguson brain suction t.
forceps t.
Frazier suction t.
Japanese suction t.
multipore suction t.
t. of posterior horn
Rhoton suction t.
Sachs brain suction t.
slotted suction t.
volar t.
Tipramine
Tirilazad Efficacy Stroke Study (TESS)
Tisseel artificial dura
Tissucol
tissue
adipose t.
Antoni A, B t.
areolar t.
autologous adrenal medullary t.
brain t.
caudate t.
cingulate t.
connective t.
cortical t.
cryopreserved t.
t. culture
t. dilator
distensible t.
epivaginal connective t.
t. factor pathway inhibitor
fetal mesencephalic t.
t. fibrin sealant
t. forceps
granulation t.
gray matter t.
t. hyperperfusion
t. implant
t. inhibitor of metalloproteinase (TIMP)
insular cortex t.
Kuhnt intermediary t.
t. magnetic susceptibility artifact
mesencephalic t.
nervous t.
occipital cortex t.
parietal t.
partial oxygen pressure of brain t. ($PbrO_2$)
peripheral t.
pharyngeal t.
pial t.
t. plane dissector
t. plasminogen activator (TPA, t-PA)
postmortem brain t.
t. respiration
spinal cord t.
splenium t.
temporal t.
thalamus t.
t. transplantation
t. welding
white matter t.
tissue-based monoamine oxidase assay
Tissue-Guard bovine pericardial patch
tissue-type
t.-t. metabolic response
t.-t. PA
titanium
t. alloy needle
t. alloy screw and rod system
t. aneurysm clip
t. cable
t. construct
t. hollow screw plate system
t. mesh cage
t. micromesh

t. micro system
t. mini bur hole cover
t. mini bur hole covering
t. miniplate
t. plate
Sugita T.
t. wire
t. wound retractor

titer
complement fixation antibody t.
Hu-Ab t.

titubation

tizanidine hydrochloride

TK2
thymidine kinase gene

^{201}Tl
thallium-201
^{201}Tl chloride
^{201}Tl scintigraphy
^{201}Tl SPECT

TLICS
Thoracolumbar Injury Classification and Severity Score

TLIF
transforaminal lumbar interbody fusion

TMB
transient monocular blindness

TMJ
temporomandibular joint
TMJ dysfunction with headache

TMP
transmembrane potential

TMS
transcranial magnet stimulation

TN
trigeminal neuralgia

TNF
tumor necrosis factor

TNF-alpha
tumor necrosis factor-alpha

TNFR
tumor necrosis factor receptor

TOAD-64 gene

tobacco-alcohol amblyopia

Tobey-Ayer test

tobramycin

tocopherol
alpha t.

TOCP
triorthocresyl phosphate

Todd
T. body
T. paresis
T. postepileptic paralysis

toddler
Checklist for Autism in T.'s (CHAT)
Modified Checklist for Autism in T.'s (M-CHAT)

Todd-Wells
T.-W. apparatus
T.-W. stereotactic frame
T.-W. technique

toe
t. clonus
t. drop
t. phenomenon
t. reflex
t. sign
striatal t.
t. walking

Toennis
T. dissecting scissors
T. dura dissector
T. dura knife
T. dural hook
T. ES standalone constant-current electrical stimulator
T. tumor forceps

Toennis-Adson dissector

toe-walking

Tofranil

Toft spinal correction treatment

togavirus infection

tokishakuyakusan treatment

tolazamide

tolbutamide

tolcapone

tolerability

tolerance
glucose t.
pain t.

tolfenamic acid

Tolinase

tolmetin

Tolosa-Hunt syndrome

tolterodine

toluidine blue-stained

tomacula

tomaculous neuropathy

tomentum

Tomkins-Horn

tomogram
open-mouthed anteroposterior t.

NOTES

tomograph
CTI-Siemens 933 t.
PC-2048B positron emission t.
tomographic
tomography
automated computed axial t.
automated computerized axial t. (ACAT)
cerebrovascular computed t.
computed t. (CT)
computed axial t. (CAT)
computerized axial t. (CAT)
cranial computed t.
dynamic single-photon emission computed t.
emission computed t.
F-labeled fluoromisonidazole positron emission t.
fluorodeoxyglucose positron emission t. (FDG-PET)
fluorodopa positron emission t.
head computed t.
helicoidal computerized t.
ictal single-photon emission computed t.
infusion computed t.
magnetic resonance t. (MRT)
optical positron emission t. (O-PET)
plain t.
positron emission t. (PET)
preoperative t.
quantitative computerized t.
single-photon emission computed t. (SPECT)
volumetric computed t.
xenon computed t.
xenon-enhanced computed t. (XeCT)
Tomoscan
Philips T.
tonaphasia
tone
airway muscle t.
dopaminergic t.
infant muscle t.
low EMG t.
muscle t.
resting t.
short-term vasomotor t.
sphincter t.
upper airway muscular t.
vascular t.
vasomotor t.
viscerosomatic t.
tongs
Cherry traction t.
Cone skull traction t.
Crutchfield-Raney skull traction t.
Crutchfield skeletal traction t.
Crutchfield skull traction t.
Edmonton extension t.
Gardner-Wells t.
Mayfield t.
Reynolds skull traction t.
Trippi Wells t.
tongue
t. base prominence
t. of cerebellum
chameleon t.
galloping t.
t. movement
t. phenomenon
t. reduction surgery
t. retainer
septum of t.
t. thrusting
trombone tremor of t.
tongue-in-groove operation
tongue-locking device
tongue-retaining device
tonic
t. block
t. contraction
t. convulsion
t. drop attack
t. epilepsy
t. inhibitor control
t. neck response
t. phase
t. pupil
t. reflex
t. seizure
t. spasm
t. status epilepticus
tonically dilated pupil
tonic-clonic
t.-c. activity
generalized t.-c. (GTC)
t.-c. seizure
t.-c. status epilepticus
tonicoclonic, tonoclonic
t. spasm
tonometry
tonotopic
tonsil
cerebellar t.
t. of cerebellum
cerebral t.
herniation of cerebellar t.
tonsilla, pl. **tonsillae**
t. cerebelli
tonsillar
t. herniation
t. nerve
t. plexus

tonus
myogenic t.
neurogenic t.
tool
communication t.
Cybon surgical navigation t.
genetic t.
insomnia assessment t.
MMS-900 balancing t.
quantitative morphometric t.
relationship t.
tooth
t. atrophy
T. disease
t. grinding
top
t. of basilar syndrome
circular laminar hook with offset t.
topagnosia
topagnosis
Topamax
top-down
t.-d. organization of memory
t.-d. regulation
topectomy
topesthesia
tophaceous gout
tophus
topical
t. clonidine
t. thrombin
topiramate monotherapy
topoanesthesia
topognosis, topognosia
topographical agnosia
topographic memory loss
topography
steady-state probe t. (SSPT)
topology
toponarcosis
toposcope
toposcopic catheter
topothermesthesiometer
toppling gait
Toradol
TORCH
toxoplasmosis, other infections, rubella, cytomegalovirus, and herpes simplex
TORCH syndrome
torch
saline t.
torcular
t. epidermoid
t. herophili
t. meningioma
Torg ratio
Torkildsen
T. operation
T. shunt
T. ventriculocisternostomy
torlone fixation pin
tornado epilepsy
Tornwaldt cyst
torpillage
torpor
torque
t. transducer
unwanted screw t.
torque-pulse perturbation
Torré syndrome
torsades
t. de pointes
t. de pointes arrhythmia
torsion
t. disease of childhood
t. dystonia
t. neurosis
ocular t.
t. spasm
t. stability
torsional
t. abnormality
t. gripping strength
t. nystagmus
t. stiffness
torsionometer
torso
t. flexion angle
t. flexion load
t. flexion posture
Torsten Sjögren syndrome
torti
pili t.
torticollar
torticollis
benign paroxysmal t.
dermatogenic t.
dystonic t.
fixed t.
hysterical t.
idiopathic t.
intermittent t.
labyrinthine t.

NOTES

torticollis *(continued)*
neurogenic t.
ocular t.
paroxysmal t.
psychogenic t.
rheumatic t.
spasmodic t.
t. spastica
spurious t.
symptomatic t.
tortipelvis
tortuosity
toruloma
TOS
thoracic outlet syndrome
Toscana virus
tosylate
daledalin t.
total
t. agenesis
t. AIMS score
t. aphasia
t. body neutron activation analysis
t. cord transection
t. emotional memory score
t. excision
t. fractional regional brain volume
t. hypophysectomy
t. monocular blindness
t. neuroleptic dosage
t. parenteral nutrition (TPN)
t. pituitary ablation
t. scale
t. symptom
t. symptom score
t. weighted sum score
totalis
alopecia capitis t.
ophthalmoplegia t.
rachischisis t.
toto
in t.
touch
t. cell
t. corpuscle
organ of t.
t. perception threshold (TPT)
t. pressure
t. receptor
Tourette
T. disease
Gilles de la T.
T. syndrome
T. Syndrome Association (TSA)
T. Syndrome Association Unified Tic Rating Scale
tourniquet
Drake t.
t. ischemia
Tournoux
atlas of Talairach and T.
tower skull
toxemia
toxic
t. amblyopia
t. delirium
t. dementia
t. disorder
t. epidermal necrolysis (TEN)
t. exposure
t. headache
t. hydrocephalus
t. hypoxia
t. metabolite
t. neuritis
t. neuropathy
t. nystagmus
t. paraplegia
t. retinoneuropathy
t. shock syndrome
t. side effect
t. spasm
t. tetanus
t. vertigo
toxicity
acute neuronal t.
alcohol t.
aluminum t.
arsenic t.
caffeine t.
central anticholinergic t.
dose-limiting t.
drug t.
epinephrine t.
glutamate t.
hexachlorophene t.
hydrazine t.
lead t.
manganese t.
mercury t.
methyl alcohol t.
neurogenic cardiac t.
norepinephrine t.
propylene glycol t.
social t.
sympathomimetic t.
thallium t.
toxicophobia
toxicus
Gambierdiscus t.
toxin
bacterial t.
botulinum t.
botulinum t. type A, B
botulism t.
chemical t.
endogenous benzodiazepine-like t.
environmental t.

manganese t.
marine t.
mercury t.
metallic t.
methyl alcohol t.
organic t.
plant t.
shiga t.
uremic t.
toxin-induced sleep disorder
Toxocara canis
toxocariasis infection
toxoid
tetanus t.
Toxoplasma gondii
toxoplasmic
t. encephalitis (TE)
t. encephalomyelitis
t. meningoencephalitis
toxoplasmosis
acquired t.
AIDS-related t.
cerebral t.
congenital t.
intramedullary t.
ocular t.
t., other infections, rubella, cytomegalovirus, and herpes simplex (TORCH)
t., other infections, rubella, cytomegalovirus infection, herpes
Toyama classification
TPA
temporal processing acuity
temporopolar artery
tissue plasminogen activator
t-PA
tissue plasminogen activator
TPJ
temporoparietal junction
T-plate
TPN
total parenteral nutrition
TPP
thyrotoxic periodic paralysis
TPT
touch perception threshold
trabecula, pl. **trabeculae**
arachnoid t.
nondecalcified t.
trabecular
t. arcade
t. bone
trabecularis
substantia t.
trace
t. conditioned reflex
dashed gray velocity t.
memory t.
solid gray velocity t.
tracer
flow t.
radioactive t.
tracheal
t. injury
t. traction
trachelagra
trachelism, trachelismus
trachelocyrtosis
trachelodynia
trachelokyphosis
trachelology
tracheostomy
tracing
dipole t.
tracker
T. Excel microcatheter
T. infusion catheter
Polaris position t.
Tracker-10, -18 catheter
tracking
eye t.
speech t.
Tracrium
tract
accessory nucleus of optic t.
aerodigestive t.
anterior corticospinal t.
anterior pyramidal t.
anterior raphespinal t.
anterior spinocerebellar t.
anterior spinothalamic t.
anterior trigeminothalamic t.
anterolateral t.
Arnold t.
ascending t.
association t.
auditory t.
Bechterew t.
Bruce t.
t. of Bruce and Muir
bulbar t.

NOTES

tract *(continued)*
bulboreticulospinal t.
Burdach t.
caerulospinal t.
central tegmental t.
cerebellorubral t.
cerebellorubrospinal t.
cerebellospinal t.
cerebellotegmental t.
cerebellothalamic t.
Collier t.
corticobulbar t.
corticohypothalamic t.
corticomesencephalic t.
corticopontine t.
corticopontocerebellar t.
corticorubral t.
corticospinal t.
crossed pyramidal t.
cuneocerebellar t.
deiterospinal t.
dentatothalamic t.
direct pyramidal t.
dorsal column sensory t.
dorsal spinocerebellar t.
dorsal trigeminothalamic t.
dorsolateral t.
external corticotectal t.
extracorticospinal t.
fastigiobulbar t.
fastigiospinal t.
fiber sensory t.
Flechsig t.
frontopontine t.
frontotemporal t.
geniculocalcarine t.
geniculostriate t.
t. of Goll
Gowers t.
habenulointerpeduncular t.
habenulopeduncular t.
Hoche t.
hypothalamohypophysial t.
hypothalamospinal t.
intermediolateral t.
internal corticotectal t.
interpositospinal t.
interstitiospinal t.
lateral corticospinal t.
lateral olfactory t.
lateral pyramidal t.
lateral raphespinal t.
lateral reticulospinal t.
lateral root of optic t.
lateral spinothalamic t.
lateral vestibulospinal t.
Lissauer t.
Loewenthal t.
mamillopeduncular t.
mamillotegmental t.
mamillothalamic t.
Marchi t.
medial reticulospinal t.
medial root of optic t.
medial vestibulospinal t.
medullary reticulospinal t.
medullary solitary t.
Meynert t.
Monakow t.
motor t.
t. of Münzer and Wiener
neospinothalamic t.
nerve t.
nigrostriatal t.
nigrostriate t.
nucleus of lateral olfactory t.
nucleus of solitary t.
occipitocollicular t.
occipitopontile t.
occipitopontine t.
occipitotectal t.
olfactory t.
olivocerebellar t.
olivocochlear t.
olivospinal t.
optic t.
pain t.
pain-transmitting t.
paraventriculohypophysial t.
parietopontine t.
pontoreticulospinal t.
posterior spinocerebellar t.
posterior trigeminothalamic t.
posterolateral t.
prepyramidal t.
pyramidal t.
reticulocerebellar t.
reticulospinal t.
retinohypothalamic t. (RHT)
rubrobulbar t.
rubropontine t.
rubroreticular t.
rubrospinal t.
Schultze comma t.
Schütz t.
t. of Schütz
semilunar t.
sensory t.
septomarginal t.
solitariospinal t.
solitary t.
spinal dermal sinus t.
spinocerebellar t.
spinocervical t.
spinocervicothalamic t.
spinoolivary t.
spinoreticular t.
spinospinalis t.

spinotectal t.
spinothalamic t.
spinovestibular t.
spiral foraminous t.
Spitzka-Lissauer t.
Spitzka marginal t.
strionigral t.
sulcomarginal t.
supraopticohypophysial t.
tectobulbar t.
tectocerebellar t.
tectopontine t.
tectospinal t.
tegmental t.
tegmentospinal t.
temporofrontal t.
temporopontine t.
testobulbar t.
thalamoolivary t.
transverse peduncular t.
triangular t.
trigeminal t.
trigeminospinal t.
trigeminothalamic t.
tuberohypophysial t.
tuberoinfundibular t.
Türck t.
urinary t.
ventral raphespinal t.
ventral spinocerebellar t.
ventral spinothalamic t.
ventral trigeminothalamic t.
vestibulocerebellar t.
vestibulospinal t.
Vicq d'Azyr t.
Waldeyer t.
white matter t.

traction
Ace Trippi-Wells tong cervical t.
Ace universal tong cervical t.
t. anchor
axial t.
bipolar vertebral t.
Bremer halo crown t.
Crile head t.
device for transverse t. (DTT)
Halter t.
t. neuritis
t. response of infant
t. spur
t. theory
tracheal t.
transverse t.

traction-type injury

tractography

tractotomy
anterolateral t.
bulbar cephalic pain t.
intramedullary t.
medullary t.
mesencephalic t.
pontine t.
pyramidal t.
Schwartz t.
Sjöqvist t.
spinal t.
spinothalamic t.
stereotactic t.
stereotactic subcaudate t. (SST)
subcaudate t.
trigeminal t.
Walker t.

tractus
t. anterolaterales
t. bulboreticulospinalis
t. caeruleospinalis
t. centralis tegmenti
t. cerebellorubralis
t. cerebellothalamicus
t. corticobulbaris
t. corticopontini
t. corticospinalis
t. corticospinalis anterior
t. corticospinalis lateralis
t. corticospinalis ventralis
t. descendens nervi trigemini
t. dorsolateralis
t. fastigiobulbaris
t. fastigiospinalis
t. frontopontinus
t. habenulointerpeduncularis
t. habenulopeduncularis
t. hypothalamohypophysialis
t. interpositospinalis
t. interstitiospinalis
t. mesencephalicus nervi trigemini
t. occipitopontinus
t. olfactorius
t. olivocerebellaris
t. olivocochlearis
t. opticus
t. paraventriculohypophysialis
t. parietopontinus

NOTES

tractus *(continued)*
t. pontoreticulospinalis
t. posterolateralis
t. pyramidalis
t. pyramidalis anterior
t. pyramidalis lateralis
t. pyramidalis ventralis
t. raphespinalis anterior
t. raphespinalis lateralis
t. reticulospinalis
t. reticulospinalis anterior
t. reticulospinalis ventralis
t. rubrobulbaris
t. rubropontinus
t. rubrospinalis
t. solitariospinalis
t. solitarius
t. solitarius medullae oblongatae
t. spinalis nervi trigeminalis
t. spinalis nervi trigemini
t. spinocerebellaris anterior
t. spinocerebellaris dorsalis
t. spinocerebellaris posterior
t. spinocerebellaris ventralis
t. spinocervicalis
t. spinoolivaris
t. spinotectalis
t. spinothalamicus
t. spinothalamicus anterior
t. spinothalamicus lateralis
t. spinothalamicus ventralis
t. spinovestibularis
t. supraopticohypophysialis
t. tectobulbaris
t. tectopontinus
t. tectospinalis
t. tegmentalis centralis
t. temporopontinus
t. trigeminospinalis
t. trigeminothalamicus
t. trigeminothalamicus anterior
t. trigeminothalamicus posterior
t. tuberoinfundibularis
t. vestibulospinalis
t. vestibulospinalis lateralis
t. vestibulospinalis medialis

traditional
t. circulatory criteria (TCC)
t. limbic circuit
t. neuroleptic
t. neuroleptic agent

tragus, pl. **tragi**
ipsilateral t.

train
orphan t.
t. of spikes

trained reflex

training
American Association of Directors of Psychiatric Residency T.
anxiety control t.
biologic t.
body weight-supported treadmill t.
habit reversal t.
speed-dependent treadmill t. (STT)
strength t.
tactile-kinesthetic t.

train-of-4 stimulus

trait
abnormal t.
t. characteristic
cluster B t.
dependence t.
egosyntonic t.
identified t.
impulsive-aggressive t.
premorbid personality t.
psychopathic t.
sickle cell t.
spike-and-wave t.

trait-level region abnormality

traitor

trajectory
behavioral t.
bullet t.
cognitive t.
emotional t.
operative t.

tramadol

tram track sign

trancelike state

tranexamic acid

transacetylase
dihydrolipoyl t.

transaminase
alanine t.
GABA t.
glutamyl t.
serum glutamic oxaloacetic t.
serum glutamic-pyruvic t.
serum glutamyl t.

transantral
t. ethmoidal approach
t. ethmoidal orbital decompression

transarterial platinum coil embolization

transarticular
t. screw
t. screw fixation

transaxillary approach

transaxonal ephaptic transmission

transbasal

transcallosal
t. band (TCB)
t. conduction delay
t. conduction time (TCT)
t. interforniceal corridor

t. interforniceal-transforaminal microsurgical approach
t. interhemispheric approach
t. transforaminal approach
transcalvarial
transcapsular gray bridge
transcarbamoylase
ornithine t.
transcarbamylase
transcardiac perfusion
transcatheter
t. obliteration
t. study
transcavernous transpetrous apex approach
transcendentalism
transcerebellar
t. diameter
t. hemispheric approach
transcervical
transchoroidal approach
transcochlear approach
transcortical
t. aphasia
t. apraxia
t. incision
t. technique
t. transventricular approach
transcranial
t. B-mode ultrasound
t. color-coded duplex sonography
t. color-coded real-time sonography
t. Doppler (TCD)
t. Doppler B mode
t. Doppler ultrasonography
t. frontofacial advancement
t. frontotemporoorbital approach
t. high-frequency repetitive electrical stimulation
t. magnetic stimulation
t. magnet stimulation (TMS)
t. motor evoked potential
t. orbital exploration
t. real-time color Doppler imaging
t. resection
t. skull-base endoscopy
transcription
broad phonemic t.
t. factor
t. factor in patterning
transcubital approach
transcutaneous
t. carbon dioxide monitoring
t. electrical nerve stimulation
t. oxygen monitoring
transcytosis
blood-brain t.
bulk flow t.
transdermal
Duragesic T.
t. methylphenidate system
t. patch
transdiaphragmatic pressure
transdominance
transducer
bur hole t.
t. cell
Combitrans t.
Drager MTC t.
force t.
intrasinus t.
nasal cannula pressure t.
neuroendocrine t.
piezoresistive t.
torque t.
Transpac IV pressure t.
transducer-measured intracranial venous pressure
transducer-tipped catheter
transduction
chemical-mechanical t.
pain t.
phospholipid-related signal t.
sensory t.
signal t.
transdural
transected axon
transection
fiber tract t.
t. hook
multiple subpial t.'s (MST)
subpial t.
total cord t.
transendothelial migration
transentorhinal region
transethmoidal encephalocele
transethmosphenoidal hypophysectomy
transfacial transclival approach
transfectant
transfected fibroblast
transfemoral
t. artery technique
t. catheter

NOTES

transfer
t. deficit
t. direct current stimulation
immunostimulatory gene t.
interdigital t.
linear energy t. (LET)
saturation t.
vector-mediated gene t.
virus-mediated gene t.
transferase
acylcholestrol acyl t. (ACAT)
chloramphenicol acetyl t. (CAT)
uridine glucuronyl t.
transference
idealizing t.
self-object t.
twinship t.
transferred sensation
transferrin
antihuman t.
carbohydrate-deficient t.
transfix
transfontanel Doppler ultrasound
transforaminal
t. herniation
t. lumbar interbody fusion (TLIF)
transform
2-dimensional Fourier t. (2DFT)
3-dimensional Fourier t. (3DFT)
fast Fourier t. (FFT)
Fourier t.
isotropic 3-dimensional Fourier t.
multidimensional Fourier t.
transformation
hemorrhagic t. (HT)
Z-score t.
transformational
transforming
t. growth factor (TGF)
t. growth factor beta
transfrontal approach
transfrontonasoorbital approach
transfusion
albumin t.
autologous blood t.
fetal t.
transgene
nonselective expression of t.
transgenic
transgress
transient
alpha t.
t. brainstem ischemia
t. cognitive impairment (TCI)
t. disorder
t. dystonia
t. emotional disturbance
t. emotional stress
t. facial paresthesia
t. flaccid paralysis
t. focal neurologic event (TFNE)
t. global amnesia (TGA)
t. hemiparesis
t. hemisphere attack
t. insomnia
t. ischemic attack (TIA)
t. leukopenia
t. monocular blindness (TMB)
t. monocular visual loss
t. mutism
t. neonatal myasthenia gravis
t. nystagmus
t. pain
t. plexus injury
positive occipital sharp t.
t. signal abnormality
t. tic disorder of childhood
t. visual phenomenon
t. voltage
t. white matter disease
transillumination
t. microscopy
skull t.
transinsular
transisthmian
transitional
t. convolution
t. gyrus
t. meningioma
t. vertebra
transitive
t. inference task
t. limb movement
transitivism
transitivity
transketolase
translabyrinthine
t. suboccipital approach
t. transotic approach
translation
coronal plane deformity sagittal t.
translational
t. fracture
t. position
translocation
reciprocal t.
robertsonian chromosome t.
transmandibular glossopharyngeal approach
transmantle pressure gradient
transmaxillosphenoidal approach
transmembrane
t. ionic shift
t. potential (TMP)
t. spanning
transmissible
t. neurodegenerative disease

t. spongiform encephalopathy (TSE)
t. spongiform viral encephalopathy

transmission
autosomal dominant t.
cholinergic t.
depolarization-dependent synaptic t.
diffusion t.
t. disequilibrium test
duplex t.
ephaptic t.
extrastriatal dopamine t.
familial t.
fetal AIDS t.
GABA-mediated inhibitory synaptic t.
genetic t.
glutamate-mediated excitatory synaptic t.
glutamatergic synaptic t.
impaired neuromuscular t.
indirect genetic t.
nerve impulse t.
neurochemical t.
neuromuscular junction t.
nonsynaptic t.
orderly nerve cell t.
transaxonal ephaptic t.
volume t.
X-linked recessive t.

transmitter
endogenous t.
inhibitory t.
miniature ultrasound t.
radiofrequency t.
t. substance
t. system

transmitter-gated ion channel

transnasal
t. approach
t. biopsy
t. septal displacement procedure

transnasoorbital approach

transneuronal
t. atrophy
t. degeneration

Transonics flow probe

transoral
t. approach
t. odontoid resection

transorbital
t. leukotomy
t. lobotomy

transosseous venography

Transpac IV pressure transducer

transpalatal approach

transparent septum

transpedicular
t. approach
t. cannulated screw
t. drill guide
t. fixation effective pedicle diameter
t. fixation system design
t. screw-rod fixation
t. spinal instrumentation

transpeptidase
gamma-glutamyl t.

transperitoneal approach

transpetrosal approach

transplant
adrenal body t.
allogenic t.
carotid body t.
chromaffin cell t.
fetal neural t.
fetal tissue t.
mesencephalic t.

transplantation
adrenal medulla t.
autologous hematopoietic stem cell t. (AHSCT)
bone marrow t.
brain t.
core assessment program for intracerebral t. (CAPIT)
fetal cell t.
intracranial-extracranial t.
liver t.
neural t.
organ t.
orthotopic liver t.
porcine cell t.
stem cell t.
tissue t.

transport
anterograde axonal t.
axonal t.
axoplasmic t.
defective glucose t.
fast axonal t.
glucose t.
retrograde t.
slow axonal t.

NOTES

transport *(continued)*
- solute t.
- substrate t.

transporter
- amino acid t.
- divalent cation t.
- dopamine t. (DAT)
- drug t.
- glutamate t.
- neurotransmitter t.
- plasma membrane dopamine t.
- t. protein

transposition
- Müller-König t.
- seventh cranial nerve t.
- vertebral artery t.

transradial cerebral angiography

transsinus approach

transsphenoidal
- t. approach
- t. bipolar forceps
- t. chiasmapexy
- t. complication
- t. curette
- t. encephalocele
- t. evacuation
- t. hook
- t. hypophysectomy
- t. meningoencephalocele
- t. removal
- t. selective adenomectomy
- t. speculum
- t. surgery

transsphenoidal cryohypophysectomy

transsternal

transsylvian
- t. approach
- t. keyhole

transsynaptic
- t. chromatolysis
- t. degeneration

transtemporal
- t. approach
- t. fissure

transtentorial
- t. approach
- t. uncal herniation

transthalamic

transthoracic
- t. approach
- t. discectomy
- t. vertebral body resection

transthyretin (TTR)
- t. mutation
- t. protein
- t. variant

transthyretin-associated neuropathic amyloidosis

transtorcular
- t. approach
- t. embolization
- t. occlusion

transuncodiscal approach

transvenous
- t. approach
- t. retrograde nidus sclerotherapy
- t. therapy

transventricular
- t. approach
- t. injury

transversa
- crista t.

transversae
- fibrae pontis t.

transversalis
- crista t.

transverse
- t. atlantal ligament
- t. bipolar montage
- t. cerebral fissure
- t. connector
- t. cord lesion
- t. crest
- t. diffusivity
- t. fasciculus
- t. fiber of pons
- t. fissure of cerebellum
- t. fissure of cerebrum
- t. fixation
- t. fixator application
- t. fornix
- t. gradient coil
- t. incision
- t. magnetization
- t. magnetization phase
- t. myelitis
- t. myelopathy
- t. nerve of neck
- t. occipital sulcus
- t. orientation
- t. pedicle angle
- t. pedicle diameter
- t. peduncular tract
- t. pontine fiber
- t. relaxation
- t. relaxation rate
- t. rhombencephalic flexure
- t. ridge
- t. septum
- t. sinus (TS)
- t. sinus of dura mater
- t. sinus occlusion
- t. stria of corpus callosum
- t. temporal convolution
- t. temporal gyri of Heschl
- t. temporal gyrus
- t. temporal sulcus

t. traction
t. tripolar epidural array
t. velum
t. vertebral body fracture
transversectomy
transversi
fasciculi t.
gyri temporales t.
sulci temporales t.
transversospinalis muscle group
transversum
velum t.
transversus
sulcus occipitalis t.
sulcus temporalis t.
transvestism
transzygomatic approach
Tranxene
tranylcypromine sulfate
trapdoor lamina
trapdoor-type flap
trapezius muscle
trapezoidal metal cage
trapezoid body
trapezoidei
nucleus anterior corporis t.
nucleus dorsalis corporis t.
nucleus lateralis corporis t.
nucleus medialis corporis t.
nucleus ventralis corporis t.
trapezoideum
corpus t.
trapped ventricle syndrome
trapping
aneurysm t.
t. of aneurysm
Traquair
junctional scotoma of T.
Trasylol
Traube-Hering-Mayer
T.-H.-M. wave
T.-H.-M. wave in cerebrospinal fluid
trauma
abdominal t.
acceleration-deceleration forces in craniocerebral t.
amnesia for t.
birth t.
cerebral t.
cervical spine t.
t. characteristic
child abuse with craniocerebral t.
circumflex nerve t.
t. coma databank (TCDB)
compression-rarefaction strain in craniocerebral t.
cranial nerve t.
t. craniocerebral
craniocerebral drug t.
t. cue
exposure to t.
facial nerve perinatal t.
head t.
intensity of t.
intestinal t.
long-term effects of t.
lumbar spine t.
maxillofacial t.
median nerve t.
nonaccidental t.
nonpenetrating t.
penetrating t.
perinatal craniocerebral t.
peripheral nerve t.
premorbid t.
psychological t.
radial nerve t.
sciatic nerve t.
severe head t.
t. spectrum disorder
spinal cord injury t.
t. survivor
thoracolumbar t.
ulnar nerve t.
ventromedial frontal lobe t.
vertebral artery t.
whiplash t.
TraumaCal
trauma-induced fistula
traumasthenia
traumatic
t. amnesia
t. anastomosis
t. anterolisthesis
t. brachial plexus disorder
t. brain injury (TBI)
t. central cord syndrome
t. cervical disc herniation
t. cervical discopathy
T. Coma Data Bank
t. degeneration
t. displacement
t. headache

NOTES

traumatic *(continued)*
t. hematoma
t. intracranial aneurysm (TICA)
t. intracranial hemorrhage
t. intracranial lesion
t. meningeal hemorrhage
t. meningocele
t. myelopathy
t. neurasthenia
t. neuritis
t. neuroma
t. neuropathy
t. neurosis
t. progressive encephalopathy
t. pseudomeningocele
t. spondylolisthesis
t. subarachnoid hemorrhage (TSAH)
t. syringomyelia
t. tap
t. tetanus
traumatica
cephalhydrocele t.
malacia t.
Traum-Ex
Trautmann triangle
Travasorb
traversal
tentorial t.
traversing segment
traxoprodil mesylate
trazodone
TRE
target registration error
Treacher Collins syndrome
treatment
acupuncture t.
asthma t.
bacterial meningitis t.
t. completion rate
t. compliance
compression rod t.
t. condition
conventional neuroleptic t.
disease-altering t.
distraction/compression scoliosis t.
dopaminergic t.
D-penicillamine t.
dual compression scoliosis t.
dystonia t.
t. effectiveness
ethanol t.
fluoxetine t.
gamma-interferon t.
t. gap
Hartel t.
hepatic encephalopathy t.
hypervolemic t.
immunoglobulin t.
insomnia t.
insulin coma t.
insulin shock t.
t. intensity parameter
intravenous immunoglobulin t.
Kleine-Levin syndrome t.
leg cramp t.
lithium t.
massage t.
Matas t.
microoperative t.
t. model
naltrexone-venlafaxine t.
neuromuscular scoliosis orthotic t.
ongoing neuroleptic t.
t. outcome
t. period
t. phase
phenylketonuria t.
physiotherapy t.
poliomyelitis t.
t. program
t. protocol
protocol-driven t.
t. regimen
t. resistant
t. response rate
Schlösser t.
short-term t.
spinal deformity t.
stereotactic radiation therapy t.
stimulant t.
t. strategy
suboptimal t.
Toft spinal correction t.
tokishakuyakusan t.
tuberculosis meningitis t.
unconventional t.
treatment-emergent
t.-e. akathisia
t.-e. asthenia
t.-e. extrapyramidal side effect
t.-e. hypertonia
t.-e. hypomania
t.-e. somnolence
treatment-intolerant patient
treatment-related complication
tree
dendritic t.
maidenhair t.
neurovascular t.
trefoil tendon deformation
trematode
t. infection
paragonimiasis t.
schistosomiasis t.
trembling
hereditary chin t.
involuntary t.
t. palsy

tremens
alcoholic delirium t.
delirium t. (DT)
tremogram
tremograph
tremor
action t.
alcoholic withdrawal t.
alternating t.
alternative t.
anticonvulsant medication-induced postural t.
arsenical t.
benign familial essential t.
cerebellar t.
cerebral t.
T. Clinical Rating Scale
coarse t.
continuous t.
defined t.
drug-induced t.
drug/toxin-induced t.
dystonic t.
enhanced physiologic t.
essential palatal t.
familial cortical t.
fibrillary t.
fine t.
flapping t.
hereditary essential t.
heredofamilial t.
Holmes t.
hysterical t.
intention t.
isometric t.
kinetic t.
limb t.
t. lingua
t. measurement
medication-induced t.
mercurial t.
metallic t.
methylxanthine-induced postural t.
t. opiophagorum
orthostatic t.
parkinsonism t.
passive t.
t. pathophysiology
persistent t.
physiologic t.
pill-rolling t.
position-specific t.
postural t.
t. potatorum
primary orthostatic t.
progressive cerebellar t.
psychogenic t.
reduced t.
rest t.
resting t.
rubral t.
saturnine t.
t. self-rating scale
senile t.
t. severity
static t.
striocerebellar t.
sustention/intention t.
symptomatic palatal t.
tardive t.
task-specific t.
t. tendinum
voice t.
volitional t.
wing-beating t.
tremorgram
tremulous
trench lung
Trendelenburg
T. gait
T. position
T. sign
T. symptom
trending
evoked potential t.
trepanation
trephination
cranial vault t.
trephine
t. craniotomy
D'Errico skull t.
DeVilbiss skull t.
Galt skull t.
Michele vertebral body t.
Scoville skull t.
Treponema
T. denticola
T. pallidum
T. pallidum immobilization
T. pallidum immobilization test
Trevor disease
Trexan
TRH
thyrotropin-releasing hormone

NOTES

triad
- t. of altered mental status
- Charcot t.
- t. of Dejerine syndrome
- Hutchinson t.
- Jacod t.
- Luciani t.
- narcoleptic t.
- t. protein

trial
- clinical t.
- controlled medication t.
- double-blind placebo t.
- double-blind placebo-controlled t.
- European Carotid Surgery T. (ECST)
- head-to-head clinical t.
- lower hook t.
- North American Symptomatic Carotid Endarterectomy T. (NASCET)
- open-label t.
- placebo-controlled t.
- randomized clinical t.
- randomized controlled t.
- tumor sensitizer t.
- upper hook t.
- VA Symptomatic T.
- t. visit

triamterene
- hydrochlorothiazide and t.

triangle
- t. of fillet
- Glasscock t.
- Gombault t.
- Gombault-Philippe t.
- Guillain-Mollaret t.
- hypoglossal t.
- interscalene t.
- Mullan t.
- opticocarotid t.
- paramedian t.
- Parkinson t.
- Philippe t.
- Reil t.
- Trautmann t.
- Wernicke t.

triangular
- t. base-transverse bar configuration
- t. crest
- t. lamella
- t. nucleus
- t. nucleus of septum
- t. part
- t. recess
- t. ridge
- t. septal nucleus
- t. syndrome
- t. tract

triangulare
- velum t.

triangularis
- crista t.
- nucleus t.
- pars t.
- recessus t.

triangulated pedicle screw

Triavil

triazolam

tribasilar synostosis

tricarboxylic acid (TCA)

triceps
- t. surae jerk
- t. surae reflex

trichalgia

trichesthesia

trichilemmoma

trichinellosis

trichinosis infection

trichlormethiazide

trichloromonofluoromethane
- dichlorodifluoromethane and t.

trichodynia

trichoepithelioma

trichoesthesia

trichoesthesiometer

trichofolliculoma

trichorrhexis nodosa

trichosis sensitiva

trichrome
- Gomori t.
- t. stain

tricortical iliac crest bone graft

tricresyl phosphate peripheral neuropathy

tricyclic
- t. drug
- t. effect

Tridione

triethanolamine salicylate

triethiodide
- gallamine t.

triethylene tetramine dihydrochloride

trifacial
- t. nerve
- t. neuralgia

trifluoperazine hydrochloride

trifluopromazine

triflupromazine

trifocal neuralgia

trifurcation of middle cerebral artery

trigeminal
- t. branch
- t. cave
- t. cavity
- t. cistern
- t. cough
- t. cranial nerve

t. crest
t. decompression
t. dermatome
t. electrode
t. eminence
t. evoked potential (TEP)
t. ganglion
t. hypesthesia
t. impression of temporal bone
t. lemniscus
t. lesioning
t. mesencephalic nucleus
t. motor dysfunction
t. motor nucleus
t. nerve neurinoma
t. neuralgia (TN)
t. neurolysis
t. neuroma
t. neuropathy
t. nucleus caudalis
t. nucleus caudalis lesioning
t. paralysis
t. rhizotomy
t. root
t. root section
t. schwannoma
t. stimulation
t. tract
t. tractotomy
t. tubercle

trigeminale
cavum t.
ganglion t.
tuberculum t.

trigeminalis
cavitas t.
lemniscus t.
nervus t.
nuclei nervi t.
nucleus inferior nervi t.
nucleus mesencephalicus t.
nucleus motorius t.
nucleus sensorius inferior nervi t.
nucleus tractus mesencephalici nervi t.
tractus spinalis nervi t.

trigemini
nuclei nervi t.
nucleus mesencephalicus nervi t.
nucleus motorius nervi t.
nucleus principalis nervi t.
nucleus sensorius principalis nervi t.
nucleus sensorius superior nervi t.
nucleus spinalis nervi t.
nucleus tractus mesencephali nervi t.
nucleus tractus spinalis nervi t.
radices nervi t.
radix sensoria nervi t.
tractus descendens nervi t.
tractus mesencephalicus nervi t.
tractus spinalis nervi t.

trigeminocerebellar artery

trigeminofacial reflex

trigeminospinalis
tractus t.

trigeminospinal tract

trigeminothalamic
t. fiber
t. tract

trigeminothalamicus
tractus t.

trigeminovascular
t. pathway
t. theory

trigeminus
descending nucleus of t.
main sensory nucleus of t.
mesencephalic nucleus of t.
motor nucleus of t.
principal sensory nucleus of t.
spinal nucleus of t.

trigger
t. area
t. finger
headache t.
kinesigenic t.
t. point
t. point muscle block
t. point neuralgia
seizure t.
visual t.
t. zone

triggered EMG

triggering
reflexive saccade t.

TriggerWheel Wand

trigona (*pl. of* trigonum)

trigone
t. of auditory nerve
cerebral t.
collateral t.

NOTES

trigone *(continued)*
t. of fillet
t. of habenula
habenular t.
hypoglossal t.
t. of hypoglossal nerve
interpeduncular t.
lateral lemniscus t.
t. of lateral lemniscus
t. of lateral ventricle
lemniscal t.
Müller t.
oculomotor t.
olfactory t.
pontocerebellar t.
Reil t.
vagal nerve t.
vagus t.
t. of vagus nerve
ventricular t.
trigonocephaly
trigonum, pl. **trigona**
t. cerebrale
t. collaterale
t. collaterale ventriculi lateralis
t. habenula
t. hypoglossale
t. lemnisci lateralis
t. lemniscus
t. nervi acustici
t. nervi hypoglossi
t. nervi vagi
t. olfactorium
t. pontocerebellare
t. vagale
t. ventriculi
trihexoside
ceramide t.
trihexosyl ceramide
trihexyphenidyl hydrochloride
triiodobenzoic acid
Trilafon
trilaminar myopathy
Trileptal
trill
vocal t.
trimeric form
trimethadione
trimethaphan
trimethobenzamide hydrochloride
trimethoprim-sulfamethoxazole
trimipramine maleate
Trimstat
trinitrate
glyceryl t.
Trinity polyaxial pedicle screw system
trinucleotide
t. repeat
t. repeat expansion
triorthocresyl
t. phosphate (TOCP)
t. phosphate neuropathy
triosephosphate isomerase deficiency
Triosil
tripelennamine
triphasic
t. slow-wave activity
t. wave
triphosphatase
adenosine t. (ATPase)
triphosphate
adenosine t.
deoxynucleoside t.
guanosine t. (GTP)
inositol t.
1,4,5-triphosphate
inositol t. (IP_3)
5′-triphosphate
adenosine 5′-t. (ATP)
triple
t. A syndrome (AAAS)
t. A syndrome gene
t. discharge
t. repeat disorder
triplegia
spastic t.
Triple-H therapy
triple-phase bone scan
triplet-repeat disease
triple-wire technique
tripoding
tripolar nerve cuff electrode
tripole
guarded t.
narrow t.
Trippi Wells tongs
triptan rebound headache
Triptil
trismic
trismoid
trismus
t. capistratus
t. dolorificus
t. nascentium
t. neonatorum
t. sardonicus
trisomy
t. C, D syndrome
t. 9 mosaic syndrome
t. 8, 13, 20, 21 syndrome
trisulfapyrimidine
triton
t. reciprocating saw
t. tumor
triventricular hydrocephalus
trivial risk
Trivittatus virus
Trk receptor

tRNA
alanine t.
trocar
brain t.
Frazier brain t.
hollow stainless-steel t.
McCain TMJ t.
Paulus t.
pyramidal t.
trochanter reflex
trochlear
t. cranial nerve
t. headache
t. nerve [CN IV]
t. nerve neoplasm
t. nerve palsy
t. nerve paralysis
t. nerve paresis
t. nucleus
trochlearis
nervus t. [CN IV]
nucleus nervi t.
trochlearium
decussatio fibrarum nervorum t.
Trolard
vein of T.
T. vein
trombone tremor of tongue
tromethamine (THAM)
ketorolac t.
Trömner
T. percussion hammer
T. reflex
trophic
t. change
t. gangrene
trophicity
trophism
trophodermatoneurosis
trophoneurosis
facial t.
lingual t.
muscular t.
Romberg t.
trophoneurotic
t. atrophy
t. leprosy
t. ulcer
trophotropic zone of Hess
tropical
t. ataxic neuropathy (TAN)
t. myeloneuropathy
t. spastic paraparesis
t. spastic paraparesis/HTLV-I-associated myelopathy
t. spastic paraplegia
tropicamide
troponin-tropomyosin complex
trough
synaptic t.
Trousseau
T. phenomenon
T. point
T. sign
T. spot
T. syndrome
T. twitching
Troyer syndrome
Tru-Cut needle biopsy
true
t. anosmia
t. aphasia
t. component
t. difference
t. dual pathology
t. neurogenic thoracic outlet syndrome
t. neuroma
t. nystagmus
truncal
t. apraxia-ataxia
t. ataxia
t. dysmetria
t. vagotomy
truncation
t. artifact
t. mutation
trunci plexus brachialis
truncus
t. arteriosus
t. corporis callosi
t. encephali
t. inferior plexus brachialis
t. lumbosacralis
t. medius plexus brachialis
t. nervi accessorii
t. nervi spinalis
t. superior plexus brachialis
t. sympatheticus
t. sympathicus
t. vagalis anterior
t. vagalis posterior
trunk
accessory nerve t.

NOTES

trunk *(continued)*
anterior vagal t.
t. ataxia
communicating branch of sympathetic t.
t. of corpus callosum
encephalic t.
ganglia of sympathetic t.
ganglion of sympathetic t.
lumbosacral t.
meningohypophysial t.
posterior vagal t.
t. posture
sympathetic t.
trunnion-guided radiosurgery
truss element
Trypanosoma
T. brucei
T. cruzi
trypanosome fever
trypanosomiasis
acute t.
African t.
American t.
chronic t.
Cruz t.
East African t.
Gambian t.
t. infection
Rhodesian t.
West African t.
tryptamine
tryptizol hydrochloride
tryptophan
t. hydroxylase
t. hydroxylase allelic genotype
TS
transverse sinus
TS system
TSA
Tourette Syndrome Association
TSAH
traumatic subarachnoid hemorrhage
TSC1 gene
TSC2 gene
T-score elevation
TSE
transmissible spongiform encephalopathy
TSH
thyroid-stimulating hormone
T-shaped
T-s. Edwards-Barbaro syringeal shunt
T-s. Edwards-Barbaro syringeal shunt table
T-s. incision
TSRH
Texas Scottish Rite Hospital
TSRH buttressed laminar hook
TSRH circular laminar hook
TSRH crosslink stabilization
TSRH double-rod construct
Galveston fixation with TSRH
TSRH implant
TSRH instrumentation
TSRH pedicle hook
TSRH pedicle screw-laminar claw construct
TSRH plate
TSRH rod fixation
TSRH universal spinal instrumentation system
Tsuji laminaplasty
tsutsugamushi
Rochalimaea t.
TTC
TTR
transthyretin
T-tube shunt
TTX
tetrodotoxin
T-type calcium channel
tubbylike protein
tube
Adson brain suction t.
air t.
alar lamina of neural t.
basal lamina of neural t.
basal plate of neural t.
blunt suction t.
Cone suction t.
Dandy suction t.
diverting shunt t.
dorsal plate of neural t.
endoneurial t.
endothelin-1 platinum-Dacron microcoil endotracheal t.
endotracheal t.
Ferguson brain suction t.
flow regulated suction t.
Frazier suction t.
Hardy suction t.
malleable multipore suction t.
medullary t.
microbore Tygon t.
nasogastric t.
neural t.
Nishizaki-Wakabayashi suction t.
Rhoton-Merz suction t.
Sachs brain suction t.
Sapporo shunt t.
Silastic t.
suction t.
tympanostomy t.
Univent endotracheal t.
ventral plate of neural t.

Yankauer suction t.
Yasargil suction t.
tuber, pl. **tubera**
t. anterius
t. cinereum
t. corporis callosi
cortical t.
t. dorsale
frontal t.
gray t.
subependymal t.
t. valvulae
t. of vermis
t. vermis
tuberales
nuclei t.
tuberalis
pars t.
tuberal nucleus
tubercle
acoustic t.
amygdaloid t.
anterior thalamic t.
ashen t.
auditory t.
Babès t.
t. bacillus
Chassaignac t.
cuneate t.
t. of cuneate nucleus
gracile t.
gray t.
intercolumnar t.
Morgagni t.
nucleus cuneatus t.
nucleus gracilis t.
t. of nucleus gracilis
olfactory t.
pharyngeal t.
posterior thalamic t.
rabic t.
Rolando t.
t. of saddle
trigeminal t.
wedge-shaped t.
tubercula (*pl. of* tuberculum)
tubercular meningitis
tuberculoma
t. en plaque
intracranial t.
tuberculosis
calvarial t.
cerebral t.
t. infection
t. meningitis
t. meningitis treatment
miliary pulmonary t.
Mycobacterium t.
t. peripheral neuropathy
pulmonary t.
spinal t.
spine t.
tuberculous
t. abscess
t. antigen
t. focus
t. meningitis
t. spondylitis
tuberculum, pl. **tubercula**
acoustic t.
t. anterius thalami
t. cinereum
t. cuneatum
t. gracile
t. hypoglossi
t. nuclei cuneati
t. nuclei gracilis
t. olfactorium
t. sella
t. sellae meningioma
t. sellae turcicae
t. trigeminale
tuberohypophysial tract
tuberoinfundibular
t. pathway
t. tract
tuberoinfundibularis
tractus t.
tuberomammillaris
nucleus t.
tuberomammillary nucleus
tuberosa
urticaria t.
tuberothalamic infarction
tuberous
t. sclerosis
T. Sclerosis Alliance
t. sclerosis monster cell
t. sclerosis railroad track appearance
t. sclerosis syndrome
Tubex gauze dressing
tubing
Intramedic PE-50 polyethylene t.

NOTES

tubular
t. aggregate myopathy
t. necrosis
tubulin assembly
tubulization
tubus medullaris
tuck position
Tuffier
T. laminectomy retractor
T. rib spreader
Tuffier-Raney retractor
tuft
dendritic t.
tufted cell
Tukey test
tulip pedicle screw
Tumarkin
otolithic crisis of T.
tumefaction
tumescence
penile t.
tumescent
tumor
acidophilic pituitary t.
acoustic nerve sheath t.
ACTH-secreting pituitary t.
adenomatoid odontogenic t.
adhesio interthalamica t.
adrenocorticotropic hormone-secreting pituitary t.
adult granulosa cell t. (AGCT)
aggressive papillary middle ear t.
angioglomoid t.
anterior cingulate gyrus t.
aortic body t.
astrocytic t.
atypical giant cell t.
atypical teratoid/rhabdoid t. (AT/RT)
basiocciput t.
basophilic pituitary t.
t. bed
benign cranial nerve t.
benign lymphoepithelial parotid t.
bone t.
brain t.
brainstem t.
t. bulk
carotid body t.
cartilaginous t.
cavernous sinus t.
t. cell
central nervous system t.
cerebellar t.
cerebellopontine angle t.
cervical dumbbell t.
cervical intramedullary t.
cervicomedullary t.
chemoreceptor t.
chiasmatic t.
childhood primitive neuroectodermal t.
chondromatous t.
chromaffin t.
Collins law of survival after brain t.
collision t.
congenital t.
t. control
convexity metastatic t.
craniopharyngeal duct t.
Cushing triad in brain t.
deep t.
dermoid t.
t. differentiating agent
diffuse fibrillary astrocytic t.
diffuse intrinsic brainstem t.
dumbbell t.
dysembryoplastic neuroepithelial t.
eighth nerve t.
endodermal sinus t.
enhancing exophytic t.
t. enucleation
ependymal t.
epidermoid t.
epidural t.
Erdheim t.
t. extension
t. extirpation
extradural t.
extrameatal intracapsular t.
extramedullary spinal cord t.
foramen jugulare t.
foramen ovale t.
foramen rotundum t.
frontal lobe t.
germ cell t.
giant cell t.
giant glomus t.
giant pituitary t.
glial t.
glomus jugulare t.
glomus vagale t.
t. grading
granular cell t.
high-grade t.
t. histology
hourglass t.
hypoglossal foramen t.
inclusion t.
infiltrating t.
infratemporal fossa t.
infratentorial Lindau t.
infratentorial neurological t.
inoperable t.
interdural t.
intracavernous t.
intracranial t.

intradural t.
intramedullary spinal cord t.
intraorbital granular cell t.
intrasellar growth hormone-secreting pituitary t.
intraspinal epidermoid t.
intraventricular t.
intrinsic brainstem t.
invasive t.
Kernohan classification of brain t.
Koenen t.
leptomeningeal t.
Lindau t.
low-grade t.
lumbar t.
lymphoepithelial parotid t.
lymphomatous t.
malignant brain t.
malignant germ cell t.
margaroid t.
t. marker
McLain-Weinstein classification of spinal t.'s
medullary t.
melanotic neuroectodermal t.
meningeal t.
metastatic brain t.
t. metastatic to spine
midline brain t.
mixed germ cell t.
mixed pineal t.
t. necrosis
t. necrosis factor (TNF)
t. necrosis factor-alpha (TNF-alpha)
t. necrosis factor receptor (TNFR)
Nelson t.
nerve sheath t.
neuroectodermal t.
neuroepithelial t.
neuronal t.
nongerminoma malignant germ cell t.
nonresectable t.
occipital lobe t.
olfactory groove t.
optic chiasm t.
optic pathway t.
orbital solitary fibrous t.
Pancoast t.
parachiasmal epidermoid t.
paranasal sinus t.
parasagittal t.
parasellar t.
parietal lobe t.
parotid t.
pearl t.
pearly t.
pediatric brain t.
pediatric supratentorial hemispheric t.
Pepper t.
peripheral nerve sheath t.
peripheral neuroectodermal t.
petroclival t.
petrous bone t.
pineal cell t.
pineal parenchymal t.
pineal region t.
pituitary t.
pontine angle t.
posterior fossa t.
Pott puffy t.
primary brain t.
primary neuroectodermal t.
primitive neuroectodermal t. (PNET)
primitive neuroepithelial t.
prolactin-secreting pituitary t.
Rathke pouch t.
recurrent t.
resectable t.
t. resection
residual t.
rhabdoid t.
right frontal craniotomy for gross total resection of t.
sand t.
sarcomatous t.
Schwann cell t.
secondary t.
sellar t.
t. sensitizer trial
sheath t.
t. shrinkage
slow-growing t.
small bowel carcinoid t.
smooth muscle t.
solitary fibrous t.
t. specimen
spinal cord t.
spindle cell t.
t. stroma
subdural t.
subependymal t.

T

NOTES

tumor *(continued)*
superior orbital fissure t.
superior pulmonary sulcus t.
t. suppressor gene
t. suppressor gene mutation
supratentorial primary malignant brain t.
supratentorial primitive neuroectodermal t.
tectal plate t.
temporal lobe t.
teratoid t.
teratoid-rhabdoid t.
thalamic t.
thoracic t.
triton t.
turban t.
t. type
t. vaccine
vascular t.
vasoformative t.
vertebral body t.
visible t.
visual system t.
t. volume
Wilms t.
tumoral calcinosis
tumor-associated rickets
tumor/cerebellum ratio
tumor/healthy tissue ratio
tumorigenesis
glial t.
tumor-infiltrating
t.-i. leukocyte (TIL)
t.-i. lymphocyte (TIL)
tumor-nerve bundle
tumorous involvement
TUNEL-positive cell
tunicate
tunicin
tuning fork test
Tun-L-Kath epidural catheter
tunnel
t. cell
cubital t.
superior-inferior submucous t.
tarsal t.
t. vision
tunnelable ventricular ICP catheter
tunneled ventriculostomy
Tuohy needle
turban tumor
turbid
turbidity
turbinectomy
turbo-spin echo
Turbo Tracker catheter
turcica
diaphragm of sella t.
sella t.
turcicae
tuberculum sellae t.
Türck
T. bundle
T. column
T. degeneration
T. fasciculus
T. tract
Turcot syndrome
Turkish-variant NCL
Turnbull method
Turner
intraparietal sulcus of T.
T. marginal gyrus
T. sulcus
T. syndrome
turning
saccadic contraversive head t.
turricephaly
Turyn sign
tussive
t. absence
t. syncope
tutamina cerebri
Tutoplast
T. anterior tibialis tendon
T. auditory ossicle
T. bone
T. costal cartilage
T. Dura patch
T. fascia lata
T. fascia temporalis
T. processed allograft
TVI
time-variance imaging
T1-weighted
T1-w. inversion recovery scan
T1-w. magnetic resonance image
T1-w. MR image
T1-w. spin echo
T1-w. spin-echo image
T2-weighted
T2-w. magnetic resonance image
T2-w. magnetic resonance scan
T2-w. MRI lesion
T2-w. MR image
T2-w. spin echo
T2-w. spin-echo image
T2-w. spin-echo sequence
T2-w. turbo-gradient image
twice-born
twice-repeated multivariate analysis of variance
twilight
t. phenomenon
t. state

twin
conjoined t.'s
dizygotic t.
monozygotic t.
t. research
Twin-K
twinship transference
twitch
Cogan lid t.
t. contraction
twitcher
twitching
facial t.
phasic t.
Trousseau t.
uremic t.
twoness
limen to t.
Tycolet
tying forceps
Tylenol
Tylox
tympana (*pl. of* tympanum)
tympani
anterior canaliculus of chorda t.
chorda t.
communicating branch of otic ganglion to chorda t.
communicating branch of otic ganglion with chorda t.
nervus musculi tensoris t.
pyramis t.
ramus communicans nervi glossopharyngei cum chorda t.
ramus communicans nervi lingualis cum chorda t.
tensor t.
tympanic
t. cavity
t. enlargement
t. ganglion
t. intumescence
t. nerve
t. swelling
tympanica
intumescentia t.
tympanici
ramus tubarius plexus t.
tympanico
ramus communicans nervi intermedii cum plexu t.
tympanicum
ganglion t.
glomus t.
tympanicus
nervus t.
plexus t.
tympanometry
tympanophonia
tympanoplasty
tympanosquamous suture
tympanostomy tube
tympanum, pl. **tympana, tympanums**
pyramid of t.
Tyndall effect
type
amyloidosis-Dutch t.
asthenic t.
Binswanger t.
choleric constitutional t.
dementia of the Alzheimer t.
dementia Alzheimer t. (DAT)
dementia frontal t.
function t.
t. 1 G_{M1} gangliosidosis
hereditary cerebral hemorrhage with amyloidosis-Dutch t. (HCHWA-D)
hypercompensatory t.
t. II curve pattern
t. II odontoid fracture
limb-girdle muscular dystrophy t. 2B (LGMD2B)
melancholic t.
paranoid t.
senile dementia of Alzheimer t. (SDAT)
sialidosis t. I
striatonigral degeneration t.
t. 2 superconductor
tumor t.
typhi
Salmonella t.
typhoid peripheral neuropathy
typhomania
typhosus
status t.
typhus
epidemic t.
t. fever
murine t.
typical
t. absence seizure
t. neuroleptic

NOTES

typify
typing
genetic t.
HLA t.
HLA-DR15 t.
leukocyte antigen t.
tyramine challenge test
tyramine-induced hypertensive crisis
tyropanoate
tyropanoic acid
tyrosine
t. hydroxylase
t. hydroxylase-positive
t. kinase
t. kinase A receptor
t. metabolism disorder
t. phosphatase
tyrosine-kinase receptor
tyrosinemia
t. aminoaciduria
premature infant t.
tyrosinosis
Tysabri
Tzanck smear

UARS
upper airway resistance syndrome
UBE3A
UBE3A gene
UBE3A mutation
ubiquitin
u. pathway
u. protein ligase
ubiquitin-activating enzyme E1
ubiquitin-conjugating enzyme E2
ubiquitin-ligase gene
ubiquitin-ligating enzyme E3
ubiquitin-proteosome system (UPS)
UCLA
University of California Los Angeles
UCLA Brain Mapping Center
uEEG ProSystem 5000
UHDRS
Unified Huntington Disease Rating Scale
UHMWPE
ultra-high molecular weight polyethylene
UHMWPE cable
Uhthoff
U. phenomenon
U. sign
UL
unit labyrinthectomy
ulcer
acute decubitus u.
Cushing u.
decubitus u.
neurogenic u.
neurotrophic u.
psychogenic duodenal u.
psychogenic gastric u.
psychogenic peptic u.
stress u.
trophoneurotic u.
ulceration
cerebrovascular u.
genital u.
oral u.
ulegyria
perisylvian u.
Ullmann line
Ullrich disease
ulnar
u. nerve
u. nerve entrapment
u. nerve lesion
u. nerve trauma
u. neuropathy
u. reflex
ulnari
ramus communicans nervi mediani com nervo u.
ulnaris
nervi digitales dorsales nervi u.
nervi digitales palmares communes nervi u.
nervi digitales palmares proprii nervi u.
nervus u.
rami musculares nervi u.
ramus dorsalis nervi u.
ramus palmaris nervi u.
ramus profundus nervi u.
ramus superficialis nervi u.
Ulrich-Turner syndrome
Ulthoff symptom
Ultracet
ultradian rhythm
Ultradol
ultra-high
u.-h. molecular weight polyethylene (UHMWPE)
u.-h. molecular weight polyethylene fiber
u.-h. molecular weight polyethylene fiber cable
UltraPower
U. basic drill system
U. bur guard
U. bur guard drill system
U. revision
U. revision drill system
U. surgical drill system
ultrasonic
u. aspirating device
u. aspiration
u. dissector
u. localizer
u. probe
u. surgical aspirator
u. therapy
u. wave
ultrasonographic
u. guidance
u. localization
ultrasonography
B-mode u.
color flow duplex u.
cranial u.
Doppler u.
sequential u.
transcranial Doppler u.
ultrasonosurgery

ultrasound
cranial u.
Doppler u.
intraoperative B-mode u.
Intrascan u.
quantification u.
TCD u.
transcranial B-mode u.
transfontanel Doppler u.
ultrasound-guided transfrontal transventricular approach
ultrastructural study
ultraterminal fiber
UMN
upper motor neuron
uncal
u. gyrus
u. infarction
u. transtentorial herniation
uncalis
vena u.
unc-33 gene
uncharacteristically
unci (*pl. of* uncus)
unciform fasciculus
uncinate
u. attack
u. aura
u. bundle of Russell
u. epilepsy
u. fasciculus of cerebellum
u. fasciculus of Russell
u. fit
u. gyrus
u. process
uncinatus
fasciculus u.
unclassified epileptic seizure
uncommon glioma
uncompensated hydrocephalus
uncomplicated
u. arteriosclerotic dementia
u. presenile dementia
u. senile dementia
unconditioned
u. reflex
u. response
u. stimulus
uncontrollable
u. motor activity
u. movement
unconventional
u. pharmaceutical
u. treatment
uncotomy
uncovertebral joint hypertrophy
uncus, pl. **unci**
arachnoid of u.
u. band of Giacomini
u. gyri fornicati
u. gyri hippocampus
u. gyri parahippocampalis
u. of temporal lobe
vein of u.
undercutting
cortical u.
u. saw
underlying
u. condition
u. mass lesion
u. sleep-disordered breathing
u. structural lesion
undifferentiated
u. cell adenoma
u. effect
undifferentiated-type
undulant fever
unexpected gait stop
ungual fibroma
unguis
u. avis
Haller u.
u. ventriculi lateralis cerebri
unicameral bone cyst
unicoronal synostosis
unidirectional nystagmus
Unified
U. Huntington Disease Rating Scale (UHDRS)
U. Parkinson Disease Rating Scale (UPDRS)
unifocal origin
uniform pore structure
Unilab Surgibone bovine bone graft
unilateral
u. anesthesia
u. chorea
u. deficit
u. dystonic posturing
u. epileptiform activity
u. facial pain syndrome
u. focus of activity
u. gliosis
u. hearing loss
u. hemilaminectomy
u. hemiparesis
u. hydrocephalus
u. hyperreflexia
u. hypophysectomy
u. interfacetal dislocation or subluxation
u. interictal focal epileptic discharge
u. laminotomy
u. megalencephaly
u. migraine
u. migraine headache
u. optic neuritis

u. pain
u. pedicle cannulation
u. pupil dilation
u. seizure
u. variable screw placement system
u. visual loss
unimodal association cortex
uninhibited neurogenic bladder
unintelligible speech
uniparental disomy
Unipen
unipolar
u. cell
u. cutting loop
u. neuron
u. patient
u. spongioblastoma
unipolare
spongioblastoma u.
unisensory
unit
afferent motor u.
AME microcurrent TENS u.
BICAP u.
Cadwell 5200A somatosensory evoked potential u.
2-component micrograp precision control suction u.
delirium u.
Dial Away Pain 400 electrotherapy u.
Eclipse TENS u.
efferent motor u.
fast motor u.
functional vertebral spinal u.
Hounsfield u. (HU)
intensive care u. (ICU)
internal pulse generating u.
u. labyrinthectomy (UL)
Leksell stereotactic gamma u.
Malis electrocoagulation u.
Maxima II TENS u.
Mayfield radiolucent base u.
motor u. (MU)
neurocritical care u. (NCCU)
neurology/neurosurgery intensive care u. (NNICU)
polyphasic motor u.
Radionics bipolar coagulation u.
reinnervated motor u.
Schwann cell u.
Sheffield gamma u.
201-source cobalt-60 gamma u.
u. spinal rod
stereotactic gamma u.
Tac gel for EMS u.
Tac gel for TENS u.
teleradiotherapy u.
valve u.
Wright Care TENS u.
ZD-Neurosurgical localizing u.
uniting
u. canal
u. duct
Univent endotracheal tube
universal
U. bone screw insertion/extraction system
U. cannulated screw system
u. flexion posture
u. instrumentation
u. phobia
U. Spine Classification
University
U. of California Los Angeles (UCLA)
U. of Pennsylvania Smell Test
U. Plate spinal attachment
unkei-to
unmyelinated
u. axon
u. fiber
u. nerve
unpleasantness
pain u.
unprovoked
u. anger
u. seizure
unresponsiveness
Full Outline of U. (FOUR)
unruptured intracranial aneurysm
unshunted hydrocephalus
unspecified
u. aneurysm
u. depression
unstable
u. fracture
u. injury pattern
u. lesion
u. posture
unsteadiness
postural u.
unstoppable flow of speech
untethering surgery

NOTES

unusual
u. sleep behavior
u. sleep movement
Unverricht
U. disease
U. myoclonus epilepsy
Unverricht-Lafora disease
Unverricht-Lundborg
U.-L. disease
U.-L. myoclonus epilepsy
U.-L. syndrome
unwanted screw torque
unyielding
u-PA
urokinase-type plasminogen activator
upbeating nystagmus
upbiting/downbiting pituitary rongeur
UPDRS
Unified Parkinson Disease Rating Scale
UPDRS scale
UPF
uvulopalatal flap
UPP
uvulopalatoplasty
upper
u. abdominal periosteal reflex
u. airway
u. airway collapse
u. airway dilating muscle
u. airway muscular tone
u. airway obstruction
u. airway reflex
u. airway resistance
u. airway resistance syndrome (UARS)
u. airway ventilation
u. bony endplate
u. cervical spine anterior construct
u. cervical spine anterior exposure
u. cervical spine fusion
u. cervical spine posterior construct
u. cervical spine procedure
u. extremity pronator sign
u. extremity scarf sign
u. hand
u. homonymous quadrantanopia
u. hook trial
u. limb areflexia
u. motoneuron
u. motor neuron (UMN)
u. motor neuron disease
u. motor neuron dysfunction
u. motor neuron impairment
u. motor neuron lesion
u. motor neuron paralysis
u. motor neuron weakness
u. pons
u. radicular syndrome
u. thoracic spine
UPPP
uvulopalatopharyngoplasty
up-regulation
receptor u.-r.
upregulation/downregulation hypothesis
UPS
ubiquitin-proteosome system
upside-down Mooney face
uptake
radioisotope u.
u. site
upward
u. gaze deficit
u. gaze paresis
Uracel
uranoschisis
uratic degeneration
urbanization
urea
u. blood level
u. cycle
u. cycle disorder
Ureaphil Injection
uremia peripheral neuropathy
uremic
u. amaurosis
u. coma
u. convulsion
u. encephalopathy
u. frost
u. neuropathy
OKT3 u.
u. polyneuropathy
u. toxin
u. twitching
uretericus
plexus u.
ureter injury
ureterolysis
urethral complex
urethrism, urethrismus
urethritis
urethrospasm
urgency
bladder u.
urinary u.
uric
u. acid
u. acid level
uridine
u. glucuronyl transferase
u. monophosphate synthase deficiency
urinary
u. creatinine
u. incontinence
u. infection in spina bifida cystica
u. porphobilinogen
u. reflex

u. sphincter
u. tract
u. tract function
u. urgency
urine
u. continence
u. coproporphyria
u. screening
u. testing
Uristix
Dextrostix U.
urocrisis, urocrisia
U-rod
compression U-r.
urogenital atrophy
Urografin
urokinase plasminogen activator receptor
urokinase-type
u.-t. PA
u.-t. plasminogen activator (u-PA)
Uro-KP-Neutral
urticaria
giant u.
u. gigans
u. gigantea
u. tuberosa
U-shaped scalp flap
Usher syndrome
ustus
Aspergillus u.
uterovaginalis
plexus u.
utricle
utricular
u. nerve
u. reflex
u. spot
utricularis
nervus u.
utriculi
macula u.
utriculoampullaris
nervus u.
utriculoampullarly nerve
utriculosaccular
u. duct
u. dysfunction
utriculosaccularis
ductus u.
utriculus
utterance
socially stigmatizing u.
uveitis
juxtapapillary u.
uveomeningeal syndrome
uveomeningoencephalic syndrome
uveomeningoencephalitis
uvula
bifid u.
u. cerebelli
u. of cerebellum
u. vermis
uvulectomy
uvulopalatal flap (UPF)
uvulopalatopharyngoplasty (UPPP)
uvulopalatoplasty (UPP)
laser u. (LUPP)
laser-assisted u. (LAUP)

NOTES

V1 halo ring
VA
ventriculoatrial
vertebral artery
VA Hospital
VA Symptomatic Trial
VAC
vacuum-assisted closure
VAC Therapy
vacant staring
vaccination
complication following measles v.
v. encephalomyelitis
v. encephalopathy
v. peripheral neuropathy
vaccine
diphtheria, tetanus toxoids, and pertussis v.
tumor v.
vaccine-associated Guillain-Barré syndrome
vaccinia
myelitis v.
Vac-Lok
V.-L. bag immobilizer
V.-L. cushion
vacuo
hydrocephalus ex v.
vacuolar
v. degeneration
v. myelopathy
vacuum
v. disc
v. headache
v. phenomenon
vacuum-assisted closure (VAC)
VaD
vascular dementia
vagal
v. attack
v. lobe
v. nerve implant
v. nerve stimulation (VNS)
v. nerve trigone
v. part of accessory nerve
vagale
glomus v.
trigonum v.
vagalis
pars v.
vagectomy
vagi (*pl. of* vagus)
vagina
v. cellulosa
v. externa nervi optici
v. interna nervi optici
vaginae
v. nervi optici
pars anterior fornicis v.
pars anterior fornix v.
pars posterior fornix v.
pars postlaminalis nervi optici v.
vaginal
v. hyperesthesia
v. nerve
v. plexus
vaginales
nervi v.
vaginismus
functional v.
vagoaccessorius
vagoaccessory-hypoglossal syndrome
vagoaccessory syndrome
vagoglossopharyngeal neuralgia
vagogram
vagolysis
vagolytic
vagomimetic
vagosplanchnic
vagosympathetic
vagotomy
bilateral v.'s
highly selective v.
parietal cell v.
posterior truncal v.
selective v.
truncal v.
vagotonia
vagotonic
vagotony
vagotropic
vagovagal
vagus, pl. **vagi**
v. area
v. cranial nerve [CN X]
dorsal motor nucleus of v.
dorsal nucleus of v.
vagi eminentia
ganglion inferius nervi v.
ganglion rostralis nervi v.
ganglion superius nervi v.
ganglion of trunk of v.
lobus v.
v. nerve examination
v. nerve jugular ganglion
v. nerve rostral ganglion
v. nerve stimulation (VNS)
v. nerve stimulation technique
v. nerve stimulator

vagus *(continued)*
v. neuropathy
nuclei nervi v.
nucleus commissuralis nevi v.
nucleus dorsalis nervi v.
nucleus posterior nervi v.
plexus pharyngeus nervi v.
rami bronchiales anteriores nervi v.
rami bronchiales posteriores nervi v.
rami cardiaci cervicales inferiores nervi v.
rami cardiaci cervicales superiores nervi v.
rami cardiaci thoracici nervi v.
rami celiaci nervi v.
rami gastrici nervi v.
rami renales nervi v.
ramus articularis nervi v.
ramus communicans nervi glossopharyngei ramo auriculari nervi v.
ramus communicans nervi glossopharyngei ramo meningeo nervi v.
ramus communicans nervi intermedii cum nervo v.
ramus meningeus nervi v.
ramus pharyngeus nervi v.
v. reflex
v. stimulator implant
v. trigone
trigonum nervi vagi

Vail
V. neuralgia
V. syndrome

Vairox high-compression vascular stockings

valacyclovir

Valentin
V. corpuscle
V. nerve
V. pseudoganglion
V. tympanic ganglion

valepotriate

valerianic acid

valinemia

Valium

vallecula, pl. **valleculae**
v. cerebelli
v. of cerebellum
sulcus valleculae
v. sylvii

Valleix point

Valleylab
V. CUSA CEM system
V. neurosurgical product

vallis

valproate

valproate-associated hyperammonemia

valproic
v. acid
v. acid and derivative
v. acid poisoning

valpromide

valrocemide

Valsalva maneuver

value
impedance v.
v. system

valve
Aesculap-Miethke v.
auxiliary v.
ball-in-cone v.
Codman Hakim programmable v.
Codman-Medos programmable v.
Codman slit v.
Cordis-Hakim v.
cruciform slit v.
CRx Diamond v.
Delta v.
Denver v.
differential pressure v.
double spring ball v.
dual-switch v.
Hakim high-pressure v.
Hakim precision v.
Heyer-Pudenz v.
Heyer-Schulte bur hole v.
Holter-Hausner v.
Holter high-pressure v.
Holter medium-pressure v.
hydrostatic v.
v. infection
Low Profile v.
Medos v.
Medos-Hakim v.
membrane v.
Miethke dual-switch v.
Mishler v.
needle v.
Novus hydrocephalic v.
Novus mini v.
v. opening pressure
Orbis-Sigma v. (OSV)
Orbis-Sigma cerebrospinal fluid shunt v.
Orbis-Sigma v. II
v. patency
pedi-gravity assisted v.
Phoenix ancillary v.
Phoenix cruciform v.
programmable v.
prosthetic heart v.
PS Medical Flow Control v.
Pudenz v.
Pudenz-Heyer-Schulte v.
v. replacement

rotating hemostatic v.
slit v.
Sophy adjustable pressure v.
Sophy mini programmable pressure v.
standard v.
Strata adjustable Delta v.
v. system
Tarin v.
Tarinus v.
v. unit
Vieussens v.
Willis v.

valve-regulated shunt

valvulae
tuber v.

valvula semilunaris tarini

valvuloplasty

van
V. Allen syndrome
V. Allen-type familial amyloid polyneuropathy
v. Bogaert-Canavan disease
v. Bogaert disease
v. Bogaert encephalitis
v. Bogaert sclerosing leukoencephalitis
v. der Knaap syndrome
v. der Kolk law

Vancocin

vanilloid VR1 receptor

vanishing
v. white matter
v. white matter disease

Vanzetti sign

variability
respiratory v.

variable
clinical v.
continuous v.
demographic v.
dynamic v.
v. heavy chain (VH)
v. positive airway pressure (VPAP)
prognostic v.
v. screw placement
v. screw placement system
v. screw placement system instrumentation
v. screw placement system-instrumented lumbar spine
v. screw placement system-plated patient
situational v.
v. spinal plating (VSP)
v. stereotactic image fusion
v. stiffness microcatheter

variance
analysis of v. (ANOVA)
analysis v.
v. assumption
multivariate analysis of v. (MANOVA)
twice-repeated multivariate analysis of v.

Vari-Angle
V.-A. aneurysm clip
V.-A. clip applier
V.-A. clip holder
V.-A. screw

variant
anatomical v.
Becker v.
benign epileptiform v.
bizarre v.
v. Creutzfeldt-Jakob disease (vCJD)
migraine v.
multiple sclerosis v.
neuroectodermal tumor desmoplastic v.
petit mal v.
primitive trigeminal artery v.
v. surface glycoprotein (VSG)
transthyretin v.
Westphal v.

variation
coefficient of v. (COV)
contingent negative v.
diurnal mood v.
genetic v.
situational tic v.

varicella
congenital v.
v. encephalitis
v. zoster encephalomyelitis
v. zoster virus
v. zoster virus infection

varicella-zoster
v.-z. virus (VZV)
v.-z. virus antigen
v.-z. virus reactivation

varices (*pl. of* varix)

varicose fiber

V

NOTES

varicosity
autonomic v.
Varidase
variegate porphyria
VariGrip spine fixation system
varimax rotation
Vario microscope
varix, pl. **varices**
orbital v.
varolii
pons v.
VAS
visual analog scale
vasa
v. recta
v. vasorum
Vasamedics laser Doppler flow probe
vascular
v. accident
v. cell adhesion molecule-1 (VCAM-1)
v. change
v. chorea
v. circle of optic nerve
v. cognitive impairment
v. decompression
v. dementia (VaD)
v. dilation
v. dissection
v. endothelial growth factor (VEGF)
v. endothelium
v. erosion
v. foot plate
v. fragility
v. groove
v. growth factor
v. hamartoma
v. headache
v. higher level gait disorder
v. immune deposit
v. injury
v. intratympanic mass
v. loop
v. malformation
v. meninx
v. myelopathy
v. occlusion
v. organ of lamina terminalis
v. Parkinson disease
v. parkinsonism
v. patch graft
v. perforation
v. plexus
v. ring
v. sensation
v. smooth muscle
v. spasm
v. steal
v. structure
v. surgery
v. tone
v. tumor
vascularis
pars v.
plexus v.
vascularity
intense v.
vascularized split calvarial cranioplasty
vasculature
CNS v.
systemic v.
vasculitic
v. mechanism
v. necrosis
v. neuropathy
vasculitis, pl. **vasculitides**
acute rheumatic fever v.
benign angiopathy of CNS v.
Churg-Strauss v.
Cogan syndrome v.
collagen vascular disease v.
cryoglobulinemic v.
headache with v.
hypersensitivity v.
hypocomplementemic urticarial v.
juvenile rheumatoid arthritis v.
Kawasaki disease v.
large vessel v.
leukocytoclastic v.
mesenteric v.
necrotizing v.
pauciimmune necrotizing v.
radiation v.
retinal v.
septic venous v.
systemic v.
Takayasu arteritis v.
Wegener granulomatosis v.
vasculitis-vasculopathy
HZV v.-v.
vasculomotor
vasculomyelinopathy
vasculopathy
HIV-associated vasculitic v.
inflammatory diabetic v.
radiation v.
radiation-induced v.
vasculosa
meninx v.
pars v.
tela v.
vasculosum
organum v.
punctum v.
vase
Rubin v.
Vaseline gauze packing

Vaseretic 10-25
vasoactive
v. intestinal peptide
v. intestinal polypeptide (VIP)
v. substance
vasoconstriction
caffeine-induced v.
sympathetic nervous system-medicated v.
vasoconstrictive action
vasoconstrictor
v. center
v. nerve
v. pathway
vasodepressor syncope
vasodilatation
hypoxic cerebral v.
mannitol-induced cerebral v.
vasodilating antihypertensive medication
vasodilation
vasodilative
vasodilator
v. center
v. headache
v. nerve
vasoformative tumor
vasogenic
v. edema
v. shock
v. theory
vasomotor
v. absence
v. ataxia
v. center
v. change
v. component
v. epilepsy
v. fiber
v. headache
v. imbalance
v. instability
v. ischemia
v. nerve
v. paralysis
v. rhinitis
v. spasm
v. syncope
v. tone
vasoneuropathy
vasoneurosis
vasopressin (VP)
arginine v.
deamino-D-arginine v.
v. receptor agonist
v. tannate
vasopressor reflex
vasoreactivity
cerebral v.
vasoreflex
vasoresponsiveness
vasorum
nervi v.
vasa v.
VasoSeal closure device
vasosensory nerve
vasospasm
angiographic v.
arterial v.
cerebral v.
delayed cerebral v.
migraine v.
symptomatic v.
vasospasm-related hydrocephalus
vasospastic attack
vasostimulant
vasotocin
arginine v.
vasovagal
v. attack
v. epilepsy
v. syncope
v. syndrome
vastus lateralis muscle biopsy
Vater corpuscle
Vater-Pacini
V.-P. body
V.-P. corpuscle
vault
cranial v.
craniosacral v. (CV)
craniosacral v. 4 (CV4)
VBR
vertebral body replacement
VCAM-1
vascular cell adhesion molecule-1
VCAM-1 receptor
VCAM1
vCJD
variant Creutzfeldt-Jakob disease
VDRL
Venereal Disease Research Laboratory
VDRL test
VDS
ventral derotation spondylodesis

NOTES

V

Vectastain ABC kit
vector
v. diagram
v. field
gene therapy v.
lentiviral v.
M v.
macroscopic magnetization v.
magnetic field v.
nuclear magnetization v.
v. phase
vector-mediated gene transfer
vector-producing cell (VPC)
VectorVision$_2$
VectorVision$_2$ENT
VectorVision$_2$Fluoro
VectorVision image-guided surgery system
VectorVision$_2$Spine
vecuronium bromide
VEE
Venezuelan equine encephalomyelitis
vegetative
v. circadian rhythmicity
v. nervous system
v. state
v. symptom
vegetotherapy
VEGF
vascular endothelial growth factor
veil
aqueduct v.
vein
aneurysm of Galen v.
anterior cerebral v.
anterior jugular v.
anterior pontomesencephalic v.
arterialized leptomeningeal v.
azygos v.
basal v.
brachiocephalic v.
bridging v.
Browning v.
carotid v.
v. of caudate nucleus
cerebellar v.
v. of cerebellum
cerebral v.
cervical intersegmental v.
choroid v.
cistern of great cerebral v.
common basal v.
v. of corpus striatum
cortical v.
deep middle cerebral v.
diencephalic v.
diploic v.
direct lateral v.
dorsal callosal v.
draining v.
emissary v.
v. of Galen
v. of Galen aneurysm
v. of Galen malformation
great cerebral v.
inferior anastomotic v.
inferior basal v.
inferior cerebral v.
inferior choroid v.
inferior thalamostriate v.
inferior ventricular v.
innominate v.
insular v.
internal cerebral v.
internal jugular v.
intradural draining v.
jugular v.
jugulocephalic v.
Labbé v.
v. of Labbé
lateral atrial v.
lateral direct v.
v. of lateral recess of fourth ventricle
lingual v.
linguofacial v.
maxillary v.
medial atrial v.
v. of medulla oblongata
meningeal v.
meningorachidian v.
mesencephalic v.
myelencephalic v.
v. of olfactory gyrus
ophthalmic v.
orbital v.
parietal v.
v. patch rupture
peduncular v.
v. of pons
pontine v.
pontomesencephalic v.
posterior callosal v.
v. of posterior horn
posterior marginal v.
posterior pericallosal v.
precentral cerebellar v.
prefrontal v.
primitive maxillary v.
radicular v.
right hepatic v.
Rosenthal v.
saphenous v.
v. of septum pellucidum
striate v.
superficial middle cerebral v.
superficial temporal v.
superior anastomotic v.

superior basal v.
superior cerebral v.
superior choroid v.
superior ophthalmic v.
superior thalamostriate v.
superior thyroid v.
surface thalamic v.
telencephalic v.
terminal v.
thalamostriate v.
thrombosed thick-walled v.
Trolard v.
v. of Trolard
v. of uncus
vertebral v.

vela (*pl. of* velum)
Velban
Veley headrest
vellicate
vellication
vellus olivae inferioris
velocardiofacial syndrome
velocimetry
laser Doppler v.
velocity
absorption v.
average v.
blood v.
blood flow v.
conduction v.
v. encoding
flow v.
glutamate transport v.
maximum saccade peak v.
motor conduction v. (MCV)
nerve conduction v. (NCV)
peak systolic v.
preserved conduction v.
v. profile
saccade v.
saccadic v.
spectral v.
spin v.
sway v.
target v.
vergence v.
velopharyngeal incompetence (VPI)
velum, pl. **vela**
anterior medullary v.
frenulum of superior medullary v.
inferior medullary v.
v. interpositum
v. medullare inferius
v. medullare superius
v. palatinum
posterior medullary v.
v. semilunare
superior medullary v.
v. tarini
v. terminale
transverse v.
v. transversum
v. triangulare

vena, pl. **venae**
v. anastomotica inferior
v. anastomotica superior
venae anteriores cerebri
v. anterior septi pellucidi
v. atrii lateralis
v. atrii medialis
v. basalis
v. cava injury
v. cerebri anterior
v. cerebri inferiores
v. cerebri internae
v. cerebri magna
v. cerebri media profunda
v. cerebri media superficialis
v. cerebri profundae
v. cerebri superficiales
v. cerebri superiores
v. choroidea inferior
v. choroidea superior
v. cornus posterioris
v. directae laterales
v. dorsalis corporis callosi
v. gyri olfactorii
v. hemispherii cerebelli inferiores
v. hemispherii cerebelli superiores
v. inferiores cerebelli
v. inferiores cerebri
v. inferior vermis
v. insulares
v. internae cerebri
v. lateralis ventriculi lateralis
v. magna cerebri
v. medialis ventriculi lateralis
v. media profunda cerebri
v. media superficialis cerebri
v. medullae oblongatae
v. mesencephalicae
v. nuclei caudati
v. parietales
v. pedunculares

V

NOTES

vena *(continued)*
v. petrosa
v. pontis
v. pontomesencephalica
v. pontomesencephalica anterior
v. posterior corporis callosi
v. posterior septi pellucidi
v. precentralis cerebelli
v. prefrontales
v. profundae cerebri
v. recessus lateralis
v. septi pellucidi anterior
v. septi pellucidi posterior
v. striatae
v. superficiales cerebri
v. superiores cerebelli
v. superiores cerebri
v. superior vermis
v. terminalis
v. thalamostriatae inferiores
v. thalamostriata superior
v. uncalis
v. ventricularis inferior
v. vermis inferior
v. vermis superior
VenaFlow compression system
venereal
V. Disease Research Laboratory (VDRL)
V. Disease Research Laboratory test
Venezuelan
V. equine encephalitis
V. equine encephalomyelitis (VEE)
venipuncture pain
venlafaxine hydrochloride
venography
digital subtraction v.
epidural v.
magnetic resonance v. (MRV)
transosseous v.
vertebral v.
venom
animal v.
venorespiratory reflex
venous
v. aneurysm
v. angioma
v. angle
v. dural sinus
v. embolism
v. hypertension
v. lake
v. lake configuration
v. malformation
v. occlusion plethysmography (VOP)
v. occlusive disease
v. outflow obstruction
v. oxygen saturation
v. plexus
v. sinus of dura mater
v. sinus thrombosis
v. stasis
v. stasis retinopathy
v. system
v. thromboembolic disease (VTED)
venous-side embolization
venous-sinus
thrombocytopenia v.-s.
ventilated
ventilation
abnormal v.
assisted v.
controlled mechanical v. (CMV)
high-frequency percussive v. (HFPV)
mechanical v.
nasal bilevel v.
negative-pressure v.
noninvasive positive pressure v.
sleep-related v.
upper airway v.
ventilation/perfusion inequality
ventilator
v. alarm
v. weaning
ventilatory support neurologic complication
Ventolin
ventral
v. acoustic stria
v. amygdalofugal pathway
v. anterior nucleus
v. anterior nucleus of thalamus
v. branch of thoracic nerve
v. column of spinal cord
v. derotation spondylodesis (VDS)
v. fasciculus proprius of spinal cord
v. funiculus
v. globus pallidus
v. horn
v. intermediate nucleus (VIM)
v. intermediate nucleus of thalamus
v. intermediate thalamic nucleus
v. lateral complex of thalamus
v. lateral geniculate nucleus
v. lateral nucleus of thalamus
v. medial complex of thalamus
v. medial mesencephalic syndrome
v. medial nucleus of oculomotor nerve
v. median fissure of medulla oblongata
v. median fissure of spinal cord
v. medullary compression
v. mesencephalic dopaminergic cell

v. mesencephalon
v. nucleus of trapezoid body
v. pallidum
v. paraflocculus
v. paralimbic region
v. part of pons
v. plate of neural tube
v. pontine infarction
v. posterior inferior (VPI)
v. posterior intermediate nucleus of thalamus
v. posterior lateral (VPL)
v. posterior lateral nucleus of thalamus
v. posterior medial (VPM)
v. posterior nucleus
v. posteroinferior nucleus
v. posterolateral (VPL)
v. posterolateral nucleus
v. posterolateral nucleus of thalamus
v. posteromedial (VPM)
v. posteromedial nucleus
v. posteromedial nucleus of thalamus
v. premammillary nucleus
v. principal nucleus
v. putamen
v. ramus
v. ramus of thoracic nerve
v. raphespinal tract
v. regimental area
v. respiratory group
v. root of spinal nerve
v. spinal artery occlusion
v. spinal cord compression
v. spinal root
v. spinocerebellar tract
v. spinothalamic tract
v. stream
v. striatum
v. tegmental area (VTA)
v. tegmental decussation
v. tegmentum
v. thalamic peduncle
v. tier thalamic nucleus
v. trigeminothalamic tract
v. white column
v. white commissure

ventrale
pallidum v.
striatum v.

ventralis
commissura supraoptica v.
v. intermedius
lamina v.
nucleus campi v.
nucleus periventricularis v.
nucleus premammillaris v.
v. oralis posterior
paraflocculus v.
pedunculus thalami v.
v. posterior lateralis
v. posteromedialis
radix v.
sulcus v.
thalamus v.
tractus corticospinalis v.
tractus pyramidalis v.
tractus reticulospinalis v.
tractus spinocerebellaris v.
tractus spinothalamicus v.

ventricle
Arantius v.
ballooned floor of v.
body of lateral v.
v. of brain
bulb of occipital horn of lateral v.
bulb of posterior horn of lateral v.
central part of lateral v.
cerebral v.
v. of cerebral hemisphere
choroid plexus of fourth v.
choroid plexus of lateral v.
choroid plexus of third v.
choroid tela of fourth v.
choroid tela of third v.
colloid cyst of third v.
cornua of lateral v.
v. of diencephalon
Duncan v.
v. effacement
fifth v.
fourth v.
inferior horn of lateral v.
lateral aperture of fourth v.
lateral recess of fourth v.
lateral vein of lateral v.
left v.
limiting sulcus of fourth v.
medial vein of lateral v.
median aperture of fourth v.
median sulcus of fourth v.

NOTES

ventricle *(continued)*
medullary stria of fourth v.
pineal v.
v. puncture
v. of rhombencephalon
right v.
roof of fourth v.
sixth v.
slit v.
spinal cord terminal v.
sylvian v.
v. of Sylvius
Sylvius v.
tela choroidea of fourth v.
tela choroidea of lateral v.
tela choroidea of third v.
tenia of fourth v.
terminal v.
third v.
trigone of lateral v.
vein of lateral recess of fourth v.
Verga v.
Vieussens v.
Wenzel v.
v. width
ventricular
v. aqueduct
v. block
v. catheter occlusion
v. catheter reservoir
v. decompression
v. dilation
v. drainage
v. enlargement
v. ependyma
v. fibrillation
v. fluid
v. ganglion
v. layer
v. needle
v. Ommaya reservoir
v. puncture
v. trigone
v. wall
ventriculitis
ventriculoamniotic shunting
ventriculoatrial (VA)
v. shunt
ventriculoatriostomy
ventriculocisternal shunt
ventriculocisternostomy
Torkildsen v.
ventriculoencephalitis
cytomegalovirus v.
ventriculofugal artery
ventriculogram
iohexol CT v.
ventriculography
air v.
cerebral v.
stereotactic anteroposterior and lateral metrizamide v.
water-soluble contrast v.
ventriculojugular (VJ)
ventriculomastoidostomy
ventriculomegaly
progressive posthemorrhagic v.
ventriculometry
ventriculoperitoneal (VP)
v. shunt
v. shunting
ventriculopleural shunt
ventriculopuncture
ventriculoscope
4-channel Aesculap v.
rigid v.
ventriculoscopy
monoportal v.
ventriculostomy
v. catheter
endoscopic third v. (ETV)
v. needle
neuroendoscopic third v.
straight-in v.
terminal v.
third v.
tunneled v.
ventriculostomy-related infection
ventriculosubarachnoid
ventriculotomy
ventriculovenous shunt
ventriculum
iter a tertio ad quartum v.
ventriculus
v. dexter cerebri
v. lateralis
v. lateralis cerebri
v.'s quarti
v. quartus
v. quartus cerebri
v. quintus
v. sinister cerebri
v. terminalis
v. terminalis medullae spinalis
v. tertius
v. tertius cerebri
trigonum v.'s
Ventrix
V. fiberoptic ventricular drainage system
V. fiberoptic ventricular monitoring system
V. SD fiberoptic subdural ICP catheter
V. tunnelable ventricular ICP monitoring and drainage system
V. tunnelable ventricular intracranial pressure monitoring system

ventrobasal
v. complex of the thalamus
v. nucleus
v. nucleus complex
ventrobasales
nuclei v.
ventrocaudal nucleus
ventrolateral (VL)
v. nuclear complex
v. sclerosis
v. sulcus
v. surface of medulla
ventrolateralis
nucleus hypothalamicus v.
v. thalamotomy
ventromedial
v. frontal leukotomy
v. frontal lobe trauma
v. hypothalamic hamartoma
v. hypothalamic nucleus
v. nucleus of hypothalamus
v. prefrontal cortex
v. prefrontal cortex of brain
ventromedialis
nucleus hypothalamicus v.
ventroposterolateral (VPL)
v. pallidotomy
ventroposteromedial (VPM)
v. pallidotomy
venturesome
venular obstruction
VEP
visual evoked potential
VEPTR
vertical expandable prosthetic titanium rib
VER
visual evoked response
vera
neuralgia facialis v.
polycythemia v.
verapamil
Veratran
Verax
verbal
v. ability
v. agraphia
v. amnesia
v. analog pain scale
v. apraxia
v. auditory agnosia
v. command
v. communication
v. cue
v. episodic memory
v. information
v. intellectual functioning
v. intervention
v. material
v. memory deficit
v. memory encoding task
v. memory exercise
v. memory impairment
v. reasoning deficit
v. recall score
v. weighted sum score
v. working memory
verbalizing
inappropriate v.
verborum
delirium v.
vergae
cavum v.
Verga ventricle
verge
anal v.
vergence
v. movement
v. system
v. velocity
Verhoeff-Van Gieson stain
veridical memory
vermal nodulus
vermian
v. artery
v. atrophy
v. medulloblastoma
v. split
vermicular sulcus
vermilion border
vermis
anterior v.
v. cerebelli
folium of v.
inferior vein of v.
medullary body of v.
nodule of v.
nodulus v.
pyramid of v.
pyramis v.
superior vein of v.
tuber v.
tuber of v.
uvula v.

V

NOTES

vermis *(continued)*
vena inferior v.
vena superior v.
Vermont
V. spinal fixator
V. spinal fixator articulation
vernal encephalitis
Vernet syndrome
Verneuil neuroma
vernoestival encephalitis
Verocay body
verocytotoxin
VersaPulse holmium laser
versatility
attachment v.
versenate
calcium disodium v.
versican proteoglycan
versicolor
membrana v.
version
Hare Psychopathy Checklist: Screening V.
versive seizure
VertAlign spinal support system
vertebra, pl. **vertebrae**
block v.
butterfly v.
cervical v.
coccygeal v.
coronal cleft v.
fish v.
inferior v.
lamina arcus vertebrae
limbus v.
lumbar v.
lumbosacral v.
sacral v.
v. spreader
thoracic v.
thoracolumbar v.
transitional v.
wedge-shaped v.
vertebral
v. angiogram
v. angiography
v. angioma
v. aplasia
v. artery (VA)
v. artery injury
v. artery occlusion
v. artery transposition
v. artery trauma
v. body anterior cortex
v. body anterior cortex penetration
v. body corpectomy
v. body decompression
v. body growth
v. body impactor
v. body replacement (VBR)
v. body tumor
v. cervical instability
v. collapse
v. column
v. column injury
v. compression deformity
v. curvature
v. dissection
v. endplate enhancement
v. exposure
facioauricular v. (FAV)
v. fascia
v. fracture
v. fusion
v. ganglion
v. hemangioendothelioma
v. hemangioma
v. level
v. marrow
v. marrow fat
v. nerve
v. origin angioplasty and stenting
v. osteosynthesis
v. osteosynthesis fusion rate
v. part
v. plate
v. plate application
v. plate bypass
v. plexus
v. pulp
v. resection
v. subluxation
v. vein
v. venography
vertebrale
ganglion v.
vertebralis
columna v.
pars v.
plexus v.
theca v.
vertebrectomy
Bohlman anterior cervical v.
cervical spondylotic myelopathy v.
microsurgical thoracoscopic v.
vertebrobasilar
v. aneurysm
v. artery
v. atherosclerosis
v. circulation
v. disease
v. infarction
v. insufficiency
v. ischemia
v. syndrome
v. system
v. transient ischemic attack

vertebrogenic
v. pain syndrome
v. symptom complex
vertebroplasty
vertex, pl. **vertices**
V. reconstruction system
v. sharp wave
vertical
v. axis
v. conflict
v. conjugate saccade
v. expandable prosthetic titanium rib (VEPTR)
v. eye movement
v. gaze
v. gaze limitation
v. gaze palsy
v. gaze paresis
v. line bisection
v. midline incision
v. migration
v. nystagmus
v. ocular deviation
v. pedicle diameter
v. plane
v. ring curette
v. sharp wave
v. suspension test
v. vertigo
verticalis
sulcus v.
vertices (*pl. of* vertex)
vertiginosus
status v.
vertiginous aura
vertigo
v. ab stomacho laeso
angiopathic v.
apoplectic v.
arteriosclerotic v.
v. attack
aural v.
benign functional v.
benign paroxysmal positional v.
benign positional paroxysmal v.
benign postural v.
central v.
cerebral v.
cervical v.
Charcot v.
chronic v.
disabling positional v. (DPV)
encephalic v.
endemic paralytic v.
epidemic v.
episodic v.
galvanic v.
gastric v.
height v.
horizontal v.
intractable v.
labyrinthine v.
laryngeal v.
lateral v.
mechanical v.
nocturnal v.
objective v.
ocular v.
organic v.
paralyzing v.
paroxysmal positional v.
peripheral v.
phobic postural v.
physiologic v.
positional v.
posttraumatic v.
postural v.
primary v.
proprioceptive v.
psychogenic v.
psychophysiologic v.
residual v.
rotary v.
sham-movement v.
somatoform v.
stomachal v.
subjective v.
systematic v.
tenebric v.
toxic v.
vertical v.
vestibular v.
visual v.
voltaic v.
verum
septum v.
very
v. high dose phenobarbital
v. low amplitude
v. low density lipoprotein receptor
v. low density syndrome
v. short Minnesota differential aphasia test

NOTES

Vesalius
canal of V.
foramen of V.
vesanique
vesical
v. center
v. plexus
v. reflex
vesicalis
plexus v.
vesicle
cerebral v.
encephalic v.
forebrain v.
hindbrain v.
lipid-containing v.
midbrain v.
ocular v.
ophthalmic v.
optic v.
pinocytotic v.
primary brain v.
synaptic v.
telencephalic v.
vesicospinal center
vesicoureteral reflux
vesicula ophthalmica
vesicular
v. eruption
v. stomatitis virus
vesiculation of the Golgi
vessel
blood v.
cerebral blood v.
collateral v.
crack-like v.
ectatic v.
v. hyperplasia
nutrient v.
opticociliary shunt v.
pain-sensitive v.
parent v.
pial cortical v.
resistance v.
telangiectatic discectomy v.
4-vessel cerebral angiogram
vest
Bremer AirFlo halo v.
halo v.
Minerva v.
Orthotrac pneumatic v.
vestibule aqueduct of v.
vestibuli aqueductus v.
vestibular
v. apparatus
v. aqueduct
v. area
v. crest
v. deficit
v. disorder
v. end-organ nystagmus
v. fissure of cochlea
v. function
v. ganglion
v. hair cell
v. labyrinth
v. membrane
v. migraine
v. migraine headache
v. nerve examination
v. nerve section
v. neurectomy
v. neuritis
v. neuronitis
v. nucleus
v. organ
v. part of vestibulocochlear nerve
v. reflex
v. root
v. root of vestibulocochlear nerve
v. schwannoma
v. sense
v. suppressant
v. system
v. vertigo
vestibulare
ganglion v.
vestibulares
nuclei v.
vestibularis
area v.
pars caudalis nervi v.
pars inferior nervi v.
pars rostralis nervi v.
pars superior nervi v.
radix v.
ramus communicans cochlearis nervi v.
vestibule
v. aqueduct of vest
crest of v.
olfactory v.
vestibuli
aqueductus v.
v. aqueductus vest
crista v.
scala v.
vestibulocerebellar
v. ataxia
v. tract
vestibulocerebellum
vestibulocochlear
v. nerve [CN VIII]
v. neurectomy
v. neuropathy
v. nucleus
v. organ

vestibulocochleare
organum v.
vestibulocochlearis
nervus v. [CN VIII]
nuclei nervi v.
pars cochlearis nervi v.
pars vestibularis nervi v.
radix cochlearis nervi v.
radix inferior nervi v.
radix superior nervi v.
radix vestibularis nervi v.
vestibuloequilibratory control
vestibulogenic
v. epilepsy
v. seizure
vestibuloocular
v. reflex (VOR)
v. reflex suppression
v. retraining
vestibulopathy
idiopathic bilateral v.
vestibulospinal
v. drive
v. influence
v. input
v. reflex
v. signal
v. tract
vestibulospinalis
tractus v.
vestibulothalamic
VGB
vigabatrin
VGCC
voltage-gated calcium channel
VGPT
visually guided pointing task
VH
variable heavy chain
VHL
von Hippel-Lindau
VHL syndrome
viability
neuronal v.
viable synapse
vibration
v. artifact
v. detection threshold
v. loss
v. sense
v. syndrome
vibratory sensibility
Vibrio parahaemolyticus
vibrometer
vibrotactile
Vicoprofen
Vicq
V. d'Azyr band
V. d'Azyr bundle
V. d'Azyr centrum semiovale
V. d'Azyr fasciculus
V. d'Azyr foramen
V. d'Azyr foramen cecum
V. d'Azyr stripe
V. d'Azyr tract
Vicryl Rapide suture
victim
primary v.
vidarabine
video
v. electroencephalographic monitoring
v. game epilepsy
v. monitoring of seizure
v. therapy
video-assisted
v.-a. endoscopic sympathectomy
v.-a. thorascopic surgery
videocamera
endoscope v.
videocassette recording
videoconference
videoconferencing
video-EEG
v.-EEG monitoring
v.-EEG recording
videofluoroscopy
videonystagmography
video-oculography (VOG)
video-polysomnographic
videosomnography
infrared v.
Videx
vidian
v. artery
v. canal
v. nerve
v. neuralgia
v. plexus
Vienna
V. encephalitis
V. reaction apparatus
Vieussens
V. ansa

NOTES

Vieussens *(continued)*
anulus of V.
V. centrum
V. ganglion
V. loop
V. valve
V. ventricle
view
field of v.
swimmer's v.
Waters v.
viewing
tachistoscopy v.
V. Wand
V. Wand image guided system
viewpoint
economic v.
genetic v.
vigabatrin (VGB)
vigil
coma v.
vigilambulism
vigilance reaction time
Vigor
Profile of Mood States, V.
Viking II nerve monitoring device
Villaret-Mackenzie syndrome
Villaret syndrome
villus, pl. **villi**
arachnoid granulation v.
choroid plexus v.
viloxazine
VIM
ventral intermediate nucleus
Vim
V. thalamotomy
V. thalamus
vimentin tumor marker
vinblastine sulfate
vinca alkaloid
vincristine
v. peripheral neuropathy
procarbazine, lomustine (CCNU), v. (PCV)
v. sulfate
vinculum, pl. **vincula**
vincula lingula
vincula lingulae cerebelli
Vineland
V. Adaptive Behavior Composite
V. Adaptive Behavior Scale
V. percentile scale
violator
violent
v. ambulation
v. behavior
v. conduct disorder
v. onset headache
violinist's cramp
Vioxx
VIP
vasoactive intestinal polypeptide
Viracept
viral
v. delivery
v. DNA
v. encephalitis
v. encephalomyelitis
v. infection
v. intracerebral arteritis
v. leukoencephalitis
v. meningitis
v. myelitis
v. particle
v. receptor
v. rhinitis
v. vector-mediated therapy
v. vector system
viral-mediated illness
Viramune
Virchow
V. disease
V. granulation
V. psammoma
Virchow-Robin
V.-R. space
V.-R. space of brain
Virgoan
viridans
Streptococcus v.
v. streptococcus
virile reflex
virilescence
virilia
virilization
virtual
v. endoscopy
v. probe
v. reality therapy
virus
Central European tick-borne encephalitis v.
cytomegalic inclusion v.
dengue v.
DNA v.
double-stranded DNA v.
ECHO v.
v. encephalomyelitis
enteric cytopathic human orphan v.
Epstein-Barr v. (EBV)
hepatropic v.
herpes simplex v. (HSV)
herpes simplex v. type 1 (HSV-1)
herpes simplex v. type 2 (HSV-2)
herpes zoster v. (HZV)
human immunodeficiency v. (HIV)
human T-cell leukemia v. (HTLV)
human T-cell lymphoma v.

human T-cell lymphotropic v.
inhibitory v.
Jamestown Canyon v. (JCV)
Japanese encephalitis v.
JC v.
Junin v.
Lassa fever v.
lymphocytic choriomeningitis v. (LCMV)
Machupo v.
measles v.
neurotropic v.
Newcastle disease v.
Nipah v.
Oklahoma tick fever v.
oncolytic v.
ONYX-015 v.
Powassan v.
rabies v.
Rio Bravo v.
RNA v.
rubella v.
Seoul v.
snowshoe hare v.
St. Louis encephalitis v. (SLEV)
Toscana v.
Trivittatus v.
varicella-zoster v. (VZV)
varicella zoster v.
vesicular stomatitis v.
WEE v.

virus-mediated gene transfer

visceral

v. afferent fiber
v. anesthesia
v. aura
v. brain
v. crisis
v. disorder
v. efferent fiber
v. emotional state
v. epilepsy
v. larva migrans
v. lobe
v. motor component
v. motor neuron
v. nerve fiber
v. nervous system
v. neurofiber
v. nucleus of oculomotor nerve
v. pain
v. plexus
v. plexus ganglion
v. reflex
v. sense
v. sensory component
v. sympathectomy

viscerale

ganglion v.

viscerales

neurofibrae v.

visceralis

nervus v.
plexus v.
ramus v.

visceralium

ganglia plexuum v.

viscerogenic

v. referred pain
v. reflex

visceromotor

v. pathway
v. reflex

viscerosensory

v. process
v. reflex

viscerosomatic tone

viscerotome

viscoelastic action

viscoelasticity

viscosity

blood v.
social v.

visible tumor

vision

abrupt loss of v.
v. assessment
blurred v.
color v.
dimness of v.
double v.
facial v.
foveal v.
funnel v.
impaired v.
v. loss
organ of v.
recovery of v.
v. restoration therapy (VRT)
stable v.
subjective v.
tunnel v.

visit

baseline v.

NOTES

visit *(continued)*
clinical v.
followup v.
post baseline v.
trial v.
visitation
conjugal v.
Vistaril
visual
v. acuity
v. acuity loss
v. agnosia
v. alexia
v. allesthesia
v. amnesia
v. analog scale (VAS)
v. aphasia
v. association area
v. association cortex
v. axis
v. blurring
v. change
v. claudication
v. constructional praxis
v. cortical area
v. disturbance
v. episodic memory
v. evoked cortical potential
v. evoked potential (VEP)
v. evoked response (VER)
v. failure
v. field cut
v. field defect
v. field deficit
v. field depression
v. field disorder
v. field testing
v. fixation
v. function monitoring
v. grasp reflex
v. hallucination
v. image movement disorder
v. inattention
v. memory impairment
v. mismatch negativity (VMMN)
v. motor processing
v. object-naming task
v. orbicularis reflex
v. organ
v. paraneoplastic syndrome
v. pathway
v. phenomenon
v. receiving area
v. receptor cell
v. reflex epilepsy
v. region
v. representation strategy
v. scanning
v. shimmering with aura
v. shining with aura
v. sparkling with aura
v. subsystem
v. symptom
v. system
v. system tumor
v. trigger
v. vertigo
visualization
endoscopic v.
visual-kinetic dissociation
visually
v. guided pointing task (VGPT)
v. guided saccade
visual-vestibular conflict
visuoauditory
visuoconstructional ability
visuoconstructive skill
visuognosis
visuomotor
v. behavior
v. problem-solving skill
v. status
visuoperceptual skill
visuopsychic area
visuosensory area
visuospatial
v. acalculia
v. agnosia
v. construction
v. constructional apraxia
v. constructive cognition
v. deficit
v. disorientation
v. function
v. functioning
v. hemineglect
v. memory
v. neglect
v. reasoning
v. skill
visus
organum v.
VitaCarn Oral
vitae
arbor v.
vital
v. capacity
v. center
v. node
Vitallium
V. equipment
V. plate
vitamin
v. B1
v. B6
v. B12
v. B1 deficiency
v. B6 deficiency

v. B12 deficiency
v. B12 deficiency dementia
v. B, D, E, K
v. B12 level
v. B12 neuropathy
v. D
v. D deficiency
v. D malabsorption
v. E
v. E deficiency
v. K-dependent clotting factor II, VII, IX, X

vitrea
lamina v.

vitrectomy

vitreous
v. hemorrhage
v. lamella
v. membrane
persistent hyperplastic primary v. (PHPV)
primary v.

vitro matrigel model

vitronectin

vituperate

vituperative

vivacious

Vivactil

vivid
v. hallucination
v. nightmare

viviparity

viviparous

vivipation

vivo
ex v.

VJ
ventriculojugular
VJ shunt

VL
ventrolateral
VL thalamotomy

VMETH
volumetric multiple-exposure transmission holography

VMMN
visual mismatch negativity

VNS
vagal nerve stimulation
vagus nerve stimulation
VNS therapy

vocabulary
auditory v.
v. skill

vocal
v. cord
v. cord paralysis
v. fold approximation
v. fold paralysis
v. motor amusia
v. tic disorder
v. trill

vocalization
nocturnal v.
orofacial movement without v.

vocational performance

VOG
video-oculography

Vogt
V. disease
V. point
V. syndrome
V. triad of seizures, mental retardation, and facial angiofibroma

Vogt-Hueter point

Vogt-Koyanagi-Harada syndrome

Vogt-Spielmeyer disease

VOI
voxel of interest

voice
discordance of v.
hallucinated v.
v. intonation
quavering v.
v. tremor

voice-verbal
eyes, motor, v.-v.

void
signal v.

Voigt line

Voit nucleus

volar tip

volatile
v. anesthetic
v. hydrocarbon

volitional
v. capacity
v. deficit
v. impairment
v. sleep deprivation
v. tremor

Volkmann contracture

NOTES

volley
antidromic v.
Volpe criteria
voltage
transient v.
voltage-activated conductance
voltage-dependent neurotransmitter release
voltage-gated
v.-g. calcium channel (VGCC)
v.-g. potassium channel
v.-g. sodium channel
v.-g. sodium channel blocker
voltage-regulated calcium channel
voltage-sensitive
v.-s. block
v.-s. protein
voltaic vertigo
volume
amygdala v.
blood flow v.
brain v.
caudate v.
cerebellar v.
cerebral blood v. (CBV)
cerebrospinal fluid v.
cortical v.
v. expansion
frontal lobe v.
hippocampal raw v.
infarction v.
v. of interest
intracranial brain v.
intracranial raw v.
ischemic lesion v.
mamillary body v.
mean corpuscular v.
mean intracranial raw v.
mean normalized whole brain v.
normalized whole brain v.
prefrontal cortical v.
raw v.
regional brain parenchymal v.
v. regulation
relative cerebral blood v. (rCBV)
v. segmentation
sensitive v.
tidal v. (VT)
total fractional regional brain v.
v. transmission
tumor v.
whole-brain raw v.
volume-averaging error
volumetric
v. analysis
v. computed tomography
v. infusion pump
v. interstitial brachytherapy
v. loss
v. multiple-exposure transmission holography (VMETH)
v. resection
v. solution (VS)
v. stereotaxy
volumetry
hippocampal v.
MRI v.
voluntary
v. movement
v. mutism
v. nystagmus
v. time-out
vomer
posterior v.
vomeronasal
v. organ
v. sensory neuron (VSN)
v. zone
vomiting
anticipatory v. (AV)
v. center
cerebral v.
cyclic v.
ictal v.
v. reflex
v. with headache
von
v. Ebner gland
v. Economo disease
v. Economo encephalitis
v. Frey hair
v. Frey monofilament
v. Frey test
v. Gierke disease
v. Graefe sign
v. Graefe strabismus hook
v. Hippel disease
v. Hippel-Lindau (VHL)
v. Hippel-Lindau disease
v. Hippel-Lindau syndrome
v. Mises stress distribution
v. Monakow diaschisis concept
v. Monakow fiber
v. Recklinghausen disease
v. Recklinghausen neurofibromatosis
v. Willebrand disease
v. Willebrand factor (vWF)
voodoo
VOP
venous occlusion plethysmography
VOR
vestibuloocular reflex
voxel
contiguous v.
v. of interest (VOI)
spectroscopy v.
voxel-based morphometry
voxel-by-voxel analysis

voxel-wise analysis
voyager
brain v. 4.0
VP
vasopressin
ventriculoperitoneal
VP shunt
VPAP
variable positive airway pressure
Sullivan VPAP III
VPC
vector-producing cell
VPI
velopharyngeal incompetence
ventral posterior inferior
VPI nucleus
VPL
ventral posterior lateral
ventral posterolateral
ventroposterolateral
VPL nucleus
VPL pallidotomy
VPM
ventral posterior medial
ventral posteromedial
ventroposteromedial
VRT
vision restoration therapy
NovaVision VRT
VS
volumetric solution
Profile VS
VSG
variant surface glycoprotein
V-shaped incision
VSN
vomeronasal sensory neuron
VSP
variable spinal plating
VSP plate instrumentation
VT
tidal volume
VTA
ventral tegmental area
VTED
venous thromboembolic disease
V-tunnel drill system
vu
déjà vu
VueLock anterior cervical spine system
VuePASS portal access surgical system
vulnerability
danger-laden schema v.
hippocampal v.
pretraumatic v.
segmental v.
Vulpian
V. atrophy
V. effect
Vulpian-Bernhardt spinal muscular atrophy
vulva, pl. **vulvae**
pruritus vulvae
vWF
von Willebrand factor
VZV
varicella-zoster virus
VZV reactivation
VZV-specific T cell

NOTES

V

Waardenburg syndrome
Wackenheim clivus canal line
Wada
W. language lateralization testing
W. language and memory testing
W. memory asymmetry
W. memory score
W. memory test
W. procedure
W. protocol
Waddell
W. sign
W. test
waddling gait
wafer
BCNU-impregnated polymer w.
Gliadel w.
polyanhydride biodegradable polymer w.
w. technology
waiter's cramp
wake
w. after sleep onset (WASO)
w. rhythm
w. switch
wakefulness
w. disorder
w. drive
neuromodulation of w.
neurotransmitter of w.
waking
w. background EEG
w. numbness
w. paralysis
waking-NREM
Waldenstrom
macroglobulinemia of W.
W. macroglobulinemia
Waldeyer
W. tract
W. zonal layer
walk
scissoring w.
Walker
W. lissencephaly
W. syndrome
W. tractotomy
Walker-Warburg syndrome
walking
w. ability
w. aid
bipedal w.
chromosome w.
heel w.
heel-toe w.
w. stance
sudden difficulty w.
w. swing phase
toe w.
wall
w. fistula
parapharyngeal w.
pharyngeal w.
ventricular w.
Wallenberg syndrome
wallerian
w. degeneration
w. law
Wallgraft endoprosthesis
Wallstent
Magic W.
W. stent
Walther ganglion
wand
3-dimensional reconstruction w.
Elekta viewing w.
ISG viewing w.
NCP programming w.
Programming W.
stylus-type sensor w.
TriggerWheel W.
Viewing W.
wandering
w. cell
episodic nocturnal w.
nocturnal paroxysmal w.
wander risk
Wangensteen needle holder
waning
w. discharge
waxing and w.
war
drug w.
injury of w.
Warburg syndrome
ward
long-stay w.
Wardrop method
Ware instrument
warfare
ABC w.
warfarin syndrome
Waring blender syndrome
warm
w. effector
W. 'n Form lumbosacral corset
w. sensitivity
w. spot
warm-sensitive neuron

warmth
w. receptor
w. sensory threshold
warmup phenomenon
warm-wire anemometer
warning
black box w.
Warrington Recognition Memory test
wart
brain w.
Wartenberg
W. disease
W. sign
W. symptom
washboard effect
washer
plate-spacer w.
washout
drug w.
WASO
wake after sleep onset
wasting
cerebral salt w.
muscle w.
nitrogen w.
w. palsy
w. paralysis
salt w.
w. syndrome
watching
repetitive w.
watchmaker's cramp
water
w. intoxication
intracerebral w.
Waterhouse-Friderichsen syndrome
Waters
W. view
W. view radiograph
watershed
w. area
w. area paresis
w. region
w. zone
w. zone infarction
water-soluble
w.-s. contrast myelography
w.-s. contrast ventriculography
watertight closure
Watson
W. angular rate sensor
W. syndrome
Watson-Schwartz test
wave
A w.
alpha w.
w. analyzer
aperiodic w.
arciform w.
axon w.
beta w.
brain w.
centrotemporal sharp w.
continuous w. (CW)
cortical fast w.
delta w.
E w.
EEG alpha w.
electroencephalographic w.
expectancy w.
flat top w.
w. form
gamma w.
generalized periodic sharp w.
H w.
Hering-Traube w.
interictal sharp w.
Jewett w.
kappa w.
lambda w.
M w.
monophasic w.
mu w.
w. number
positive sharp w.
random w.
rho w.
R1, R2 w.
sawtooth w.
sharp w.
slow-frequency w.
square w.
theta w.
Traube-Hering-Mayer w.
triphasic w.
ultrasonic w.
vertex sharp w.
vertical sharp w.
waveform
abnormal w.
w. amplitude
apiculate w.
dampened w.
ICP w.
monophasic w.
nondampened w.
out-of-phase w.
signal voltage w.
w. of sleep
wavelength
wavelet entropy
wavenumber
wavering light with aura
waveshape
wax
bone w.
Horsley bone w.
waxing and waning

1-way flow mechanism
Wayne laminectomy seat
wayward
WBC
white blood cell
WBI
whole-brain irradiation
WBRT
whole-brain radiation therapy
weakness
abduction w.
adduction w.
arm w.
asymmetric flaccid w.
bulbar muscle w.
diaphragmatic w.
eye muscle w.
facial w.
hemifacial w.
infranuclear w.
intercostal muscle w.
limb w.
myopathic w.
neck w.
pharyngeal w.
psychological w.
pyramidal w.
residual w.
sternocleidomastoid muscle w.
sudden w.
upper motor neuron w.
weaning
ventilator w.
wearing-off phenomenon
Weary
W. cordotomy knife
W. nerve hook
W. nerve root retractor
web
subsynaptic w.
web-based neuropsychological test protocol
Weber
W. esthesiometer
W. human genome screening set
W. sign
W. syndrome
W. test
Weber-Christian disease
Weber-Fergusson incision
Weber-Leyden syndrome
webspace incision
Webster needle holder
Weck clip
Wedensky
W. effect
W. facilitation
W. inhibition
W. phenomenon
wedge
Duo-Cline bed w.
wedge-compression fracture
wedge-shaped
w.-s. astrocyte
w.-s. fasciculus
w.-s. tubercle
w.-s. vertebra
WEE
western equine encephalomyelitis
WEE virus
weekend headache
weeping
overt w.
Wegener
W. granulomatosis (WG)
W. granulomatosis-associated neuropathy
W. granulomatosis vasculitis
Weibel-Palade body
Weigert staining
weight
w. gain potential
w. loss
w. regulation
w. sense
target w.
weighted sum score
weighting
proton density w.
T1 w.
T2 w.
weight-loss surgery
weight-neutral psychotic medication
Weil-Blakesley intervertebral disc rongeur
Weinberg rib spreader
Weingrow reflex
Weinstein Enhanced Sensory test
Weiss sign
Weitbrecht cord
Weitlaner-Beckman retractor
Weitlaner retractor
Welander
W. disease

NOTES

W

Welander *(continued)*
W. muscular dystrophy
W. syndrome
welding
laser tissue w.
tissue w.
welfare
w. system
well-being
global w.-b.
subjective w.-b.
well-circumscribed lesion
Wellcovorin
well-defined focal brain lesion
well-formed electroencephalogram rhythm
wellness
w. principle
sense of w.
Wells stereotactic apparatus
Wenzel ventricle
Werdnig-Hoffmann
W.-H. disease
W.-H. spinal muscular atrophy
Wermer syndrome
Wernekinck
W. commissure
W. decussation
Wernicke
W. aphasia
W. center
W. dementia
W. disease
W. dysphasia
W. encephalopathy
W. field
W. hemianopic pupillary phenomenon
mirror of W.
W. radiation
W. reaction
W. region
W. second motor speech area
W. sign
W. syndrome
W. triangle
W. zone
Wernicke-Korsakoff
W.-K. encephalopathy
W.-K. syndrome
Wernicke-Mann spastic hemiplegia
West
W. African sleeping sickness
W. African trypanosomiasis
W. hand and foot nerve tester
W. Nile encephalitis
W. Nile fever
W. Nile virus-induced paralysis
W. syndrome (WS)
Westco Neurostat-Mark II
Westergren method
westermani
Paragonimus w.
western
W. Aphasia Battery
W. blot analysis
W. blot test
W. equine encephalitis
W. equine encephalitis virus infection
w. equine encephalomyelitis (WEE)
w. medicine
Weston Hurst disease
Westphal
W. disease
W. nucleus
W. phenomenon
W. pseudosclerosis
W. pupillary reflex
W. sign
W. variant
W. zone
Westphal-Erb sign
Westphal-Piltz phenomenon
Westphal-Strümpell pseudosclerosis
wet
w. beriberi
w. bipolar system
w. brain
Wever-Bray phenomenon
WFNS
World Federation of Neurosurgical Societies
WFNS scale
WG
Wegener granulomatosis
wheelchair dependency
whiplash
acute w.
cervical w.
w. injury
w. shaken infant syndrome
w. trauma
Whipple
W. disease
W. disease peripheral neuropathy
whispering dystonia
Whitacre spinal needle
white
w. atrophy
w. blood cell (WBC)
w. blood cell count
w. column of spinal cord
w. commissure
w. commissure of spinal cord
w. iritis
w. lamina of cerebellum
w. layer of cerebellum

w. matter
w. matter of centrum ovale
w. matter change
w. matter degeneration
w. matter degenerative disease
w. matter hyperintensity
w. matter hypodensity
w. matter infarction
w. matter ischemia
w. matter lactate
w. matter lactate level
w. matter lesion (WML)
w. matter pathology
w. matter region
w. matter signal abnormality
w. matter structure
w. matter tissue
w. matter tract
w. noise masking
W. and Panjabi criteria
w. rami communicantes
w. ramus
w. softening
w. substance
w. substance of cerebellum
w. substance of spinal cord

white-out syndrome
Whitesides-Kell cervical technique
WHO
World Health Organization
WHO astrocytoma classification
WHO instrument

whole
w. cranial headache
w. focus orientation

whole-body
w.-b. activity
w.-b. cooling

whole-brain
w.-b. atrophy
w.-b. blood flow
w.-b. boundary
w.-b. coverage
w.-b. irradiation (WBI)
w.-b. mapping database
w.-b. radiation therapy (WBRT)
w.-b. radiotherapy
w.-b. raw volume

whole-cell
w.-c. patch-clamp
w.-c. patch clamp technique
w.-c. recording

whole-cortex MEG/EEG system
whole-head neuromagnetometer
wholeness
sense of w.

whole-spine MRI
whorl
storiform w.

whorling pattern
Whytt disease
wick
Silastic w.

wicket
w. rhythm
w. spike

wide area network
wide-based posture
wide-blade laminar hook
wide-necked aneurysm
widened interspinous gap
widespread
w. beta activity
w. distribution of activity

width
line w.
pulse w.
third ventricle w.
ventricle w.

Wiener
tract of Münzer and W.

Wigraine
Wilbrand
W. knee
W. knee injury

Wilcoxon rank sum test
Wilde cord
Wildervanck syndrome
wild-type (WT)
w.-t. allele
w.-t. protein

will
concept of w.

Williams
W. sequestrectomy
W. syndrome

Willis
arterial circle of W.
W. centrum nervosum
circle of W.
W. circle aneurysm
W. circle developmental anomaly
W. cord
W. headache

W

NOTES

Willis *(continued)*
W. nerve
posterior circle of W.
spontaneous occlusion of circle of W.
W. valve
willisii
accessorius w.
chordae w.
Wilms tumor
Wilson
W. disease
W. frame
W. hepatolenticular degeneration
W. rib spreader
W. syndrome
Wiltberger
W. anterior cervical approach
W. fusion
W. spinous process spreader
Wiltse
W. paraspinal approach
W. system
W. system aluminum master rod
W. system cross-bracing
W. system double-rod construct
W. system H construct
W. system single-rod construct
W. system spinal rod
Wiltse-Gelpi retractor
wind contusion
window
acoustic bone w.
CT bone w.
wind-up
spinal w.-u.
wing
ashen w.
w. of central lobule
central lobule w.
w. of crista galli
gray w.
w. plate
sphenoid w.
wing-beating tremor
wingless gene
wink
anal w.
w. reflex
Winkelman disease
winking
jaw w.
w. spasm
Winquist tibial/femoral extraction system
Winslow concept
Winston-Lutz method
Wintrobe method
wire
Amplatz exchange length w.
Bentson exchange length w.
Choice PT exchange w.
w. contour preparation
Drummond w.
w. extrusion
Fast Dasher 14 w.
Kirschner w.
Luque w.
Mullan w.
w. osteosynthesis
w. passage
w. penetration depth
w. removal technique
spinous process w.
w. stabilization
sublaminar w.
w. thrombosis
titanium w.
Wisconsin interspinous w.
Wisconsin spinous process w.
wiring
facet fracture stabilization w.
facet subluxation stabilization w.
posterior interspinous w.
spinous process w.
sublaminar w.
Wisconsin
W. interspinous wire
W. Sleep Cohort Study
W. spinous process wire
withdrawal
alcohol w.
amphetamine w.
caffeine w.
cocaine w.
w. effect
w. emergent syndrome
ethanol w.
w. headache
hypnotic w.
neonatal opiate w.
newborn drug w.
nicotine w.
opioid w.
w. process
w. reflex
sedative w.
withdrawal-emergent dyskinesia
WML
white matter lesion
wnt gene
Wohlfart-Kugelberg-Welander
W.-K.-W. disease
W.-K.-W. syndrome
Wolf endoscope

Wolff
W. headache
W. vasogenic theory
Wolf-Hirschhorn syndrome
Wolf-Orton body
Wolfram
W. needle electrode
W. syndrome
Wollaston theory
Wolman disease
women
parkinsonian postmenopausal w.
physiology of w.
Women's Health Initiative Insomnia Rating Scale
woodcutter's encephalitis
Woodson
W. dural separator
W. dural separator-spatula
W. dura packer
modification or W.
word
w. blindness
w. deafness
w. discrimination
w. generation
w. list learning
w. processing
w. production
w. recall
w. recognition
w. retrieval
stimulus w.
word-finding difficulty
3-word recall test
word-selection anomia
work
bright light reexposure for shift w.
w. evaluation systems technology
w. performance
working
w. ability
w. capacity
w. memory
w. memory function
workload
mental w.
work-related task
workstation
MKM w.
Sun w.
world
W. Federation of Neurological Surgeons scale
W. Federation of Neurosurgical Societies (WFNS)
W. Health Organization (WHO)
inner w.
intrapsychic w.
wormian bone
worrying symptom
worsening
symptom w.
Wort
St. John's W.
wound
dehisced w.
entry w.
exit w.
gunshot w.
penetrating neck w.
psychic w.
shrapnel w.
stab w.
through-and-through gunshot w.
Wound-Evac drain
W-P
wrist-palm
wrap
cotton w.
Dura-Kold ice w.
wrapping of aneurysm
wrench
Texas Scottish Rite Hospital w.
T-handle nut w.
T-handle screw w.
Wright
W. Care TENS unit
W. syndrome
Wrisberg
W. ganglion
nerve of W.
W. nerve
wrist
w. clonus
w. clonus reflex
w. drop
wrist-drop
wrist-palm (W-P)
wrist-to-abductor pollicis brevis
writer's cramp

W

NOTES

writing
compulsive w.
w. hand
wrong-way deviation
wry neck, wryneck
WS
West syndrome
WT
wild-type
Würzburg
W. implant system
W. titanium plating system
Wyatt screening
Wyburn-Mason
W.-M. arteriovenous malformation
W.-M. syndrome
Wyler cylindrical subdural electrode

X
X chromosome
X inactivation
X Knife
X25 PCR
Xanax
xanchromatic
xanthine
x. oxidase
x. oxidase inhibitor
xanthoastrocytoma
pleomorphic x. (PXA)
xanthochromatic
xanthochromia of cerebrospinal fluid
xanthochromic
xanthocyanopsia
xanthogranuloma
xanthogranulomatous cyst
xanthoma
choroidal x.
xanthomatosis
cerebrotendinous x.
xanthomatous
x. astrocytoma
x. Rathke cleft cyst
xanthosarcoma
Xe
xenon
Xe clearance method
^{133}Xe
xenon-133
^{133}Xe intravenous injection technique
XeCT
xenon-enhanced computed tomography
XeCT CBF study
XeCT scanning
XenoDerm
xenogeneic
x. chromaffin cell
x. graft
xenograft
glioblastoma x.
xenon (Xe)
x. computed tomography
x. CT
x. CT cerebral blood flow
x. CT measurement
x. CT scanning
x. inhalation
x. method
xenon-133 (^{133}Xe)
xenon-CT
xenon-enhanced
x.-e. computed tomography (XeCT)
x.-e. CT
x.-e. CT scanning
xeroderma pigmentosum
XeScan
^{133}XeSPECT contrast medium
***x* gradient**
Xia
X. hook system
X. spinal system
xiphodynia
xiphoidalgia
XKnife
XK-PRO100 high-speed drill system
XL illuminator
X-linked
X-l. abnormality
X-l. adrenoleukodystrophy
X-l. anophthalmia
X-l. Charcot-Marie-Tooth disease
X-l. cortical migration disorder
X-l. hydrocephalus
X-l. lissencephaly
X-l. lymphoproliferative syndrome
X-l. recessive bulbospinal neuronopathy
X-l. recessive muscular dystrophy
X-l. recessive transmission
X-l. spastic paraparesis
X-l. spinobulbar muscular atrophy
Xomed Nerve Integrity Monitor-2
X-O test
Xp21 myopathy
Xphoria
Xpress 100 disposable perforator bur hole drill
x-ray
artifact on x-r.
x-r. exposure
intraoperative x-r.
x-r. irradiation
isocentric linear accelerator x-r.
x-r. localization
orthogonal x-r.
plain x-r.
x-r. therapy (XRT)
XRT
x-ray therapy
X-Trel spinal cord stimulation system
X-Trozine
XXX syndrome
Xyrem
xyrospasm
XYY karyotype

X

^{90}Y
radioactive yttrium
Yale
Y. brace
Y. Global Tic Severity Scale (YGTSS)
Y. Tic Severity Scale
Yankauer suction tube
Yasargil
Y. arachnoid knife
Y. artery forceps
Y. bayonet forceps
Y. bayonet scissors
Y. carotid clamp
Y. clip-applying forceps
Y. craniotomy
Y. cross-legged clip
Y. elevator
Y. flat serrated ring forceps
Y. hypophysial forceps
Y. instrument
Y. knotting forceps
Y. Leyla retractor arm
Y. ligature carrier
Y. ligature guide
Y. microclip
Y. microcurette
Y. microdissector
Y. micro forceps
Y. microforceps
Y. microrasp
Y. microscissors
Y. microvascular knife
Y. needle holder
Y. OptiMat floor stand
Y. pituitary rongeur
Y. rasp
Y. retractor
Y. scoop
Y. spring hook
Y. suction tube
Y. tissue lifter
Y. titanium aneurysm clip
Y. tumor forceps
Y. vessel clip
Yasargil-Aesculap
Y.-A. instrument
Y.-A. spring clip
Yasargil-Leyla
Y.-L. brain retractor
Y.-L. brain retractor z-gradient coil
yaw plane sign
year
Functional Fitness Assessment for Adults over 60 Y.'s
yellow
y. fever
y. fever encephalitis
y. ligament
y. softening
y. spot
Yersinia
Y. enterocolitica
Y. pestis
***y* gradient**
YGTSS
Yale Global Tic Severity Scale
Y incision
yoke
double y.
Young-Helmholtz trichromacy theory
young spine
yo-yo syndrome
Y-shaped reference arc
yttrium
radioactive y. (^{90}Y)
yttrium-90

Y

Z
Z coordinate
Z disc
zalcitabine
Zaleplon
zaleplon
Zanaflex
Zantac
Zantryl
Zaraflex
Zarit burden interview
Zarontin
Zaroxolyn
Zavesca
ZD
ZD frame
ZD stereotactic system
Z-disc disorder
ZD-Neurosurgical localizing unit
zebra
z. body
z. body myopathy
Zeiss
Z. Axiovert microscope
Z. IIIRS photomicroscope
Z. Image Guided System
Z. MKM microscope
Z. operating microscope
Z. OPMI Neuro/NC4 surgical microscope
Z. stereotactic tool navigator system
Z. STN surgical tool navigator
Z. Super Lux 40 light source
Zeiss-Contraves operating microscope
zeitgeber
Zelapar
Zeldox
Zellweger syndrome
Zenker
Z. paralysis
Z. solution
Zephir anterior cervical plate system
Zeppelin micro-motor system
zero
z. cerebral pseudotumor cerebri
z. drift of sensor
z. ICP ventricle shunt
physiologic z.
protein z.
zero-order elimination kinetics
Zestoretic
zeta/beta
receptor protein tyrosine phosphatase z./b.
RPTP z./b.
zeta-glucosaminide
zeta method
zeugmatography
Fourier transformation z.
z-gradient
z-g. coil
z-g. field
zic gene
zidovudine and lamivudine
Ziehen-Oppenheim disease
Zielke
Z. bifid hook
Z. instrument
Z. instrumentation
Z. VDS implant
Ziemssen motor point
zifrosilone
Zika fever
Zimmer
Z. caudal hook
Z. clip
Z. microsaw
Zimmerlin atrophy
zinc
z. acetate
z. protoporphyrin level
zinc-finger
z.-f. family
z.-f. gene
Zinn
anulus of Z.
Z. corona
Z. vascular circle
Zinn-Haller
circle of Z.-H.
Zinsser-Cole-Engman syndrome
ziprasidone
z. HCl
z. hydrochloride
z. mesylate
Zocor
zolazepam
Zollinger-Ellison syndrome
zolmitriptan
Zoloft
zolpidem tartrate
Zomaril
Zomax
zombie-like
zometapine
Zomig nasal spray

Zomig-ZMT
ZON
zonisamide
zona, pl. **zonae**
z. dermatica
z. epithelioserosa
z. hypothalamicae
z. incerta
z. lateralis
z. medialis
z. medullovasculosa
z. ophthalmica
z. periventricularis
z. rolandica
zonal
z. layer of cerebral cortex
z. layer of superior colliculus
z. layer of thalamus
zonale
stratum z.
zone
active z.
anaplastic z.
arterial border z.
chemosensitive z.
dolorogenic z.
dorsal root entry z. (DREZ)
embryologic z.
entry z.
ependymal z.
epileptogenic z.
Flechsig primordial z.
H z.
head z.
hyperalgesic z.
z. of hypothalamus
ictal onset z.
intermediate gray z.
irritative z.
language z.
latent z.
lateral z.
Lissauer marginal z.
Marchant z.
marginal z.
medial z.
medullary inhibitory z.
motor z.
Obersteiner-Redlich z.
z. of partial preservation
periventricular z.
primary epileptogenic z.
reflexogenic z.
root entry z.
spike-initiation z.
Spitzka marginal z.
subplate z.
subventricular z.
tender z.
trigger z.
vomeronasal z.
watershed z.
Wernicke z.
Westphal z.
Zonegran capsule
zonesthesia
zonifugal
zonipetal
zonisamide (ZON)
z. capsule
zonular layer
zoogonous
zoogony
zoom microscope
zoophile
zoophilic
zopiclone
ZORprin
zoster
z. encephalomyelitis
herpes z.
z. immune globulin
measles, rubella and z. (MRZ)
ophthalmic z.
z. paresis
z. sine herpete
z. virus infection
Zostrix
zotepine
Z-plate
Z-p. anterior thoracolumbar instrumentation
Z-p. fixation system
Z-score
Z-s. map
Z-s. transformation
z-touch laser device
Zuckerkandl
Z. convolution
organ of Z.
zuclopenthixol
Zülch
giant cell monstrocellular sarcoma of Z.
Zung
Z. Anxiety Scale
Z. Self-Rating Depression Scale
Zung Anxiety Scale
Zyban
Zydis
Z. drug delivery technology
Zyprexa Z.
zygal fissure
zygapophysial
z. joint
z. joint damage
z. joint laxity
zygoma

zygomatic
z. fracture
z. nerve
z. reflex
z. resection approach
zygomatici
ramus zygomaticofacialis nervi z.
ramus zygomaticotemporalis nervi z.
zygomatico
ramus communicans nervi lacrimalis cum nervo z.
zygomaticofacial branch of zygomatic nerve
zygomaticoorbital artery
zygomaticotemporal branch of zygomatic nerve
zygomaticus
nervus z.
zygomycosis
rhinocerebral z.
zygon
zygosis
zygosity
zygote
Zyprexa Zydis

NOTES

Contents: The Appendices

Appendix 1
Anatomical Illustrations

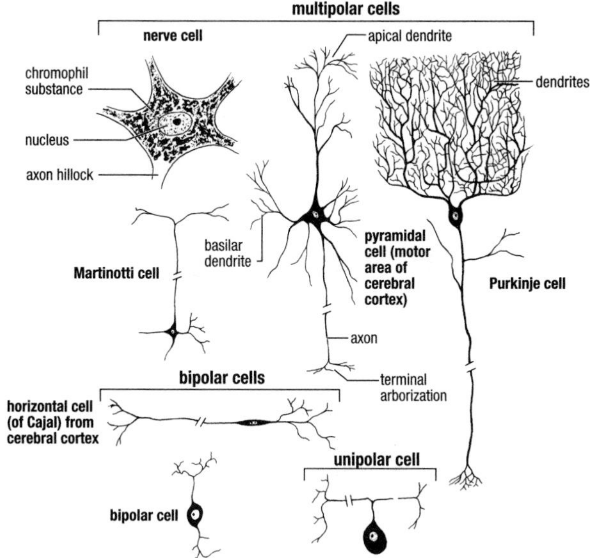

types of neurons

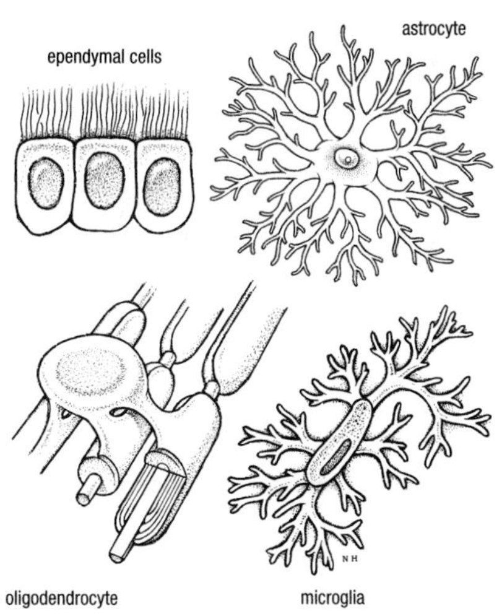

neuroglia: supporting structures of the nervous system

Anatomical Illustrations

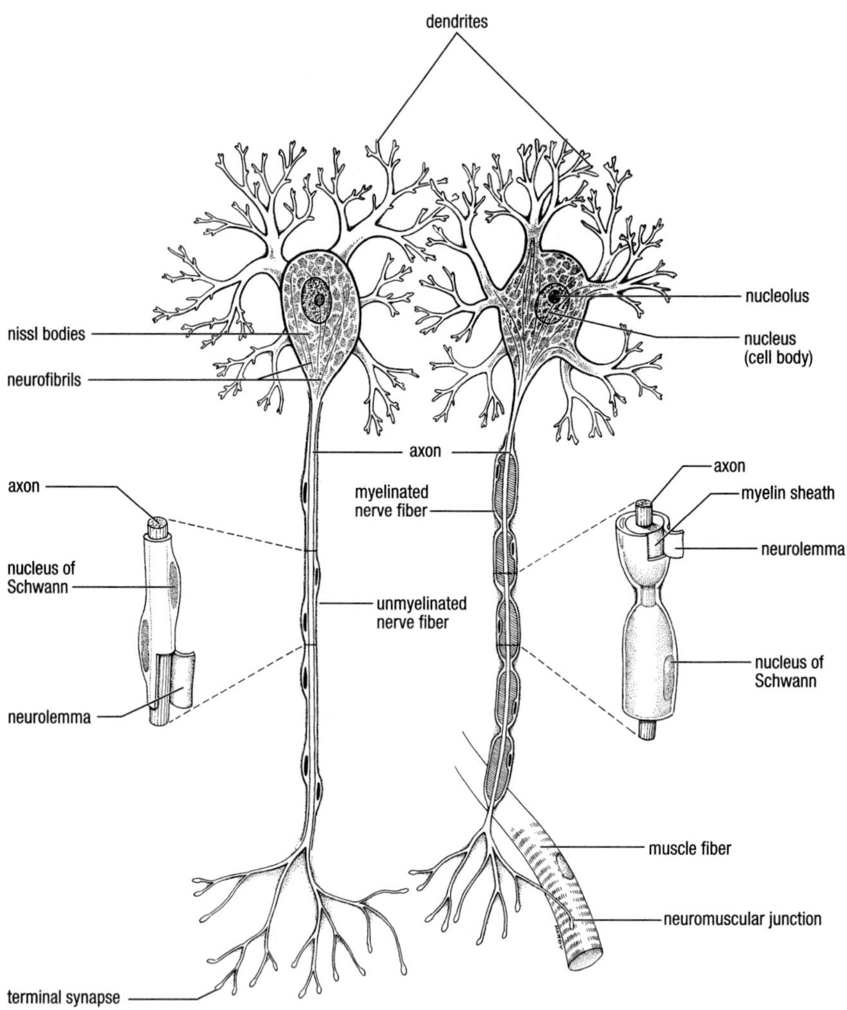

myelinated and unmyelinated neurons

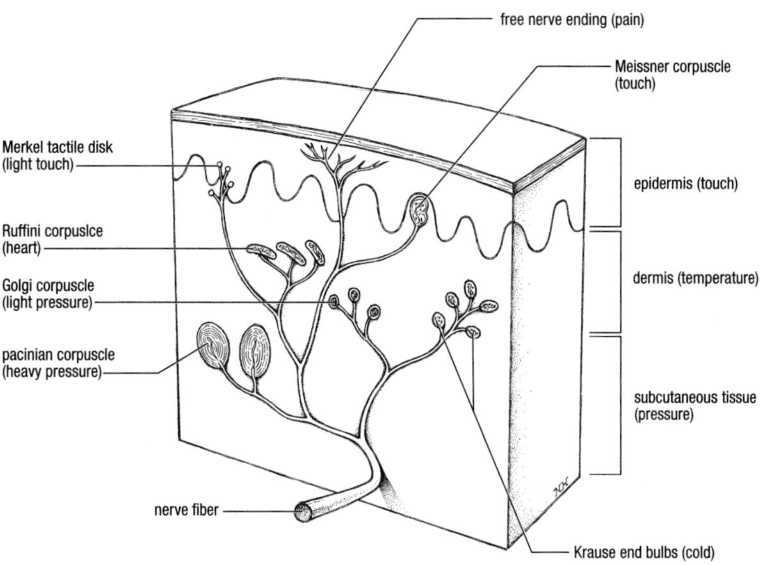

sensory nerves and bodies

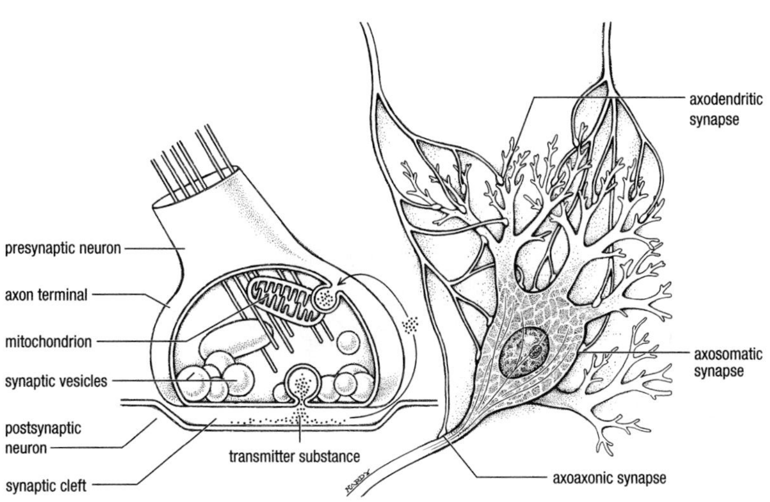

nerve synapse

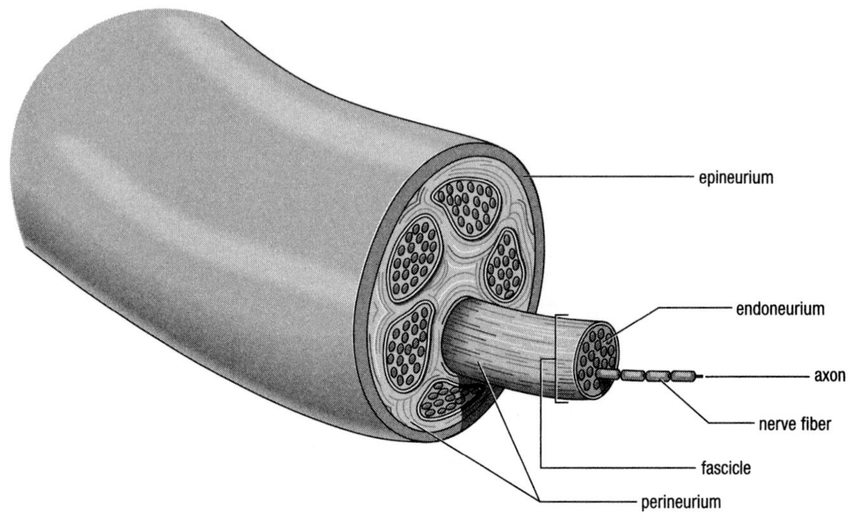

peripheral nerve: outside surface or surrounding area of an organ or structure

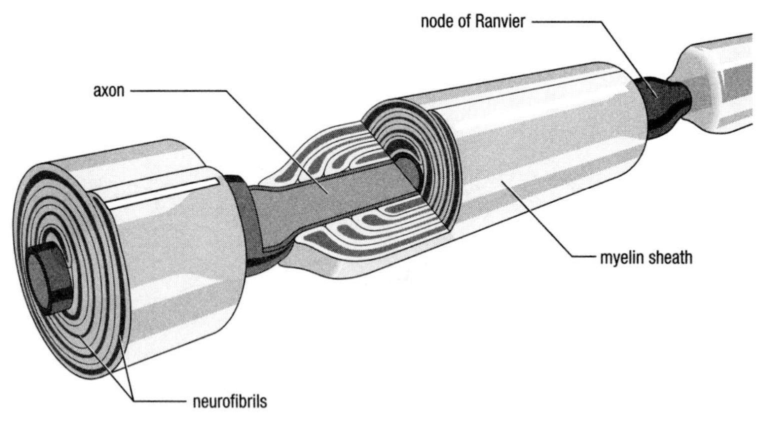

axon, myelin sheath, and node of Ranvier

nerve fiber groups					
diameter of fiber thickness	**histology**	**fiber groups**		**conduction speed**	**function**
1–22 m			α	80–120 m/sec	motor impulses, afferent impulses from muscle spindles and tendon organs
			β	60 m/sec	tactile impulses of the skin
3–20 m	thick fibers with relatively thick myelin sheaths	A	γ	40 m/sec	efferent impulses to the contractile portions of intrafusal muscle fibers
			δ	20 m/sec	mechanoreceptor impulses; cold, warm, and painful sensations of the skin (fast)
1–3 m	thin fibers or thin myelin sheaths	B		10 m/sec	preganglionic vegetative fibers
1 m	fibers without sheaths	C		1 m/sec	postganglionic vegetative fibers and afferent fibers of the sympathetic trunk, impulses of mechanoreceptors, cold and warm receptors (slow)

nerve fiber groups

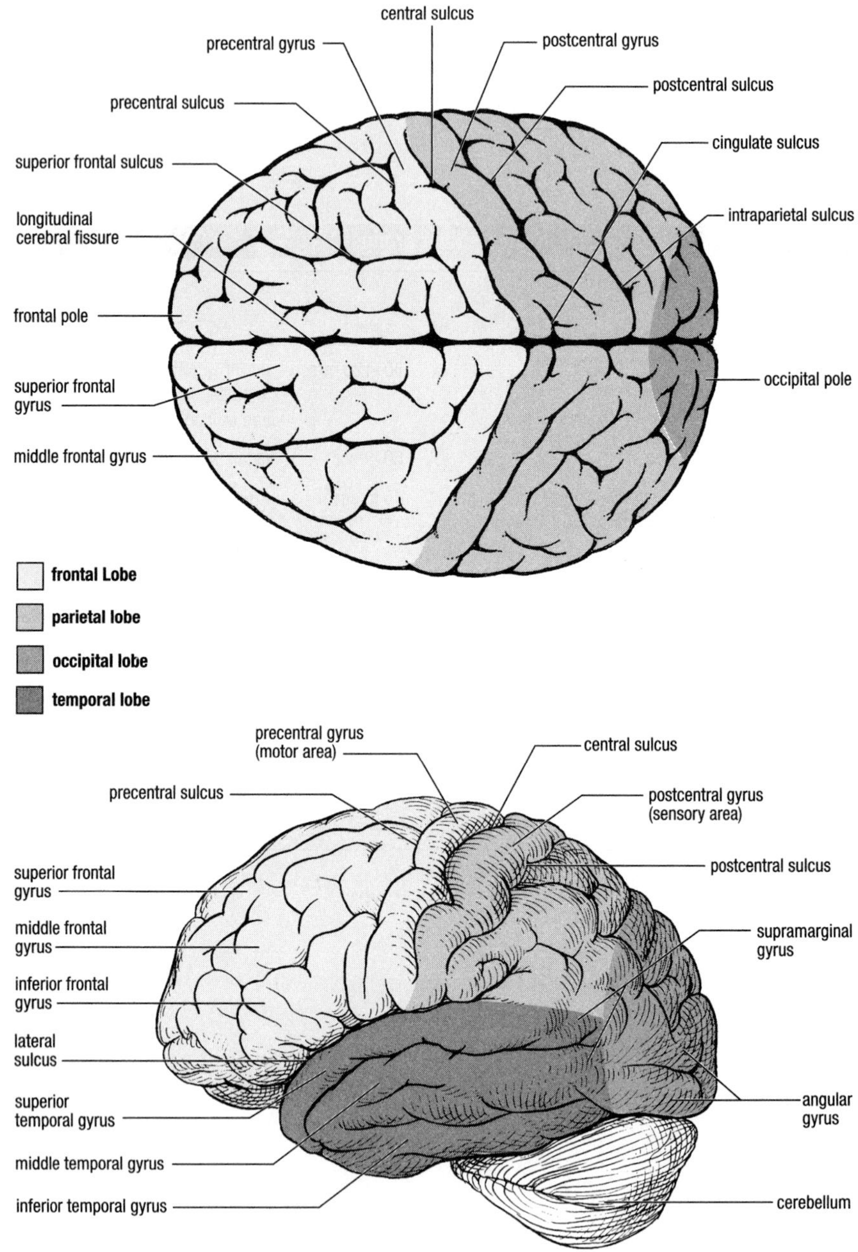

brain: superior view (top) and lateral view (bottom)

Anatomical Illustrations

choroid plexus

thalamus

splenium of corpus callosum

parietooccipital sulcus (fissure)

pineal body (gland)

calcarine sulcus (visual area)

cerebral aqueduct

4th ventricle

cerebellum

choroid plexus

median aperture

central canal

cerebrum

body of corpus callosum

septum pellucidum

genu of corpus callosum

fornix

anterior commissure

interventricular foramen

massa intermedia

hypothalamus

mamillary body

brainstem

midbrain

pons

medulla oblongata

brain, median section

A7

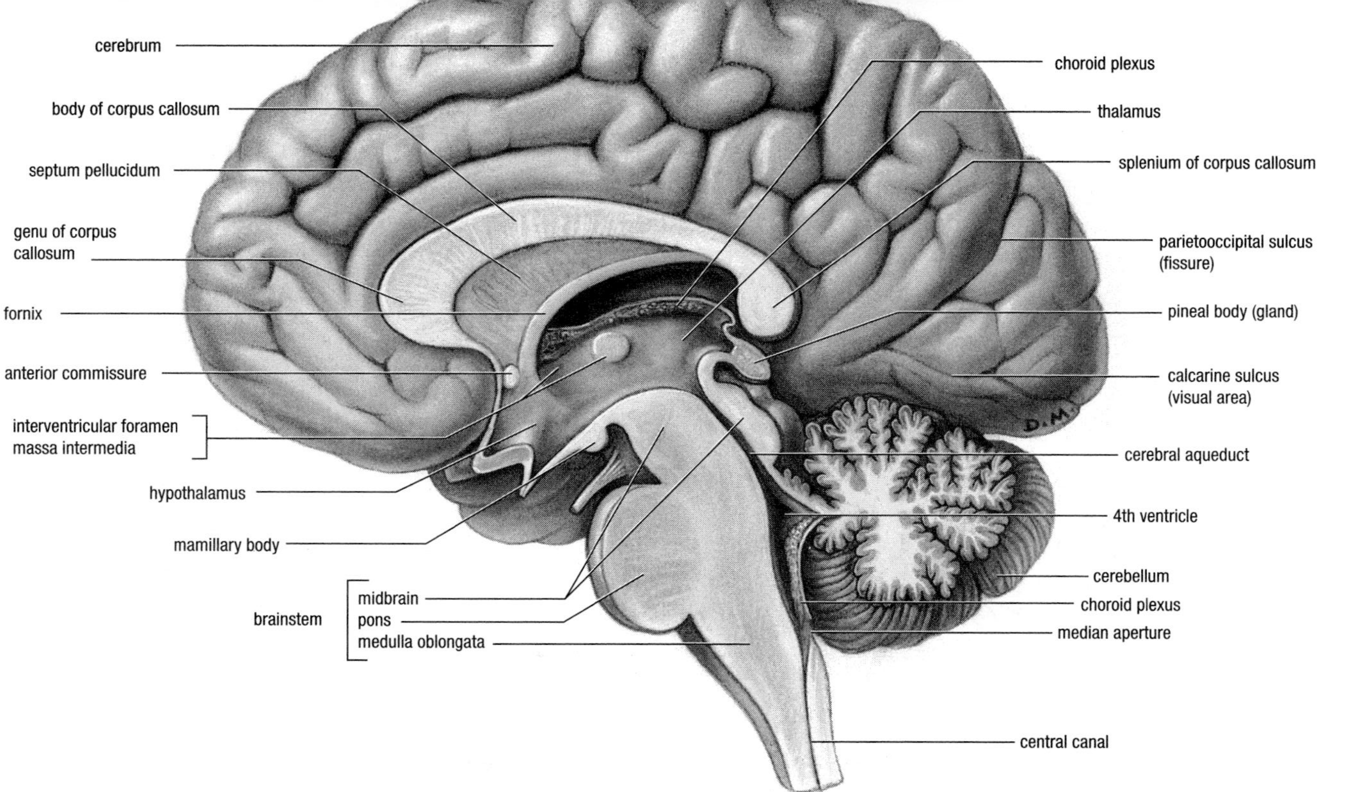

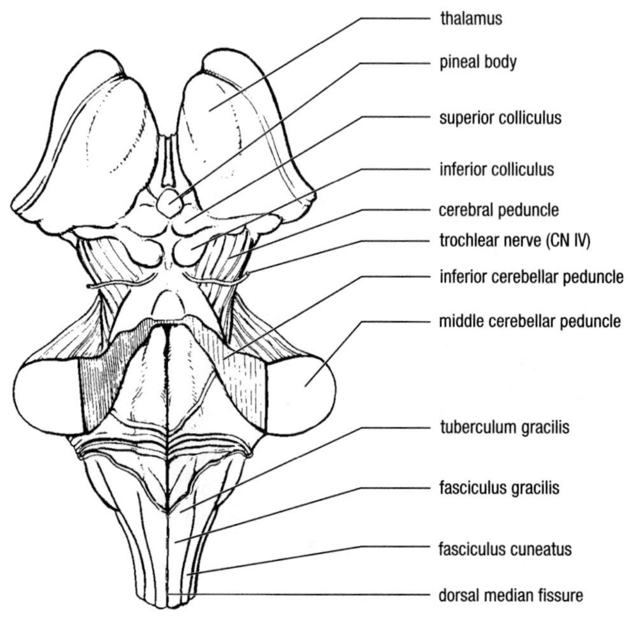
thalamus
pineal body
superior colliculus
inferior colliculus
cerebral peduncle
trochlear nerve (CN IV)
inferior cerebellar peduncle
middle cerebellar peduncle
tuberculum gracilis
fasciculus gracilis
fasciculus cuneatus
dorsal median fissure

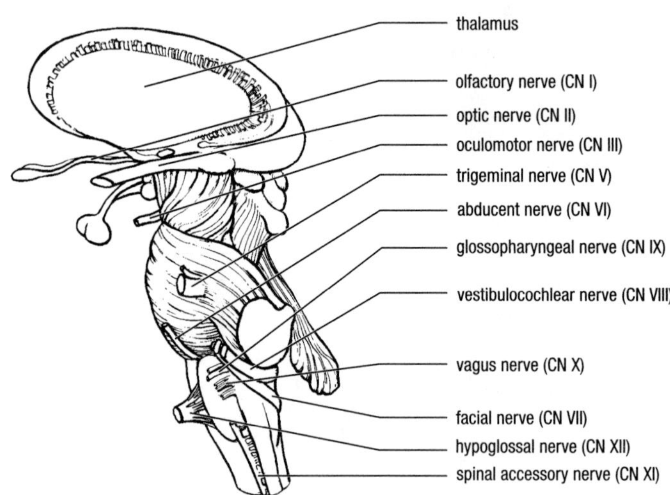
thalamus
olfactory nerve (CN I)
optic nerve (CN II)
oculomotor nerve (CN III)
trigeminal nerve (CN V)
abducent nerve (CN VI)
glossopharyngeal nerve (CN IX)
vestibulocochlear nerve (CN VIII)
vagus nerve (CN X)
facial nerve (CN VII)
hypoglossal nerve (CN XII)
spinal accessory nerve (CN XI)

brainstem: dorsal view (top) and lateral view (bottom)

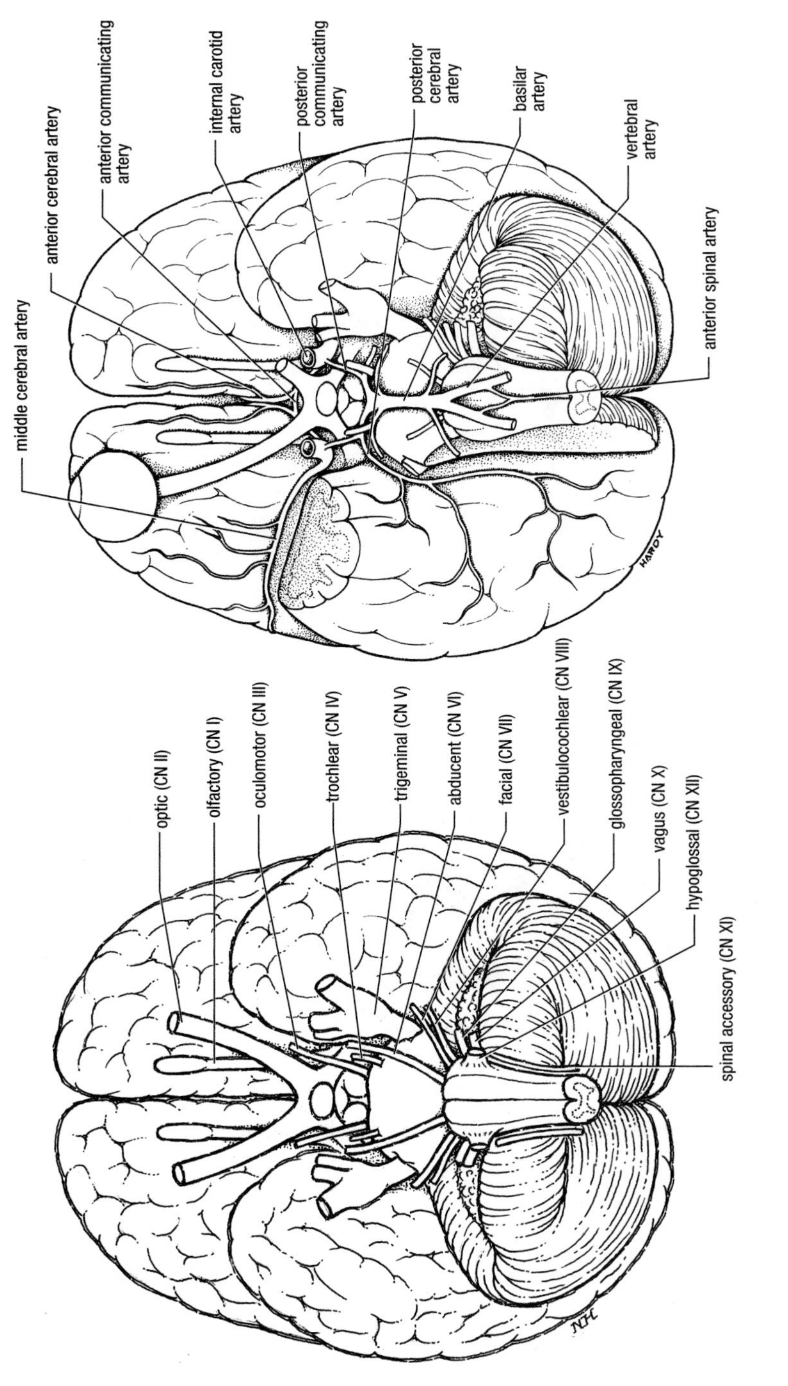

vascular network at the base of the brain

cranial nerves

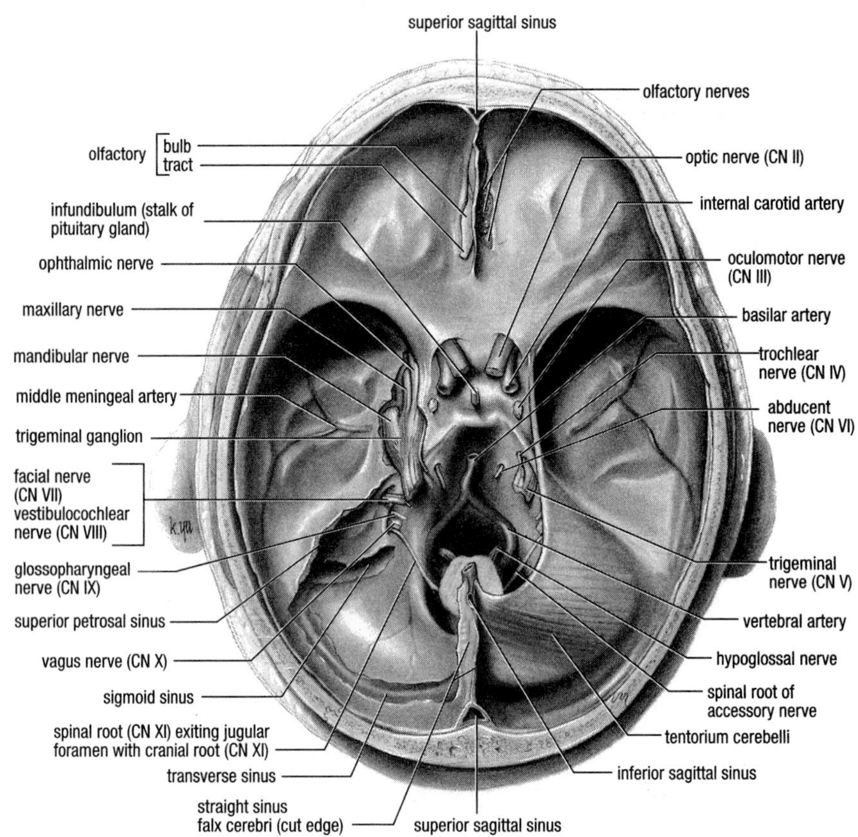
superior sagittal sinus
olfactory nerves
olfactory
bulb
tract
optic nerve (CN II)
infundibulum (stalk of pituitary gland)
internal carotid artery
ophthalmic nerve
oculomotor nerve (CN III)
maxillary nerve
basilar artery
mandibular nerve
trochlear nerve (CN IV)
middle meningeal artery
abducent nerve (CN VI)
trigeminal ganglion
facial nerve (CN VII)
vestibulocochlear nerve (CN VIII)
glossopharyngeal nerve (CN IX)
trigeminal nerve (CN V)
superior petrosal sinus
vertebral artery
vagus nerve (CN X)
hypoglossal nerve
sigmoid sinus
spinal root of accessory nerve
spinal root (CN XI) exiting jugular foramen with cranial root (CN XI)
tentorium cerebelli
transverse sinus
inferior sagittal sinus
straight sinus
falx cerebri (cut edge)
superior sagittal sinus

nerves and vessels of the interior of base of skull, superior view

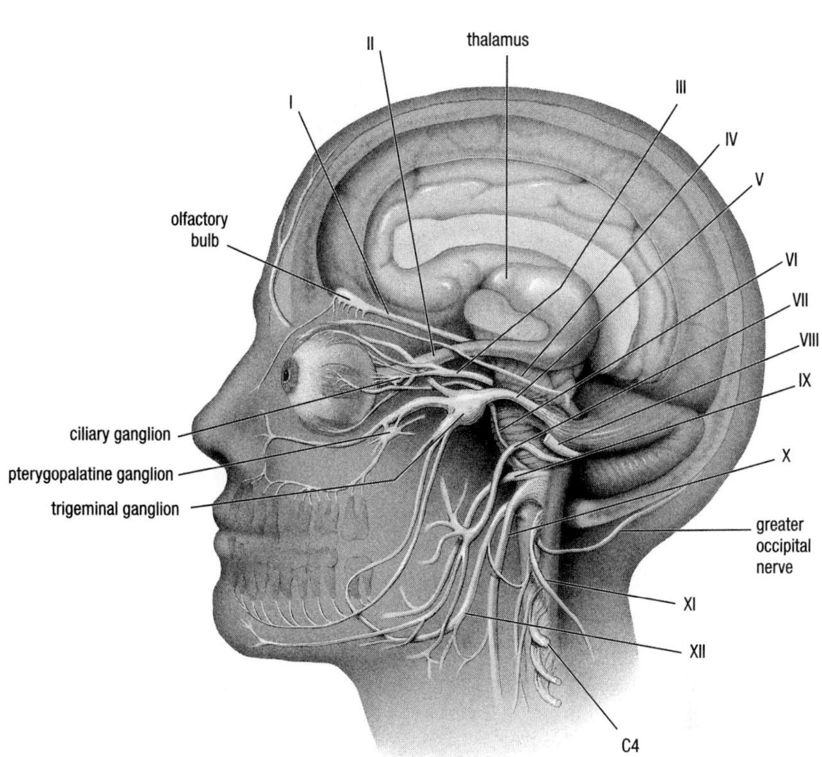

key

cranial nerves

I	olfactory nerve	**VI**	facial nerve
II	optic nerve	**VIII**	vestibulocochlear nerve
III	oculomotor nerve	**IX**	glossopharyngeal nerve
IV	trochlear nerve	**X**	vagus nerve
V	trigeminal nerve	**XI**	accessory nerve
VI	abducens nerve	**XII**	hypoglossal nerve

cranial nerves, lateral view

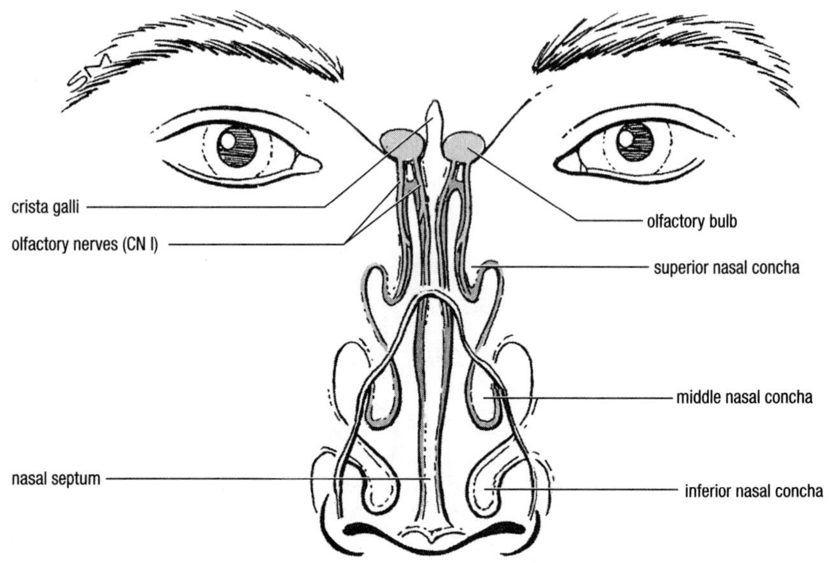

olfactory nerves (CN I), anterior view

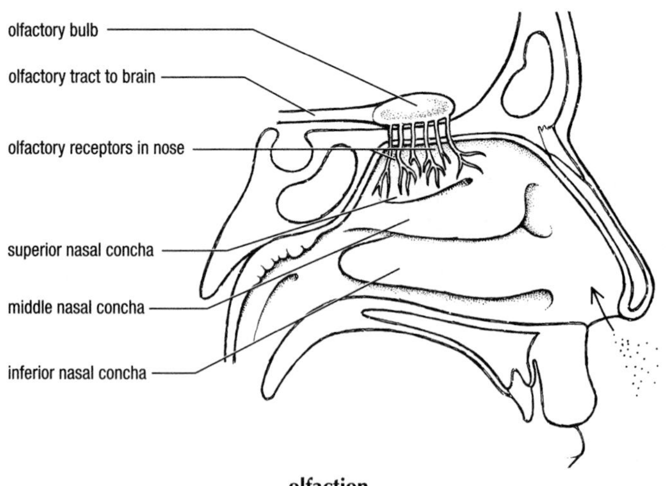

olfaction

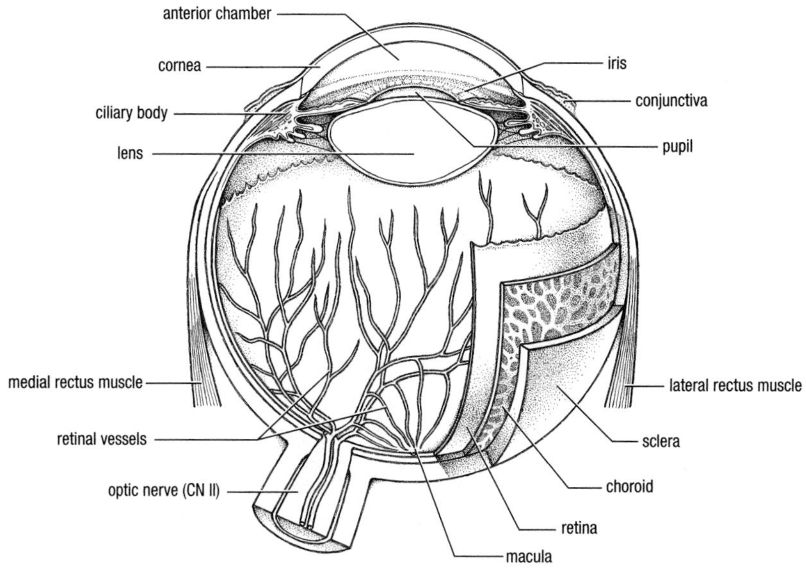

optic nerve (CN II) and structures of the eye

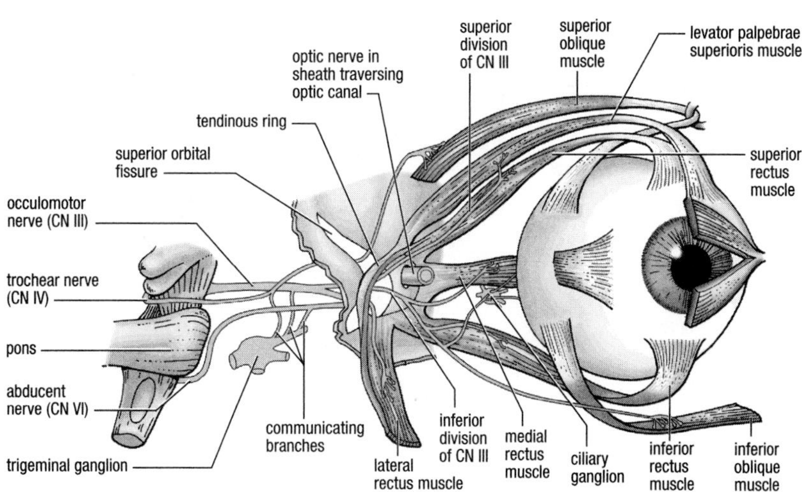

oculomotor nerve (CN III), trochlear nerve (CN IV), and abducent nerve CN VI)

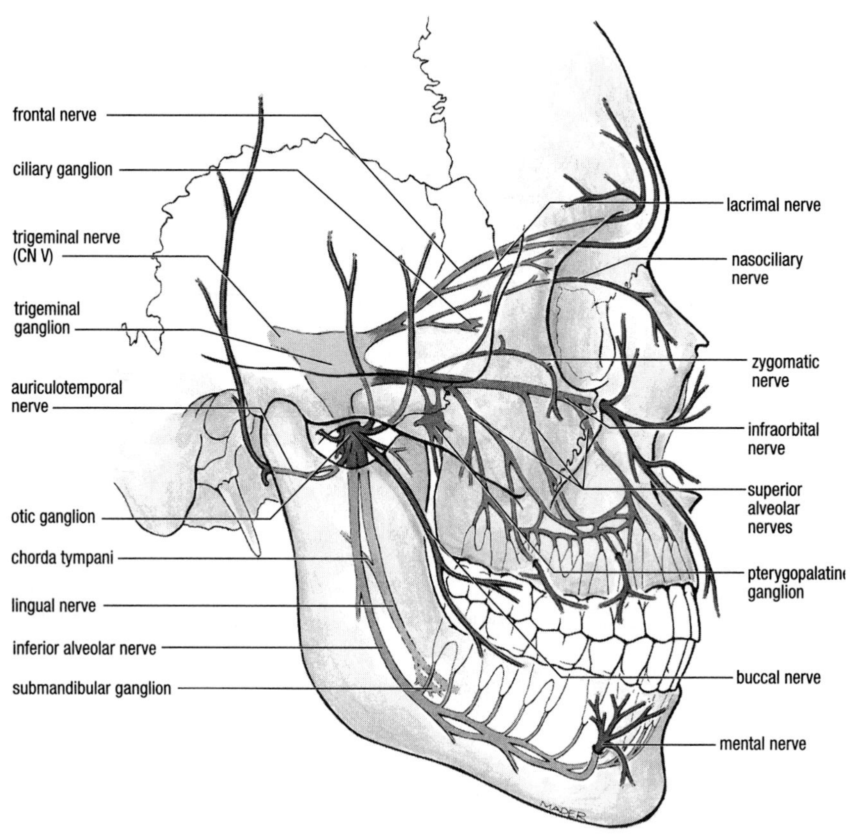

distribution of the trigeminal nerve (CN V)

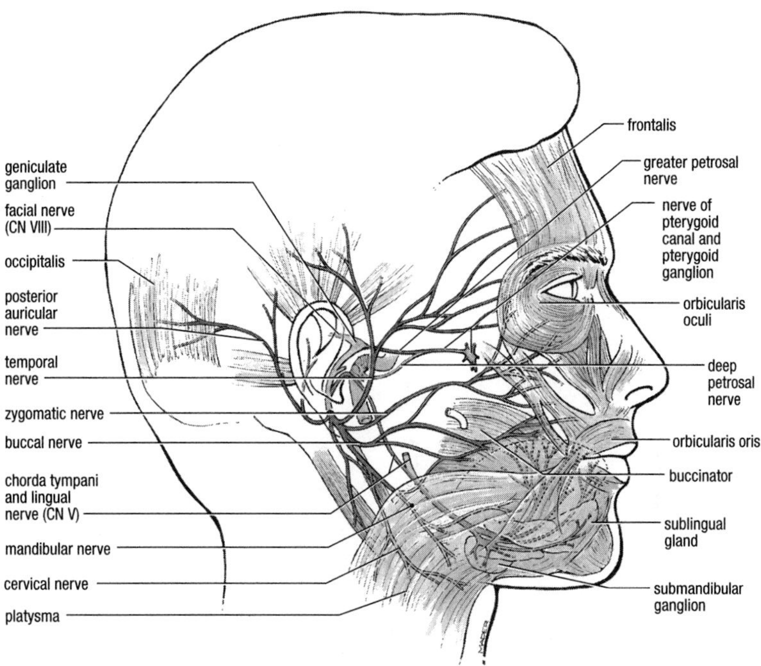
frontalis
geniculate ganglion
greater petrosal nerve
facial nerve (CN VIII)
nerve of pterygoid canal and pterygoid ganglion
occipitalis
posterior auricular nerve
orbicularis oculi
temporal nerve
deep petrosal nerve
zygomatic nerve
buccal nerve
orbicularis oris
chorda tympani and lingual nerve (CN V)
buccinator
sublingual gland
mandibular nerve
cervical nerve
submandibular ganglion
platysma

facial nerve (CN VII)

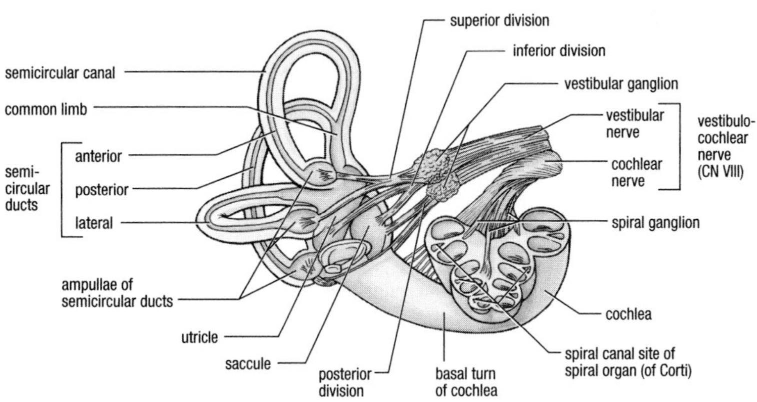
superior division
inferior division
semicircular canal
vestibular ganglion
common limb
vestibular nerve
vestibulo-cochlear nerve (CN VIII)
anterior
semi-circular ducts
cochlear nerve
posterior
lateral
spiral ganglion
ampullae of semicircular ducts
cochlea
utricle
spiral canal site of spiral organ (of Corti)
saccule
posterior division
basal turn of cochlea

vestibulocochlear nerve (CN VIII)

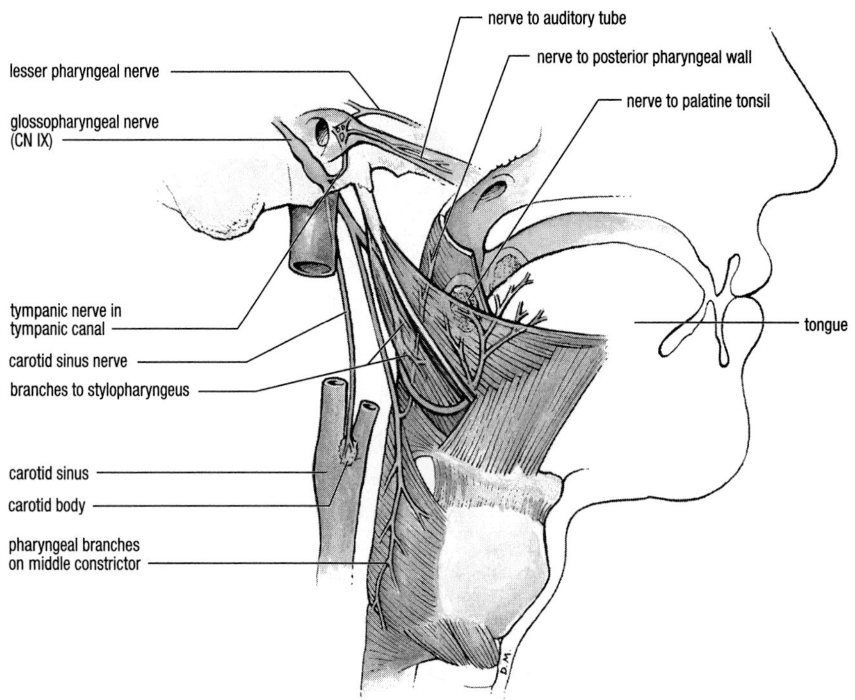
nerve to auditory tube
nerve to posterior pharyngeal wall
nerve to palatine tonsil
lesser pharyngeal nerve
glossopharyngeal nerve
(CN IX)
tympanic nerve in
tympanic canal
carotid sinus nerve
branches to stylopharyngeus
tongue
carotid sinus
carotid body
pharyngeal branches
on middle constrictor
D.M.

glossopharyngeal nerve (CN IX)

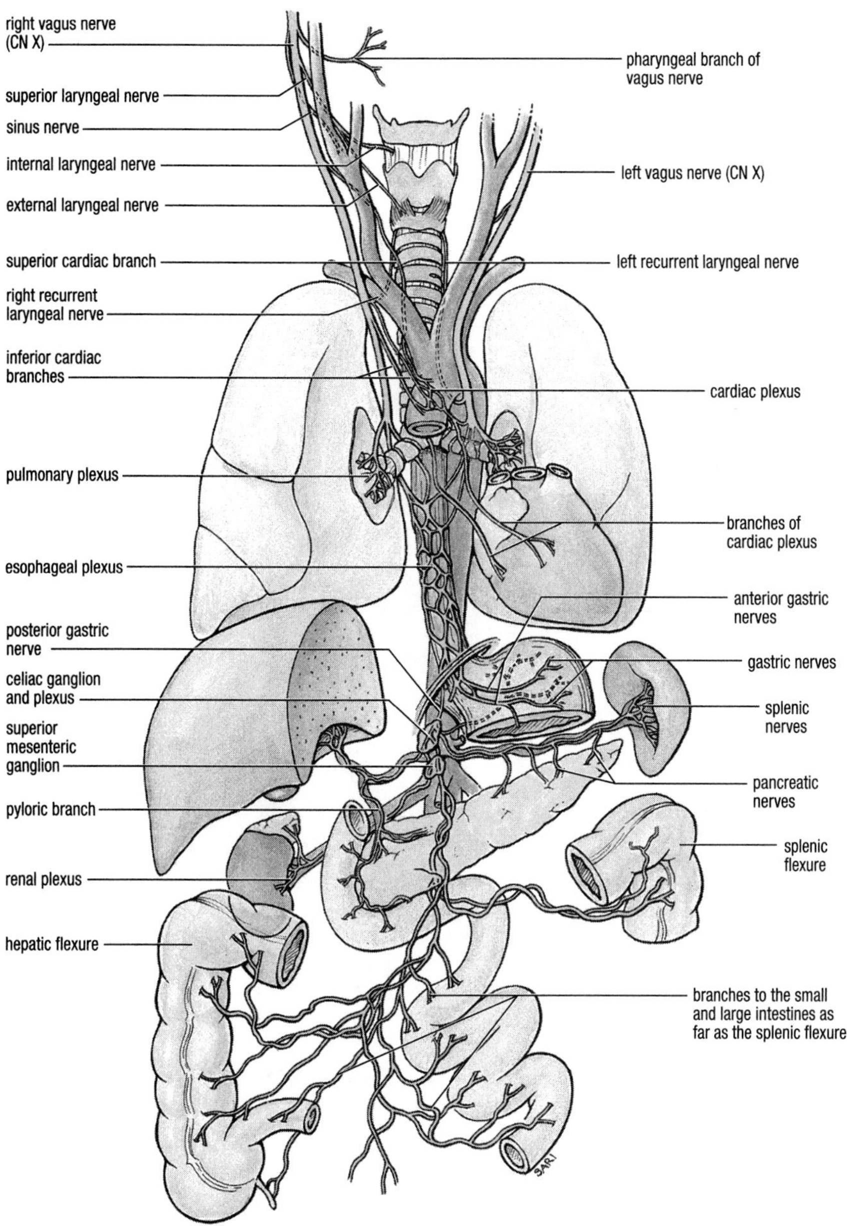
right vagus nerve (CN X)
superior laryngeal nerve
sinus nerve
internal laryngeal nerve
external laryngeal nerve
superior cardiac branch
right recurrent laryngeal nerve
inferior cardiac branches
pulmonary plexus
esophageal plexus
posterior gastric nerve
celiac ganglion and plexus
superior mesenteric ganglion
pyloric branch
renal plexus
hepatic flexure
pharyngeal branch of vagus nerve
left vagus nerve (CN X)
left recurrent laryngeal nerve
cardiac plexus
branches of cardiac plexus
anterior gastric nerves
gastric nerves
splenic nerves
pancreatic nerves
splenic flexure
branches to the small and large intestines as far as the splenic flexure
SARI

distribution of the vagus nerve (CN X)

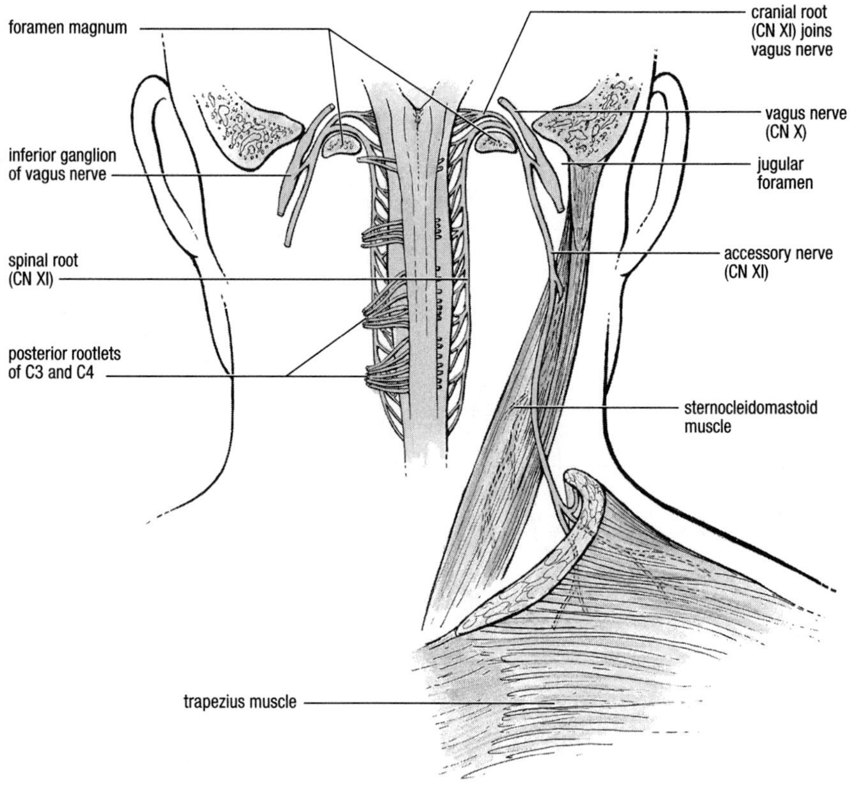

distribution of the accessory nerve (CN XI)

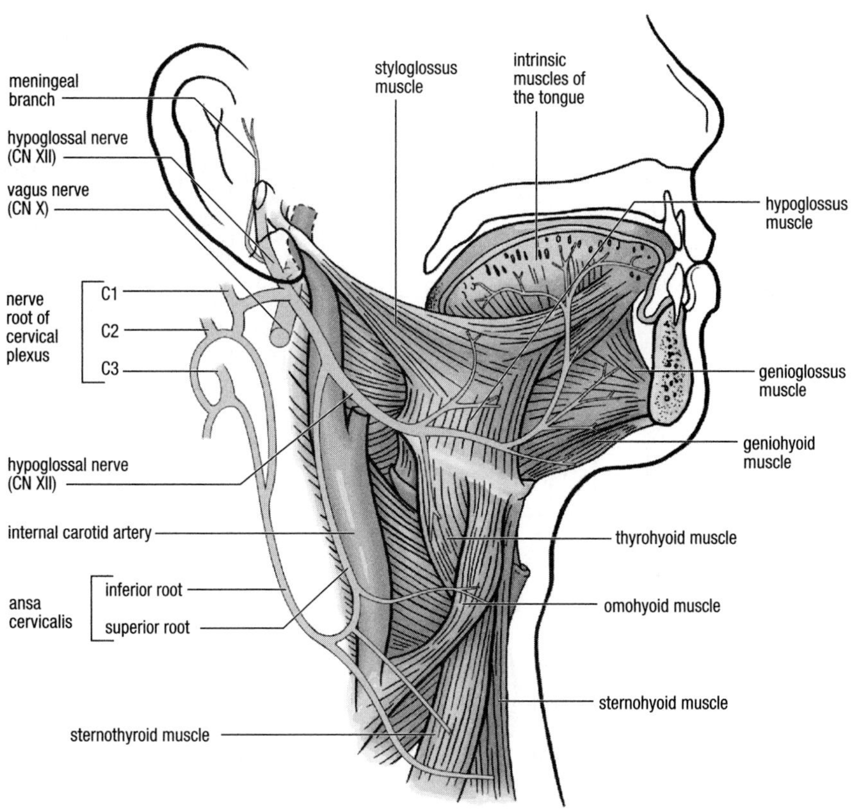

distribution of the hypoglossal nerve (CN XII)

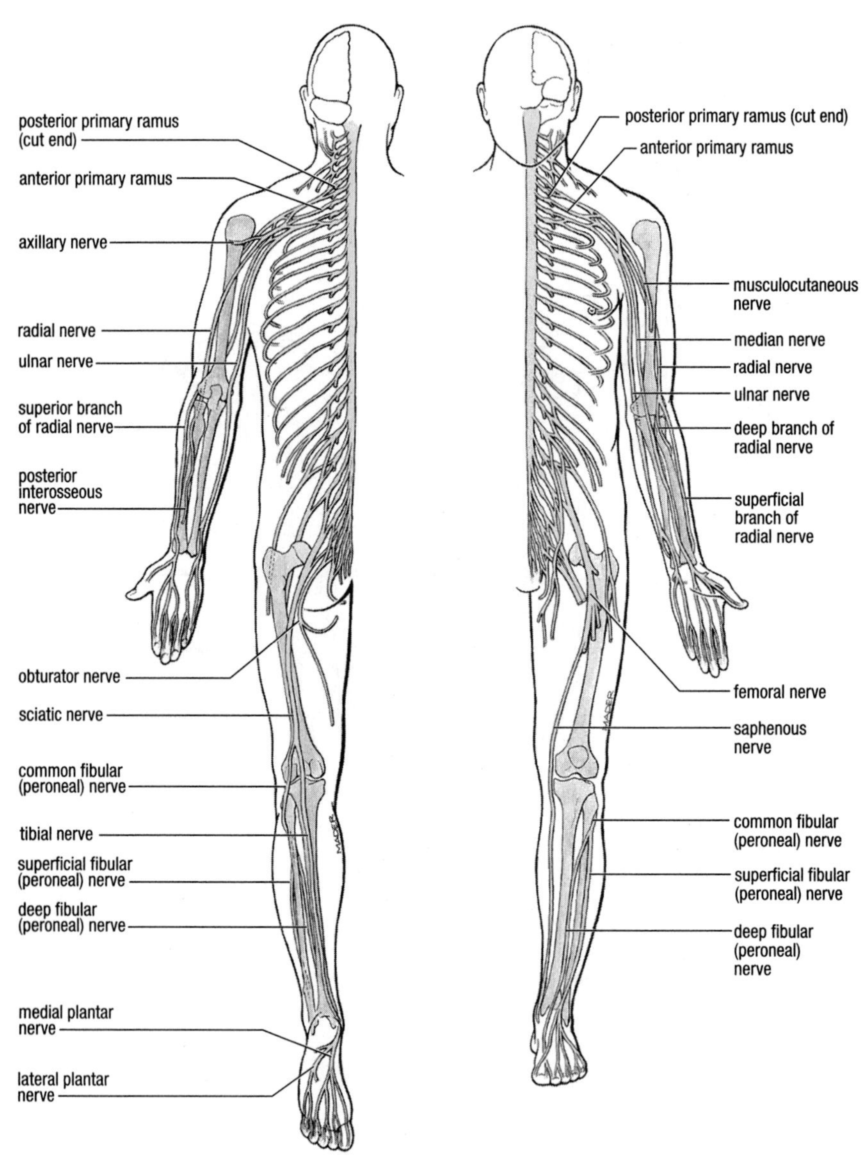

overview of the nervous system: posterior view (left) and anterior view (right)

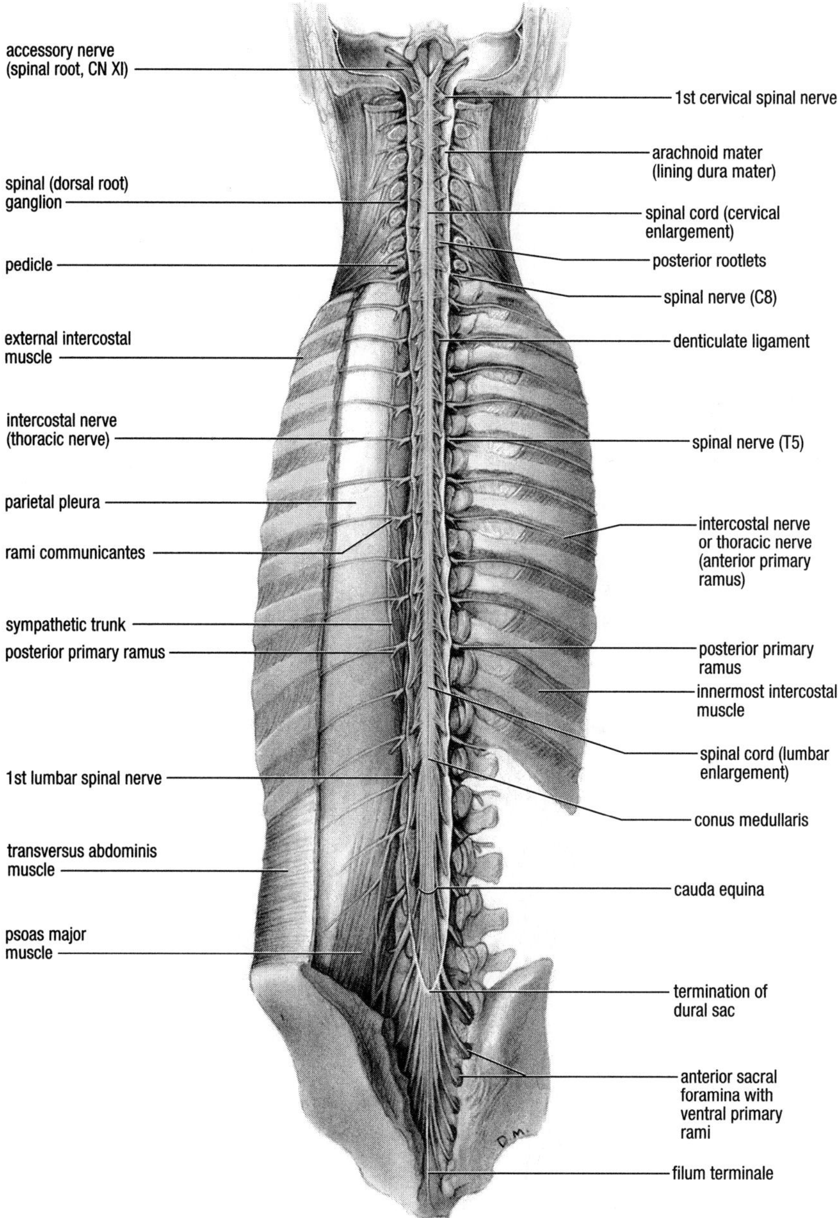
accessory nerve
(spinal root, CN XI)
1st cervical spinal nerve
arachnoid mater
(lining dura mater)
spinal (dorsal root)
ganglion
spinal cord (cervical
enlargement)
pedicle
posterior rootlets
spinal nerve (C8)
external intercostal
muscle
denticulate ligament
intercostal nerve
(thoracic nerve)
spinal nerve (T5)
parietal pleura
intercostal nerve
or thoracic nerve
(anterior primary
ramus)
rami communicantes
sympathetic trunk
posterior primary ramus
posterior primary
ramus
innermost intercostal
muscle
spinal cord (lumbar
enlargement)
1st lumbar spinal nerve
conus medullaris
transversus abdominis
muscle
cauda equina
psoas major
muscle
termination of
dural sac
anterior sacral
foramina with
ventral primary
rami
filum terminale
D.M.

spinal cord and surrounding structures, posterior view

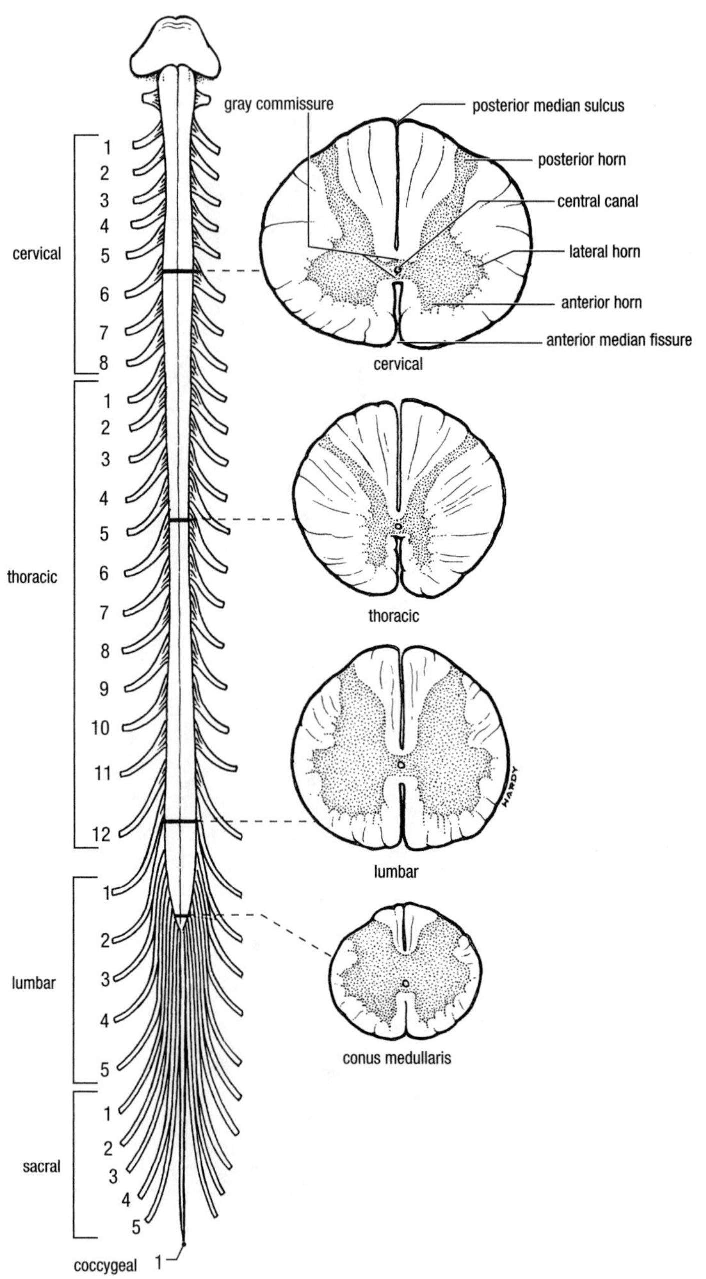

spinal cord showing cross-sections at various levels

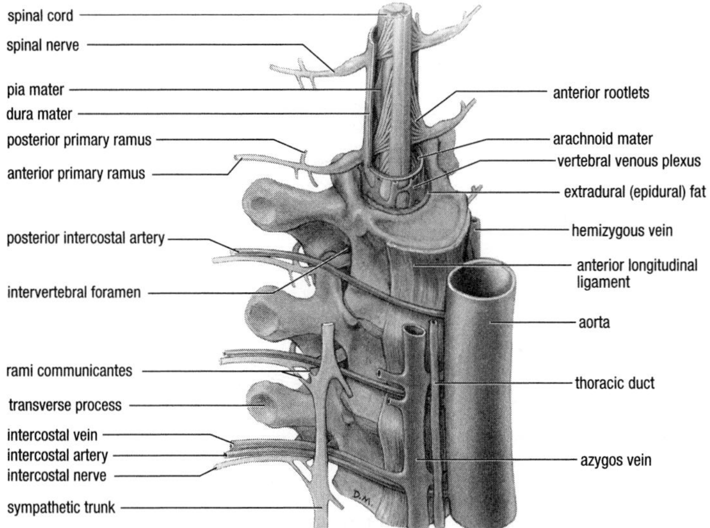

spinal cord and prevertebral structures

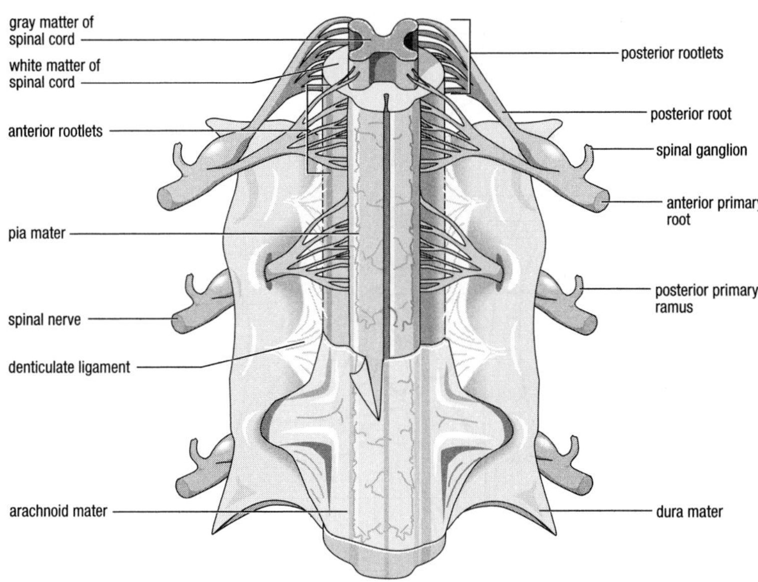

open view of the compartments of the spinal cord showing the various meninges and the spinal nerves

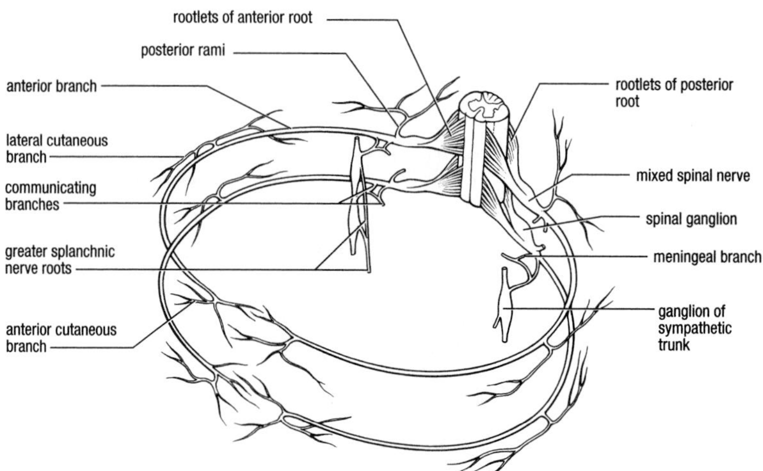
rootlets of anterior root
posterior rami
anterior branch
lateral cutaneous branch
communicating branches
greater splanchnic nerve roots
anterior cutaneous branch
rootlets of posterior root
mixed spinal nerve
spinal ganglion
meningeal branch
ganglion of sympathetic trunk

spinal nerves, with roots and branches

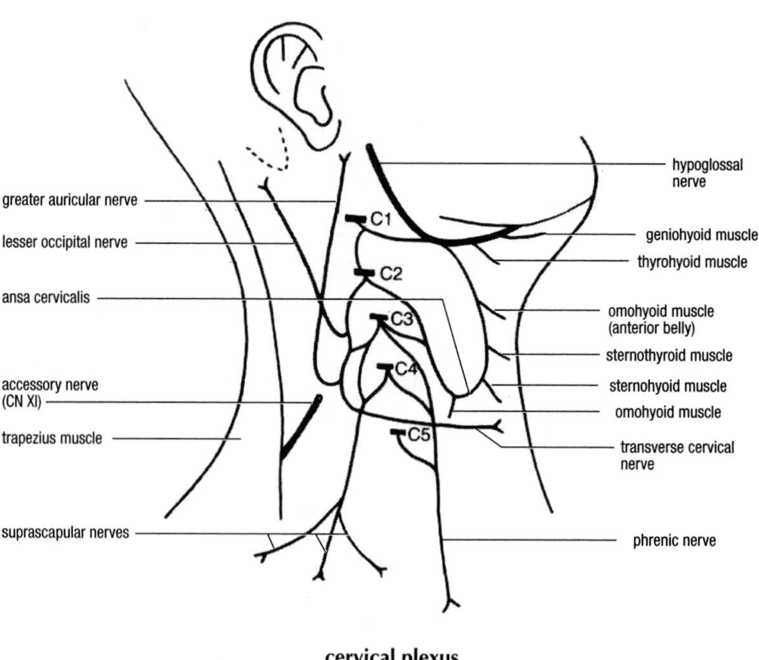
greater auricular nerve
lesser occipital nerve
ansa cervicalis
accessory nerve (CN XI)
trapezius muscle
suprascapular nerves
C1
C2
C3
C4
C5
hypoglossal nerve
geniohyoid muscle
thyrohyoid muscle
omohyoid muscle (anterior belly)
sternothyroid muscle
sternohyoid muscle
omohyoid muscle
transverse cervical nerve
phrenic nerve

cervical plexus

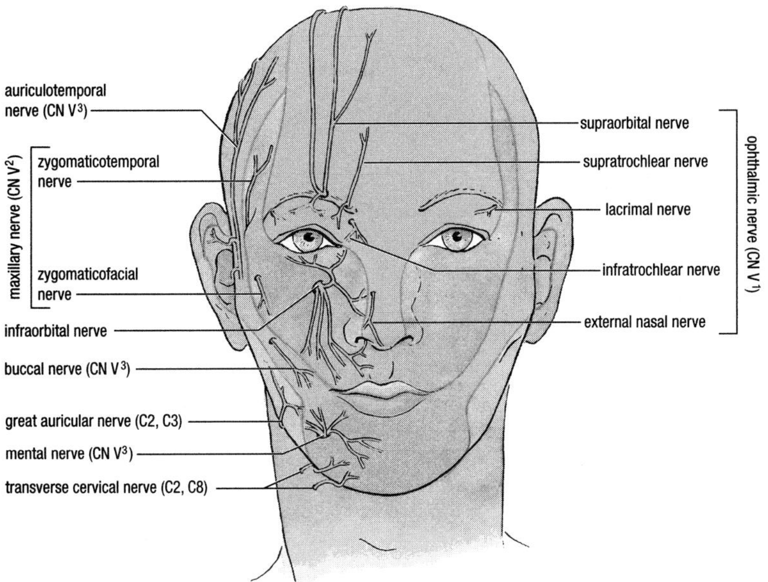

sensory nerves of the face and scalp, anterior view

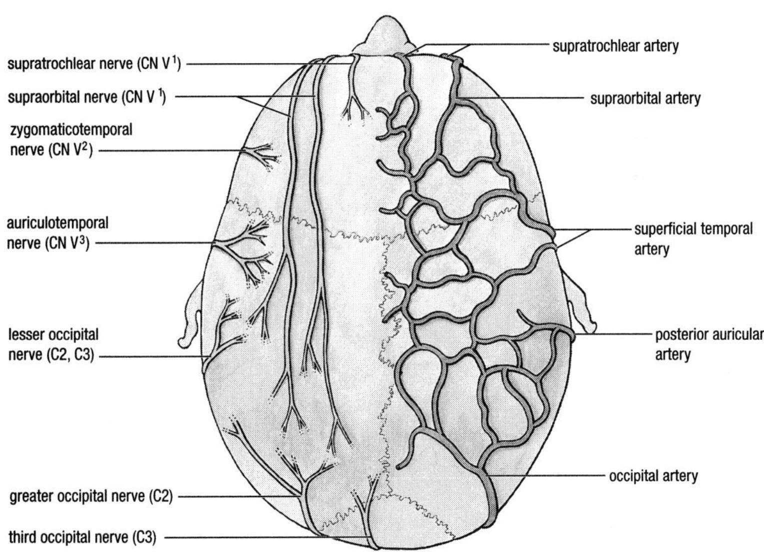

sensory nerves and arteries of the face and scalp, superior view

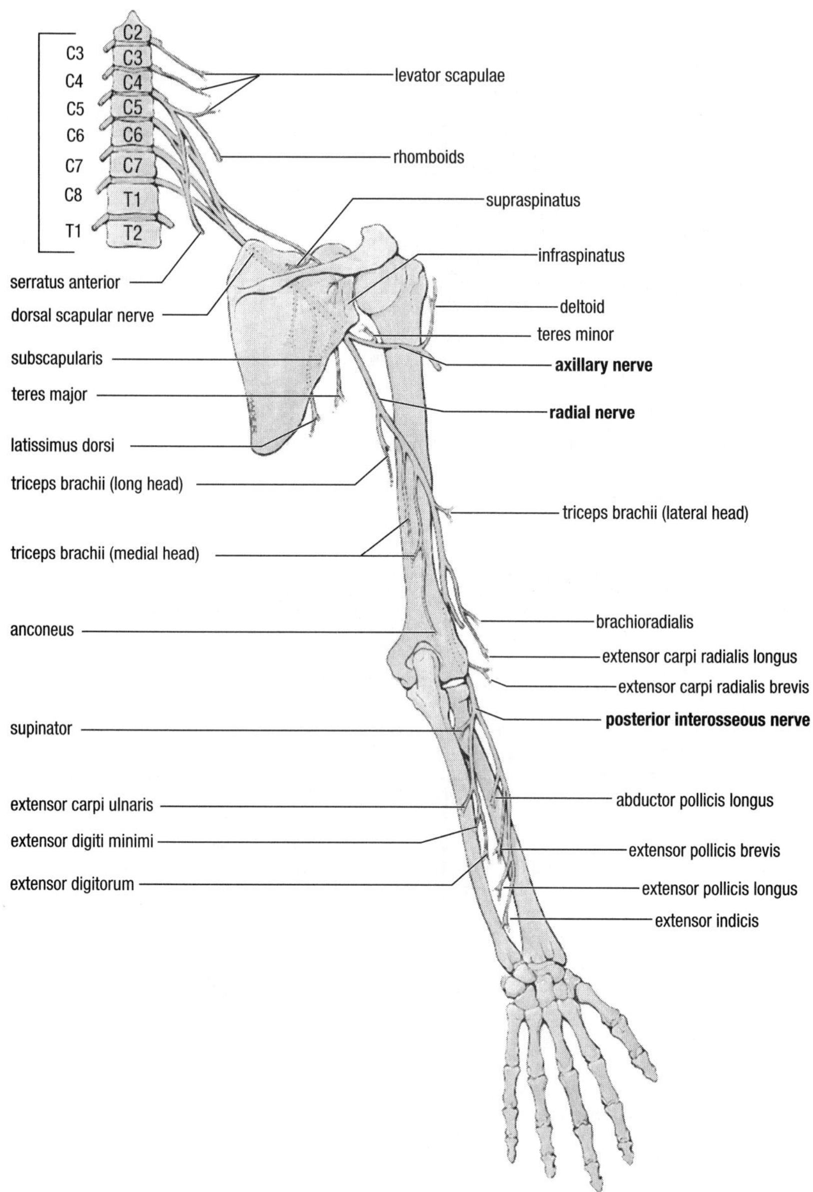
C2
C3
C4
C5
C6
C7
C8
T1
T1
T2
levator scapulae
rhomboids
supraspinatus
infraspinatus
serratus anterior
dorsal scapular nerve
deltoid
teres minor
subscapularis
axillary nerve
teres major
radial nerve
latissimus dorsi
triceps brachii (long head)
triceps brachii (lateral head)
triceps brachii (medial head)
brachioradialis
anconeus
extensor carpi radialis longus
extensor carpi radialis brevis
posterior interosseous nerve
supinator
abductor pollicis longus
extensor carpi ulnaris
extensor digiti minimi
extensor pollicis brevis
extensor digitorum
extensor pollicis longus
extensor indicis

innervation of the upper limb muscles, radial nerve

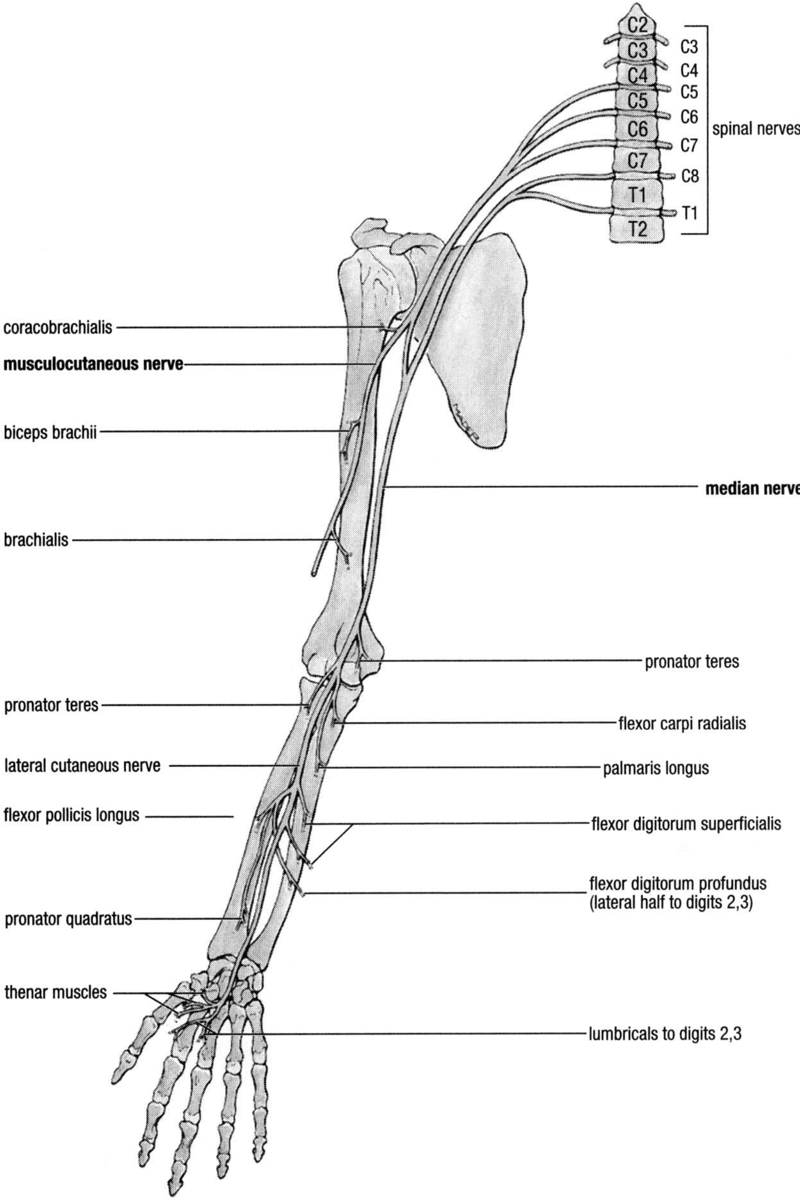

innervation of the upper limb muscles, median and musculocutaneous nerves

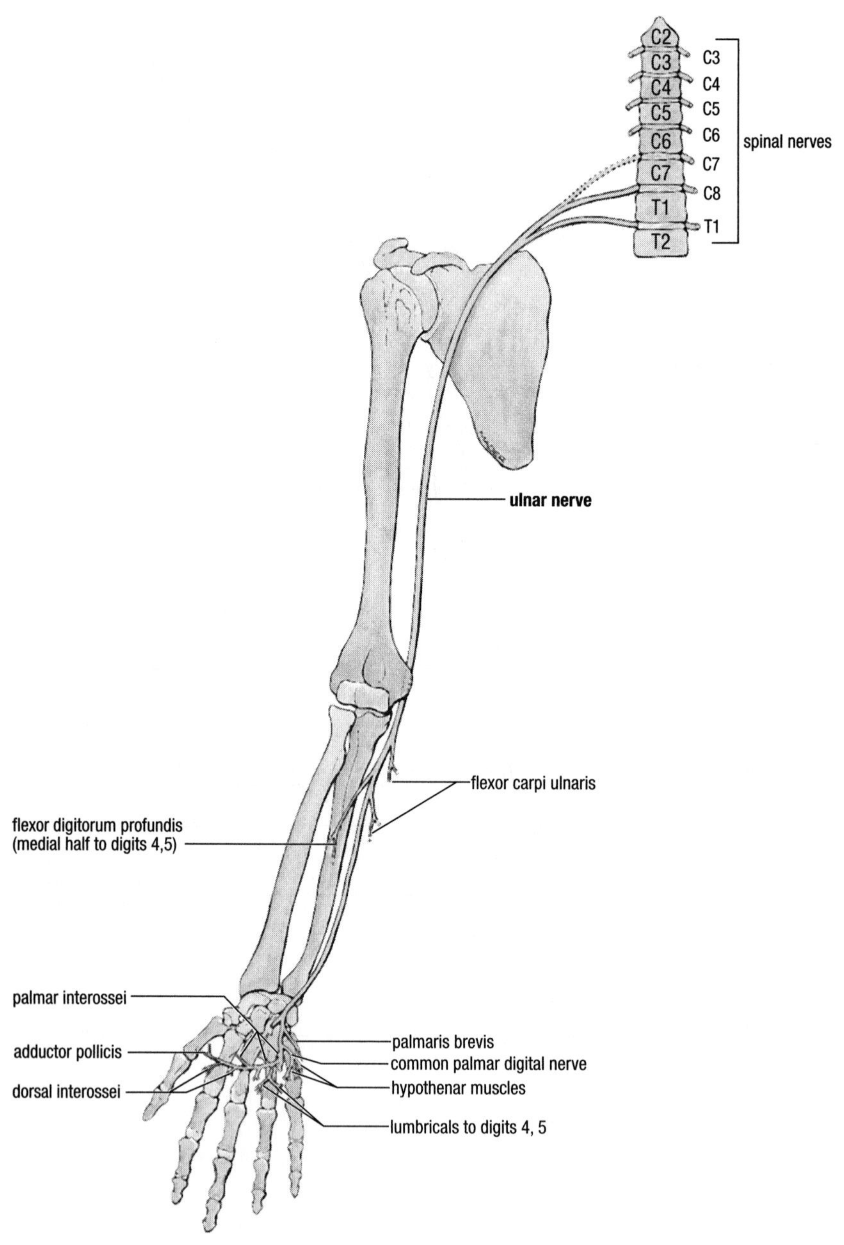

innervation of the upper limb muscles, ulnar nerve

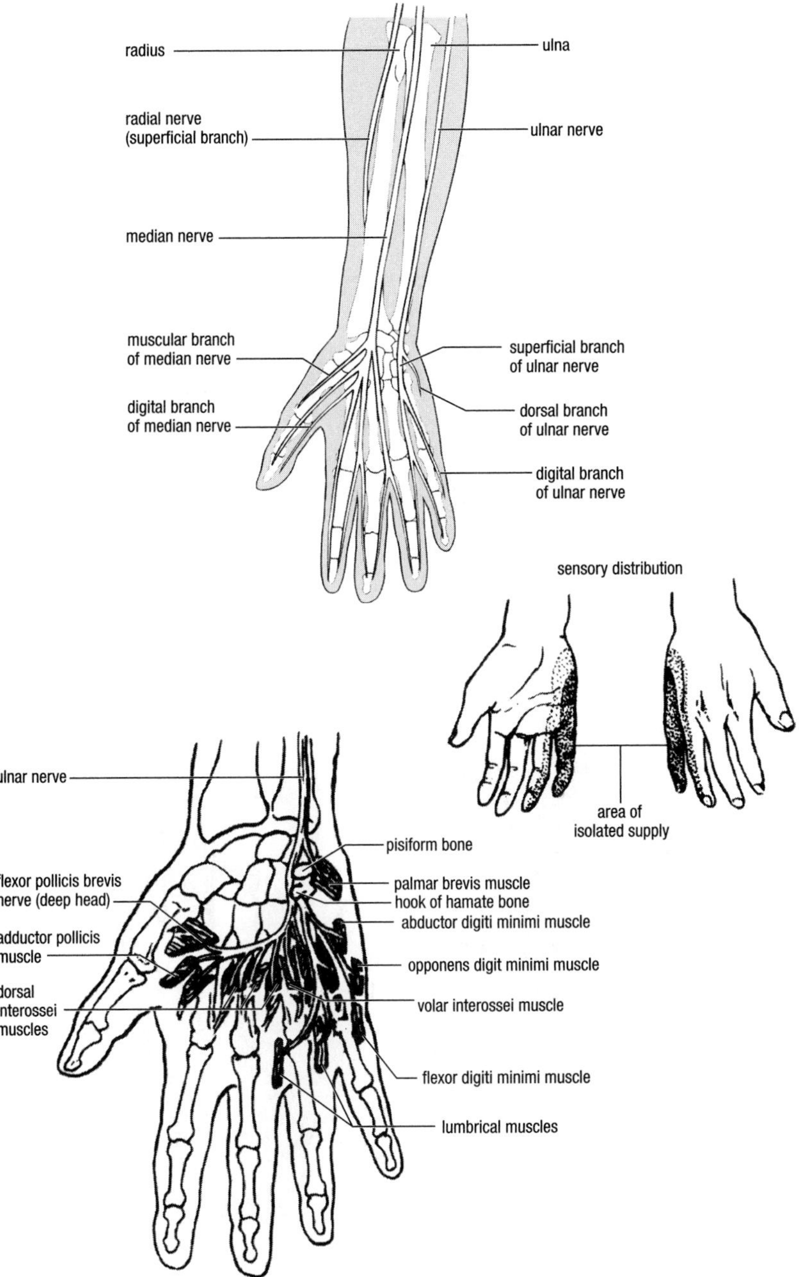
radius
ulna
radial nerve
(superficial branch)
ulnar nerve
median nerve
muscular branch
of median nerve
superficial branch
of ulnar nerve
digital branch
of median nerve
dorsal branch
of ulnar nerve
digital branch
of ulnar nerve
sensory distribution
area of
isolated supply
ulnar nerve
pisiform bone
flexor pollicis brevis
nerve (deep head)
palmar brevis muscle
hook of hamate bone
abductor digiti minimi muscle
adductor pollicis
muscle
opponens digit minimi muscle
dorsal
interossei
muscles
volar interossei muscle
flexor digiti minimi muscle
lumbrical muscles

nerves of the hand and sensory distribution

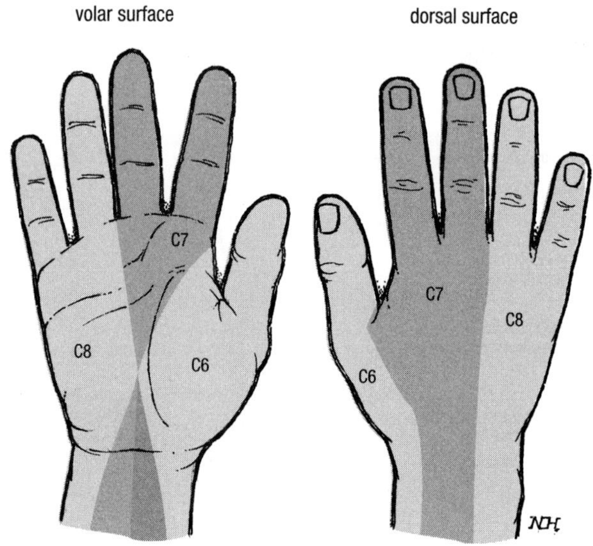

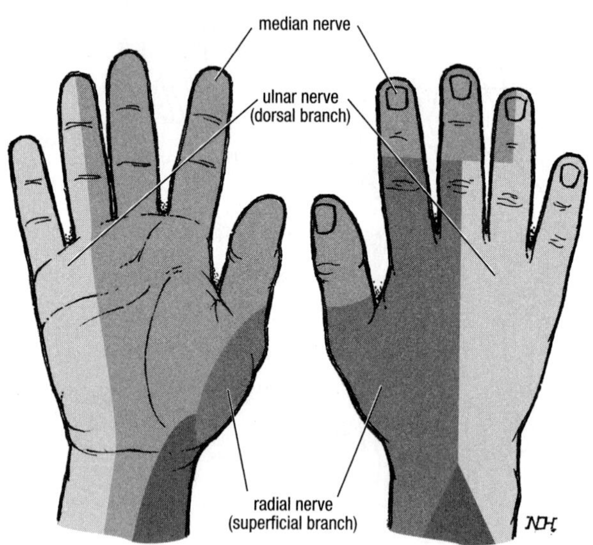

innervation of hand

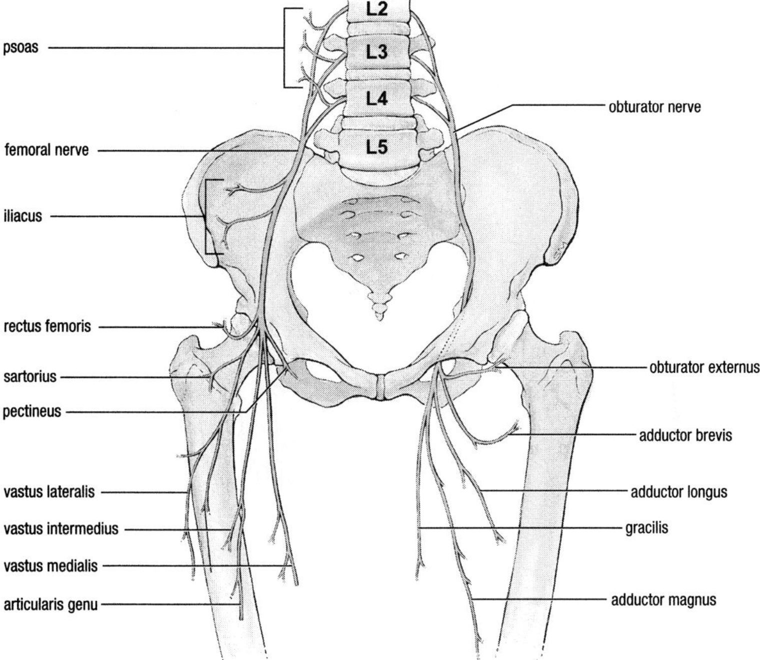

motor distribution of lower limb nerves, femoral and obturator nerves

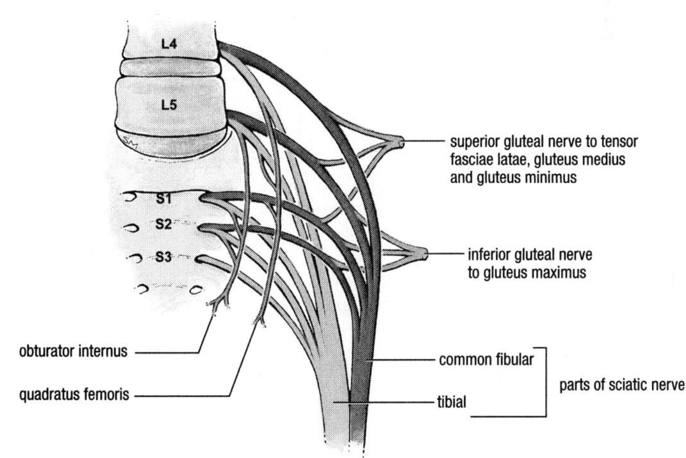

motor distribution of lower limb nerves, sciatic nerve

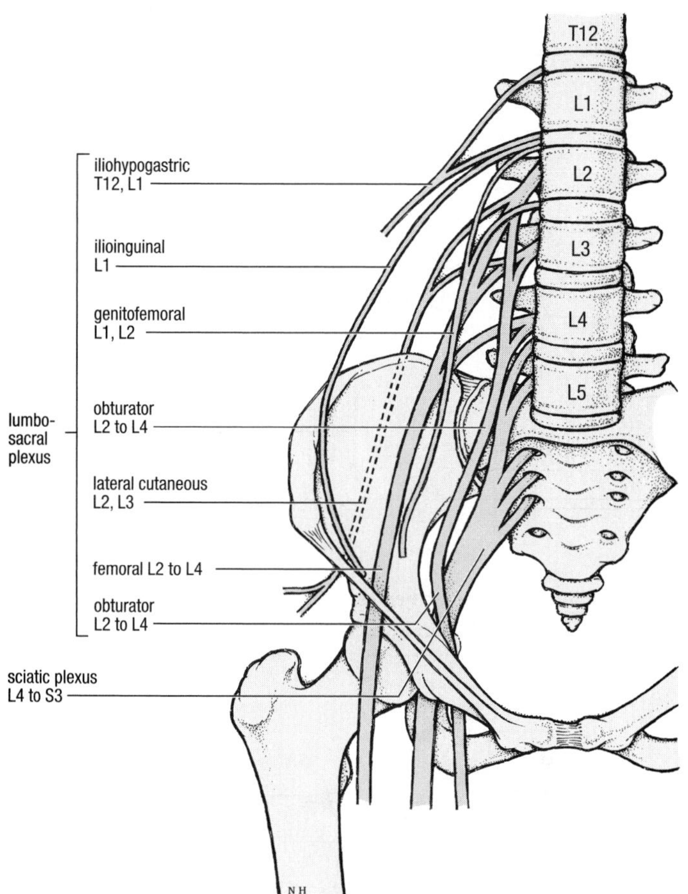

lumbosacral plexus and sciatic plexus

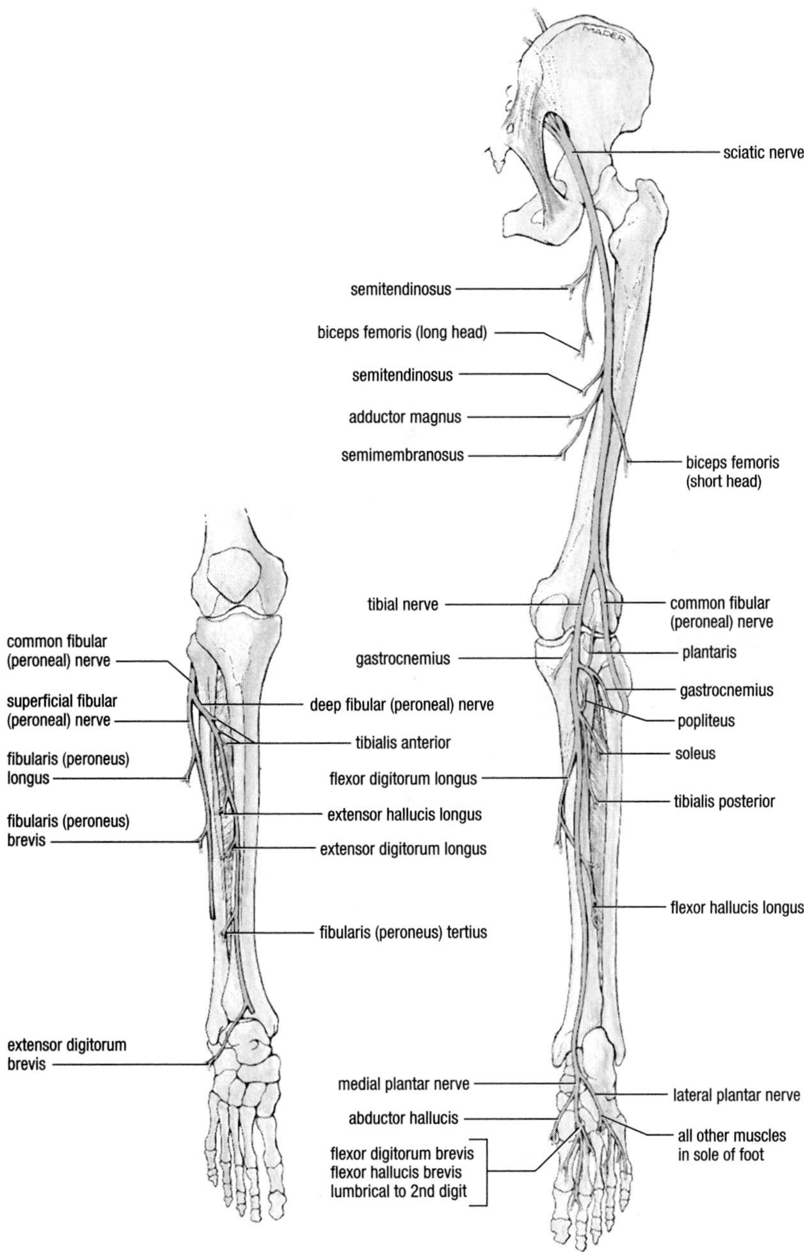

motor distribution of lower limb nerves: common fibular (peroneal) nerve (left) and sciatic nerve (right)

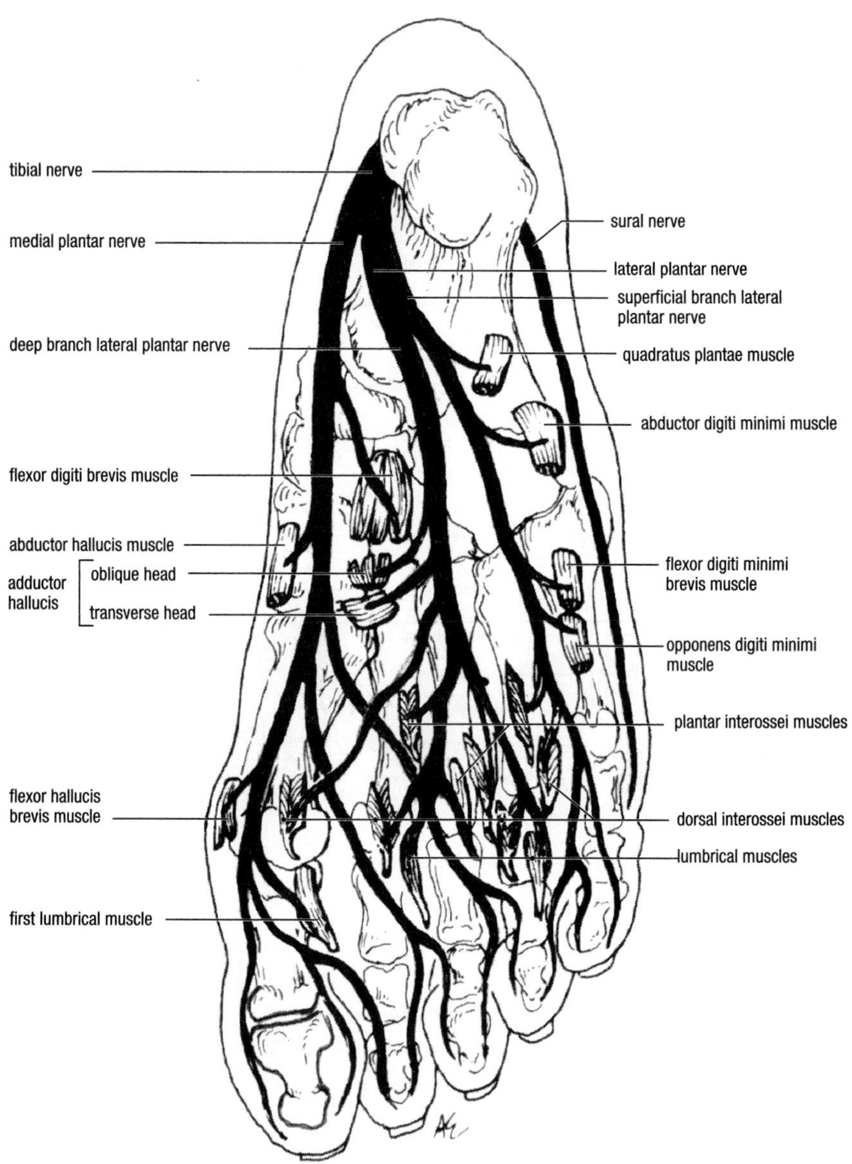
tibial nerve
medial plantar nerve
deep branch lateral plantar nerve
flexor digiti brevis muscle
abductor hallucis muscle
adductor hallucis
oblique head
transverse head
flexor hallucis brevis muscle
first lumbrical muscle
sural nerve
lateral plantar nerve
superficial branch lateral plantar nerve
quadratus plantae muscle
abductor digiti minimi muscle
flexor digiti minimi brevis muscle
opponens digiti minimi muscle
plantar interossei muscles
dorsal interossei muscles
lumbrical muscles

nerves of the foot

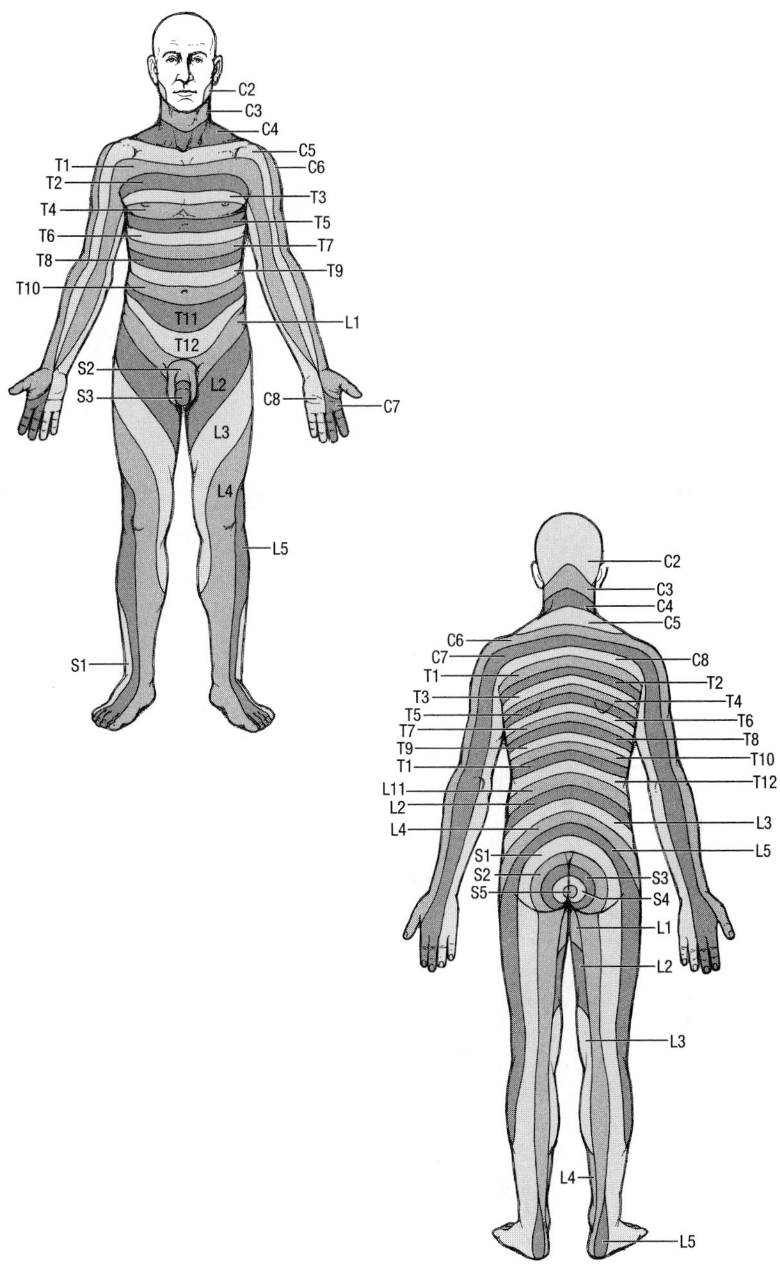

dermatomes: anterior view (left) and posterior view (right). C1 nerve lacks a significant afferent component and does not supply the skin.

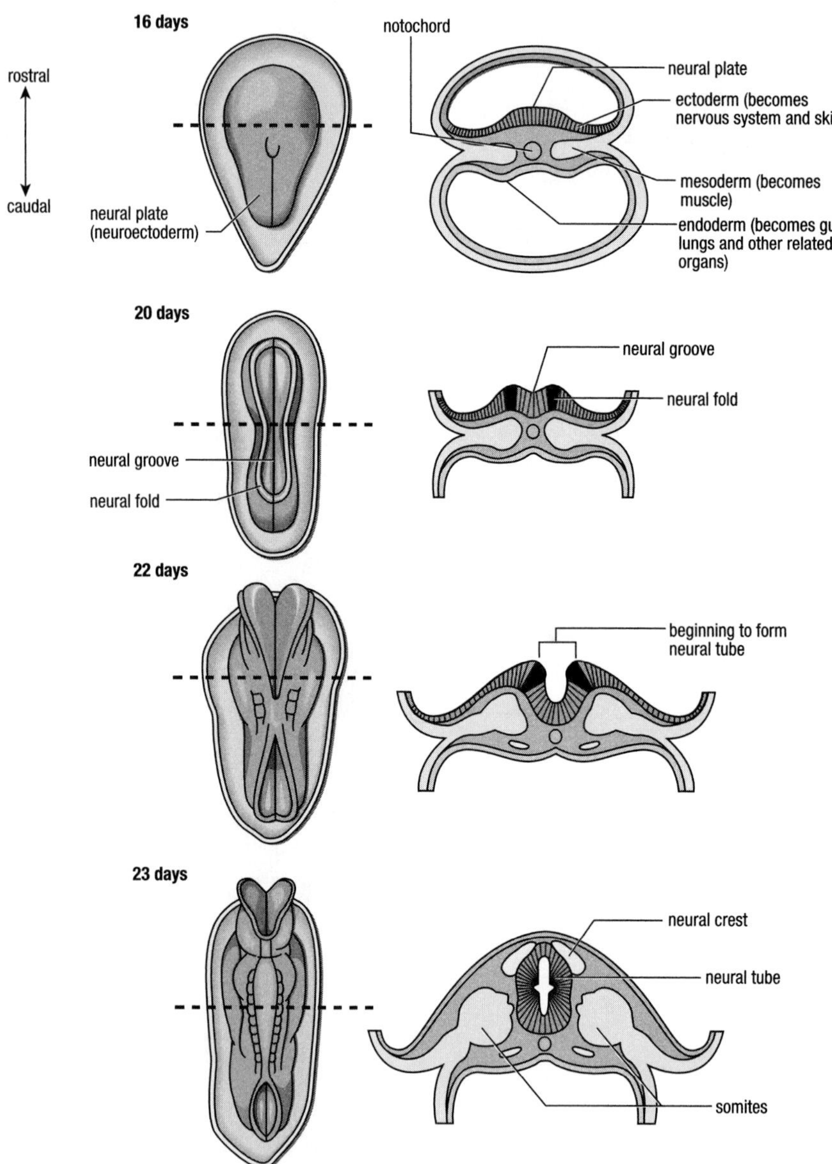

progressive formation of the neural tube

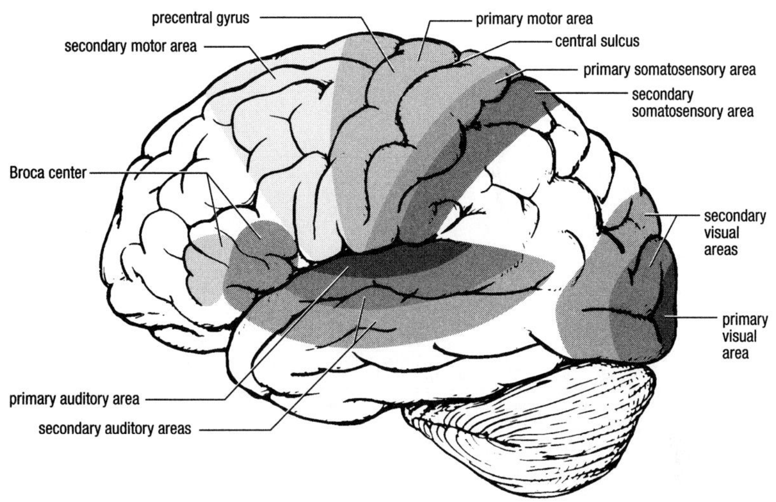

cerebral cortex and its major functional areas

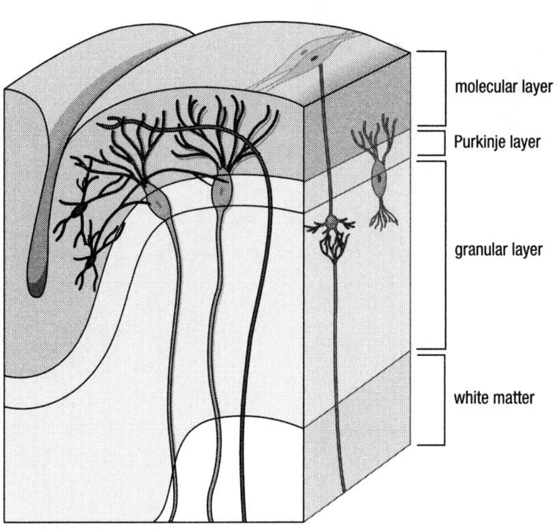

cross-section of cerebellar cortex

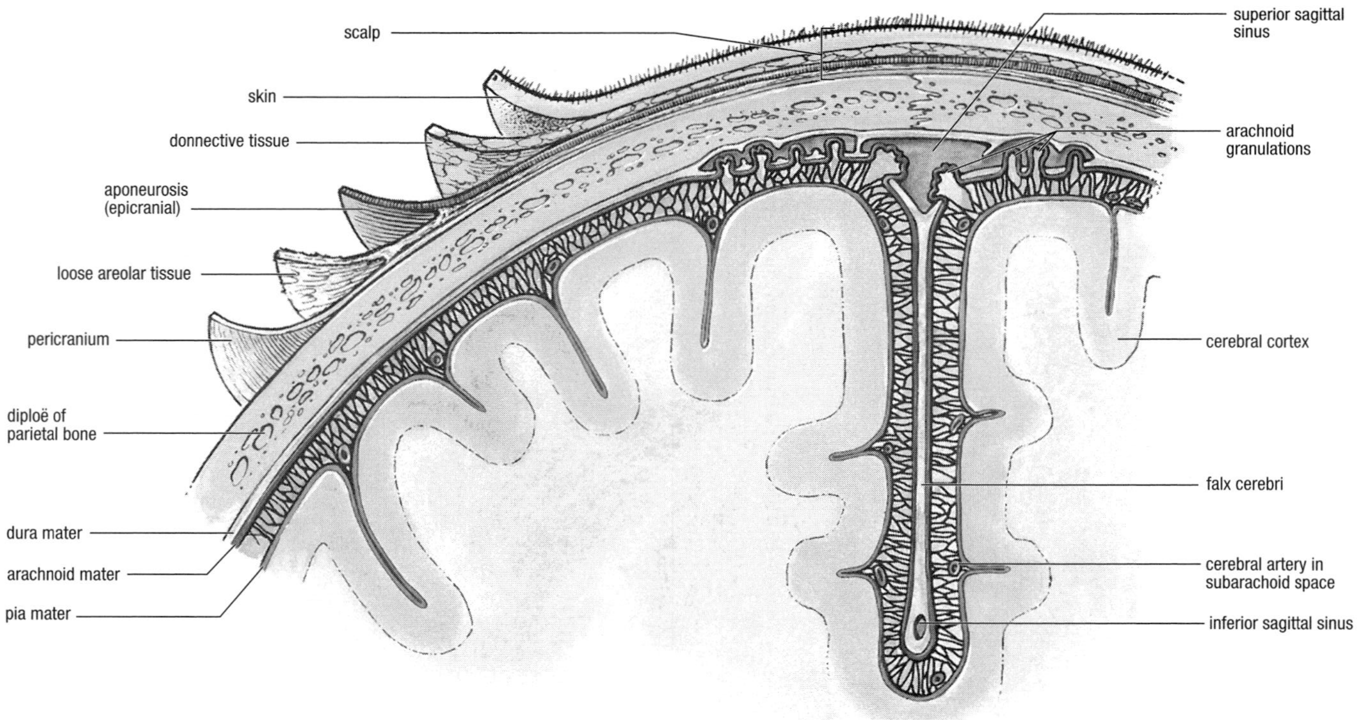
scalp
skin
donnective tissue
aponeurosis (epicranial)
loose areolar tissue
pericranium
diploë of parietal bone
dura mater
arachnoid mater
pia mater
superior sagittal sinus
arachnoid granulations
cerebral cortex
falx cerebri
cerebral artery in subarachoid space
inferior sagittal sinus

scalp, skull, and meninges

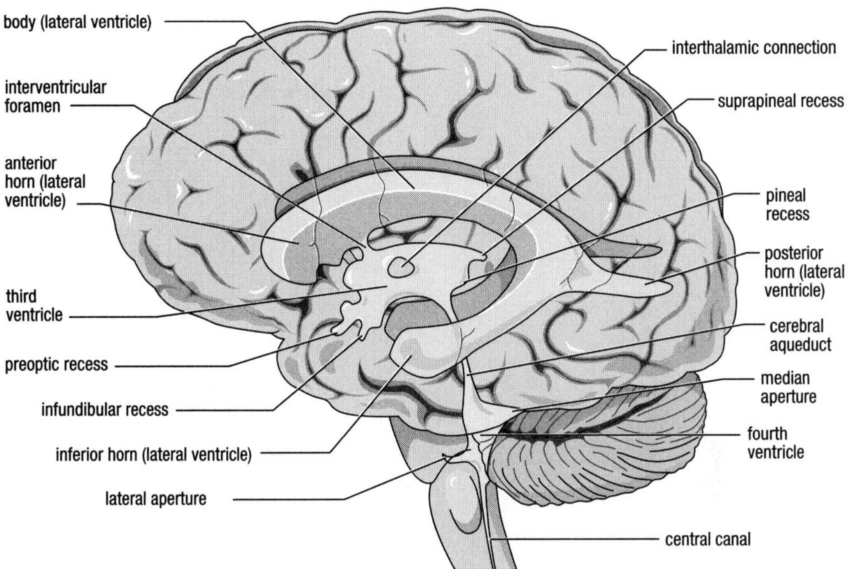

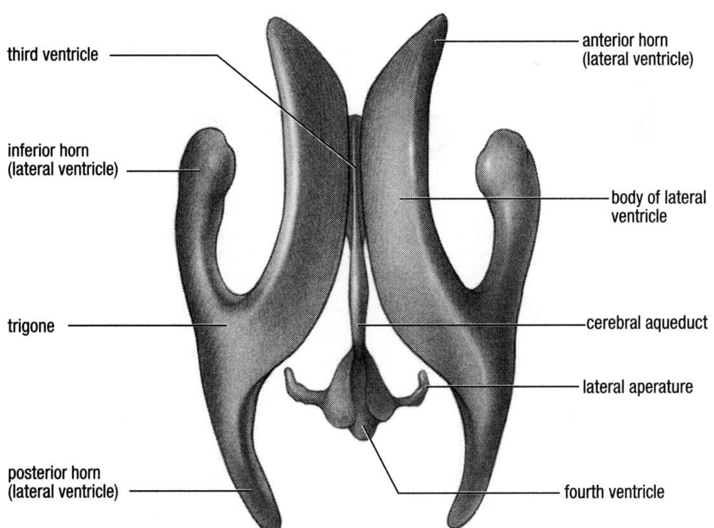

ventricles of the brain: lateral view (top) and superior view (bottom)

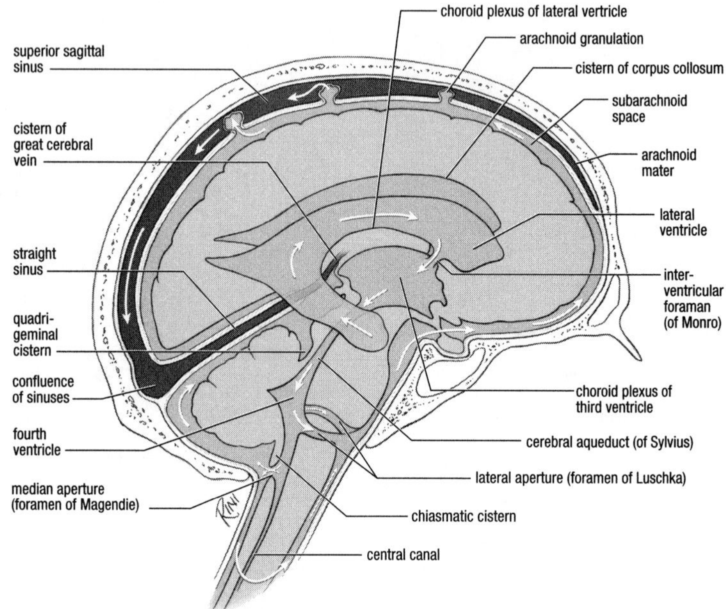

circulation of cerebrospinal fluid

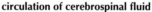

human cerebrospinal fluid (CSF)	
(average measurements, mg/dL)	
volume	120 – 200 ml
specific gravity	1.006 – 1.008
reaction	pH ca. 7.5
freezing point depression	0.55 (0.52 – 0.58)
pressure (lumbar, subject reclining)	60 – 150 mm H_2O
protein	15 – 25
glucose	50 – 75 mg/100mL
phosphatidic acid	ca. 1.0
cholesterol	0.3 – 0.6
chloride	100 – 130 mEq/liter
phosphate	3 – 5
blood	meg/pst
cell count	0 – 5 mononuclear cells
protein	
lumbar	15 – 456
total	15 – 45
cisternal	15 – 25 mg/100 mL
ventricular	5 – 15 mg/100 mL

human cerebrospinal fluid

Anatomical Illustrations

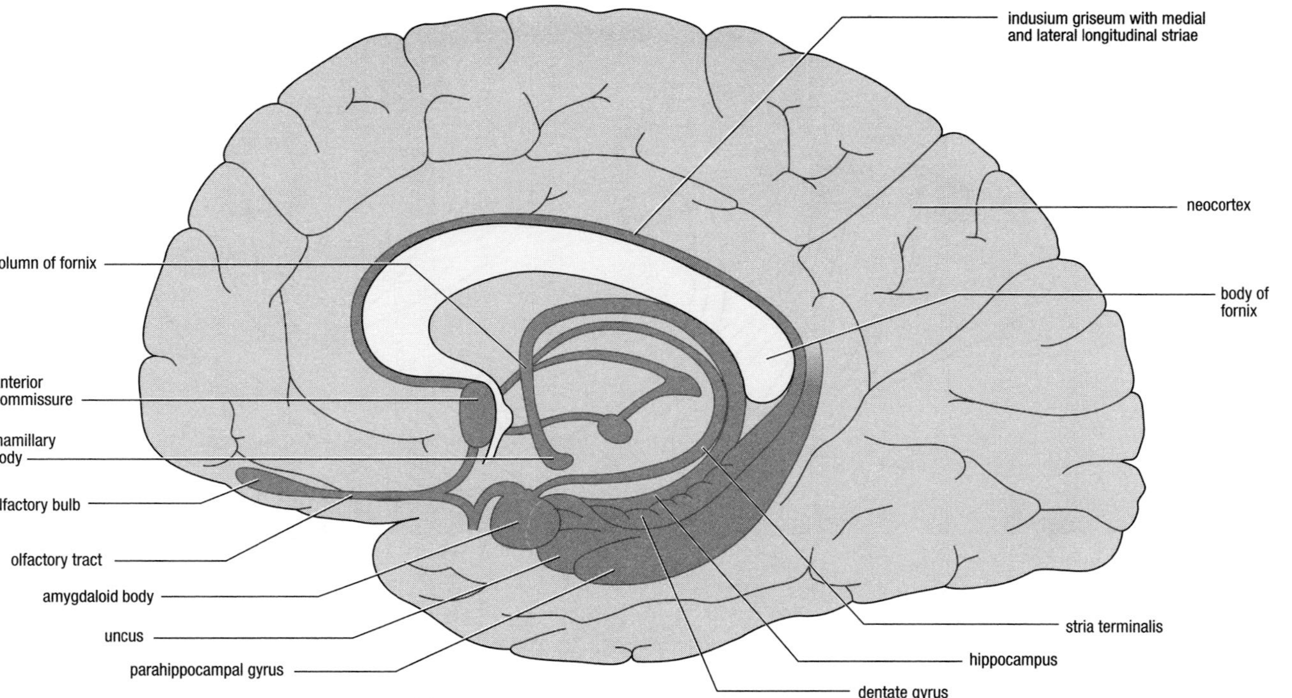

limbic system (the center of emotions)

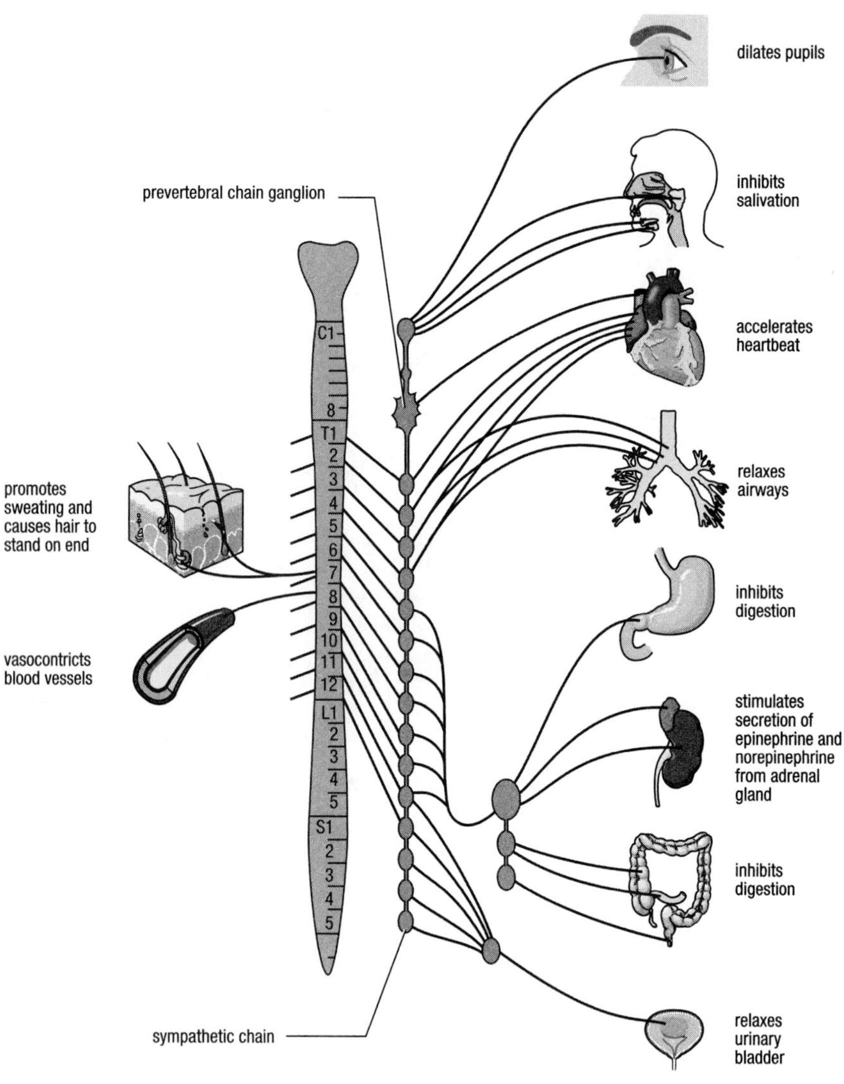

components of the sympathetic nervous system and the spinal nerves and the organs they innervate

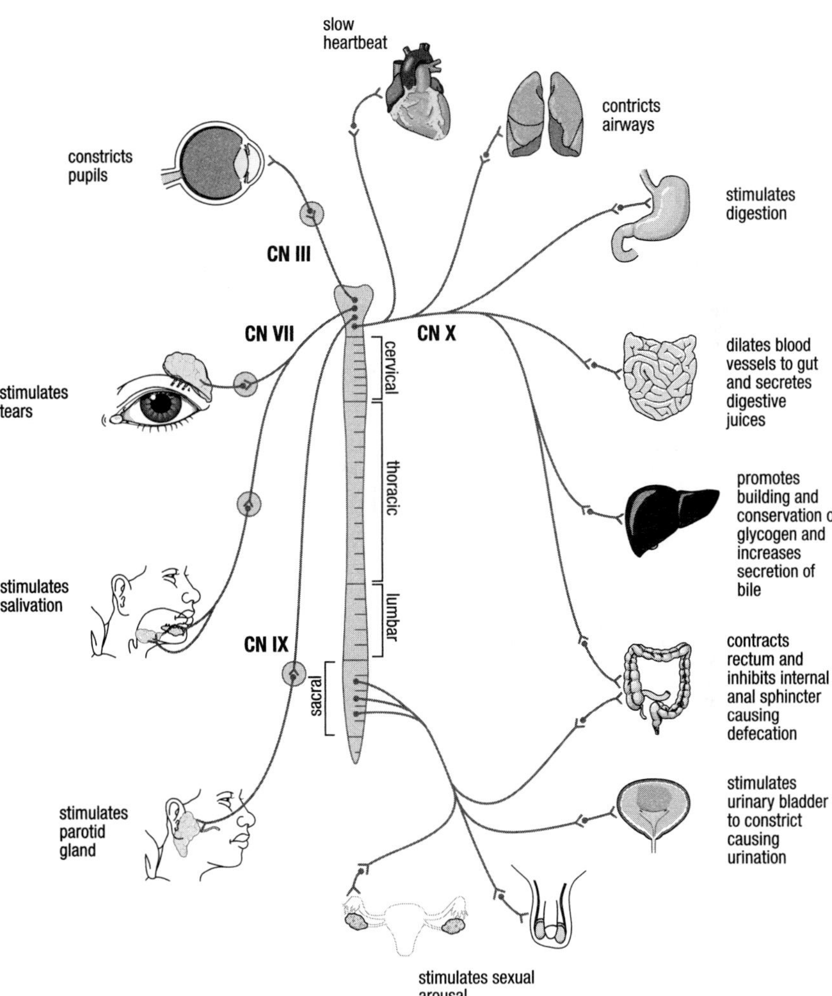

the parasympathetic nervous systems and the organs that are innervated by each nerve

autonomic nervous system				
organ	**function of sympathetic nervous system**	**sympathetic nerve(s)**	**function of parasympathetic nervous system**	**parasympathetic nerve(s)**
eye	pupil dilation, contraction of ciliary muscle for accommodation	postganglionic fibers from superior cervical ganglion (internal carotid nr.)	constriction of pupil	postganglionic fibers from ciliary ganglion via short ciliary nerves
lacrimal gland	slight or no effect	postganglionic fibers from superior cervical ganglion (external carotid nr.)	secretion	postganglionic fibers from pterygopalatine ganglion via zygomatico-temporal nerve
salivary glands	thick, viscous secretion	external carotid nerve	abundant, watery secretion	postganglionic fibers from submandibular ganglion and from otic ganglion
heart	increase of rate and strength of heartbeats, dilation of coronary vessels (indirectly), reduction of conduction time	cervical cardiac and thoracic cardiac nerves	contraction of coronary vessels (indirectly), increase of conduction time	postganglionic fibers from terminal/intramural ganglia via vagus nerve
lungs	bronchodilation, inhibition of secretion	pulmonary nerves	bronchial constriction, stimulation of secretion	postganglionic fibers from terminal/intramural ganglia via vagus nerve
digestive tract	peristaltic inhibition, vasoconstriction	greater, lesser, least splanchnic nerves and branches from celiac, superior mesenteric, and inferior mesenteric ganglia	stimulation of peristalsis and secretion	postganglionic fibers from terminal/intramural ganglia via vagus and pelvic nerves
liver and gallbladder	release of glucose	branches from celiac ganglion	excretion of bile	postganglionic fibers from terminal/intramural ganglia via vagus nerve
adrenal medulla	secretion of epinephrine	lesser splanchnic nerve	no connection	no nerves
kidney	vasoconstriction, inhibition of urine formation	branches from cortico-renal ganglion	no effect	no nerves
bladder	retention of urine	branches from inferior mesenteric ganglion (via hypogastric plexus)	release of urine	postganglionic fibers from terminal/intramural ganglia via pelvic nerves
genitalia	ejaculation	branches from inferior mesenteric ganglion (via hypogastric plexus)	penile and clitoral erections	postganglionic fibers from terminal/intramural ganglia via pelvic nerves
sweat glands	secretion	postganglionic fibers from sympathetic chain ganglia	no connection	no nerves
peripheral blood vessels	constriction of smooth muscle	postganglionic fibers from sympathetic chain ganglia	no connection, apart from dilation in the genital area	no nerves
skeletal muscle	constriction of smooth muscles in blood vessels	postganglionic fibers from sympathetic chain ganglia	dilation	no nerves

autonomic nervous system

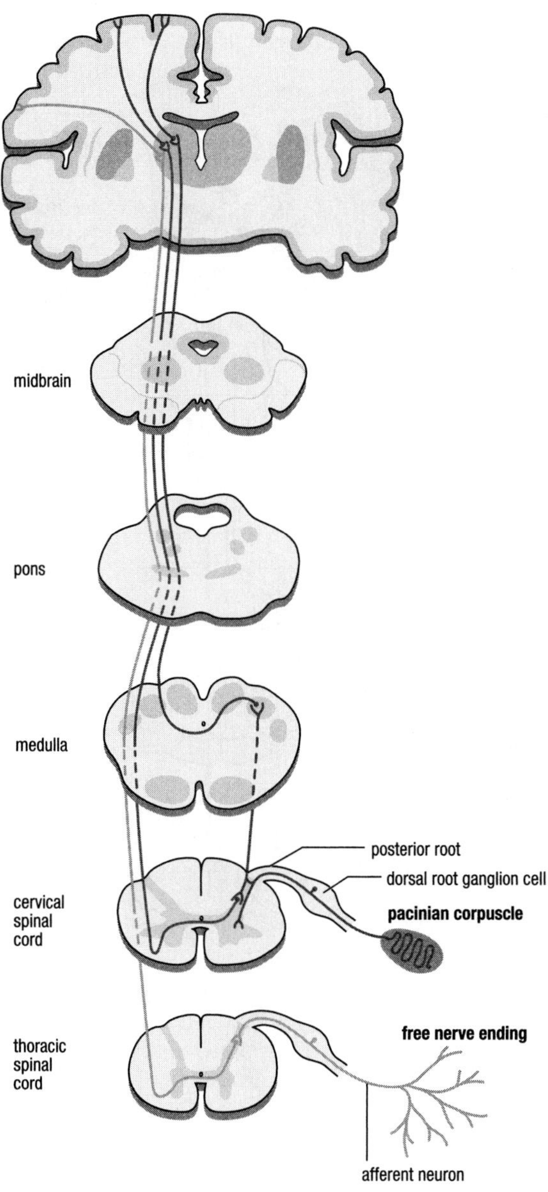

afferent sensory tracts

posterior limb of
internal capsule

motor cortex of cerebellum
(motor area)

corticospinal fibers

red nucleus (subcortical
relay center)

medulla

corticospinal fibers

lateral corticospinal tract

anterior corticospinal
tract

descending subcortical
motor pathway,
rubrospinal tract

lower motor neuron

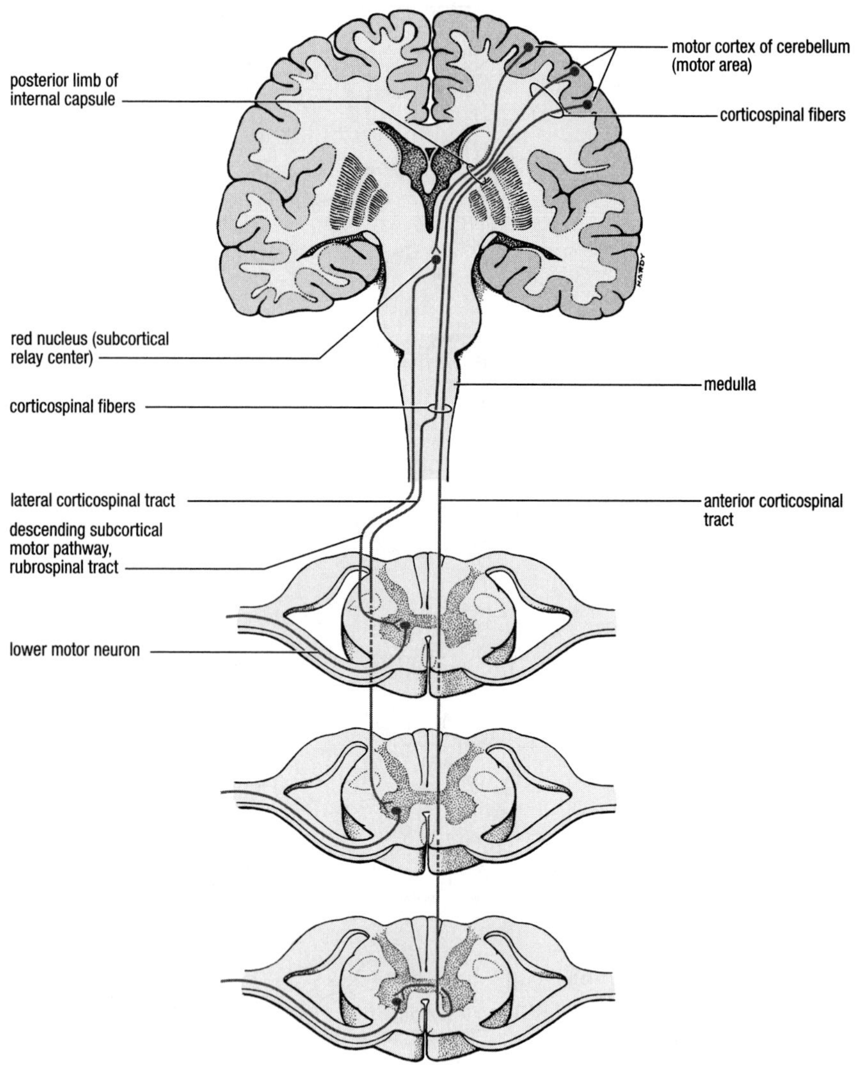

corticospinal tract

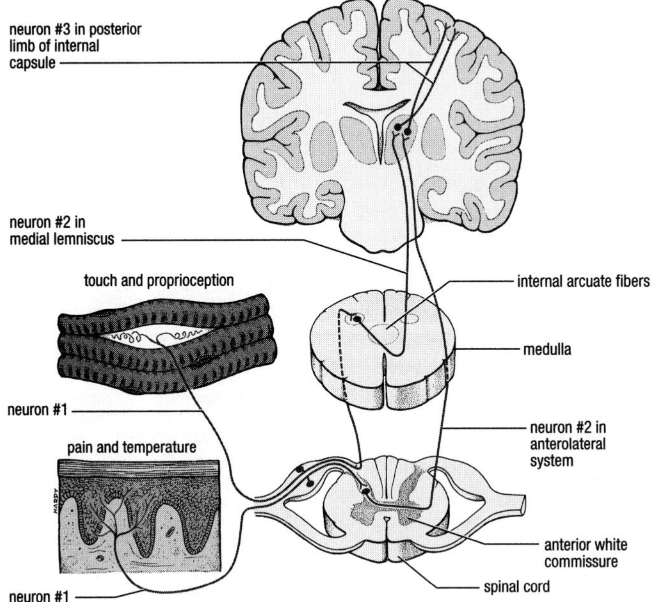

decussation of nerve fibers

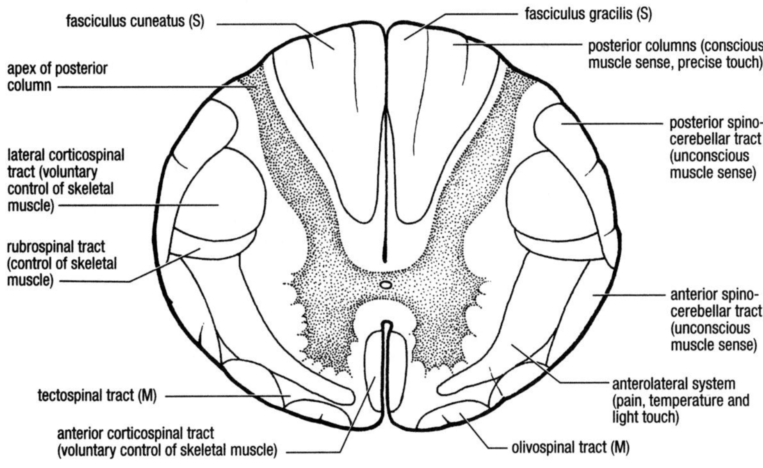

principal fiber tracts of the spinal cord: sensory (S), motor (M)

sensation			
modality of sensation	**object of perception**	**nature of stimuli**	**receptor type**
sense of sight	brightness, darkness, colors	electromagnetic radiation 4000–7000 Å	photo-receptors
sense of temperature	cold, heat	electromagnetic radiation 7000–9000 Å, convective heat transport	thermo-receptors
tactile sense of skin	pressure, touch		
sense of hearing	sound frequencies		
statokinetic sense	absolute body position, speed of body, relative body position and movement of body parts and joints, sense of strength	modification of mechano-receptors by solid objects or transmission of air-pressure changes	mechano-receptors
sense of smell	odors	chemical substances	
sense of taste	sour, salty, sweet, bitter	ions	chemo-receptors
sense of pain	pain	mechanical tissue injury	nociceptors

sensation

Anatomical Illustrations

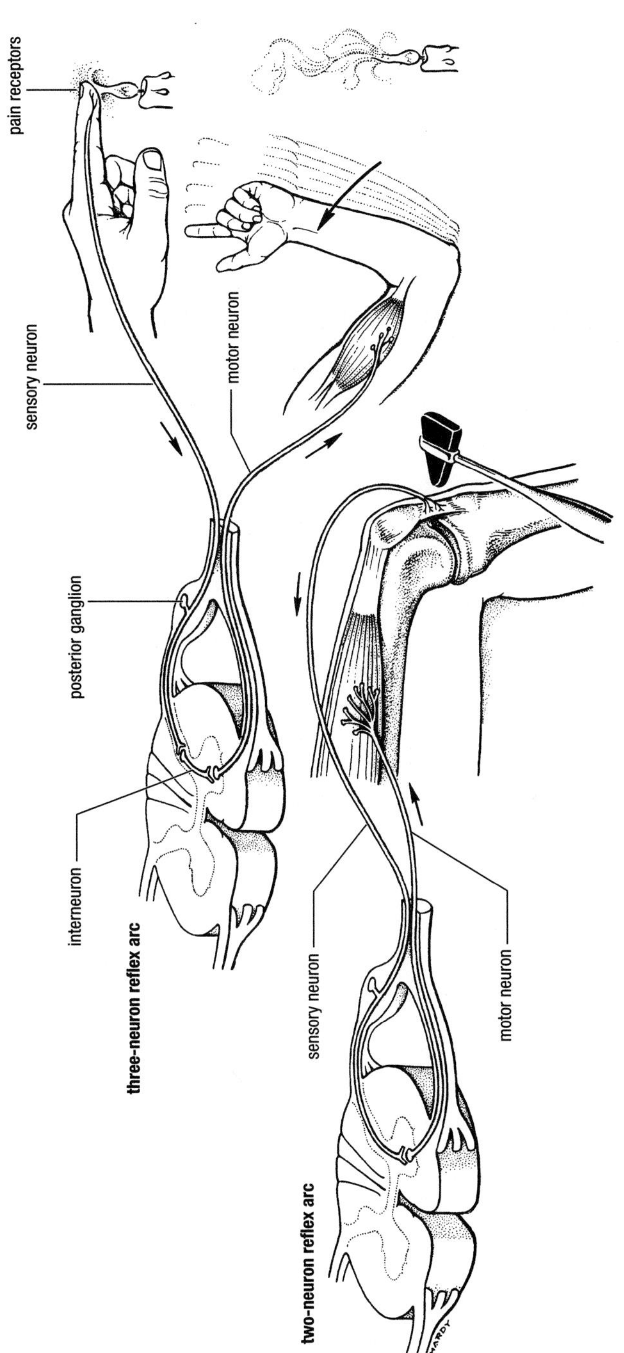

reflex arcs: flexor reflex (top) and stretch reflex (bottom)

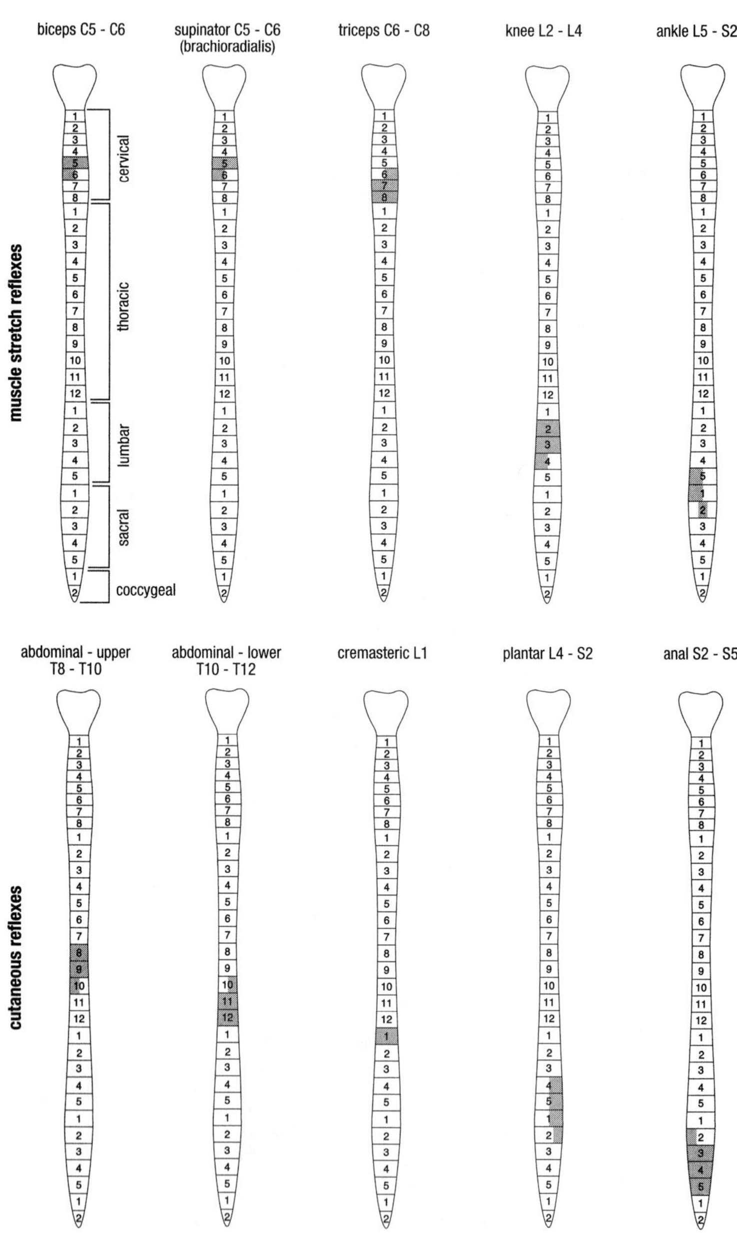

spinal nerves responsible for muscle stretch reflexes and cutaneous reflexes

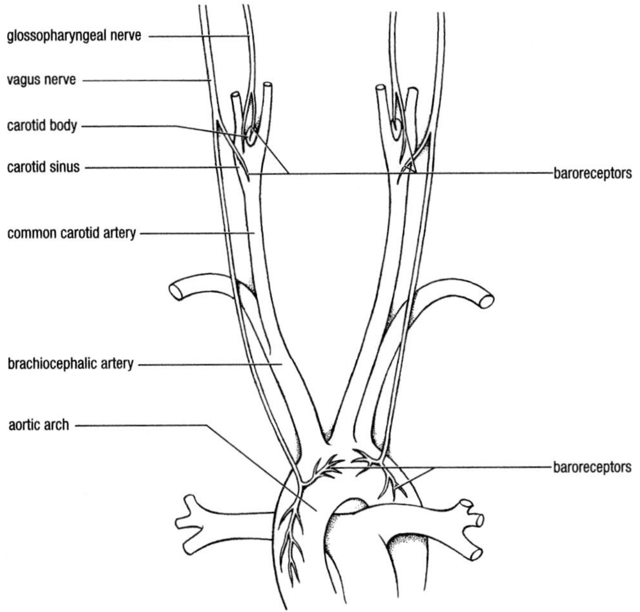

baroreceptors

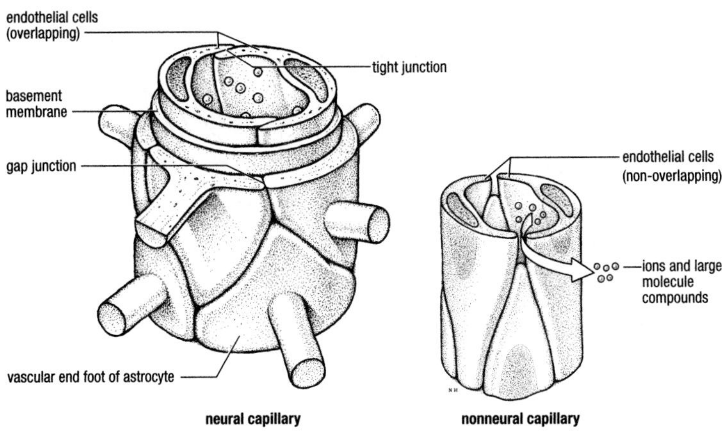

blood-brain barrier

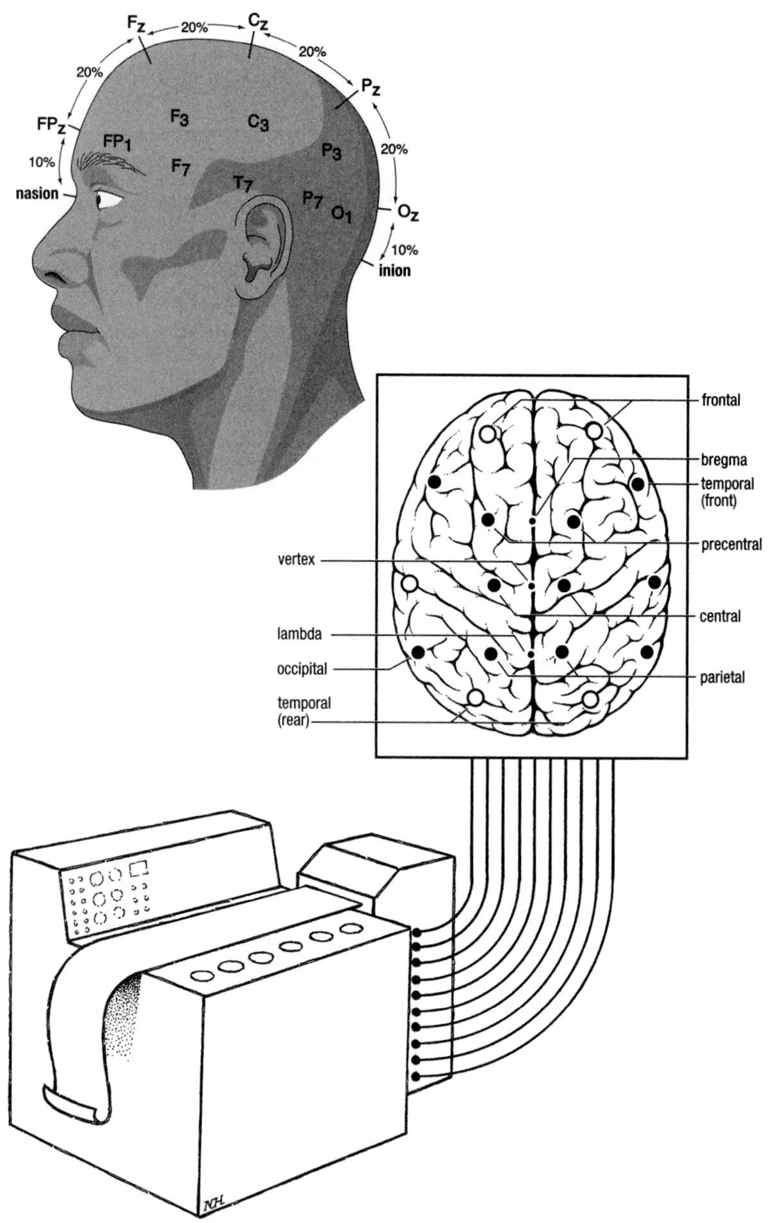

electroencephalogram (EEG) and lateral view of the head showing proper EEG electrode placement

electroencephalogram						
				physiologic variations of potential		
type of wave	shape	frequency per sec.	amplitude in V	in waking EEG		in sleeping EEG
				adult	child	all ages
beta	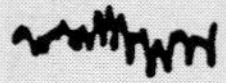	14 – 30	5 – 50	frontal and precentral prominent, in clusters	seldom prominent	beta-activity ("spindles") sign of light sleep
alpha	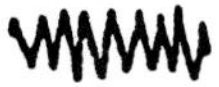	8 – 13	20 – 120	predominant activity	predominant activity, age 5 and above	not a sign of sleep
theta	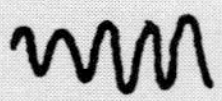	4 – 7	20 – 100	constant, not prominent	predominant activity, from 18 mos. to 5 yrs.	normal sign of sleep
delta	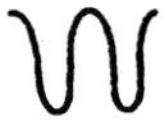	0.5 – 3	5 – 250	not prominent	predominant activity until 18 mos.	concomitant sign of deep sleep
gamma	—	31 – 60	– 10	laws governing predominance and localization not fully known		

electroencephalogram

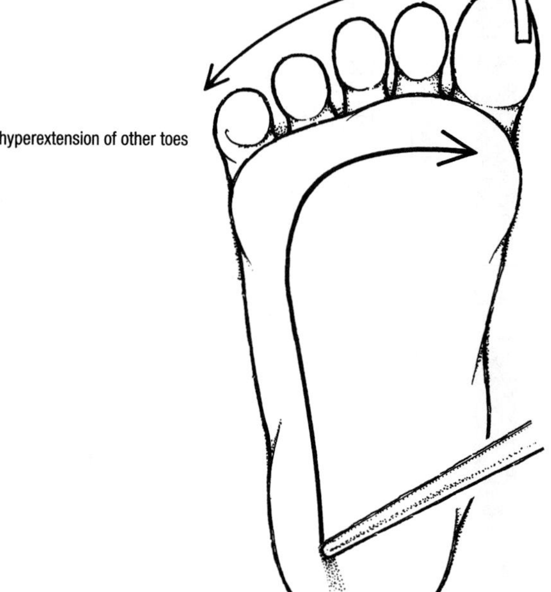

Babinski sign

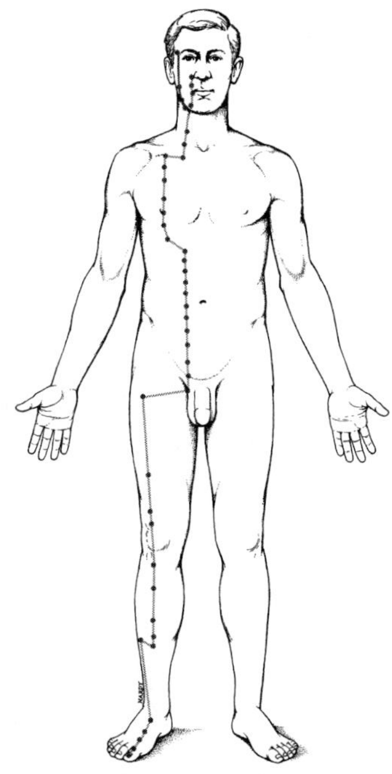

acupuncture meridians

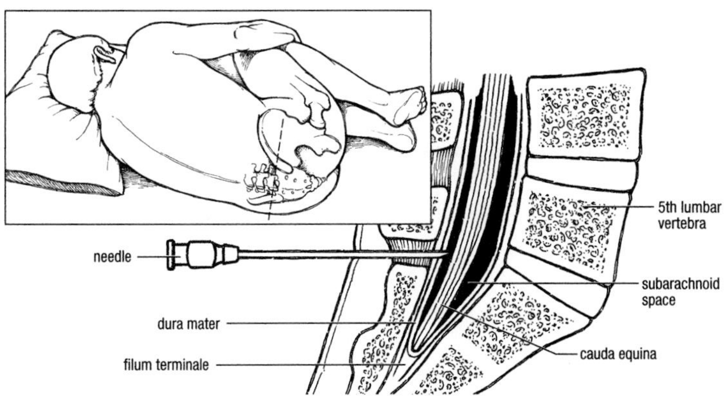

lumbar puncture

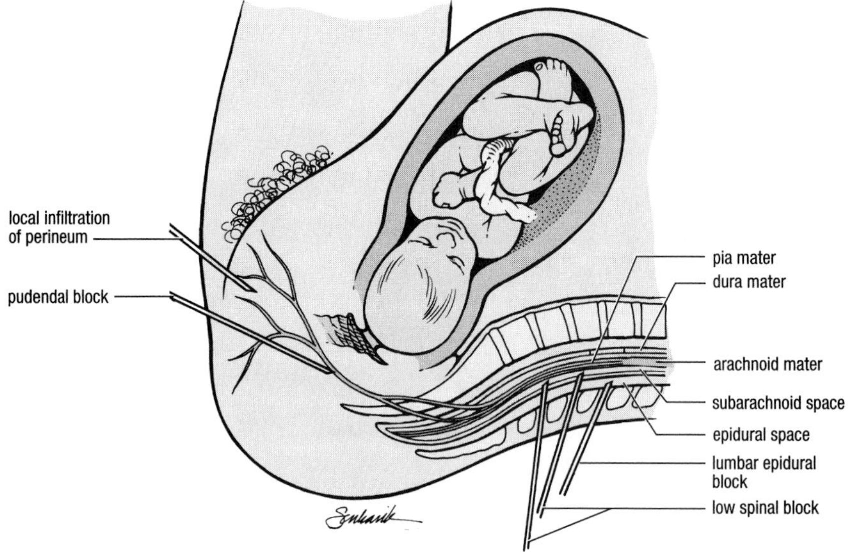

regional anesthesia for childbirth (sites of injection)

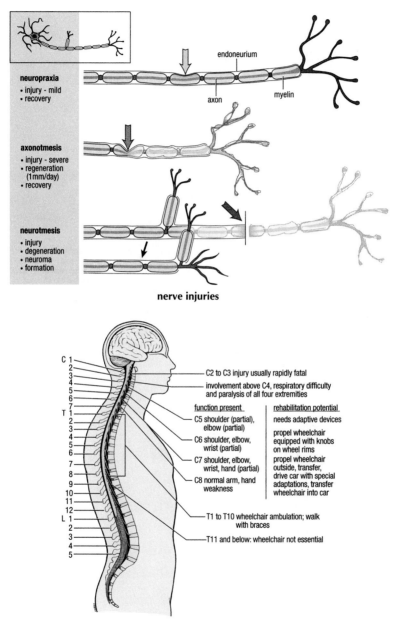

Anatomical Illustrations

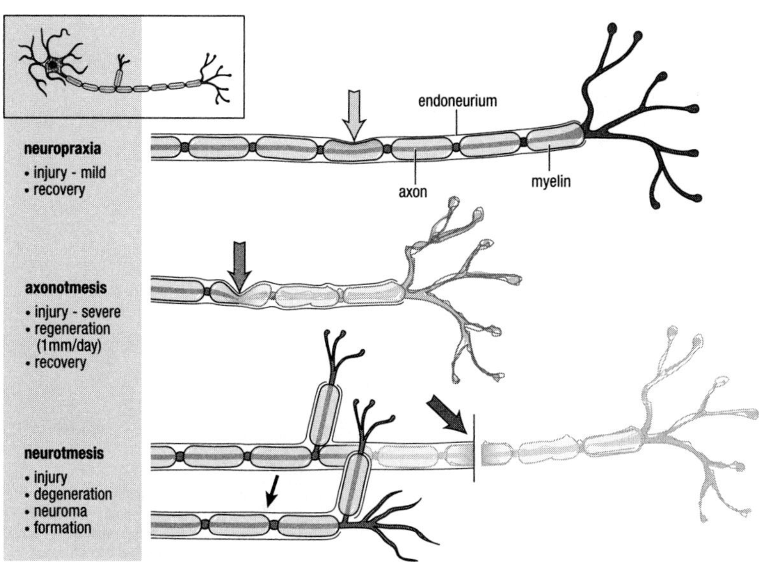

nerve injuries

C 1, 2, 3, 4, 5, 6, 7
T 1, 2, 3, 4, 5, 6, 7, 8, 9, 10, 11, 12
L 1, 2, 3, 4, 5

C2 to C3 injury usually rapidly fatal

involvement above C4, respiratory difficulty and paralysis of all four extremities

function present	rehabilitation potential
C5 shoulder (partial), elbow (partial)	needs adaptive devices
C6 shoulder, elbow, wrist (partial)	propel wheelchair equipped with knobs on wheel rims
C7 shoulder, elbow, wrist, hand (partial)	propel wheelchair outside, transfer,
C8 normal arm, hand weakness	drive car with special adaptations, transfer wheelchair into car

T1 to T10 wheelchair ambulation; walk with braces

T11 and below: wheelchair not essential

spinal cord injuries

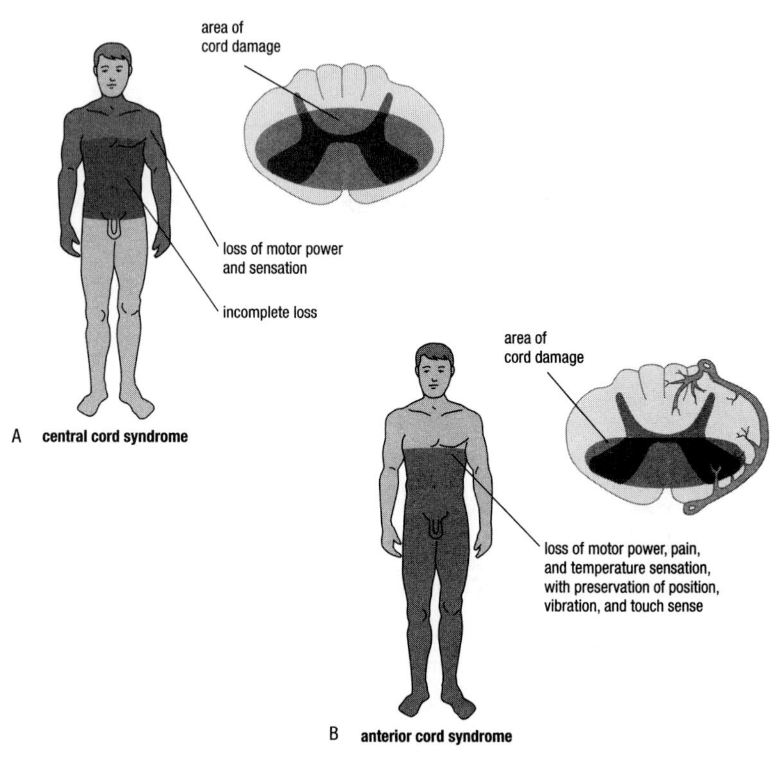

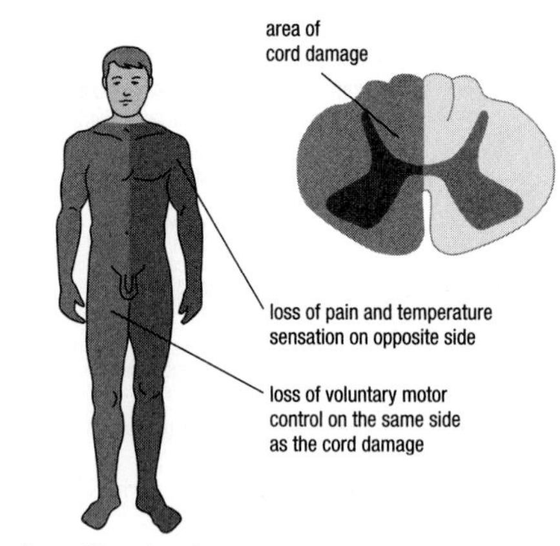

spinal cord injuries: (A) central cord syndrome; (B) anterior cord syndrome; (C) Brown-Séquard syndrome

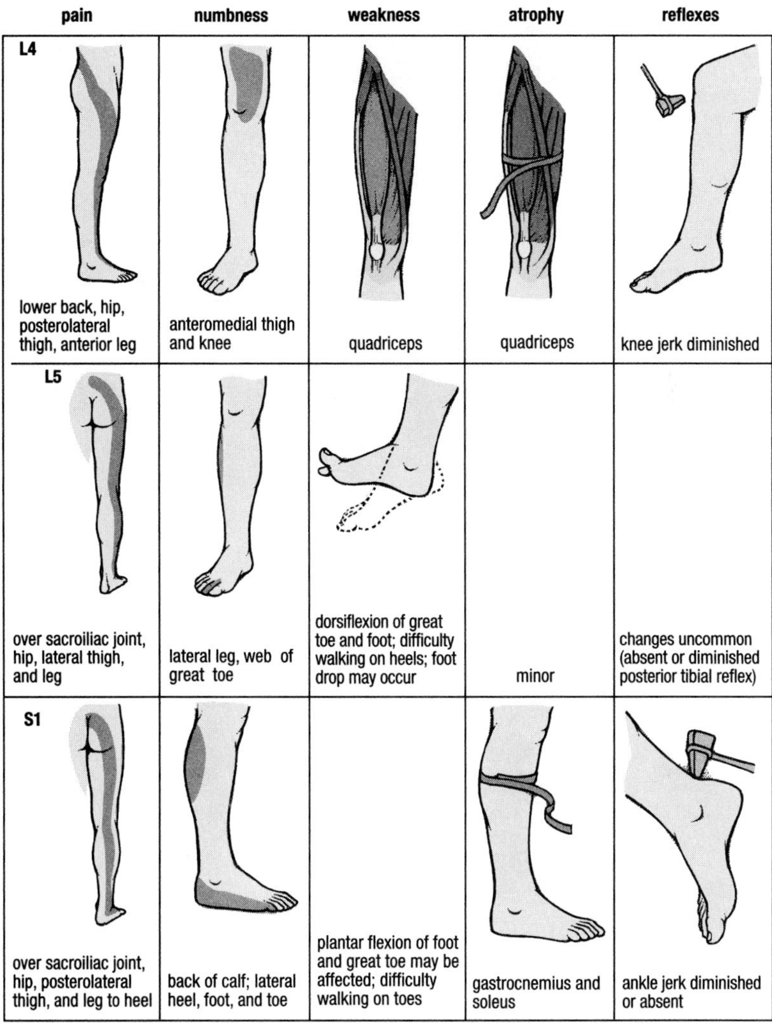

	pain	numbness	weakness	atrophy	reflexes
L4	lower back, hip, posterolateral thigh, anterior leg	anteromedial thigh and knee	quadriceps	quadriceps	knee jerk diminished
L5	over sacroiliac joint, hip, lateral thigh, and leg	lateral leg, web of great toe	dorsiflexion of great toe and foot; difficulty walking on heels; foot drop may occur	minor	changes uncommon (absent or diminished posterior tibial reflex)
S1	over sacroiliac joint, hip, posterolateral thigh, and leg to heel	back of calf; lateral heel, foot, and toe	plantar flexion of foot and great toe may be affected; difficulty walking on toes	gastrocnemius and soleus	ankle jerk diminished or absent

intervertebral disk herniation (nerves compressed: L4, L5, and S1)

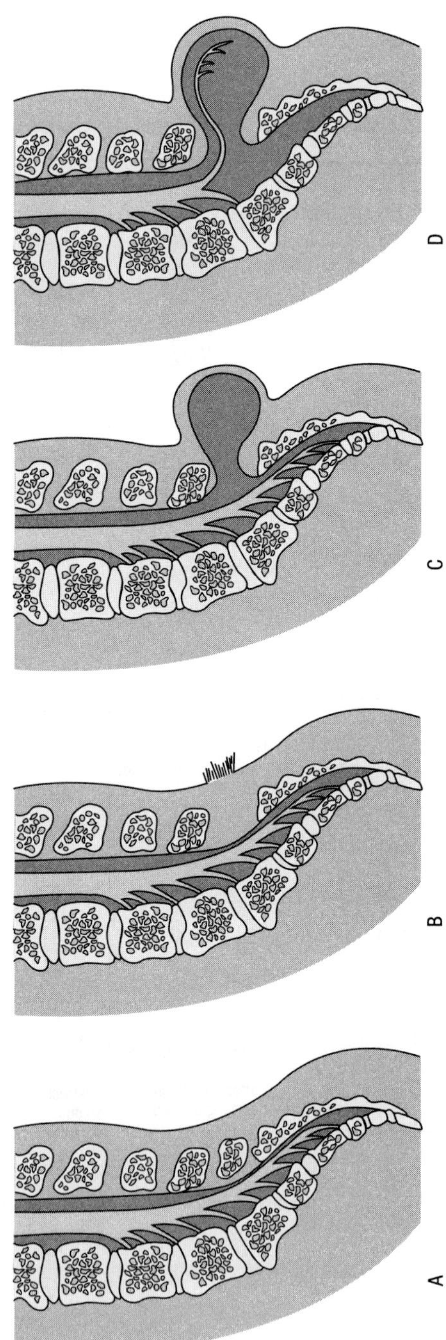

four degrees of spinal cord anomalies: (A) normal spinal cord; (B) spina bifida occulta; (C) meningocele; (D) myelomeningocele

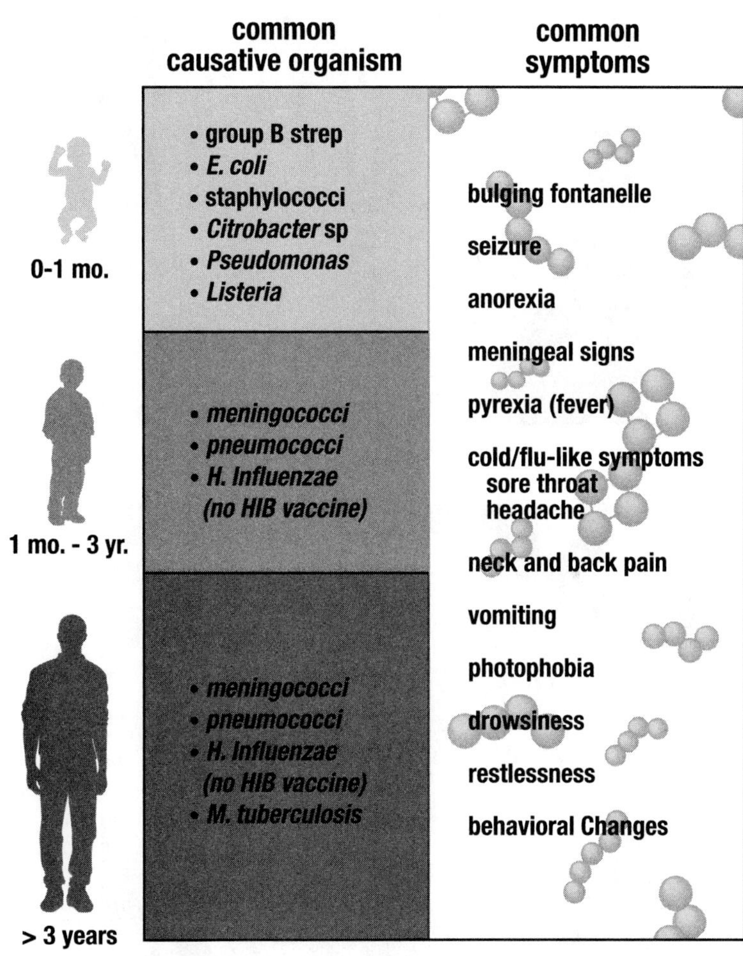

causative organisms and symptoms of bacterial meningitis, arranged according to patient's age

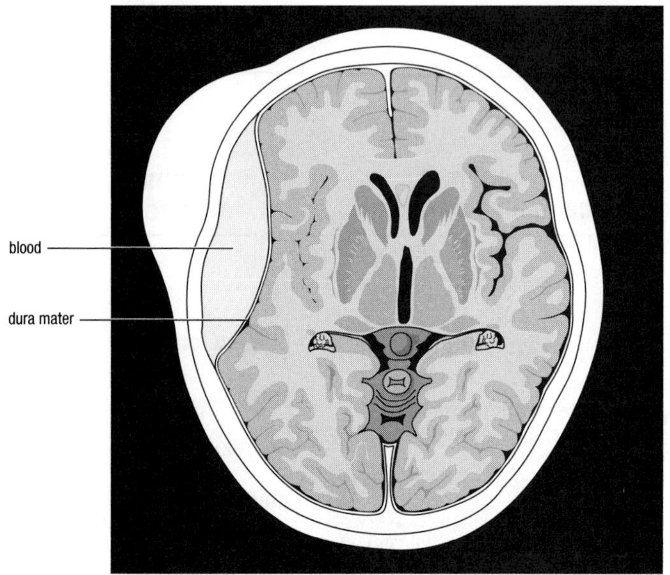

epidural hematoma

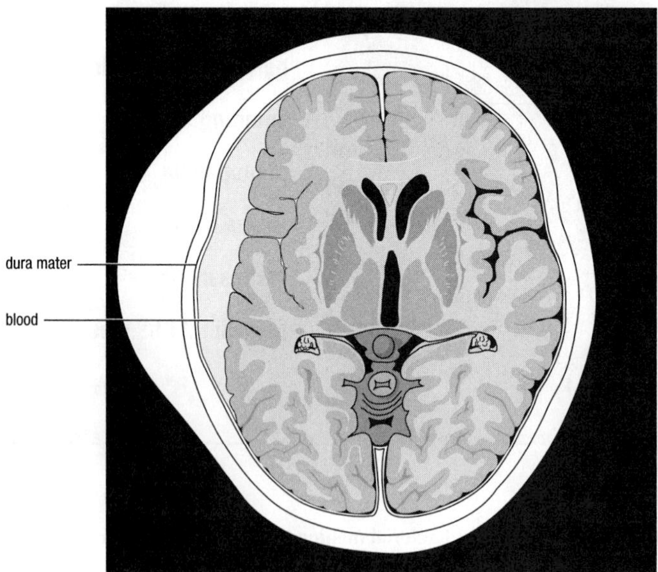

subdural hematoma

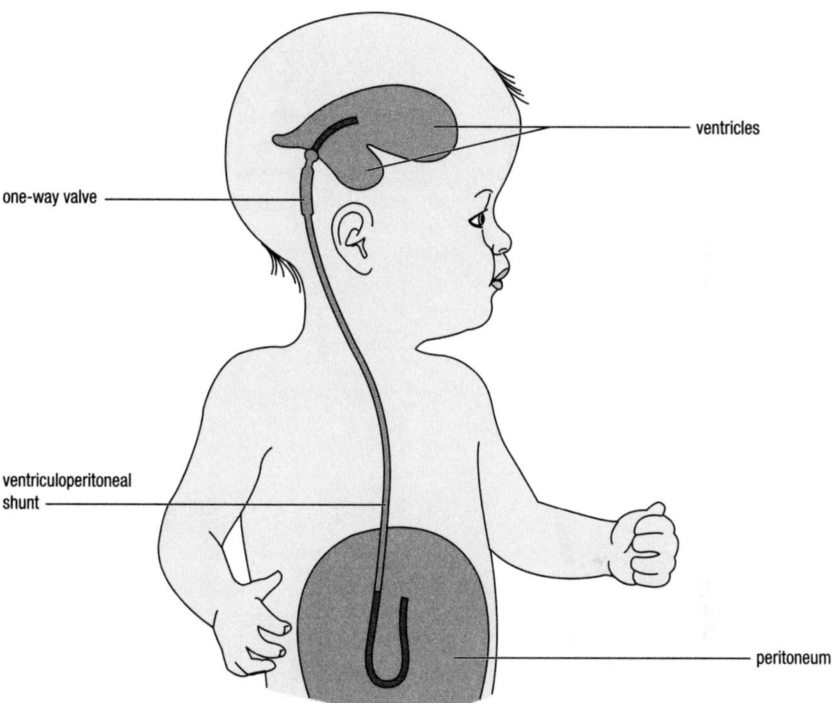

infant with ventriculoperitoneal shunt: excess cerebrospinal fluid is drained from the ventricles to the peritoneum with a one-way valve, located behind the ear, to prevent backflow

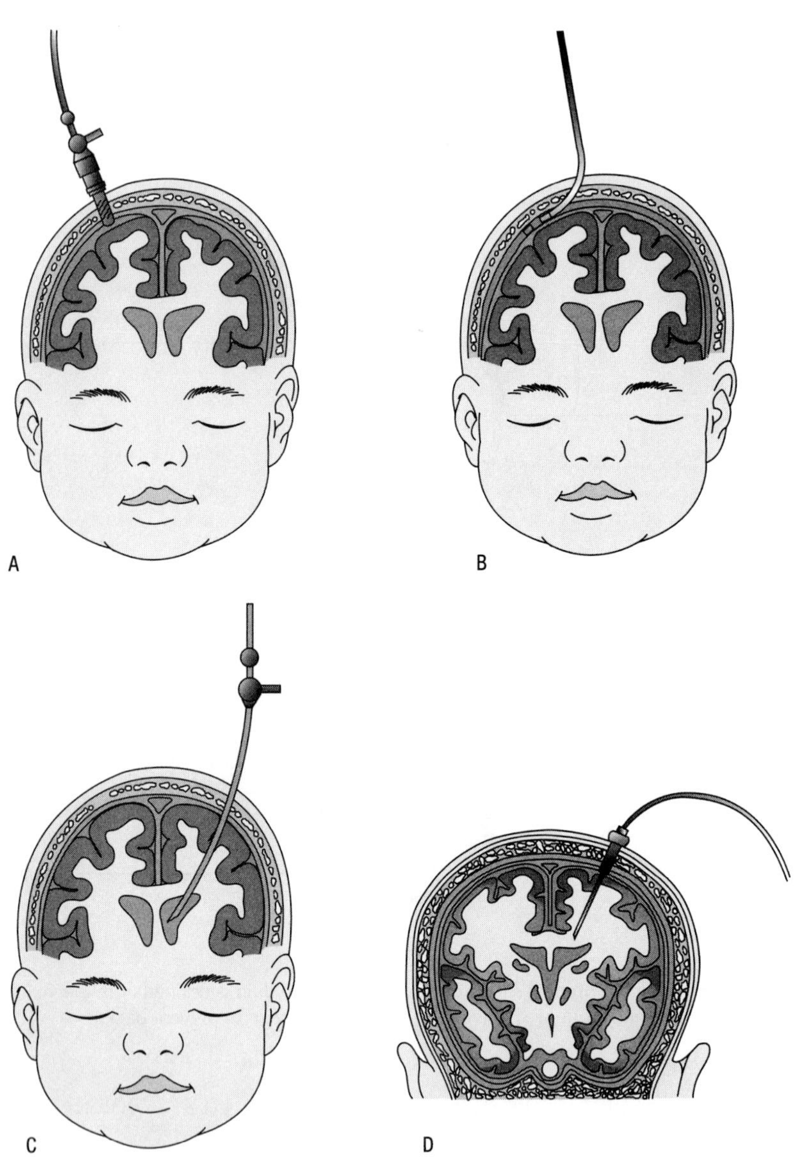

placement of intracranial pressure monitor: (A) a subarachnoid screw passes through a bur hole in the skull ending in the epidural space; (B) a fiberoptic sensor is implanted into the epidural space; (C) an intraventricular catheter is inserted through the anterior fontanelle and threaded into the lateral ventricle; (D) a fiberoptic transducer-tipped catheter is inserted through a subarachnoid bolt into the white matter of the brain

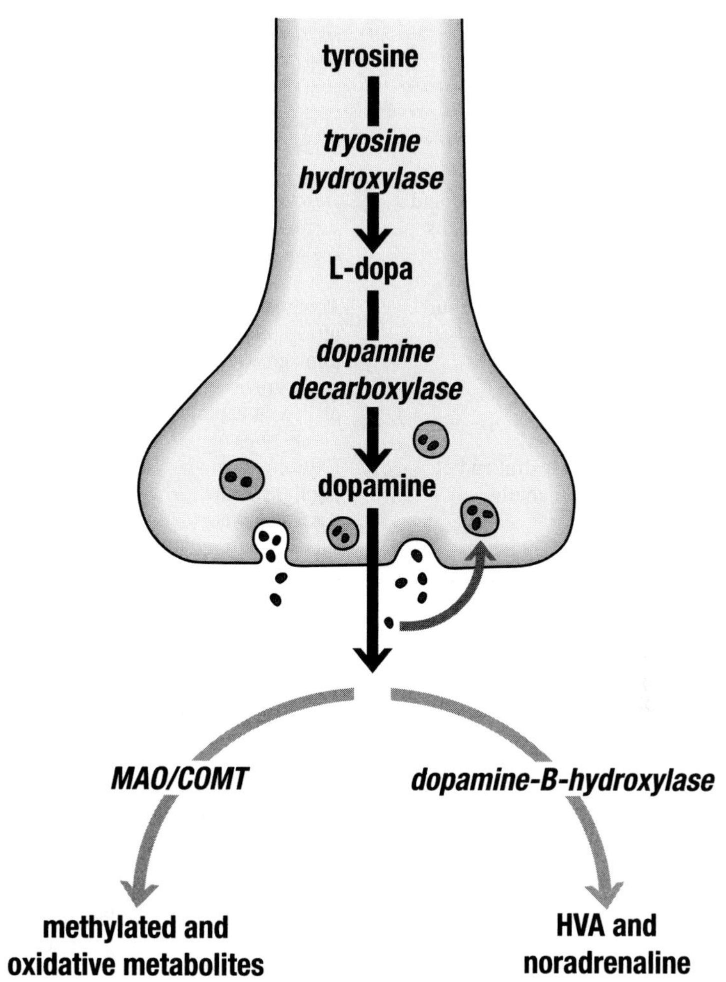

process of dopamine metabolism at terminal end of axon

Appendix 2

Table of Nerves

1. Nerves of the Head and Neck Region

Nerve	Origin	Course	Innervation
Abducent	Pons	Intradural on clivus; traverses cavernous sinus and superior orbital fissure to enter orbit	Lateral rectus
Ansa cervicalis	Hypoglossal and cervical plexus	Descends on external surface of carotid sheath	Omohyoid, sternohyoid, and sternothyroid
Deep petrosal	Internal carotid plexus	Traverses cartilage of foramen lacerum, joins greater petrosal nerve at entrance of pterygoid canal	Lacrimal gland, mucosa of nasal cavity, palate, and upper pharynx
Glossopharyngeal	Rostral end of medulla	Exits cranium via jugular foramen, passes between superior and middle constrictors of pharynx to tonsillar fossa, enters posterior third of tongue	Somatic to stylopharyngeus; visceral to parotid gland; posterior two thirds of tongue, pharynx, tympanic cavity, auditory tube,carotid body, and sinus
Great auricular	Cervical plexus	Ascends over sternocleidomastoid; anterior and parallel to external jugular	Skin of auricle, adjacent scalp over angle of jaw; parotid sheath
Greater petrosal	Genu of facial nerve	Exits facial canal via hiatus for greater petrosal nerve	Pterygoid ganglion for innervation of lacrimal, nasal, palatine, and upper pharyngeal mucous glands
Hypoglossal	Between pyramid and olive of myelencephalon	Hypoglossal canal, medial to angle of mandible, between mylohyoid and hypoglossus to muscles of tongue	Intrinsic and extrinsic muscles of tongue

(continued)

Nerve	Origin	Course	Innervation
Intermediate	Facial nerve	Internal acoustic meatus, merging with larger facial nerve	Pterygopalatine and submandibular ganglia via greater petrosal nerve, chorda tympani; tongue and palate
Lesser occipital	Cervical plexus	Parallel to anterosuperior border of sternocleidomastoid	Skin of posterior surface of auricle and adjacent scalp
Lesser petrosal	Tympanic plexus	Tympanic cavity into middle cranial fossa; descends through sphenopetrosal fissure or foramen ovale	Otic ganglion for secretomotor innervation of parotid gland
Long thoracic	Anterior rami	Distally on external surface of serratus anterior	Serratus anterior
Nerve to mylohyoid	Inferior alveolar nerve	Inferior alveolar nerve outside mandibular foramen to groove on medial aspect of ramus of mandible	Mylohyoid and anterior belly of digastric muscle
Nerve to tensor tympani	Otic ganglion	Cartilaginous portion of pharyngotympanic tube to hemicranial of tensor tympani	Tensor tympani
Nerve to tensor veli palatini	Anterior trunk mandibular nerve	Branch of nerve to medial pterygoid	Tensor veli palatini
Olfactory	Olfactory cells in olfactory epithelium of roof of nasal cavity	Foramen of cribriform plate of ethmoid to olfactory bulbs	Olfactory mucosa

(continued)

Nerve	Origin	Course	Innervation
Phrenic	Cervical plexus	Superior thoracic aperture between mediastinal pleura and pericardium	Diaphragm; pericardial sac, mediastinal and diaphragmatic pleura, diaphragmatic peritoneum
Posterior inferior nasal	Greater palatine	Greater palatine canal through plate of palatine bone	Mucosa of inferior concha and walls of inferior and middle meatuses
Subclavian	Brachial plexus	Posterior to clavicle, anterior to brachial plexus and subclavian artery	Subclavius; sternoclavicular joint
Supraclavicular	Cervical plexus	Center or posterior border of sternocleidomastoid; fan out as they descend onto lower neck, upper thorax, and shoulder	Skin of lower anterolateral neck, uppermost thorax, and shoulder
Supraorbital	Frontal nerve	Supraorbital foramen, breaks up into small branches	Mucous membrane of frontal sinus, conjunctivae, and skin of forehead
Suprascapular	Brachial plexus	Posterior triangle of neck; under superior transverse scapular ligament	Supraspinatus, infraspinatus muscles; superior and posterior glenohumeral joint
Supratrochlear	Frontal nerve	Supraorbital nerve, divides into two or more branches	Skin in middle of forehead to hairline
Transverse cervical	Cervical plexus	Posterior border of sternocleidomastoid muscle; runs anteriorly across muscle	Skin overlying anterior triangle of neck

(continued)

Nerve	Origin	Course	Innervation
Trochlear	Dorsolateral aspect of mesocephalon below inferior colliculus	Passes around brainstem to enter dura in edge of tentorium close to posterior clinoid process; runs in lateral wall of cavernous sinus, entering orbit via superior orbital fissures	Superior oblique muscle
Upper subscapular	Brachial plexus	Posteriorly enters subscapularis	Superior portion of subscapularis

2. Nerves of the Facial Region

Nerve	Origin	Course	Innervation
Auriculotemporal	Mandibular nerve	Passes between neck of mandible and external acoustic meatus to accompany superficial temporal artery	Skin anterior to auricle, posterior temporal region, tragus, helix of auricle, exterior acoustic meatus, upper tympanic membrane
Buccal	Mandibular nerve	Infratemporal fossa, passes anteriorly to reach cheek	Skin and mucosa of cheek, buccal gingiva
Chorda tympani	Facial nerve	Traverses tympanic cavity, passes between incus and malleus; exits temporal bone via petrotympanic fissure; enters infratemporal fossa, merges with lingual nerve	Submandibular and sublingual glands; taste sensation from anterior two thirds of tongue
Deep temporal	Mandibular nerve	Temporal fossa deep to temporalis muscle	Temporalis; periosteum of temporal fossa

(continued)

Nerves

Nerve	Origin	Course	Innervation
External nasal	Anterior ethmoidal nerve	Runs in nasal cavity and emerges on face between nasal bone and lateral nasal cartilage	Skin on dorsum of nose, including tip of nose
Facial	Posterior border of pons	Runs through internal acoustic meatus and facial canal of petrous part of temporal bone, exiting via stylomastoid foramen; forms intraparotid plexus	Stapedius, posterior belly of digastric, stylohyoid, facial and scalp muscles; skin of external acoustic meatus
Greater palatine	Branch of pterygopalatine ganglion (maxillary nerve)	Passes inferiorly through greater palatine canal and foramen	Palatine glands; mucosa of hard palate
Inferior alveolar	Terminal branch of posterior mandibular nerve	Lateral and medial pterygoid muscles of infratemporal fossa to enter mandibular canal of mandible	Lower teeth, periodontium, periosteum, and gingiva of lower jaw
Infraorbital	Terminal branch of maxillary nerve	Runs in floor of orbit and emerges at infraorbital foramen	Skin of cheek, lower lid, lateral side of nose and inferior septum and upper lip, upper premolar incisors and canine teeth; mucosa of maxillary sinus and upper lip
Lesser palatine	Pterygopalatine ganglion	Passes inferiorly through palatine canal and lesser palatine foramen	Glands of soft palate; mucosa of soft palate
Lingual	Terminal branch of posterior mandibular nerve	Joins chorda tympani, passes anteroinferiorly between lateral and medial pterygoid muscles, enters oral cavity	Submandibular ganglion for submandibular and sublingual salivary glands; anterior two thirds of tongue, floor of mouth, lingual mandibular gingiva

(continued)

Nerve	Origin	Course	Innervation
Mandibular	Trigeminal ganglion	Foramen ovale into infratemporal fossa, divides into anterior and posterior trunks, ramifying into smaller branches, bifurcating into lingual and inferior alveolar nerve	Muscles of mastication, mylohyoid, anterior belly of digastric, tensor tympani, tensor veli palatini; skin overlying mandible, lower half of mouth, and temporomandibular joint
Masseteric	Mandibular nerve	Passes laterally through mandibular notch	Masseter; temporomandibular joint
Maxillary	Trigeminal nerve	Anteriorly through foramen rotundum, into pterygopalatine fossa, sensory roots to pterygopalatine ganglion; continues anteriorly through infraorbital fissures as infraorbital nerve	Pterygopalatine ganglion, lacrimal gland, mucosal glands of nasal cavity, palate and upper pharynx; skin overlying maxilla, mucosa of posteroinferior nasal cavity and maxillary sinus; upper half of mouth
Mental	Terminal branch of inferior alveolar nerve	Mandibular canal at mental foramen	Skin of chin; skin and mucosa of lower lip
Nasopalatine	Pterygopalatine ganglion	Exits pterygopalatine fossa via sphenopalatine foramen; runs anteroinferiorly across nasal septum, through incisive foramen to palate	Mucosal glands of nasal septum; mucosa of nasal septum, anterior-most hard palate
Nerve to lateral/ medial pterygoid	Anterior mandibular nerve	Arises in infratemporal fossa, inferior to foramen ovale	Lateral and medial pterygoid muscles

(continued)

Nerves

Nerve	Origin	Course	Innervation
Nerve to pterygoid canal	Formed by merger of greater and deep petrosal nerves	Traverses pterygoid canal, to pterygopalatine ganglion in pterygopalatine fossa	Pterygopalatine ganglion
Nerve to stapedius	Facial nerve	Arises as facial nerve descends posterior to muscle in facial canal	Stapedius
Pharyngeal	Pterygopalatine ganglion	Passes posteriorly through palatovaginal canal	Supplies mucosa of nasopharynx posterior to the pharyngotympanic tubes
Superior alveolar	Maxillary nerve	Emerges from pterygomaxillary fissure into infratemporal fossa to posterior aspect of maxilla; arises from infraorbital nerve of maxillary sinus, descends walls of sinus	Mucosa of maxillary sinus, maxillary teeth and gingiva
Trigeminal	Lateral surface of pons by two roots; motor and sensory	Crosses medial part of crest of petrous part of temporal bone, trigeminal cave of dura mater lateral to body of sphenoid and cavernous sinus; motor root passes ganglion to become part of mandibular nerve	Muscles of mastication, mylohyoid, anterior belly of digastric, tensor tympani, tensor veli palatini; dura of anterior and middle cranial fossa, skin of face, teeth, gingiva, mucosa of nasal cavity, paranasal sinuses and mouth

(continued)

Nerve	Origin	Course	Innervation
Zygomatic	Maxillary nerve	Arises in floor of orbit, divides into zygomaticofacial and zygomaticotemporal nerves, traverses foramina of same; communicating branch joins lacrimal nerve	Skin over zygomatic arch, anterior temporal region; conveys secretory postsynaptic parasympathetic fibers from pterygopalatine ganglion to lacrimal gland

3. Nerves of the Eye Region

Nerve	Origin	Course	Innervation
Anterior ethmoidal	Nasociliary nerve	Arises in orbit, passes via anterior ethmoidal foramen to cranial cavity then cribriform plate of ethmoid to nasal cavity	Dura of anterior cranial fossa; mucous membranes of sphenoidal sinus, ethmoid cells and upper nasal cavity
Ciliary	Nasociliary nerve; ciliary ganglion	Passes to posterior aspect of eyeball	Cornea, conjunctiva; ciliary body and iris
Frontal	Ophthalmic nerve	Crosses orbit on superior aspect of levator palpebrae superioris; divides into supraorbital and supratrochlear branches	Skin of forehead, scalp, upper eyelid, and nose; conjunctiva of upper lid and mucosa of frontal sinus
Infratrochlear	Nasociliary nerve	Follows medial wall of orbit to upper eyelid	Skin, conjunctiva of upper eyelid
Lacrimal	Ophthalmic nerve	Palpebral fascia of upper eyelid near lateral angle of eye	Small area of skin and conjunctiva of lateral part of upper eyelid

(continued)

Nerves

Nerve	Origin	Course	Innervation
Nasociliary	Ophthalmic nerve	Arises in superior orbital fissure, anteromedially across retrobulbar orbit, providing sensory root to ciliary ganglion, terminates as infratrochlear nerve and nasal branches	Branches of ciliary ganglion convey postsynaptic sympathetic and parasympathetic to ciliary body and iris; tactile sensation from eyeball; mucous membrane of ethmoid cells, anterosuperior nasal cavity; skin of root dorsum and apex of nose
Oculomotor	Interpeduncular fossa of mesencephalon	Dura lateral to posterior clinoid process, lateral wall of cavernous sinus, enters orbit through superior orbital fissure and divides into superior and inferior branches	All extraocular muscles except superior oblique and lateral rectus; presynaptic parasympathetic fibers to ciliary ganglion for ciliary body and sphincter pupillae
Ophthalmic	Trigeminal ganglion	Anteriorly in lateral wall of cavernous sinus to enter orbit through superior orbital fissure, branching into frontal, nasociliary, and lacrimal nerve	General sensation from eyeball; mucous membrane of ethmoid cells, frontal sinus, dura of anterior cranial fossa, falx cerebri, and tentorium cerebelli, anterosuperior nasal cavity; skin of forehead, upper lid root, dorsum and apex of nose

(continued)

Nerve	Origin	Course	Innervation
Optic	Ganglion cells of retina	Exits orbit via optic canals; fibers from nasal half of retina, crosses to contralateral side at chiasm; passes via optic tracts to geniculate bodies, superior colliculus, and pretectum	Vision from retina
Posterior ethmoidal	Nasociliary	Leaves orbit via posterior ethmoidal foramen	Supplies ethmoidal and sphenoidal paranasal sinuses

4. Nerves of the Ear Region

Nerve	Origin	Course	Innervation
Cochlear	Division of vestibulocochlear nerve	Traverses internal acoustic meatus, enters modiolus with spiral ganglia and peripheral processes in spiral lamina	Spiral organ
Posterior auricular	As first extracranial branch of facial nerve	Passes posterior to ear, sending branch to occipital region	Posterior auricular muscle and intrinsic auricular muscles, occipital belly of occipitofrontalis
Tympanic	As first extracranial branch of glossopharyngeal nerve, from inferior glossopharyngeal ganglion	Passes into tympanic canaliculus, enters tympanic cavity, ramifies on promontory of labyrinthine wall as tympanic plexus	Otic ganglion for secretomotor innervation of parotid gland; mucosa of tympanic cavity, mastoid cells, and pharyngotympanic tube
Vestibular	As a division of the vestibulocochlear nerve	Traverses internal acoustic meatus to vestibular ganglion at fundus; branches pass to vestibule of bony labyrinth	Cristae of ampullae of semicircular ducts, maculae of saccule and utricle

(continued)

Nerve	Origin	Course	Innervation
Vestibulocochlear	Groove between pons and myelencephalon	Traverses internal acoustic meatus, dividing into cochlear and vestibular nerve	Spiral organ and cristae of ampullae of semicircular ducts, maculae of saccule and utricle

5. Nerves of the Thoracic Region

Nerve	Origin	Course	Innervation
Abdominopelvic splanchnic	Lower thoracic and lumbar segments of sympathetic trunk	Passes medially and inferiorly to prevertebral ganglion of paraaortic plexus	Abdominopelvic blood vessels and viscera
Cardiac plexus	Cervical and cardiac branches of vagus nerve and cardiopulmonary splanchnic nerve from sympathetic trunk	From arch of aorta, posterior surface of heart, extends along coronary arteries and to SA node	SA nodal tissue, coronary arteries; parasympathetic fibers slow rate, reduce force of heartbeat, constrict arteries; sympathetic fibers have opposite effect
Cardiopulmonary splanchnic	Cervical and upper thoracic ganglia of sympathetic trunk	Descends anteromedially to cardiac, pulmonary and esophageal plexuses	Conveys postsynaptic sympathetic fibers to nerve plexuses of thoracic viscera
Cervical splanchnic	Cervical ganglia of sympathetic trunk	Pass medially and inferiorly to cardiac and pulmonary plexuses	Conducting tissue and coronary arteries
Esophageal plexus	Vagus nerve; sympathetic ganglia, greater splanchnic nerve	Tracheal bifurcation, Vagus, and sympathetic nerve form plexus around esophagus	Vagal and sympathetic fibers to smooth muscles and glands of inferior two thirds of esophagus
Greater splanchnic	Thoracic sympathetic ganglia	Highest abdominopelvic splanchnic nerve; anteromedially passes on bodies of thoracic vertebrae, through diaphragm to celiac trunk	Celiac ganglia, innervation of celiac arteries

(continued)

Nerve	Origin	Course	Innervation
Intercostal	Anterior rami of T1-T11 nerves	Intercostal spaces between internal and innermost layers of intercostal muscles	Intercostal muscles; muscles of anterolateral abdominal wall; skin overlying pleura/peritoneum deep to muscles
Lateral pectoral	Brachial plexus	Clavipectoral fascia to deep surface of pectoral muscles	Pectoralis major, medial pectoral nerve that innervates pectoralis minor
Least splanchnic	12th thoracic ganglion of sympathetic trunk	Diaphragm with sympathetic trunk, ends in renal plexus	Renal arteries and derivatives
Lesser splanchnic	10th and 11th thoracic ganglia of sympathetic trunk	Descends anteromedially to perforate diaphragm to reach aorticorenal ganglion	Prevertebral ganglia; visceral afferents from upper GI tract
Lumbar splanchnic	Lumbar ganglia of sympathetic trunk	Passes anteromedially on bodies of lumbar vertebrae to prevertebral ganglia of paraaortic plexus	Lower abdominal wall and pelvic viscera; visceral afferents from same
Medial pectoral	Medial cord of brachial plexus	Passes between axillary artery and vein, enters deep surface of pectoralis minor	Pectoralis minor and part of pectoralis major
Pulmonary plexus	Vagus nerve, cardiopulmonary splanchnic nerve from sympathetic trunk	Forms on primary bronchi, extends along root of lung and bronchial subdivisions	Parasympathetic fibers constrict bronchioles; sympathetic fibers dilate them
Recurrent laryngeal	Vagus nerve	Subclavian on right; left runs around aortic arch, ascends in tracheoesophageal groove	Intrinsic muscles of larynx (except cricothyroid); inferior to level of vocal cords

(continued)

Nerve	Origin	Course	Innervation
Subcostal	Anterior ramus of T12 spinal nerve	Inferior border of 12th rib in same manner as intercostal nerves	Muscles of anterolateral abdominal wall; lateral cutaneous branch supplies skin inferior to anterior iliac crest
Superior laryngeal	Vagus nerve	Descends in parapharyngeal space; lateral to thyroid cartilage divides into internal and external laryngeal nerves; inferior pierces thyrohyoid membrane; runs inferomedially to gap between cricoid and thyroid cartilages	Cricothyroid muscle; supraglottic
Thoracic splanchnic	Thoracic ganglia of sympathetic trunk	Anteromedially on thoracic vertebrae as lower cardiopulmonary splanchnic nerve to thoracic plexus; upper abdominopelvic splanchnic nerves to prevertebral ganglia of paraaortic plexuses	1st–5th splanchnic nerves; 6th–12th splanchnic nerves; thoracic ganglia; presynaptic sympathetic fibers to prevertebral ganglia
Thoracoabdominal	Lower intercostal nerve	Costal margin between 2nd and 3rd layers of abdominal muscles	Anterolateral abdominal muscles; overlying skin, underlying peritoneum, periphery of diaphragm
Thoracodorsal	Posterior cord of brachial plexus	Between upper and lower subscapular nerves, runs inferolaterally along posterior axillary wall to latissimus dorsi	Latissimus dorsi

(continued)

Nerve	Origin	Course	Innervation
Vagus	Via 8–10 rootlets from medulla of brainstem	Superior mediastinum posterior to sternoclavicular joint and brachiocephalic vein; gives rise to recurrent laryngeal nerve; continues into abdomen	Voluntary muscle of larynx and upper esophagus; involuntary muscle/glands of tracheobronchial tree, gut, and heart via pulmonary, esophageal, and cardiac plexuses; pharynx, larynx, reflex afferents from same areas as above

6. Nerves of the Back and Spinal Region

Nerve	Origin	Course	Innervation
Accessory	Medulla and cervical spinal cord	Spinal root ascends into cranial cavity via foramen magnum; exits via jugular foramen; traverses posterior triangle of neck	Sternocleidomastoid and trapezius
Dorsal scapular	Anterior ramus of C5 with contribution from C4	Scalenus medius, descends deep to levator scapulae, enters deep surface of rhomboids	Rhomboids and occasionally supplies levator scapulae
Greater occipital	Medial branch of posterior ramus of spinal nerve C2	Deep muscles of neck and trapezius to ascend posterior scalp to vertex	Multifidus cervicis, semispinalis capitis; posterior scalp
Suboccipital	Posterior ramus of C1 spinal nerve	Between occipital bone and atlas, inferior to transverse part of vertebral artery, into suboccipital triangle; communicates with occipital nerve	Suboccipital muscles

(continued)

Nerves

7. Nerves of the Shoulder and Arm Region

Nerve	Origin	Course	Innervation
Anterior interosseous	Median nerve in distal cubital fossa	Inferiorly on interosseous membrane	Flexor digitorum profundus, flexor pollicis longus, pronator quadrates
Axillary	Terminal branch of posterior cord of brachial plexus	Posterior aspect of arm with posterior circumflex humeral artery; winds around surgical neck of humerus; gives rise to brachial cutaneous nerve	Teres minor and deltoid; shoulder joint and skin over inferior part of deltoid
Deep branch of radial nerve	Radial nerve distal to elbow	Neck of radius in supinator; posterior compartment of forearm, becomes posterior interosseous nerve	Extensor carpi radialis brevis and supinator
Deep branch of ulnar nerve	Ulnar nerve at wrist, passes between pisiform and hamate	Deep between muscles of hypothenar eminence, across palm with deep palmar arch	Hypothenar muscles, lumbricals of digits 4 and 5, all interossei, adductor pollicis and deep head of flexor pollicis brevis
Lateral cutaneous nerve of forearm	Musculocutaneous nerve	Descends along lateral border of forearm to wrist	Skin of lateral aspect of forearm
Lower subscapular	Posterior cord of brachial plexus	Passes inferolaterally to subscapular artery and vein, to subscapularis and teres major	Inferior portion of subscapularis and teres major
Medial cutaneous nerve of arm	Medial cord of brachial plexus	Runs along medial side of axillary vein; communicates with intercostobrachial nerve	Skin on medial side of arm
Medial cutaneous nerve of forearm	Medial cord of brachial plexus	Runs between axillary artery and vein	Skin over medial side of forearm

(continued)

Nerve	Origin	Course	Innervation
Musculocutaneous	Lateral cord of brachial plexus	Deep surface of coracobrachialis, descends between biceps brachii and brachialis	Flexor muscles of arm; lateral antebrachial cutaneous nerve
Palmar cutaneous branch of ulnar nerve	Arises from ulnar nerve near middle of forearm	Ulnar artery, perforates deep fascia in the distal third of forearm	Skin at base of medial palm, overlying medial carpals
Posterior cutaneous nerve of forearm	Arises in arm from radial nerve	Perforates lateral head of triceps, descends along lateral side of arm and posterior aspect of forearm to wrist	Skin of distal posterior arm, posterior aspect of forearm
Posterior interosseous	Terminal branch of deep branch of radial nerve	Between superficial and deep layers of posterior forearm; between extensor pollicis longus and interosseous membrane	Extensor carpi ulnaris, extensors of digits, abductor pollicis longus
Radial	Terminal branch of posterior cord of brachial plexus	Descends posterior to axillary artery; radial groove with deep brachial artery; passes between long and medial head of triceps; bifurcates in cubital fossa into superficial and deep radial nerve	Triceps brachii, anconeus, brachioradialis, extensor carpi radialis longus muscles; skin on posterior aspect of arm and forearm via posterior cutaneous nerve of arm and forearm
Superficial branch of ulnar nerve	Arises from ulnar nerve at wrist, passes between pisiform and hamate bones	Palmaris brevis, divides into two common palmar digital nerve	Palmaris brevis; skin of the palmar and distal dorsal aspects of digit 5 and medial side of digit 4, proximal portion of palm

(continued)

Nerve	Origin	Course	Innervation
Ulnar	Terminal branch of medial cord of brachial plexus	Runs down medial aspect of arm; does not branch in the brachium	Majority of intrinsic muscles of hand; deep head of flexor pollicis brevis; medial lumbricales for digits 4 and 5; skin of palmar and distal dorsal aspects of medial 1–1/2 digits and adjacent palm

8. Nerves of the Hand

Nerve	Origin	Course	Innervation
Common palmar digital	Median and superficial branch of ulnar nerve	Runs distally between long flexor tendons of palm, bifurcating in distal palm	Proper palmar digital nerve; skin and joints of palmar and dorsal aspect of fingers
Dorsal branch of ulnar nerve	Ulnar nerve about 5 cm proximal to flexor retinaculum	Passes distally deep to flexor carpi ulnaris, dorsally to perforate deep fascia, medial side of dorsum of hand, dividing into 2 or 3 dorsal digital nerve	Skin of medial aspect of dorsum of hand, proximal portions of little and medial half of ring finger; adjacent sides of proximal portion of ring and middle fingers
Lateral branch of median nerve	Median nerve as it enters palm of hand	Runs laterally to palmar thumb and radial side of index finger	First lumbrical; skin of palmar and distal dorsal aspects of thumb, radial half of index finger
Medial branch of median nerve	Median nerve as it enters palm	Runs medially to adjacent sides of index, middle and ring fingers	Second lumbrical; skin of palmar and distal dorsal aspects of adjacent sides of index, middle and ring fingers

(continued)

Nerve	Origin	Course	Innervation
Median	Arises by two roots; one from lateral cord of brachial plexus, one from medial cord; root joins lateral to axillary artery	Medial side of brachial artery; cubital fossa, between heads of pronator teres, intermediate and deep layers of anterior forearm; becomes superficial proximal to wrist; passes deep to flexor retinaculum	Flexor muscles in forearm; thenar muscles, lateral lumbricals; skin of palmar and distal dorsal aspects of lateral 3–1/2 digits and palm
Palmar cutaneous branch of ulnar nerve	Arises from ulnar nerve, near middle of forearm	Ulnar artery and deep fascia in distal third of forearm	Skin at base of medial palm overlying medial carpals
Recurrent branch of median nerve	Median nerve distal to flexor retinaculum	Distal border of flexor retinaculum, enters thenar muscles	Abductor pollicis brevis, opponens pollicis, superficial head of flexor pollicis brevis
Superficial branch of radial nerve	Radial nerve	Anterior to pronator teres, to brachioradialis; deep fascia at wrist, passes onto dorsum of hand	Skin of lateral half of dorsum of hand and thumb, proximal portions of digits 2, 3, and lateral half of 4

9. Nerves of the Abdomen and Pelvic Regions

Nerve	Origin	Course	Innervation
Cavernous nerve	Parasympathetic fibers of prostatic nerve plexus	Perforates perineal membrane to reach erectile bodies of penis	Helicine arteries of cavernous bodies; stimulation produces engorgement at arterial pressure

(continued)

Nerve	Origin	Course	Innervation
Clunial	Posterior rami of L1, L2, and L3; posterior rami of S1, S2, and S3; posterior cutaneous nerve of thigh	Superior nerves cross iliac crest: middle nerves exit through posterior sacral foramina, entering gluteal region; inferior nerves curve around inferior border of gluteus maximus	Skin of buttock or gluteal region as far as greater trochanter
Coccygeal	Conus medullaris of spinal cord	Anterior and posterior rami join adjacent rami of S4 and S5; anterior rami form coccygeal plexus, gives rise to anococcygeal nerve	Skin over coccyx
Genitofemoral	Lumbar plexus	Descends on anterior surface of psoas major, divides into genital and femoral branches	Femoral branch supplies skin over femoral triangle; genital branch supplies scrotum or labia majora; genital branch to cremaster muscle
Hypogastric	Superior hypogastric plexus into pelvis	Sacrum within hypogastric sheath, merges with pelvic splanchnic nerve in inferior hypogastric plexus	Pelvic viscera; intraperitoneal pelvic viscera
Iliohypogastric	Lumbar plexus	Traverses abdominal muscle; external oblique aponeurosis to reach inguinal and pubic regions	Internal oblique and transverse abdominal muscles; superolateral quadrant of buttock; skin over iliac crest and hypogastric region

(continued)

Nerve	Origin	Course	Innervation
Ilioinguinal	Lumbar plexus	Passes between 2nd and 3rd layers of abdominal muscles; inguinal canal, divides into femoral and scrotal or labial branches	Lower part of internal oblique, transverse abdominal muscles; skin over femoral triangle; mons pubis, adjacent skin of labia majora or scrotum
Inferior anal	Pudendal nerve	Pudendal canal, medially through ischioanal fat pad to anal canal	External anal sphincter; perianal skin
Inferior gluteal	Sacral plexus	Pelvis through greater sciatic foramen inferior to piriformis, divides into several branches	Gluteus maximus
Lateral cutaneous nerve of thigh	Lumbar plexus	Deep to inguinal ligament, medial to anterior superior iliac spine	Skin on anterior and lateral aspects of thigh
Nerve to obturator internus	Sacral plexus	Gluteal region, greater sciatic foramen, inferior to piriformis; descends posterior to ischial spine; lesser sciatic foramen, to obturator internus	Superior gemellus and obturator internus
Quadratus femoris	Sacral plexus	Leaves pelvis through greater sciatic foramen deep to sciatic nerve	Inferior gemellus and quadratus femoris; hip joint
Obturator	Lumbar plexus	Enters thigh through obturator foramen, divides into anterior and posterior branches	Adductor longus, adductor brevis, gracilis, and pectineus; obturator externus, adductor magnus; skin of medial thigh above knee

(continued)

Nerve	Origin	Course	Innervation
Pelvic splanchnic	Sacral plexus	Runs anteriorly and inferiorly to merge with inferior hypogastric plexus	Parasympathetic fibers for pelvic viscera, descending and sigmoid colon; subperitoneal pelvic viscera
Perineal	Terminal branch of pudendal nerve	Pudendal nerve from pudendal canal to superficial perineum dividing into superficial cutaneous and deep motor branch	Urogenital triangle; skin of posterior urogenital triangle
Posterior cutaneous nerve of thigh	Sacral plexus	Leaves pelvis through greater sciatic foramen inferior to piriformis, deep to gluteus maximus	Skin of buttock; skin over posterior aspect of thigh and calf; lateral perineum, upper medial thigh
Posterior labial	Perineal nerve	Pudendal canal and ramifies in subcutaneous tissue	Skin of posterior portion of labium majus
Pudendal	Sacral plexus	Enters gluteal region through greater sciatic foramen inferior to piriformis; descends to sacrospinous ligament; perineum through lesser sciatic foramen	Most motor and sensory innervation to perineum
Sciatic	Sacral plexus	Enters gluteal region through greater sciatic foramen inferior to piriformis; descends along posterior aspect of thigh, divides proximal to knee into tibial and common fibular peroneal nerves	Hamstrings; provides articular branches to hip and knee joints

(continued)

Nerve	Origin	Course	Innervation
Superior gluteal	Sacral plexus	Leaves pelvis through greater sciatic foramen, superior to piriformis, runs between gluteus medius and minimus	Gluteus medius, gluteus minimus, tensor fasciae latae

10. Nerves of the Legs and Feet

Nerve	Origin	Course	Innervation
Anterior femoral cutaneous	Femoral nerve	Arises in femoral triangle, fasciae latae of thigh along path of sartorius muscle	Skin on medial and anterior aspects of thigh
Calcaneal branches	Tibial and sacral nerves	Passes from distal part of posterior aspect of leg to skin on heel	Skin of heel
Common fibular	Terminal branch of sciatic nerve	Begins at apex of popliteal fossa; follows medial border of biceps femoris muscle to posterior aspect of head of fibula; bifurcates into superficial and deep fibular nerves	Skin on lateral part of posterior aspect of leg; knee joint via articular branch; short head of biceps femoris
Common plantar digital	Medial and lateral plantar nerves	Runs anteriorly in sole of foot between flexor tendons; bifurcates in distal sole	Proper plantar digital nerves; skin and joints of plantar and distal dorsal aspect of toes
Deep fibular	Common fibular nerve	Arises between fibularis longus and neck of fibula; extensor digitorum longus; extensor retinaculum; distal end of tibia, enters dorsum of foot	Muscles of anterior compartment of leg, dorsum of foot; skin of first interdigital cleft; sends articular branches to the joints it crosses

(continued)

Nerves

Nerve	Origin	Course	Innervation
Femoral	Lumbar plexus	Passes deep to midpoint of inguinal ligament; lateral to femoral vessels, divides into muscular and cutaneous branches	Anterior thigh muscles; hip and knee joints; skin on anteromedial side of thigh and leg
Lateral plantar	Smaller terminal branch of tibial nerve	Passes laterally in foot between quadratus plantae, flexor digitorum brevis muscles, divides into superficial and deep branches	Quadratus plantae, abductor digiti minimi, flexor digiti minimi brevis; plantar and dorsal interossei, lateral three lumbricals, adductor hallucis; skin on sole lateral to a line splitting 4th digit
Medial cutaneous nerve of leg	Saphenous nerve	Descends medial side of leg with greater saphenous vein	Skin of antero-medial side of leg and medial side of foot
Medial dorsal cutaneous nerve	Superficial fibular nerve	Descends across ankle anteriorly running onto medial aspect of dorsum of foot	Most of skin of dorsum of foot, proximal portion of toes, except for web between great and 2nd toes
Medial plantar	Terminal branch of the tibial nerve	Passes distally in foot between abductor hallucis and flexor digitorum brevis; divides into muscular and cutaneous branches	Abductor hallucis, flexor digitorum brevis, flexor hallucis brevis and first lumbrical; skin of medial side of sole of foot and sides of first three digits
Saphenous	Femoral nerve	Descends with femoral vessels through femoral triangle and adductor canal, descends with great saphenous vein	Skin on medial side of leg and foot

(continued)

Nerve	Origin	Course	Innervation
Superficial fibular	Common fibular nerve	Arises between fibularis longus and neck of fibula, descends in lateral compartment of leg; deep fascia at distal third of leg, becomes cutaneous and sends branches to foot and digits	Fibularis longus and brevis; skin on distal third of anterior surface of leg, dorsum of foot and all digits except lateral side of 5th and adjoining sides of 1st and 2nd digits
Sural	Arises from medial and lateral sural cutaneous nerves	Descends between heads of gastrocnemius, becomes superficial at middle of leg; descends with small saphenous vein, passes posterior to lateral malleolus to lateral side of foot	Skin on posterior and lateral aspects of leg and lateral side of foot
Tibial	Sciatic nerve	Forms as sciatic, bifurcates at apex of popliteal fossa; descends through same, lies on popliteus; runs inferiorly on tibialis posterior with posterior tibial vessels; terminates beneath flexor retinaculum, dividing into medial and lateral plantar nerves	Muscles of posterior compartment of thigh; popliteal fossa, posterior compartment of leg, sole of foot; knee joint, skin of leg, sole of foot

Appendix 3
Cranial Nerves: Functions & Common Tests

There are 12 pairs of cranial nerves. These nerves control the 5 senses and are necessary for bodily function. The cranial nerves include sensory/afferent, motor/efferent, and mixed/ sensory and motor. Sensory nerves receive information from the eyes, ears, nose, skin, and internal organs. Motor nerves innervate voluntary and involuntary muscles of the body. Cranial nerves may be affected by various conditions such as trauma, infection, aneurysm, tumor, inflammation, and ischemia.

Cranial Nerve	Innervation	Main Function	Common Tests
1st – olfactory nerve	sensory	smell	identify odors
2nd – optic nerve	sensory	sight/vision	visual acuity
3rd – oculomotor nerve	motor	extraocular eye movement, upper lid evaluation, accommodation, pupillary reactions	extraocular range of motion, pupillary constriction
4th – trochlear nerve	motor	superior oblique muscle	extraocular range of motion
5th – trigeminal nerve	motor/ sensory	teeth, chewing muscles, scalp	corneal reflex, jaw/ palate clench, pain/light touch comparison
6th – abducens nerve	motor	lateral rectus muscle	eye abduction
7th – facial nerve	motor/ sensory	facial expression muscles, taste, anterior two thirds of tongue	forehead wrinkle, shut-eye pry, smile symmetry comparison, taste tests
8th – vestibulocochlear nerve	sensory	hearing, balance	hearing-Rinne test, balance-Weber test
9th – glossopharyngeal nerve	motor/ sensory	tongue/pharynx, taste, anterior one third of tongue	gag reflex
10th – vagus nerve	motor/ sensory	pharynx, tongue, larynx, thoracic/ abdominal viscera, trachea, esophagus	gag reflex
11th – accessory nerve	motor	trapezius, sternomastoid muscles	shoulder shrug, head-turn against resistance
12th – hypoglossal nerve	motor	tongue muscles	tongue test for deviation

Appendix 4

Types of Brain and Spinal Cord Tumors

Type	Location
Astrocytoma	A glioma that arises most frequently in the cerebrum of adults. Arises in the brain stem, cerebrum, and cerebellum of children. Astrocytomas can be classified as low-grade well-differentiated, anaplastic, pilocytic, and glioblastoma multiforme.
Brainstem glioma	Occurs in the lowest portion of brain.
Chordoma	Spinal cord tumor that develops from remnants of early fetal spine-like structure, which is later replaced by the spinal cord.
Craniopharyngioma	Occurs near hypothalamus, in the pituitary gland region. Usually benign, but can be considered malignant because of potential damage to the hypothalamus from pressure, affecting vital functions.
Ependymoma	Commonly develops in the lining of the ventricles; can also develop in spinal cord.
Ganglioneuroma	Occurs in the brain or spinal cord.
Germ cell tumor	Arises from developing sex cells.
Glioblastoma multiforme	Also called grade 4 astrocytoma; originates in glial cells.
Hemangioblastoma	Arises from blood vessels of the brain and spinal cord.
Medulloblastoma	Usually develops in the cerebellum, but may occur in other areas as well.
Meningioma	Develops in the medulla and can spread to the spine or to other parts of the body.
Mixed oligoastrocytoma	Comprised of oligodendrocytes and astrocytes; originates in glial cells.

Oligodendroglioma	Usually arises in the cerebrum; fewer than 10% are malignant.
Optic nerve glioma	Occurs on or near the nerves that travel between the eye and brain vision centers.
Pineal region tumor	Occurs in the pineal gland region.
Pituitary adenoma	Occurs in the pituitary gland, generally arising in adenohypophysis.
Schwannoma	May originate from a peripheral or sympathetic nerve, or from various cranial nerves, particularly the eighth nerve.

Appendix 5

Common Neurologic Disorders

Disorder/Disease	Symptoms	Tests	Treatments
Alzheimer disease	progressive cognitive difficulties, aggressive behavior, depression, impaired memory	memory tests, blood tests, brain scan	medications, family counseling
cerebral palsy	infants—developmental delay, abnormal muscle tone, unusual posture	MRI, CT, ultrasound of brain, motor skill tests	behavior therapy, physical therapy, counseling, muscle surgery, mechanical aides, medications
spastic	muscles permanently contracted, stiff		
athetoid/dyskinetic	uncontrolled, slow movements		
ataxic	rare form with wide-based gait, motor difficulties		
mixed form	combination of symptoms		
chronic fatigue syndrome	tender lymph nodes, sore throat, headaches, joint pain, muscle pain, extreme fatigue, cognitive impairment	no definitive test	no curative treatment, symptoms may be treated with medications, rest, nutrition, exercise
epilepsy	convulsions, blackouts, blank staring, fainting with loss of bladder/ bowel control, dazed behavior, muscle jerks, sensory perception changes,unusual/ inappropriate movements, unprovoked fear, anger, or panic	EEG, MRI, CT scan, PET scan	medications, diet, vagus nerve stimulation (VNS)
Huntington disease	tics, twitches, mood changes, clumsiness, depression, chorea, slurred speech, dementia	genetic testing, physical exam	medications to control symptoms, family counseling

Disorder/Disease	Symptoms	Tests	Treatments
multiple sclerosis	numbness, tingling, burning, itching in face, extremities, trunk; fatigue, mood swings, euphoria, depression, apathy, cognitive problems, visual disturbances, loss of bowel and bladder control, Lhermitte sign, muscle weakness and spasticity, dementia	physical exam, lab tests, spinal tap, MRI, ophthalmoscopy	corticosteroids, other medications, exercise
Parkinson disease	tremor, gait/balance disturbances, limb/ trunk rigidity, bradykinesia	neurological exam, MRI, urine/blood tests, CT scan	medications,family/ patient counseling
Tourette syndrome	motor and vocal tics, obsessive/compulsive behavior, attention deficit hyperactivity disorder (ADHD), aggressive/injurious behaviors	no definitive test; EEG, MRI, CT used to rule out other disorders	stimulant medications, family/patient counseling, psychotherapy

Appendix 6

Manual Muscle Testing Rating Scale

Manual muscle testing (MMT) is a standardized system of measuring and recording muscle strength. MMT can be used to test virtually all palpable skeletal muscles and is a crucial part of diagnosing diseases of the muscles, connective tissue, and nervous system. To assess the strength of a muscle, a numbering system is used to grade muscle strength based on manual testing. The numerical score (0-5) is dependent on the quality of muscle strength in relation to whether there is movement against resistance with or without gravity eliminated. If strength falls between 2 categories, plus (+) and minus (-) may be used with the number.

0	No muscle contraction detectable.
1	Trace muscle contraction.
2	Active muscle movement without gravity.
3	Muscle moveable against gravity, not against resistance.
4	Muscle movement against some resistance.
5	Normal muscle movement. Overcomes all resistance.

Appendix 7
Sleep Medicine Terminology

acoustic signature event (ASI)
adjustment sleep disorder
adolescent narcolepsy
advanced sleep-phase syndrome
age-related sleep physiology
alcohol-dependent sleep disorder
alcohol-induced insomnia
altitude insomnia
anxiety disorder
apnea
apnea index (AI)
apnea-hypopnea index (AHI)
autonomic change in sleep
auto-titrating continuous positive airway pressure (APAP)
behavior disorder
benign neonatal sleep myoclonus
bilevel positive airway pressure (BiPAP)
body mass index (BMI)
cardioballistic artifact
cataplexy
central alveolar hypoventilation syndrome
central sleep apnea (CSA)
cephalometric analysis
cephalometric radiograph
chronic insomnia
chronic obstructive pulmonary disease (COPD)
circadian rhythm
comorbid sleep disorder
confusional arousal
congenital central hypoventilation syndrome
continuous positive airway pressure (CPAP)
cycle of sleep
daytime consequences of sleeplessness
daytime fatigue
delayed sleep-phase syndrome
dementia insomnia
desaturation index (DI)
digital polysomnography
disorders of excessive sleepiness
disorders of initiation and maintenance of sleep
drug-induced insomnia
dyssomnia
early final awakening
electrical status epilepticus of sleep
electrocardiogram (EKG)
electrode pop artifact
electroencephalogram (EEG)
electrooculography (EOG)
endocrine disorder
endocrine secretion
environmental influence
environmental sleep disorder
epilepsy insomnia
epilepsy with daytime sleepiness
Epworth Sleepiness Scale (ESS)
excessive daytime sleepiness
excessive sleep inertia
exhalation positive airway pressure
exhalation positive airway pressure (EPAP)
extraocular movements (EOM)
fatal familial insomnia
fiberoptic nasopharyngolaryngoscopy
first night effect
flow-limitation arousal
focal akathisia
focal seizure
food allergy insomnia
free-running circadian sleep disorder
frontal seizure
full-night polysomnography
function of sleep

functional outcomes of sleep questionnaire (FOSQ)
gasping for breath
generalized anxiety disorder(GAD)
genioglossus advancement
genioglossus muscle
habitual sleep episode
head banging
60-hertz artifact
6-hertz spike
high arousal threshold
high-altitude illness
hippocampal pattern
histamine 2 antagonist
histamine antagonist
histaminergic neuron
HLA typing
Horne-Ostberg questionnaire
24-hour ambulatory monitoring
human lymphocyte antigen (HLA)
human sleep characteristic
hyoid advancement
hyoid muscle
hypercapnic ventilatory response (HCVR)
hypernychthemeral syndrome
hypersomnia parkinsonism
hypersomnolence
hypertension with insomnia
hypnagogic hallucination
hypnagogic hypersynchrony
hypnogenic paroxysmal dystonia
hypnogram
hypnopompic hypersynchrony
hypnotic intoxication
hypnotic medication
hypnotic withdrawal
hypnotic-dependent insomnia
hypnotic-dependent sleep disorder
hypocapnic ventilatory response
hypocretin system
hypomania associated with sleep disturbance
hypopnea
idiopathic central sleep apnea
idiopathic hypersomnia
idiopathic insomnia
induced hypocapnic central apnea
infant REM sleep
infant sleep
infant sleep apnea
infant sleep staging
infrared videosomnography
in-phase deflection
insomnia
insomnia assessment tool
insomnia treatment
insomnia with steroids
insomnia-related panic disorder
inspiratory positive airway pressure (IPAP)
insufficient sleep syndrome
irregular sleep-wake disorder
irregular sleep-wake pattern
isocapnic hypoxia
Johns Hopkins Severity Scale
Karolinska Sleepiness Scale
Kleine-Levin syndrome
laser uvulopalatoplasty (LUPP)
laser-assisted uvulopalatoplasty (LAUP)
lateral cephalometric radiography
lateral hypothalamus
Leeds Sleep Evaluation Questionnaire (LSEQ)
leg cramp
leg movement
leg movement monitoring
levator palatini
light effect on circadian rhythm
limit-setting sleep disorder
load compensation
long sleeper
loose-belt artifact
low-amplitude circadian rhythm
lowest saturation of oxygen
lymphangioleiomyomatosis
maintenance of wakefulness test (MWT)
major depression disorder

mandibular advancing oral appliance
maxillomandibular advancement (MMA)
maxillomandibular expansion (MME)
mechanical receptor
medication-induced insomnia
medication-induced seizure
medication-related sleepiness
memory reinforcement theory
mental status examination
Minnesota Multiphasic Personality Inventory (MMPI)
3-minute rule
misplaced thermocouple artifact
mixed sleep apnea
Moebius syndrome
molecular feedback
mood disorder
movement disorder
multiple sleep latency test (MSLT)
muscle artifact
muscular circulation
narcolepsy
nasal bilevel ventilation
nasal cannula pressure transducer
nasal congestion
nasal continuous positive airway pressure (NCPAP, nCPAP)
nasal reconstruction
nasal septal deviation
neck circumference
neurobiology of sleep
neurocognitive dysfunction
neurologic illness insomnia
neuromodulation of sleep
neuromodulation of wakefulness
neuromuscular disorder
neurotransmitter of sleep
neurotransmitter of wakefulness
newborn REM
newborn sleep
nicotine withdrawal
nicotine-induced insomnia
nightmare
nighttime pain
nocturnal angina
nocturnal cardiac ischemia
nocturnal dyspnea
nocturnal eating syndrome
nocturnal event
nocturnal frontal lobe epilepsy
nocturnal leg cramp
nocturnal pain
nocturnal paroxysmal dystonia
nocturnal paroxysmal wandering
nocturnal polysomnography
nocturnal reflux
nocturnal sleep disturbance
nocturnal wandering
non-24-hour sleep-and-wake disorder
non-24-hour sleep phase syndrome
nonapneic sleep disorder
nonentrained sleep-wake disorder
noninvasive ventilation
nonrapid eye movement sleep
normal human physiology
normal sleep
normal sleep cycle
obesity hypoventilation syndrome (OHS)
obstructive apnea (OA)
obstructive arrhythmia
obstructive dementia
obstructive sleep apnea (OSA)
obstructive sleep apnea syndrome (OSAS)
obstructive sleep apnea-hypopnea (OSAH)
obstructive sleep apnea-hypopnea syndrome (OSAHS)
opioid intoxication
opioid withdrawal
oral appliance guideline
oral appliance side effect
oral appliance therapy
orexin
orexin A
orexin B

orexin-containing neuron
oropharyngeal reconstruction
out-of-phase deflection
oximetry
oxygen desaturation index (ODI)
painful erection
panic disorder
parasomnia
partial arousal event
pavor nocturnes
pediatric daytime sleepiness scale (PDSS)
pediatric polysomnography
pediatric respiratory definition
pediatric sleep questionnaire (PSQ)
pediatric sleep survey
periodic breathing
periodic limb movement (PLM)
periodic limb movement disorder (PLMD)
periodic limb movements of sleep
pharmacology of sleep
phylogeny of sleep
pneumatic splint mechanism
polysomnography (PSG)
positional obstructive sleep apnea
positional therapy
positive airway pressure (PAP)
posttraumatic insomnia
primary insomnia
primary snoring
primary snoring disorder (PSD)
prior sleep
problem sleepiness
progressive muscle relaxation
psychogenic event
psychometric testing of sleeplessness
psychophysiologic insomnia
pulmonary medication
quality of life (QOL)
quiet sleep
quiet sleep characteristic
rapid eye movement (REM)
rebound effect
rebound insomnia
recovery sleep
rectus spike artifact
recurrent insomnia
repeated test of sustained wakefulness (RTSW)
respiration supplemental resistance
respiratory arousal index (RAI)
respiratory arousal response
respiratory disturbance index (RDI)
respiratory effort amplitude
respiratory effort-related arousal
respiratory event arousal (REA)
respiratory inductance plethysmography
respiratory monitoring
respiratory rate
respiratory variability
restless leg syndrome (RLS)
restrictive lung disease
retinohypothalamic tract (RHT)
reversible uvulopalatal flap
rhythmic kicking movement
rhythmic midtemporal burst of drowsiness
rhythmic movement disorder
salivation
saturation of oxygen (SaO2)
schizophrenia-related sleep disturbance
screamer
seasonal affective disorder (SAD)
secondary insomnia
secondary narcolepsy
secondary periodic leg movement of sleep
secondary restless leg syndrome
sedative hypnotic
sedative intoxication
sedative withdrawal
seizure classification
seizure in sleep
seizure-related behavior
short sleeper

short-term insomnia
sinus arrest
sinus bradycardia
sleep apnea (SA)
sleep apnea syndrome (SAS)
sleep architecture
sleep attack
sleep bruxism
sleep center referral
sleep characteristic
sleep choking syndrome
sleep deprivation
sleep disorder associated with mental disorder
sleep disorder facility
sleep disturbance associated with mania
sleep disturbance in major depression
sleep drunkenness
sleep hallucination
sleep history
sleep hygiene
sleep hyperhidrosis
sleep hypopnea syndrome (SHS)
sleep inertia
sleep log
sleep montage
sleep onset of rapid eye movement
sleep onset period (SOP)
sleep paralysis
sleep period time
sleep restriction
sleep spindle
sleep start
sleep state misperception
sleeptalking
sleep terror
sleep timing questionnaire (STQ)
sleepiness consequence
sleepiness countermeasure
sleeping sickness
sleeplessness analysis
sleeplessness log
sleep-onset association disorder
sleep-onset rapid eye movement period (SOREMP)
sleep-related abnormal swallowing
sleep-related asthma
sleep-related breathing disorder (SRBD)
sleep-related epilepsy
sleep-related gastroesophageal reflux
sleep-related headache
sleep-related oxygenation
sleep-related painful erection
sleep-related ventilation
sleep-wake activity inventory (SWAI)
sleep-wake oscillator
sleep-wake pattern
sleep-wake rhythm
sleep-wake schedule
sleep-wake transition disorder
sleepwalking
slow eye movement (SEM)
slow sharp spike of sleep (SSSS)
slow-wave sleep (SWS)
snoring
sodium channel 5A mutation
somatic skeletal muscle
somniloquy
somnolence
splanchnic circulation
St. Mary's Hospital Sleep Questionnaire (SMHSQ)
stage 2 sleep
stage 3 sleep
stage 4 sleep
staged surgical approach
stamp test
Starling resistor model of upper airway
stereotypic movement disorder
stimulant-dependent sleep disorder
substance abuse
substance dependence
subwakefulness syndrome
sudden infant death syndrome (SIDS)

sudden unexplained nocturnal death syndrome (SUNDS)
supplemental oxygen
surgery evaluation
sweat artifact
teeth grinding
tensor palatini
terminal insomnia
terrifying hypnagogic hallucination
tongue base prominence
tooth grinding
toxin-induced sleep disorder
tracheal traction
transient insomnia
twitcher
ultradian rhythm
unintelligible speech
unusual sleep behavior
unusual sleep movement
upper airway
upper airway dilating muscle
upper airway resistance syndrome (UARS)
upper airway ventilation
uvulopalatal flap (UPF)
uvulopalatopharyngoplasty (UPPP)
uvulopalatoplasty (UPP)
velopharyngeal incompetence (VPI)
vibration artifact
violent ambulation
volitional sleep deprivation
wake rhythm
wakefulness
wakefulness drive
waveform of sleep
weight-loss surgery
Women's Health Initiative Insomnia Rating Scale (WHIIRS)
Zeitgeber

Appendix 8
Sample Reports

CERVICAL LAMINECTOMY, REMOVAL EPIDURAL HEMATOMA

PREOPERATIVE DIAGNOSIS: Postoperative epidural hematoma with spinal cord compression.

POSTOPERATIVE DIAGNOSIS: Postoperative epidural hematoma with spinal cord compression.

ANESTHESIA: General endotracheal.

DESCRIPTION OF PROCEDURE: The patient was taken to the operating room. After placement of appropriate intravenous lines for cardiovascular monitoring, the patient was induced with adequate general endotracheal anesthesia. The patient was turned to the right lateral position. Head was placed on the donut headrest in a neutral position. The midline incision was opened after removal of the surgical staples. Weitlaner retractor was placed. The paraspinal and subcutaneous tissues were dissected. The midline ligamentum nuchae sutures were removed which revealed an epidural hematoma. The hematoma appeared to have come beneath the ligamentum nuchae and the paraspinal muscles. There was a subcutaneous hematoma as well. The Weitlaner retractor was in the muscles, and a very large epidural hematoma was encountered in the epidural space with spinal cord compression. This was completely removed, and following this, good pulsations were noted of the cervical cord. Hemostasis was assured in all lateral gutters. Bone wax was placed on the lateral edge of the laminectomy, and hemostasis was assured. Gelfoam was placed in the epidural space. Several drains were placed. A medium Hemovac drain was placed in the epidural space and exited via a separate stab incision. A subcutaneous Hemovac was placed after closure of the paraspinal muscles in the ligamentum nuchae. The subcutaneous tissues were closed with 3-0 Dexon, and skin staples were applied to the skin. Sterile dressing was applied.

The patient was returned to the supine position, reversed from general endotracheal anesthesia, and taken to the recovery room in satisfactory condition. The patient tolerated the procedure well with no intraoperative complications. Blood loss was not replaced intraoperatively.

ESTIMATED BLOOD LOSS: 250 mL.

CRANIOTOMY, EVACUATION OF CLOT, AND TEMPORAL LOBECTOMY

PREOPERATIVE DIAGNOSIS: Left temporoparietal clot.

POSTOPERATIVE DIAGNOSIS: Left temporoparietal clot.

PROCEDURE PERFORMED: Left frontotemporal parietal craniotomy for evacuation of left temporoparietal clot and temporal lobectomy.

DESCRIPTION OF PROCEDURE: The patient was brought to the operating room, having been previously intubated, and was placed under general anesthesia. The patient was placed in Mayfield head clamps with the temporal part of the head on the left hand side basically parallel to the floor. A shoulder roll was placed under the left shoulder to allow this rotation. The hair was shaved and the surgical area prepped and draped in the usual sterile fashion.

A curvilinear incision was carried out 1 fingerbreadth anterior to the tragus at the level of the zygoma and carried out superiorly, posteriorly around the pinna and then superiorly along the hairline anteriorly to the edge of the hairline. This was made down to subperiosteum. The musculocutaneous flap was developed. A subperiosteal dissection was performed with the Bovie cautery to expose the whole frontotemporal parietal region. Perforating towel clamps were then used with rubber bands to hold back the musculocutaneous flap. A bur hole was made in the temporal region with the keyhole on the left-hand side down to dura. The dura was dissected epidurally with a Bentall tool, and a B14 attachment to the device was then used to go circularly around the created temporoparietal frontal craniotomy. Basically the flap was dissected from the dura and removed and cracked basically at the attachment of the temporal anterior region.

At that point we coagulated the epidural space and the bleeders. We waxed the bone edge, and we performed a subtemporal decompression by performing a temporal craniectomy using Leksell rongeur and Kerrison punches. We thinned down the sphenoid ridge. At that point we saw the floor of the middle cranial fossa. We then irrigated and opened up the dura in a horseshoe fashion from bur hole to bur hole and flapped it inferiorly, stayed with 4-0 Surgilon. At that point we saw a very large amount of hemorrhagic material over the temporal lobe as well as a small subdural. The temporal lobe was extremely hemorrhagic, swollen, and angry appearing. We used bipolar cautery to enter the middle temporal gyrus basically midway along the temporal lobe. We popped into a large clot cavity, and we evacuated the clot cavity of some liquified clot and removed a massive clot from the temporal lobe and then superiorly into the parietal area as well. We evacuated this clot and irrigated copiously. Then using a suction coagulation technique, we performed an inferior and middle temporal lobectomy approximately 6 cm from the temporal tip and basically went along the tentorial edge. We saw the 3rd nerve in the cistern and basically stopped at that point. Hemostasis was achieved using hydrogen peroxide-soaked cotton balls, Surgicel, and coagulation technique. The brain was completely compressed and temporal fossa was completely opened, and we were satisfied with our result.

At that point we irrigated copiously. We then loosely applied the dura and placed Gelfoam and Oxycel in the temporal fossa. We reapplied the bone flap with miniplates, placed a Hemovac in the epispinal space and reapproximated the temporalis muscle with 0 Vicryl and subcutaneous Vicryl for the subgaleal region, staples for the skin, 3-0 nylon for the drain, and dry sterile dressing and Kerlix wrap for the actual dressing. The patient was then brought to the recovery room, intubated and in stable condition.

Lumbar Fusion

Preoperative Diagnosis: Segmental instability L5-S1.

Postoperative Diagnosis: Segmental instability L5-S1.

Procedure Performed: L5-S1 posterior lumbar interbody fusion with interbody allograft spacers with segmental instrumentation, posterolateral fusion L5-S1 with morcellized allograft and local autograft.

Description of Procedure: The patient was brought to the operating room, positioned supine, and with general endotracheal anesthesia, the patient was rotated onto the Wilson frame. The lumbar region was prepped and draped in the usual sterile fashion.

Then through a midline incision this was carried down to the lumbodorsal fascia, centered over the area of interest. A subperiosteal dissection was carried out, exposing the laminae of L3, L4, L5, and S1 bilaterally. The transverse process of L5 bilaterally and the sacral alae bilaterally were exposed, and the soft tissue intervening was removed and separated. Basically at that point, the self-retaining retractors were deepened. We performed a laminectomy of L5 using Leksell rongeur including inferior processes. We dissected a plane between the remaining bone and the ligamentum. We removed the remainder of the bone and the inferior process with Kerrison rongeur, and then we exposed the L5 nerve roots bilaterally and S1 nerve roots bilaterally. The annulus was exposed by coagulating the epidural space and medially tracking each S1 nerve root bilaterally. The anulus was exposed, and anulotomies were performed after nerve root retraction was performed. This was removed completely using various different instruments from the Synthes PLIF set. When that was performed we distracted the interspace up to 13 mm, and then we inserted the interbody allograft spacer provided by the Synthes PLIF system; 13 x 22-mm grafts bilaterally. These were countersunk well, and fluoroscopy confirmed excellent position of these. At that point we irrigated copiously, placed Gelfoam in the epidural space, and under fluoroscopic guidance we drilled into each pedicle of L5 and S1 bilaterally. Then using sequential maneuvers of pedicle finder, pedicle probe, and testing to make sure that the bone was not breached in any sort of fashion within the pedicle tap, 6.2 x 45-mm screws were inserted at L5 and 7 x 40-mm screws were inserted at S1 bilaterally with excellent purchase and excellent positioning. At this point we decorticated the intertransverse region between the L5 and S1 sacral alae. We harvested fresh femoral head and reamed out the intramedullary bone and used that in conjunction with the bone that was harvested from the laminectomy as well as morcellized allograft and demineralized bone matrix and then packed that in the intertransverse region. After that was performed we placed the rotating heads on the pedicle screws. Rods were placed within the cups of the actual rotating heads, and we placed a locking cap over that and tightened it to appropriate tension.

We irrigated copiously, placed new Gelfoam in the epidural space, placed a drain in the epispinal space, tunneled out subcutaneously, and sutured with 3-0 nylon. We closed the fascia in interrupted fashion with 0 Vicryl, subcutaneous with 3-0 Vicryl, and staples for the skin. Dry sterile dressing was placed. The patient was then rotated back onto the stretcher. We used Cell Saver throughout the operation, and we retrieved 300 mL of Cell Saver blood. After extubation, the patient was noted to be in stable condition moving all 4 extremities.

Lumbar Hemilaminectomy

Preoperative Diagnosis: Left L5-S1 herniated disk.

Postoperative Diagnosis: Left L5-S1 herniated disk.

Procedure Performed: Left L5-S1 hemilaminectomy for diskectomy and removal of herniated disk.

Description of Procedure: The patient was brought to the operating room, positioned supine, and underwent general endotracheal anesthesia. The patient was rotated onto the Wilson frame. The lumbar region was prepped and draped in the usual sterile fashion.

An incision was made in the midline centered over the area of interest in the lumbar dorsal fascia. Self-retaining retractors were placed, and a subperiosteal dissection was carried out on the left side to expose the laminae of L5 and S1 out to the facet capsule. An intraoperative x-ray confirmed our level as being at L5-S1. We used a Leksell rongeur to thin out the lamina of L5. Then an upbiting curette was used to go underneath the lamina of L5, dissecting a plane and sweeping it laterally underneath the medial aspect of the facet capsule. After that was performed, we used a Kerrison punch to remove the inferior aspect of the L5 lamina and also perform medial fasciectomy. The dura immediately came into view, and this was followed inferiorly along the S2 nerve root out through its foramina. We retracted the S1 nerve root. We saw large segments of disk herniation with inferior migration. We entered the axial angles after the nerve root was medially retracted and removed the disk material piecemeal. We also removed a large fragment that was at the level of the S1 pedicle and swept it superiorly into the disk space and removed it. It appeared that part of it was calcified, and part of it was cartilaginous as well. We emptied the disk space, irrigated it out, decompressed the S1 nerve root completely and we were satisfied.

We irrigated the area. We placed Gelfoam into the epidural space and then placed Depo-Medrol over that. We then placed a Hemovac in the epispinal space, tunneled out subcutaneously, and sutured it with 3-0 nylon. We then closed the fascia in interrupted fashion with 0 Vicryl, subcutaneous with 3-0 Vicryl, and staples for the skin. Dry sterile dressing was placed. The patient was rotated back onto the stretcher, extubated, and noted to be in stable condition moving all extremities.

Neurological Symptoms and Weakness: Chart Note

This patient is a 53-year-old female who had no specific neurological symptoms before. She described one incident a year or so ago when she briefly felt a generalized weak sensation, but nothing came out of it. On October 17, 20XX, she had 3 episodes the same day a few hours apart. She was up and about but not necessarily doing any strenuous activity with these episodes. Generally speaking, the episodes were brief, from 5 to 30 minutes, and they were characterized initially with the left hand and left face tingling and then subsequently by a tingling sensation to the left side of the face, arm, and leg. There was no corresponding motor loss. There was no actual numbness per se. None of the episodes were accompanied by difficulties with vision, speech, blackout, chest pain, palpitations, and so on. On October 23, 20XX, similar symptoms returned, and she thinks they have sort of persisted in the sense that they never really cleared, but on the other hand she has not experienced further motor difficulties with them. She did have a mild headache on the day she went to the emergency room, but other than that she is not subject to headaches. She has been started on Aggrenox, and earlier in the month she was started on a mild diuretic for possible fluctuation in blood pressure.

When she went to the emergency room, some blood work was done, which is pretty well unremarkable. However, we are waiting for some further cholesterol results. CT scan showed an encephalic cyst, which is most likely a porencephalic cyst in the left occipital area, which is not an uncommon thing, but no additional intracranial pathology was described, and the ultrasound Doppler carotid study was essentially unremarkable as well.

On examination, I do not hear specific bruits in the neck or over the precordium. In spite of her symptoms, there is really no sensory or motor loss, particularly on the left side, that can be demonstrated.

At the moment, the evidence is very minimal in terms of structural disease, but I would suggest doing an MR scan. I think Aggrenox is fine. I will also suggest a 2D echocardiogram be looked into, and she tells me that her family doctor in fact has arranged it, and that is great. We will see what the blood work looks like, and obviously if it shows even a marginal increase in cholesterol, then it needs to be managed aggressively with medications. We will see what the MR scan looks like. If the 2D echocardiogram is abnormal, then additional steps may be indeed required.

NEUROTRAUMA GUNSHOT WOUND: DISCHARGE SUMMARY

This 19-year-old male sustained a gunshot wound to his left neck on October 7, 20XX. He was subsequently brought to this institution where he has been until the present time.

On arrival at the emergency department, the patient was hypoxemic with minimal ventilatory effort and was therefore intubated. The patient had sustained a gunshot wound to the neck, as mentioned above. There was a wound to the left neck just below the angle of the mandible. The patient was quadriplegic at the time of presentation and has remained in this state since that time.

Evaluation, which included a CT head, C-spine, and CT angiogram of his neck, revealed a small comminuted fracture of the angle of the left mandible and a fracture of the left facet of C3 as well as the right lamina of C4. The bullet fragment was present in the paraspinal soft tissues adjacent to C4 on the right side. The CT angiogram did not reveal any evidence of a vascular injury in the area of the wound.

The patient was subsequently admitted to the neurotrauma intensive care unit. From a neurologic/neurosurgical standpoint, he has remained quadriplegic since that time. He is awake and can communicate by mouthing words. He has no sensation below his clavicles. He is not able to initiate breath on the ventilator. He has been fully ventilated throughout his stay in the intensive care unit. He was tried on pressure support ventilation once but became hypoxemic after approximately 1 to 1-1/2 hours.

He was hypotensive during his initial days following admission and required dopamine to maintain his blood pressure. His heart rate has been well maintained, although he has had some episodes of bradycardia and even asystole with suctioning. However, these have seemed to resolve, as he has not had a problem with his heart rate on suctioning or other maneuvers for quite a number of days.

He has had an upright C-spine x-ray, which revealed good alignment of the C-spine. He also underwent flexion and extension views of his C-spine, which revealed only approximately 1 mm of subluxation at the C3-4 level on flexion. Therefore, the neurosurgical team deemed that he does not require any operative fixation, and he can be maintained without a cervical collar.

His hospital course has been complicated by a number of issues. Most significantly, he was experiencing episodes of hypoxemia during his admission. He also had some abdominal distention at the same time, and a CT scan revealed free air in the abdomen. He was subsequently taken to the operating room on October 14, 20XX, where a perforation of his transverse colon was found. He underwent a subtotal colectomy with an ileostomy and mucous fistula. Subsequent to this, he developed a collection in his left lower quadrant, which was enhancing on a contrast-enhanced CT scan. Therefore, an ultrasound-guided percutaneous drain was inserted by interventional radiology. This drain was removed on October 31, 20XX. He also has recently developed an abdominal wound infection. The lower end of the wound was therefore opened and is being packed with saline-soaked gauze. There is a small 1-cm area in the upper two thirds of the incision that is also open and that is also being packed.

The patient has had recurrent episodes of desaturation associated with lobar, segmental, and subsegmental collapse. He has undergone a number of bronchoscopies for mucous plugging but has not had any bronchoscopies for over a week. His chest x-ray from November 2, 20XX, revealed some collapse of the right lower lobe and a small infiltrate of the right middle and right lower lobes. His white blood count was 10.5, he has not had a fever, and he has therefore not been started on any antibiotics.

The patient had a tracheostomy performed on October 16, 20XX. The nurse pointed out to me today that there is an area of skin breakdown inferior to the tracheostomy. This did not appear to be infected, but certainly this will need to be observed closely.

He had a PEG tube inserted on October 31, 20XX. Initially, GI had seen him and was going to put in a PEG tube. They noted severe esophagitis but also could not locate the stomach when they were inserting their finder needle. They, therefore, abandoned their attempts. He had his PEG tube inserted by radiology on October 31, 20XX, without any problems. He has been tolerating his feeds since then and is at his goal rate of 65 mL an hour of TraumaCal.

His current lines include a right radial arterial line, a right PICC line, his tracheostomy, and his Foley catheter. As mentioned above, he also has an ileostomy and a mucous fistula. The ileostomy has been functioning well.

His current medications include Fragmin 5000 units subcutaneously once a day and Prevacid 30 mg via PEG tube twice a day. The plan for this is to continue at this dose for 12 weeks, which would end on February 25, 20XX, and then switch him to 30 mg once a day. This is because of his severe esophagitis. He is also on gabapentin 300 mg via the PEG tube 3 times a day. He is also on nortriptyline 25 mg via PEG tube each night. He has also been taking Percocet for neck pain, and we have been in the process of weaning that down. He was to be given Percocet 2 tablets every 8 hours via PEG tube for 5 days and then starting November 4, 20XX, we were going to drop him to 1 tablet every 6 hours for 5 days, and then down to every 8 hours for 5 days, then every 12 hours for 5 days, and then hopefully discontinue. He has not complained of any increased neck pain while we have been weaning the Percocet.

His most recent laboratory work was from November 2, 20XX. This revealed a white blood count of 10.5, hemoglobin of 98, and platelets of 575,000. His INR was 1.24 with a PTT of 25.4. His last blood gas was 7.43, 37, 40, and 97, and that was done at 0500 hours on November 2, 20XX. His ventilation parameters at that point were PRVC of 600 mL at a rate of 12 breaths per minute with an FIO2 of 0.6 and a PEEP of 10. Since that time, he has come down to an FIO2 of 0.4 with all the other parameters being the same. His saturations have been excellent on those settings.

To continue his lab work, his last sodium was 137, potassium 4.5, chloride 102, total CO2 of 27, random glucose 5.8, urea 3.8, and creatinine 46. His phosphorus has been mildly elevated at 1.6, his magnesium was 0.78, and his calcium was 2.29 with an albumin of 27.

I believe that summarizes the patient's course to the present. If you have any questions at all, please feel free to contact us at the neurotrauma intensive care unit. Thank you very much for accepting this patient in transfer. It is very much appreciated.

Sample Reports

OCCIPITOCERVICAL FUSION FROM OCCIPUT TO C5

PREOPERATIVE DIAGNOSES: Occipitocervical instability, syringomyelia C2-C4.

POSTOPERATIVE DIAGNOSES: Occipitocervical instability, syringomyelia C2-C4.

PROCEDURE PERFORMED: Occipitocervical fusion from occiput to C5.

DESCRIPTION OF PROCEDURE: My part of the operation included basically exposing the cervical spine by subperiosteal dissection from occiput down to C7. We went out to the lateral and to the facet capsules bilaterally to the rounded portion. We cleaned all the soft tissue off the joints, and we noticed that the C4-5 joint had been completely disrupted; C2 and C3 were fused. C1 was assimilated to occiput.

I did use an awl technique to go in the center of the lateral mass and then, through the technique described in the literature, placed awl holes at C3, C4, and C5 and also bilaterally. I drilled a 14-mm drill hole into each lateral mass, then tapped and then placed vertex 3.5 x 14-mm screws in C3, C4, and C5 bilaterally with excellent purchase. I also used a Cahill T-plate from Sofamor Danek which was placed in the sub occiput at the keyhole level. Three 10-mm screws sequentially below the inion were placed in the midline. We used the awl, then drilled 10 mm and then tapped, and a 10-mm cancellous screw was then screwed in with excellent purchase, basically at all 3 levels of the plate. A vertex with a connector system to the actual Cahill T-plate was then bent accordingly from the occiput to cervical region, and a machine screw was placed into the connector of the occiput area, then placed over the rotating heads of the vertex system, and then the locking cap was tightened at C3, C4, and C5. On the opposite side, only C4 and C5 could be used because of the nature of the significant acute angle of the actual occiput cervical region, and we purchased it as well.

We then decorticated the occipital and cervical regions throughout over the facet capsules and occiput area. We took the harvested bone from the laminectomy, cleaned it of all subperiosteal attachments and also morcellized allograft and packed it laterally and occipitally for our fusion. It was then irrigated copiously, and the drain was placed. Closure was initiated with subfascial 0 Vicryl in a watertight fashion and then 3-0 Vicryl and staples for the skin. A dry sterile dressing was placed.

The patient was rotated back onto the stretcher, extubated and noted to be in stable condition moving all 4 extremities. Dr. Blank will be dictating the procedure of the decompressive laminectomy, suboccipital craniectomy and syringotomy, and syringosubarachnoid shunt.

OPEN REDUCTION THORACIC SPINE FRACTURE

PREOPERATIVE DIAGNOSES: T8 and T10 compression fractures.

POSTOPERATIVE DIAGNOSES: T8 and T10 compression fractures.

PROCEDURE PERFORMED: T8 and T10 open reduction of compression fracture, application of prosthetic device as well as deep open biopsy of the vertebral bodies of T8 and T10.

DESCRIPTION OF PROCEDURE: The patient was brought to operating room, positioned supine, and underwent general endotracheal anesthesia. The patient was rotated onto bolsters. Under fluoroscopic guidance, the operation was conducted. The thoracic region was prepped and draped in the usual sterile fashion. Then a needle localization was performed localizing the level of T8 under fluoroscopic guidance with a 22-gauge needle.

Starting on the right side, we then made a stab incision over the area of T8 pedicle on the right, and we made the incision down to subcutaneous fat. We then directed an 11-gauge Tuohy needle into the pedicle of T8 and directed it transcuticular. The trajectory was going medial into the vertebral body fracture. After this was performed, we exchanged it with a guidewire, and an osseous introducer was placed in the posterior cortex of the vertebral body. Then we used a bone-filling device without the stylet to direct the needle anteriorly into the vertebral body fracture. On AP view it was noted that the trajectory was quite medial to the midline. We decided to go unilateral as our approach. We put the stylet back into the bone-filling device, cleared a channel, and then placed a balloon into the actual vertebral body and blew it up to 300 psi, filled it to approximately 2 mL, deflated it, and then we placed methylmethacrylate impregnated with antibiotics into the void that was created by the balloon tamp through a bone-filling device and directed that into the vertebral body which was filled very well. Approximately 3 mL were actually delivered into the vertebral body with excellent filling.

After that was completed we then did the same exact procedure at T10 bilaterally with excellent filling. During the T8 procedure we also took a vertebral biopsy by directing the bone-filling device anteriorly. We took a core biopsy of the actual bone and sent it for pathology. We did the exact same procedure at T10. In terms of filling, we filled approximately 3 mL on either side with excellent filling of the vertebral body. We also had a biopsy taken at that level as well. After that was completed, we irrigated copiously, and then placed a staple along the incision line at each level. We had x-rays performed to confirm our postoperative procedure, and then we placed dry sterile dressing. The patient was rotated onto the stretcher, extubated, and noted to be in stable condition moving all 4 extremities.

Optical Tracking System Supratentorial Reopening of Craniotomy for Resection of Temporal Lobe Tumor

Preoperative Diagnosis: Large temporal tumor.

Postoperative Diagnosis: Large temporal tumor.

Procedure Performed: Supratentorial reopening of craniotomy for resection of temporal lobe tumor using optical tracking system stereotaxis.

Indications for Procedure: This patient is a 34-year-old woman who previously had a craniotomy in India, and she said that "dead tissue" was removed and her headaches improved. Two weeks prior to the admission she noted increased symptoms with vomiting, shoulder pain, and her right eye turning outward. CT showed a large temporal tumor. Informed consent was obtained and she was taken to surgery.

Description of Procedure: The patient was placed under adequate general anesthesia. An endotracheal tube, arterial line, central line, and Foley catheter were placed. OTS stereotaxis was employed and Sugita 4-point head pin fixation. Registration was done; it was accepted and confirmed visually.

She had had an incision from her previous procedure, and we basically used this incision other than the part that was going down on her face and crossing her facial nerve. We reopened the previous craniotomy and exposed the brain, and there was clearly abnormal-looking tissue and expanded gyri and sulci.

We used the neuronavigational system to get us down to the tumor, and then we began an internal debulking of this very large lesion. Quick section diagnosis showed a "high-grade glial tumor." We debulked the tumor as best as possible. I believe there was some going up to the sylvian fissure, and there was the possibility of some residual left there. We debulked as much as possible. At one point there was small entry into the ventricle, but this was immediately covered with Gelfoam.

Once we had completed the resection, we obtained excellent hemostasis. The dura was then closed, the bone replaced with miniplates, and the scalp closed in the usual fashion in multiple layers and dressings were applied.

In the recovery room, she was awake and following commands x4 without any drift. All counts were correct and there were no complications.

Reexploration Posterior Cervical Area with Hardware Removal

Preoperative Diagnosis: C3-C4 and C4-C5 cervical spinal stenosis.

Postoperative Diagnosis: C3-C4 and C4-C5 cervical spinal stenosis.

Procedure Performed: Reexploration posterior cervical area with removal of hardware C5, C6, and C7 bilaterally, bilateral decompressive laminectomy L3-L4 and L4-L5, axis titanium screw plate segmental fixation C3, C4, C5, C6, and C7 bilateral, arthrodesis interfacet C3-C4, C4-C5 bilateral.

Anesthesia: General endotracheal.

Description of Procedure: In the operating room routine monitoring devices were placed. General anesthesia and endotracheal intubation were carried out. Baseline somatosensory evoked potentials obtained. Three-pin Mayfield headrest was then placed, Foley catheter was in place, prophylactic antibiotics and IV steroids were given. The patient was turned to the prone position and all dependent areas were padded. The head, neck, and body were in neutral position. Lateral cervical spine films show excellent normal alignment from C5 up. The patient was known to have a fusion from C5 through C7.

The posterior cervical wound was opened and extended superiorly and careful dissection carried out, as there was no lamina at C5, C6, and C7. The spinous processes at C3 and C4 and the lamina and facet complexes were completely exposed and inferior exposure spanned down to the level of T1. The axis plates in the bilateral C5, C6, and C7 areas were now exposed. The screws at C5, C6, and C7 were then removed allowing removal of the plate. A solid interfacet fusion was apparent from C5 to C7.

Now a laminectomy was carried out in usual fashion at C3-C4 and C4-C5 with Leksell and 2-mm Kerrison. This was carried out to the level of the pedicles bilaterally. A total neural decompression was thus achieved. Now reapplication of the fixation device was undertaken first with drilling of the facet joint at C4-C5 and C3-C4 bilaterally. Next drill holes were made roughly in the middle of the facets at C3 and C4 on the right side, and then an awl was used in a superolateral direction paralleling roughly the screws placed at C5, C6, and C7. Once drilling was begun, it was continued to 14 mm at C4 and 12 mm at C3. This was done correspondingly on the left side. The depth gauge was used to ascertain that bicortical purchase was now possible with screw placement at these depths. A 6-hole axis plate was obtained, trimmed down to a 5-level plate, and recontoured to fit flat over the facet complexes from C3 to C7 bilaterally. Now the previously removed screws at C5, C6, and C7, which were 14-mm screws, were now placed. A tap was used to screw the screw holes at C3 and C4, and then a 12-mm screw was placed at C3, and 14-mm screws were placed at C4 bilaterally. All screws yielded excellent purchase. The plate-and-screw construct was quite solid bilaterally. It should be noted that prior to placement of the plate, however, the drilled-out interfacet joints at C3 and C4-C5 were stuffed with autologous bone harvested during the laminectomy. Bone was also placed lateral to the decorticated facet complexes at C3-C4 and C4-C5.

Once the construct and arthrodesis were completed, thorough irrigation was carried out. Gelfoam was placed over the exposed dura and an extradural Hemovac exited through a separate wound and attached to a self-suctioning device. The wound was then closed in anatomical layers with a multilayer closure of the ligamentum nuchae, followed by a multilayer closure of the fascia and the skin was finally closed with skin staples and a sterile dressing. The patient tolerated the procedure well. The evoked potentials remained stable throughout the case. The patient was awake, alert, extubated, moving all his extremities, and following commands with normal strength prior to leaving the operating room. He was taken to the recovery room in stable condition.

DRAINS: One extradural Hemovac.

ESTIMATED BLOOD LOSS: 250 mL.

REPEAT CRANIOTOMY, VASCULAR ABNORMALITY RESECTION, ICP MONITOR PLACEMENT

PREOPERATIVE DIAGNOSIS: Obstructive hydrocephalus due to cerebellar hematoma.

POSTOPERATIVE DIAGNOSES: Obstructive hydrocephalus due to cerebellar hematoma; occult vascular abnormality.

PROCEDURE PERFORMED: Repeat craniotomy for clot, resection of vascular abnormality. Intracranial pressure monitor.

INDICATIONS FOR PROCEDURE: The patient was admitted with obstructive hydrocephalus due to posterior fossa cerebellar hematoma. He was treated shortly following admission with emergency suboccipital craniotomy for evacuation of the clot. Postoperatively he appeared improved initially, but then deteriorated neurologically, and followup imaging studies demonstrated persistence of the obstructive hydrocephalus with cerebellar hematoma. After discussing the rationale, risks, and procedure of surgery, the following operation was undertaken.

Description of Procedure: With the patient generally anesthetized, prone on the bolster frame, and head in pin fixation, previous suboccipital craniectomy site was reopened.

The bony removal was extended across the midline and down to the foramen magnum. Previous dural opening was extended, and the hematoma presenting at the cortical surface was suctioned away, and the removal of the clot led to a deeper cavity from which persistent arterial hemorrhage was encountered.The operating microscope was wheeled into place, and the remainder of the dissection was performed using microneurosurgical technique.

Further resection of clot from the depths of the cavity led to identification of a cluster of abnormal vessels which appeared to have been the origin of the hematoma. We spent considerable time systematically coagulating the abnormal vessels to eventually secure careful hemostasis.

Once we were satisfied that the clot had been adequately evacuated and that meticulous hemostasis had been achieved, we irrigated the wound with hydrogen peroxide and with Ringer lactate before closing the dura, leaving a subdural intracranial pressure monitoring catheter in place.

The scalp wound was closed in layers in the usual fashion, and the suboccipital muscles were approximated and the skin closed with staples.

At the conclusion of the procedure, the patient was discharged from the operating room in good condition.

Revision Ventriculoperitoneal Shunt

Preoperative Diagnosis: Ventriculoperitoneal shunt requiring replacement.

Postoperative Diagnosis: Ventriculoperitoneal shunt requiring replacement.

Procedure Performed: Revision of ventriculoperitoneal shunt, insertion of new ventriculoperitoneal shunt, bur hole and removal of foreign body from the ventricle and repair of cerebrospinal fluid leak, all under magnification vision, advancement flap and plastic repair of the skin for a distance of 5 cm removing 2.5-cm scar.

Description of Procedure: With the patient under adequate general endotracheal anesthesia, he was placed supine on the operating table, head turned to the left, and prepped and draped in the usual fashion for ventriculoperitoneal shunt. The skin was infiltrated with 0.5% Xylocaine with 1:200,000 epinephrine and the abdominal incision opened. We came upon a catheter that was large, within muscle and subcutaneous tissue, and once free of this tissue did drain clear fluid. It was a slit-valve catheter, and we could not maintain a competent shunt without totally replacing the distal catheter and placing an appropriate pressure shunt on the cranium; a medium pressure Codman shunt adult size was chosen.

We then created an incision in the posterior temporooccipital region on the right side close to the path of the shunt and parallel to the flushing chambers of the inner shunt. We isolated this. It was difficult because of the scarring and calcifications that occurred but we isolated it, placed a clamp proximal to the flushing chambers in order to occlude the shunt and then transected the flushing chambers from the proximal end. We attempted to remove the entire system from the distal end unsuccessfully. We then passed a passer from the cranial to the abdominal incision and passed down the catheter and removed the passer. We created a subgaleal pocket for the pumping mechanism of the shunt. A bur hole was placed at the site of the incision and the dura cauterized and incised, the pia arachnoid seared and incised. The ventricular catheter passed on the first pass; 8 cm into the right lateral ventricle, and crystal-clear fluid came out. This was collected and sent for appropriate studies. A curved plastic holder was sutured to the periosteum with 4-0 silk. The entire apparatus set well, pumped well, and emptied very nicely.

We attempted to remove the LeRoy reservoir from this incision but were unable to do so, and therefore we went to the cranial incision which had healed with a widened scar. We infiltrated this with 0.5% Xylocaine with 1:200,000 epinephrine. An incision was made excising the entire scar which was on the anterior border of the curvilinear incision. Meticulous hemostasis was obtained. We cut down upon a LeRoy reservoir that had been partially enclosed in cranium, and it was easily removed, but CSF came out of the hole through which the catheter of the reservoir passed. We irrigated and demonstrated no blood. A pledget of Gelfoam was placed within the passage of the catheter, gained access to the cranium, and then bone was pressed down over this. A watertight seal was achieved. We then created a flap of periosteum that was secured on the medial side and sewed this down over the hole that had been filled with Gelfoam and treated with bone wax. This was secured with multiple 4-0 Vicryl sutures.

We then turned our attention to the skin where an incision was made through the dermis of the scar, and then the posterior margins of the galea were dissected off the skin and the scar removed. We then sutured galea and skin together with inverted 4-0 Vicryl and closed the skin with running subcuticular 4-0 Monocryl obtaining watertight and cosmetic closure. We now turned our attention to the distal end and demonstrated the peritoneal cavity which was then opened between clamps using sharp dissection and passed the distal end of the catheter into the peritoneal cavity under direct vision after checking and demonstrating excellent flow.

The wound was then closed in layers with pursestring 4-0 Vicryl to the peritoneum, interrupted 4-0 Vicryl to rectus sheath and fascia, subcutaneous 4-0 Vicryl, and running 4-0 Monocryl subcuticularly. Dressings of Bacitracin ointment and Steri-Strips were applied. The patient tolerated the procedure well. All counts were correct at the end of the procedure, and the patient was returned to the recovery room in excellent condition.

SUBDURAL DRAIN PLACEMENT

PROCEDURE PERFORMED: Subdural drain placement.

ANESTHESIA: Local and neuroleptic anesthesia.

DRAIN: Subdural drain.

SPECIMEN: Nil.

COMPLICATIONS: Nil.

BLOOD TRANSFUSION: Nil.

BLOOD LOSS: Minimal.

CLINICAL HISTORY: The patient is a 45-year-old lady with past medical history of migraine. She is not on any blood thinner, and 10 days ago she developed sudden-onset right-sided headache. No history of nausea. No history of vomiting. Headache was worse with changing posture. No history of weakness, seizure, or change in vision. There was no history of trauma. The patient had a CT at another hospital which showed right subdural hematoma, and she was transferred to our hospital.

On exam, the patient was neurologically intact. CT showed right subacute subdural hematoma with mass effect and midline shift. A discussion was held with the family regarding surgical intervention, and risks and benefits were explained. The plan was, because of absence of clear cause for the hematoma, to arrange some investigations after the evacuation.

OPERATIVE REPORT: The patient was brought to the OR. She was put in the supine position, head tilted to the left side. Head was put on a donut headrest. We identified the place for the incision, about 3 cm above the right ear and 4 cm in front of the ear, just above the origin of the temporalis muscle. A small strip of hair was shaved. Lidocaine 5 mL with epinephrine was injected, and the skin was prepped and draped in the usual sterile manner.

The anesthetist started giving the patient a dose of neuroleptic medication. We made the skin incision with a straight incision about 3 cm straight to the skull. Bleeding from the skin was controlled using bipolar. The pericranium was elevated using a periosteal elevator. Using the pneumatic drill, one bur hole was made. Upon exposure of the dura, there was a vessel of the dura which was coagulated. The rest of the dura was coagulated. Small bleeding was coming from the epidural space beneath the bone edges, which was coagulated. Dura was opened in cruciate incision without opening the membrane of the hematoma and the edges of the dura were sewn together. Then we coagulated the membrane of the hematoma, and a small incision was made, and the liquefied hematoma started to come out. We applied pressure to prevent air entry. Meanwhile, a subdural drain was passed through the skin to exit at a point about 5 cm in front of the site of incision and, with the help of Adson, the drain was inserted inside the subdural space. After inserting the drain, it was tested by attaching it to empty bulb suction, and this system was working. After that a small piece of Gelfoam was put in the bur hole. Hemostasis was secured with bipolar. Hemostasis was satisfactory. After that the galea was closed with 3 interrupted absorbable stitches. The scalp was closed with staples.

The patient tolerated the procedure and was transferred to recovery in stable condition.

Appendix 9

Common Terms by Procedure

Cervical Laminectomy, Removal Epidural Hematoma

3-0 Dexon
bone wax
cervical laminectomy
epidural hematoma
epidural space
Gelfoam
hemostasis
Hemovac drain
lateral gutter
ligamentum nuchae
ligamentum nuchae suture
paraspinal muscle
skin staple
spinal cord compression
stab incision
subcutaneous hematoma
Weitlaner retractor

Craniotomy, Evacuation of Clot, and Temporal Lobectomy

0 Vicryl
3-0 nylon
4-0 Surgilon
B14 attachment
Bentall tool
bipolar cautery
bleeders
Bovie cautery
bur hole
cistern
clot cavity
cranial fossa
craniotomy
curvilinear incision
dura
epispinal space
frontotemporal parietal craniotomy
frontotemporal parietal region
Gelfoam
gyrus
hemorrhagic
Hemovac
Kerlix wrap
Kerrison punch
keyhole
Leksell rongeur
Mayfield head clamp
miniplates
musculocutaneous flap
Oxycel
perforating towel clamp
pinna
shoulder roll
sphenoid ridge
subcutaneous Vicryl
subgaleal region
subperiosteal dissection
subperiosteum
subtemporal decompression
Surgicel
temporal fossa
temporal gyrus
temporal lobectomy
temporalis muscle
temporoparietal clot
tentorial edge
tragus
zygoma

Lumbar Fusion

0 Vicryl
3-0 nylon
3-0 Vicryl
annulotomy
annulus
Cell Saver blood

decorticate
demineralized bone matrix
epidural space
extubate
femoral head
fluoroscopic guidance
fluoroscopy
Gelfoam
interbody allograft spacer
interspace
intertransverse region
intramedullary bone
Kerrison rongeur
lamina
laminectomy
Leksell rongeur
ligamentum
local autograft
locking cap
lumbar interbody fusion
lumbodorsal fascia
morcellized allograft
pedicle
pedicle finder
pedicle probe
pedicle screw
pedicle tap
rotating head
sacral ala
subperiosteal dissection
Synthes PLIF set
Wilson frame

Lumbar Hemilaminectomy

0 Vicryl
3-0 nylon
3-0 Vicryl
axial angle
cartilaginous
Depo-Medrol
disk space
diskectomy
dural
endotracheal anesthesia
epidural space
epispinal space
facet capsule
fascia
fasciectomy
foramina
Gelfoam
hemilaminectomy
Hemovac
herniated disk
Kerrison punch
lamina
Leksell rongeur
lumbar dorsal fascia
nerve root
pedicle
self-retaining retractor
staple
subperiosteal dissection
upbiting curette
Wilson frame

Neurological Symptoms and Weakness: Chart Note

2D echocardiogram
Aggrenox
blackout
bruit
diuretic
encephalic cyst
intracranial pathology
motor loss
MR scan
occipital area
porencephalic cyst
precordium
structural disease
ultrasound Doppler carotid study

Neurotrauma Gunshot Wound: Discharge Summary

abdominal distention
asystole
bradycardia
bronchoscopy
cervical collar
clavicle
collection
comminuted fracture
contrast-enhanced CT scan
C-spine
CT angiogram
desaturation
dopamine
esophagitis
facet
finder needle
Foley catheter
Fragmin
free air
gabapentin
hypotensive
hypoxemic
ileostomy
interventional radiology
intubate
lamina
lobar collapse
mandible
mucous fistula
mucous plugging
neurosurgical
neurotrauma intensive care unit
nortriptyline
operative fixation
paraspinal soft tissue
PEG tube
Percocet
PICC line
Prevacid
quadriplegic
radial arterial line
saline-soaked gauze
segmental collapse
subluxation
subsegmental collapse
subtotal colectomy
tracheostomy
transverse colon
TraumaCal
ultrasound-guided percutaneous drain
upright C-spine x-ray
vascular injury
ventilation parameter
ventilator
ventilatory effort

Occipitocervical Fusion from Occiput to C5

3-0 Vicryl
awl hole
awl technique
Cahill T-plate
cancellous screw
cervical spine
connector system
decorticate
facet capsule
harvested bone
inion
keyhole level
laminectomy
locking cap
machine screw
morcellized allograft
occipitocervical fusion
occipitocervical instability
occiput
purchase
staple
subfascial 0 Vicryl

subperiosteal attachment
subperiosteal dissection
syringomyelia
vertex
vertex system

Open Reduction Thoracic Spine Fracture

11-gauge Tuohy needle
22-gauge needle
balloon
balloon tamp
bolster
bone-filling device
compression fracture
core biopsy
endotracheal anesthesia
fluoroscopic guidance
guide wire
localization needle
methylmethacrylate
open biopsy
open reduction
osseous introducer
pedicle
posterior cortex
prosthetic device
stab incision
stylet
subcutaneous fat
thoracic region
trajectory
transcuticular
vertebral biopsy
vertebral body

Optical Tracking System Supratentorial Reopening of Craniotomy for Resection of Temporal Lobe Tumor

arterial line
central line
craniotomy
dura
endotracheal tube
Foley catheter
Gelfoam
glial tumor
gyrus
hemostasis
internal debulking
miniplate
neuronavigational system
optical tracking system (OTS)
registration
resection
stereotaxis
Sugita 4-point head pin
sulcus
supratentorial reopening
sylvian fissure
temporal lobe tumor
temporal tumor
ventricle

Reexploration Posterior Cervical Area with Hardware Removal

3-pin Mayfield headrest
5-level plate
6-hole axis plate
arthrodesis
autologous bone
awl
axis plate
axis titanium screw plate
bicortical purchase
cervical spinal stenosis
decompressive laminectomy
decorticated facet complex
depth gauge
drill hole
dura
endotracheal intubation

extradural Hemovac drain
facet complex
facet joint
fascia
fixation device
Foley catheter
Gelfoam
interfacet fusion
interfacet joint
IV steroid
Kerrison
lamina
laminectomy
Leksell
ligamentum nuchae
multilayer closure
neural decompression
pedicle
plate-and-screw construct
prophylactic antibiotic
segmental fixation
self-suctioning device
skin staple
somatosensory evoked potential
spinous process
tap

Repeat Craniotomy, Vascular Abnormality Resection, ICP Monitor Placement

arterial hemorrhage
bolster frame
cerebellar hematoma
cortical surface
craniotomy
dissection
dural opening
foramen magnum
hemostasis
hydrogen peroxide
ICP monitor
microneurosurgical technique
obstructive hydrocephalus
occult vascular abnormality
operating microscope
pin fixation
posterior fossa
resection
Ringer lactate
subdural intracranial pressure monitoring catheter
suboccipital craniotomy
suboccipital muscle

Revision Ventriculoperitoneal Shunt

0.5% Xylocaine
4-0 Monocryl
4-0 silk
4-0 Vicryl suture
advancement flap
Bacitracin ointment
bur hole
calcification
catheter
clear spinal fluid (CSF)
Codman shunt
cosmetic closure
cranium
CSF leak
curved plastic holder
curvilinear incision
dermis
distal catheter
dura
endotracheal anesthesia
epinephrine
flushing chamber
galea
Gelfoam
hemostasis
LeRoy reservoir
magnification vision
passer

periosteum
peritoneal cavity
pia arachnoid
plastic repair
pledget
posterior temporooccipital region
pumping mechanism
pursestring 4-0 Vicryl
rectus sheath
slit-valve catheter
Steri-Strips
subcutaneous tissue
subgaleal pocket
ventricle
ventricular catheter
ventriculoperitoneal shunt
watertight seal

Subdural Drain Placement

Adson
air entry
bipolar
bone edge
bur hole
coagulate
cruciate incision
CT
donut headrest
dura
empty bulb suction
epidural space
epinephrine
Gelfoam
hematoma
hemostasis
interrupted absorbable stitch
lidocaine
liquefied hematoma
mass effect
midline shift
neuroleptic anesthesia
neuroleptic medication
pericranium
periosteal elevator
pneumatic drill
staple
subdural drain
subdural hematoma
subdural space
temporalis muscle

Appendix 10

Drugs by Indication

ALZHEIMER DISEASE

Acetylcholinesterase Inhibitor
- Aricept® [US/Can]
- Cognex® [US]
- donepezil
- Exelon® [US/Can]
- rivastigmine
- tacrine

Acetylcholinesterase Inhibitor (Central)
- galantamine
- Reminyl® [US/Can]

Cholinergic Agent
- Exelon® [US/Can]
- rivastigmine

Ergot Alkaloid and Derivative
- ergoloid mesylates
- Hydergine® [Can]

N-Methyl-D-Aspartate Receptor Antagonist
- memantine
- Namenda™ [US]

AMYOTROPHIC LATERAL SCLEROSIS (ALS)

Anticholinergic Agent
- Atropine

Cholinergic Agent
- Mestinon®-SR [Can]
- Mestinon® Timespan® [US]
- Mestinon® [US/Can]
- pyridostigmine

Miscellaneous Product
- Rilutek® [US/Can]
- riluzole

Skeletal Muscle Relaxant
- Apo-Baclofen® [Can]
- baclofen
- Gen-Baclofen [Can]
- Lioresal® [US/Can]
- Liotec [Can]
- Nu-Baclo [Can]
- PMS-Baclofen [Can]

BEHÇET SYNDROME

Immunosuppressant Agent
- Alti-Azathioprine [Can]
- Apo-Azathioprine® [Can]
- Apo-Cyclosporine® [Can]
- Azasan® [US]
- azathioprine
- cyclosporine
- Gen-Azathioprine [Can]
- Gengraf® [US]
- Imuran® [US/Can]
- Neoral® [US/Can]
- Restasis™ [US]
- Rhoxal-cyclosporine [Can]
- Sandimmune® I.V. [Can]
- Sandimmune® [US]

CEREBRAL PALSY

Skeletal Muscle Relaxant
- Dantrium® [US/Can]
- dantrolene

CLAUDICATION

Blood Viscosity Reducer Agent
- Albert® Pentoxifylline [Can]
- Apo-Pentoxifylline SR® [Can]
- Nu-Pentoxifylline SR [Can]
- pentoxifylline
- Pentoxil® [US]
- ratio-Pentoxifylline [Can]
- Trental® [US/Can]

CUSHING SYNDROME

Antineoplastic Agent
- aminoglutethimide
- Cytadren® [US]

CUSHING SYNDROME (DIAGNOSTIC)

Diagnostic Agent
- Metopirone® [US]
- metyrapone

DEEP VEIN THROMBOSIS (DVT)

Anticoagulant (Other)
- Apo-Warfarin® [Can]
- Coumadin® [US/Can]
- dalteparin
- danaparoid
- enoxaparin
- Fragmin® [US/Can]
- Gen-Warfarin [Can]
- Hepalean® [Can]
- Hepalean® Leo [Can]
- Hepalean®-LOK [Can]
- heparin
- Hep-Lock® [US]
- Innohep® [US/Can]
- Lovenox® HP [Can]
- Lovenox® [US/Can]
- Orgaran® [Can]
- Taro-Warfarin [Can]
- tinzaparin
- warfarin

Factor Xa Inhibitor
- Arixtra® [US/Can]
- fondaparinux

Low Molecular Weight Heparin
- Fraxiparine™ [Can]
- Fraxiparine™ Forte [Can]
- nadroparin (Canada only)

DYSTONIA

Neuromuscular Blocker Agent, Toxin
- botulinum toxin type B
- Myobloc® [US]

EPICONDYLITIS

Nonsteroidal Antiinflammatory Drug (NSAID)
- Advil® Children's [US-OTC]
- Advil®Infants' [US-OTC]
- Advil® Junior [US-OTC]
- Advil® [US-OTC/Can]
- Aleve® [US-OTC]
- Anaprox® DS [US/Can]
- Anaprox® [US/Can]
- Apo-Ibuprofen® [Can]
- Apo-Indomethacin® [Can]
- Apo-Napro-Na® [Can]
- Apo-Napro-Na DS® [Can]
- Apo-Naproxen® [Can]
- Apo-Naproxen SR® [Can]
- EC-Naprosyn® [US]
- Gen-Naproxen EC [Can]
- Genpril® [US-OTC]
- Ibu-200 [US-OTC]
- ibuprofen
- Indocid® [Can]
- Indocid® P.D.A. [Can]
- Indocin® SR [US]
- Indocin® [US/Can]
- Indo-Lemmon [Can]
- indomethacin
- Indotec [Can]
- I-Prin [US-OTC]
- lansoprazole and naproxen
- Menadol® [US-OTC]
- Midol® Maximum Strength Cramp Formula [US-OTC]
- Motrin® Children's [US-OTC/Can]
- Motrin® IB [US-OTC/Can]
- Motrin® Infants' [US-OTC]
- Motrin® Junior Strength [US-OTC]
- Motrin® [US/Can]
- Naprelan® [US]
- Naprosyn® [US/Can]
- naproxen
- Naxen(R) [Can]

Novo-Methacin [Can]
Novo-Naprox EC [Can]
Novo-Naprox [Can]
Novo-Naprox Sodium [Can]
Novo-Naprox Sodium DS [Can]
Novo-Naprox SR [Can]
Novo-Profen® [Can]
Nu-Ibuprofen [Can]
Nu-Indo [Can]
Nu-Naprox [Can]
Rhodacine® [Can]
Riva-Naproxen [Can]
Ultraprin [US-OTC]

EPILEPSY

Anticonvulsant
acetazolamide
Alti-Clobazam [Can]
Alti-Divalproex [Can]
Apo-Acetazolamide® [Can]
Apo-Carbamazepine® [Can]
Apo-Clobazam® [Can]
Apo-Divalproex® [Can]
Apo-Gabapentin® [Can]
Apo-Lamotrigine® [Can]
carbamazepine
Carbatrol® [US]
Celontin® [US/Can]
clobazam (Canada only)
Depacon® [US]
Depakene® [US/Can]
Depakote® Delayed Release [US]
Depakote® ER [US]
Depakote® Sprinkle(R) [US]
Diamox® [Can]
Diamox® Sequels® [US]
Epitol® [US]
Epival® ER [Can]
Epival® I.V. [Can]
ethosuximide
felbamate
Felbatol® [US]
Frisium® [Can]
gabapentin
Gabitril® [US/Can]
Gen-Carbamazepine CR [Can]
Gen-Divalproex [Can]
Lamictal® [US/Can]
lamotrigine
magnesium sulfate
methsuximide
Neurontin® [US/Can]
Novo-Carbamaz [Can]
Novo-Clobazam [Can]
Novo-Divalproex [Can]
Novo-Gabapentin [Can]
Nu-Carbamazepine® [Can]
Nu-Divalproex [Can]
Nu-Gabapentin [Can]
PMS-Carbamazepine [Can]
PMS-Clobazam [Can]
PMS-Gabapentin [Can]
PMS-Lamotrigine [Can]
PMS-Valproic Acid [Can]
PMS-Valproic Acid E.C. [Can]
ratio-Lamotrigine [Can]
Rhoxal-valproic [Can]
Sabril® [Can]
Taro-Carbamazepine Chewable [Can]
Tegretol® [US/Can]
Tegretol®-XR [US]
tiagabine
Topamax® [US/Can]
topiramate
valproic acid and derivatives
vigabatrin (Canada only)
Zarontin® [US/Can]

Anticonvulsant, Miscellaneous
Keppra® [US/Can]
levetiracetam
oxcarbazepine
Trileptal® [US/Can]

Anticonvulsant, Sulfonamide
Zonegran™ [US/Can]
zonisamide

Antidepressant
- Alti-Clobazam [Can]
- Apo-Clobazam® [Can]
- clobazam (Canada only)
- Frisium® [Can]
- Novo-Clobazam [Can]
- PMS-Clobazam [Can]

Barbiturate
- amobarbital
- Amytal® [US/Can]
- Apo-Primidone® [Can]
- Luminal® Sodium [US]
- Mebaral® [US/Can]
- mephobarbital
- Mysoline® [US/Can]
- phenobarbital
- PMS-Phenobarbital [Can]
- primidone

Benzodiazepine
- Alti-Clonazepam [Can]
- Apo-Clonazepam® [Can]
- Apo-Clorazepate® [Can]
- Apo-Oxazepam® [Can]
- Clonapam [Can]
- clonazepam
- clorazepate
- Gen-Clonazepam [Can]
- Klonopin® [US/Can]
- Novo-Clonazepam [Can]
- Novo-Clopate [Can]
- Novoxapam® [Can]
- Nu-Clonazepam [Can]
- Oxazepam
- Oxpram® [Can]
- PMS-Clonazepam [Can]
- PMS-Oxazepam [Can]
- Rho-Clonazepam [Can]
- Rivotril® [Can]
- Serax® [US]
- Tranxene® SD(TM)-Half Strength [US]
- Tranxene® SD(TM) [US]
- Tranxene® [US]
- T-Tab® [US]

Hydantoin
- Cerebyx® [US/Can]
- Dilantin® [US/Can]
- ethotoin
- fosphenytoin
- Peganone® [US/Can]
- Phenytek™ [US]
- phenytoin

EXTRAPYRAMIDAL SYMPTOMS

Anticholinergic Agent
- Akineton® [US/Can]
- Apo-Benztropine® [Can]
- Apo-Trihex® [Can]
- benztropine
- biperiden
- Cogentin® [US/Can]
- Kemadrin® [US]
- PMS-Procyclidine [Can]
- Procyclid™ [Can]
- procyclidine
- trihexyphenidyl

GAUCHER DISEASE

Enzyme
- alglucerase
- Ceredase® [US]
- Cerezyme® [US/Can]
- imiglucerase

Enzyme Inhibitor
- miglustat
- Zavesca® [US]

GLIOMA

Antineoplastic Agent
- CeeNU® [US/Can]
- lomustine

Antiviral Agent
- interferon alfa-2b and ribavirin combination pack
- Rebetron® [US/Can]

Biological Response Modulator
- interferon alfa-2b
- interferon alfa-2b and ribavirin combination pack
- Intron® A [US/Can]
- Rebetron® [US/Can]

GUILLAIN-BARRÉ SYNDROME

Immune Globulin
- Carimune™ [US]
- Flebogamma® [US]
- Gamimune® N [US/Can]
- Gammagard® S/D [US/Can]
- Gammar®-P I.V. [US]
- Gamunex® [US/Can]
- immune globulin (intravenous)
- Iveegam EN [US]
- Iveegam Immuno® [Can]
- Octagam® [US]
- Panglobulin® [US]
- Polygam® S/D [US]
- Venoglobulin®-S [US]

HARTNUP DISEASE

Vitamin, Water Soluble
- niacinamide

HEAVY METAL POISONING

Antidote
- deferoxamine
- Desferal® [US/Can]
- PMS-Deferoxamine [Can]

HUNTINGTON CHOREA

Monoamine Depleting Agent
- tetrabenazine (Canada only)

INTERMITTENT CLAUDICATION

Platelet Aggregation Inhibitor
- cilostazol
- Pletal® [US/Can]

INTRACRANIAL PRESSURE

Barbiturate
- Pentothal® [US/Can]
- Thiopental

Diuretic, Osmotic
- mannitol

JAPANESE ENCEPHALITIS

Vaccine, Inactivated Virus
- Japanese encephalitis virus vaccine (inactivated)
- JE-VAX® [US/Can]

LEAD POISONING

Chelating Agent
- BAL in Oil® [US]
- Calcium Disodium Versenate® [US]
- Chemet® [US/Can]
- Cuprimine® [US/Can]
- Depen® [US/Can]
- dimercaprol
- edetate calcium disodium
- penicillamine
- succimer

MARFAN SYNDROME

Rauwolfia Alkaloid
- reserpine

MÉNIÈRE DISEASE

Antihistamine
- Antivert® [US/Can]
- betahistine (Canada only)
- Bonamine™ [Can]
- Bonine® [US-OTC/Can]
- Dramamine® Less Drowsy Formula [US-OTC]
- meclizine
- Serc® [Can]

MERCURY POISONING

Chelating Agent
- BAL in Oil® [US]
- Dimercaprol

MULTIPLE SCLEROSIS

Antigout Agent
- colchicine
- ratio-Colchicine [Can]

Biological, Miscellaneous
- Copaxone® [US/Can]
- glatiramer acetate

Biological Response Modulator
- Avonex® [US/Can]
- Betaseron® [US/Can]
- interferon beta-1a
- interferon beta-1b
- Rebif® [US/Can]

Skeletal Muscle Relaxant
- Apo-Baclofen® [Can]
- baclofen
- Dantrium® [US/Can]
- dantrolene
- Gen-Baclofen [Can]
- Lioresal® [US/Can]
- Liotec [Can]
- Nu-Baclo [Can]
- PMS-Baclofen [Can]

MUSCARINE POISONING

Anticholinergic Agent
- atropine

MYASTHENIA GRAVIS

Cholinergic Agent
- ambenonium
- edrophonium
- Enlon® [US/Can]
- Mestinon®-SR [Can]
- Mestinon® Timespan® [US]
- Mestinon® [US/Can]
- Mytelase® [US/Can]
- neostigmine
- Prostigmin® [US/Can]
- pyridostigmine
- Reversol® [US]

NARCOLEPSY

Adrenergic Agonist Agent
- ephedrine

Amphetamine
- Adderall® [US]
- Adderall XR™ [US]
- Desoxyn® [US/Can]
- Dexedrine® [US/Can]
- dextroamphetamine
- dextroamphetamine and amphetamine
- Dextrostat® [US]
- methamphetamine

Central Nervous System Stimulant, Nonamphetamine
- Alertec®[Can]
- Concerta® [US/Can]
- Cylert® [US]
- Metadate® CD [US]
- Metadate™ ER [US]
- Methylin™ ER [US]
- Methylin™ [US]
- methylphenidate
- modafinil
- PemADD® CT [US]
- PemADD® [US]
- pemoline
- PMS-Methylphenidate [Can]
- Provigil® [US/Can]
- Ritalin® LA [US]
- Ritalin-SR® [US/Can]
- Ritalin® [US/Can]

NERVE BLOCK

Local Anesthetic
- AK-T-Caine™ [US]
- Ametop™ [Can]
- Anestacon® [US]
- Band-Aid® Hurt-Free™ Antiseptic Wash [US-OTC]
- Betacaine® [Can]
- bupivacaine

Burnamycin [US-OTC]
Burn Jel [US-OTC]
Burn-O-Jel [US-OTC]
Carbocaine® [Can]
Cepacol Viractin® [US-OTC]
chloroprocaine
Citanest® Plain [US/Can]
LidaMantle® [US]
lidocaine
lidocaine and epinephrine
Lidodan™ [Can]
Lidoderm®[US/Can]
LidoSite™ [US]
L-M-X™ 4 [US-OTC]
L-M-X™ 5 [US-OTC]
Marcaine® Spinal [US]
Marcaine® [US/Can]
mepivacaine
Nesacaine®-CE [Can]
Nesacaine®-MPF [US]
Nesacaine® [US]
Novocain® [US/Can]
Opticaine® [US]
Polocaine® MPF [US]
Polocaine® [US/Can]
Pontocaine® [US/Can]
Pontocaine® With Dextrose [US]
Premjact® [US-OTC]
prilocaine
procaine
Sensorcaine®-MPF [US]
Sensorcaine® [US/Can]
Solarcaine® Aloe Extra Burn Relief [US-OTC]
tetracaine
tetracaine and dextrose
Topicaine® [US-OTC]
Xylocaine® MPF [US]
Xylocaine® MPF With Epinephrine [US]
Xylocaine® [US/Can]
Xylocaine® Viscous [US]
Xylocaine® With Epinephrine [Can]
Xylocard® [Can]
Zilactin® [Can]
Zilactin-L® [US-OTC]

NEURALGIA

Analgesic, Topical
Antiphlogistine Rub A-535 Capsaicin [Can]
Antiphlogistine Rub A-535 No Odour [Can]
ArthriCare® for Women Extra Moisturizing [US-OTC]
ArthriCare® for Women Multi-Action [US-OTC]
ArthriCare® for Women Silky Dry [US-OTC]
ArthriCare® for Women Ultra Strength [US-OTC]
Capsagel® [US-OTC]
capsaicin
Capzasin-HP® [US-OTC]
Mobisyl® [US-OTC]
Myoflex® [US-OTC/Can]
Sportscreme® [US-OTC]
triethanolamine salicylate
Zostrix®-HP [US-OTC/Can]
Zostrix® [US-OTC/Can]

Nonsteroidal Antiinflammatory Drug (NSAID)
Asaphen [Can]
Asaphen E.C. [Can]
Ascriptin® Extra Strength [US-OTC]
Ascriptin® [US-OTC]
Aspercin Extra [US-OTC]
Aspercin [US-OTC]
aspirin
Bayer® Aspirin Extra Strength [US-OTC]
Bayer® Aspirin Regimen Adult Low Strength [US-OTC]
Bayer® Aspirin Regimen Children's [US-OTC]

Bayer® Aspirin Regimen Regular Strength [US-OTC]
Bayer® Aspirin [US-OTC]
Bayer® Extra Strength Arthritis Pain Regimen [US-OTC]
Bayer® Plus Extra Strength [US-OTC]
Bayer® Women's Aspirin Plus Calcium [US-OTC]
Bufferin® Extra Strength [US-OTC]
Bufferin® [US-OTC]
Buffinol Extra [US-OTC]
Buffinol [US-OTC]
Easprin® [US]
Ecotrin® Low Strength [US-OTC]
Ecotrin® Maximum Strength [US-OTC]
Ecotrin® [US-OTC]
Entrophen® [Can]
Halfprin® [US-OTC]
Novasen [Can]
St Joseph® Adult Aspirin [US-OTC]
Sureprin 81™ [US-OTC]
ZORprin® [US]

NEURITIS (OPTIC)

Adrenal Corticosteroid

A-HydroCort® [US]
A-methaPred® [US]
Apo-Prednisone® [Can]
Aristocort® Forte Injection [US]
Aristocort® Intralesional Injection [US]
Aristocort® Tablet [US/Can]
Aristospan® Intraarticular Injection [US/Can]
Aristospan® Intralesional Injection [US/Can]
betamethasone (systemic)
Celestone® Soluspan® [US/Can]
Celestone® [US]
Cortef® Tablet [US/Can]
cortisone acetate
Cortone® [Can]
Decadron® [US/Can]
Deltasone® [US]
Depo-Medrol® [US/Can]
Dexamethasone Intensol® [US]
dexamethasone (systemic)
DexPak® TaperPak® [US]
Diodex® [Can]
hydrocortisone (systemic)
Hydrocortone® Phosphate [US]
Kenalog® Injection [US/Can]
Medrol® [US/Can]
methylprednisolone
Orapred™ [US]
Pediapred® [US/Can]
PMS-Dexamethasone [Can]
Prednicot® [US]
prednisolone (systemic)
Prednisol® TBA [US]
prednisone
Prednisone Intensol™ [US]
Prelone® [US]
Solu-Cortef® [US/Can]
Solu-Medrol® [US/Can]
Sterapred® DS [US]
Sterapred® [US]
triamcinolone (systemic)
Winpred™ [Can]

NEUROLOGIC DISEASE

Adrenal Corticosteroid

A-HydroCort® [US]
A-methaPred® [US]
Apo-Prednisone® [Can]
Aristocort® Forte Injection [US]
Aristocort® Intralesional Injection [US]
Aristocort® Tablet [US/Can]
Aristospan® Intraarticular Injection [US/Can]
Aristospan® Intralesional Injection [US/Can]
betamethasone (systemic)
Celestone® Soluspan® [US/Can]
Celestone® [US]

Cortef® Tablet [US/Can]
corticotropin
cortisone acetate
Cortone® [Can]
Decadron® [US/Can]
Deltasone® [US]
Depo-Medrol® [US/Can]
Dexamethasone Intensol® [US]
dexamethasone (systemic)
DexPak® TaperPak® [US]
Diodex® [Can]
H.P. Acthar® Gel [US]
hydrocortisone (systemic)
Hydrocortone® Phosphate [US]
Kenalog® Injection [US/Can]
Medrol® [US/Can]
methylprednisolone
Orapred™ [US]
Pediapred® [US/Can]
PMS-Dexamethasone [Can]
Prednicot® [US]
prednisolone (systemic)
Prednisol® TBA [US]
prednisone
Prednisone Intensol™ [US]
Prelone® [US]
Solu-Cortef® [US/Can]
Solu-Medrol® [US/Can]
Sterapred® DS [US]
Sterapred® [US]
triamcinolone (systemic)
Winpred™ [Can]

OSTEODYSTROPHY

Vitamin D Analog
Calciferol™ [US]
Calcijex® [US]
calcitriol
DHT™ Intensol™ [US]
DHT™ [US]
dihydrotachysterol
Drisdol® [US/Can]
ergocalciferol
Hytakerol® [US/Can]
Ostoforte® [Can]
Rocaltrol® [US/Can]

OSTEOMALACIA

Vitamin D Analog
Calciferol™ [US]
Drisdol® [US/Can]
ergocalciferol
Ostoforte® [Can]

OSTEOMYELITIS

Antibiotic, Miscellaneous
Alti-Clindamycin [Can]
Apo-Clindamycin® [Can]
Cleocin HCl® [US]
Cleocin Pediatric® [US]
Cleocin Phosphate® [US]
Cleocin® [US]
Clindoxyl® [Can]
Dalacin® C [Can]
Novo-Clindamycin [Can]
Vancocin® [US/Can]
vancomycin
Antifungal Agent, Systemic
Fucidin® [Can]
Fucithalmic® [Can]
fusidic acid (Canada only)
Carbapenem (Antibiotic)
imipenem and cilastatin
meropenem
Merrem® I.V. [US/Can]
Primaxin® [US/Can]
Cephalosporin (First Generation)
Ancef® [US]
cefazolin
cephalothin
Cephalosporin (Second Generation)
Apo-Cefuroxime® [Can]
Cefotan® [US/Can]
cefotetan
cefoxitin
Ceftin® [US/Can]

cefuroxime
Kefurox® [Can]
Mefoxin® [US/Can]
ratio-Cefuroxime [Can]
Zinacef® [US/Can]
Cephalosporin (Third Generation)
Cefizox® [US/Can]
cefotaxime
ceftazidime
ceftizoxime
ceftriaxone
Claforan® [US/Can]
Fortaz® [US/Can]
Rocephin® [US/Can]
Tazicef® [US]
Penicillin
ampicillin and sulbactam
dicloxacillin
Dycill® [Can]
nafcillin
Nallpen® [Can]
oxacillin
Pathocil® [Can]
ticarcillin and clavulanate potassium
Timentin® [US/Can]
Unasyn® [US/Can]
Unipen® [Can]
Quinolone
ciprofloxacin
Cipro® [US/Can]
Cipro® XL [Can]
Cipro® XR [US]

OSTEOPOROSIS

Bisphosphonate Derivative
alendronate
Aredia® [US/Can]
Didronel® [US/Can]
etidronate disodium
Fosamax® [US/Can]
Gen-Etidronate [Can]
Novo-Alendronate [Can]
pamidronate

Electrolyte Supplement, Oral
calcium glubionate
calcium lactate
calcium phosphate (tribasic)
Posture® [US-OTC]
Estrogen and Progestin Combination
estrogens (conjugated/equine) and medroxyprogesterone
Premphase® [US/Can]
Premplus® [Can]
Prempro™ [US/Can]
Estrogen Derivative
Alora® [US]
Cenestin® [US/Can]
C.E.S.® [Can]
Climara® [US/Can]
Congest [Can]
Delestrogen® [US/Can]
Depo®-Estradiol [US/Can]
Esclim® [US]
Estrace® [US/Can]
Estraderm® [US/Can]
estradiol
Estradot® [Can]
Estrasorb™ [US]
Estratab® [Can]
Estring® [US/Can]
EstroGel® [US/Can]
estrogens (conjugated A/synthetic)
estrogens (conjugated/equine)
estrogens (esterified)
ethinyl estradiol
Femring™ [US]
Gynodiol® [US]
Menest® [US/Can]
Menostar™ [US]
Oesclim(R) [Can]
Premarin® [US/Can]
Vagifem® [US/Can]
Vivelle-Dot® [US]
Vivelle® [US/Can]

Mineral, Oral
ACT® [US-OTC]
Fluor-A-Day [US-OTC/Can]
fluoride
Fluorigard® [US-OTC]
Fluorinse® [US]
Fluotic® [Can]
Flura-Drops® [US]
Flura-Loz® [US]
Gel-Kam® Rinse [US]
Gel-Kam® [US-OTC]
Lozi-Flur™ [US]
Luride® Lozi-Tab® [US]
Luride® [US]
NeutraCare® [US]
NeutraGard® [US-OTC]
Pediaflor® [US]
Pharmaflur® 1.1 [US]
Pharmaflur® [US]
Phos-Flur® Rinse [US-OTC]
Phos-Flur® [US]
PreviDent® 5000 Plus™ [US]
PreviDent® [US]
Stan-Gard® [US]
Stop® [US]
Thera-Flur-N® [US]
Polypeptide Hormone
Calcimar® [Can]
calcitonin
Caltine® [Can]
Miacalcin® NS [Can]
Miacalcin® [US]
Selective Estrogen Receptor Modulator (SERM)
Evista® [US/Can]
raloxifene

OSTEOSARCOMA

Antineoplastic Agent
Adriamycin® [Can]
Adriamycin PFS® [US]
Adriamycin RDF® [US]
Apo-Methotrexate® [Can]
cisplatin
doxorubicin
methotrexate
Platinol®-AQ [US]
ratio-Methotrexate [Can]
Rheumatrex® [US]
Rubex®[US]
Trexall™ [US]

PAGET DISEASE OF BONE

Bisphosphonate Derivative
alendronate
Aredia® [US/Can]
Didronel® [US/Can]
etidronate disodium
Fosamax® [US/Can]
Gen-Etidronate [Can]
Novo-Alendronate [Can]
pamidronate
Skelid® [US]
tiludronate
Polypeptide Hormone
Calcimar® [Can]
calcitonin
Caltine® [Can]
Miacalcin® NS [Can]
Miacalcin® [US]

PARKINSONISM

Anti-Parkinson Agent
Akineton® [US/Can]
amantadine
Apo-Benztropine® [Can]
Apo-Bromocriptine® [Can]
Apo-Trihex® [Can]
benserazide and levodopa (Canada only)
benztropine
biperiden
bromocriptine
Cogentin® [US/Can]
Comtan® [US/Can]
Endantadine® [Can]

entacapone
Kemadrin® [US]
Parlodel® [US/Can]
PMS-Amantadine [Can]
PMS-Bromocriptine [Can]
PMS-Procyclidine [Can]
Procyclid™ [Can]
procyclidine
Prolopa® [Can]
Requip® [US/Can]
ropinirole
Symmetrel® [US/Can]
Tasmar® [US]
tolcapone
trihexyphenidyl

Anti-Parkinson Agent, COMT Inhibitor
levodopa, carbidopa, and entacapone
Stalevo™ [US]

Anti-Parkinson Agent (Dopamine Agonist)
levodopa, carbidopa, and entacapone
Stalevo™ [US]

Dopaminergic Agent (Anti-Parkinson)
Apo-Levocarb® [Can]
Apo-Selegiline® [Can]
carbidopa
Eldepryl® [US/Can]
Endo®-Levodopa/Carbidopa [Can]
Gen-Selegiline [Can]
levodopa and carbidopa
Lodosyn® [US]
Mirapex® [US/Can]
Novo-Levocarbidopa [Can]
Novo-Selegiline [Can]
Nu-Levocarb [Can]
Nu-Selegiline [Can]
pergolide
Permax® [US/Can]
pramipexole
selegiline
Sinemet® CR [US/Can]
Sinemet® [US/Can]

Reverse COMT Inhibitor
Comtan® [US/Can]
entacapone

POLIOMYELITIS

Vaccine, Live Virus and Inactivated Virus
IPOL® [US/Can]
poliovirus vaccine (inactivated)

POLYCYTHEMIA VERA

Antineoplastic Agent
busulfan
Busulfex® [US/Can]
mechlorethamine
Mustargen® [US/Can]
Myleran® [US/Can]

POLYMYOSITIS

Antineoplastic Agent
Apo-Methotrexate® [Can]
chlorambucil
cyclophosphamide
Cytoxan® [US/Can]
Leukeran® [US/Can]
methotrexate
Procytox® [Can]
ratio-Methotrexate [Can]
Rheumatrex® [US]
Trexall™ [US]

Immunosuppressant Agent
Alti-Azathioprine [Can]
Apo-Azathioprine® [Can]
Azasan® [US]
azathioprine
Gen-Azathioprine [Can]
Imuran® [US/Can]

REYE SYNDROME

Diuretic, Osmotic
mannitol
Osmitrol® [US/Can]
Resectisol® [US]

Ophthalmic Agent, Miscellaneous
glycerin
Osmoglyn® [US]
Vitamin, Fat Soluble
AquaMEPHYTON® [Can]
Konakion [Can]
Mephyton® [US/Can]
Phytonadione

RHEUMATIC DISORDERS

Adrenal Corticosteroid
A-HydroCort® [US]
A-methaPred® [US]
Apo-Prednisone® [Can]
Aristocort® Forte Injection [US]
Aristocort® Intralesional Injection [US]
Aristocort® Tablet [US/Can]
Aristospan® Intraarticular Injection [US/Can]
Aristospan® Intralesional Injection [US/Can]
betamethasone (systemic)
Celestone® Soluspan® [US/Can]
Celestone® [US]
Cortef® Tablet [US/Can]
corticotropin
cortisone acetate
Cortone® [Can]
Decadron® [US/Can]
Deltasone® [US]
Depo-Medrol® [US/Can]
Dexamethasone Intensol® [US]
dexamethasone (systemic)
DexPak® TaperPak® [US]
Diodex® [Can]
H.P. Acthar® Gel [US]
hydrocortisone (systemic)
Hydrocortone® Phosphate [US]
Kenalog® Injection [US/Can]
Medrol® [US/Can]
methylprednisolone
Orapred™ [US]
Pediapred® [US/Can]
PMS-Dexamethasone [Can]
Prednicot® [US]
prednisolone (systemic)
Prednisol® TBA [US]
prednisone
Prednisone Intensol™ [US]
Prelone® [US]
Solu-Cortef® [US/Can]
Solu-Medrol® [US/Can]
Sterapred® DS [US]
Sterapred® [US]
triamcinolone (systemic)
Winpred™ [Can]

RICKETS

Vitamin D Analog
Calciferol™ [US]
Drisdol® [US/Can]
ergocalciferol
Ostoforte® [Can]

SPASTICITY

Alpha2-Adrenergic Agonist Agent
tizanidine
Zanaflex® [US/Can]
Benzodiazepine
Apo-Diazepam® [Can]
diazepam
Valium® [US/Can]
Skeletal Muscle Relaxant
Apo-Baclofen® [Can]
baclofen
Dantrium® [US/Can]
dantrolene
Gen-Baclofen [Can]
Lioresal® [US/Can]
Liotec [Can]
Nu-Baclo [Can]
PMS-Baclofen [Can]

SPINAL CORD INJURY

Skeletal Muscle Relaxant
- Dantrium® [US/Can]
- dantrolene

SPONDYLITIS (ANKYLOSING)

Nonsteroidal Antiinflammatory Drug (NSAID)
- Apo-Diclo® [Can]
- Apo-Diclo Rapide® [Can]
- Apo-Diclo SR® [Can]
- Apo-Piroxicam® [Can]
- Cataflam® [US/Can]
- diclofenac
- Diclotec [Can]
- Feldene® [US/Can]
- Gen-Piroxicam [Can]
- Novo-Difenac® [Can]
- Novo-Difenac-K [Can]
- Novo-Difenac® SR [Can]
- Novo-Pirocam® [Can]
- Nu-Diclo [Can]
- Nu-Diclo-SR [Can]
- Nu-Pirox [Can]
- Pennsaid® [Can]
- Pexicam® [Can]
- piroxicam
- PMS-Diclofenac [Can]
- PMS-Diclofenac SR [Can]
- Riva-Diclofenac [Can]
- Riva-Diclofenac-K [Can]
- Solaraze™ [US]
- Voltaren Rapide® [Can]
- Voltaren® [US/Can]
- Voltaren®-XR [US]

STATUS EPILEPTICUS

Barbiturate
- amobarbital
- Amytal® [US/Can]
- Luminal® Sodium [US]
- Nembutal® Sodium [Can]
- Nembutal® [US]
- pentobarbital
- phenobarbital
- PMS-Phenobarbital [Can]

Benzodiazepine
- Apo-Diazepam® [Can]
- Apo-Lorazepam® [Can]
- Ativan® [US/Can]
- Diastat® [US/Can]
- Diazemuls® [Can]
- diazepam
- Diazepam Intensol® [US]
- lorazepam
- Lorazepam Intensol® [US]
- Novo-Lorazem® [Can]
- Nu-Loraz [Can]
- PMS-Lorazepam [Can]
- Riva-Lorazepam [Can]
- Valium® [US/Can]

Hydantoin
- Dilantin® [US/Can]
- Phenytek™ [US]
- phenytoin

STROKE

Antiplatelet Agent
- Alti-Ticlopidine [Can]
- Apo-Ticlopidine® [Can]
- Asaphen [Can]
- Asaphen E.C. [Can]
- aspirin
- Bayer® Aspirin Extra Strength [US-OTC]
- Bayer® Aspirin Regimen Regular Strength [US-OTC]
- Bayer® Aspirin [US-OTC]
- Bayer® Plus Extra Strength [US-OTC]
- Easprin® [US]
- Ecotrin® Maximum Strength [US-OTC]
- Ecotrin® [US-OTC]
- Entrophen® [Can]

Gen-Ticlopidine [Can]
Novasen [Can]
Novo-Ticlopidine [Can]
Nu-Ticlopidine [Can]
PMS-Ticlopidine [Can]
Rhoxal-ticlopidine [Can]
St Joseph® Adult Aspirin [US-OTC]
Sureprin 81™ [US-OTC]
Ticlid(R) [US/Can]
ticlopidine

Fibrinolytic Agent
Activase® rt-PA [Can]
Activase® [US]
alteplase
Cathflo™ Activase® [US/Can]

Skeletal Muscle Relaxant
Dantrium® [US/Can]
dantrolene

SUDECK ATROPHY

Calcium Channel Blocker
Adalat® CC [US]
Adalat® XL(R) [Can]
Apo-Nifed® [Can]
Apo-Nifed PA® [Can]
Nifedical™ XL [US]
nifedipine
Novo-Nifedin [Can]
Nu-Nifed [Can]
Procardia® [US/Can]
Procardia XL® [US]

SYPHILIS

Antibiotic, Miscellaneous
chloramphenicol
Chloromycetin® [Can]
Chloromycetin® Sodium Succinate [US]
Diochloram® [Can]
Pentamycetin® [Can]

Penicillin
Bicillin® L-A [US]
penicillin G benzathine
penicillin G (parenteral/aqueous)
penicillin G procaine
Permapen® Isoject® [US]
Pfizerpen-AS® [Can]
Pfizerpen® [US/Can]
Wycillin® [Can]

Tetracycline Derivative
Adoxa™ [US]
Apo-Doxy® [Can]
Apo-Doxy Tabs® [Can]
Apo-Tetra® [Can]
Doryx® [US]
Doxy-100® [US]
Doxycin [Can]
doxycycline
Doxytec [Can]
Monodox® [US]
Novo-Doxylin [Can]
Novo-Tetra [Can]
Nu-Doxycycline [Can]
Nu-Tetra [Can]
Sumycin® [US]
tetracycline
Vibramycin® [US]
Vibra-Tabs® [US/Can]
Wesmycin® [US]

TOURETTE DISEASE

Antipsychotic Agent, Butyrophenone
Apo-Haloperidol® [Can]
Apo-Haloperidol LA® [Can]
Haldol® Decanoate [US]
Haldol® [US]
haloperidol
Haloperidol-LA Omega [Can]
Haloperidol Long Acting [Can]
Novo-Peridol [Can]
Peridol [Can]
PMS-Haloperidol LA [Can]

Neuroleptic Agent
Orap™ [US/Can]
pimozide

Phenothiazine Derivative

Apo-Chlorpromazine® [Can]
chlorpromazine
Largactil® [Can]
Novo-Chlorpromazine [Can]

VERTIGO

Antihistamine

Aler-Dryl [US-OTC]
Allerdryl® [Can]
AllerMax® [US-OTC]
Allernix [Can]
Antivert® [US/Can]
Apo-Dimenhydrinate(R) [Can]
Banophen® [US-OTC]
Benadryl® Allergy [US-OTC/Can]
Benadryl® Dye-Free Allergy [US-OTC]
Benadryl® Gel Extra Strength [US-OTC]
Benadryl® Gel [US-OTC]
Benadryl® Injection [US]
Bonamine™ [Can]
Bonine® [US-OTC/Can]
Compoz® Nighttime Sleep Aid [US-OTC]
dimenhydrinate
Diphen® AF [US-OTC]
Diphen® Cough [US-OTC]
Diphenhist [US-OTC]
diphenhydramine
Diphen® [US-OTC]
Dramamine® Less Drowsy Formula [US-OTC]
Dramamine® [US-OTC]
Genahist® [US-OTC]
Gravol® [Can]
Hydramine® Cough [US-OTC]
Hydramine® [US-OTC]
Hyrexin-50® [US]
meclizine
Novo-Dimenate [Can]
Nytol® Extra Strength [Can]
Nytol® Maximum Strength [US-OTC]
Nytol® [US-OTC/Can]
PMS-Diphenhydramine [Can]
Siladryl® Allergy [US-OTC]
Silphen® [US-OTC]
Simply Sleep® [Can]
Sleepinal® [US-OTC]
Sominex® Maximum Strength [US-OTC]
Sominex® [US-OTC]
TripTone® [US-OTC]
Tusstat® [US]
Twilite® [US-OTC]
Unisom® Maximum Strength SleepGels® [US-OTC]

WILSON DISEASE

Chelating Agent

Syprine® [US/Can]
trientine